Noise-Induced Hearing Loss

Armand L. Dancer, Ph.D.
Director
Physiology Laboratory
Maitre de Recherches
French-German Research Institute of Saint-Louis
Saint-Louis, France

Donald Henderson, Ph.D.
Professor and Chairman
Department of Communicative Disorders and Sciences
State University of New York at Buffalo
Buffalo, New York

Richard J. Salvi, Ph.D.
Professor
Department of Communicative Disorders and Sciences
Hearing Research Laboratory
State University of New York at Buffalo
Buffalo, New York

Roger P. Hamernik, Ph.D.
Professor
Departments of Physics and Speech and Hearing
State University of New York at Plattsburgh
Plattsburgh, New York

Mosby Year Book

St. Louis Baltimore Boston Chicago London Philadelphia Sydney Toronto

Mosby Year Book

Dedicated to Publishing Excellence

Editor: David Marshall
Developmental Editor: Ellen Thomas
Project Manager: Kimberly A. LoDico
Designer: Barbara Torode

Printed in the United States of America.

Mosby-Year Book, Inc.
11830 Westline Industrial Drive
St. Louis, MO 63146

Library of Congress Cataloging-in-Publication Data
Noise-induced hearing loss / [edited by] Armand L. Dancer . . . [et al.].
p. cm.
Based on a conference held in Beaune, France in May 28-30, 1990.
Includes bibliographical references and index.
ISBN 1-55664-321-7
1. Deafness, Noise-induced—Congresses. I. Dancer, Armand L.
[DNLM: 1. Cochlea—physiopathology—congresses. 2. Ear Protective Devices—congresses. 3. Hearing Loss, Noise-Induced—congresses. 4. Noise—adverse effects—congresses. WV 270 N784 1990]
RF293.5N65 1991
617.8'071—dc20
DLC 91-19784
for Library of Congress CIP

Contributors

Richard A. Altschuler, Ph.D.
Associate Professor,
Kresge Hearing Research Institute,
University of Michigan,
Ann Arbor, Michigan

Jean-Marie Aran, Ph.D.
Director of Research,
Experimental Audiology Laboratory,
Institut Nationale de la Santé et de la Recherche Medicale,
Bordeaux, France

C. Aurousseau
Research Technician, Experimental Audiology Laboratory,
Institut National de la Santé et de la Recherche Medicale,
Bordeaux, France

Alf Axelsson, M.D.
Professor and Chief,
Department of Audiology,
University of Göteborg,
Göteborg, Sweden

Brian R. Bancroft, M.A.
Research Scientist,
Hearing Research Laboratory,
State University of New York at Buffalo,
Buffalo, New York

Marie-Louise Barrenäs, M.D.
Associate Professor,
Department of Occupational Audiology,
University of Göteborg,
Göteborg, Sweden

Elliott H. Berger, M.S., Mem. INCE
Manager, Acoustical Engineering,
Cabot Safety Corporation,
Indianapolis, Indiana

Richard P. Bobbin, Ph.D.
Professor, Otolaryngology Department,
Louisiana State University School of Medicine,
New Orleans, Louisiana

Flint A. Boettcher, Ph.D.
Research Assistant Professor,
Hearing Research Laboratory,
State University of New York at Buffalo,
Buffalo, New York

Barbara A. Bohne, Ph.D.
Professor, Department of Otolaryngology,
Washington University School of Medicine,
St. Louis, Missouri

Erik Borg, M.D., Ph.D.
Professor and Physician,
Department of Physiology II,
Karolinska Institute,
Stockholm, Sweden

Arjan Bosman, Ph.D.
Assistant Professor, Experimental Audiology,
Utrecht University,
Utrecht, The Netherlands

Marie-Claire Botte, Ph.D.
Director of Research, Experimental Psychology Laboratory,
Institut Nationale de Recherches et de Securité,
Paris, France

Michael B. Calford, B.Sc., Ph.D.
Senior Research Fellow, VTHRC,
Department of Physiology and Pharmacology,
University of Queensland,
St. Lucia, Queensland, Australia

Pierre Campo, Ph.D.
Research Scientist,
Institut Nationale de Recherches et de Securité,
Vandoeuvre, France

Barbara Canlon, Ph.D.
Docent, Department of Physiology II,
Karolinska Institute,
Stockholm, Sweden

William W. Clark, Ph.D.
Senior Research Scientist,
Central Institute for the Deaf,
St. Louis, Missouri

Ann E. Clock, M.A.
Research Scientist, Hearing Research Laboratory,
State University of New York at Buffalo,
Buffalo, New York

Alan R. Cody, Ph.D.
Lecturer, Department of Physiology,
University of Queensland,
St. Lucia, Queensland, Australia

H. Steven Colburn, Ph.D.
Professor of Biomedical Engineering,
Boston University,
Boston, Massachusetts

Vittorio Colletti, M.D.
Professor, Department of Otolaryngology,
Polyclinic Borgo Roma,
Verona, Italy

Armand L. Dancer, Ph.D.
Director of Research,
Physiology Laboratory
French-German Research Institute of Saint-Louis,
Saint-Louis, France

Claude J. Dechesne, Ph.D.
Research Scientist
Laboratory of Sensory Neurophysiology
Institut Natinale de Recherches et de Securité,
Montpellier, France

Laurent Décory, Ph.D.
Research Scientist,
Physiology Laboratory
French-German Research Institute of Saint-Louis,
Saint-Louis, France

David F. Dolan, Ph.D.
Research Investigator,
Kresge Hearing Research Institute,
University of Michigan,
Ann Arbor, Michigan

D. Dulon
Research Scientist,
Experimental Audiology Laboratory,
Institut Nationale de la Santé et de la Recherche Medicale,
Bordeaux, France

Berit Engström, M.D., Ph.D.
Staff, Department of Physiology II,
Karolinska Institute,
Stockholm, Sweden

J. P. Erre
Research Engineer,
Experimental Audiology Laboratory,
Institut Nationale de la Santé et de la Recherche Medicale,
Bordeaux, France

Francesco Fiorino, M.D.
Department of Otolaryngology,
Hospital of Borgo Roma,
Verona, Italy

Åke Flock, M.D., Ph.D.
Professor and Chairman,
Department of Physiology II,
Karolinska Institute,
Stockholm, Sweden

George M. Gerken, Ph.D.
Visiting Professor, Department of Otorhinolaryngology,
University of Texas Southwestern Medical Center at Dallas,
Dallas, Texas

Michael Anne Gratton, Ph.D.
Assistant Professor,
Department of Otolaryngology,
Medical University of South Carolina,
Charleston, South Carolina

A. Guilhaume
Research Engineer,
Experimental Audiology Laboratory,
Institut Nationale de la Santé et de la Recherche Medicale,
Bordeaux, France

Ervin R. Hafter, Ph.D.
Professor, Department of Psychology,
University of California at Berkeley,
Berkeley, California

Roger P. Hamernik, Ph.D.
Professor,
Departments of Physics and Speech and Hearing,
State University of New York at Plattsburgh,
Plattsburgh, New York

Duane O. Hartshorn, M.D.
Resident, Department of Otolaryngology,
University of Michigan,
Ann Arbor, Michigan

Eri Hashino, M.S.
Research Assistant Professor,
Department of Communication,
Tokyo Woman's Christian University,
Tokyo, Japan

T. Hayashida
Student, Experimental Audiology Laboratory,
Institut Nationale de la Santé et de la Recherche Medicale,
Bordeaux, France

Robert H. Helfert, Ph.D.
Research Investigator, Kresge Hearing Research Institute,
University of Michigan,
Ann Arbor, Michigan

Per-Anders Hellström
Engineer, Chalmers University of Technology;
Research Engineer, Hearing Research Laboratory,
Lindholmen Development,
Göteborg, Sweden

Donald Henderson, Ph.D.
Professor and Chairman,
Department of Communicative Disorders and Sciences,
State University of New York at Buffalo,
Buffalo, New York

Raymond Hétu, Ph.D.
Professor and Director,
Acoustic Department,
University of Montreal,
Montreal, Quebec, Canada

H. Hiel
Student, Experimental Audiology Laboratory,
Institut de la Santé et de la Recherche Medicale,
Bordeaux, France

Manfried Hoke, M.D., Ph.D.
Director, Institute of Experimental Audiology,
University of Münster,
Münster, Germany

Dexter R. F. Irvine, B.A., Ph.D.
Reader, Department of Psychology,
Monash University,
Clayton, Australia

Marjorie D. Jung, M.S.
Assistant Professor and Chief of Audiology Section,
Division of Otolaryngology,
Department of Surgery,
University of Connecticut School of Medicine,
Farmington, Connecticut

Shyam M. Khanna, Ph.D.
Professor of Auditory Biophysics,
Columbia University College of Physicians and Surgeons,
New York, New York

D. O. Kim, D.Sc.
Professor and Director of Research,
Division of Otolaryngology,
Department of Surgery,
University of Connecticut School of Medicine,
Farmington, Connecticut

Hung N. Kim, M.D.
Clinical Resident,
Department of Otolaryngology,
Baylor College of Medicine,
Houston, Texas

Chantal Laroche, Ph.D.
Research Scientist, Acoustic Department,
University of Montreal,
Montreal, Quebec, Canada

Robert Lataye
Research Scientist,
Institut Nationale de Recherches et de Securité,
Vandoeuvre, France

Klaus Lehnertz
Clinic of Epileptology,
University of Bonn,
Bonn, Germany

Gerald Leonard, M.D.
Associate Professor, Division of Otolaryngology,
Department of Surgery,
University of Connecticut School of Medicine;
Chief, Division of Otolaryngology,
University of Connecticut Health Center,
Farmington, Connecticut

Bernadette Lepage, M.O.A.
Research Assistant, National Acoustics Laboratories,
Chatswood, Australia

Eric L. Lepage, Ph.D.
Doctor, Senior Research Scientist, and Head of Hearing Conservation Unit,
National Acoustics Laboratories,
Chatswood, Australia

Zhi'an Liang, M.D.
Professor and Chief of Laboratory of Audition,
Shanghai Institute of Physiology,
Academia Sinica,
Shanghai, China

M. Charles Liberman, Ph.D.
Associate Professor,
Department of Otology and Laryngology,
Harvard Medical School,
Boston, Massachusetts

Fredrik Lindgren, Ph.D.
Consultant in Audiology and Acoustics,
Cabot Safety Corporation,
Indianapolis, Indiana

Paula Löfstrand, B.S.
Department of Physiology II,
Karolinska Institute,
Stockholm, Sweden

Bernd Lütkenhöner, M.D.
Senior Scientist,
Institute of Experimental Audiology,
University of Münster,
Münster, Germany

Richard L. McKinley, B.S., M.S.
Biomedical Engineer, Bioacoustics and Biocommunications,
Harry G. Armstrong Aerospace Medical Research Laboratory,
Dayton, Ohio

William Melnick, Ph.D.
Professor, Department of Otolaryngology,
Ohio State University,
Columbus, Ohio

Josef M. Miller, Ph.D.
Professor and Director,
Kresge Hearing and Research Institute,
University of Michigan,
Ann Arbor, Michigan

John H. Mills, Ph.D.
Professor, Department of Otolaryngology,
Medical University of South Carolina,
Charleston, South Carolina

Sabine Mönikheim
Research Scientist,
Experimental Psychology Laboratory,
Institut Nationale de Recherches et de Securité,
Paris, France

Giancarlo Z. Montresor, M.D.
Research Scientist,
Laboratory of Sensory Neurophysiology,
Institut Nationale de la Santé et de la Recherche Medicale
Montpellier, France

David B. Moody, Ph.D.
Research Scientist,
Kresge Hearing Research Institute,
University of Michigan,
Ann Arbor, Michigan

Jean K. Moore, Ph.D.
Staff,
House Ear Institute,
Los Angeles, California

John K. Niparko, M.D.
Assistant Professor,
Department of Otolaryngology,
University of Michigan,
Ann Arbor, Michigan

Charles W. Nixon, Ph.D.
Chief, Bioacoustics and Biocommunications,
Harry G. Armstrong Aerospace Medical Research Laboratory,
Dayton, Ohio

Christo Pantev, Ph.D.
Senior Scientist,
Institute of Experimental Audiology,
University of Münster,
Münster, Germany

James H. Patterson, Jr., Ph.D.
Sensory Research Division,
U.S. Army Aeromedical Research Laboratory,
Fort Rucker, Alabama

Robert Patuzzi, B.Eng., Ph.D.
Research Fellow, Department of Physiology,
University of Western Australia,
Nedlands, Australia

Nicholas L. Powers, B.S.
Research Scientist,
Hearing Research Laboratory,
State University of New York at Buffalo,
Buffalo, New York

G. Richard Price, Ph.D.
Research Team Leader,
Behavioral Research Directorate,
United States Army Human Engineering Laboratory,
Aberdeen Proving Ground, Maryland

Cindy A. Prosen, Ph.D.
Research Investigator,
Kresge Hearing Research Institute,
University of Michigan,
Ann Arbor, Michigan

Jean-Luc Puel, Ph.D.
Research Scientist,
Laboratory of Auditory Neurobiology,
Institut Nationale de Recherches et de Securité,
Montpellier, France

Rémy Pujol, Ph.D.
Professor and Director,
Laboratory of Auditory Neurobiology,
Institut Nationale de la Santé et de la Recherche Medicale,
Montpellier, France

Hung Tran Quoc, Ing.
Engineer, Acoustic Department
University of Montreal,
Montreal, Quebec, Canada

Ramesh Rajan, B.Sc.(Hons.), Ph.D.
Wright Research Fellow,
Department of Psychology,
Monash University,
Clayton, Victoria, Australia

Yehoash Raphael, Ph.D.
Post-Doctoral Affiliate,
Kresge Hearing Research Institute,
University of Michigan,
Ann Arbor, Michigan

Edwin W. Rubel, Ph.D.
Professor,
Hearing Development Laboratories,
University of Washington,
Seattle, Washington

Ian J. Russell, Ph.D.
Professor, School of Biological Sciences,
University of Sussex, Falmer,
Brighton, United Kingdom

Josée St.-Vincent, M.O.A.
Audiologist,
St.-Vincent de Paul Hospital
Quebec, Canada

Richard J. Salvi, Ph.D.
Professor,
Department of Communicative Disorders and Sciences,
Hearing Research Laboratory,
State University of New York at Buffalo,
Buffalo, New York

Samuel S. Saunders, M.A.
Research Scientist,
Hearing Research Laboratory,
State University of New York at Buffalo,
Buffalo, New York

Robert S. Schlauch, Ph.D.
Assistant Professor,
Department of Communication Disorders,
University of Minnesota,
Minneapolis, Minnesota

Richard A. Schmiedt, Ph.D.
Associate Professor,
Department of Otolaryngology,
Medical University of South Carolina,
Charleston, South Carolina

Mark E. Schneider
Senior Staff Fellow,
National Institutes of Health,
Bethesda, Maryland

Bradley A. Schulte, Ph.D.
Associate Professor,
Department of Pathology,
Medical University of South Carolina,
Charleston, South Carolina

Guido F. Smoorenburg, Ph.D.
Professor of Experimental Audiology,
TNO Institute for Perception,
Soesterberg;
Staff, University Hospital,
Utrecht University,
Utrecht, The Netherlands

Jacek Smurzynski, Ph.D.
Post-Doctoral Fellow, Division of Otolaryngology,
Department of Surgery,
University of Connecticut Health Center,
Farmington, Connecticut

Masahiro Sokabe, Ph.D.
Associate Professor, Department of Physiology,
Nagoya University School of Medicine,
Nagoya, Japan

Vlasta Spongr, M.S.
Research Scientist,
Hearing Research Laboratory,
State University of New York at Buffalo,
Buffalo, New York

Joseph W. Steuver, B.S.E.E.
Electronics Engineer,
Bioacoustics and Biocommunications,
Harry G. Armstrong Aerospace Medical Research Laboratory,
Dayton, Ohio

Malini Subramaniam, Ph.D.
Staff, Hearing Research Laboratory,
State University of New York at Buffalo,
Buffalo, New York

Yasuo Tanaka, M.D.
Professor, Department of Otolaryngology,
Dokkyo University School of Medicine,
Koshigaya Hospital,
Koshigaya, Saitama, Japan

Constantine Trahiotis, Ph.D.
Professor of Surgery and Neuroscience,
University of Connecticut Health Center,
Farmington, Connecticut

Mats Ulfendahl, Ph.D.
Staff, Department of Physiology II,
Karolinska Institute,
Stockholm, Sweden

Marcel Van Der Venne, Dr.Sc.
Commission of the European Communities,
Luxembourg

Patrick Vassout, Ph.D.
Research Scientist,
Physiology Laboratory,
French-German Research Institute of Saint-Louis,
Saint-Louis, France

Giuseppe Verlato, M.D., Ph.D.
Researcher, Department of Otolaryngology,
Hospital of Borgo Roma,
Verona, Italy

Robert J. Wenthold, Ph.D.
Section Chief,
National Institutes of Health,
Bethesda, Maryland

J. Patrick Wilson, B.Sc., Ph.D., F.I.O.A.
Honorary Senior Research Fellow,
Department of Communication, and
Neuroscience Lecturer, Electronic Engineering Group,
Department of Physics,
University of Keele,
Staffordshire, England

Lisa Z. Wise, B.Sc., Ph.D.
Senior Tutor, Department of Psychology,
Monash University,
Claxton, Australia

Preface

Noise-induced hearing loss (NIHL) continues to be a significant public health problem. In 1987, the National Institute of Occupational Safety and Health rated NIHL as one of the United States' top 10 work-related problems, involving at least 11 million workers (NIOSH, 1987). The problem is even more severe in the military. In 1986, the Veteran's Administration paid over $167 million for compensation claims related to NIHL. The problem is equally serious in Europe, where over 15 million people work in potentially dangerous noise environments. While these statistics are alarming, they do not begin to reflect the personal hardship, the diminished quality of life, and the loss in personal productivity associated with NIHL.

Fortunately, the problem of NIHL has not been ignored by the scientific community and, over the past decade, considerable progress has been made in understanding many of the important issues. The current volume is intended to provide the reader with an overview of many of the important advances that have been made in understanding the basic science and applied aspects of noise-induced hearing loss in recent years. For example, scientists are beginning to reveal the cellular mechanism of noise-induced hearing loss; how acquired hearing loss is exacerbated by other environmental factors; how digital electronics can be used in the next generation of acoustic monitoring devices; and, most recently, how individuals might be screened for susceptibility to NIHL. These issues and solutions require the coordinated efforts of scientists from quite diverse disciplines. For society to use the new information and for scientists to continue to make progress, it is important to have a forum in which progress can be discussed and integrated to develop directions for new research.

In 1975, members of the Organizing Committee, with support from NIOSH, hosted an international conference on the problem of NIHL. The conference brought together experts from most of the disciplines concerned with NIHL. Each participant presented a critical review of a topic along with the individual's own recent contributions. The papers and discussions of the symposium were published and became a standard reference. Since then, two international conferences have been held, one in 1980 and another in 1985. Collectively, the proceedings from these conferences have become one of the most definitive sources of information on NIHL and have had a direct impact on noise legislation.

In the five years since the last conference, significant advances have been made in understanding both the basic science and the applied aspects of NIHL. The most recent conference was held in Beaune, France, May 28–30, 1990, and the proceedings of the conference forms the basis of this book. The papers contained in this volume have been divided into seven sections, which focus on important basic science and applied issues described below.

1. ***Cochlear Mechanisms of NIHL.*** Basic scientists working on the mechanics and biochemistry of the cochlea have begun to study the changes associated with NIHL. The application of laser interferometry is beginning to reveal the complicated interrelation between the vibrational pattern of the cellular subsystems within the cochlea and how they change with NIHL. Auditory physiologists continue to document the complex set of changes in the neural code from cochleas damaged by noise, while other laboratories are studying the physiology of hair cells from noise-damaged

cochleas. Research on cochlear echoes in normal and pathologic ears can now be interpreted in terms of controlled changes in cochlear mechanics. Collectively, these results have important implications for understanding the cochlear changes associated with NIHL.

2. ***Central Changes in NIHL.*** The effects of noise are typically thought to be limited to cochlear function. However, recent anatomic and physiologic data suggest that peripheral hearing loss may influence central auditory processing. This information may be important for both compensation and rehabilitation strategies.

3. ***Co-factors in NIHL.*** The relation between a given noise exposure and the degree of hearing loss is not simple. It is partially mediated by other nonacoustic variables such as vibration, ototoxic drugs, and certain airborne pollutants. A better appreciation of these potential interactions is critical for minimizing the risk of NIHL in the workplace. Also, the effects of intense noise exposure may be partially mediated by the developmental status of the subject. Data from animal studies point to a "critical" period in auditory development that coincides with increased susceptibility to the effects of noise. Other studies with aged animals suggest that elderly subjects are more vulnerable to the effects of noise. It is important to integrate this information and explore the relevance to noise standards for humans.

4. ***Performance Changes in NIHL.*** The problem of NIHL has captured the interest of psychoacoustics, and the field has moved beyond correlating cochlear pathology with changes in pure tone thresholds. Psychoacousticians have begun to document a wide range of suprathreshold hearing deficits that affect frequency selectivity, temporal resolution, intensity coding, and sound localization. These deficits almost certainly contribute to poor speech perception and need to be considered when designing and fitting hearing aids.

5. ***Hearing Protection.*** The current noise standards are limited to some extent by noise measurement. Recent developments in digital electronics have made possible the design of more valid monitoring systems which could be useful in estimating the traumatic power of impulse and impact noise. In addition, personal hearing protection devices are not used as extensively as they might be because of design problems. Active hearing protection devices may prove extremely useful when communication is needed in noisy environments.

6. ***Susceptibility and Resistance to Noise.*** Historically, studies of individual susceptibility have focused on such variables as eye color, sex, smoking, and heart disease. Although each of these may have some predictive value, they contribute only a small part to the range of susceptibility seen in studies in NIHL. Recent data suggest that the efferent system to the cochlea and the acoustic reflex may protect the auditory system from NIHL. Individual differences in either of these protective mechanisms may contribute significantly to the determination of susceptibility to NIHL. Of particular interest is the possibility that certain noise exposures can protect the auditory system from future traumatic exposures.

7. ***Parameters of the Exposure.*** Parametric studies of continuous, impulse, impact, and intermittent noise continue to clarify the importance of the acoustic parameters in NIHL. Several laboratories have reported on the differences (both audiologically and histologically) between impulse/impact noise and continuous noise. These results are critical for the evaluation of noise standards. In addition, studies of isolated hair cells may pro-

vide a perspective on the changes in the mechanical properties of the hair cells that are caused by exposure to traumatic and nontraumatic noise.

Important advances made in each of the seven topic areas are provided by a team of internationally recognized experts from a broad range of disciplines. It is hoped that this book will serve as a source of up-to-date material that will be used to educate and inform government officials and the public as well as to stimulate further research that will provide new insights into the basic science and applied aspects of noise-induced hearing loss.

ARMAND L. DANCER, Ph.D.
DONALD HENDERSON, Ph.D.
RICHARD J. SALVI, Ph.D.
ROGER P. HAMERNIK, Ph.D.

Acknowledgments

The IVth International Symposium on the Effects of Noise was held in Beaune, France, May 28–30, 1990. The symposium brought together a distinguished group of scientists and clinicians from all the disciplines related to noise-induced hearing loss. The conference was organized by Flint Boettcher, Vittorio Colletti, Armand Dancer, Roger Hamernik, Donald Henderson, John Mills, Richard Salvi, and Samuel Saunders. The conference was supported by a number of agencies and programs. We interpret the enthusiastic support as evidence of the widespread concern for the problems of excessive noise and a vote of confidence that scientists are making progress in understanding the problem. Our thanks and gratitude go to the following supporters:

Société Française d'Acoustique (SFA), France

Bruel & Kjaer, France

Direction des Etudes et Recherches de l'Electricite de France

Direction des Recherches, Etudes et Techniques (DRET), France

Institut Franco-Allemand de Recherches de Saint-Louis, France

Institut National de la Santé et de la Recherche Medicale (INSERM), France

Secretariat d'Etat charge de l'Environment, France

Ville de Beaune, France

Commission des Communautes Européennes (CEE), Luxembourg

Project Lindholmen, Sweden

U.S. Air Force European Office of Aerospace Research and Development (EOARD), England

U.S. Army Research Standardization & Development Group (USARSDG), England

E.A.R. Division, U.S.A.

National Institute on Deafness & Other Communicative Disorders, U.S.A.

National Institute of Occupational Safety & Health (NIOSH), U.S.A.

U.S. Army Medical Research & Development Command, U.S.A.

The manuscripts contained in this book represent survey papers presented at the International Symposium. The papers have been edited and organized around seven key topic areas that have both practical and theoretical significance. This volume will provide students, educators, researchers and government officials with a comprehensive, up-to-date review of basic science and applied aspects of noise-induced hearing loss.

Contents

SECTION ONE

Cochlear Mechanisms

CHAPTER 1

Mechanical Analysis in the Cochlea at the Cellular Level

SHYAM M. KHANNA
ÅKE FLOCK
MATS ULFENDAHL

The use of an optical sectioning microscope and a heterodyne interferometer in combination has allowed us to measure the individual cellular mechanical responses in a guinea pig temporal bone preparation in response to sound applied to the ear. The initial observations in this preparation were reported earlier (ITER, 1989). The original method had several limitations, and we have tried to reduce or eliminate them in a systematic way. Some of these limitations were as follows: (1) because the preparation was immersed in tissue culture medium, it was connected to the sound source with a long tube; therefore the sound pressure could not be measured near the tympanic membrane (Khanna et al, 1989c); (2) the carrier-to-noise ratio of the interferometer was adequate for the measurements on the Hensen's cells, which had higher reflectivity, but only marginal for other structures; (3) the dipping cone used on the objective lens for vibration measurements in the cochlea did not have sufficient working distance for measurements of malleus vibration, needed as a reference for the cochlear vibratory response.

These limitations were removed by the following improvements in the measuring system: (1) the length of the tube connecting the acoustic transducer to the preparation was shortened to a minimum, and a flexible probe microphone tube was designed so that sound pressure could be measured at the entrance of the bony meatus within a few millimeters of the tympanic membrane; (2) the interferometer performance was improved by a series of steps that included (a) use of a lens of higher numerical aperture, (b) reduction of internal light losses in the interferometer to maximize the power reaching the photodetector, (c) use of a detector with lower noise, (d) improvement in the alignment technique, and (e) incorporation of a piezoelectric translator system so that micrometric adjustments of the position of the temporal bone could be made during the measurements. This system allows us to maintain the carrier level near the maximum value throughout the experiment.

These improvements enable us to regularly measure the vibratory response of cochlear structures of low reflectivity, such as the outer hair cells and the basilar membrane. The measurements are highly repeatable and can now be made over a wider frequency and amplitude range.

One of the most puzzling issues raised by our previous measurements was the relationship between the outer hair cell and the basilar membrane vibrations (Khanna et al, 1989a). This issue can now be investigated further using the improved technique of measurement.

Methods

Young, pigmented guinea pigs were used for the measurements. The technique of preparing the temporal bone and opening the cochlea was described earlier (Ulfendahl et al, 1989a,b). The temporal bone, immersed in oxygenated tissue culture medium, was mounted on a holder and attached to the micropositioning system of the microscope-interferometer. The cochlear structures were viewed through an objective lens (Olympus ULWD MS PLAN 20×) with a custom-built dipping cone (for immersion) at a 6-mm working distance.

The cochlea was viewed with the optical sectioning microscope (Koester et al, 1989),

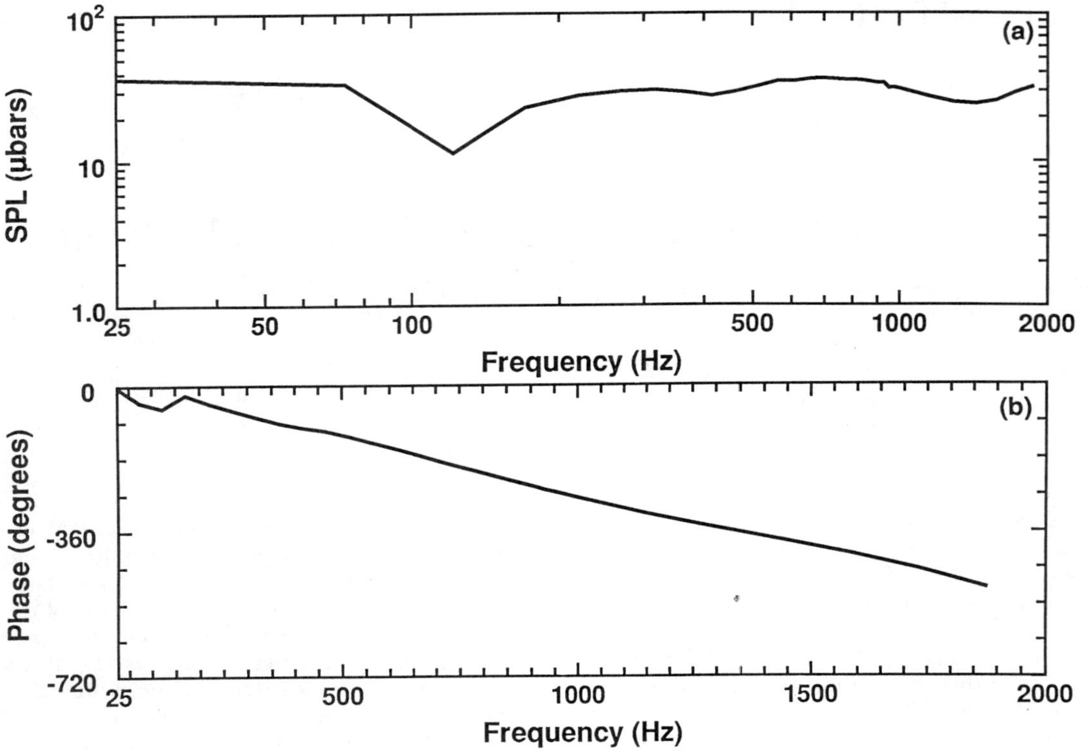

Figure 1-1 Sound pressure amplitude in microbars (*A*), and phase in degrees (*B*), measured as a function of frequency at the entrance to the bony ear canal for a constant input voltage of 2V peak applied to the acoustic system.

and the cellular vibrations were measured with the heterodyne interferometer (Willemin et al, 1989), in response to sinusoidal acoustic signals applied to the ear. The signals were generated, recorded, and analyzed digitally (Lund and Khanna, 1989).

The x, y, and z coordinates of the measurement points were determined with 1-μm resolution, using a Mitutoyo position measuring system connected to the micropositioning system (Khanna et al, 1989d). The position of the measuring beam with respect to cellular structures could then be compared with the anatomically measured distances between these structures (Kelly, 1989a,b; Kelly et al, 1989).

The measurements were made from the left temporal bone in the third turn at a position approximately 16 mm from the base of the cochlea. The results reported here are from one experiment, but data supporting these findings are available from several other experiments. It has been shown that the response of the cells deteriorates with time (Ulfendahl et al, 1989c); thus, the first response was measured within 1 hour of the time of decapitation, and measurements were continued for another hour.

Observations

Acoustic Measurements

The sound pressure generated at the entrance of the bony auditory meatus when a sinusoidal signal of 2 V peak amplitude is applied to the acoustic system is shown in Figure 1-1*A*. The frequency response in the temporal bone preparation is relatively flat over the 2-kHz frequency region. However, the notch at 120 Hz is not regularly seen. The maximum value of the sound pressure that can be produced by our present acoustic transducer is about 104 dB SPL.

The phase of the acoustic signal with reference to the phase of the electrical input to the sound system is shown in Figure 1-1*B*. The linear slope of the curve is −0.265 degrees per Hz. This is mainly due to the propagation time in the sound tubes connecting the acoustic transducer to the ear canal of the preparation. Because the probe tube measuring the

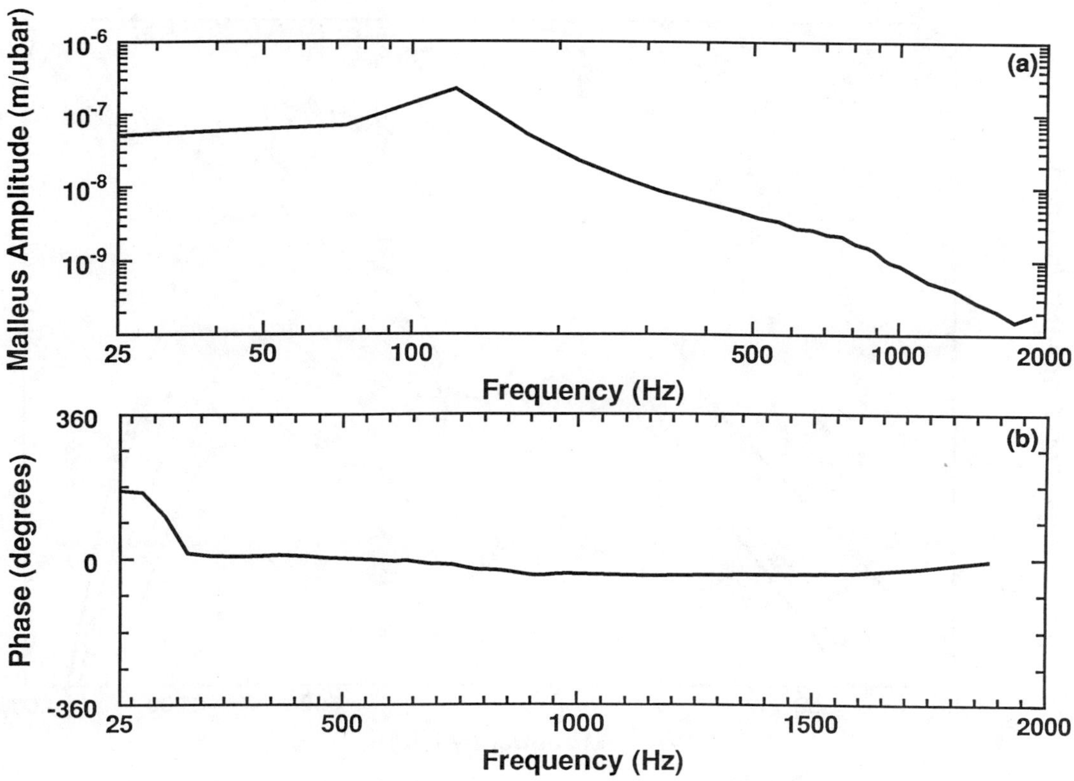

Figure 1-2 *A,* Malleus vibration amplitude in meters per microbar. *B,* Phase in degrees measured as a function of frequency.

sound pressure is now located close to the tympanic membrane, the effects of these tubes on the measurements can be accounted for. A two-channel recording system allows the vibration measurements with the interferometer to be recorded simultaneously with the sound pressure; therefore, the acoustic input can be used as a convenient reference to describe the vibratory response.

The immersion of the middle ear in the fluid, however, alters the vibratory response at any given sound pressure level and frequency from the normal condition—i.e., when the middle ear cavity is filled with air (Decraemer, unpublished observation). To take this change into account, it is important to have an additional reference that reflects the actual middle ear vibration whether the cavity is fluid filled or not.

Malleus Vibration Characteristics

Malleus vibration amplitude measured as a function of sound pressure level at the entrance of the bony meatus can be employed as a reference for the vibratory response measured in the cochlea under the same experimental conditions. The inner-ear responses can then be described in terms of the malleus vibrations.

In the guinea pig ear, it is anatomically impossible to view from the middle-ear side the manubrium of the malleus at an angle perpendicular to its direction of vibration, because the cochlea blocks this view (Khanna et al, 1989c). With the new long-working-distance (6 mm) dipping cone, the manubrium of the malleus can be observed at the best possible viewing angle. However, at these oblique angles, the response shape is highly angle-dependent. The use of the malleus vibration as a reference therefore contains a variable that varies from preparation to preparation. Experiments are now under way to determine the magnitude of this angle-dependent variability.

The malleus vibration amplitude calculated for a constant sound pressure level of 1 μbar at the entrance of the ear canal is shown in Figure 1-2*A*. The response amplitude in-

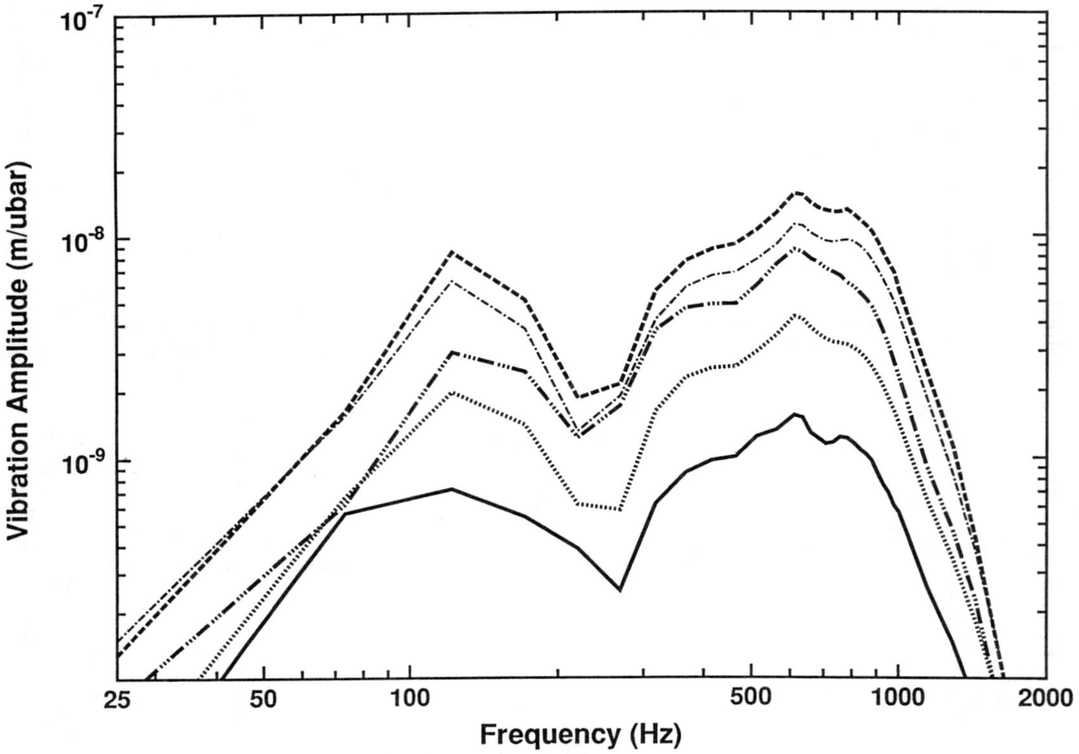

Figure 1-3 Vibration amplitude measured in meters per microbar as a function of frequency. Measurements were made in a radial direction moving from the outer bony edge of the cochlea inwards. Input voltage to the acoustic system was maintained constant at 2.0 V peak. Basilar membrane, 0 μm (solid line). Basilar membrane closer to the Hensen's cell edge, +25 μm (dotted line). Hensen's cell outer edge, +58 μm (dashed line). Hensen's cell inner edge, +111 μm (dashed dotted line). Second-row outer hair cell, +187 μm (dashed triple dotted line).

creases with frequency from 25 Hz, reaching a peak in the 120-Hz region. Thereafter, the response decreases with increasing frequency at a rate of roughly 12 dB per octave.

The malleus vibration phase measured with reference to the sound pressure phase at the entrance of the auditory meatus is shown in Figure 1-2*B*. The phase angle decreases from +180 degrees to 0 degrees from 25 to 170 Hz and remains at nearly 0 degrees up to 1900 Hz.

Cellular Vibration Characteristics

The vibration amplitude measured from selected cells is shown as a function of frequency in Figure 1-3 for a constant sound pressure of 1 μbar. The measurements can be made along a radial track, moving inward from the peripheral part of the basilar membrane across the organ of Corti towards the modiolus. In this experiment, the vibration was measured (1) at two locations on the peripheral part of the basilar membrane, attempting to make the second measurement as close to the border formed by the outer edge of the Hensen's cells as technically possible; (2) at two locations at the Hensen's cell region, near the outer edge and close to the inner edge; and (3) at a second-row outer hair cell.

The vibration amplitude increases progressively on the basilar membrane as we move inward, reaching a maximum at the outer edge of the Hensen's cell region. The vibration amplitude of the Hensen's cells at the outer edge is about four times higher than that of the basilar membrane just below it. The vibration amplitude of the cells on the reticular lamina decreases progressively as we move further inwards. These observations confirm those previously reported (Khanna et al, 1989a,b). As reported before, the shapes of the tuning curves at all points measured are similar.

The basilar membrane vibration amplitude increases as we move inward, closer to the Hensen's cells. At present, we are unable to measure the basilar membrane vibrations

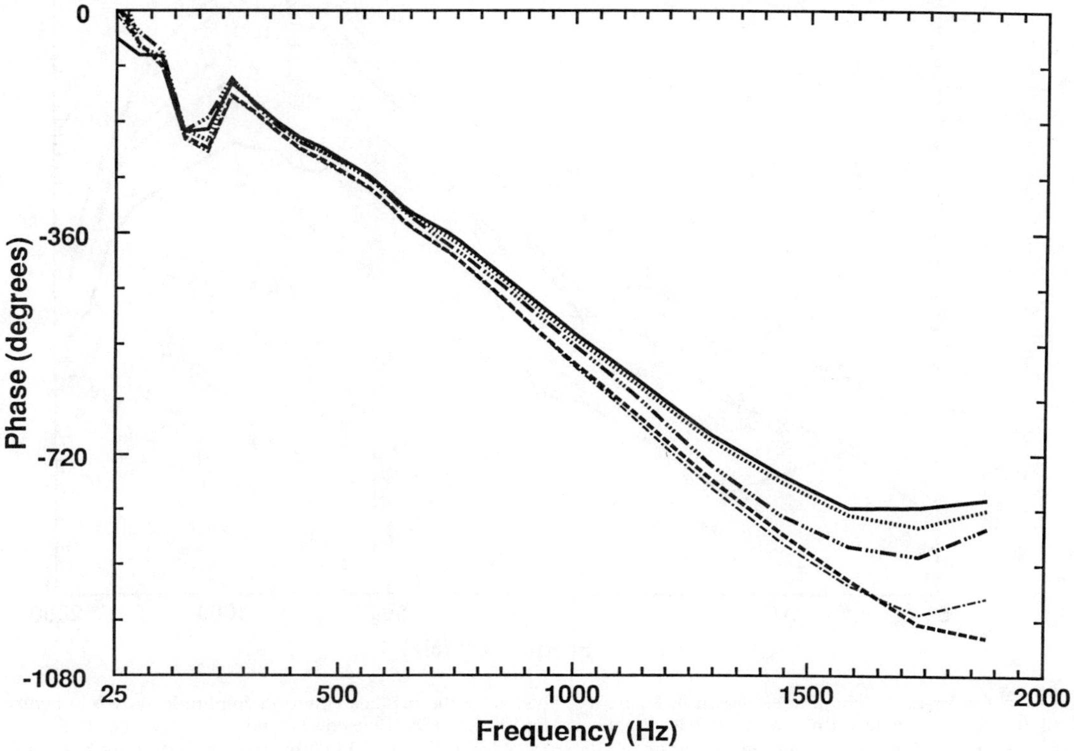

Figure 1-4 Vibration phase corresponding to the amplitude curve shown in Figure 1-3 (reference phase acoustical signal). Basilar membrane, 0 μm (solid line). Basilar membrane closer to the Hensen's cell edge, +25 μm (dotted line). Hensen's cell outer edge, +58 μm (dashed line). Hensen's cell inner edge, +111 μm (dashed dotted line). Second-row outer hair cell, +187 μm (dashed triple dotted line).

further inward, i.e., at the part underlying the organ of Corti, because the interferometer signal becomes too weak as the measuring beam penetrates the cell layers overlying the membrane.

Vibration phase corresponding to the amplitude curves of Figure 1-3 is shown in Figure 1-4. The reference in these figures is the sound pressure phase. The slope is approximately linear. In the region of 250 to 1300 Hz, its value for the basilar membrane curve is −0.55 degrees per Hz. The slope is progressively steeper for outer hair cells and Hensen's cells. Beyond 1300 Hz, the slope of the curve begins to decrease. In this region, the phase curves diverge more from each other.

Ratio of Cellular Amplitude and Malleus Amplitude

The cellular vibration amplitudes shown in Figure 1-3 were divided by the malleus vibration amplitude shown in Figure 1-2*A*. The results are shown in Figure 1-5. The peak of the response is at 940 Hz. The response increases with frequency between 50 and 200 Hz with a shallow slope (≈ 12 dB per octave) and then with a steeper slope of varying degree as it approaches the resonance peak. Beyond the resonance peak, the response drops off and the slope becomes progressively steeper with increasing frequency.

Curves obtained by subtracting the malleus vibration phase (Fig. 1-2*B*) from cellular vibration phase (Fig. 1-4) are shown in Figure 1-6. These curves show the same characteristics discussed with Figure 1-4.

Relationship Between the Outer Hair Cell and Basilar Membrane Response

The basilar membrane vibration amplitude was divided by the outer hair cell vibration amplitude (Fig. 1-3); the results are shown in Figure 1-7. In the region nearest to the Hensen's cell (dotted line), the ratio is nearly 1:1 at 70 Hz and above 1600 Hz. The

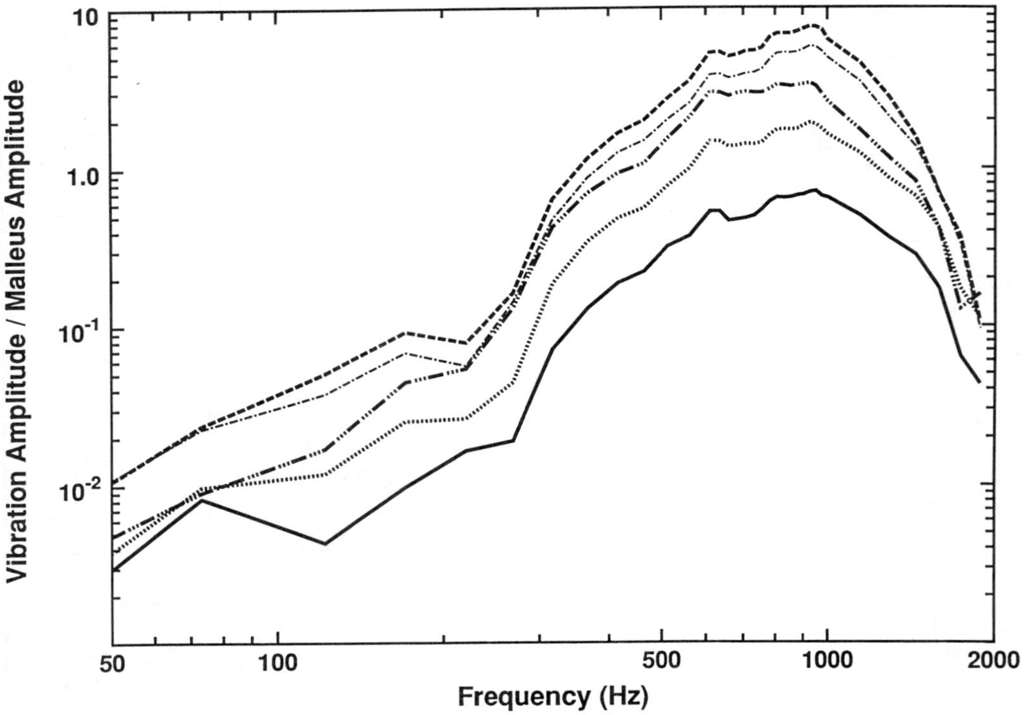

Figure 1-5 Vibration amplitudes shown in Figure 1-3 divided by the malleus vibration amplitude shown in Figure 1-2. Basilar membrane, 0 μm (solid line). Basilar membrane closer to the Hensen's cell edge, +25 μm (dotted line). Hensen's cell outer edge, +58 μm (dashed line). Hensen's cell inner edge, +111 μm (dashed dotted line). Second-row outer hair cell, +187 μm (dashed triple dotted line).

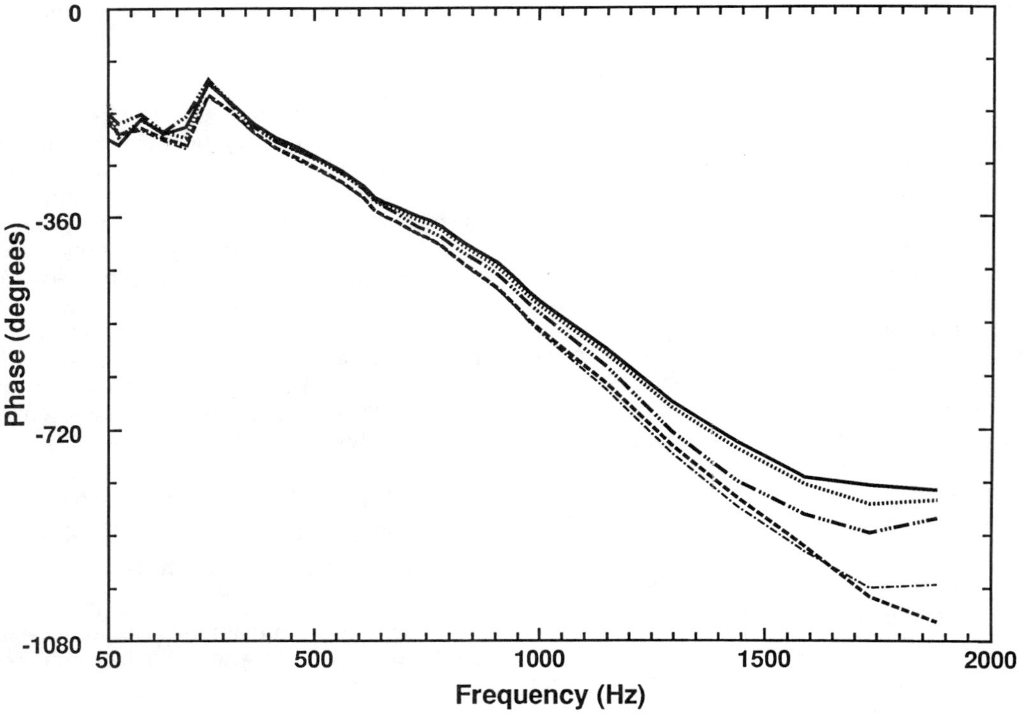

Figure 1-6 Vibration phase shown in Figure 1-4, referred to the malleus vibration phase. Basilar membrane, 0 μm (solid line). Basilar membrane closer to the Hensen's cell edge, +25 μm (dotted line). Hensen's cell outer edge, +58 μm (dashed line). Hensen's cell inner edge, +111 μm (dashed dotted line). Second-row outer hair cell, +187 μm (dashed triple dotted line).

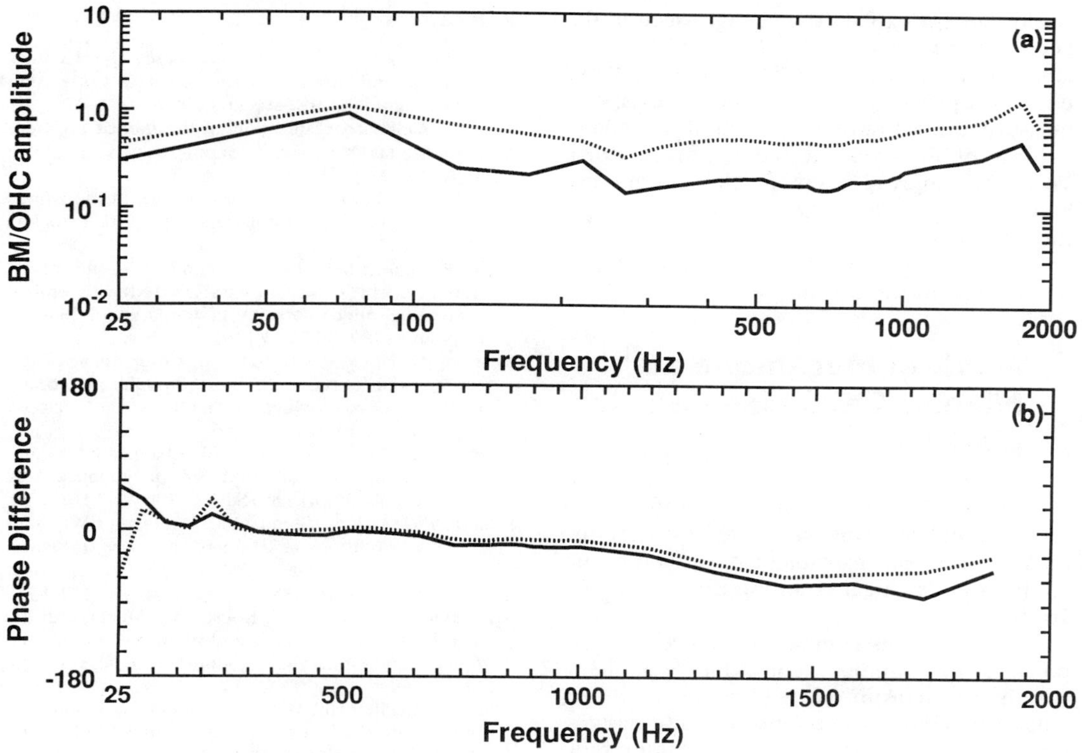

Figure 1-7 *A,* Ratio of the basilar membrane vibration amplitude to the second-row outer hair cell vibration amplitude and *B,* the difference in their vibration phases, shown for two positions on the basilar membrane. Dotted line, close to the outer edge of the Hensen cells; solid line, near the Hensen edge but not as close to it.

ratio is about 1:2 in the region between 200 and 900 Hz. The curve for the position towards the outer edge follows a similar pattern, although the ratios are lower in magnitude.

The phase difference between the basilar membrane vibrations and the outer hair cell vibrations is shown in Figure 1-7*B*. The difference is nearly 0 degrees between 150 and 650 Hz. It increases with frequency and reaches a maximum value of −90 degrees at 1750 Hz (solid line). The phase difference is position-dependent—i.e., it is smaller at the peripheral position on the basilar membrane (dotted line).

Discussion

The close similarity between the frequency responses of the vibrations of the outer hair cell and the vibrations of the basilar membrane, and the nearly zero phase angle between them, clearly indicate that the two responses are closely tied together. The change in the ratio of the basilar membrane vibration amplitude to the outer hair cell vibration amplitude with frequency suggests that the driving is more efficient near the resonance frequency and less efficient at frequencies both below and above the peak frequency. This ratio is different in each experiment and changes with time in the same population.

The basilar membrane vibration amplitude increases as the point of measurement moves inward. We do not know if this amplitude continues to increase as we move further inwards underneath the Hensen's cell and outer hair cell regions. If the basilar membrane vibration were to increase under these cells to a magnitude comparable to that of the Hensen's cells and they both vibrated with the same phase, it would suggest that the basilar membrane is driving the organ of Corti. In this case we may not be able to explain why the direction of maximum vibration is along the axis of the outer hair cells (Khanna et al, 1989e), because this axis is inclined at an angle of approximately 27 degrees to the plane of the basilar membrane (Kelly, 1989b). We could also not explain the changes seen in the cellular tuning along the radial axis of the cochlea (Khanna et al, 1989b). To answer these questions properly, it would be necessary to measure the vibrations at both the top and bottom of the cells in the organ of Corti. Technical improvements in the system are now under way to make it feasible to relate the vibration pattern of the cells of the organ of Corti to the motion of the basilar membrane beneath the organ.

Analyse Mécanique au Niveau Cellulaire dans la Cochlée

La mesure de la réponse mécanique au niveau cellulaire dans la cochlée est devenue possible avec un instrument qui combine un microscope confocal et un interféromètre hétérodyne.

Les vibrations cellulaires mesurées en réponse à un stimulus acoustique appliqué à l'oreille révèlent un mélange complexe de réponses non-linéaires continues et alternatives. Ces réponses varient avec: (1) la position radiale; (2) la position longitudinale; (3) la profondeur; (4) l'angle de mesure; (5) la fréquence du signal; (6) l'amplitude du signal; (7) la condition métabolique de la cellule. Bien que de nombreuses expériences soient encore nécessaires pour comprendre l'origine de ces réponses et pour les caractériser, une image préliminaire émerge selon laquelle la transduction auditive serait un procédé hautement dynamique qui comprendrait les effets combinés des réponses cellulaires de différents types.

ACKNOWLEDGMENTS

This research was supported by program project grant NS 22334 from the National Institute of Deafness and Communicative Disorders, and by the Emil Capita Foundation, the Torsten and Ragnar Söderberg Foundation, the Foundation Tysta Skolan, the Swedish Medical Research Council (02461), the Wenner-Gren Foundation, and the Karolinska Institute.

References

ITER (International Team for Ear Research). Cellular vibration and motility in the organ of Corti. Acta Otolaryngol [Suppl], (Stockh) 1989; 467:1-279.

Kelly JP. Cellular organization of the guinea pig's cochlea. Acta Otolaryngol [Suppl], (Stockh) 1989a; 467:97-112.

Kelly JP. Morphometry of the apical turn of the guinea pig's cochlea. Acta Otolaryngol [Suppl], (Stockh) 1989b; 467:113-122.

Kelly JP, Khanna SM, Flock Å, Ulfendahl M. Interpretation of cochlear structures visualized with optical sectioning microscopy. Acta Otolaryngol [Suppl], (Stockh) 1989; 467:123-129.

Khanna SM, Flock Å, Ulfendahl M. Comparison of the tuning of outer hair cells and the basilar membrane in the isolated cochlea. Acta Otolaryngol [Suppl], (Stockh) 1989a; 467:151-156.

Khanna SM, Flock Å, Ulfendahl M. Changes in cellular tuning along the radial axis of the cochlea. Acta Otolaryngol [Suppl], (Stockh) 1989b; 467:163-173.

Khanna SM, Flock Å, Ulfendahl M, Decraemer WF. Middle ear vibrations and sound pressure measurements in the isolated cochlea preparation. Acta Otolaryngol [Suppl], (Stockh) 1989c; 467:131-137.

Khanna SM, Rosskothen H, Koester CJ. Mechanical design of the measurement and micropositioning systems. Acta Otolaryngol [Suppl], (Stockh) 1989d; 467:51-59.

Khanna SM, Ulfendahl M, Flock Å. Modes of cellular vibration in the organ of Corti. Acta Otolaryngol [Suppl], (Stockh) 1989e; 467:183-188.

Koester CJ, Khanna SM, Rosskothen H, Tackaberry RB. Incident light optical sectioning microscope for visualization of cellular structures in the inner ear. Acta Otolaryngol [Suppl], (Stockh) 1989; 467:27-33.

Lund D, Khanna SM. A digital system for the generation of acoustic stimuli and the analysis of cellular vibration data. Acta Otolaryngol [Suppl], (Stockh) 1989; 467:77-89.

Ulfendahl M, Flock Å, Khanna SM. A temporal bone preparation for the study of cochlear micromechanics at the cellular level. Hear Res 1989a; 40:55-64.

Ulfendahl M, Flock Å, Khanna SM. Isolated cochlea preparation for the study of cellular vibrations and motility. Acta Otolaryngol [Suppl], (Stockh) 1989b; 467:91-96.

Ulfendahl M, Khanna SM, Flock Å. Changes in the vibratory responses of Hensen's cells with time. Acta Otolaryngol [Suppl], (Stockh) 1989c; 467:145-149.

Willemin JF, Khanna SM, Dändliker R. Heterodyne interferometer for cellular vibration measurement. Acta Otolaryngol [Suppl], (Stockh) 1989; 467:35-42.

CHAPTER 2

Effects of Intense Acoustic Stimulation on the Nonlinear Properties of Mammalian Hair Cells

ALAN R. CODY
IAN J. RUSSELL

In the mammalian cochlea, two forces act to reduce the ability of the primary mechanoreceptor to produce voltage responses to high-frequency acoustic stimuli. First, frictional forces in the fluid-filled compartments damp the vibration of the cochlea partition. Second, the capacitive electrical properties of the hair cell membranes effectively low-pass filter the phasic or AC components of the receptor potential at the rate of approximately 6 dB per octave above about 1 kHz (Russell and Sellick, 1978; Russell and Palmer, 1986). In theory, the combination of these two forces should make it progressively more difficult for an animal to detect acoustic stimuli above 1 kHz. The fundamental problem of detecting high-frequency sounds appears to have been overcome in the mammalian cochlea by two separate nonlinear mechanisms, both of which oppose or reduce these effects and act to establish the high degrees of frequency selectivity and sensitivity that are features of the cochlea. One source of nonlinearity is the transducer conductance of the hair cell. In response to sinusoidal stimuli delivered either as an acoustic stimulus to the cochlea or as a direct displacement of the stereocilia of the individual hair cell, the receptor potential becomes asymmetrical, which results in a steady-state or DC component (Russell and Sellick, 1978; Russell et al, 1986; Hudspeth and Corey, 1977). This potential is not influenced by the capacitive electrical properties of the cell membrane; therefore, the hair cell can produce excitatory potentials to high-frequency stimuli.

Another source of nonlinear behavior in the cochlea is that associated with the vibration of the cochlear partition. Direct measurements of basilar membrane micromechanics reveal that for any single position along the cochlear duct, the displacement of the membrane is highly tuned (Khanna and Leonard, 1982; Sellick et al, 1982). This tuning is labile and susceptible to cochlear insult in the form of loud sounds, anoxia, and specific damage to the outer hair cells (see Patuzzi and Robertson, 1988, for a review). More recently, this group of cells has been shown to have motile properties when placed in an alternating electrical field (Brownell et al, 1985) or during intracellular injection of AC or DC current (Ashmore, 1987). This evidence, coupled with the observation that the cochlea can emit sound (Kemp, 1979), has led to the proposal that outer hair cells (OHCs) in the mammalian cochlea may, through their motile properties, inject mechanical energy back into the basilar membrane in a frequency- and phase-dependent manner that acts to enhance the displacement of the partition (Neely and Kim, 1986; Weiss, 1982; McMullen and Mountain, 1985). This effectively counteracts the viscous damping forces in the cochlea. It would appear, therefore, that the cochlea has solved the two fundamental problems relating to the detection of high-frequency acoustic stimuli.

After overstimulation, the cochlea's ability to detect high-frequency stimuli is reduced (Cody and Johnstone, 1980). Presumably, this means that either the cochlear micromechanics or the nonlinear properties of the hair cell, or a combination of the two, have been modified. Thus, the supposition is that a loss of the nonlinear properties of the cochlea after acoustic overstimulation may contribute to, or underlie, noise-induced hearing loss. Intracellular data from both inner and outer hair cells recorded in the basal coil of the guinea pig cochlea tend to support this supposition in that the responses of these two hair cell groups to acoustic stimulation become increasingly linear during and after exposure to loud sound.

Methods

The specific methods for the intracellular recording of responses from mammalian hair cells have been extensively documented in a number of previous publications (Russell and Sellick, 1978; Cody and Russell, 1985). Access to the hair cells is via a small hole shaved in the bony wall of the basal turn or high-frequency end of the cochlea, where best frequencies for receptors usually fall between 16 and 22 kHz. Glass micropipettes with nominal impedances of between 80 and 120 MΩ (3 M KCl) are advanced under visual guidance through the undrained perilymph of the scala tympani into the organ of Corti. Receptor cell types are usually classified according to their responses to shaped acoustic tone bursts, their location with respect to the inner sulcus (radial aspect), and the depth of the recording site while one moves from the scala tympani to the scala media (vertical aspect). The raw data were stored on magnetic tape and then digitized for off-line analysis. Cellular harmonic responses to pure tones were determined using the fast Fourier transform and in some cases a lock-in amplifier.

Intracellular stability of the recording is a particular problem in studies of noise-induced hearing loss, presumably because of the larger excursions of the organ of Corti at high sound pressure levels. For this reason, the duration of the traumatizing tone (which is presented half an octave below the estimated characteristic frequency—CF—of the cell) was restricted to periods of either 15 or 30 seconds at a level not exceeding 110 dB SPL (SPL re 20 μPa). These restrictions meant that the levels of hair cell desensitization were low and that the recovery periods were accelerated when compared to cochlear desensitizations induced by louder and longer overstimulations. This reduced the amount of data that could be collected in any single run. To maximize the information recorded from the hair cell, multiple presentations of the stimuli and averaging of the cellular responses have not been attempted. As a result, the data tend to be noisier and more variable. In addition, hair cell responses to any single stimulus depend on the frequency and intensity of the preceding stimuli. Multiple presentations of stimuli, particularly at high levels, can result in a modified response of the cell when compared to responses to single stimuli. This problem was reduced by not attempting multiple presentations of the stimulus, and by adjusting the interval between the presentations of the test tone, so that the cellular response was not influenced by the preceding tone.

Results

Hair Cell Responses to Acoustic Stimuli

Typical hair cell responses to low- and high-frequency tones before and after exposure to a loud tone (110 dB SPL, 12.5 kHz) are shown in Figure 2-1. In the sensitive cochlea, the inner hair cell (IHC) response to a low-frequency tone (600 Hz, 65 dB SPL) demonstrates a depolarizing asymmetry of the receptor potential (Fig. 2-1*A*). This asymmetry is recorded at all levels of the stimulus and facilitates the identification of the IHC. Receptor potentials in these cells can approach 30 mV peak-to-peak for sound pressure levels of 70 to 100 dB, and there is a substantial DC component. In contrast, the OHC demonstrates a predominantly hyperpolarizing receptor potential when stimulated at the same intensity and frequency (Fig. 2-1*B*). However, the symmetry of the receptor potential is level-dependent, changing from symmetrical at low stimulus levels to hyperpolarizing and then reversing to grow in the depolarizing phase for stimulus intensities above about 70 dB SPL (Russell et al, 1986). Maximal peak-to-peak potentials approach only 8 to 10 mV, and the DC component of the receptor potential is small in comparison with that recorded for the IHC, even at the highest intensities. When the stimulus is delivered at higher frequencies (18 kHz, 65 dB SPL), the IHC response (Fig. 2-1*C*) is then seen only as a DC potential, because the phasic component of the potential has been filtered by the low-pass electrical properties of the cell membrane and the recording electrode (Russell and Sellick, 1978). For stimuli at 18 kHz and similar levels, the OHC shows only a small (1 mV) depolarizing DC receptor potential, with maximum ampli-

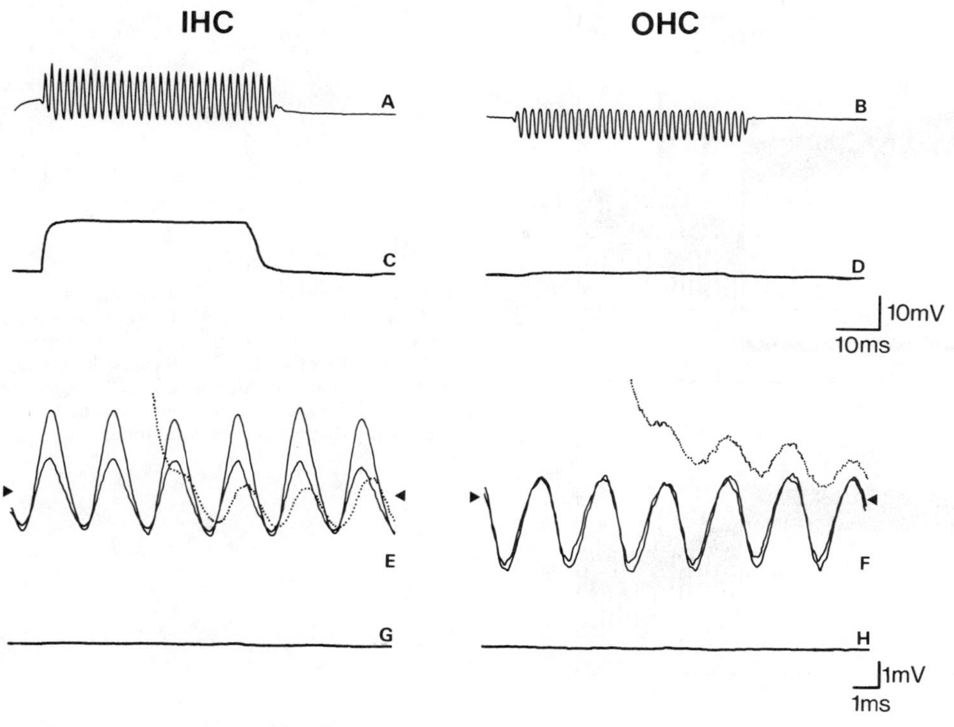

Figure 2-1 Hair cell responses to low stimulus (*A*, IHC—600 Hz, 68 dB; *B*, OHC—600 Hz, 78 dB) and high stimulus (*C*, IHC—18 kHz, 68 dB; *D*, OHC—18 kHz, 78 dB) frequencies. *E*, IHC receptor potential to a 600-Hz (85 dB SPL) tone before (solid lines) and immediately after (dotted line) exposure to a loud tone. *F*, The OHC response to the same acoustic stimuli. In this portion of the figure, the arrows at either end of the trace indicate the pretrauma membrane potential of the cell. The traces shown in *G* and *H* are the receptor potentials generated by the same stimuli used for the IHC and OHC in *C* and *D*, respectively, immediately following the loud tone.

tudes reaching only 3 to 4 mV at sound pressures of 110 to 115 dB (Fig. 2-1*D*).

A summary of the OHC and IHC responses produced in different animals to acoustic overstimulation is shown in the lower half of Figure 2-1. Immediately following the loud tone, both the IHC (Fig. 2-1*E*) and the OHC (Fig. 2-1*F*) show a decrease in the amplitude of the receptor potentials in response to a 600-Hz tone (dotted line). The IHC also demonstrates a phase lag of approximately 60 degrees following the loud tone, which recovers within a few cycles. The OHC shows an elevation of the membrane potential that is not seen in the IHC, but there is no obvious change in the phase of the receptor potential. The loss in amplitude of the IHC receptor potential is restricted to the depolarizing phase. In the OHC it is difficult to determine symmetry because of the repolarization of the membrane potential (Fig. 2-1*F*). For higher-frequency test tones (18 kHz, 65 dB SPL), it is apparent that the DC component of the receptor potential was abolished for both cell groups (Fig. 2-1*G,H*).

The response of the OHC and the IHC during the loud tone is seen more clearly in Figure 2-2. The most striking feature of this figure is the difference in behavior of the two cell types to the loud tone. OHCs show an increasing depolarization during the tone that, in this example, plateaus after about 20 seconds. At the end of the tone, the membrane potential remains elevated but recovers within 15 seconds at a rate of 0.166 mV per second. The recovery is not linear but can be approximated by a single exponential function with a time constant of about 4.5 seconds. In contrast, the IHC shows classic "adaptation" for the duration of the loud tone and hyperpolarizes at the offset. Repolarization takes place with a similar time constant to that recorded for the repolarization of the OHC. For the IHC the adaptation is intensity- and frequency-dependent, and is generally seen only for exposure durations exceeding a few hundred milliseconds. The resistance change recorded in the IHC during the loud tone mirrors the adaptation of the receptor potential, suggesting that this phenomenon is not an intrinsic prop-

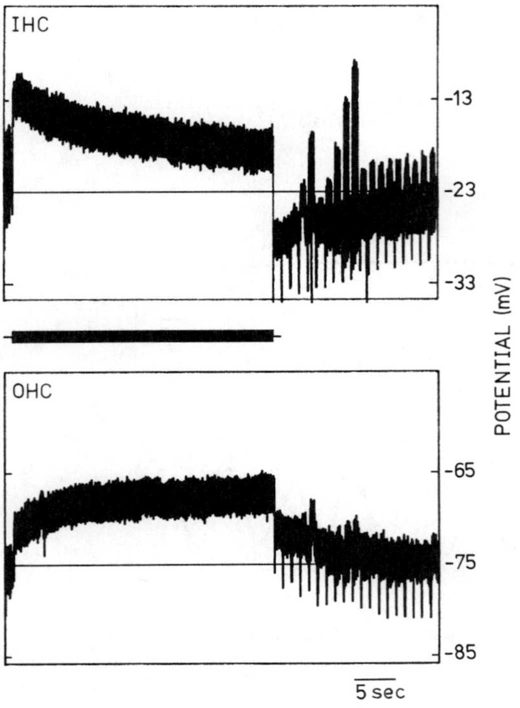

Figure 2-2 Inner hair cell (IHC) and outer hair cell (OHC) responses to a 12.5-kHz continuous tone delivered at 110 dB SPL for 30 seconds. The horizontal line in the middle of each part indicates the resting membrane potential recorded in the cell before the loud tone was presented. The bar between the two parts indicates the duration of the loud tone.

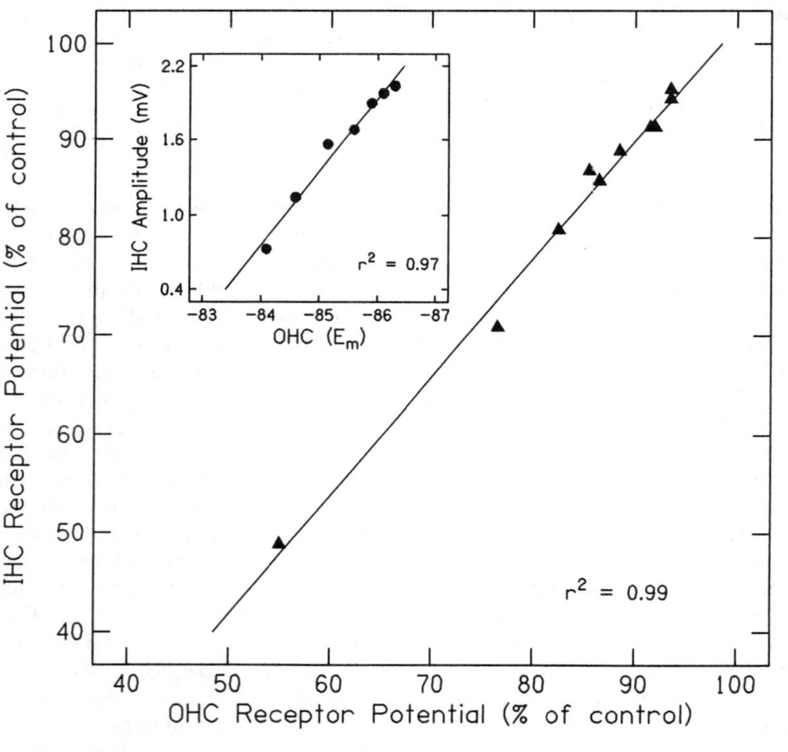

Figure 2-3 Receptor potential amplitude plotted as a percentage of pre-exposure control levels for an IHC and an OHC. Each point (solid triangles) represents the receptor potential amplitude determined at 200-ms intervals following the loud tone. The inset figure reflects the same data, but the IHC receptor potential amplitude is plotted as a function of the OHC membrane potential (solid circles). The 12.5-kHz exposure tone was presented for 225 ms.

erty of the hair cell, but rather a result of decreasing mechanical displacement of its stereocilia.

The elevation of the OHC membrane potential would appear to be intimately related to cochlear sensitivity, as shown in Figure 2-3. The recovery of the IHC DC responses to tones at their CF (see Figure 2-3, inset) is closely correlated ($r^2 = 0.97$) with the recovery of the OHC membrane potential. The recovery of the low-frequency peak-to-peak amplitude of the receptor potential for both hair cells is also closely correlated ($r^2 = 0.99$). Because the IHC and the OHC responses to test tones recover at a similar rate, the original loss in sensitivity of both hair cell groups may arise from a common mechanism or site.

Hair Cell Tuning

One of the features of the mammalian cochlea is the high degree of frequency selectivity of its receptors. This is shown in Figure 2-4 in the isoamplitude tuning curves for the AC and DC components of the hair cell receptor potential for the IHC and the OHC. Isoamplitude in this case is the amplitude of the receptor potential recorded intracellularly at the threshold of detectability for the compound action potential (CAP) of the auditory nerve. At a single recording location along the cochlea partition, both the IHC and the OHC show similar tuning properties with a high degree of selectivity for stimulus frequencies at and around the CF of the cell. It is obvious from Figure 2-4 that the AC component is highly tuned and little different between the IHC and the OHC. However, the DC component recorded from the two cell types is significantly different, particularly in terms of its level dependence. In the most sensitive animals, IHCs will produce DC receptor potentials to CF tones at sound pressure levels as low as 0 dB SPL. In the OHC, significant depolarizing DC receptor potentials are not recorded until stimulus levels reach 70 to 80 dB SPL. At this point, the AC component of the receptor potential is showing signs of saturation. In view of this disparity, the amplitude used to construct the DC tuning curve for the OHC in Figure 2-4 has been fixed at the amplitude used for the IHC (0.8 mV). Around the CF, the OHC does show a degree of tuning similar to that of the IHC, but the curve is elevated by about 55 dB in this frequency range, whereas little difference is seen for the "tail" or low-frequency regions of the tuning curve.

Following the loud tone, a change in cell sensitivity is recorded for both the IHC and the OHC in the AC component of the receptor potential, and for the IHC in the DC component of the receptor potential. This is seen as a loss in sensitivity that is maximal around the CF of the cell, with minimal changes in the "tail" sensitivity or, as is shown in Figure 2-4, small increases in sensitivity. However, it is apparent from this figure that there is little change in the OHC DC component. This finding is complicated by the fact that the DC tuning of the OHC demonstrates a level dependence not recorded in the IHC. Figure 2-5 shows two different iso-SPL, rather than isoamplitude, tuning curves for an OHC recorded in the basal turn of the guinea pig cochlea before and after acoustic overstimulation. At relatively low average SPLs (55 dB), the tuning of the DC receptor potential is complex, showing a triphasic character below and around the presumed CF of the cell. If the iso-SPL is raised to 85 dB, then the DC component of the hair cell demonstrates simpler tuning, similar to that shown in Figure 2-4. Following acoustic overstimulation (lower panel), the low-level triphasic response is lost, whereas the structure for the higher level iso-SPL curve has been maintained, although reduced in amplitude. This complex tuning (if it can be called tuning) has been recorded in all OHCs to date, although cells vary significantly. In some respects, the triphasic nature of the curve demonstrates a remarkable similarity to the frequency-dependent basilar membrane bias shown by Le Page (1987).

Hair Cell Responses to Acoustic Overstimulation

If a low-frequency tone and the high-frequency traumatizing tone are delivered simultaneously, the hair cells' response to the low-frequency tone is seen to be substantially altered by the trauma. This is shown in Figure 2-6 for an IHC. The amplitude of the receptor potential is substantially reduced and, more importantly, the depolarizing asymmetry of the receptor potential is lost and even reversed to become predominantly hyperpolarizing for all but the highest stimulus levels. In Figure 2-7, the AC components (fundamental component, first even and first odd harmonic components) and the DC component of the receptor potential for the hair cell shown in Figure 2-6 are plotted as a function of intensity for a stimulus frequency of 270 Hz both

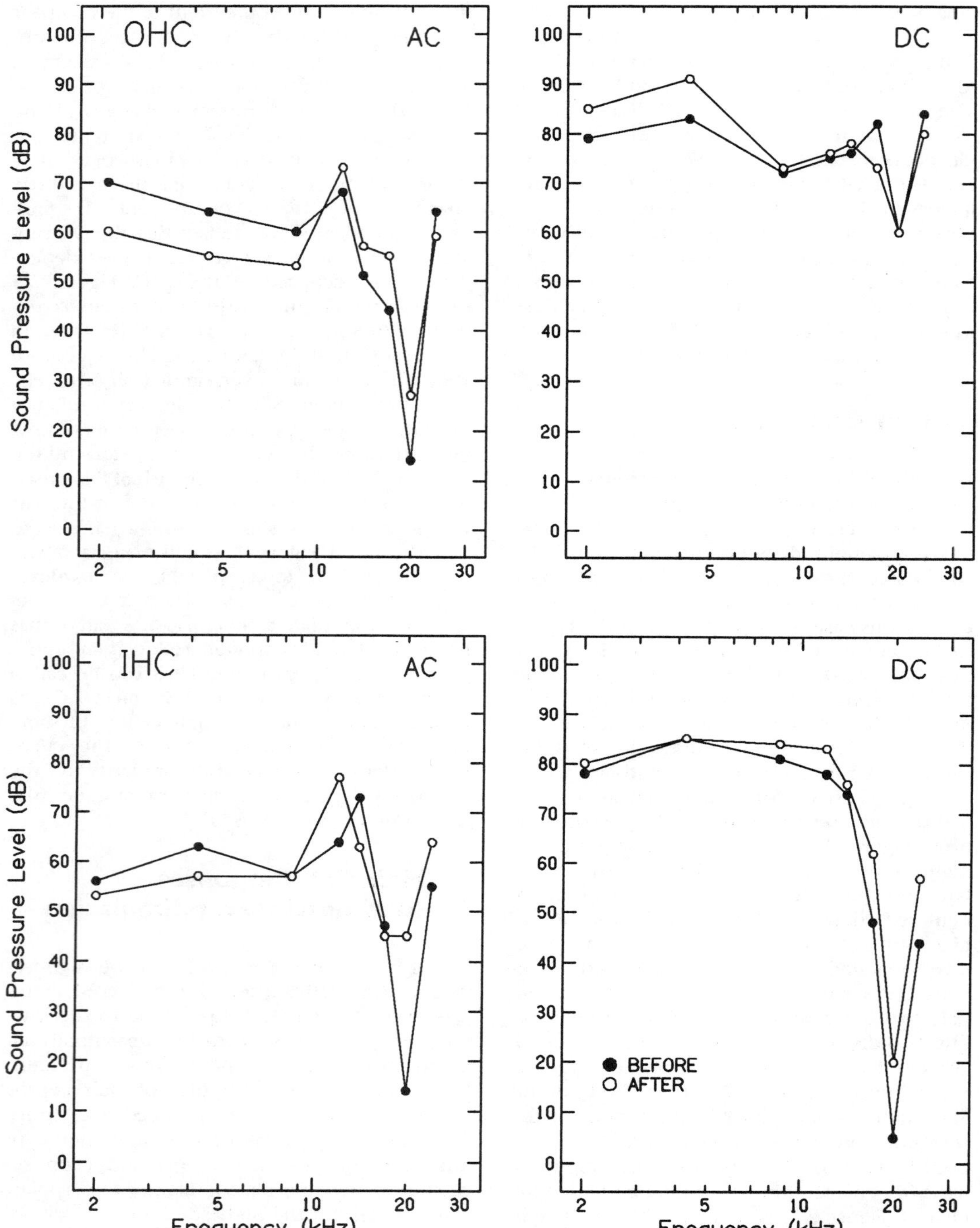

Figure 2-4 Isoamplitude tuning curves for an outer hair cell (OHC) (AC, 0.5 mV; DC, 0.8 mV) and an inner hair cell (IHC) (AC, 0.5 mV; DC, 0.8 mV) before (solid circles) and following (open circles) exposure of the cochlea to a 12.5-kHz tone for 15 seconds at a level of 110 dB SPL. A frequency-selective loss of sensitivity centered around the characteristic frequency of the cell is apparent for all but the OHC DC tuning curves.

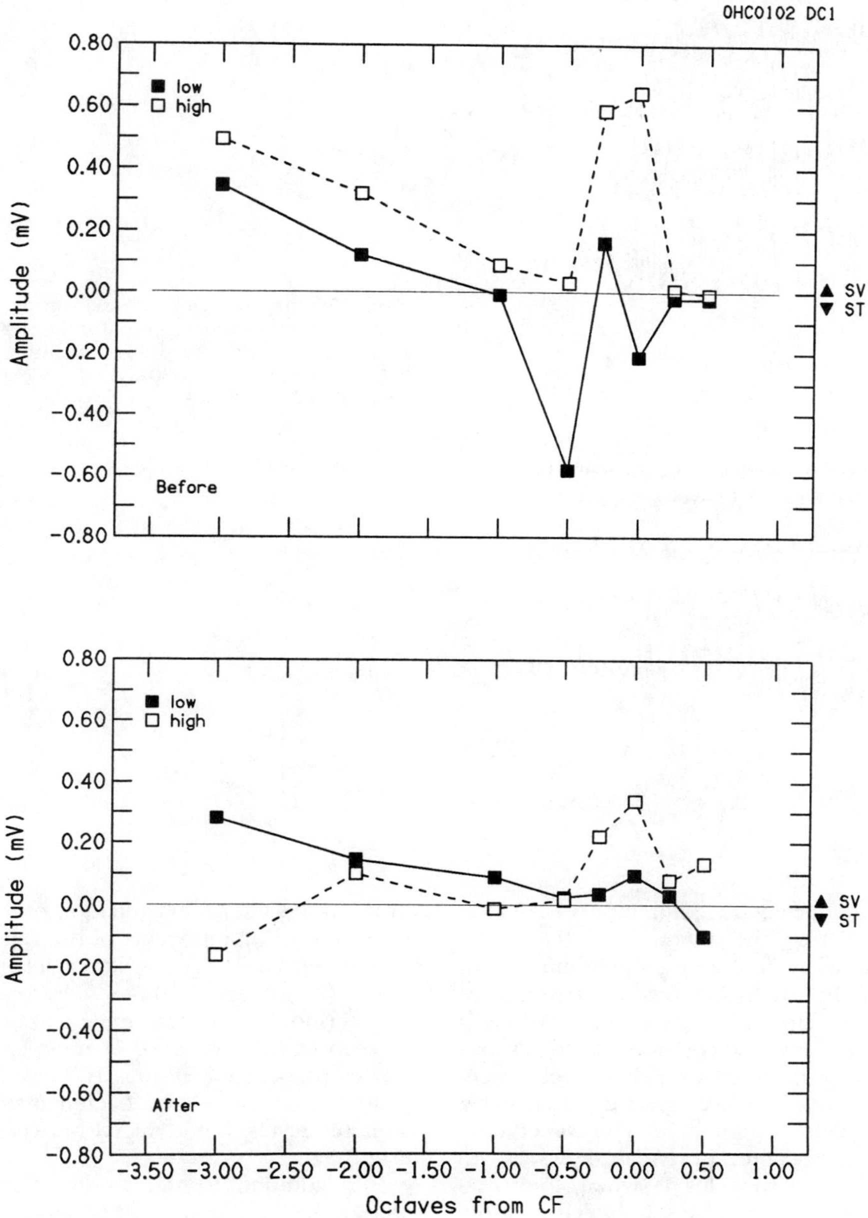

Figure 2-5 Iso-sound pressure level, DC tuning curves for an OHC recorded before (upper panel) and following (lower panel) the presentation of a 12.5-kHz, 30-second, 110-dB SPL tone. The solid squares in each panel indicate the DC tuning at a low average SPL (55 dB); the open squares denote the DC tuning at a high average SPL (85 dB). The solid arrows to the right of each panel indicate the predicted direction of movement of the cochlear partition (SV = scala vestibuli; ST = scala tympani) that would be required to produce the depolarizing (+ve) or hyperpolarizing (−ve) DC receptor potentials.

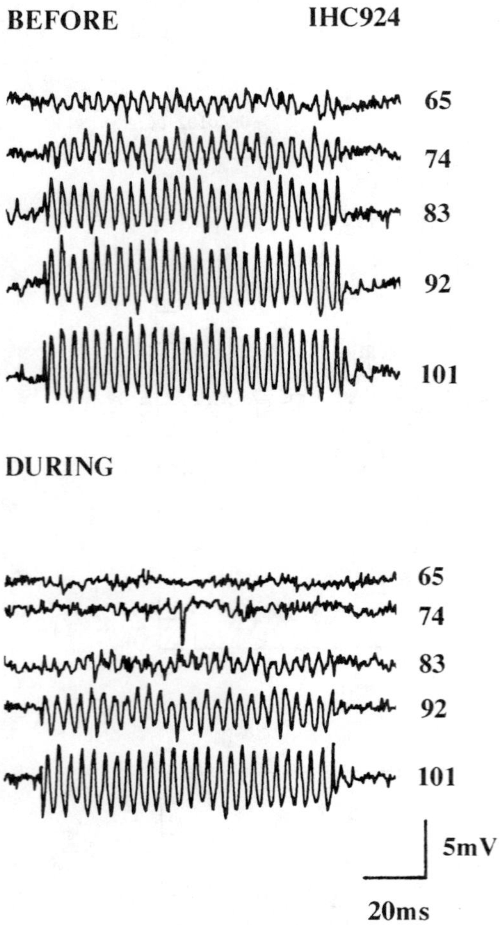

Figure 2-6 IHC receptor potentials generated in response to a 270-Hz tone delivered at the SPLs indicated to the right of each trace, before and during the simultaneous presentation of a 30-second, 13.5-kHz, 110-dB SPL loud tone.

before and during the loud tone (12.5 kHz, 110 dB SPL). At the lowest SPLs, the fundamental component shows a significant loss of sensitivity, but at higher levels (101 dB) approaches the pretrauma peak amplitudes. On average, the harmonic components are also reduced during the loud tone, but level dependence for them is not as clear-cut as it is for the fundamental component. The DC component of the receptor potential shows an increase at the lowest levels when compared with pretrauma amplitudes, followed by a decrease at higher levels, finally reversing to grow again at 101 dB SPL. This trend mirrors the changing symmetry of the receptor potential shown in the raw data plotted in Figure 2-6.

For the OHC (Fig. 2-8), the greater loss in amplitude is obvious when compared with the IHC, and it is only at the highest level that the structure of the receptor potential can be seen in the raw data. An examination of the behavior of the AC components of the receptor potential (Fig. 2-9) reveals similar changes during the loud tone to those seen for the IHC: the harmonic and fundamental components are substantially reduced at most amplitudes. In this particular cell, the DC component appears to be relatively unaffected at the highest stimulus levels, but reduced between 70 and 80 dB SPL.

In addition to the modifications of the amplitudes of the AC components of the receptor potential, the fundamental and the harmonic components of the receptor potential show significant phase changes during the loud tone (Fig. 2-10). For both the IHC and the OHC, the phase of the fundamental component remains relatively stable at all stimulus levels in the pretrauma period. During the loud tone, the phase of this component changes substantially with increasing

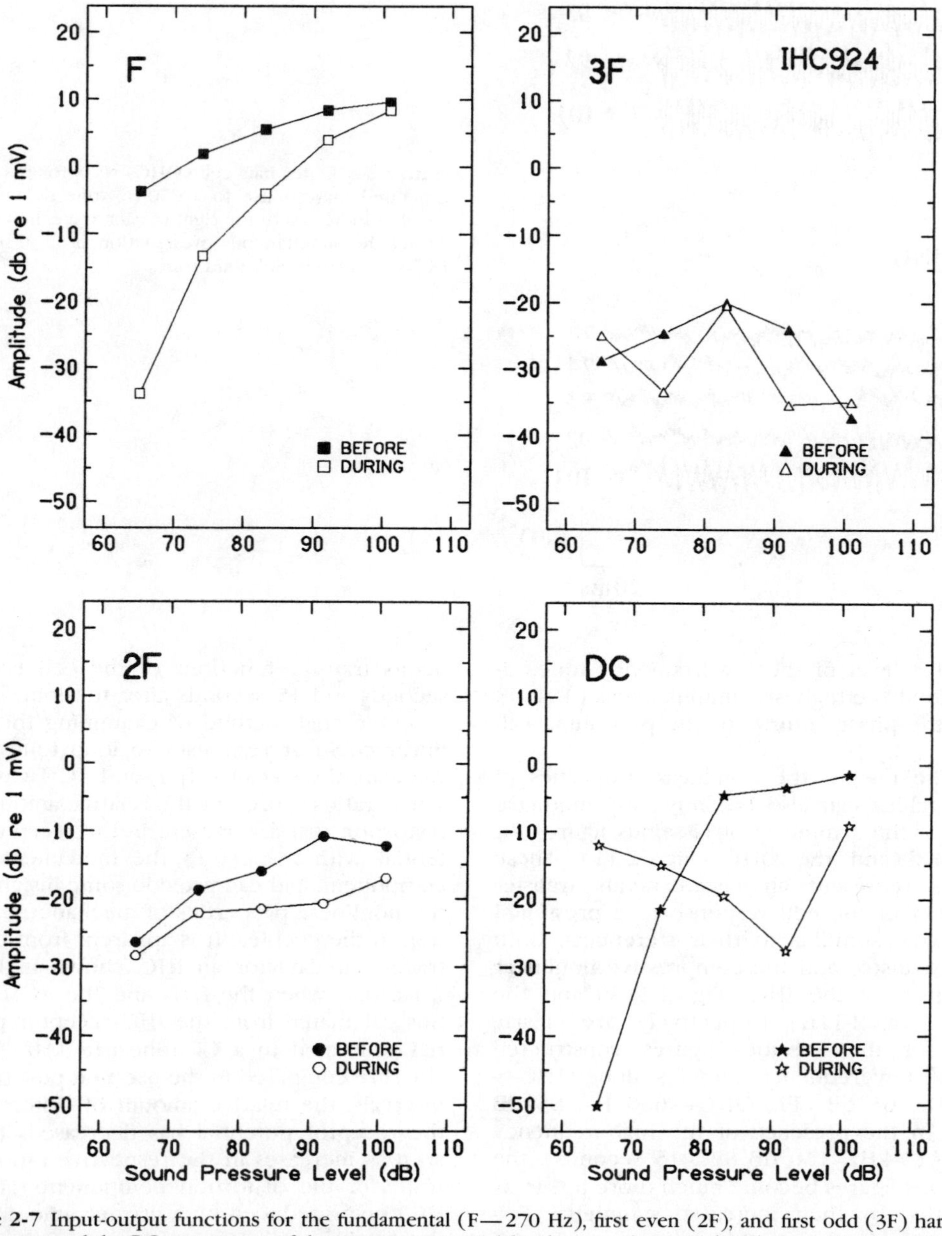

Figure 2-7 Input-output functions for the fundamental (F—270 Hz), first even (2F), and first odd (3F) harmonic components and the DC component of the receptor potential for the inner hair cell (IHC) shown in Figure 2-6. The solid and open symbols are the respective responses before and during the presentation of the loud tone.

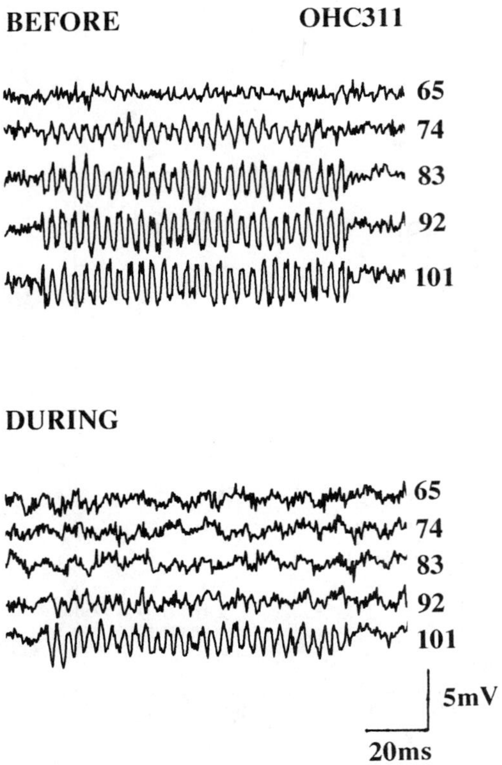

Figure 2-8 Outer hair cell (OHC) receptor potentials generated in response to a 270-Hz tone delivered at the SPLs indicated to the right of each trace, before and during the simultaneous presentation of a 30-second, 13.5-kHz, 110-dB SPL loud tone.

stimulus level of the low-frequency tone, although at the highest stimulus levels (101 dB SPL) the phase returns to the pretrauma values.

The loss of the nonlinear properties of the cochlea can also be shown by modifications of the symmetry of Lissajous figures for the IHC and the OHC (Fig. 2-11). These figures represent an instantaneous transfer function of the cell response to a presumed sinusoidal stimulus to their stereocilia. Both the expansive and the compressive nonlinear responses of the IHC (Fig. 2-11*A*) and the OHC (Fig. 2-11*B*), respectively, are clearly seen for the Lissajous figures constructed for the low-frequency stimulus alone (IHC—600 Hz, 65 dB SPL; OHC—600 Hz, 85 dB SPL). In the presence of the high-frequency tone (13 kHz, 110 dB SPL, 15 seconds), the Lissajous figures become much more linear, as indicated by their increased symmetry. Following the loud tone, the nonlinear properties of the OHC (Fig. 2-11*D*) and the nonlinear properties of the IHC (Fig. 2-11*C*) show a rapid recovery, although the IHC amplitude has not fully recovered. (The individual traces in Fig. 2-11*C* and *D* represent the instantaneous transfer functions of the cell taken 5 seconds and 15 seconds after the loud tone.)

One final method of examining the nonlinear cochlear responses to loud tones is to calculate the so-called $f_1:f_2$ and AC:DC ratios. These ratios represent the relative amounts of distortion that are present in the receptor potential with respect to the fundamental AC component, and can provide some insight into the nonlinear properties of mechanotransduction in the cochlea. It is apparent from the intracellular data for an IHC, shown in Figure 2-12, that when the $f_1:f_2$ and the AC:DC ratios calculated from the IHC receptor potential generated to a CF tone (18 kHz, 55 dB SPL) are compared in the pre- and post-trauma intervals, the relative amount of distortion in the receptor potential has decreased. This is seen as increases in the respective ratios as a result of the distortion components (f_2 and DC) being reduced by a greater amount than the fundamental AC component. That is, the hair cell response to the tone has become more linear. In this particular example, in which the high-intensity tone was only delivered for 200 ms, the ratios recovered within approximately 300 ms.

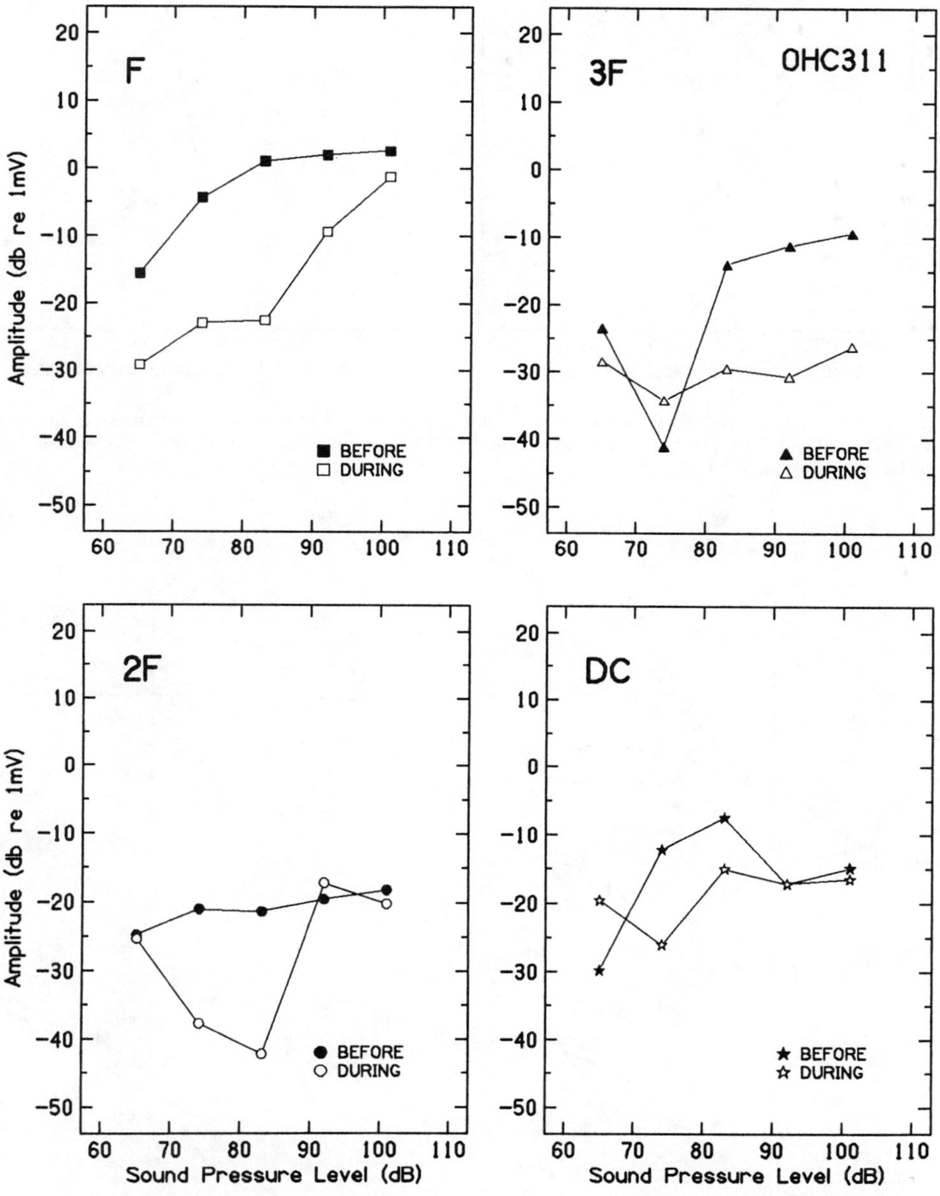

Figure 2-9 Input-output functions for fundamental (F—270 Hz), first even (2F), and first odd (3F) harmonic components and the DC component of the receptor potential for the OHC shown in Figure 2-8. The solid and open symbols are the respective responses before and during the simultaneous presentation of the loud tone.

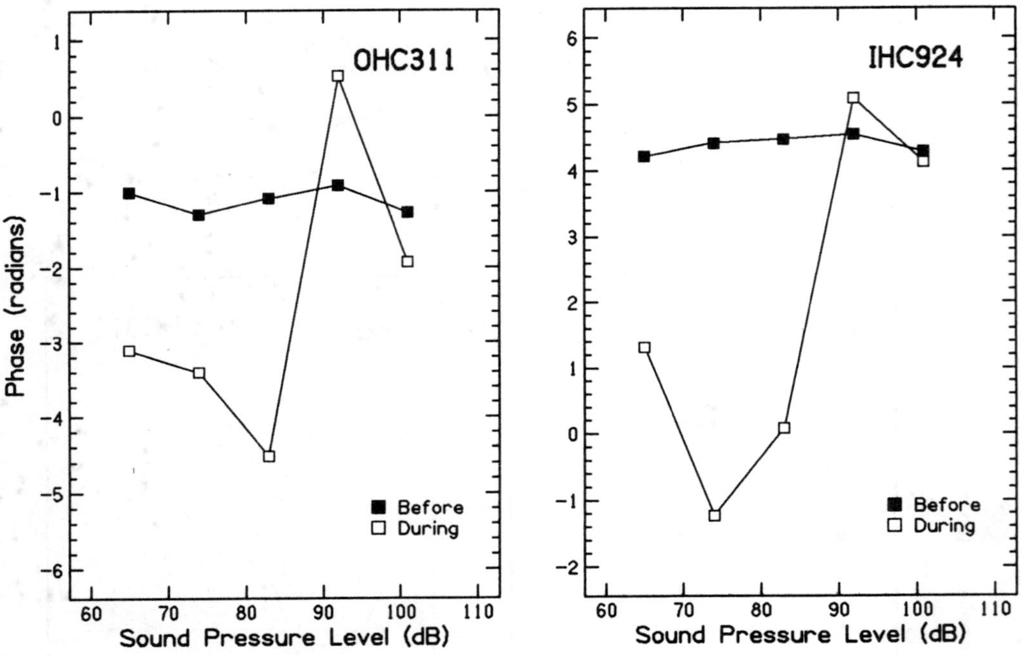

Figure 2-10 Phase changes recorded in the fundamental component of the receptor potential for the inner hair cell (IHC) and the outer hair cell (OHC) shown in Figures 2-6 and 2-8 before (filled symbols) and during (open symbols) the presentation of the loud tone.

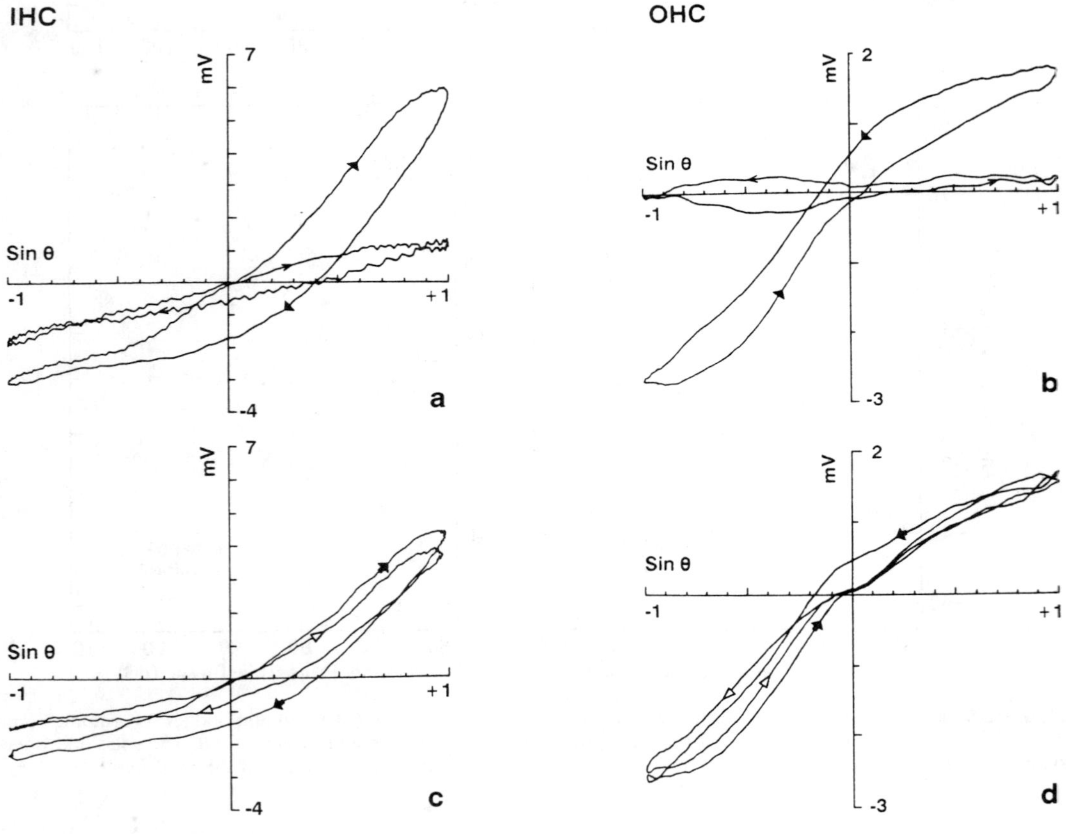

Figure 2-11 Lissajous figures constructed by plotting the instantaneous amplitude of the inner hair cell (IHC) *(a* and *c)* and outer hair cell (OHC) *(b* and *d)* receptor potentials as a function of Sin θ (i.e., a sinusoidal displacement of the stereocilia of the cell) before (*a* and *b*—solid arrows) and during (*a* and *b*—open arrows) exposure of the cochlea to a 14.5-kHz tone for 15 seconds at 110 dB SPL. The Lissajous figures were also plotted for the receptor potential recorded 5 (*c* and *d*—open triangles) and 15 (*c* and *d*—solid arrows) seconds after the loud tone. Low-frequency tone, 265 Hz, 70 dB SPL.

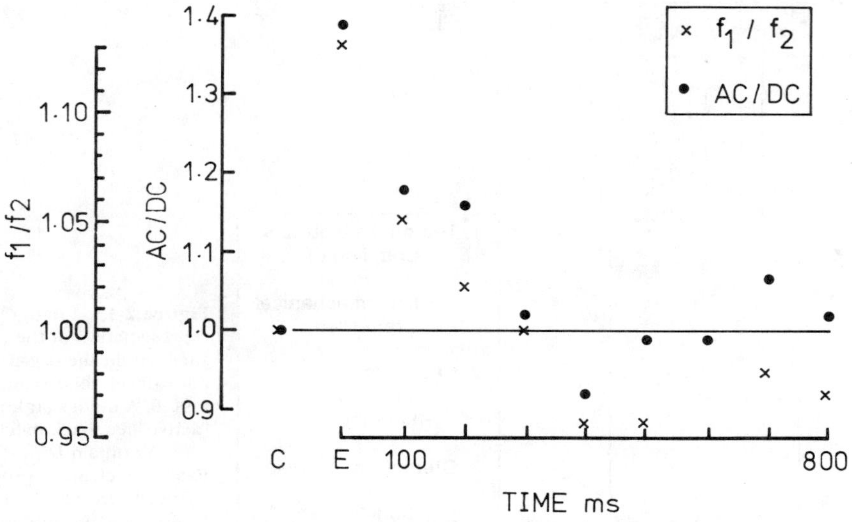

Figure 2-12 AC:DC and $f_1:f_2$ ratios for an IHC following an exposure to a 12.5-kHz, 110-dB SPL tone. C = normalized pre-exposure ratio; E = ratio at the end of the exposure.

Discussion

The data presented in the results suggest that exposure of the cochlea to loud sound results in a linearization of the hair cell response to acoustic stimuli. Because there are several possible sources of nonlinear behavior in the cochlea, it is difficult to pinpoint the origin of these losses. By eliminating some sites or mechanisms it may be possible to narrow the field. Figure 2-13*A* shows the possible sites for losses in sensitivity in the cochlea.

It is important to note that Figure 2-13 relates to low-level threshold losses after short, loud tones, and does not include possible mechanisms following large, permanent losses of sensitivity, which are usually accompanied by obvious morphologic changes of the hair cell. In this respect, direct disruption of either the paracrystalline array of actin filaments contained within the individual stereocilia or the stereocilial rootlets (Liberman et al, 1986) are not expected (Fig. 2-13*A*). In addition, stereocilial fusion, loss of tip links, or disruptions of the lateral crosslinks between stereocilia are usually seen only after prolonged exposures at higher stimulus levels (Pickles et al, 1987).

Another important structure that may play a role in cochlear desensitization is the tectorial membrane (TM) (Fig. 2-13*A*). The membrane is a complex structure composed of at least three types of collagen (II, V, and IX) and at least three noncollagenous glycosolated polypeptides, which form striated sheets within the matrix of the membrane (Hasko and Richardson, 1988). The high degree of organization of this matrix is sensitive to low Ca^{++} levels and is disrupted when the Ca^{++} chelating agents EGTA and EDTA are added to the medium; this has the functional correlate of significant reductions in the cochlea microphonic (Tanaka et al, 1980). The TM is also susceptible to the addition of Na^{+}, which induces irreversible shrinkage (Kronester-Frei, 1978). Little is known about the micromechanical properties of the TM, but some preliminary data suggest that the membrane is approximately four times stiffer in the longitudinal direction than in the radial direction (Zwislocki et al, 1988). This would correlate with the apparent morphologic asymmetry in the matrix of the membrane (Hasko and Richardson, 1988). On the basis of a recent finding that the radial stiffness of the TM is substantially less than that of the OHC stereocilia, Zwislocki and Cefaratti (1989) have proposed that the mass of the TM and the stiffness of the stereocilia behave as a resonant element with a significant role in cochlear frequency selectivity. Any change to the mechanical properties of the TM that increases its damping, or any change in the stiffness of the OHC stereocilia, will, according to Zwislocki and Cefaratti, result in a loss of sensitivity and tuning.

Frictional forces in the fluid-filled scalae of the cochlea act to reduce the displacement of the partition during acoustic stimulation. This problem increases with increasing stimulus frequencies. With the discovery that OHCs in vitro demonstrate cell motility under certain

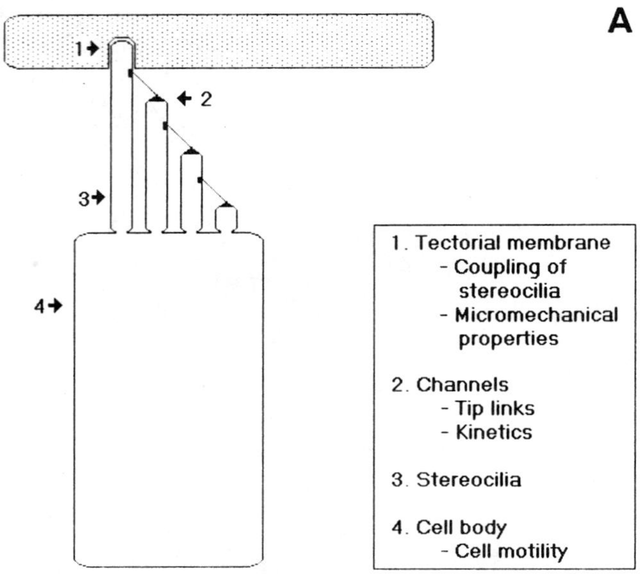

Figure 2-13 *A,* Diagrammatic representation of the possible sites within the organ of Corti for a low-level noise-induced hearing loss. *B,* A model outlining the "active" feedback mechanism. After Mountain DC. Electromechanical properties of hair cells. In: Altschuler RA, Hoffmann DW, Bobbin RP, eds. Neurobiology of hearing: the cochlea. New York: Raven Press, 1986:77.

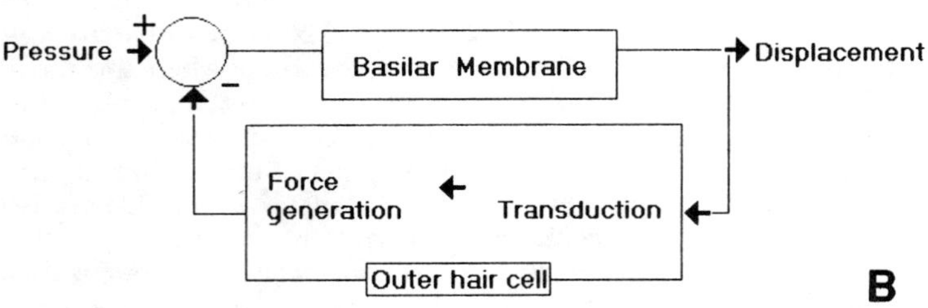

conditions (Brownell et al, 1985), and that mechanical energy can be recorded in the ear canal (Kemp, 1979), it has been proposed that OHCs generate mechanical forces in response to sound-induced current flows through their apical conductances. The resultant potential changes in the cell evoke small (2 to 15 nm per millivolt, according to Santos-Sacchi, 1989) but rapid changes in cell length (at least to 5 kHz, according to Ashmore, 1987). It is proposed that this "fast" component of cell motility acts to oppose viscous damping in the cochlea and enhances the displacement of the cochlear partition. The "slow" or tonic components of cell motility, which are seen after increasing extracellular levels of K^+ or acetylcholine (the presumptive efferent transmitter) or after the initiation of cellular contractile protein activity, are not thought to contribute to force generation of OHCs on a cycle-by-cycle basis, but may well play a role in setting the position or DC bias of the basilar membrane (Zenner et al, 1985).

In vitro experiments on the cell motility of isolated OHCs suggest that any active force-generating mechanisms postulated as essential for cochlear sensitivity and tuning are extremely robust. Cell length changes in response to injected current are still recorded in the presence of inhibitors of ATP, in the absence of calcium, and in the presence of agents acting against intracellular contractile proteins and cytoplasmic microtubules (Holley and Ashmore, 1988). This suggests that the cell force-generating mechanism does not appear to depend directly on ATP or other known cellular mechanisms that could give rise to cell motility. This evidence suggests that force-generation in OHCs may not be impaired following acoustic overstimulation and may not contribute to temporary hearing losses. However, the most recent work of

Evans (1990) suggests that morphologic changes in the subsurface cisternae of the OHC after transmembranous electrical stimulation could play a role in modifying the force-generating mechanism.

The most likely site for a noise-induced hearing loss is the transducer conductance of the OHC. As discussed in the introduction, this group of mechanotransducers appears to be essential for the frequency selectivity and sensitivity of the cochlea, and probably forms part of a feedback loop that acts to enhance the displacement of the basilar membrane. Figure 2-13*B* is a representative model of this feedback mechanism as proposed by Mountain (1986). In this model, pressure-induced displacement of the basilar membrane stimulates the OHC (mechanoelectrical transduction), which produces voltage-dependent movements of the cell (electromechanical transduction). At high frequencies, resultant force-generation acts in an amplitude- and phase-dependent manner to enhance the displacement of the basilar membrane. A number of points in the loop are crucial for its operation. The first is the force-generating mechanism of the OHC that, from the previously discussed evidence, would appear to be extremely robust and therefore probably does not contribute to low-level hearing losses in the cochlea. The second is the coupling of this force to the displacement of the basilar membrane. If there is a reduction of the coupling between the OHC stereocilia and the tectorial membrane, then both the mechanoelectrical and the electromechanical elements of the OHC will be modified. However, it is difficult to distinguish between the two elements, because they are interdependent. The third possibility is the transducer conductance. Any alteration in the functional properties of this element in the feedback loop will reduce the electrical drive to the OHC force-generating mechanism. In a previous study (Cody and Russell, 1985), current injection in OHCs following the loud tone did not reveal any obvious change in the access resistance of the cell, which suggests that there is little alteration in the number of functional apical conductances. Additionally, the data presented in this paper show that the maximum hair cell receptor potentials differed little whether recorded during or following the acoustic overstimulation (Figs. 2-7 and 2-9), whereas at the lower stimulus levels there were substantial reductions in the amplitudes of the AC and DC components of the receptor potentials. This suggests that the mechanoelectrical portion of the feedback loop (the transducer) is intact and functional, at least for these exposure conditions. In contrast, the extensive data of Patuzzi et al (1989a,b) suggest that a percentage of the OHC transducer conductances have closed following exposure of the cochlea to a loud tone. Hence, the drive to the force-generating mechanism of the OHC will be reduced, and the displacement of the cochlear partition substantially altered. However, in that series of experiments the traumatizing tone was significantly louder (115 dB SPL) and longer (30 to 150 seconds). Thus, their findings may represent an extension of the low-level threshold shifts described in this paper. It is interesting to note that pure tone exposure levels of 115 dB SPL and above in the basal turn of the guinea pig cochlea, for periods of 1 hour, produce a loss of cochlear sensitivity and obvious damage to the stereocilia of the hair cell, particularly the first row of the OHC (Cody et al, 1980). Pure tones presented for the same period, but at levels similar to those of the present study, produce much less obvious damage of the hair cell, and the threshold losses are much more variable. If the level of the tone is more critical than its duration for cochlear desensitization, then the mechanism proposed by Patuzzi and coworkers may operate above 110 dB SPL: full stop. However, the mechanism is not yet clear.

Propriétés Non Linéaires des Cellules Ciliées Internes et Externes des Mammifères Pendant et après une Exposition a un Son Fort

Chez les mammifères, les réponses non-linéaires de la cochlée en réponse à une stimulation acoustique, jouent un rôle central dans sa sélectivité en fréquence et sa sensibilité. Les non-linéarités sont particulièrement importantes dans la détection des stimulations de haute fréquence. Ceci est la conséquence directe des propriétés de filtre électrique passe-bas des membranes des cellules ciliées qui agissent pour atténuer les composantes phasiques ou alternatives des potentiels de récepteur ou des stimulations de haute fréquence. Cependant, l'asymétrie de la dépolarisation inhérente à la conductance de transduction de la cellule ciliée interne en réponse à des stimulations acoustiques symétriques signifie qu'une composante continue est générée qui n'est pas influencée par les propriétés de filtre passe-bas de la membrane cellulaire. La cellule ciliée peut donc produire des potentiels excitateurs en réponse à des stimulations de haute fréquence. Si par contre la réponse des cellules ciliées devient plus linéaire, le courant continu de dépolarisation sera réduit. Ceci implique une réduction de la probabilité de sécrétion du neurotransmetteur et, par conséquent, un abaissement du taux de décharge des potentiels d'action des fibres afférentes faisant synapse avec cette cellule. Ceci correspond à une perte de sensibilité ou, au niveau psychophysique, à une perte auditive. On peut ainsi supposer qu'une perte auditive provoquée par un bruit peut être le résultat d'une augmentation de la linéarité de la réponse de la cochlée à une stimulation acoustique.

Des mesures du mouvement de la membrane basilaire montrent que la sensibilité et le comportement non-linéaire sont substantiellement réduits après l'exposition de la cochlée à un son fort. Ceci est probablement le résultat d'une modification des stimulations mécaniques appliquées aux cellules ciliées internes avec lesquelles la majorité des fibres nerveuses auditives font synapse. La vulnérabilité de la mécanique de la membrane basilaire au traumatisme, ainsi que les preuves de plus en plus nombreuses que les cellules ciliées externes pourraient, grâce à leur contractibilité, augmenter les propriétés d'accord et de sensibilité de la micromécanique de la membrane basilaire, désignent ces cellules ciliées externes comme les candidats les plus sérieux pour être à l'origine des propriétés non-linéaires de la cochlée. Par conséquent, ces cellules seraient à l'origine des pertes auditives induites par le bruit. Des données obtenues par l'enregistrement intracellulaire des cellules ciliées internes et externes du tour basal de la cochlée du cobaye tendent à renforcer cette hypothèse car les réponses de ces deux groupes de cellules ciliées à une stimulation acoustique deviennent de plus en plus linéaires pendant et après une exposition de la cochlée à des sons forts.

References

Ashmore JF. A fast motile response in guinea pig outer hair cell: The cellular basis for the cochlear amplifier. J Physiol 1987; 338:323-347.

Brownell WE, Bader CR, Bertrand D, de Ribaupierre Y. Evoked mechanical responses of isolated cochlear hair cells. Science 1985; 227:194-196.

Cody AR, Johnstone BM. Single auditory neuron response during acute acoustic trauma. Hear Res 1980; 3:3-16.

Cody AR, Russell IJ. Outer hair cells in the mammalian cochlea and noise-induced hearing loss. Nature 1985; 315:662-665.

Evans BN. Fatal contractions: ultrastructural and electromechanical changes in outer hair cells following transmembranous electrical stimulation. Hear Res 1990; 45:265-282.

Hasko JA, Richardson GP. The ultrastructural organization and properties of the mouse tectorial membrane matrix. Hear Res 1988; 35:21-38.

Holley MC, Ashmore JF. On the mechanism of a high-frequency force generator in outer hair cells isolated from the guinea pig cochlea. Proc R Soc Lond [Biol] 1988; 232:413-429.

Hudspeth AJ, Corey DP. Sensitivity, polarity and conductance change in the response of the vertebrate hair cells to controlled mechanical stimuli. Proc Natl Acad Sci U S A 1977; 74:2407-2411.

Kemp DT. Evidence of mechanical nonlinearity and frequency selective wave amplification in the cochlea. Arch Otorhinolaryngol 1979; 224:37-45.

Khanna SM, Leonard DGB. Basilar membrane tuning in the cat cochlea. Science 1982; 215:305-306.

Kronester-Frei A. Sodium dependent shrinking properties of the tectorial membrane. Scanning Electron Microsc 1978b; 2:943-948.

Le Page EL. Frequency dependent self-induced bias of the basilar membrane and its potential for controlling sensitivity and tuning in the mammalian cochlea. J Acoust Soc Am 1987; 82:139-154.

Liberman MC, Dodds LW, Learson DA. Structure-function correlation in noise-damaged ears: A light and electron-microscopic study. In: Salvi RJ, Henderson D, Hamernik RP, Colletti V, eds. Basic and applied aspects of noise-induced hearing loss. New York: Plenum Press, 1986:163.

McMullen TA, Mountain D. Model of dc potentials in the cochlea: Effects of voltage dependent stiffness. Hear Res 1985; 17:127-141.

Mountain DC. Electromechanical properties of hair cells. In: Altschuler RA, Hoffman DW, Bobbin RP, eds. Neurobiology of hearing: the cochlea. New York: Raven Press, 1986:77.

Neely ST, Kim DO. An active cochlear model showing sharp tuning and high sensitivity. Hear Res 1983; 9:123-130.

Patuzzi R, Robertson D. Tuning in the mammalian cochlea. Physiol Rev 1988; 68:1009-1082.

Patuzzi RB, Yates GK, Johnstone BM. Changes in cochlear microphonic and neural sensitivity produced by acoustic trauma. Hear Res 1989a; 39:189-202.

Patuzzi RB, Yates GK, Johnstone BM. Outer hair cell receptor current and sensorineural hearing loss. Hear Res 1989b; 42:47-72.

Pickles JO, Osborne MP, Comis SD. Vulnerability of tip links between stereocilia to acoustic trauma in the guinea pig. Hear Res 1987; 25:173-183.

Russell IJ, Sellick PM. Intracellular studies of hair cells in the mammalian cochlea. J Physiol 1978; 284:261-290.

Russell IJ, Palmer A. Filtering due to the inner hair cell membrane properties and its relation to the phase-locking limit in cochlear nerve fibres. In: Moore

BCJ, Patterson RD, eds. Auditory frequency selectivity. New York: Plenum Press, 1986:199.

Russell IJ, Cody AR, Richardson GP. The responses of inner and outer hair cells in the basal turn of the guinea pig cochlea and in the mouse cochlea grown in vitro. Hear Res 1986; 22:199-216.

Santos-Sacchi J. Asymmetry in voltage-dependent movements of isolated outer hair cells from the organ of Corti. J Neurosci 1989; 9:2954-2962.

Sellick PM, Patuzzi R, Johnstone BM. Measurement of basilar membrane motion in the guinea pig using the Mössbauer technique. J Acoust Soc Am 1982; 72:131-141.

Tanaka Y, Asanuma A, Yanagisawa K. Potentials of outer hair cells and their membrane properties in cationic environments. Hear Res 1980; 2:431-438.

Weiss TF. Bidirectional transduction in the vertebrate hair cells: A mechanism for coupling mechanical and electrical vibrations. Hear Res 1982; 7:353-360.

Zenner HP, Zimmermann U, Schmitt U. Reversible contraction of isolated mammalian cochlear hair cells. Hear Res 1985; 18:127-133.

Zwislocki JJ, Slepecky NB, Cefaratti LK. Tectorial membrane stiffness and hair cell stimulation. XIth Midwinter Meeting, Association for Research in Otolaryngology, 1970, Clearwater Beach, Florida.

Zwislocki JJ, Cefaratti LK. Tectorial membrane. II. Stiffness measurements in vivo. Hear Res 1989; 42:211-228.

CHAPTER 3

Putative Biochemical Processes in Noise-Induced Hearing Loss

ROBERT J. WENTHOLD
MARK E. SCHNEIDER
HUNG N. KIM
CLAUDE J. DECHESNE

The elucidation of the molecular mechanisms underlying damage to the auditory system due to overstimulation presents a formidable challenge. In the biochemical analysis of the cochlea, we are faced with a very small, delicate, and complex system that includes numerous cell types that may all respond differently to this damage. Knowledge of the molecular events that occur in the cochlea because of noise damage is basic to understanding the pathogenesis of noise-induced hearing loss (NIHL), because molecular changes undoubtedly precede observable structural changes. It is reasonable to assume that the reversible stages in NIHL will be primarily detectable as molecular changes rather than structural changes. The development of any type of drug therapy to prevent or minimize trauma due to overstimulation will also rely on a knowledge of the molecular processes. Over the years several laboratories have measured a variety of common biochemical parameters after noise-induced damage (reviewed briefly below) in attempts to better understand the molecular events that take place in the cochlea. A continued effort in these types of studies using controlled stimulus conditions should give insights into the biochemistry of noise damage.

Our research has focussed on changes in specific proteins and their mRNAs that accompany or precede structural damage to the inner ear from noise, ototoxic drugs, and genetic lesions. We have divided the molecular events associated with NIHL into four stages that can be correlated with the morphological and physiological changes known to occur following NIHL (Table 3-1). Much of the existing information on molecular aspects of NIHL, as reviewed below, can be placed into these four stages. This scenario proposes that there will be changes in proteins in the organ of Corti at Stage II, when detectable morphologic changes are minimal. Proteins that undergo changes in expression at this stage may serve as sensitive molecular markers of cellular damage. Such proteins may also play roles in protecting the cell from further damage, as has been suggested for the function of stress-induced proteins. Later stages involve extensive cell damage that can extend beyond the organ of Corti, and include, for example, spiral ganglion cells. Analysis of cochlear tissue at these stages may identify proteins involved in such functions as cellular repair, trophic maintenence of auditory neurons, and regeneration. Two approaches are available for studying cochlear proteins. The first is the analysis of proteins that have been characterized previously in other tissues and have a well-known function. The list of such proteins is extensive and ranges from growth factors, to structural proteins, to proteins that may be markers of cellular damage in other systems. These proteins have been purified, antibodies have been made to them, and probes for in situ localization of their mRNAs are available. Two proteins that we have studied in this category are the 70-kD heat shock protein (discussed later) and the neurofilament subunits (Dau and Wenthold, 1989). The second approach is to use a screening technique, such as two-dimensional gel electrophoresis, to identify cochlear proteins that appear particularly important because of, for example, their abundance, localization, or response to a perturbation of the

TABLE 3-1 **Hypothetical Sequence of Molecular Changes in the Organ of Corti Associated with Noise-Induced Hearing Loss**

STAGE	MORPHOLOGY	PHYSIOLOGY	MOLECULAR CHANGES
I	Normal	Normal	Changes in metabolite and ion flux; enzyme induction.
II	Normal to slight edema of hair cells and afferent terminals	TTS	Small molecule depletion, e.g., metabolites, neurotransmitters; large molecule changes, e.g., protein denaturation, actin depolymerization; stress and repair mechanisms activated; e.g., heat shock protein synthesis
III	Permanent damage to stereocilia and reticular lamina	PTS	Extensive protein and lipid changes; stress response and repair mechanisms continue; transneuronal changes
IV	Cell death	PTS	Proteolytic enzyme synthesis; regeneration? Transneuronal changes

Morphological criteria are based on the limited resolution of light and electron microscopic observations; Stage I refers to the onset of overstimulation, in which the steady state is perturbed

system. Using this approach we have identified two spiral ganglion cell proteins whose levels of synthesis appear dependent on the presence of hair cells.

Review of Biochemical Studies Related to Noise-Induced Hearing Loss

A number of biochemical analyses, generally involving common metabolites, enzymes, or ions, have been carried out on the inner ear after noise exposure (Tables 3-2 and 3-3). These studies have addressed the general hypothesis that NIHL involves disruption of classic energy metabolism or ion homeostasis and that the resulting imbalance can be detected with suitable techniques. Three analytical methods have been used to compare noise-exposed and normal animals: (1) direct measurements of tissue metabolites or enzyme total capacities in noise-exposed animals; (2) perfusion of the perilymphatic space during or after noise exposure and subsequent analysis of the perfusate for metabolites, other soluble small molecules, and enzymes; and (3) direct measurements of ion activities during noise exposure using ion-selective microelectrodes. As a group, these studies suffer from a lack of consistency with respect to stimulus exposures, experimental animals, sampling conditions, and methods of chemical analysis. Consequently, it is difficult to draw any general conclusions from them. Some of the changes reported would clearly be expected in any cells that have been damaged from mechanical, thermal, or chemical insult. For example, the release of soluble enzymes from the cell cytoplasm, such as lactate dehydrogenase (LDH), is a common result of cell damage, and injury to any structure in the cochlea would cause an elevation of the amount of such enzymes in the perilymph (Schacht, 1982). Although such studies may give clues as to changes in metabolism and increases in enzyme activity, these analyses tell little about the biochemical mechanisms of noise damage.

Because molecular changes must precede visible structural changes, an important consideration for designing stimulus parameters for this type of experiment is to define conditions that cause a minimum of structural changes accompanying a measurable hearing loss. Such conditions are notoriously difficult to ascertain, even for an individual animal. There are enormous unexplained variances in numerous measurements of cochlear function and biochemistry in a population of animals (Robertson et al, 1980), so that biochemical analysis is further complicated by interanimal variability and species differences.

TABLE 3-2 **Analysis of Enzymes in Cochlear Tissues After Noise Exposure**

ENZYME, SPECIES	CONDITIONS	RESULTS	AUTHORS
LDH, esterases, ATPase, acid and alkaline phosphatases, phatases, cytochrome oxidase, succinic dehydrogenase, kangaroo rat	500–3000 Hz, 95–131 dB, 0.5–2 hours histochemistry	No changes seen	Stack and Webster, 1971
SDH, guinea pig	White noise, 110 dB, 63 hours histochemistry	Reduction in IHC and OHC	Quade and Geyer, 1973
LDH, guinea pig	White noise, 115 dB, 10 min. to 72 hours histochemistry and biochemistry	1-hour exposure causes increase, longer exposure shows return to normal	Ishida, 1973
Succinate dehydrogenase, guinea pig	Impulse noise, 8 days, 9 hours/day, histochemistry	Decrease in hair cell SDH Effect greater in OHC than IHC	Guttmacher et al, 1973
Lysosomal enzymes, guinea pig	120 dB, 1 hour/day for 10 days	Mostly no change—phosphatase increased	Schaetzle, 1976
LDH, glucose-6-phosphate dehydrogenase, guinea pig	95 dB, 500 Hz, 48 hours biochemistry	No changes in OHC	Thalman, 1976
LDH, rabbit	100 dB, 2 kHz, 2 hours histochemistry	OHC—Increase in basal turn, decrease in lower half of turn 2, normal in upper half	Omata et al, 1979

TABLE 3-3 **Analysis of Enzymes, Ions, and Small Molecules in Cochlear Fluids After Noise Exposure**

SUBSTANCE, SPECIES	CONDITIONS	RESULTS	AUTHORS
Na, K, guinea pig	100 dB, 2 minutes, 2000 Hz	Endolymph Na increase, K decrease	Nakashima et al, 1970a
Na, K, guinea pig	100–140 dB, white noise	Endolymph Na increase, K decrease in 15 seconds	Nakashima et al, 1970b
Lactate, guinea pig	90–105 dB, white noise, 1 hour	Lactate increase in perilymph	Schnieder, 1974
Na, glucose, aldolase, LDH, aldolase, phosphohexose isomerase, protein, guinea pig	100 dB, 8 kHz, 1 hour	No changes	Gershbein et al, 1974
LDH, MDH, chinchilla	123 dB, 700–2800 Hz, 30 minutes	Rapid increase to 24 hours, then decrease	Juhn and Ward, 1979
Na, K, Cl, guinea pig	95–125 dB, 7 days, 16 hours/day	Increase in K and Cl, decrease in Na in endolymph	Konishi et al, 1979
Na, K, Cl, guinea pig	95–105 dB, 20 minutes	With 4.2 kHz and WBN endolymph K increased, Na decreased; at 380 Hz, K decreased	Salt and Konishi, 1979
K, guinea pig	142 dB, 1 kHz, 1 hour	Decrease in endolymph K; return to normal in 5 days	Melichar et al, 1980
Glucose, lactate, pyruvate, guinea pig	100 dB, white noise, 10 minutes	No change	Lotz et al, 1981
LDH	140 dB, wide band noise, 10 minutes	No change	Haupt et al, 1983

The onset of NIHL, as it is related to temporary threshold shift (TTS) and permanent threshold shift (PTS) conditions, is a dynamic process. Frequently, in studies aimed at assessing biochemical changes, conditions and sampling times have been chosen that fall within this transitional stage at which the processes of repair and injury are not steady-state. Although steady-state conditions can be approached using exposures that cause asymptotic threshold shift, long recovery durations, or both, biochemical analyses of the organ of Corti of animals with asymptotic threshold shifts failed to see changes in LDH capacity, glucose 6-phosphate dehydrogenase capacity, ATP, and several neurotransmitter candidates (Thalmann, 1976).

Over the years, the results of biochemical measurements from similar experiments have been inconsistent (see Tables 3-2 and 3-3); such inconsistencies could be due to limitations of the analytical methods. The cochlea presents several problems for a biochemist; for example, the analysis of tissue made up of several cell types is difficult, and one cannot rule out the possibility that opposing changes in two cell types would cancel each other if the whole tissue was assayed. The rapidity with which tissues from the inner ear can be harvested is of crucial significance when attempting to capture metabolite levels in their steady state. For instance, tissue ATP/ADP and Pi ratios measured after fast freezing and with conventional enzymologic tests are two times less than when measured using in vivo P-31 nuclear magnetic resonance (NMR) imaging (Veech et al, 1979; Ingwall, 1982).

An alternative measurement of cellular bioenergetics involves the measurement of glucose metabolism using the radiolabeled nonmetabolizable glucose analog, 2-deoxyglucose (2DG). This technique measures glucose uptake and allows the calculation of glucose use on the basis of normative rate constants. The direct application of this method is difficult because the appropriate rate constants are difficult to measure in the cochlea, and the results cannot be generalized because the data for the mouse and gerbil indicate species differences to noise exposure. In the mouse cochlea, noise exposures up to 85 dB SPL induce a 230 percent increase in radiolabeled 2DG uptake in cochlear tissues (Canlon and Schacht, 1983; Canlon et al, 1984). Conversely in the gerbil, a barely detectable increase was seen at exposures up to 105 dB SPL (Goodwin et al, 1984).

The majority of data summarized in Tables 3-2 and 3-3 do not support a role for impaired energy metabolism in early events in NIHL. However, it is possible that the experiments have been conducted using wrong sound exposure parameters. Since 1985, the role of the outer hair cell and its ability to display two kinds of motility has led to a renewed emphasis of Gold's hypothesis (Gold, 1949) of an active cochlear amplifier/second filter. Biologically, the amplifier would be required at sound pressure levels near threshold. As shown below, all researchers have chosen sound levels that result in some degree of NIHL. It is possible that changes in energy flux (also reflected in changes of the steady-state levels of metabolites) could be measured at low sound levels in a sound-dependent manner. Alternatively, the energy necessary for these active mechanisms could be found in the large electrical gradients present across the reticular lamina (endocochlear potential and summating potential).

Biochemical and molecular studies are now branching out from a number of well-controlled anatomic and physiologic studies of NIHL. Recently, the structural organization of the stereocilium has been elucidated, and several studies have implicated this structure as the site of early changes leading to NIHL (Tilney et al, 1980). One current hypothesis is that initial events involve damage to a variety of structural proteins of the stereocilia and cuticular plate (Tilney et al, 1982). Many studies have correlated NIHL with structural changes in the stereocilia and cuticular plate (Saunders et al, 1985). Liberman and colleagues (Liberman, 1984; Liberman and Dodds, 1984a,b; Liberman and Kiang, 1984; Liberman and Mulroy, 1982) were able to assess the cochlea histopathologically at the light and ultrastructural levels and compare these data with the physiologic properties of individual afferent neurons that innervated the hair cell under study. Measuring the physiologic disease in an animal, they could predict the nature and degree of anatomical disruption. Their findings suggested that in stimulus conditions likely to lead to moderate PTS, the stereocilia rootlets were damaged, whereas the hair cell exhibited no pathological signs. Following exposures likely to lead to TTS, stereocilia were normal, except for a shorter supracuticular plate rootlet. In addition, hair cells and afferent terminals often appeared "swollen." These results suggest that the proteins of the stereocilia core, cuticular plate, and rootlet, which are primarily actin, fimbrin, and an as yet unidentified protein, are irreversibly damaged in PTS conditions and are functionally altered with less severe or reversible trauma (Tilney et al, 1989). Among the many observations of stereocilia trauma reported (Saunders et al., 1985), the consensus emerged that the rootlet disease is correlated with physiologic deficits; these include fracturing the core filaments of each stereocilium, depolymerization of the actin core, or both.

The biophysical consequences of mechanical overstimulation of the hair bundle were examined in vitro using isolated pieces from the guinea pig cochlea (Saunders and Flock, 1986). The hair bundle's displacement for a given stimulus energy increased as a function of overexposure. Saunders and Flock (1986) expressed their results using the conventional threshold shift terminology; thus, overexposure induced a threshold shift that was linearly related to noise exposure. Interestingly, the damaged hair bundle could recover from as much as a 5 to 7 dB threshold shift; this recovery depended on the presence of metabolically "healthy" tissues. These authors concluded that a dynamic active process counteracts the loss of stiffness caused by overstimulation.

An ultrastructural examination of the hair bundles in these experiments was not undertaken and, consequently, the type of stereocilia injury in these cases is not known. Mechanisms of stereocilia injury include fracture of individual stereocilia, depolymerization of core filaments, and disruption of the extracellular links that cross-link the bundle (Saunders et al, 1986). Thus, in addition to examining the structural changes in vitro, experiments designed to measure biochemical changes in the proteins (actin or fimbrin) may yield new information concerning the mechanisms involved in injury to the hair bundle.

Biochemical analysis will also be important in elucidating the structures involved in transduction. The nature of the transducer gating spring is unknown; this molecule would also be an important target during mechanical overstimulation. A popular model assigns the tip link structures linking adjacent rows of stereocilia to the transducer gating spring; however, it has been noted that the data supporting this model are circumstantial at best (Hudspeth, 1989). Biophysical data provided by Howard and Hudspeth (1988) suggest that the resistance to displacement of the hair bundle over the physiologically relevant range is dominated by the tension in the mechanism gating the transducer channel. For these reasons, extensive characterization of the proteins of the stereociliary membrane, reticular laminar surface, and the core proteins of the stereocilium and cuticular plate are needed. Shepherd et al. (1989) have presented evidence that a small complement of proteins is found in these structures. But progress will be hindered by the small amounts of tissue available and the limited sensitivity of the analytical techniques. A central goal of many researchers in the future will be to assign molecular identities to the mechanical analogs of various mechanoelectric transduction models.

Heat Shock Proteins

When exposed to elevated temperatures, organisms respond by the synthesis of a group of proteins known as heat shock proteins (hsps) (Lindquist, 1986; Lindquist and Craig, 1988; Welch et al, 1989). Initially observed in *Drosophila,* these proteins have been found in all animals, plants, and bacteria and are highly evolutionarily conserved. Although hyperthermia is commonly used to induce these proteins, hsps can be induced by any condition that stresses the cell and, therefore, are also referred to as stress proteins. Cellular responses to stress are rapid: increases in mRNA are seen within 1 hour, and increases in protein within a few hours. Based on their similar properties, hsps can be divided into several families; in eukaryotes there are at least three families, including the hsp90 family, hsp70 family, and hsp20 family. The number refers to the approximate molecular weight in kilodaltons of the proteins of the family. In addition to these main groups, there are numerous reports of proteins that are synthesized under stress conditions but which have not been thoroughly characterized. One of the more extensively studied families in mammals is the hsp70 family, which is composed of at least four members in humans and three in rats. The major heat-inducible member of this family is hsp70, a 70-kD protein that is usually expressed in low levels, but that is expressed at dramatically higher levels after hyperthermia. Because of its increased synthesis, as well as the decrease in synthesis of normal cellular proteins, hsp70 is the major translation product after stress. As in the other hsp families, some proteins of the hsp70 family are expressed at high levels in unstressed tissues. The most abundant of these is a 73-kD protein, referred to as the constitutive 70-kD stress protein, or p72, which is expressed at high levels in most tissues; its synthesis increases only slightly following hyperthermia. These two members of the hsp70 family are structurally similar but are distinct gene products and regulated differently (Lindquist, 1986).

Several studies suggest that a major function of hsps is to facilitate cellular repair and protect the cell from further injury (Lindquist and Craig, 1988; Welch et al, 1989). The fact that these proteins are widely distributed and respond rapidly to changing conditions is consistent with the basic emergency response of cells. The protective function of hsps is supported by studies linking the induction of these proteins with the acquisition of thermotolerance in cultured cells from a number of organisms. Cells rapidly subjected to increased temperature died much more quickly than those that were first subjected to a modest temperature increase to induce the synthesis of hsps and then subjected to the higher temperature. The protective role of hsps was more directly demonstrated by the microinjection of antibodies to the hsp70 family of proteins into fibroblasts (Riabowol et al, 1988). Cells containing the injected antibodies, which presumably inactivated hsp70 proteins, were killed by brief heat shock, whereas control cells survived. These studies suggest that an organ about to experience a potentially lethal condition might be protected by a previous induction of heat shock proteins. Such an effect has been demonstrated in the mammalian retina, where exposure to intense light normally causes photoreceptor degeneration. Prior induction of heat shock proteins by hyperthermia greatly reduced the damage due to light treatment (Barbe et al, 1988).

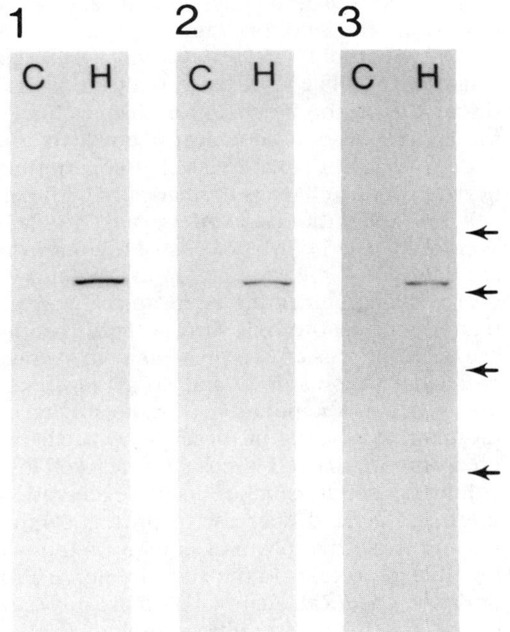

Figure 3-1 Immunoblots of (1) rat cerebellum, (2) cochlear nucleus, and (3) spiral ligament/stria vascularis stained with anti-hsp70 antibodies under normal conditions (C) and hyperthermia (H). Tissue was obtained 6 hours after a heat shock of 42.5° C.

The molecular mechanism by which hsps exert their protective effects is not fully known but is believed to involve the binding of the hsp to an already damaged protein to prevent further damage or reverse denaturation. Hsps expressed in the absence of stress have been shown to bind to precursor forms of proteins and aid in their proper folding and unfolding (Dashaies et al, 1988).

The mammalian central nervous system responds with the synthesis of hsps to a variety of stresses including hyperthermia (Sprang and Brown, 1987; Masing and Brown, 1989; Brown and Rush, 1990), ischemia (Nowak, 1985; Dienel et al, 1986; Vass et al, 1988; Dwyer et al, 1989; Nowak et al, 1990), physical trauma (Brown et al, 1989), axotomy (New et al, 1989), and neurotoxin treatment (Uney et al, 1988). Both neurons and glia can express hsp70, but the response appears to be related to the nature of the stress to which the tissue is subjected, and some neurons may be more likely to synthesize hsps than others. In the gerbil brain following transient ischemia, hsp70 induction is restricted to neurons; the protein's presence was most prominent in the hippocampus. In contrast, in rabbit and rat brain, hyperthermia greatly increased hsp70 in glial cells throughout the brain (Sprang and Brown, 1987; Marini et al, 1990). Application of the neurotoxin, kainic acid, has its greatest effect on hsp70 induction in neurons (Uney et al, 1988), whereas trauma causes hsp70 increase in both neurons and glia near the site of injury (Brown et al, 1989).

These findings raised the possibility that hsps could also protect the auditory periphery from damage due to noise, ototoxic drugs, or trauma. Recent studies showing that cells from aged animals produce less hsp70 mRNA and protein in response to hyperthermia than do cells from young animals (Fargnoli et al, 1990) suggest that hsps may also play a role in presbycusis. We have begun a study of hsp70 in the rodent inner ear. Cochlear tissue from the rat was dissected, and proteins were analyzed by SDS polyacrylamide gel electrophoresis and immunoblotting using monoclonal antibodies specific for hsp70. Control animals and animals that had been previously subjected to heat shock (a body temperature increase to 42.5° C) were analyzed. In all cochlear tissue analyzed, hsp was not detected in the unstressed animal. Heat shock, however, produced a single intense band migrating at M_1 = 70,000 as seen in gels of rat spiral ligament, cochlear nucleus, and cerebellum (Fig. 3-1).

Analysis of Cochlear Proteins by Metabolic Labeling and Acrylamide Gel Electrophoresis

Many of the most interesting and informative molecular changes taking place in the ear under conditions such as NIHL and ototoxic drug damage may involve proteins that are expressed only or predominantly in the ear. Therefore, information concerning these ear-specific proteins cannot be obtained by using other tissues, but must be obtained by biochemical analysis of inner ear tissue under various experimental conditions. The size and accessibility of this tissue limit the approaches that can be used. Several laboratories have found that proteins from the inner ear can be analyzed using one- and two-dimensional gel electrophoresis with sensitive staining techniques or after biosynthetically labeling the proteins with radioactive amino acids (Thalmann et al, 1987; Shepherd et al, 1989; Tilney et al, 1989; Thalmann et al, 1990). Proteins identified in this way can be used for the production of specific antibodies or for obtaining amino acid sequence, with the final objective of isolating cDNA clones encoding the proteins. With such tools, the proteins can then be characterized with respect to structure, function, and distribution. A sensitive technique that will help us with the identification and characterization of ear-specific proteins is to biosynthetically label the proteins with radioactive precursors (Wenthold and McGarvey, 1982a,b; Wenthold, 1985). The advantage of this method is twofold. The proper choice of radioactive precursor can offer higher sensitivity than the standard silver stain method; ^{35}S-methionine is often used as a precursor because most proteins contain methionine and ^{35}S is of sufficiently high energy to produce autoradiographs of gels in a reasonable time. Under optimal conditions with two-dimensional gels, more than 1,000 separate proteins can be detected. Cochlear proteins can be labeled in vivo with ^{35}S-methionine by exchanging the perilymph with artificial perilymph containing the radioactive amino acid. This technique minimizes trauma to the tissue and allows characterization of protein synthesis under nearly normal physiologic conditions. An alternative method, which may increase the specific labeling of the proteins and also give greater control over concentration of precursor and time of incorporation, is to incubate dissected tissue in vitro in solutions containing radioactive amino acids (Matchinski, personal communication). This method, however, is limited in that significant damage occurs when the tissue is dissected; as found in other systems, such damage could alter the normal pattern of protein synthesis. Both techniques allow the use of more-specific precursors, such as sugars that label only glycoproteins.

A second advantage of radioactive labeling of proteins is that it reflects synthesis that occurs over a defined period, whereas a stain simply reflects the total amount of a particular protein. Therefore, a dramatic change in protein in response to an experimental condition may not be seen by staining if a large, slowly metabolized pool of the protein is present. For example, under conditions of NIHL, this approach would allow the analysis of proteins that are synthesized in cochlear tissues at various times after presentation of the stimulus. Intervals as short as 15 to 30 minutes should be sufficient to produce labeling of the major proteins. Identification of these proteins may give clues concerning the molecular processes that are most affected by the stimulus.

Using this labeling protocol, we have characterized a number of proteins that are synthesized by spiral ganglion cells and transported in the auditory nerve (Tytell et al, 1980; Wenthold and McGarvey, 1982a,b; Wenthold, 1985). Especially relevant to this discussion on the biochemical changes occuring in response to cochlear damage is the finding that the synthesis of two auditory nerve proteins changes dramatically with hair cell loss (Wenthold and McGarvey, 1982a,b; Wenthold, 1985). If hair cells of a guinea pig are damaged—for example, in the genetically deaf waltzing guinea pig or in normal animals treated with an ototoxic drug—there is an increased synthesis of two proteins with average molecular weights of 27 and 36 kD in the auditory nerve. Quantitation of radioactivity indicates that labeling of these two proteins increases more than six times after hair cell loss. Following spiral ganglion cell degeneration, there is a general decrease in protein synthesis, and these two proteins emerge as the major labeled proteins in the auditory nerve. Preliminary chemical analysis of these proteins shows that they are glycoproteins. Peptide mapping of the multiple forms of each protein indicate that they are closely related, consistent with the differences arising from various degrees of glycosylation. Furthermore, the peptide mapping studies show that the 27-kD and 36-kD proteins may be similar, suggesting that they are different forms of the same protein or related subunits of the same protein complex.

The function of the 27-kD and 37-kD proteins remains to be determined. One hypothesis is that they are stress proteins produced by the spiral ganglion cells as they lose synaptic contact with hair cells and begin to degenerate. Such proteins may play a role in the survival of a small population of spiral ganglion cells, which are present several months after hair cell loss. This idea is supported by the finding that the 27-kD and 36-kD proteins continue to be expressed at high levels after most spiral ganglion cell degeneration is complete and a stable population remains.

Conclusion

It is apparent from a review of the literature that little is known about the molecular processes involved in NIHL. To fully understand these processes a knowledge of the normal biochemistry of the cochlea is necessary. Until the critical molecular mechanisms of the cochlea are defined, it is impossible to test whether or not they are affected in NIHL. The substantial amount of information known about the physiologic and morphologic aspects of NIHL provides a background for molecular studies. Although the structural characteristics of the cochlea preclude standard biochemical approaches to its analysis, the overwhelming amount of information available on molecular techniques and processes offers several promising avenues for studing the cochlea. Antibodies are now available to proteins with a wide spectrum of functions, and these can be applied to determine the localization of these proteins in the cochlea. Similarly, genes encoding a large number of proteins have now been cloned, with the number increasing daily, and these can be studied in the cochlea with in situ hybridization and related techniques. Furthermore, new antibody technology and micromolecular biology techniques can now be applied to the study of proteins expressed exclusively or primarily in the cochlea.

Processus Biochimiques et Deficits Auditifs

S'il existe peu d'informations concernant les changements biochimiques induits au niveau cochléaire par le trauma acoustique, ces changements devraient être importants, et pour la plupart d'entre eux, non spécifiques de l'oreille interne. En effet, la plupart des changements moléculaires intervenant au niveau des cellules cochléaires exposées à un traumatisme sont probablement les mêmes que ceux développés dans toutes les autres cellules sévèrement "stressées." Aussi, utiliser une telle approche au niveau de la cochlée pourrait être intéressant pour caractériser les dommages induits par un bruit ou par des drogues ototoxiques.

Nous nous sommes donc intéressés à la caractérisation de deux catégories de protéines. La première inclut des protéines dont la synthèse est induite lors de dommages cellulaires et qui ont e'té caractérisées dans d'autres systemes. La seconde catégorie inclut des protéines qui ont été spécifiquement identifiées dans la cochlée lors d'une exposition au bruit, après administration de drogues ototoxiques ou après des dommages mécaniques.

Dans la première catégorie, nous avons étudié deux protéines, la "heat shock protein 70" (hsp70) et les sous-unités de neurofilaments. La hsp70 fait partie de la famille des protéines connues comme étant des protéines du stress. Ces protéines se retrouvent en très faible quantité dans la plupart des tissus des mammifères, mais leur synthese de manière importante lorsque les cellules sont soumises à un "stress." Originellement identifiées lors d'une hyperthermie, ces protéines du "stress" sont connues pour répondre à d'autres types de "stress" dont l'ischémie, les dommages mécaniques ou les neurotoxines. Plusieurs fonctions leur ont été attribuées dont la plus intéressante serait un rôle protecteur en cas de dommages. Elles pourraient donc aussi jouer un rôle protecteur au niveau des cellules de l'oreille interne lors de dommages causés par une exposition sonore ou par l'administration de drogues ototoxiques. Les neurofilaments sont le composant majeur du cytosquelette neuronal et sont composés de trois sous-unités dont le poids moléculaire est d'environ 200, 160, et 68 kD. Chez le cobaye, ces 3 sous-unités sont abondamment présentes dans les corps cellulaires des cellules ganglionnaires de type II (Dau et Wenthold, 1989) alors que les cellules de type I ne possèdent que la sous-unité de 200 kD. Si après administration de néomycine, les cellules ganglionnaires de type II demeurent fortement immunoréactives aux 3 sous-unités, l'immunoréactivité des cellules ganglionnaires de type I augmente pour les sous-unités de 160 kD et de 68 kD, et diminue pour l'unité de 200 kD.

Pour le second groupe de protéines, nous avons décrit 2 sortes de protéines présentes en faible quantité au niveau des cellules ganglionnaires. Toutefois, leur quantité augmente après des dommages cellulaires et persiste après dégénérescence de ces cellules. Ces résultats laissent entrevoir la possibilité que ces protéines pourraient jouer un rôle dans la survie des cellules ganglionnaires restantes.

ACKNOWLEDGMENTS

We thank Drs. J. Fex and N. Slepecky for critically reading this manuscript, and Dr. T. Nowak for his collaboration on the heat shock protein study.

References

Barbe MF, Tytell M, Gower DJ, Welch WJ. Hyperthermia protects against light damage in the rat retina. Science 1988; 241:1817-1820.

Brown IR, Rush SJ. Expression of heat shock genes (hsp70) in the mammalian brain: Distinguishing constitutively expressed and hyperthermia-inducible mRNA species. J Neurosci Res 1990; 25:14-19.

Brown IR, Rush SJ, Ivy GO. Induction of a heat shock gene at the site of tissue injury in the rat brain. Neuron 1989; 2:1559-1564.

Canlon B, Schacht J. Acoustic stimulation alters deoxyglucose uptake in the mouse cochlea and inferior colliculus. Hear Res 1983; 10:217-226.

Canlon B, Takada A, Schacht J. Glucose utilization in the auditory system: Cochlear dysfunction and species differences. Comp Biochem Physiol 1984; 78A:43-47.

Dashaies RJ, Kock BD, Werner-Washburne M, Craig EA, Schekman R. A subfamily of stress proteins facilitates translocation of secretory and mitochondrial precursor polypeptides. Nature 1988; 332:800-810.

Dau J, Wenthold RJ. Immunocytochemical localization of neurofilament subunits in the spiral ganglion of normal and neomycin-treated guinea pigs. Hear Res 1989; 42:253-264.

Dienel GA, Kiessling M, Jacewicz M, Pulsinelli WA. Synthesis of heat shock proteins in rat brain cortex after transient ischemia. J Cereb Blood Flow Metab 1986; 6:505-510.

Dwyer BE, Nishimura RN, Brown IR. Synthesis of the major heat inducible heat shock protein in rat hippocampus after neonatal hypoxia-ischemia. Exp Neurol 1989; 104:28-31.

Fargnoli J, Kunisada T, Fornace AJ, et al. Decreased expression of heat shock protein 70 mRNA and protein after heat treatment in cells of aged rats. Proc Natl Acad Sci USA 1990; 87:846-850.

Gershbein LL, Manshio DT, Shurrager PT. Biochemical parameters of guinea pig perilymph sampled according to scala and following noise exposure. Environ Health Perspect 1974; 8:157-164.

Gold T. Hearing II. The physical basis of the action of the cochlea. Proc R Soc Lond [Biol] 1949; 135:492-498.

Goodwin PC, Ryan AF, Goodwin P, et al. Auditory stimulation alters the pattern of 2-deoxyglucose uptake: Relationship to stimulus intensity. Hear Res 1984; 15:215-224.

Guttmacher H, Quade R, Geyer G. Histochemical activity of succinate dehydrogenase in guinea pig cochlea after impulse stimulation. Acta Otolaryngol 1973; 76:323-327.

Haupt H, Scheibe F, Bergmann K. Total lactate dehydrogenase activity of perilymph, plasma and cerebrospinal fluid in unstressed and noise stressed guinea pigs. Arch Otorhinolaryngol 1983; 238:77-85.

Howard J, Hudspeth AJ. Compliance of the hair bundle associated with gating of mechanoelectrical transduction channels in the bullfrog's saccular hair cell. Neuron 1988; 1:189-199.

Hudspeth AJ. How the ear works. Nature 1989; 341:397-404.

Ingwall JW. Phosphorous nuclear magnetic resonance spectroscopy of cardiac and skeletal muscles. Am J Physiol 1982; 242:H729-H744.

Ishida M. Lactate dehydrogenase (LDH) activity in the inner ear under acoustic overstimulation. Annu Rep Ctr Adult Dis Japan 1973; 13:41-49.

Juhn SK, Ward WD. Alteration of oxidative enzymes (LDH and MDH) in perilymph after noise exposure. Arch Otorhinolaryngol 1979; 222:103-108.

Konishi T, Salt AN, Hamrick PE. Effects of exposure to noise on ion movement in guinea pig cochlea. Hear Res 1979; 1:325-342.

Liberman MC. Single-neuron labeling and chronic cochlear pathology. I. Threshold shift and characteristic frequency shift. Hear Res 1984; 16:33-41.

Liberman MC, Dodds LW. Single-neuron labeling and chronic cochlear pathology. II. Stereocilia damage and alterations of spontaneous discharge rates. Hear Res 1984; 16:43-53.

Liberman MC, Dodds LW. Single-neuron labeling and chronic cochlear pathology. III. Stereocilia damage and alterations of threshold tuning curves. Hear Res 1984; 16:55-74.

Liberman MC, Kiang NYS. Single-neuron labeling and chronic cochlear pathology. IV. Stereocilia damage and alterations in rate- and phase-level functions. Hear Res 1984; 16:75-90.

Liberman MC, Mulroy MJ. Acute and chronic effects of acoustic trauma: Cochlear pathology and auditory nerve pathophysiology. In: Hamernik RP, Henderson D, Salvi R, eds. New perspectives on noise-induced hearing loss. New York: Raven Press, 1982: 105.

Lindquist S. The heat shock response. Annu Rev Biochem 1986; 55:1151-1191.

Lindquist S, Craig EA. The heat-shock proteins. Annu Rev Genet 1988; 22:631-677.

Lotz P, Jakobi H, Kuhl KD, Haberland EJ. The physiological influence of sound on the cochlea metabolism. Acta Otolaryngol 1981; 91:445-450.

Marini AM, Kozuka M, Lipsky RH, Nowak TS. 70-kilodalton heat shock protein induction in cerebellar astrocytes and cerebellar granule cells in vitro: comparison with immunocytochemical localization after hyperthermia in vivo. J Neurochem 1990; 54:1509-1516.

Masing TE, Brown IR. Cellular localization of heat shock gene expression in rabbit cerebellum by in situ hybridization with plastic-embedded tissue. Neurochem Res 1989; 14:725-731.

Melichar I, Syka J, Ulehliva L. Recovery of the endocochlear potential and potassium concentrations in the cochlear fluids after acoustic trauma. Hear Res 1980; 2:55-63.

Nakashima T, Sullivan MJ, Snow JB Jr et al. Sodium and potassium changes in inner ear fluids: an in vivo study with glass microelectrodes. Acta Otolaryngol 1970a; 92:1-6.

Nakashima T, Meiring NL, Snow JB Jr. Cations in the endolymph of the guinea pig with noise-induced deafness. Surg Forum 1970b; 21:489-491.

New GA, Hendrickson BR, Jones KJ. Induction of heat shock protein 70 mRNA in adult hamster facial nuclear groups following axotomy of the facial nerve. Metab Brain Dis 1989; 4:273-279.

Nowak TS. Synthesis of a stress protein following transient ischemia in the gerbil. J Neurochem 1985; 45:1635-1641.

Nowak TS, Bond U, Schlesinger MJ. Heat shock RNA levels in brain and other tissues after hyperthermia and transient ischemia. J Neurochem 1990; 54:451-458.

Omata T, Ohtani I, Ohtsuki K et al. Electron microscopic and histochemical studies of outer hair cells in acoustically exposed rabbits. Arch Otorhinolaryngol 1979; 222:127-132.

Quade R, Geyer G. Demonstration of SDH by a perfusion method in the cochlea of the guinea pig during normal conditions and during noise. Acta Otolaryngol 1973; 75:45-54.

Riabowol KT, Mizzen LA, Welch WJ. Heat shock is lethal to fibroblasts microinjected with antibodies against hsp70. Science 1988; 242:432-436.

Robertson D, Johnstone BM, McGill RJ. Effects of loud sounds in the guinea pig cochlea. Hear Res 1980; 2:39-53.

Salt AN, Konishi T. Effects of noise on cochlear potentials and endolymph potassium concentration recorded with potassium-selective electrodes. Hear Res 1979; 1:343-363.

Saunders JC, Flock A. Recovery of threshold shift in hair-cell stereocilia following exposure to intense stimulation. Hear Res 1986; 23:233-243.

Saunders JC, Canlon B, Flock A. Changes in stereocilia micromechanics following overstimulation in metabolically blocked hair cells. Hear Res 1985; 24:217-225.

Schacht J. Biochemical aspects of noise-induced hearing loss. In: Hamernik RP, Henderson D, Salvi R, eds. Perspectives on noise-induced hearing loss. New York: Raven Press, 1982:95.

Schaetzle W. Distribution and possible function of lysosomal enzymes in the inner ear under normal and pathophysiological conditions. Arch Otorhinolaryngol 1976; 212:77-84.

Schnieder EA. A contribution to the physiology of the perilymph. Part III: On the origin of noise-induced hearing loss. Ann Otol Rhinol Laryngol 1974; 83:406-412.

Shepherd GMG, Barres BA, Corey DP. Bundle blot purification and initial protein characterization of hair cell stereocilia. Proc Natl Acad Sci USA 1989; 86:4973-4977.

Sprang GK, Brown IR. Selective induction of a heat shock gene in fiber tracts and cerebellar neurons of the rabbit brain detected by in situ hybridization. Mol Brain Res 1987; 3:89-93.

Stack CR, Webster DB. Glycogen content in the outer hair cells of kangaroo rat (D. spectabilis) cochlea prior to and following auditory stimulation. Acta Otolaryngol 1971; 71:483-493.

Thalmann R. Quantitative biochemical techniques for studying normal and noise damaged ears. In: Henderson D, Hamernik RP, Dosanjh DS, Mills JH, eds. The effects of noise on hearing. New York: Raven Press, 1976:129.

Thalmann I, Takahashi K, Varghese J et al. Biochemical features of major organ of Corti proteins (OPC-I and OPC-II) including partial amino acid sequence. Laryngoscope 1990; 100:99-105.

Thalmann I, Thallinger G, Crouch EC et al. Composition and supramolecular organization of the tectorial membrane. Laryngoscope 1987; 97:357-367.

Tilney LG, DeRosier DJ, Mulroy MJ. The organization of actin filaments in the stereocilia of cochlear hair cell. J Cell Biol 1980; 86:244-259.

Tilney LC, Saunders JC, Engelman E, DeRosier DJ. Changes in the organization of actin filaments in the stereocilia of noise-damaged lizard cochleae. Hear Res 1982; 7:181-197.

Tilney MS, Tilney LG, Stephens RE et al. Preliminary biochemical characterization of the stereocilia and cuticular plate of hair cells of the chick cochlea. J Cell Biol 1989; 109:1711-1723.

Tytell M, Gulley RL, Wenthold RJ, Lasek RJ. Fast axonal transport in auditory neurons in the guinea pig: A rapidly turned-over glycoprotein. Proc Natl Acad Sci (USA) 1980; 77:3042-3046.

Uney JB, Leigh PN, Marsden CD, et al. Stereotacic injection of kainic acid into the striatum of rats induces synthesis of mRNA for heat shock protein 70. FEBS Lett 1988; 235:215-218.

Vass K, Welch WJ, Nowak TS. Localization of 70 kDa stress protein induction in gerbil brain after ischemia. Acta Neuropathol 1988; 77:128-135.

Veech RL, Lawson JWR, Cornell NW, Krebs HA. Cytosolic phosphorylation potential. J Biol Chem 1979; 254:6538-6547.

Welch WJ, Mizzen LA, Arrigo AP. Structure and function of mammalian stress proteins. In: Pardue ML, Feramisco JR, Lindquist S, eds. Stress-induced proteins. New York: Alan R. Liss, 1989:187.

Wenthold RJ. Auditory nerve proteins. In: Drescher DG, ed. Auditory biochemistry. Springfield: Charles C Thomas, 1985:336.

Wenthold RJ, McGarvey ML. Different polypeptides are rapidly transported in auditory and optic neurons. J Neurochem 1982a; 39:27-35.

Wenthold RJ, McGarvey ML. Changes in rapidly transported proteins in the auditory nerve after hair cell loss. Brain Res 1982b; 253:263-269.

CHAPTER 4

Pharmacologic Approach to Acoustic Trauma in the Cochlea

RICHARD P. BOBBIN

Many chemicals have been explored for their ability to interact with cochlear damage induced with intense sound: vitamins, vasodilators, tranquilizers, stimulants, antibiotics, steroids, and nonsteroidal anti-inflammatory agents (Bobbin and Gondra, 1976; Bobbin et al, 1976; Kisiel and Bobbin, 1981a,b; Brown et al, 1981). Several chapters in this book address the interaction of intense sound with particular drugs. I will attempt to ascribe mechanisms to the interaction of intense sound with several different drugs: kynurenic acid, cytochalasin, salicylate, quinine, and nimodipine.

Hair Cell to Afferent Nerve Synapse

It is known that intense sound exposure induces swelling of the afferent dendrites at the level of the inner hair cells (Robertson, 1983). Thus it appears possible that during intense sound exposure, excess neurotransmitter is released from the inner hair cells which, in turn, damages the afferent nerve endings. Because an excitatory amino acid (EAA), such as glutamic acid or aspartic acid, may be the hair cell transmitter (Bledsoe et al, 1988), it is reasonable to suppose that an EAA induces the swelling observed after intense sound exposure. In the central nervous system EAAs are neurotoxic (Koh et al, 1990). Pujol et al. (1985) demonstrated that EAAs (kainic acid) induce swelling of the afferent nerve endings in the cochlea. Therefore we tested whether an EAA antagonist would reduce the effects of intense sound exposure in the cochlea (Puel et al, 1988).

Briefly, anesthetized and artificially respired guinea pigs with sectioned middle-ear muscles were used. Various agents were perfused through the perilymph compartment of the cochlea before, during, and after intense sound exposure (Fig. 4-1). The intense sound exposure consisted of a 6-kHz, 95-dB SPL, 15-minute continuous pure tone. The EAA antagonist we studied was kynurenic acid. The cochlear potentials (cochlear microphonics [CM], summating potential [SP], compound action potential of the auditory nerve [CAP], N1 latency) were monitored from a wire in the basal turn scala vestibuli in response to tone bursts (8,484 Hz). The intense sound induced several interesting effects (see Chapter 36): (1) the greatest reduction in the CAP and SP was localized one-half octave higher (8,484 Hz) than the intense tone exposure (see the review of McFadden, 1986), and (2) only the low-intensity portions of the intensity functions were affected.

The effects of kynurenic acid and its interaction with the intense sound are illustrated in Figure 4-2. The drug reduced both high- and low-intensity CAP; this effect was readily reversed with artificial perilymph. The effects of the drug added to the effects of the intense sound. When the drug was washed out, the added effect of the drug was removed, exposing the effects of the intense sound. We therefore concluded that the drug exhibited simple additive effects with the intense sound.

Generally, investigators feel that the low-intensity CAP and SP reflect the active process—mechanical or electrical events or both—utilized by the cochlea to achieve its sensitivity. Most guess that the outer hair cells (OHCs) are the anatomic basis of the active process (Brownell, 1990). We observed a suppression of only low-intensity-evoked CAP and SP, so we conclude that the intense sound that we used only damaged the active process. Others explain this damage to the active pro-

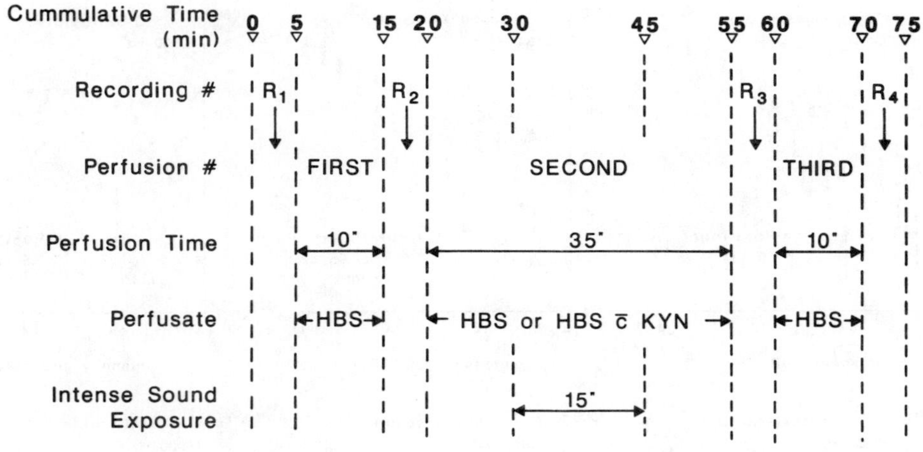

Figure 4-1 Schematic diagram of the timing of events for the experiments studying the interaction of intense sound and kynurenic acid (HBS, artificial perilymph). (From Puel J-L, Bobbin RP, Fallon M. The active process is affected first by intense sound exposure. Hear Res 1988; 37:53-64.)

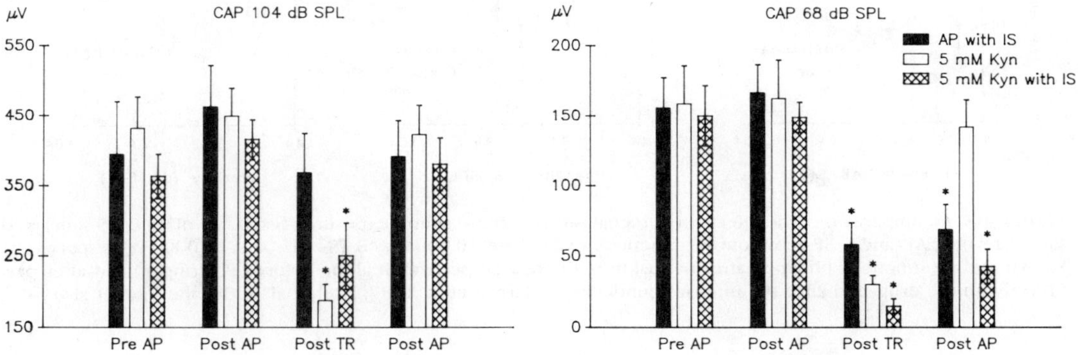

Figure 4-2 Results of the experiment utilizing the scheme illustrated in Figure 4-1 in three groups of five animals each. This figure illustrates the effect of (1) intense sound (IS) exposure combined with artificial perilymph perfusion (AP); (2) kynurenate (5 mm) perfusion alone; and (3) intense sound exposure combined with kynurenate (5 mm) perfusion. The IS was a 6-kHz, 95-dB SPL tone with a duration of 15 min. Shown are the mean and S.E. ($n = 5$) values for a compound action potential (CAP) of the auditory nerve obtained in response to 8,484-Hz tone-bursts of 104 and 68 dB SPL before any perfusions (Pre AP), after the first perfusion with artificial perilymph (Post AP), and after three different treatments (Post TR). AP with IS, intense sound during artificial perilymph perfusion; 5 mm Kyn, 5-mm kynurenic acid perfusion without intense sound; 5 mm Kyn with IS, 5-mm kynurenic acid perfusion with the intense sound exposure. The last set of bars shows the data obtained after the last perfusion with artificial perilymph (Post AP) alone. (From Puel J-L, Bobbin RP, Fallon M. The active process is affected first by intense sound exposure. Hear Res 1988; 37:53-64.)

cess by intense acoustic stimulation as damage to the stereocilia of the OHCs (Nielsen and Slepecky, 1986). Kynurenic acid is thought to act only at the EAA receptors on the afferents (Bledsoe et al, 1988). Therefore, our data indicate that there was no apparent interaction between the damaging effects of the intense sound at the stereocilia and the action of kynurenic acid at the EAA receptors. Our data indicating that the high-intensity CAP was unaffected suggest that the tone exposure we used was not of sufficient intensity to induce afferent swelling. This is consistent with the results of Robertson (1983), who showed that to obtain afferent nerve swelling one must use a tone greater than 110 dB SPL.

Drugs That Act Like Intense Sound on Cochlear Potentials

Figure 4-3 compares the effects of cytochalasin D, salicylate, and intense sound on the CAP and negative SP (−SP). Cytochalasin

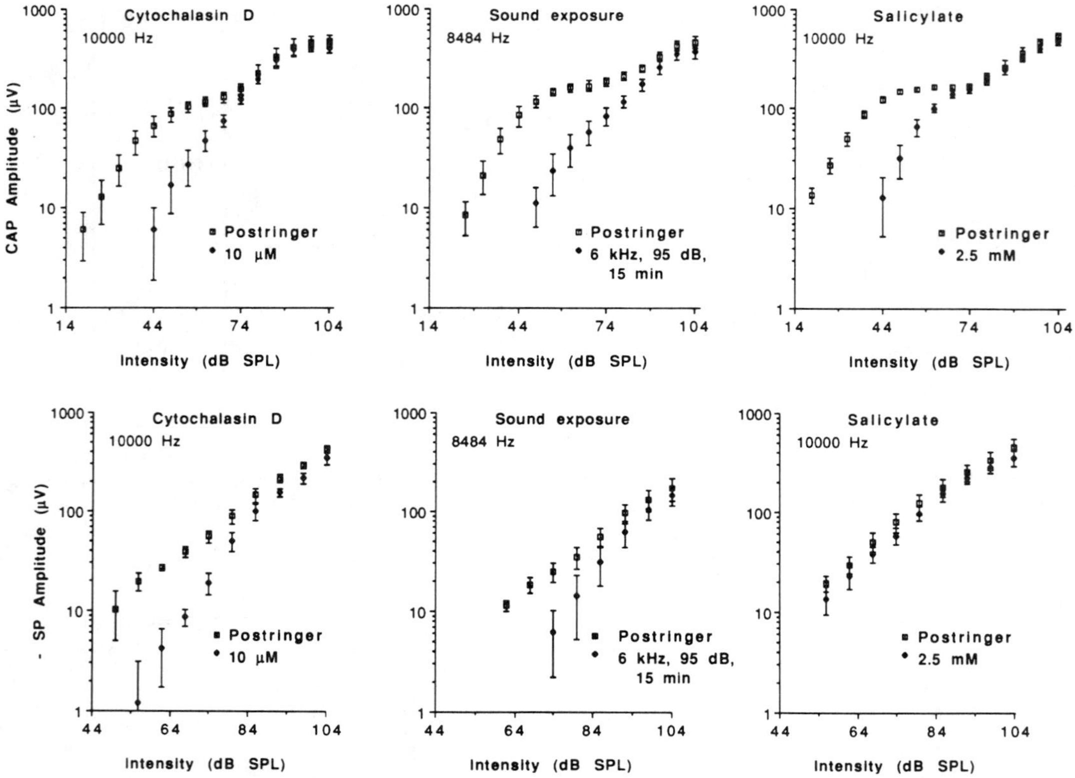

Figure 4-3 A comparison of the effects of cytochalasin D, intense sound exposure (6 kHz, 95 dB SPL, 15 min), and salicylate on CAP and −SP input/output functions evoked by 10,000 Hz, 8,484 Hz, and 10,000 Hz, respectively. Shown are the functions obtained after perfusion with artificial perilymph alone before (Postringer) and after perfusion with the drug, and after the intense sound. (From Barron et al, 1987; Puel et al, 1988; and Puel et al, 1990.)

D suppresses only the low-intensity CAP and SP, as does intense sound (Barron et al, 1987). Conversely, in both of our studies with salicylate, we found that it does not change the −SP, but suppresses the low-intensity CAP (Puel et al, 1989, 1990). Our CM and SP results conflict with the results reported by Stypulkowski (1989). Stypulkowski reported that intravenously administered salicylate decreased the magnitude of the round-window-recorded SP and increased CM. One major difference between Stypulkowski's preparation and ours is that in our preparation we avoided systemic effects such as changes in blood pressure and respiration induced by salicylate. In addition, we were able to demonstrate reversal of the salicylate effects (Puel et al, 1990), whereas Stypulkowski did not. We therefore concluded that either Stypulkowski's results reflect the changes in the physiologic state of the animal, or we measured different −SP and CM potentials.

However, the point to emphasize is that salicylate-induced CAP alterations are similar to those induced by intense sound, but different in terms of the −SP, according to Puel et al (1989, 1990). On the other hand, the actions of cytochalasin D are similar to those of intense sound on both potentials. Cytochalasin is thought to act on actin polymerization, so we speculated that it acts on the active process, possibly the stereocilia (Barron et al, 1987). Salicylate, in contrast, has a much greater effect on the CAP than on the −SP. This led us to speculate that the drug acted at a different site than intense sound—not the stereocilia of the OHCs. Stypulkowski (1989), Brownell (1990), and Brownell et al (1990) present evidence that salicylate acts on the OHCs. In contrast, in our experiments salicylate suppresses spontaneous activity before it affects evoked activity in the afferent nerve fibers, and it antagonizes the action of glutamate (Puel et al, 1989). Because the −SP is an electrical event originating from the OHCs and IHCs, and because of the lack of effect of

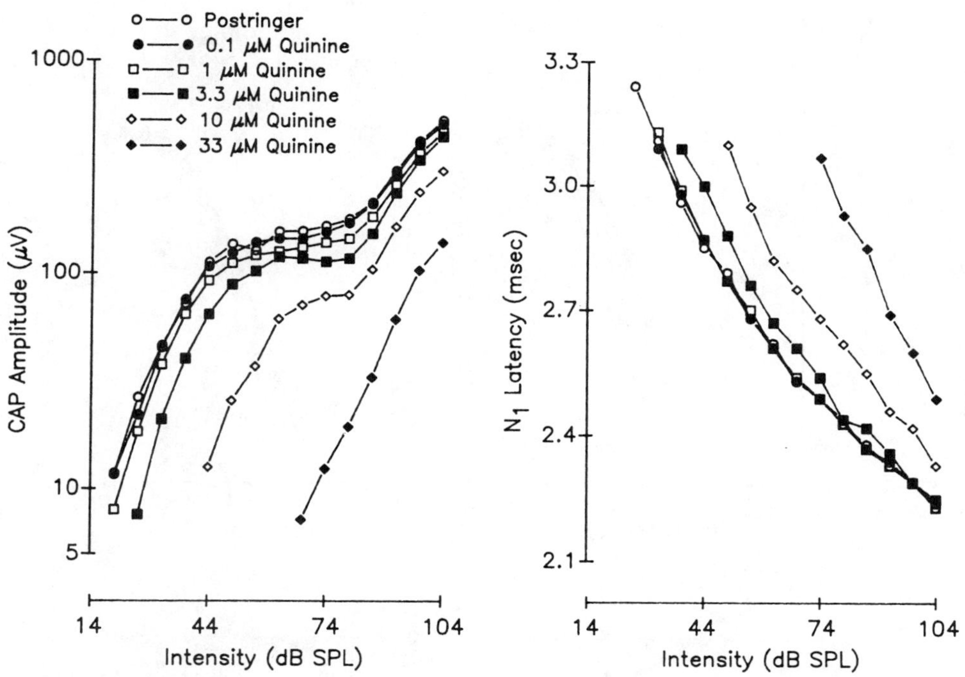

Figure 4-4 Effect of perfusion of quinine (n = 5) through the perilymphatic compartment on CAP and N1 latency as a function of intensity. Shown are functions recorded after predrug artificial perilymph perfusion (Postringer) and after perfusion of various concentrations of quinine. (From Puel J-L, Bobbin RP, Fallon M. Salicylate, mefenamate, meclofenamate, and quinine on cochlear potentials. Otolaryngol Head Neck Surg 1990; 102:66-73.)

salicylate on the −SP, our evidence generally indicates that the drug acts at "expression" of the active process. This could be the junction of the hair cell to nerve fiber (Puel et al, 1989, 1990). We suggest that salicylate acts at the transmitter release mechanism at the IHCs or at the transmitter receptor cites on the afferent endings.

What are the effects of these drugs in combination with intense sound? Cytochalasin has not been investigated in combination with intense sound, although it would be an interesting experiment given the possibility that the two may act at the stereocilia. On the other hand, McFadden and Plattsmier (1983) present evidence that salicylate potentiates the action of intense sound. It appears to me that salicylate simply adds to the effects of intense sound in a manner similar to kynurenic acid. I base this assertion on the electrophysiologic evidence presented above, which indicates that the drugs (kynurenic acid, salicylate) and intense sound act at different sites in the cochlea, and that the effect of the drugs at one site does not appear to interact with the effect of intense sound at the other site.

Thus, in general, any drug that acts at a site different from one acted on by intense sound may simply add to the effects of the intense sound. Of course here we are referring only to those cases in which the sound is at an intensity that affects the active process or acts on the stereocilia, and in which the drugs are reversibly ototoxic.

Drugs That Act Differently from Intense Sound on Cochlear Potentials

Figure 4-4 illustrates the effects of quinine perfused through the cochlea (Puel et al, 1990). The effects of quinine on CAP and N1 latency are similar to the effects of kynurenic acid. In general, the CAP input/output curve shows a "parallel" shift to the right and down, whereas the latency curve is shifted to the right and up. There is little evidence that the drug selectively suppresses the low-intensity portion of the CAP or the active process. If anything, the drug affects both the active and passive processes together.

Another major characteristic of quinine is the drug's large, but approximately equal, ef-

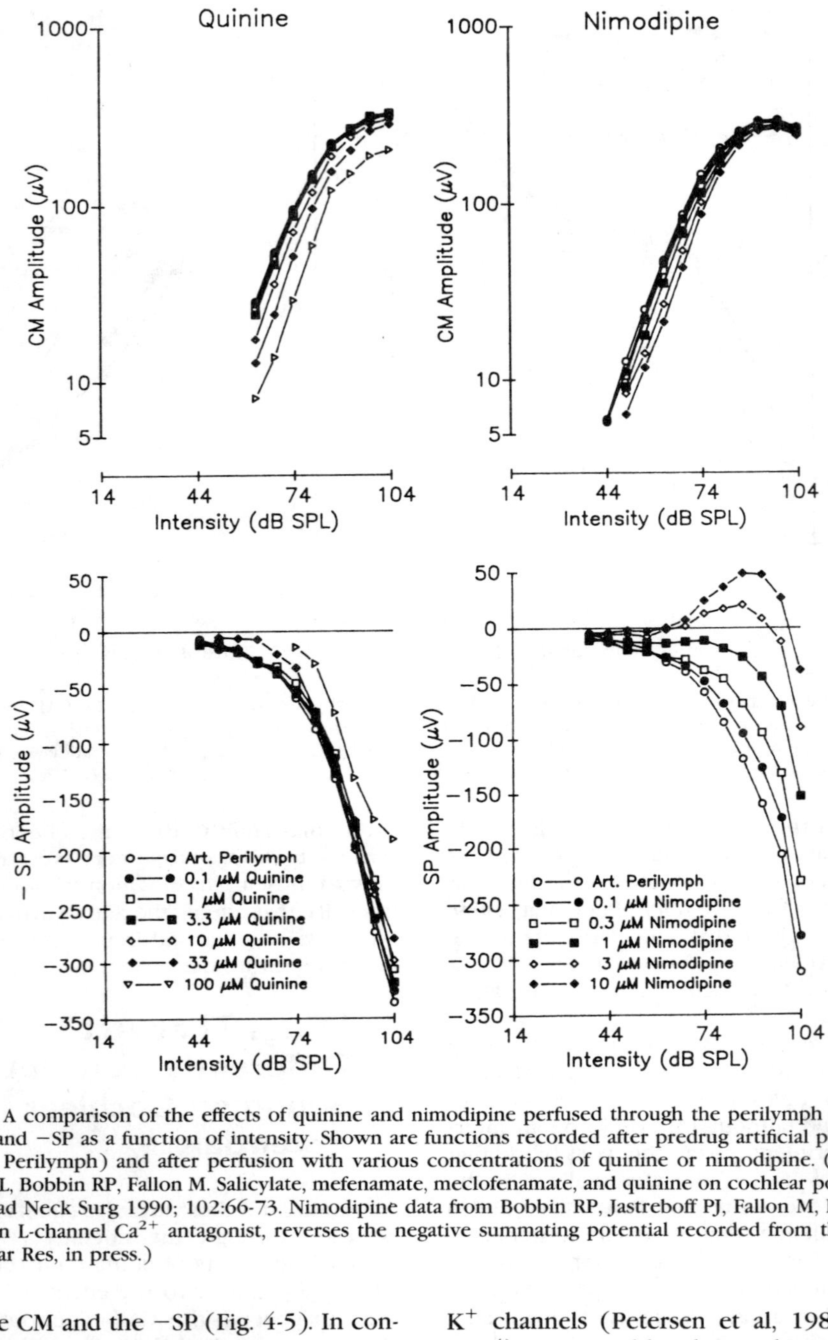

Figure 4-5 A comparison of the effects of quinine and nimodipine perfused through the perilymph compartment on the CM and −SP as a function of intensity. Shown are functions recorded after predrug artificial perilymph perfusion (Art. Perilymph) and after perfusion with various concentrations of quinine or nimodipine. (Quinine data from Puhl J-L, Bobbin RP, Fallon M. Salicylate, mefenamate, meclofenamate, and quinine on cochlear potentials. Otolaryngol Head Neck Surg 1990; 102:66-73. Nimodipine data from Bobbin RP, Jastreboff PJ, Fallon M, Littman T. Nimodipine, an L-channel Ca^{2+} antagonist, reverses the negative summating potential recorded from the guinea pig cochlea. Hear Res, in press.)

fect on the CM and the −SP (Fig. 4-5). In contrast is the action of nimodipine, an L-type Ca^{2+} channel antagonist, which has a much greater effect on the −SP than on CM, as shown in Figure 4-5 (Bobbin et al, 1990). The effect of nimodipine on CAP and N1 latency is similar to that of quinine. The effects of both drugs are readily reversible.

Quinine is thought to act by blocking ATP-dependent and Ca^{2+}-dependent outward K^+ channels (Petersen et al, 1986; Ohmori, 1984). Presumably these channels are involved in the movement of K^+ out of the hair cell. Because CM is thought to be predominately a K^+ current, the large effect of quinine on CM is in accordance with its known actions. The effect on SP is a result of the action of the drug on CM.

In contrast to quinine, nimodipine is known as a Ca^{2+} channel antagonist. These results then suggest a role for Ca^{2+} in the production of the −SP. Many possible mechanisms may explain the dramatic effect of nimodipine on the −SP. These include the blockade of a Ca^{2+} current, a Ca^{2+}-dependent K^+ current, and a Ca^{2+}-dependent shortening and lengthening of OHCs (Bobbin et al, 1990). Conversely, Ca^{2+} channel antagonists are known to have many actions other than blockade of Ca^{2+} L-channels (Zernig, 1990). For instance, Sato (1989) observed a reduction in the endocochlear potential (EP) with nifedipine, another organic Ca^{2+} channel antagonist. However, we did not detect a change in EP with nimodipine. In addition, Sato did not duplicate the effect of nifedipine on the EP with 10 mm EGTA, which probably means that the change in EP by nifedipine was not related to Ca^{2+}.

We predict that, like salicylate and kynurenic acid, quinine will simply add to the effects of an intense sound that damages the active process or the stereocilia. In contrast, nimodipine may reduce the effects of intense sound on the active process. The literature suggests that this may be the case (Mann et al, 1987). Such a reduction may come about if nimodipine reduces the contractual pull of the OHCs on their own stereocilia.

Up to this point, the discussion has centered on an intense sound exposure that affects only the active process and in particular appears to damage the stereocilia. On the other hand, if the sound is intense enough to affect the hair cell itself or to induce swelling of the afferents, then the above drugs may have different interactions with the sound. For instance, kynurenic acid and salicylate may prevent the damage to the afferents. By blocking an outward K^+ channel, quinine may potentiate the effects of such an intense sound by inducing an additional depolarization of the cell.

Conclusion

Overall, it appears that the pharmacology of drug action in the ear is becoming clearer. We are beginning to understand the mechanism of action of aspirin, quinine, and other classic ototoxic drugs, and new drugs are proving useful tools. In addition, there is new knowledge of the mechanism of action of intense sound. With this new knowledge in these two areas, we can make predictions as to whether the drugs will or will not interact with intense sound in damaging the cochlea.

Approche Pharmacologique du Traumatisme Sonore Cochléaire

Historiquement, plusieurs substances chimiques ont été utilisées dans le but d'augmenter ou de réduire les dommages cochléaires induits par un traumatisme acoustique. Ces substances appartiennent à toutes les classes d'agents pharmacologiques: vitamines, vaso-dilatateurs, tranquillisants, stimulants, antibiotiques ou anti-inflammatoires non stéroïdiens.

Notre laboratoire a utilisé plusieurs approches expérimentales afin de tester des substances susceptibles d'interagir ou de prévenir les effets d'un traumatisme acoustique. Tout d'abord, nous avons examiné l'aspect "stress" grâce à un pré-traitement à la réserpine, une drogue qui abolit l'action du système nerveux sympathique. Un tel traitement n'avait aucun effet sur les dommages anatomiques induits par un son intense de 4 kHz. Ensuite nous avons essayé de prévenir l'effet traumatique de ce même son intense en utilisant l'acide amino-oxyacétique connu pour réduire de manière réversible le potentiel endocochléaire. Ce traitement atténuait la perte des cellules ciliées induite par le son traumatique. Toutefois, les résultats n'étaient pas aussi clairs lorsque cette étude fut reprise en utilisant des techniques électrophysiologiques (Kisiel et Bobbin, 1981).

D'autres données indiquent que le traumatisme acoustique ainsi que le glutamate (le neurotransmetteur présumé des cellules ciliées internes) provoquent des gonflements des terminaisons afférentes sous les cellules ciliées. Dans le système nerveux central, le glutamate est impliqué dans la mort neuronale. Aussi, nous avons testé l'effet d'un antagoniste du glutamate, l'acide kynurénique, lors d'une exposition à un traumatisme acoustique (Puel et coll., 1988). Les résultats étaient négatifs et indiquaient que le son intense utilisé n'affectait que les mécanismes actifs (probablement les stéréocils). Ces résultats indiquent aussi que l'intensité du son traumatique utilisée n'était pas suffisante pour provoquer des gonflements des terminaisons nerveuses afférentes. De nouvelles études devront être effectuées en utilisant un traumatisme acoustique plus intense.

La nimodipine, un bloqueur des canaux calciques, abolit le potentiel de sommation négatif (Bobbin et coll., 1989). Ceci indique

que le potentiel de sommation négatif reflète un courant calcique dans les cellules ciliées et/ou les propriétés contractiles des cellules ciliées externes. Aussi il n'est pas surprenant que les antagonistes calciques puissent réduire l'effet d'un traumatisme acoustique (Mann et coll., 1987).

En résumé, il semble que plus on avance dans le domaine de la biologie et de la pharmacologie cochléaire mieux l'interaction de différentes drogues avec le traumatisme acoustique est comprise.

ACKNOWLEDGMENTS

Thanks to Maureen Fallon and Jenny Crist for help in conducting the experiments described in this chapter and in preparing the figures. Special thanks to Jean-Luc Puel, Ph.D., who conducted many of the experiments. Preparation of this chapter was supported in part by NIH grant DC00379.

References

Barron SE, Bobbin RP, Guth P, Norris C. Cytochalasin D suppresses sound-evoked potentials in guinea pig cochlea. Hear Res 1987; 31:147-154.

Bledsoe SC Jr, Bobbin RP, Puel J-L. Neurotransmission in the inner ear. In: Jahn AF, Santos-Sacchi JR, eds. Physiology of hearing. New York: Raven Press, 1988:385.

Bobbin RP, Gondra MI. Effect of nicotine on cochlear function and noise-induced hair cell loss. Ann Otol Rhinol Laryngol 1976; 85:247-254.

Bobbin RP, Guth MS, Mines AB. An examination of an electrochemical mechanism for noise-induced hair cell loss, i.e., noise with aminooxyacetic acid. Trans Am Acad Ophthalmol Otolaryngol 1976; 82:299-304.

Bobbin RP, Jastreboff PJ, Fallon M, Littman T. Nimodipine, an L-channel Ca^{2+} antagonist, reverses the negative summating potential recorded from the guinea pig cochlea. Hear Res 1990; 46:277-288.

Brown RD, Penny JE, Henley CM, et al. Ototoxic drugs and noise. In: Evered D, Lawrenson G, eds. Tinnitus. London: Pitman Books, 1981:151.

Brownell WE. Outer hair cell electromotility and otoacoustic emissions. Ear Hear 1990; 11:82-92.

Brownell WE, Shehata WE, Imredy JP. Slow electrically and chemically evoked volume changes in guinea pig outer hair cells. In: Akkas N, ed. Biomechanics of active movement and deformation of cells. Berlin: Springer-Verlag, 1990:493.

Kisiel DL, Bobbin RP. Miscellaneous ototoxic agents. In: Brown RD, Daigneault EA, eds. Pharmacology of hearing. New York: Wiley, 1981a:231.

Kisiel D, Bobbin RP. Interaction of aminooxyacetic acid and ethacrynic acid with intense sound at the level of the cochlea. Hear Res 1981b; 6:129-140.

Koh J-Y, Goldberg MP, Hartley DM, Choi DW. Non-NMDA receptor-mediated neurotoxicity in cortical culture. J Neurosci 1990; 10:693-705.

Mann W, Pilgramm M, Lohle E, Beck C. Calciumantagonisten und die Schadigung des cortischen organs bei knalltrauma. HNO 1987; 35:203-207.

McFadden D. The curious half-octave shift: Evidence for a basalward migration of the traveling-wave envelope with increasing intensity. In: Salvi RJ, Henderson D, Hamernik RP, Colletti V, eds. Basic and applied aspects of noise-induced hearing loss. New York: Plenum, 1986:295.

McFadden D, Plattsmier HS. Aspirin can potentiate the temporary hearing loss induced by intense sounds. Hear Res 1983; 9:295-316.

Nielsen DW, Slepecky N. Stereocilia. In: Altschuler RA, Bobbin RP, Hoffman DW, eds. Neurobiology of hearing: the cochlea. New York: Raven Press, 1986:23.

Ohmori H. Studies of ionic currents in the isolated vestibular hair cell of the chick. J Physiol (Lond) 1984; 350:561-581.

Petersen OH, Findlay I, Suzuki K, Dunne MJ. Messenger-mediated control of potassium channels in secretory cells. J Exp Biol 1986; 124:33-52.

Puel J-L, Bledsoe SC Jr, Bobbin RP, et al. Comparative actions of salicylate on the amphibian lateral line and guinea pig cochlea. Comp Biochem Physiol 1989; 93C:73-80.

Puel J-L, Bobbin RP, Fallon M. The active process is affected first by intense sound exposure. Hear Res 1988; 37:53-64.

Puel J-L, Bobbin RP, Fallon M. Salicylate, mefenamate, meclofenamate, and quinine on cochlear potentials. Otolaryngol Head Neck Surg 1990; 102:66-73.

Pujol R, Lenoir M, Robertson D, et al. Kainic acid selectively alters auditory dendrites connected with cochlear inner hair cells. Hear Res 1985; 18:145-151.

Robertson D. Functional significance of dendrite swelling after loud sounds in the guinea pig cochlea. Hear Res 1983; 9:263-278.

Sato Y. Effects of a calcium channel blocker and calcium chelating agents on cochlear electrical activity in the guinea pig. Acta Otolaryngol (Stockh) 1989; 108:76-82.

Stypulkowski PH. The mechanism(s) of salicylate (aspirin) induced hearing loss and tinnitus. Abstracts of the 12th Midwinter Research Meeting, Association for Research in Otolaryngology, St. Petersburg, Florida, February 5–9, 1989, p 189.

Zernig G. Widening potential for Ca^{2+} antagonists: Non–L-type Ca^{2+} channel interaction. TiPS 1990; 11:38-44.

CHAPTER 5

Effect of Noise on Auditory Nerve Responses

ROBERT PATUZZI

Clinical Changes in Human Noise-Induced Hearing Loss

Following noise exposure in human beings, audiograms often show a characteristic decrease in sensitivity in the 2- to 8-kHz region, commonly termed a "noise-notch" (Bilger, 1976) (Fig. 5-1). For those not already familiar with the physiology of noise-induced deafness, it is useful to catalogue the most common features of the noise-notch. These are:

1. The hearing loss is frequency-specific.
2. The loss does not always occur at the frequency of the traumatic exposure (McFadden, 1986).
3. Within the notch the frequency selectivity is reduced (Tyler and Tye-Murray, 1986).
4. The ear's ability to cope with a wide range of sound intensities is reduced. This is commonly termed "recruitment" (McFadden and Plattsmier, 1982).
5. There is commonly a distorted sense of pitch within or at the edges of the lesion termed "diplacusis" (McFadden and Plattsmier, 1982).
6. In a normal cochlea there are interactions between the frequency components of a complex stimulus. If two pure tones are presented simultaneously, the response to one can be reduced by the presence of the other. Following acoustic trauma this "two-tone suppression" is reduced (Mills, 1982; Salvi et al, 1982; Schmiedt et al, 1980a,b; Smoorenburg, 1980).
7. In a normal cochlea, two pure-tone stimuli can also interact to generate other tones, known as "distortion" or "combination" tones. These tones are clearly audible to the subject and can be detected in the external ear canal using a sensitive microphone (Wilson, 1980; Zurek, 1985). Following acoustic trauma, the distortion tones are reduced or abolished (Smoorenburg, 1980).

Correlates of Human Data in Primary Afferent Responses

These changes can also be observed in the response of the primary afferent neurons innervating the cochlea. For example, the loss of sensitivity within the noise-notch is due directly to the loss of sensitivity of the neurons innervating the site of the lesion (Cody and Johnstone, 1980; Kiang et al, 1986; Liberman and Mulroy, 1982; Lonsbury-Martin and Meikle, 1978; Robertson, 1982; Salvi et al, 1982; Schmiedt et al, 1980). In Figure 5-2*A*, a range of single-fiber frequency tuning curves (FTCs) is shown, which was obtained in experiments in a normal cat. Each of the curves is the equivalent of a "pure-tone audiogram" for a single afferent fiber, in that the threshold of neural firing is plotted versus the frequency of the pure-tone stimulus. Each curve possesses a sensitive tip region, centered around the most sensitive or characteristic frequency (CF) for each fiber, and a relatively insensitive, low-frequency tail region. The CF of each fiber is correlated with its site of innervation along

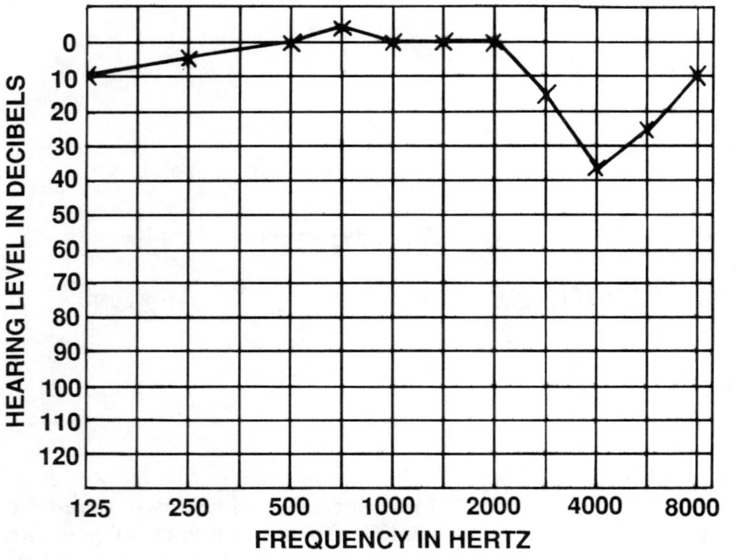

Figure 5-1 A typical human audiogram after exposure to industrial noise. The reduction in sensitivity in the region of 2 to 8 kHz is commonly termed a "noise-notch."

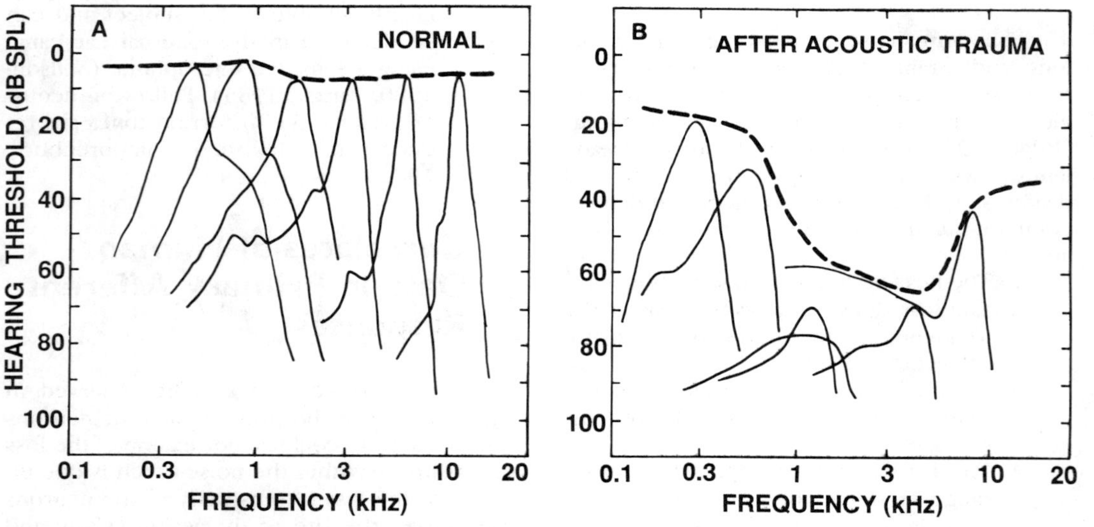

Figure 5-2 *A,* Typical frequency threshold curves (FTCs) for single primary afferent neurons in the cat. The gross audiogram (dashed line) is defined by the tips of the collection of individual FTCs. *B,* After acoustic trauma (narrow-band noise, 115 dB SPL, 30 min), a localized reduction in threshold is observed similar to the human noise-notch. This is due to loss of sensitivity at the FTC tip. (Redrawn from Liberman and Mulroy, 1982.)

the cochlear length, in accordance with an approximately logarithmic place-frequency map (Robertson and Johnstone, 1979; Liberman, 1982). The gross pure-tone audiogram, as measured clinically, is defined by the tips of the thousands of individual single-fiber FTCs across the frequency range, and is represented in Figure 5-2 by a dashed line. Note that the results of Figure 5-2 are essentially in the format of the typical pure-tone audiogram for human subjects, except that the frequency range in the cat is wider and sound pressure is in units of absolute sound pressure level (dB SPL) rather than the normalized units used clinically (dB HL).

After exposure to a traumatic sound, a noise-notch can be produced in experimental animals that is similar to that seen in man, as illustrated in Figure 5-2*B.* In this case, the traumatic acoustic stimulus was narrow-band noise lasting 30 minutes. The loss of sensitivity in the notch region can be seen to be due to a loss of the sensitive tip region around the CF of each FTC.

This frequency-dependent change after acoustic trauma can be seen in more detail in Figure 5-3, *A*, which shows FTCs before and after acoustic trauma for a *single* afferent neuron of the spiral ganglion in the high-frequency region of the guinea pig cochlea (Cody and Johnstone, 1980). The curves in Figure 5-3, *A* are plotted in the more typical format of physiologic reports, i.e., upside-down relative to the normal clinical audiogram. Before acoustic trauma, the FTC possessed the typical sensitive tip region around the 21-kHz CF, and a low-frequency tail region that was about 75 dB less sensitive than the tip. After acoustic trauma, in this case a 15.75-kHz pure-tone exposure at 100 dB SPL for 7 minutes, the tip thresholds were elevated by about 40 dB, and the CF changed from 21 kHz before trauma to 14 kHz after trauma. This drop in CF is a typical feature of noise trauma (Liberman, 1984). Notice also that the thresholds in the low-frequency tail region changed little. Changes on the tail are normally only seen after more prolonged exposures, which produce dramatic threshold elevation near CF. This is also illustrated in Figure 5-3, *A*. After 31 minutes of exposure to the traumatic stimulus the FTC of the neuron was elevated further around CF, and threshold elevation was also observed on the low-frequency tail region. In such cases, it is difficult to assign a CF because of the irregular shape of the FTC. This progressive change in neural tuning is typical of changes observed after pure-tone exposures, although it is possible to elevate neural threshold relatively evenly over the whole FTC with a suitable choice of traumatic stimulus (Liberman et al, 1986).

The change in sharpness or tuning of the FTC can be quantified by the Q_{10dB} value, which is defined as the CF of the neuron divided by the width of the curve 10 dB above its CF point. In a normal cochlea, this ratio can be as high as 10, but following noise-trauma it can be reduced to values below 2. For example, in Figure 5-3, *A*, the Q_{10dB} value was 10 before trauma, but was reduced to 1.2 following the 7-minute exposure.

Mechanical Component of Noise-Induced Hearing Loss

Many of the response properties of the primary afferent fibers can be explained by the vibration of the organ of Corti within the cochlea (Patuzzi, 1986). This is illustrated in Figure 5-3*B*, where isodisplacement FTCs for the vibration of the organ of Corti at a particular location in the high-frequency region of the guinea pig cochlea are presented (Sellick et al, 1982). Three curves are shown: the normal FTC obtained in a cochlea with near-normal neural thresholds; a curve obtained after general deterioration of the preparation, and a curve obtained after death. In the normal condition, the mechanical FTC is highly sensitive and tuned, which explains the normal primary afferent response (Patuzzi and Robertson, 1988). However, after general deterioration of the preparation, the mechanical sensitivity is reduced most near the tip region of the tuning curve, with relatively small changes on the low-frequency tail. After death the mechanical sensitivity is reduced further near CF, but again minimal changes are seen on the low-frequency tail.

Because these mechanical changes are similar to the changes in the neural response after loud sound, it is tempting to propose that the neural changes have a mechanical origin. Certainly, the change in mechanical sensitivity is closely correlated with elevation of neural threshold after general deterioration of cochlear condition, as can be seen in Figure 5-3, *C*. Here, the sound pressure required to produce a fixed neural response (a just-detectable compound action potential from the auditory nerve) is plotted against the sound pressure required to produce a fixed mechanical response (0.04 mm per second vibration of the organ of Corti at CF).

This circumstantial evidence for a mechanical component in noise-induced hearing loss is supported by other observations. For example, it is known that the mechanical properties of the cochlea influence the movement of the eardrum through the middle ear ossicles, thereby modifying the acoustic properties of the ear canal. If two pure tones are presented to the external ear canal, the distorted movement of the eardrum caused by the distorted vibration within the cochlea produces sounds in the ear canal that are not present in the original stimulus. Most prominently, two tones at frequencies of f_1 and f_2 produce another tone at a frequency of $2f_1 - f_2$. Known as the "cubic difference tone," this acoustic distortion is reduced following loud sound that elevates neural threshold, indicating a change in the vibration within the cochlea (Johnstone et al, 1990; Lonsbury-Martin et al, 1987; Schmiedt, 1986; Siegel and Kim, 1982). Figure 5-3*D* shows the correlation between the reduction in gross neural sensitivity (compound action potential threshold) after

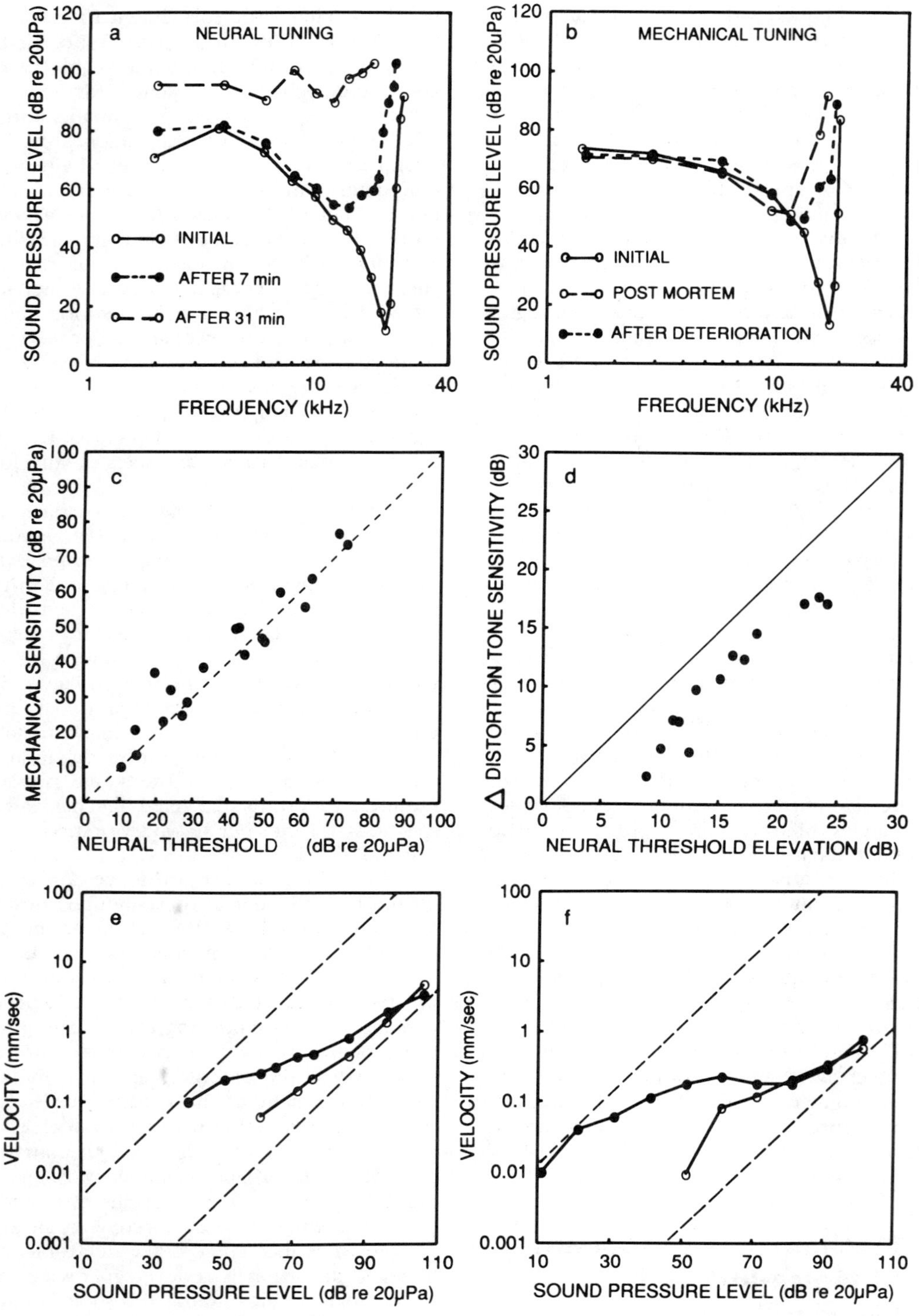

Figure 5-3 Evidence supporting a mechanical component to noise-induced threshold shifts. *A,* Frequency threshold curve (FTC) of a single afferent neuron before and after acoustic trauma (after Cody and Johnstone, 1980). *B,* FTC for 0.35-nm vibration of the organ of Corti before and after deterioration of preparation (after Sellick et al, 1982). *C,* Correlation between neural and mechanical sensitivity after general deterioration of a preparation (after Sellick et al, 1982). *D,* Correlation between changes in neural and distortion tone sensitivities after acute acoustic trauma (after Johnstone et al, 1990). *E* and *F,* Examples of the growth of vibration of the organ of Corti before (●) and after (○) acoustic trauma (after Sellick et al, 1982; Patuzzi et al, 1984).

exposure to a pure-tone traumatizing stimulus, and the change in the level of the f_1 and f_2 tones required to produce a fixed level of $2f_1-f_2$ distortion tone in the ear canal. Although this is not a simple measure of the change in organ vibration, these results do indicate that noise-induced hearing loss can be associated with changes in vibration within the cochlea.

The simplest indication that vibration is changed by acoustic trauma comes from direct measurement of vibration before and after acoustic trauma. Figure 5-3*E* and *F* shows two examples of the increase in vibration amplitude of the organ of Corti with an increase in the intensity of a pure-tone CF stimulus. As the sound pressure is increased, the vibration amplitude grows, but not in proportion with stimulus amplitude. In particular, the amplitude increases by only about 0.5 dB with each decibel of increase in the stimulus. This nonlinear growth or "compression" of vibration amplitude is a normal feature of the mechanical response of the organ of Corti to stimuli in the tip region of the tuning curve, and is crucial to the ear's ability to cope with a wide range of sound intensity. However, after prolonged, intense stimulation, the vibration becomes less sensitive to low stimulus levels, but the sensitivity is relatively unchanged at high intensities. In other words, the growth of vibration amplitude with stimulus level is less compressive, or more linear, after trauma. It is interesting to note here that the small change in vibration amplitude at high intensities after trauma argues against any suggestion that temporary threshold shift after acoustic trauma is in some way a protective mechanism in the ear: from a mechanical point of view, it offers no protection at all.

Noise Trauma, Vibration, and Active Process

The most widely accepted explanation for these observations is that the response properties of the primary afferent neurons are determined by the release of neurotransmitter from the basolateral walls of the inner hair cells, and that the inner hair cell response is determined relatively simply by the vibration of the organ of Corti (Patuzzi and Robertson, 1988). Complications in understanding normal cochlear function arise because the vibration of the organ of Corti appears to be assisted in its vibration at low stimulus levels, but not at higher levels. It now seems that the outer hair cells (OHCs) of the organ of Corti apply forces in synchrony with the vibration that partially or wholly cancel the inherent viscous damping that would otherwise limit sensitivity. These forces are commonly termed "active" forces because they appear to require metabolic energy, and the physiological process that generates them is commonly termed the "active process." Its action in canceling viscous damping is also referred to as "negative damping." Importantly, the active process and the generation of these forces appear to be controlled by the receptor currents through the OHCs, or by the receptor potentials these currents produce. In this sense, the active process is thought to be "electromechanical" (Ashmore, 1987; Brownell, 1983; Mountain, 1986; Santos-Sacchi and Dilger, 1988).

This scheme is shown in Figure 5-4, in which a sound stimulus produces pressure fluctuations in the fluids within the cochlea, producing vibration of the organ and deflection of the hair bundles of the OHCs and inner hair cells (IHCs). In both cell types this oscillation of the hair bundles opens and closes ionic "mechanoelectrical transduction channels" at the apex of the hair cells, producing receptor currents through these cells, and consequently the receptor potentials within them (Holton and Hudspeth, 1986). In the case of the IHCs, the intracellular receptor potential simply produces release of neurotransmitter and neural firing. In contrast, the receptor potential within the OHCs appears to control the active forces that assist vibration of the organ, increasing mechanical sensitivity near CF. The major stages of transduction have been numbered in Figure 5-4 to simplify the discussion of the effects of acoustic trauma on the mechanical and neural responses.

Loss of OHC Receptor Current Produces Loss of Vibration

If the active process *is* controlled by the receptor currents through the OHCs, then one obvious explanation for noise trauma is the reduction of these currents by the acoustic overstimulation (stage 2 of Fig. 5-4). This would starve the active process of the electrical drive that seems to be necessary for mechanical and neural sensitivity near CF. This proposal has been investigated in the high-frequency region of the guinea pig cochlea (Patuzzi et al, 1989b), using the gross neural response to tone bursts as a measure of the vi-

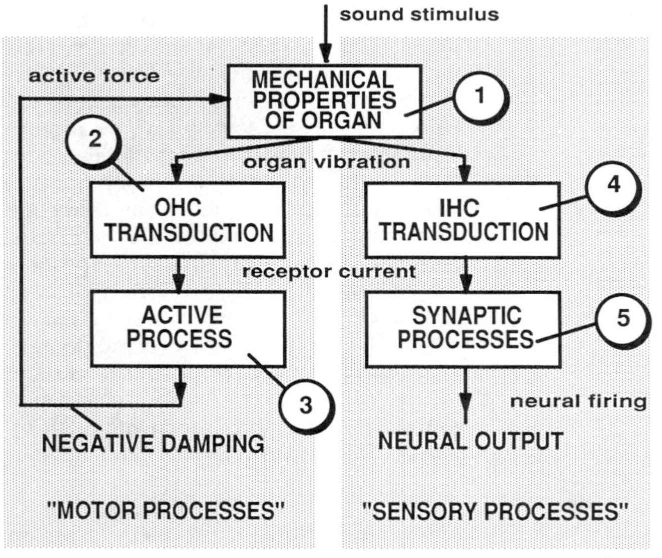

Figure 5-4 Schematic representation of the major stages of transduction within the mammalian cochlea. Each numbered stage is a possible site of disruption producing changes in the neural response. As argued in the text, the most vulnerable stage of transduction appears to be the production of the high-frequency receptor current through the outer hair cells (stage 2). IHC = inner hair cell. OHC = outer hair cell.

bration at CF in that region (Sellick et al, 1982), and the low-frequency microphonic potential in the extracellular fluid as a measure of the efficiency with which OHCs produce receptor current relative to normal. There appears to be a strong correlation between neural threshold and the efficiency of OHCs, as shown in Figure 5-5*A*. When the transduction process producing the OHC receptor currents is impaired, neural sensitivity falls, presumably because of a drop in mechanical sensitivity at the tip of the FTC (as in Fig. 5-3*A* and *B*). This relationship between mechanical gain at CF (relative to a passive cochlea with no active process) and the remaining fraction of OHC receptor current, expressed as a fractional efficiency relative to normal, OHC_{effic}, is given by the empirical expression (Patuzzi et al, 1989b)

$$GAIN(OHC_{effic}) = 55\ dB.OHC_{effic}/(1 - 0.85(1 - OHC_{effic})) \quad (1)$$

Rearranging this expression, we can write an expression for the hearing loss, HL, as

$$HL(OHC_{effic}) = 100\ dB/(0.85 + 1/(1 - OHC_{effic})) \quad (2)$$

At first glance, the large change in neural sensitivity observed for a relatively small change in the OHC receptor currents might suggest that the reduction in receptor current was not the causative change. In fact, this critical dependence on OHC receptor current is precisely the relationship we *would* expect if the OHCs were acting to cancel viscosity (Mountain, 1986; Neely and Kim, 1986; Patuzzi et al, 1989b). Importantly, if the reduction of OHC receptor current (stage 2 of Fig. 5-4) can adequately explain the loss of sensitivity near CF, then by exclusion, other changes, such as a disruption of the active process per se (stage 3 of Fig. 5-4), are unlikely.

Why does the OHC receptor current drop after acoustic trauma? A number of observations suggest that the proteins that presumably form the ionic channels that allow the flow of receptor current (Holton and Hudspeth, 1986) inactivate into a closed state. In particular, the shape of the sigmoidal curve relating hair bundle angle or displacement of the organ of Corti to the amount of receptor current seems to be scaled in amplitude following moderate noise trauma in a way consistent with such a closure (Fig. 5-5*B*) (Patuzzi et al, 1989a). There are also characteristic changes in potentials and potassium levels within the organ of Corti, which are consistent with this view (Johnstone et al, 1988; Salt and Konishi, 1979).

The normally compressive (nonlinear) growth of organ vibration with increasing stimulus intensity at CF (Fig. 5-3*E* and *F*) may also be explained by the fact that the high-frequency receptor current through the OHCs saturates for relatively large displacements of the organ of Corti; the closure of the transduction channels may also account for the loss of compression and the reduction in two-tone interactions after acoustic trauma. Because these two aspects of trauma are fundamental to the

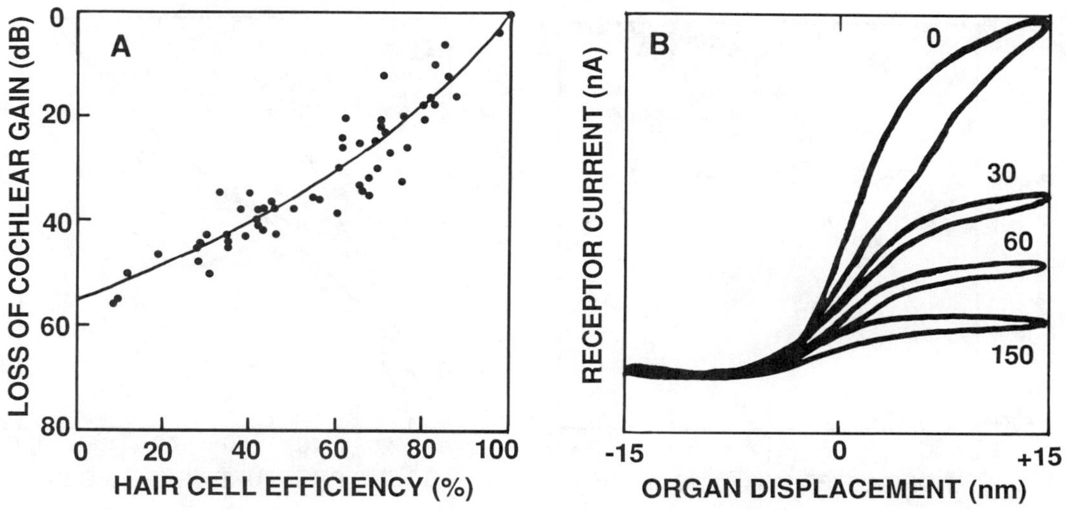

Figure 5-5 *A*, Correlation between fall in the efficiency of production of OHC receptor current (OHC_{effic}) relative to normal and loss of cochlear amplification at characteristic frequency. Cochlear amplification was estimated using compound action potential threshold to tone bursts. (After Patuzzi RB, Yates GK, Johnstone BM. Changes in cochlear microphonic and neural sensitivity produced by acoustic trauma. Hear Res 1989a; 39:189-202.) *B*, The sigmoidal relationship between transverse displacement of the organ of Corti in the guinea pig and receptor current through the OHCs. Curves are derived from recordings of extracellular microphonic potential. The parameter is duration of exposure to a pure-tone traumatizing stimulus (10 kHz, 115 dB SPL). After exposure the relationship is scaled in a way consistent with closure of mechanoelectrical transduction channels at the apex of the outer hair cells.

clinical changes after noise trauma, it is worth investigating the effects of the proposed channel closure in some detail.

Mechanical Growth Functions at Characteristic Frequency Before Trauma

Consider the growth of vibration amplitude with the level of a CF tone stimulus, before and after noise trauma. Before trauma, the sigmoidal relationship between organ displacement and OHC receptor current (Fig. 5-5*B*) results in an approximately hyperbolic growth of OHC receptor current amplitude (Fig. 5-6*A*) (Patuzzi et al, 1989b). That is, if the organ of Corti vibrates sinusoidally with an amplitude A, then the amplitude of the OHC receptor current would be given by $I_{ohc} = I_{sat} \cdot A/(A + A_{sat})$. Here, A_{sat} is the vibration amplitude at which the amplitude of the receptor current reaches half its saturation value, I_{sat}. This half-saturation displacement is estimated to be about 10 nm (Patuzzi, 1987). At low levels of the stimulus, receptor current grows approximately linearly, but as vibration amplitude grows, the efficiency with which OHCs produce receptor current decreases such that $OHC_{effic} = A_{sat}/(A + A_{sat})$. By combining this expression for OHC_{effic} with equation 2, we can estimate the loss in mechanical sensitivity as a function of vibration amplitude, A, as

$$HL(A) = 100\ dB/(0.85 + (A + A_{sat})/A) \qquad (3)$$

This drop in sensitivity with increasing vibration amplitude is the normal loss of mechanical sensitivity at high sound levels that produces compression within the ear, and does *not* correspond to an acoustic trauma. This result allows us to predict the compressive growth function for vibration in a normal ear at CF by using equation 3 to correct a linear growth function that had full amplification over the entire stimulus range, as shown by the solid line in Figure 5-6*B*. Also shown are all experimentally measured growth functions presently available (Sellick et al, 1982; Patuzzi et al, 1984; Robles et al, 1986). It can be seen from this comparison that the growth predicted using this simple analysis is similar to the measured mechanical growth functions—surprisingly so, considering the vastly different experimental results that have been used in the analysis.

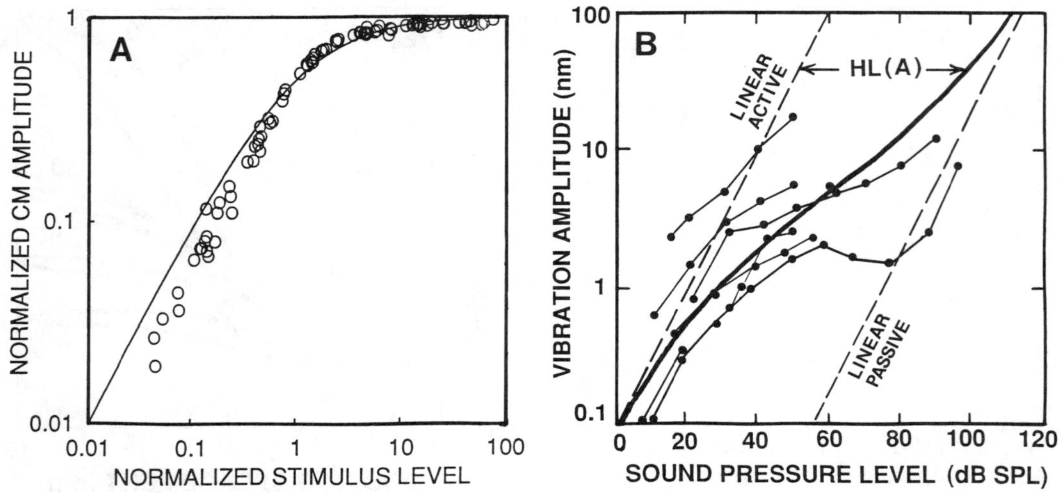

Figure 5-6 *A,* Hyperbolic growth of amplitude of OHC receptor current with level of a 200-Hz pure-tone stimulus. Data were obtained from measurements of extracellular microphonic in the first turn of the guinea pig cochlea in 14 normal preparations. Amplitude is normalized to maximal response at high intensities, whereas stimulus is normalized to the level giving half the maximal response. *B,* Predicted growth function for vibration of organ of Corti in the first turn of the guinea pig cochlea based on the hyperbolic saturation of outer hair cell receptor current and equation 3. Data points show experimental growth functions in the high-frequency regions of guinea pig and chinchilla cochlea. (After Patuzzi RB, Yates GK, Johnstone BM. Changes in cochlear microphonic and neural sensitivity produced by acoustic trauma. Hear Res 1989a; 39:189-202.)

Mechanical Growth Functions at Characteristic Frequency After Trauma

Consider, now, a traumatized ear in which the OHC receptor currents are reduced by a fraction, n, but the sigmoidal relationship between organ displacement is preserved (Fig. 5-5*B*). In this case, the hyperbolic growth of receptor current (Fig. 5-6*A*) would also be maintained, but scaled vertically by the factor n. As a result, the efficiency of the OHCs in producing receptor current would be $OHC_{effic} = n \cdot A_{sat}/(A + A_{sat})$. Substitution of this expression into equation 2 yields a more general expression for the loss of mechanical sensitivity as vibration amplitude is increased, which includes saturation of OHC current *and* closure of channels. That is,

$$HL(A, n) = 100\ dB/(0.85 + (n \cdot (A + A_{sat})/A) \quad (4)$$

Some mechanical growth functions calculated on this basis are illustrated in Figure 5-7*A* for various values of the fractional closure of channels. They are similar to the growth functions observed experimentally (Sellick et al, 1982) (Fig. 5-3*E* and *F*).

Can Loss of OHC Receptor Current Explain "Recruitment"?

If the neural growth functions became less compressive after noise trauma, as a result of the changes in vibration (Fig. 5-3*E* and *F*), then much of the clinical phenomenon of "recruitment" could be explained by closure of the transduction channels. Increasing the intensity of a pure-tone stimulus would progressively stimulate more and more neurons as the stimulus crossed each neuron's FTC, increasing its firing rate above spontaneous activity. In a normal ear, with its extremely sharp FTCs and its nonlinear growth of vibration amplitude, this process of recruiting nerve fibers into activity would occur relatively slowly as the stimulus level was increased (Fig. 5-8*A*). In an ear that had suffered acoustic trauma, however, the tuning curves would generally be broader, and the growth of vibration with stimulus level would be more rapid, as described earlier. As a result, the rate at which fibers were recruited as stimulus level was increased would be much greater in the traumatized ear, and lead to an abnormally rapid growth in perceived loudness of the stimulus (Fig. 5-8*B*).

Although this view of noise trauma seems

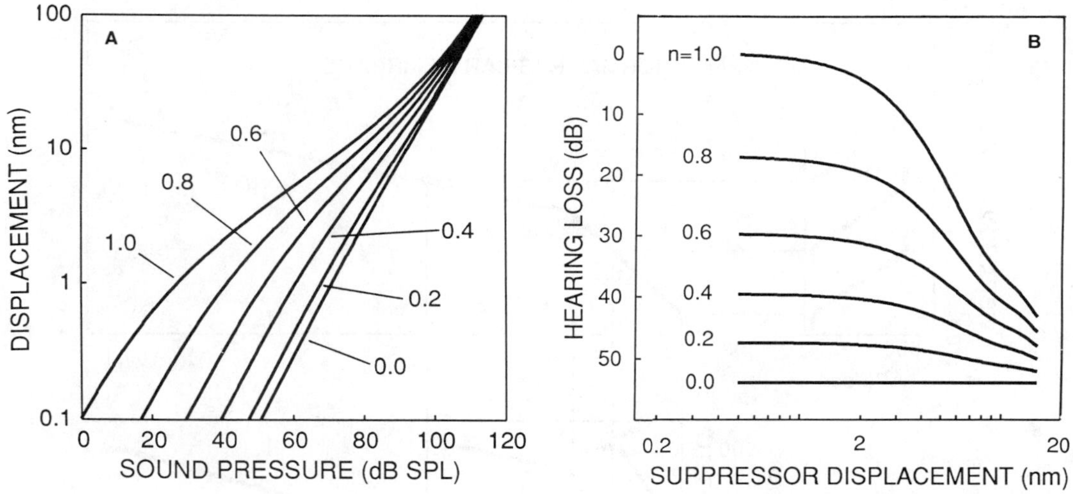

Figure 5-7 *A*, Predicted growth functions for vibration amplitude in the first turn of the guinea pig based on equation 2. Parameter is fraction of remaining outer hair cell (OHC) transduction channels. (After Patuzzi RB, Yates GK, Johnstone BM. Changes in cochlear microphonic and neural sensitivity produced by acoustic trauma. Hear Res 1989a; 39:189-202.) *B*, Predicted variation of hearing loss (drop in cochlear gain at characteristic frequency) with amplitude of low-frequency suppressor tone vibration. Parameter is fraction of remaining OHC transduction channels.

internally consistent, until recently there has been little experimental evidence that the growth rate for firing of the afferent neurons is significantly altered by noise trauma (Liberman, 1984; Schmiedt et al, 1980a,b). This is somewhat odd: it would seem inescapable that such changes should occur if the mechanical stimulus to the IHCs and neurons changed so dramatically. However, more recent reports indicate that the variation in the shape of normal neural rate-intensity functions is greater than was previously thought (Sachs et al, 1989; Winter et al, 1990; Yates et al, 1990), suggesting that previous reports may have missed the more subtle changes in neural rate-intensity functions. Briefly, variations in the properties of the IHCs or afferent synapses or both probably result in different neurons with similar CFs being stimulated over a different range of organ displacement. Because the growth of vibration at CF is nonlinear, the resultant rate-intensity function for these neurons has a different shape (Fig. 5-8*A*). After trauma, however, when the growth function for vibration becomes less sensitive and linear, the neural growth functions should all converge to a similar sigmoidal shape (Fig. 5-8*B*).

Given these complications, it now seems likely that the absence of a reported change in the neural rate-intensity functions with acoustic trauma is due to the limited dynamic range of the primary afferent neurons, the initial linear portion of the vibration growth function at CF, and other experimental complications (possibly microelectrode characteristics). Future investigations of neural rate-intensity functions before and after noise trauma may find changes consistent with the changes already observed in organ vibration, and may produce a simple explanation based on the broadening of FTCs and less compressive growth of a CF stimulus.

Two-Tone Suppression Before and After Noise Trauma

Suppression by a Tone Below CF

At least some of the reduction in two-tone interactions after cochlear trauma (Salvi et al, 1982; Schmiedt et al, 1980; Robertson, 1976, 1981), notably two-tone suppression, may also be explained by a reduction in OHC receptor current. First, nonlinearity in the active process, whether it is in the current drive to the process, or the force generation stage per se, would result in "intermodulation distortion" when more than one pure-tone stimulus was presented simultaneously. Essentially, the presence of a second, "suppressor" tone interferes with, or "jams," the high-frequency receptor current necessary to drive the active process that assists vibration at CF. As already described, only a small reduction in the effi-

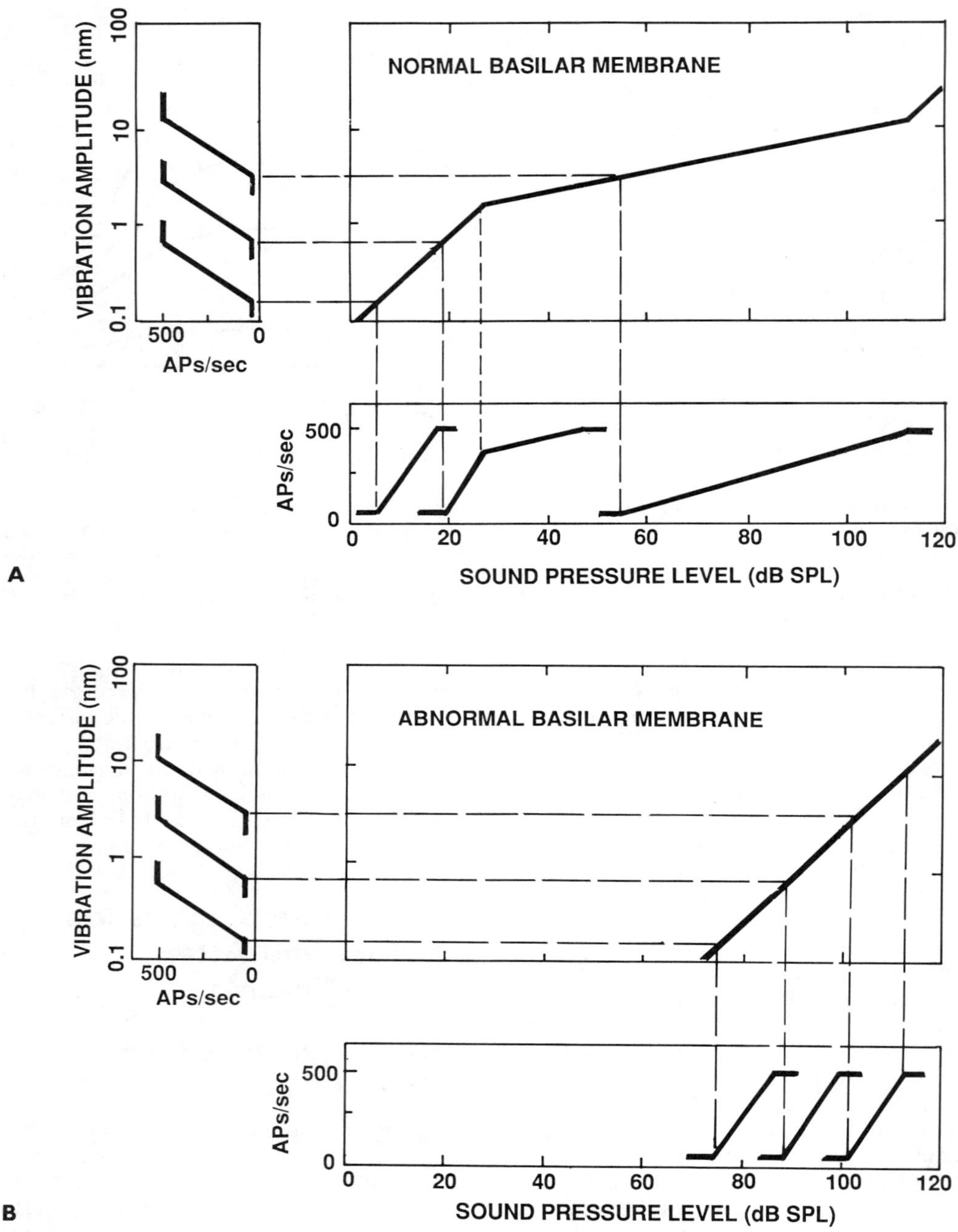

Figure 5-8 *A,* Depending on the sensitivity of a particular IHC-afferent synapse combination, the nonlinear growth of organ vibration at characteristic frequency can produce neural rate-intensity functions with different shapes. If the combination is very sensitive, the neural rate-intensity function may only reflect the initial linear portion of the mechanical growth function. Conversely, a less-sensitive hair cell–synapse combination may only reflect the highly nonlinear part of the mechanical growth function, producing a sloping rate-intensity curve. *B,* After trauma, when the mechanical growth function becomes less sensitive and linear (Fig. 5-3, *E* and *F*), all the rate-intensity functions for the hair cell–synapse combinations should change, and converge to the more commonly reported sigmoidal growth function.

ciency of receptor current generation would reduce the gain of the cochlea significantly for frequencies near the tip of the tuning curve. This effect is most easily understood when the stimulus or probe tone is presented at the CF of a neuron, while the suppressor tone is presented at a frequency on the low-frequency tail. Because vibration of the organ of Corti at tail frequencies is not significantly influenced by the active process, neither noise trauma nor nonlinear interactions would significantly affect the vibration produced by the low-frequency suppressor. The influence of a low-frequency suppressor on the response to a CF tone, however, would be profound. When the active process is intact, mechanical and neural sensitivity at CF is high, and even a small change in the efficiency with which the OHCs generate negative damping forces would greatly reduce sensitivity at CF.

The influence of this interference in reducing the efficiency of OHCs in producing receptor current can be estimated from the shape of the OHC transfer curve (Engebretson and Eldrege, 1968; Patuzzi et al, 1989b) (Fig. 5-5*B*). This is also the case after acoustic trauma when only a fraction, n, of the transduction channels remain operative, and the transfer curve (Fig. 5-5*B*) is scaled vertically by the same fraction. Using equation 4, we can estimate the reduction in active amplification at CF produced by a suppressor tone, before and after trauma. Figure 5-7*B* shows the loss of sensitivity at CF that would be predicted over a range of amplitude of suppressor tone vibration and channel closure. Notice that for small suppressor amplitudes the suppression curves start from different hearing losses, as a result of the hearing loss induced by channel closure, but that for high suppression amplitudes they all converge to the same loss (close to 55 dB). In essence, disruption of the active process, whether by channel closure or nonlinear interference of receptor current by a suppressor tone, cannot produce more than a total loss of active assistance. As hearing is lost through channel closure, the amount of suppression that can be produced is reduced, and the suppressor vibration required to produce a fixed amount of suppression increases. This is consistent with the clinical and experimental observations that two-tone interactions such as suppression are reduced after noise trauma. This is not to say that two-tone suppression cannot occur in a traumatized cochlea. There are clearly other nonlinearities in the transduction chain that produce suppression in a traumatized cochlea (Geisler and Greenberg, 1986).

Suppression by a Tone Above Characteristic Frequency

If two-tone suppression *is* due to a reduction in the OHC receptor current at CF caused by the suppressor tone, how can we explain the classic observation that a tone *above* CF, which produces no vibration at the CF site (Sellick et al, 1982), can produce suppression (Sachs and Kiang, 1968)? Conversely, how can such two-tone suppression be abolished if sensitivity and tuning remain (Robertson and Johnstone, 1981)? The easiest explanation for these apparent anomalies is that the vibration of the organ of Corti at the peak of the traveling wave does not rely on the action of OHCs *at that site*, but on OHCs slightly more basalward, towards the stapes (de Boer, 1983; Geisler et al, 1990). This peculiar aspect of two-tone suppression emphasizes that the processes within the cochlea that produce sensitivity, tuning, and two-tone interactions are not simple point-processes, but are probably distributed along the cochlear length.

Threshold Changes on the Low-Frequency Tail of the Frequency Threshold Curve (FTC)

As already mentioned, neural sensitivity on the low-frequency tail portion of the FTC can be reduced following intense, prolonged stimulation (Fig. 5-3*A*). Such changes on the tail are most likely due to disruption of the IHCs, synaptic mechanisms that detect organ vibration (stage 4 or 5 of Fig. 5-4), or both, or to changes in the passive mechanical properties of the organ of Corti, unrelated to the active process (stage 1 of Fig. 5-4) (Zwislocki, 1982; Neely and Kim, 1986; Liberman and Dodds, 1984). Because mechanical sensitivity for tail frequencies seems relatively robust (Fig. 5-3*B*), it seems unlikely that the early changes on the tail can be explained by changes in the passive mechanical properties. Moreover, in some cases neural sensitivity on the tail can actually improve following overstimulation (Liberman and Dodds, 1984). It has been suggested that this tail hypersensitivity may be related to an increased vibration of the organ of Corti at these frequencies, due to a reduced stiffness of the OHC stereocilia (Liberman and Dodds, 1984; Neely and Kim, 1986). A drop in the stiffness of the stereocilia has been observed in extirpated cochleas overstimulated in vitro (Saunders and Flock, 1986), but it is not yet clear how these results relate to the disruptive processes in vivo. Similarly, although it is also known that the high-frequency neurons of the guinea pig cochlea change their response to very low frequency tones in a complicated way after acute acoustic trauma (Patuzzi and Sellick, 1983), it is not clear how these changes relate to the normal function at more physiologic frequencies.

If disruption of the OHC hair bundles reduces stiffness of the organ of Corti and actually increases vibration, what elevates the low-frequency tail? The simplest explanations would be disruption of the detection of organ vibation by the IHCs, disruption of transmitter release and action potential initiation in the afferent neurons (stages 4 and 5 of Fig. 5-4), or both. Although disruption of the afferent dendrites has been observed (Spoendlin, 1976; Lim et al, 1982; Hunter-Duvar et al, 1982; Robertson, 1983), postsynaptic disruption is unlikely to be the prime origin of temporary threshold elevation following noise trauma. Animals exposed to traumatic stimuli while the synapse was blocked pharmacologically suffer the same hearing loss as those without this block (Puel et al, 1988). Threshold elevation on the tail of the FTC would therefore seem to be due to either disruption of transmitter release or changes in the mechanoelectrical transduction in the IHCs (Cody and Russell, 1985, 1988). Neither disruption has been fully investigated.

Additivity of Noise-Induced Hearing Loss—"Motor Processes" and "Sensory Processes"

The analysis of noise-induced hearing loss presented here suggests a way of approaching another fundamental issue in noise trauma: How do sensorineural hearing losses add? and Is an ear that is already damaged by noise more (or less) susceptible to further damage? We can limit our attention initially to only those hearing losses that reduce the OHC receptor current, either by reducing the biological voltages that drive the current (e.g., by anoxia and various ototoxic drugs), or by blocking the transduction channels (e.g., by acoustic trauma or drugs). Furthermore, we can make the simplifying assumption that the *fractional* loss of current produced by one trauma is unchanged by the occurrence of a prior trauma. In such a case, the fraction of remaining receptor current after two successive traumas would be the product of the fractions remaining after each trauma alone. That is, if one trauma on its own left only the fraction n_1 of OHC receptor current remaining and produced the hearing loss HL_1 (calculated from equation 2), and another trauma on its own left only the fraction n_2 of current, producing the hearing loss HL_2, then the total residual current if both traumas were combined would be $n_1 \cdot n_2$. By substituting this fractional receptor current into equation 2 we can predict the hearing loss, HL_{tot}, expected when both traumas are combined. This addition of such hearing losses is summarized graphically in Figure 5-9. The contours of the total hearing loss, HL_{tot}, have been generated using equation 2, so that the combined loss can be estimated graphically. An important point to note is that the hearing losses do *not* add arithmetically (in decibel or linear units); rather, the hearing loss saturates at 55 dB, when all active assistance to vibration is abolished. As an example, a noise exposure that produced a 50% closure of channels would produce a 35-dB hearing loss. If presented again it may produce a further 50 percent reduction in operative channels, to give a total of 25 percent remaining. Simplistically it might be expected that the total loss would be 70 dB = 35 dB + 35 dB; however, the loss predicted on the basis of equation 2 would be 46 dB. Such a loss due to a drop in OHC receptor current and loss of vibration at CF might usefully be termed a "motor loss."

The fact that noise-induced hearing losses can be greater than 55 dB (the maximum loss due to total abolition of the active process) is presumably due to impairment of IHC and neural function. As already described, any such loss that was *not* associated with a loss of OHC receptor current would not add in the manner predicted by equation 2. For example, decibel hearing losses that were associated with the IHCs or neurons or both would probably add arithmetically to the loss predicted on the basis of Figure 5-9. These losses could presumably be recognized by the changes they produced on the low-frequency tail of the FTC (Liberman and Dodds, 1984; Siegel and Relkin, 1987). Such losses might usefully be termed "sensory losses." As an example, imagine that the noise trauma described previously also produced a 90 percent reduction in the efficiency of synaptic transmission at the eighth nerve synapse, producing on its own a 20-dB drop in neural sensitivity across the

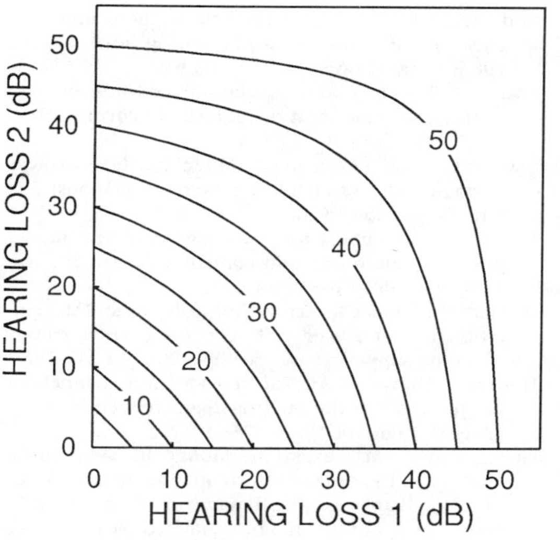

Figure 5-9 Iso-loss contours showing total loss of cochlear sensitivity at characteristic frequency predicted on the basis of equation 2 when two traumatic influences, each producing hearing losses of hearing loss 1 and hearing loss 2 separately, are combined within the one cochlea.

whole FTC, including a 20-dB elevation of threshold on the FTC tail. We would then expect a total loss of 66 dB equal to the sum of the loss of active gain (motor loss = 46 dB) and the synaptic component (sensory loss = 20 dB). This issue of additivity of sensorineural loss, and noise trauma in particular, is of obvious importance on epidemiologic, experimental, and medicolegal grounds. Preliminary experiments indicate that the model for addition presented here is adequate to predict the total hearing loss after many combined cochlear lesions (Patuzzi and Rajan, 1990).

Finally, it should be pointed out that the arguments and analysis presented in this chapter have been based on findings in the high-frequency regions of the guinea pig cochlea. It appears that the role of the active process in the low-frequency regions of the cochlea is less pronounced (Patuzzi and Robertson, 1988), and that changes in neural responses in these regions are more likely to be due to disruptions of transduction stages other than the OHC receptor current or the active force generation process (stages 2 and 3 of Fig. 5-4). The changes in transduction in the low-frequency regions are therefore likely to be similar to those changes producing threshold elevation on the tail of the FTC in high-frequency regions (stages 1, 4, and 5 of Fig. 5-4). It must also be stressed that the changes described here are mostly associated with acute acoustic trauma, and are likely to represent the first stages of noise-induced hearing loss. Apart from the obvious difference of actual loss of neurons and hair cells in chronic noise trauma, it seems likely that many of the changes discussed would also occur after chronic noise exposure.

Effets du Bruit sur les Réponses du Nerf Auditif

La réponse du nerf auditif à des stimulations acoustiques est le résultat d'une série complexe de processus siégeant dans la cochlée. Dans cette présentation, différents types d'altération de la réponse nerveuse induits par des bruits seront passés en revue et discutés en fonction des connaissances actuelles sur la physiologie cochléaire. Les sujets abordés incluront le décalage d'une demi-octave, la perte de sensibilité, la sélectivité fréquentielle et l'interaction de deux sons dans la réponse neuronale ainsi que l'origine du recrutement et de la diplacousie après un traumatisme sonore. Ces modifications seront discutées en termes d'altération des cellules ciliées et des processus synaptiques. L'additivité de l'élévation de seuil sera également discutée.

References

Ashmore JF. A fast motile response in guinea pig outer hair cells: The cellular basis of the cochlear amplifier. J Physiol 1987; 388:323-347.

Bilger RC. The audiometric profile of noise-induced hearing loss. In: Henderson D, Hamernik RP, Dosanjh OS, Mills JH, eds. Effects of noise on hearing. New York: Raven Press, 1976:457.

de Boer E. No sharpening? A challenge for cochlear mechanics. J Acoust Soc Am 1983; 73:567-573.

Brownell WE. Observations of a motile response in isolated outer hair cells. In: Webster WR, Aitkin LM, eds. Mechanisms of hearing. Clayton, Australia: Monash University Press, 1983:5.

Cody AR, Johnstone BM. Single auditory neuron response during acute acoustic trauma. Hear Res 1980; 3:3-16.

Cody AR, Russell IJ. Outer hair cells in the mammalian cochlea and noise-induced hearing loss. Nature 1985; 315:662-665.

Cody AR, Russell IJ. Acoustically induced hearing loss: Intracellular studies in the guinea pig cochlea. Hear Res 1988; 35:59-70.

Engebretson AM, Eldredge DH. Model for the nonlinear characteristics of cochlear potentials. J Acoust Soc Am 1968; 44:548-554.

Geisler CD, Greenberg S. A two-stage nonlinear model possesses automatic gain control. J Acoust Soc Am 1986; 80:1359-1363.

Geisler CD, Yates GK, Patuzzi RB, Johnstone BM. Saturation of outer hair cell receptor current causes two-tone suppression. Hear Res 1990; 44:241-256.

Holton T, Hudspeth AJ. The transduction channels of the hair cells of the bullfrog characterized by noise analysis. J Physiol 1986; 375:195-227.

Hunter-Duvar IM, Suzuki M, Mount RJ. Anatomical changes in the organ of Corti after acoustic stimulation. In: Hamernik RP, Henderson D, Salvi R, eds. New perspectives on noise-induced hearing loss. New York: Raven Press, 1982:3.

Johnstone BM, Kapadia S, Gleich B, et al. Some properties of the cubic distortion tone emission in guinea pigs. Adv Audiol 1990; 7:57.

Johnstone BM, Patuzzi R, Syka J, Sykova E. Stimulus-related potassium changes in the organ of Corti of guinea pig. J Physiol 1988; 408:77-92.

Kiang NY-S, Liberman MC, Sewell WF, Guinan JJ. Single unit clues to cochlear mechanisms. Hear Res 1986; 22:171-182.

Liberman MC. The cochlear frequency map for the cat: Labeling auditory-nerve fibers of known characteristic frequency. J Acoust Soc Am 1982; 72:1441-1449.

Liberman MC. Single-neuron labeling and chronic cochlear pathology. I. Threshold shift and characteristic frequency shift. Hear Res 1984; 16:33-41.

Liberman MC, Dodds LW. Single-neuron labeling and chronic cochlear pathology. III. Stereocilia damage and alterations of threshold tuning curves. Hear Res 1984; 16:55-74.

Liberman MC, Dodds W, Learson DA. Structure-function correlation in noise-damaged ears: a light and electron-microscopic study. In: Salvi RJ, Henderson D, Hamernik RP, Colletti V, eds. Basic and applied aspects of noise-induced hearing loss. New York: Plenum Press, 1986:163.

Liberman MC, Kiang NY-S. Single neuron labeling and chronic cochlear pathology. V. Stereocilia damage and alterations in rate- and phase-level functions. Hear Res 1984; 16:75-90.

Liberman MC, Mulroy MJ. Acute and chronic effects of acoustic trauma: Cochlear pathology and auditory nerve pathophysiology. In: Hamernik RP, Henderson D, Salvi R, eds. New perspectives on noise-induced hearing loss. New York: Raven Press, 1982:105.

Lim DJ, Dunn DE, Ferraro JA, Lempert BL. Anatomical changes found in cochleas of animals exposed to typical industrial noise. In: Hamernik RP, Henderson D, Salvi R, eds. New perspectives on noise-induced hearing loss. New York: Raven Press, 1982:23.

Lonsbury-Martin BL, Martin GK, Probst R, Coats AC. Acoustic distortion products in rabbit ear canal. I. Basic features and physiological vulnerability. Hear Res 1987; 28:173-189.

Lonsbury-Martin BL, Meikle MB. Neural correlates of auditory fatigue. Frequency dependent changes in activity of single cochlear nerve fibres. J Neurophysiol 1978; 41:987-1006.

McFadden D. The curious half-octave shift: Evidence for a basalward migration of the traveling-wave envelope with increasing intensity. In: Salvi RJ, Henderson D, Hamernik RP, Colletti V, eds. Basic and applied aspects of noise-induced hearing loss. New York: Plenum Press, 1986:295.

McFadden D, Plattsmier HS. Suprathreshold after-effects of exposure to intense sounds. In: Hamernik RP, Henderson D, Salvi R, eds. New perspectives on noise-induced hearing loss. New York: Raven Press, 1982:347.

Mills JH. Effects of noise on auditory sensitivity, psychophysical tuning curves, and suppression. In: Hamernik RP, Henderson D, Salvi R, eds. New perspectives on noise-induced hearing loss. New York: Raven Press, 1982:249.

Mountain DC. Active filtering by hair cells. In: Allen JB, Hall JL, Hubbard A, Neely ST, Tubis A, eds. Peripheral auditory mechanism. Berlin: Springer-Verlag, 1986:179.

Neely ST, Kim DO. A model for active elements in cochlear biomechanics. J Acoust Soc Am 1986; 79:1472-1480.

Patuzzi R. Mechanical correlates of noise trauma in the mammalian cochlea. In: Salvi RJ, Henderson D, Hamernik RP, Colletti V, eds. Basic and applied aspects of noise-induced hearing loss. New York: Plenum Press, 1986:123.

Patuzzi R. A model of the generation of the cochlear microphonic with nonlinear hair cell transduction and nonlinear basilar membrane mechanics. Hear Res 1987; 30:73-82.

Patuzzi R, Johnstone BM, Sellick PM. The alteration of the vibration of the basilar membrane produced by loud sound. Hear Res 1984; 13:99-100.

Patuzzi RB, Rajan R. Additivity of sensorineural hearing loss. (In preparation)

Patuzzi R, Robertson D. Tuning in the mammalian cochlea. Physiol Rev 1988; 68:1005-1082.

Patuzzi R, Sellick PM. The alteration of the low frequency response of primary auditory afferents by cochlear trauma. Hear Res 1983; 11:125-132.

Patuzzi RB, Yates GK, Johnstone BM. Changes in cochlear microphonic and neural sensitivity produced by acoustic trauma. Hear Res 1989a; 39:189-202.

Patuzzi RB, Yates GK, Johnstone BM. Outer hair cell receptor current and sensorineural hearing loss. Hear Res 1989b; 42:47-72.

Puel JL, Bobbin RP, Fallon M. The active process is affected first by intense pure sound. Hear Res 1988; 37:53-64.

Robertson D. Correspondence between sharp tuning and two-tone inhibition in primary auditory neurons. Nature 1976; 259:477-478.

Robertson D. Effects of acoustic trauma on stereocilia structure and spiral ganglion cell tuning properties in the guinea pig cochlea. Hear Res 1982; 7:55-74.

Robertson D. Functional significance of dendritic swelling after loud sounds in the guinea pig cochlea. Hear Res 1983; 9:263-278.

Robertson D, Johnstone BM. Aberrant tonotopic organization in the inner ear damaged by kanamycin. J Acoust Soc Am 1979; 66:466-469.

Robertson D, Johnstone BM. Primary auditory neurons: Nonlinear responses altered without changes in sharp tuning. J Acoust Soc Am 1981; 69:1096-1098.

Robles L, Ruggero MA, Rich NC. Basilar membrane mechanics at the base of the chinchilla cochlea. I. Input-output functions, tuning curves, and phase responses. J Acoust Soc Am 1986; 80:1364-1374.

Sachs MB, Kiang NYS. Two-tone inhibition in auditory nerve fibers. J Acoust Soc Am 1968; 43:1120-1128.

Sachs MB, Winslow RL, Sokolowski BHA. A computational model for rate-level functions from cat auditory-nerve fibers. Hear Res 1989; 41:61-70.

Salt AN, Konishi T. Effects of noise on cochlear potentials and endolymph potassium concentration recorded with potassium-selective electrodes. Hear Res 1979; 1:343-363.

Salvi RJ, Perry J, Hamernik RP, Henderson D. Relationship between cochlear pathologies and auditory nerve and behavioral responses. In: Hamernik RP, Henderson D, Salvi RJ, eds. Perspectives on noise-induced hearing loss. New York: Raven Press, 1982:165.

Santos-Sacchi J, Dilger JP. Whole cell currents and mechanical responses from isolated outer hair cells. Hear Res 1988; 35:143-150.

Saunders JC, Flock A. Recovery of threshold shift in hair cell stereocilia following exposure to intense stimulation. Hear Res 1986; 23:233-243.

Schmiedt RA. Acoustic distortion in the ear canal. I. Cubic difference tones: Effects of acute noise injury. J Acoust Soc Am 1986; 79:1481-1490.

Schmiedt RA, Zwislocki JJ. Effects of hair cell lesions on responses of cochlear nerve fibers. II. Single- and two-tone intensity functions in relation to tuning curves. J Neurophysiol 1980a; 43:1390-1405.

Schmiedt RA, Zwislocki JJ, Hamernik RP. Effects of hair cell lesions on responses of cochlear nerve fibers. I. Lesions, tuning curves, two-tone inhibition, and response to trapezoidal-wave patterns. J Neurophysiol 1980b; 43:1367-1389.

Sellick PM, Patuzzi RB, Johnstone BM. Measurement of basilar membrane motion in the guinea pig using the Mossbauer technique. J Acoust Soc Am 1982; 72:131-141.

Siegel JH, Kim DO. Cochlear biomechanics: vulnerability to acoustic trauma and other alterations as seen in neural responses and ear-canal sound pressure. In: Hamernik RP, Henderson D, Salvi R, eds. New perspectives on noise-induced hearing loss. New York: Raven Press, 1982:137.

Siegel JH, Relkin EM. Antagonistic effects of perilymphatic calcium and magnesium on the activity of single cochlear afferent neurons. Hear Res 1987; 28:131-147.

Smoorenburg GF. Effects of temporary threshold shift on combination tone generation and on two-tone suppression. Hear Res 1980; 2:347-356.

Spoendlin H. Anatomical changes following various noise exposures. In: Henderson D, Hamernik RP, Dosanjh DS, Mills JH, eds. Effects of noise on hearing. New York: Raven Press, 1976:69.

Tyler RS, Tye-Murray N. The relationship between speech perception and psychoacoustical measurements in noise-induced hearing loss subjects. In: Salvi RJ, Henderson D, Hamernik RP, Colletti V, eds. Basic and applied aspects of noise-induced hearing loss. New York: Plenum Press, 1986:323.

Wilson JP. The combination tone, 2f1 − f2, in psychophysics and ear canal recording. In: van den Brink G, Bilsen FA, eds. Psychophysical, physiological and behavioural studies in hearing. Delft, Netherlands: Delft University Press, 1980:43.

Winter IM, Robertson D, Yates GK. Diversity of characteristic frequency rate-intensity functions in the guinea pig auditory nerve fibres. Hear Res 1990; 45:191-202.

Yates GK, Winter IM, Robertson D. Basilar membrane nonlinearity determines auditory nerve rate-intensity functions and cochlear dynamic range. Hear Res 1990; 45:203-220.

Zurek PM. Acoustic emissions from the ear: A summary of results from humans and animals. J Acoust Soc Am 1985; 78:340-344.

Zwislocki JJ. Micromechanics of the cochlea and possible changes caused by intense noise. In: Hamernik RP, Henderson D, Salvi R, eds. New perspectives on noise-induced hearing loss. New York: Raven Press, 1982:209.

CHAPTER 6

Acoustic Stimulation and Overstimulation in the Cochlea: A Comparison Between Basal and Apical Turns of the Cochlea

RICHARD A. ALTSCHULER
YEHOASH RAPHAEL
CINDY A. PROSEN
DAVID F. DOLAN
DAVID B. MOODY

There is now considerable evidence of differences between the apical and the basal turns of the cochlea. Much of this difference seems to relate to differences in outer hair cells (OHCs). One conspicuous difference is in the size of OHCs and their stereocilia in basal and apical turns. There are also many other important differences, such as that of medial efferent innervation: basal turn OHCs receive a much greater cholinergic input, and apical turns receive a much greater gamma-aminobutyric acid (GABA) immunoreactive input (Altschuler and Fex, 1986). Apical turn OHCs receive a much greater afferent input (Spoendlin, 1969, 1979), which may have different characteristics than the afferent input at the base, based on reaction to kainic acid (Pujol et al, 1985). There are also developmental differences: basal OHCs mature first and perhaps reach a higher degree of differentiation (Pujol et al, 1980). In the guinea pig there are differences in cytoskeletal organization, with OHCs of apical turns having a greater infracuticular network of actin (Thorne et al, 1987). They also have more rows of subsurface cisternae along their lateral wall (unpublished observations). ^{32}P-labeling of phosphoinositides is significantly higher in the apex than in the base of the guinea pig cochlea (Niedzielski and Schacht, 1990). There are also differences between base and apex in sensitivity to ototoxic agents: basal OHCs are generally more likely to be lost following ototoxic insults (Hawkins, 1976). Major physiologic differences in response properties are seen in DC responses between OHCs of basal and apical turns. OHCs in the basal turn of the guinea pig cochlea do not show significant DC receptor potentials to high-frequency stimulation (less than 90 dB SPL) appropriate for this region of the cochlea (Cody and Russell, 1987). In contrast, OHCs from more-apical regions (third turn) show DC receptor potentials at low sound levels and low frequencies (Dallos, 1985).

In addition, there are several differences in the frequency turning curves (FTCs) between auditory nerve fibers innervating the basal and apical turns of the cochlea. High–characteristic frequency (CF) fibers are more sharply tuned (higher Q_{10dB} values) than low-CF (less than 1.0 kHz) fibers. High-CF fibers show "tail" regions on the low-frequency side of the FTC, whereas tail regions are seen on the high-frequency side of the FTC for fibers with CFs below 1.0 kHz (Kiang et al, 1965; Liberman and Kiang, 1978).

Differences of the Base and Apex in Processing

In light of these differences between the basal and apical turns of the cochlea, it is not surprising that there are differences in the processing of auditory signals between the apex and the base (Schuknecht and Neff, 1952; Clark and Bohne, 1986; Smith et al, 1987; Prosen et al, 1990). These studies suggest that there is a redundancy of encoding mechanisms in the mammalian cochlea for low-frequency signals, so that the loss of apical hair cells has less effect on hearing than the loss of an equivalent number of basal hair cells. Figures 6-1 through 6-3 illustrate this point. The upper half of Figure 6-1 depicts the cytocochleogram of a guinea pig treated with 200 mg per kilogram per day of kanamycin for 23 days; the lower half of this figure shows the resulting behaviorally assessed hearing loss. Thresholds at the high frequencies shifted by 40 to 60 dB correspond to complete OHC loss and partial inner hair cell (IHC) loss in the base of the cochlea. A number of researchers (Ryan and Dallos, 1975; Hawkins et al, 1977; Prosen et al, 1978; Stebbins et al, 1987) concur that substantial basal OHC loss is commonly accompanied by a 40 to 60 dB high-frequency hearing loss.

In contrast to these basal hair cell loss data, when damage is restricted to the apex of the cochlea, little hearing loss is noted in any frequency region. Figure 6-2 depicts histopathologic and psychophysical data from a guinea pig exposed to a 0.25-kHz octave band of noise. Although most of the OHCs were destroyed in the apical 20 percent of the cochlea, no substantial threshold shift was reported at any frequency. The effects of a more substantial apical hair cell loss on hearing are seen in Figure 6-3. The upper half of this figure displays the cytocochleogram from a chinchilla whose apical hair cells were destroyed with a liquid-nitrogen-cooled cryoprobe; the filled circles in the lower half of this figure show the corresponding hearing loss determined for this chinchilla. Complete destruction of receptor cells in the apical cochlea caused threshold shifts of 20 dB or less. This again illustrates that nearly normal absolute hearing may occur despite substantial apical receptor cell destruction.

A masking experiment was conducted to check if, in the absence of apical hair cells, basal hair cells can be responsible for the remaining low-frequency sensitivity (Fig. 6-3). Open circles in the lower half of Figure 6-3 depict threshold shift data from a cryolesioned chinchilla measured in the presence

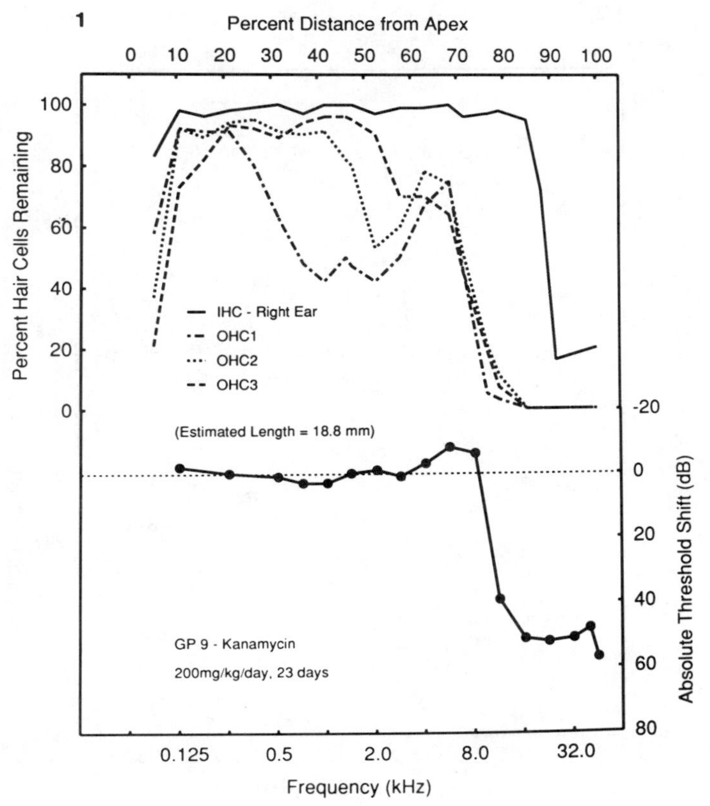

Figure 6-1 Cytocochleogram (top) of hair cell loss, and behaviorally determined auditory threshold shift function (bottom) from a kanamycin-deafened guinea pig.

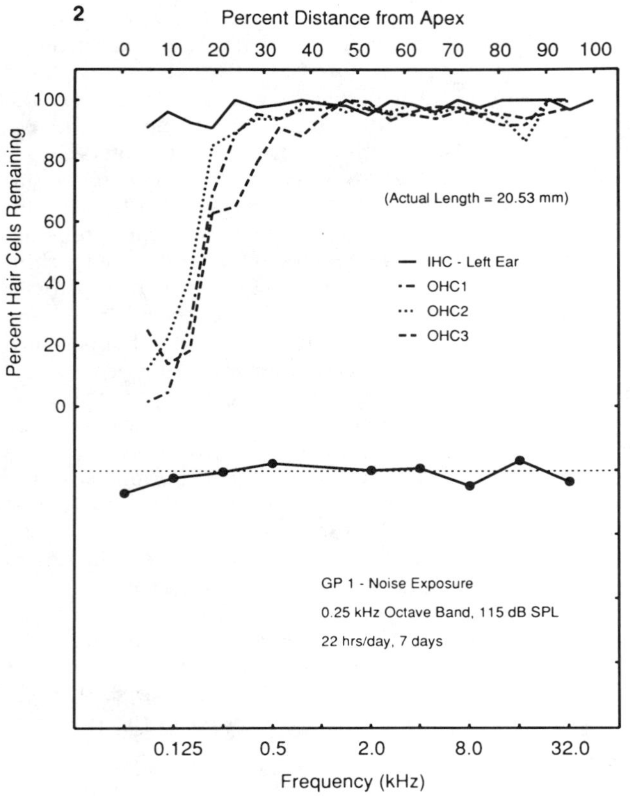

Figure 6-2 Cytocochleogram (top) of hair cell loss, and behaviorally determined auditory threshold shift function (bottom) from a guinea pig exposed to a 0.25 kHz OBN at 115 dB SPL, 22 hours per day for 7 days.

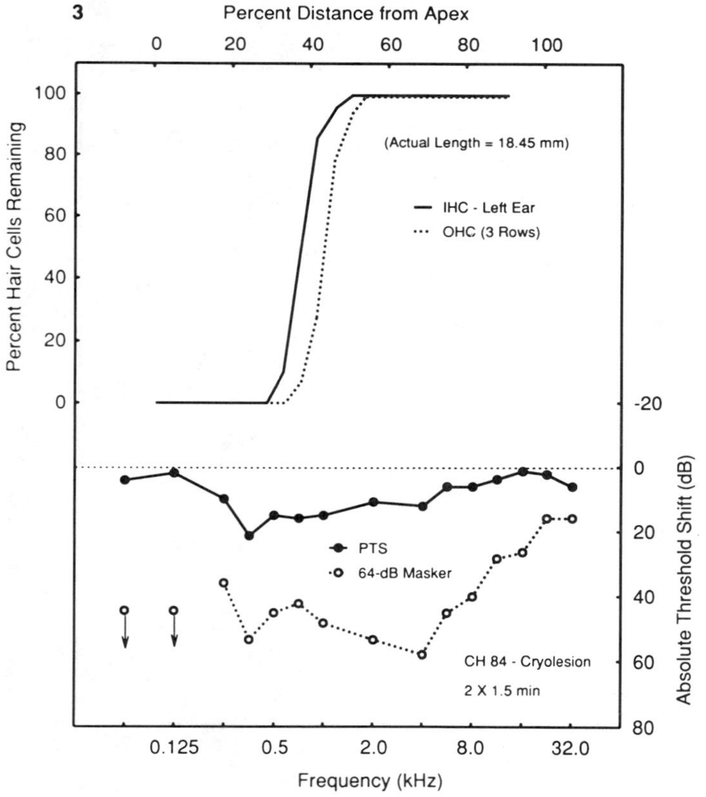

Figure 6-3 Cytocochleogram (top) of hair cell loss, and behaviorally determined auditory threshold shift function (bottom) from a chinchilla with a lesion caused by a cryoprobe applied to the apex of the bony wall of the cochlea.

of a high-pass noise masker (710-Hz cutoff). In both normal and damaged ears, a high-pass masker should increase the thresholds of frequencies within the pass band. However, in ears with apical hair cell destruction, if more basally-located cells detect low-frequency signals, thresholds for the low frequencies also should be elevated in the presence of the masker. Data in Figure 6-3 suggest that mid- or basal-turn fibers detect low-frequency stimuli when all apical cells have been destroyed: in the presence of the high-pass masker, thresholds at *all* frequencies were elevated. In summary, these data suggest that multiple mechanisms exist for detecting the low-frequency stimuli but not the high-frequency stimuli.

Thus, there is evidence that high-frequency and low-frequency stimulations of the cochlea are processed differently. One might therefore expect that overstimulation might have different effects at different frequencies. Bohne et al (1985) and Clark et al (1986) have, in fact, suggested differences in the patterns of hair cell loss after high-frequency versus low-frequency noise exposure. This might be due to (1) the different type of sound wave formed on the basilar membrane by high frequencies versus low frequencies; (2) the fact that hair cells of different rows and turns have different sensitivities to noise overstimulation; or (3) both of the above.

We compared the effects of high- and low-frequency acoustic overstimulation. Guinea pigs were exposed to either a 0.5-kHz or a 4.0-kHz octave band noise of 117 dB SPL, 14 hours per day for 10 days. We chose 117 dB SPL because, in guinea pigs, there appears to be a considerable increase in effect at this intensity over 112 db SPL (Prosen et al, 1990). Auditory brain stem responses (ABRs) were measured prior to the first noise exposure, after 5 days, and at the end of the last exposure session. Several animals from each group were immediately sacrificed, whereas others survived for an additional week (without sound stimulation) and then were tested for ABRs and sacrificed. Animals were perfused systemically followed by local intrascalar fixation. Cochleae fixed with 3 percent paraformaldehyde were processed for molecular analysis using antibodies or probes to actin, intermediate filaments, and other cytoskeletal components. Cochleae fixed with 3 percent glutaraldehyde and 2 percent paraformaldehyde followed by osmium and hafnium chloride postfixation were processed for cytocochleograms and ultrastructural analysis.

Auditory Brain Stem Response

Threshold shifts derived from auditory brain stem response (ABR) measurements for 500-Hz and 4-kHz exposures are shown in Figure 6-4. Overstimulation of 500 Hz caused a 20-dB or greater threshold shift at all frequencies tested. The mildest shift (25 to 35 dB) was at 2.0 kHz, whereas the largest was 20 to 70 dB, at 16.0 kHz. With the 4.0-kHz overstimulation, threshold shifts were generally greater at all frequencies, compared to the 500-Hz exposure. Threshold shifts of 20 to 60 dB at 2.0 kHz, 30 to 70 dB at 4 kHz, 50 to 90 dB at 8.0 and 16.0 kHz, and 40 to 50 dB at 30.0 kHz were measured.

Outer Hair Cell

Histochemically processed surface preparations proved useful for counting damaged hair cells. Detection of early changes in cytoskeletal and junctional proteins provided a sensitive measure for damage during early stages of hair cell degeneration.

Exposure of 500 Hz

The pattern of hair cell loss with 500-Hz overstimulation is seen in the top half of Figure 6-5. The most extensive (and consistent) OHC loss was observed in the third turn. Loss ranged from a low of 25 percent at either end to almost 50 percent through the middle two-thirds. The surrounding fourth and second turn regions showed more variability. Apical turn loss of OHCs averaged 30 percent in most animals. There was little difference in the extent of damage between OHC rows. The higher-frequency turns (second, first, and hook) had minimal OHC loss. The shapes of OHC bodies appeared distorted in areas surrounding OHC loss.

Exposure of 4 kHz

The pattern of OHC loss from the 4-kHz exposure is seen in the lower half of Figure 6-5. Loss of OHCs was most extensive in the second turn and upper basal turn regions. Often a region of 20 percent loss would abruptly turn into a region of 100 percent loss within 0.24 mm and then return to the less-disturbed pattern again. There was little difference be-

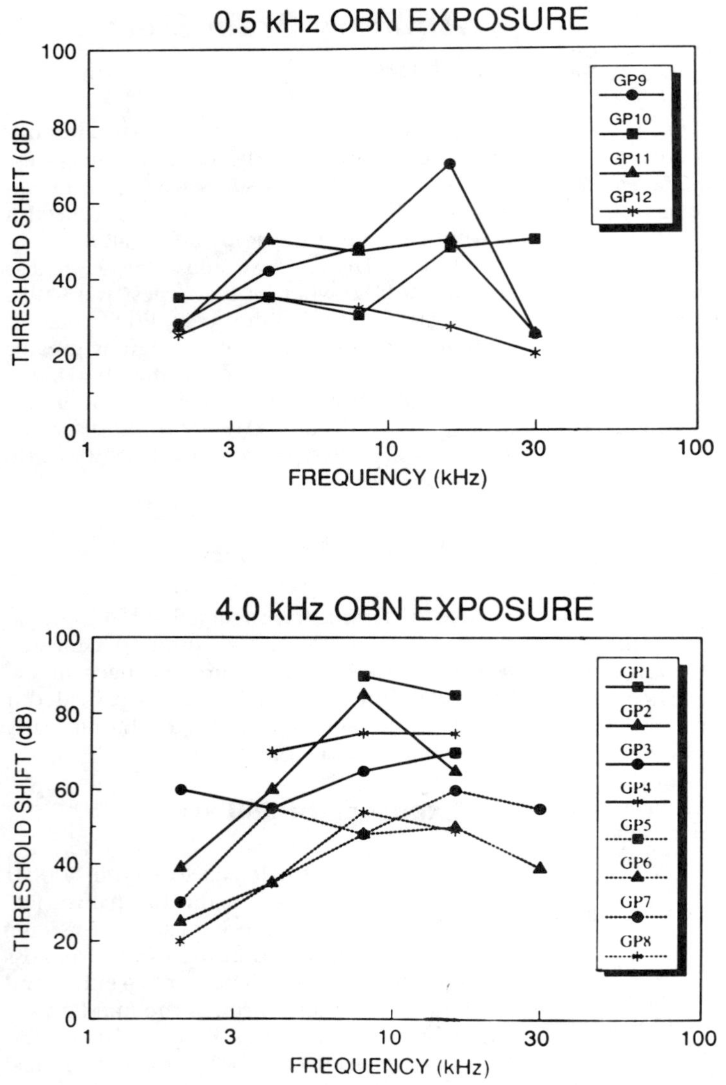

Figure 6-4 Auditory brain-stem responses showing threshold shifts from guinea pigs exposed to 0.5-kHz (top) or 4.0-kHz (bottom) noise overstimulation (117 dB SPL, 14 hours per day for 10 days).

tween the three rows of hair cells. Swelling of OHCs was seen in regions close to areas of lesion. Distorted body shape of OHCs was less notable in the 4-kHz exposure than in the 500-Hz exposure.

Variability between animals was much greater with the 500-Hz exposures. Although the differences in the magnitude of damage from high- and low-frequency exposures may be related to middle-ear transfer functions, this does not completely explain the differences in the degree of spread.

Inner Hair Cells

Inner hair cell (IHC) loss was minimal with the 500-Hz exposure, with only scattered loss (3 to 5 percent) in the third turn, in regions where OHC loss was greatest. In the second turn swollen IHCs were periodically spaced (Fig. 6-6). Swelling was also seen in extreme apical and basal turns, but here there was no periodicity. With the 4-kHz exposure IHC loss of roughly 10 percent was seen in the second and third turns, correlating with areas of greatest OHC loss. No swelling of IHCs was observed in neighboring regions.

The region of IHC loss corresponded to the frequency of overstimulation better than it did for OHC with both frequencies tested. OHC loss was much more extended along the cochlear spiral in both frequencies of overstimulation; however, the spread and magnitude of OHC damage was much greater with the higher-frequency overstimulation.

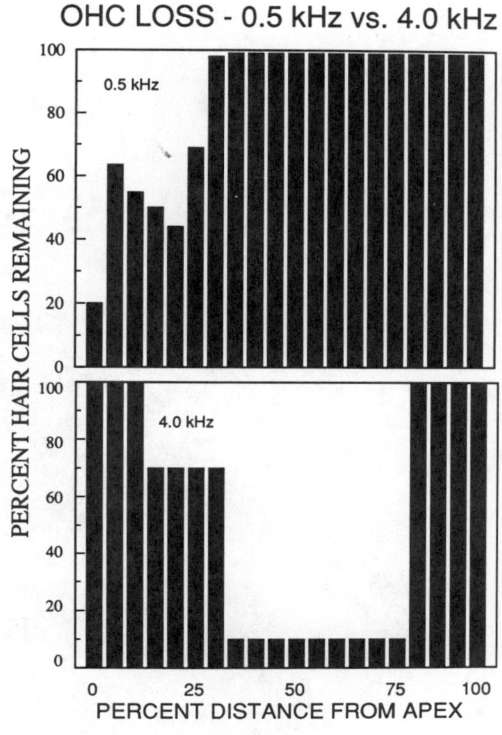

Figure 6-5 Representative cytocochleograms of OHC loss in guinea pigs exposed to 0.5-kHz (above) or 4.0-kHz (below) noise overstimulation (117 dB SPL, 14 hours per day for 10 days).

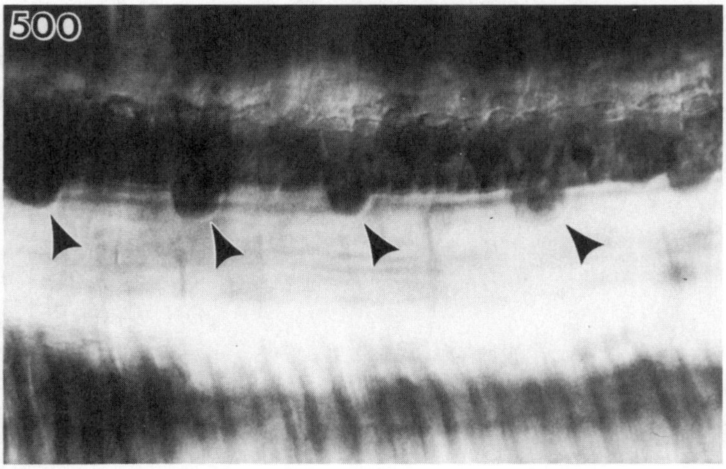

Figure 6-6 Surface preparation from the second turn of the cochlear spiral of a guinea pig sacrificed immediately after exposure to 0.5-kHz noise (117 dB SPL, 14 hours per day for 10 days) showing swollen inner hair cells (arrows).

Ultrastructure

Changes in the apical domain of OHCs and IHCs, similar to those described by Liberman (1987) and Liberman and Dodds (1984, 1987), were observed in areas of damage from both high- and low-frequency exposures. As Liberman (1987) reported, stereociliar fusion was accompanied by perturbation of the cuticular plate (Fig. 6-7*A*). Often a perturbation of subsurface cisternae was also observed in OHCs (Fig. 6-7*B, C*).

Afferent Dendrites

Many vacuoles and spaces were seen by the bases of IHCs in regions of OHC loss. These are commonly interpreted as swollen afferents (Spoendlin, 1971; Robertson, 1983),

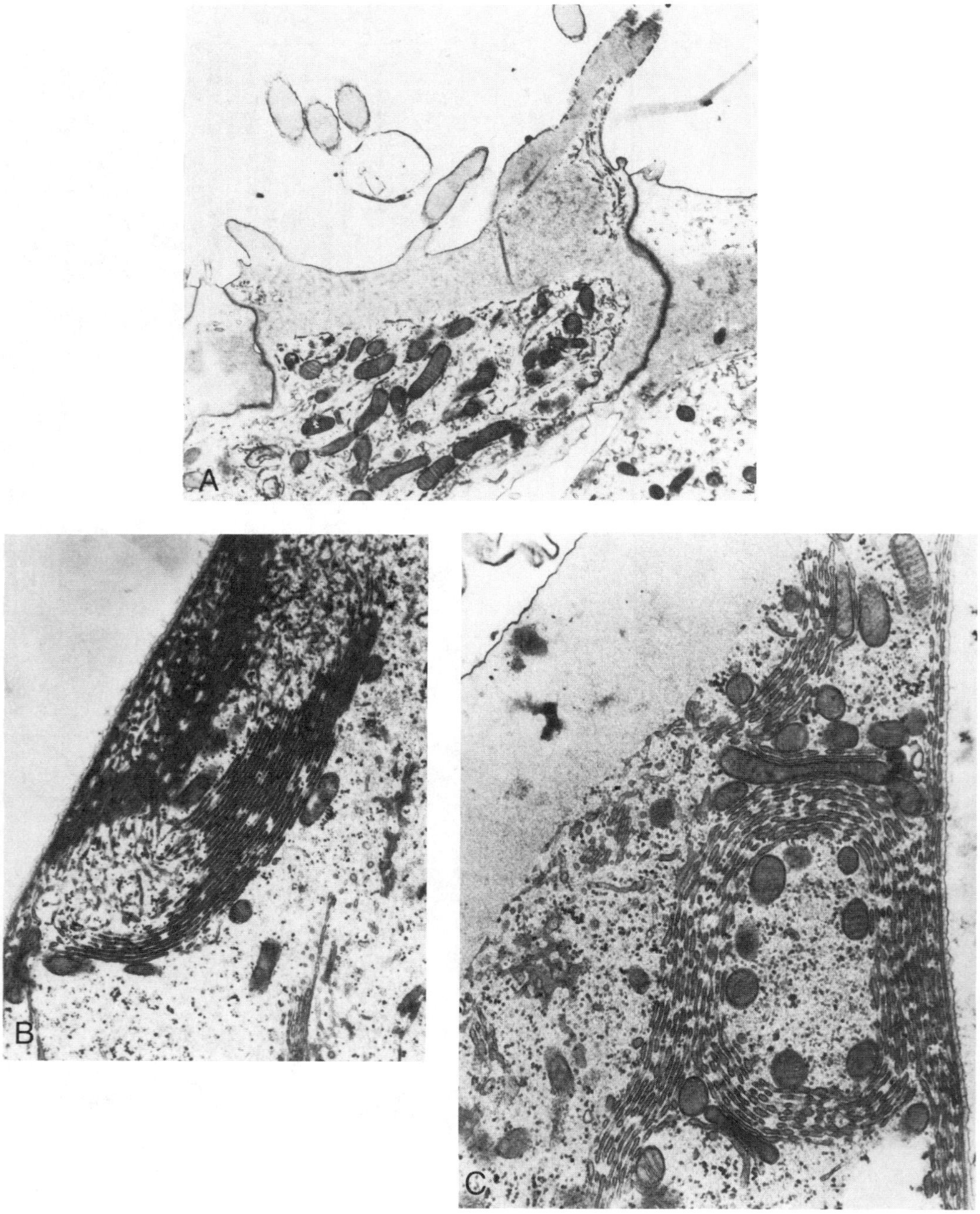

Figure 6-7 Electron micrographs showing perturbation of cuticular plate and fused stereocilia of apical domain of an inner hair cell *A*, and perturbation of the subsurface cisternae of an outer hair cell *B,C*, from an animal sacrificed 2 hours after cessation of 4.0-kHz noise overstimulation (117 dB SPL, 14 hours per day for 10 days).

although Liberman and Dodds (1987) suggested that they may also reflect vacuolization and blebbing of IHCs. In our material, these vacuoles and spaces appeared to reflect a large loss of the unmyelinated portions of radial afferents (Fig. 6-8*A, B*); an example is a missing afferent terminal being replaced by an efferent terminal (Fig. 6-8, *B*). Within Rosenthal's canals, myelinated peripheral processes of auditory nerve were observed in normal numbers.

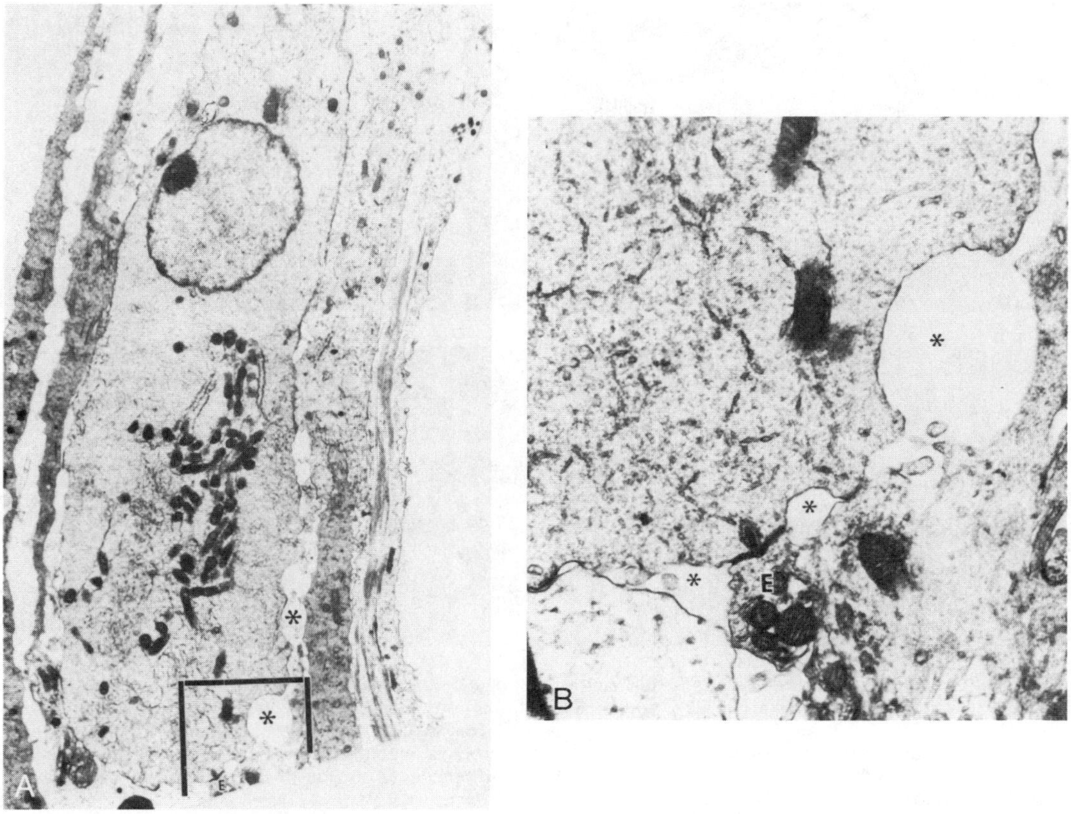

Figure 6-8 Electron micrographs showing loss of afferent dendrites (*) at the base of an inner hair cell *A*, of a guinea pig sacrificed 1 week after cessation of 4.0-kHZ noise overstimulation (117 dB SPL, 14 hours per day for 10 days). *B*, In a higher magnification of a portion from the inner hair cell base, the replacement of a lost afferent by an efferent (E) can be seen apposing a synaptic bar.

Swelling and loss of afferent dendrites at IHC bases was apparent with both high- and low-frequency exposures. The loss of afferent dendrites corresponded closely to regions of OHC loss. IHCs usually looked normal. This suggests that auditory nerve dysfunction could be a component of both temporary and permanent threshold shifts.

Scar Formation

The distributions of microfilaments (actin), cytokeratins, vimentin, and tight junction-specific proteins were studied, in order to elucidate the structural and molecular basis that underlies the dynamics and mechanism of phalangeal scar formation in different cochlear regions. Collecting data from animals that were sacrificed at various intervals after the noise made it possible to reconstruct the spatial and temporal sequence of changes that occur during scar formation.

Analysis at the molecular level did not reveal major differences in the pattern of scar formation between different turns of the cochlea or with the different frequencies of overstimulation. In the OHC region, the phalangeal process of outer pillar cells forms scars for first-row OHCs, whereas first- and second-row Deiters' cells form scars for second- and third-row OHCs, respectively. Minor differences appeared between the shape of the scar in the first row of OHCs and the other two rows, probably reflecting the difference in shape between the phalangeal process of outer pillar cells and such processes of Deiters' cells. Actin appeared to be an important element in the apical domain of the cells in the process of hair cell degeneration and scar formation. Actin-specific staining in the cuticular plate and the stereocilia (Fig. 6-9*A*) decreased significantly in noise-damaged cells (Fig. 6-9*B*). Within a few hours of noise exposure, an actin-rich band, which we term "bridge," formed under the apical membrane

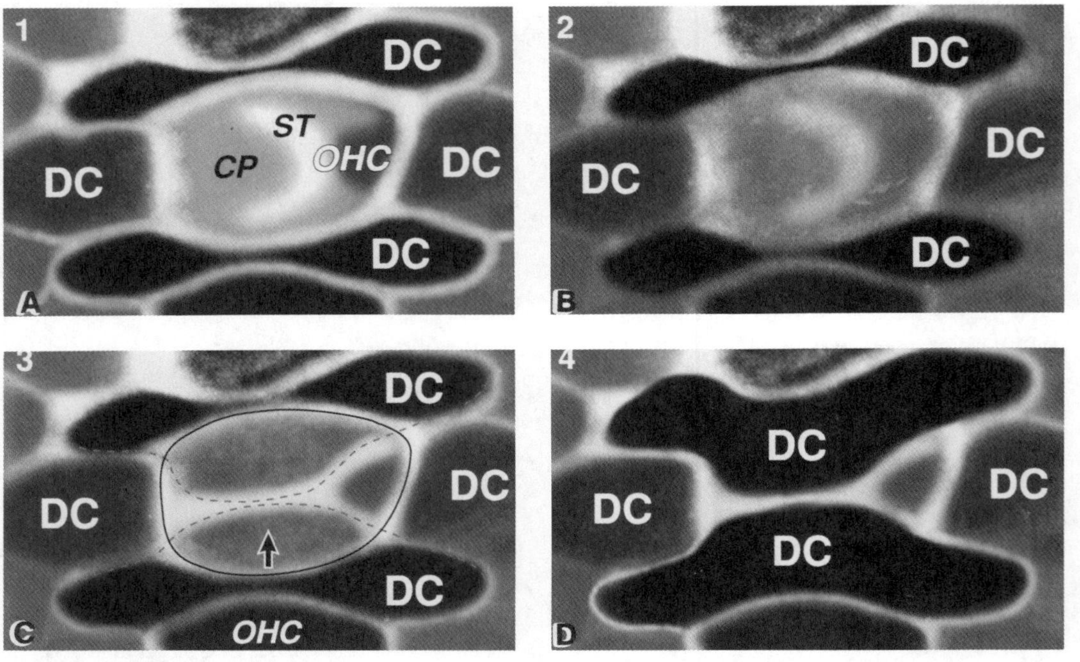

Figure 6-9 Diagram of the process of scar formation from digitized surface preparations stained for actin. *A*, The first stage (1) shows the normal appearance with staining at junctions and of the OHC stereocilia (ST) and cuticular plate (CP). *B*, The second stage (2) shows a loss of actin with less staining in the stereocilia and cuticular plate. *C*, The third stage (3) shows the Deiters' cells (DC) above and below meeting (dotted lines) under the remaining apical portion of the hair cell (outlined by black line). *D*, The remaining portion of the hair cell is then lost (4), exposing the two Deiters' cells below. OHC, outer hair cell; CP, cuticular plate; ST, stereocilia.

of the degenerating hair cells, in a plane perpendicular to the modiolus (Figs. 6-9*C*, 6-10*A*). The bridge later becomes a new adherens junction, along the attachment line of the two supporting cells that compose a scar (Fig. 6-9*D*, 6-10*A*). In early stages of the scarring process, the adherens junction of the degenerating hair cell was still faintly stained for actin (Figs. 6-9*C*, 6-10*A*), but later it disintegrated entirely (Fig. 6-9*D*). No significant differences could be detected between the changes in actin organization in scars forming in the base and such changes in the apex of the cochlea, or between the two different frequencies used as stimuli.

The expression of cytokeratins in the organ of Corti is normally restricted to nonsensory cells (Fig. 6-10*C*) (Raphael et al, 1987). After the noise exposure, the distribution of cytokeratin immunolabeling in the reticular lamina was altered. Simultaneous with the reorganization of actin, the area in the reticular lamina previously occupied by the hair cell became cytokeratin-positive, as two adjacent supporting cells filled the space of the hair cell (Fig. 6-10*D*). We have recently found a quantitative difference in the distribution of cytokeratins between basal and apical supporting cells: more cytokeratin immunostaining occurs in the apical processes of pillar cells of basal turns. No difference, however, was observed in the pattern of cytokeratin distribution in the scars of first-turn OHCs (which involve pillar cell processes) between basal and apical turns.

The apical membranes of hair cells and supporting cells, and the tight junctions between these cells, help maintain the ionic barrier between endolymph and perilymph. To find out if scar formation modulates the expression of tight junctions in a different way in basal compared to apical turns, we used tight junction-specific anticingulin antibodies (Citi et al, 1988). The pattern of anticingulin staining in whole mounts of the organ of Corti revealed a circumferential belt that surrounded all the undamaged cells (Fig. 6-10*B*). In damaged or missing hair cells, a new cingulin-positive line appeared, oriented in a fashion similar to that of the actin-rich bridge (Fig. 6-10*B*). Here again, no difference could be discerned between the base and the apex of the cochlea.

Vimentin, a protein expressed in scar-

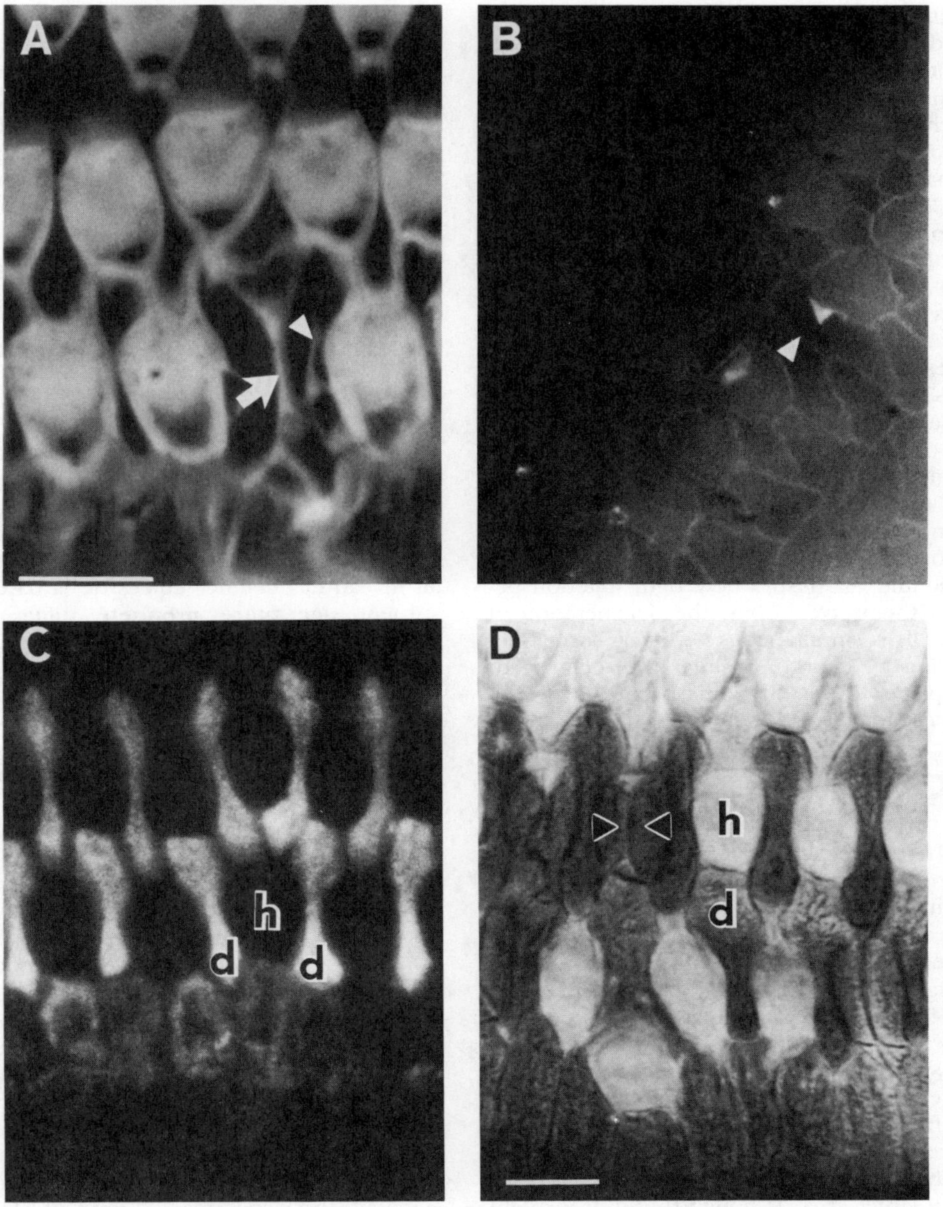

Figure 6-10 Whole mounts showing the distribution of actin, cingulin, and cytokeratin in surface view of the reticular lamina. *A,* Phalloidin labeling showing actin in the cuticular plate and adherens junctions of hair cells in the second turn. An actin-rich bridge is seen in the midline of a scar in the third row (arrow). Residual actin labeling is present where the original adherens junction had been (arrowhead). *B,* Cingulin-specific immunolabeling is restricted to the tight junctions between all cells at the reticular lamina. Cingulin is present in the midline of the phalangeal scar in a second-row OHC (arrow). *C,* Fluorescence preparation showing that cytokeratin-specific immunolabeling is restricted to the dumbbell-shaped phalangeal processes of supporting cells (d), whereas hair cells (h) are not labeled. *D,* Third-turn organ of Corti after noise-induced hair cell damage. Phalangeal scars (arrows) in second and third OHC rows are cytokeratin-positive, as are supporting cells (d), but hair cells (h) are not. The bar in *D,* which is representative for *B* through *D,* equals 10 μm.

forming cells in other tissues, was not detected in the phalangeal scar. Vimentin is present in the third-row Deiters' cells and in the inner pillars (Raphael and Osterle, 1989), but these cells do not seem to be incorporated into the scar at the level of the reticular lamina.

Comparing the changes observed in surface preparations with staining patterns in immunolabeled light-microscopic sections helped us to understand the dynamics of changes in the cytoarchitecture when scars are formed. It appeared that two specific supporting cells are predestined to form a scar for a given hair cell. The supporting cells gradually expand in volume and invade or constrict the subapical region of the hair cell. Consequently, the basolateral domain of the hair cell is separated from the apical domain. The latter seems to degenerate only after the two scar-forming supporting cells attach to each other at the bridge and establish a new tight junction between themselves. Thus, the degeneration of hair cells is simultaneous with scar formation, allowing a "smooth" cellular replacement to take place, so that the ionic barrier in the reticular lamina is maintained.

Conclusion

There appear to be differences in the processing of high- and low-frequency acoustic stimulation. Low-frequency input is probably processed in both basal and apical turns. There are also differences in the toxic effects of high- and low-frequency overstimulation. High-frequency overstimulation produces loss of greater magnitude both in terms of number and spread. This may be because there is greater resonance and transfer function for high-frequency stimulation, or because of the nature of the wave formed on the basilar membrane, with low frequencies dissipating over a larger area. Although these ideas might explain the greater hair cell loss from high-frequency overstimulation, they do not explain the greater spread.

Along with the different effects of high- and low-frequency overstimulation, and the differences in processing, differences between base and apex are also seen in the effects of rest periods (Clark and Bohne, 1986).

Although differences are seen in the effects of stimulation and overstimulation, the apical and basal reactions to overstimulation appear to have many similarities. Swelling of afferent dendrites occurs in the region of best frequency; some of the swelling is nonreversible. This may lead to loss of spiral ganglion cells, as Juiz et al. (1989) report, after kainic acid–induced swelling. OHCs also swell and exhibit apical distortions and disorganization. Scar formation and the replacement of damaged OHCs proceed in the same orderly fashion in basal and apical turns after high- or low-frequency overstimulation.

Différences de Réponses au Traumatisme Sonore entre la Base et l'Apex de la Cochlée

De nombreuses évidences indiquent que les cellules ciliées des tours basaux et apicaux différent aussi bien sur le plan physiologique que morphologique. Les dommages causés par les drogues ototoxiques, beaucoup plus forts au niveau des cellules ciliées de la base, constituent une autre propriété différentielle. Avec le trauma acoustique, quelques résultats indiquent aussi une différence base-apex. Le présent travail a pour but d'analyser ces différences en comparant les dégâts causés par des sons très intenses de fréquence élevée ou basse. Cette comparaison est basée sur une analyse des pertes de cellules ciliées et sur la cicatrisation consécutive de la lame réticulaire.

Des cobayes sont exposés à un bruit de bande d'une octave (autour soit de 0,5, soit de 4 kHz) de 117 dB SPL, 14 h par jour, pendant 10 jours. Les réponses évoquées du tronc cérébral (ABR) sont enregistrées avant l'exposition au bruit, au cinquième jour et à la fin de la dernière séance. Une partie des animaux de chaque groupe est immédiatement sacrifiée, les autres ont un délai de récupération d'une semaine et font l'objet d'un nouvel ABR avant le prélèvement des cochlées. Tous ont une double perfusion (intra-cardiaque et intracochléaire) soit avec 3 percent de paraformaldéhyde (immunocytochimie des composants du cytosquelette), soit avec un mélange 3 percent de glutaraldéhyde et de 2 percent de paraformaldéhyde suivie d'une post-fixation à l'acide osmique/chlorure d'hafnium (cytocochléogrammes et microscopie électronique).

Avec le trauma à 4 kHz, on observe des pertes auditives de 50 dB ou plus sur toutes les fréquences testées (de 2 à 30 kHz). Le trauma à 0,5 kHz provoque des pertes de 5 à 10 dB à 30 kHz, de 15 à 25 dB à 16 kHz et de 25 à 35 dB à 8, 4 et 2 kHz (avec un maximum à 4 kHz).

Les cytocochléogrammes provenant des animaux traumatisés à 4 kHz présentent des pertes cellulaires minimes au niveau de l'extrême base, comme à celui du quatrième tour et de l'apex. Ces pertes sont encore faibles dans la première moitié du premier tour; mais ailleurs elles atteignent 50% ou plus pour les cellules ciliées externes (CCE) avec un maximum dans le deuxième tour. Les pertes de cellules ciliées internes (CCI) sont de 10 percent et limitées aux deuxième et troisième tours. Le trauma de 0,5 kHz provoque une perte importante de CCE dans les deuxième, troisième et quatrième tours, avec un maximum dans le troisième. Les pertes en CCI (5 à 10 percent) sont limitées au deuxième tour; cependant les CCI du troisième tour sont hypertrophiées.

Pour les deux sortes de trauma, on note que la localisation des pertes en CCI correspond plus à la fréquence traumatique que celle des pertes en CCE. L'extension des pertes en CCE est beaucoup plus grande avec le trauma de fréquence élevée. L'immunocytochimie ne révèle pas de différence significative dans la cicatrisation de la lame réticulaire au niveau des différents tours de spire, mais quelques particularités sont notées entre la première rangée des CCE et les deux autres rangées.

L'analyse de la dégénérescence des CCE et celle de la cicatrisation à ses différents stades est poursuivie.

ACKNOWLEDGMENTS

We would like to thank Ms. Christine Sheridan for expert assistance in histologic assessments. This work was supported by NIH grants PO1-DC-05785 and RO1-DC-00442.

References

Altschuler RA, Fex J. Efferent neurotransmitters. In: Altschuler RA, Bobbin RP, Hoffmann DW, eds. Neurobiology of hearing: the cochlea. New York: Raven Press, 1986:383.

Bohne BA, Zahn SJ, Bozzay DG. Damage of the cochlea following interrupted exposure to low frequency noise. Ann Otol Rhinol Laryngol 1985; 94:122-128.

Citi S, Sabanay H, Jakes R, Geiger B, Kendrick-Jones J. Cingulin, a new peripheral component of tight junctions. Nature 1988; 333(6170):272-276.

Clark WW, Bohne BA. Effect of periodic rest on hearing loss and cochlear damage following exposure to noise. J Acoust Soc Am 1986; 82:1253-1264.

Clark WW, Bohne BA, Boettcher FA. Cochlear damage: audiometric correlates? In: Collins MJ, Glattke TJ, Harker LA, eds. Sensorineural hearing loss: mechanisms, diagnosis, treatment. Iowa City, IA: The University of Iowa, 1986:59.

Cody AR, Russell IJ. The response of hair cells in the basal turn of the guinea pig cochlea to tones. J Physiol 1987; 383:551-569.

Dallos P. Membrane potentials and response changes in mammalian outer hair cells during intracellular recording. J Neurosci 1985; 5:1609-1615.

Hawkins JE. Drug ototoxicity. In: Keidel WD, Neff WD, eds. Handbook of sensory physiology. Vol V: Auditory system. 1976:707.

Hawkins JE, Stebbins WC, Johnsson L-G, et al. The patas monkey as a model for dihydrostreptomycin ototoxicity. Acta Otolaryngol 1977; 83:123-129.

Juiz JM, Rueda J, Merchan J, Sala MC. The effects of kainic acid on the cochlear ganglion of the rat. Hear Res 1989; 40:65-74.

Kiang NYS, Watanabe T, Thomas EC, Clark LF. Discharge patterns of single fibers in the cat's auditory nerve. Cambridge, MA: MIT Press, 1965.

Liberman MC. Chronic ultrastructural changes in acoustic trauma: serial-section reconstruction of stereocilia and cuticular plates. Hear Res 1987; 26:65-88.

Liberman MC, Dodds LW. Single-neuron labeling and chronic cochlear pathology. III. Stereocilia damage and alterations of threshold tuning curves. Hear Res 1984; 16:55-74.

Liberman MC, Dodds LW. Acute ultrastructural changes in acoustic trauma: Serial-section reconstruction of stereocilia and cuticular plates. Hear Res 1987; 26:45-64.

Liberman MC, Kiang NY. Acoustic trauma in cats. Cochlear pathology and auditory nerve activity. Acta Otolaryngol 1978; 358:1-63.

Niedzielski A, Schacht J. Phosphoinositide metabolism in the guinea pig cochlea: differences between base and apex. Neurosci Abstr 1990; 16:873.

Prosen CA, Moody DB, Stebbins WC, et al. Apical hair cells and hearing. Hear Res 1990; 44:179-194.

Prosen CA, Peterson MR, Moody DB, Stebbins WC. Auditory thresholds and kanamycin-induced hearing loss in the guinea pig assessed by a positive reinforcement procedure. J Acoust Soc Am 1978; 63:559-566.

Pujol R, Carlier E, Lenoir M. Ontogenic approach to inner and outer hair cell function. Hear Res 1980; 423:30.

Pujol R, Lenoir M, Robertson D, et al. Kainic acid selectively alters auditory nerve dendrites connected with cochlear inner hair cells. Hear Res 1985; 18:145-153.

Raphael Y, Marshak G, Barash A, Geiger B. Modulation of intermediate filament expression in the developing cochlear epithelium. Differentiation 1987; 35:151-162.

Raphael Y, Oesterle EC. The distribution of intermediate filaments in the organ of Corti. Abstracts, Mid-Winter Meeting of the Association for Research in Otolaryngology, St. Petersburg Beach, FL, 1989.

Robertson D. Functional significance of dendritic swelling after loud sounds in the guinea pig cochlea. Hear Res 1983; 9:263-278.

Ryan A, Dallos P. Effect of absence of cochlear outer hair cells on behavioral auditory threshold. Nature 1975; 253:44.

Schuknecht HF, Neff WD. Hearing after apical lesions in the cochlea. Acta Otolaryngol 1952; 42:263-274.

Smith DW, Brown JN, Moody DB, et al. Cryoprobe-induced apical lesions in the chinchilla. II. Effects on

behavioral auditory thresholds. Hear Res 1987; 26:311-317.
Spoendlin H. Innervation patterns in the organ of Corti of the cat. Acta Otolaryngol 1969; 67:239-259.
Spoendlin H. Degeneration behavior of the cochlear nerve. Arch Klin Exp Ohrnaskehlkopfheilk 1971; 200:275.
Spoendlin H. Neural connections of the outer hair cell system. Acta Otolaryngol 1979; 87:381-387.
Stebbins WC, Moody DB, Hawkins JE, et al. The species-specific nature of the ototoxicity of dihydrostreptomycin in the patas monkey. Neurotoxicology 1987; 8:33-44.
Thorne PR, Carlisle L, Zajic G, et al. Differences in distribution of F-actin in hair cells along the guinea pig organ of Corti. Hear Res 1987; 30:253-265.

CHAPTER 7

Species Differences and Mechanisms of Damage

LAURENT DECORY
ARMAND L. DANCER
JEAN-MARIE ARAN

Noise-induced hearing loss has been widely studied in various animal species. The physiologic and anatomic consequences of identical overstimulation can be very different from one species to another (Dancer, 1981). For example a pure tone of 1 kHz at 120 dB SPL presented for 12 minutes to the chinchilla induces more threshold shift (TS) than the same stimulus presented for 12 hours to the squirrel monkey (Hunter-Duvar and Bredberg, 1974). The aim of our study was to determine the physiologic and anatomic consequences of identical acoustic overstimulation in three species of mammals widely used in auditory studies (cat, chinchilla, and guinea pig) and to relate the interspecies differences in noise susceptibility to the characteristics of the peripheral mechanical system (external and middle ear), or of the inner ear, or of both for each species.

Our first step was to apply continuous pure-tone overstimulation under the same experimental conditions in all three species. The physiologic auditory effects of this overstimulation were evaluated by electrocochleography (compound action potential—CAP—audiograms), and the anatomical alterations of the organ of Corti were assessed by scanning electron microscopy (SEM). Our second step was to measure the transfer function of the middle ear in all three species and to compare the physiological and anatomical effects of overstimulation as a function of the acoustic input level and acoustic power at the entrance to the cochlea. We will present a tentative mechanical interpretation of the origin (or origins) of the cochlear part of the interspecies differences in susceptibility to noise.

Cochlear Impairment

Methods

Young animals of both sexes that were free of middle-ear infection were used in this study. After premedication with a sedative and anticholinergic agents, the animals were deeply anesthetized with ketamine (guinea pigs and chinchillas) or pentothal (cats). The pinna was sectioned and the bulla exposed. In all three species the bulla was widely opened (the septum was left intact in the cat) and an electrode was implanted on the round window. Precautions were taken to prevent cooling of the animal and especially of its cochlea during the experiment. The animals were placed in an earbar head-holder system. A hollow cone allowed the insertion of different sound sources, and a probe microphone was used to measure the acoustic level in front of the tympanum (about 1.5 mm) (Décory et al, 1989a). This experimental setup allowed us to get rid of the interspecies differences that could originate from the outer-ear transfer functions.

A pre-exposure audiogram was obtained in each animal by averaging the CAP in response to tone-pips over the frequency range of 1 to 32 kHz. Each animal was then exposed to a continuous 2-, 4-, or 8-kHz pure tone for 20 minutes. The level of this pure tone ranged from 82 to 132 dB SPL at the tympanum. Twenty minutes after the end of the stimulation another CAP audiogram was measured to obtain the short-term TSs. Immediately after the second audiometric measurement the cochlea was prepared for SEM. Cochlear frequency maps for the guinea pig (Wilson and

Johnstone, 1975; Johnstone, 1977; Cody et al, 1980), chinchilla (Eldredge et al, 1981), and cat (Liberman, 1982) were used to relate anatomic location to stimulus frequency. All normal looking, altered, and missing hair cells were counted.

Results

Forty cats, 84 chinchillas, and 128 guinea pigs were exposed to acoustic overstimulation at 2, 4, or 8 kHz. Short-term TSs were measured in each of these animals, and about 200 cochleas were observed under SEM.

Threshold Shifts (CAP)

Some of the mean TSs measured in each species after exposure to 8-kHz pure tones (from 80 to 132 dB SPL) are presented in Figure 7-1 (groups of 5 to 10 animals were used for each exposure condition). The maximum TS occurs towards the high frequencies when the stimulus level increases. A phenomenon of the same kind can be observed for the exposures at 2 and 4 kHz (Décory et al, 1989a). The maximum TSs recorded from each animal of each species as a function of stimulus level (for the 2-, 4-, and 8-kHz exposures) are shown in Figure 7-2. For all exposure conditions these findings indicate an increase in auditory susceptibility from the cat to the guinea pig and from the guinea pig to the chinchilla. The slopes of the regression lines are close to each other in all three species: about +1.6 dB TS for each decibel of stimulus. For a given stimulus level, the maximum TS increases with the exposure frequency. When the exposure frequency is high, the TSs are also more restricted. We can define a Q_{20dB}, which represents the ratio between the frequency for which the maximum TS is equal to 50 dB and the range of frequencies for which the TSs vary from 50 to 30 dB. The values of this Q_{20dB} are almost the same in the three species: 0.13 at 2 kHz, 0.3 at 4 kHz, and 0.7 at 8 kHz. The higher the stimulation frequency, the smaller the frequency range of the audiogram affected by the acoustic stimulation.

Hair Cell Lesions (SEM)

We thoroughly examined 164 cochleas using SEM; the breakdown is as follows:

20 in the cat (6 at the stimulation frequency of 2 kHz, 6 at 4 kHz, and 8 at 8 kHz)

59 in the chinchilla (12 at 2 kHz, 13 at 4 kHz, and 34 at 8 kHz)

85 in the guinea pig (13 at 2 kHz, 11 at 4 kHz, and 61 at 8 kHz)

On the cochleograms shown in Figures 7-3, 7-4, and 7-5 we have presented the average results obtained in the three species for the three exposure frequencies (2, 4, and 8 kHz) and for the three stimulus levels (112, 120, and 132 dB). (Normal-looking cells correspond to the black areas, cells with damaged stereocilia correspond to the dotted areas, and missing cells correspond to the white areas.) At these frequencies the length of the organ of Corti corresponding to an octave band is equal to 2.5 mm in the guinea pig and the chinchilla, and to 3.5 mm in the cat, but the number of cells is almost identical per unit of length in these three species. For this reason, the number of injured hair cells in the cat has been multiplied by a conversion factor ($^{2.5}/_{3.5} \approx 0.7$) in order to present the results as if each species had the same number of cells per octave along the organ of Corti.

For a given stimulus level, the amount of damage increases with the exposure frequency. For example, in the three species the first row of outer hair cells (OHC 1) is the most sensitive, as previously described by Robertson and Johnstone (1980). Concerning the first lesions, a 0.3- to 0.5-octave shift can be observed between the stimulation frequency and the characteristic frequency (CF) corresponding to the area of maximum stereocilia damage. When the stimulus level increases, this shift diminishes progressively. Missing hair cells are observed at a CF location corresponding to the stimulation frequency (Cody and Robertson, 1983).

The shift of the first stereocilia damage can be explained by the theory of the cochlear amplifier of Davis (1983), according to which the damage corresponds to the maximum amplitude of the traveling wave (located towards the base when compared to the location of the active processes corresponding to a given CF). Nevertheless, with regard to this theory it is difficult to understand how, at the highest levels, the hair cell damage occurs at a location corresponding to the CF of the stimulation frequency. Other explanations, taking into account variations of cochlear damping as a function of stimulus level, have also been proposed (Dancer and Franke, 1987, 1990).

It is interesting to note that as the stimulation level increases, the changes in the position of the hair cell damage (towards the apex) are just the opposite of the changes in the frequency of the maximum short-term TS (at the high frequencies) (see Figs. 7-1 and 7-5). According to the observations of Robert-

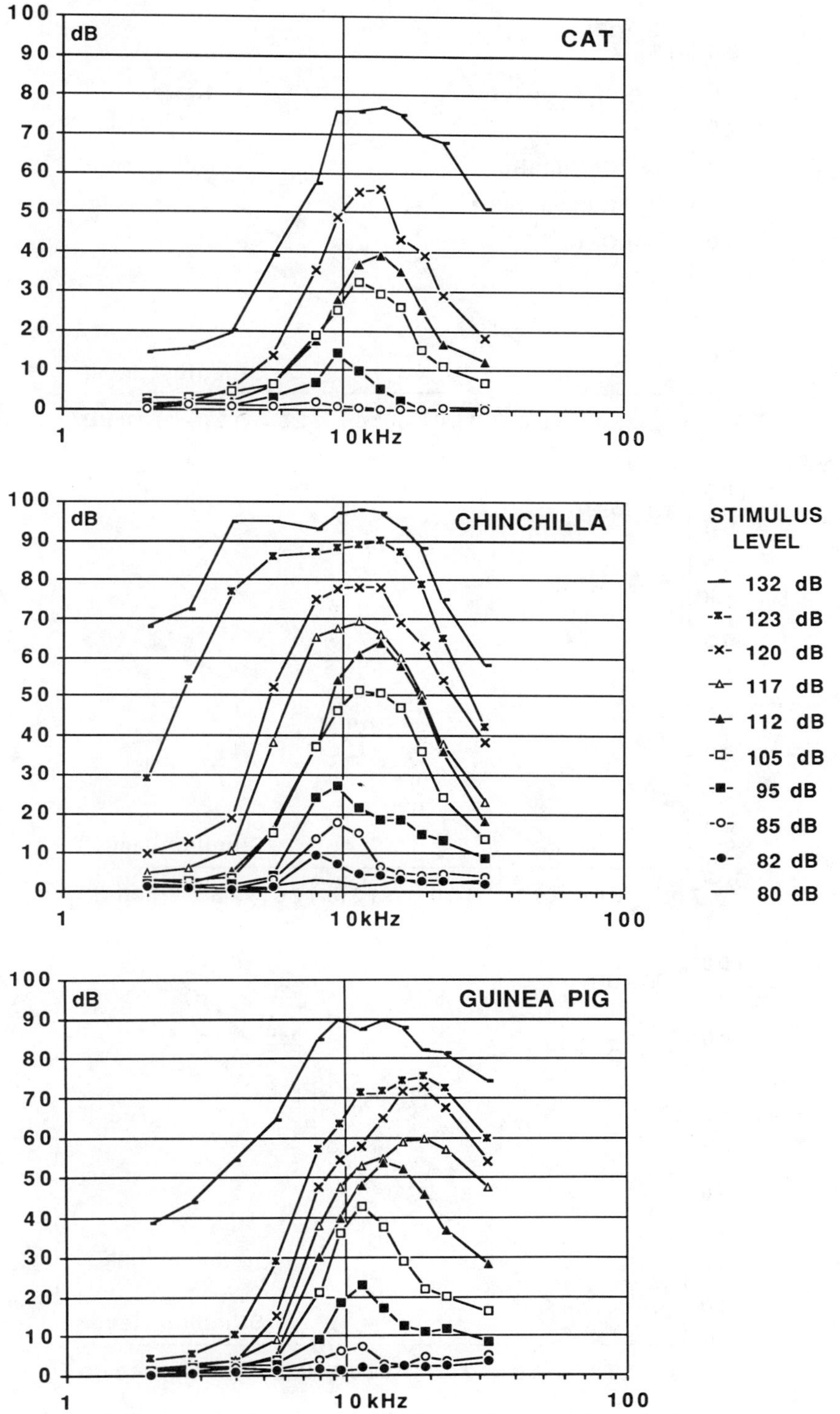

Figure 7-1 Amplitude of the short-term threshold shift measured in the cat, the chinchilla, and the guinea pig as a function of the audiometric frequency following exposure to an 8-kHz pure tone (stimulus levels range from 80 to 132 dB SPL).

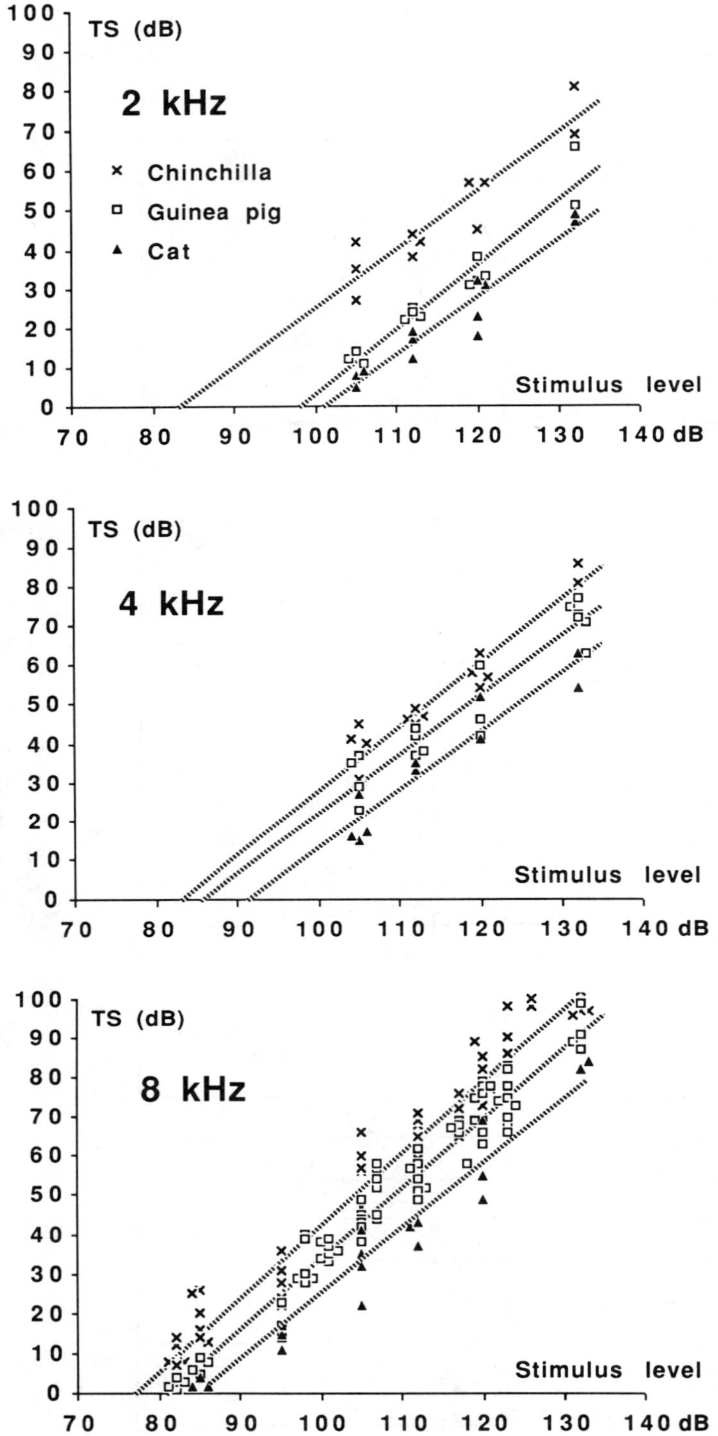

Figure 7-2 Maximum short-term threshold shift recorded from each animal of each species as a function of the stimulus level (for the 2, 4, and 8 kHz pure-tone exposures. Dotted lines correspond to regression lines; $r > 0.9$).

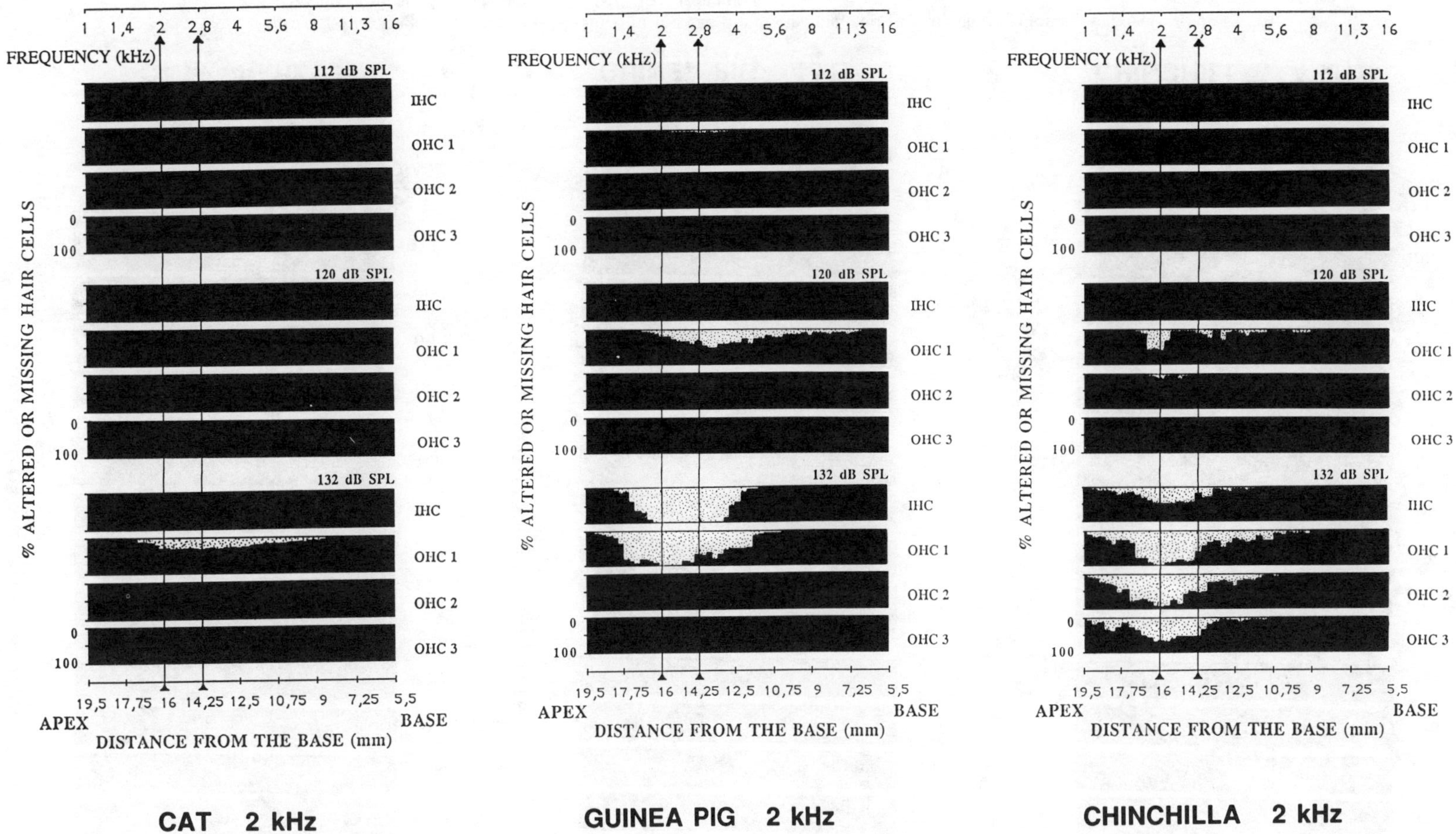

Figure 7-3 Average cochleograms obtained in the cat, the guinea pig, and the chinchilla following exposure to a 2-kHz pure tone at 112, 120, and 132 dB SPL for 20 minutes.

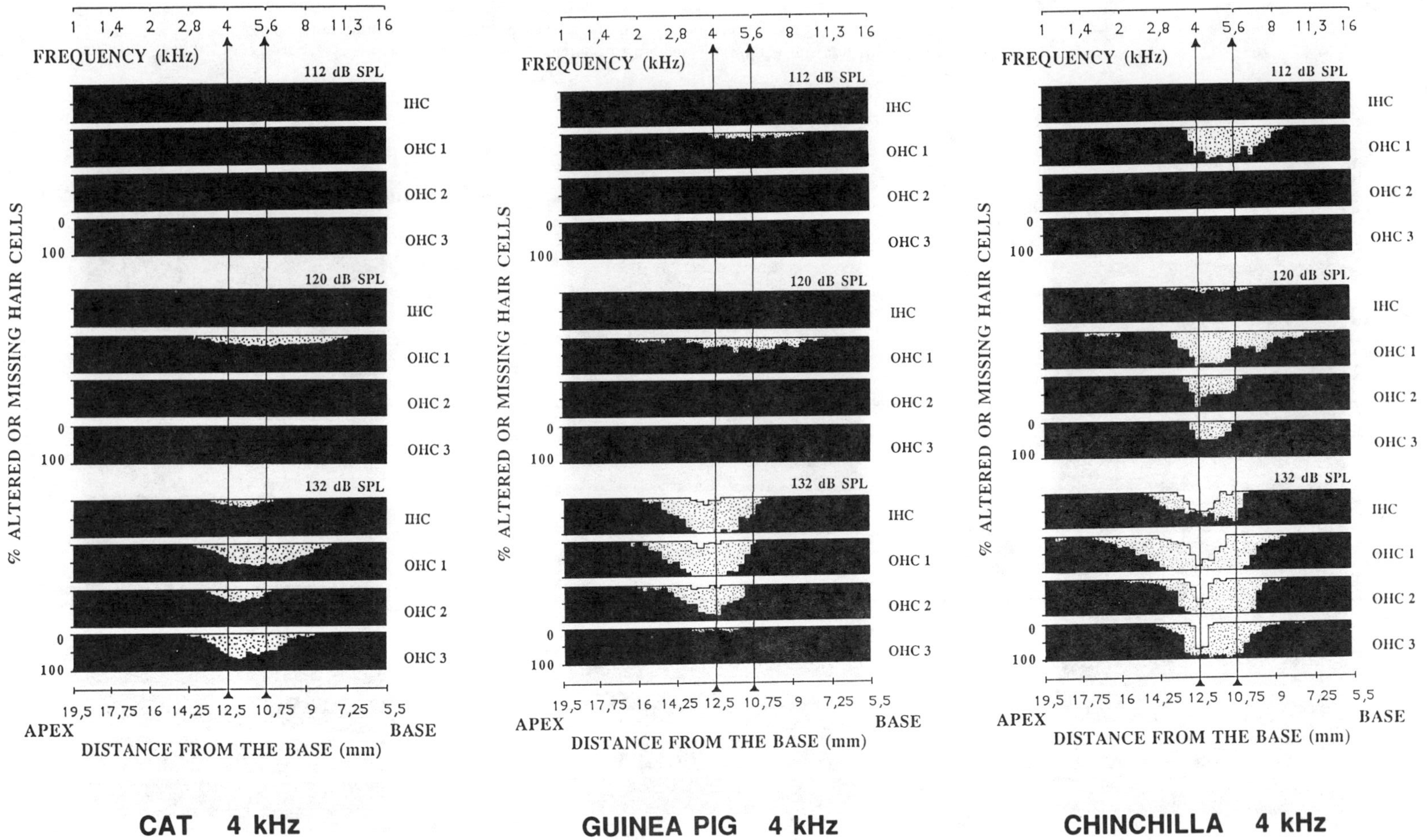

Figure 7-4 Average cochleograms obtained in the cat, the guinea pig, and the chinchilla following exposure to a 4-kHz pure tone at 112, 120, and 132 dB SPL for 20 minutes.

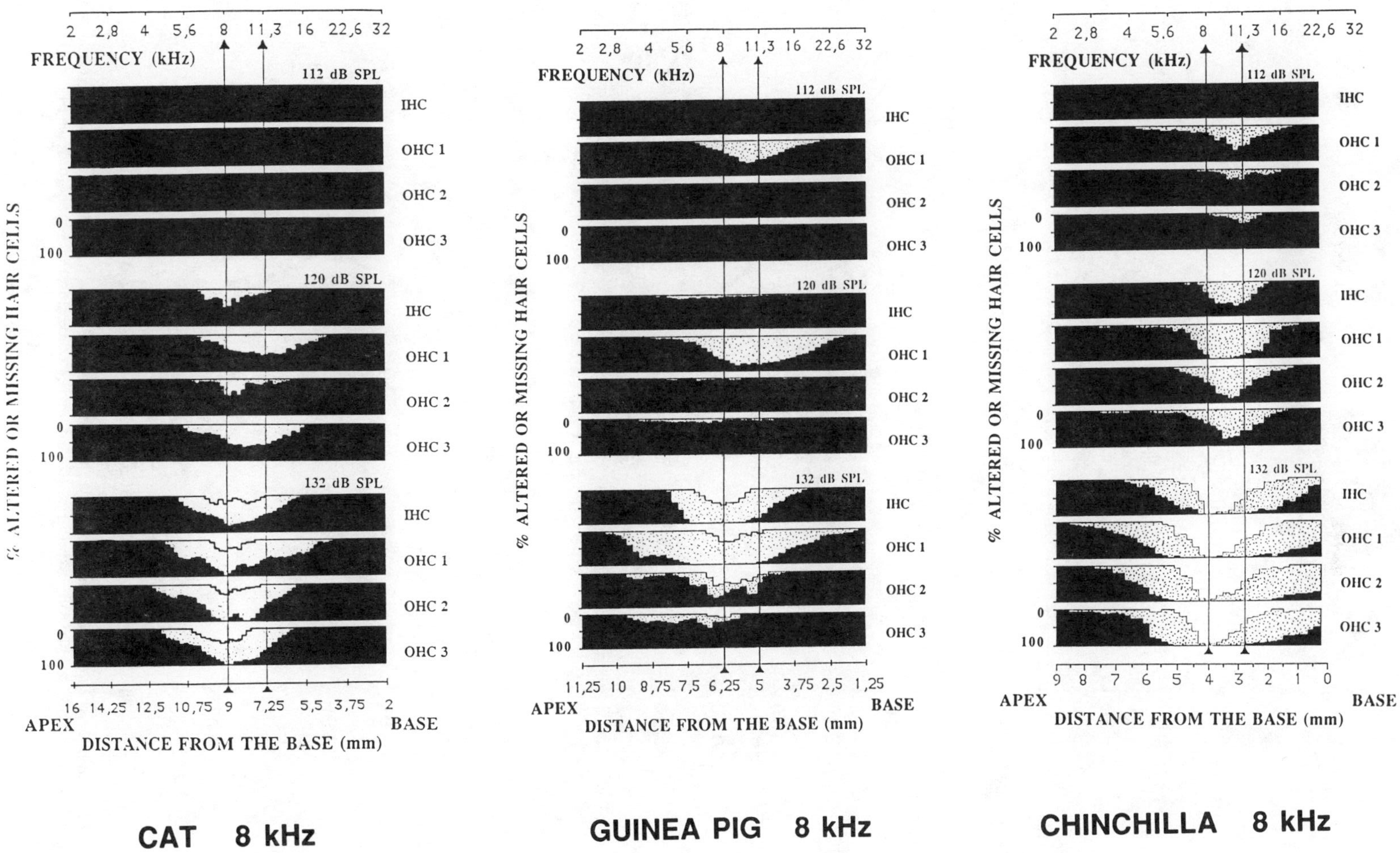

Figure 7-5 Average cochleograms obtained in the cat, the guinea pig, and the chinchilla following exposure to an 8-kHz pure tone at 112, 120, and 132 dB SPL for 20 minutes.

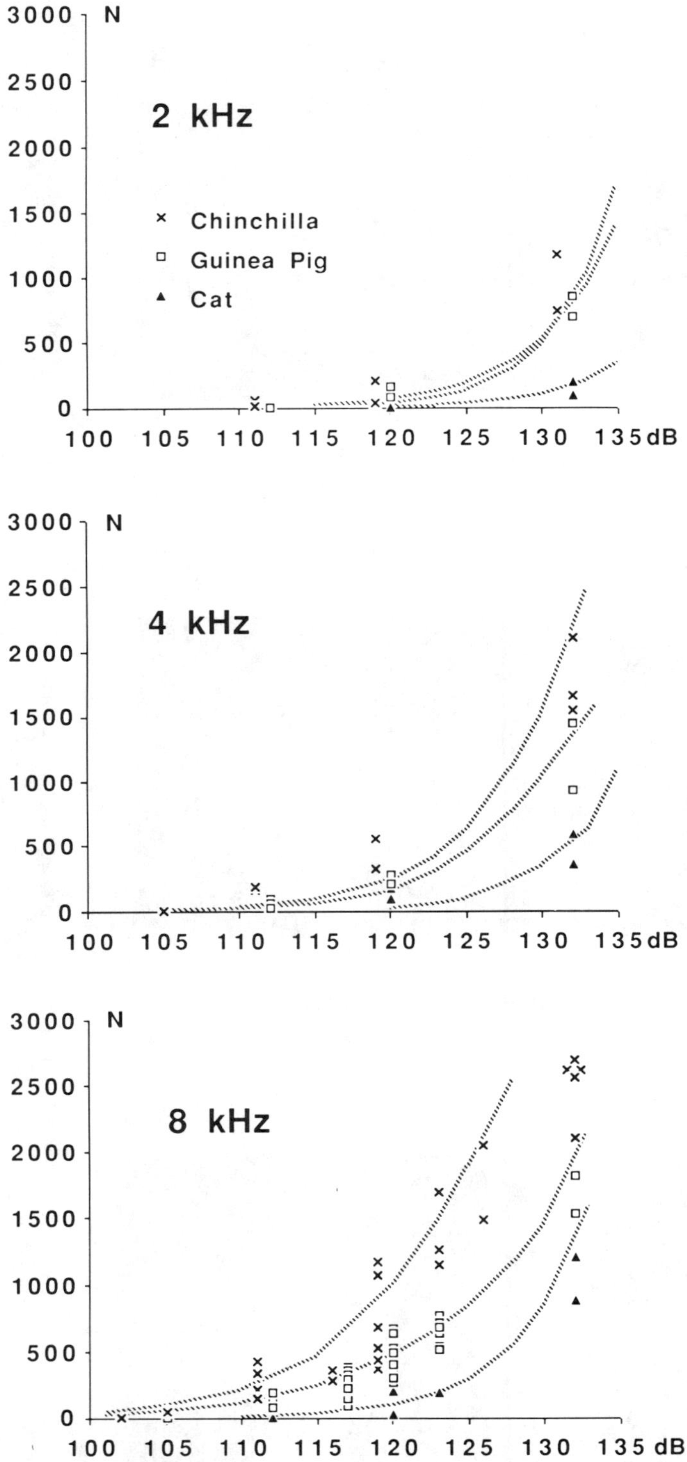

Figure 7-6 Total number of injured and missing hair cells in each animal of each species as a function of the stimulus level of the 2, 4, and 8 kHz pure-tone exposures. Dotted curves correspond to regression curves.

son et al. (1980), Robertson (1983), Liberman (1984), and Liberman and Dodds (1984a,b, 1987), that difference is due to the fact that CAP changes and morphological changes do not have quite the same origin. The TS measured 20 minutes after the end of the exposure is partially reversible, whereas the hair cell lesions observed with SEM (30 minutes after the end of the exposure) are definitive. In fact the correlation between the TS measured a few days or a few weeks after the end of the exposure and the cochlear damage would probably be exact (Cody and Robertson, 1983). In our experiments the TS includes a temporary component that does not correspond to the damage observable in SEM, and that originates from a different part of the organ of Corti. Figure 7-6 shows the total number of injured and missing hair cells (OHC 1, OHC 2, OHC 3, and inner hair cell—IHC) measured in each animal as a function of the stimulus level for the 2-, 4-, and 8-kHz exposures. These findings confirm the general increase in auditory susceptibility from the cat to the guinea pig and from the guinea pig to the chinchilla.

In our well-defined experimental conditions we have observed significant interspecies differences in auditory susceptibility for pure tones between the cat, the chinchilla, and the guinea pig. These differences can only be attributed to the conditions of transmission of the acoustic stimulus from the eardrum to the cochlea; to the anatomical, mechanical, biochemical, and physiological properties of the cochlea; or to both. To try to clear up this problem, we decided to measure, in the same experimental conditions and in each species, the transfer function of the middle ear in order to be able to compare the interspecies differences as a function of the acoustic pressure level and of the acoustic power of the stimulus at the entrance to the cochlea.

Transfer Function of the Middle Ear in the Cat, the Chinchilla, and the Guinea Pig

For a given stimulus applied at the tympanic membrane (TM), the sound pressure at the base of the scala vestibuli (SV), and hence the amplitude of the transfer function of the middle ear (TFME), has been recorded from 100 Hz to 20 kHz.

Methods

The acoustic stimulation (pure tones) is produced and controlled as previously discussed. The stimulation levels range from 70 to 120 dB SPL. The intracochlear sound pressure measurements are taken using a miniature piezoresistive transducer (Kulite) equipped with a probe filled with silicon fluid (Franke et al, 1982). The acoustic input impedance of the probe (about 10^{14} $N{\cdot}s{\cdot}m^{-5}$ at 1 kHz) is much higher than that of the guinea pig's cochlea (about 10^{11} $N.s.m^{-5}$) (Dancer and Franke, 1980), and should not modify the acoustic pressure inside the cochlea. The transducer is calibrated in a closed coupler filled with the same fluid and driven by a quartz disc; thus we obtain the frequency response of the probe in the 20 Hz to 20 kHz range with good accuracy. The animals are prepared as previously discussed. The bulla is widely opened (the septum being left intact in the cat). A hole (about 0.3 mm) is drilled into the SV of the basal turn at the most accessible part, which is—in the cat, guinea pig, and chinchilla, respectively—at 8, 7.2, and 5.5 mm from the base. The probe is put into place: its conical shape allows a good seal. The animal is then exposed to a frequency-swept pure tone (100 Hz to 20 kHz). The signal-to-noise ratio is improved by means of a narrow-band tracking filter. All the following data correspond to the amplitude of the intracochlear sound pressure referenced to the amplitude of the sound pressure in front of the TM. Whichever species is considered, the intracochlear sound pressure can be considered to be linear across the whole range of stimulation (70 to 120 dB SPL).

Results

The sound pressure was measured in the SV of the first turn of the cochlea in eight cats, nine chinchillas, and eleven guinea pigs.

Figure 7-7 shows the average amplitude of the sound pressure measured in the first turn of the SV in the cat, chinchilla, and guinea pig (with reference to sound pressure at the TM). Between 500 Hz and 10 kHz the amplitudes are close in the three species: the observed differences are less than or equal to one standard deviation (less than 10 dB). The principal difference among them is the negative peak appearing at 3 kHz in cat; this peak is due to the secondary cavity of the bulla in the cat (measurements in animals with septum re-

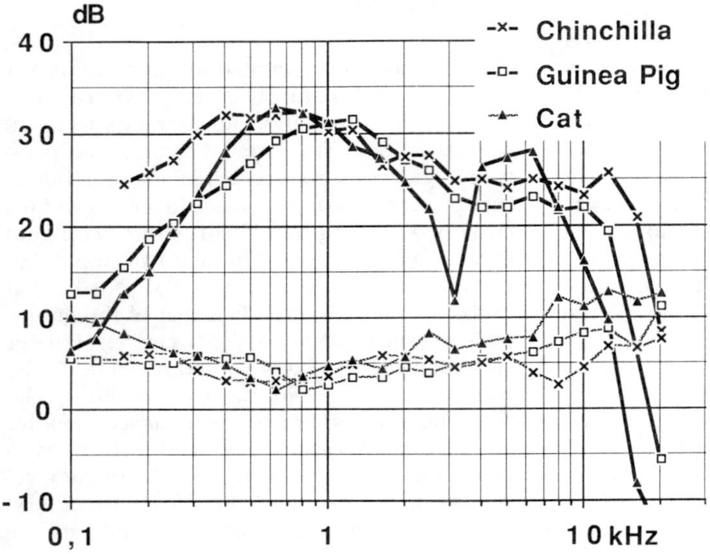

Figure 7-7 Average amplitude (continuous lines) and standard errors (dotted lines) of the sound pressure in the first turn of scala vestibuli (with reference to sound pressure at the TM) in the three species.

moved have given results comparable to those of Guinan and Peake, 1967, and Nedzelnitsky, 1980; see Décory et al, 1989b). In our experimental conditions, the amplitude of the TFME is maximal (31 to 33 dB) at 600 Hz in the cat and the chinchilla, and at 1.2 kHz in the guinea pig. In the cat, our average curve is close to the maximum values recorded by Nedzelnitsky (1980).

As mentioned earlier, these measurements were feasible only at a certain distance from the oval window. Measurements performed in scala tympani (Décory et al, 1990) indicate that the curves of Figure 7-7 actually represent the TFME only in a frequency range limited to 9 kHz in the cat, 5 kHz in the chinchilla, and 11 kHz in the guinea pig. According to previous experiments (Dancer and Franke, 1980, 1982), the actual amplitude of the TFME in the chinchilla at 8 kHz is probably larger (at most by 6 dB).

Interspecies Differences in Auditory Sensitivity

Obtaining Constant Amplitude of the Acoustic Stimulus at the Entrance to the Cochlea

With the help of the intracochlear acoustic pressure recordings we can compare the TS measurements and the SEM observations from one species to another for a given amplitude of the acoustic stimulus at the entrance to the cochlea. For each stimulation frequency we used four different criteria: the threshold of TS; the isomaximum TS (50 dB); the threshold of stereocilia damage; and isocellular injury (1,500 injured hair cells) (Décory et al, 1989b). With the help of these different electrophysiologic and anatomic criteria it is possible to make a rough evaluation (in decibels) of the average differences in auditory susceptibility of the cochlea between the three species for a constant amplitude of the acoustic stimulus at the entrance to the cochlea. Under these conditions the interspecies differences are especially noticeable between the cat and the two other species, and less remarkable between the chinchilla and the guinea pig.

Obtaining Constant Acoustic Power at the Entrance to the Cochlea

It is also possible to compare the interspecies differences as a function of the amount of mechanical energy dissipated per unit of time inside the cochlea. At the input of the cochlea when driven by a pure tone, the active acoustic power is given by the equation

$$W_c = P_c \cdot U_c \cdot \cos\varphi$$

where P_c is the rms sound pressure at the input of the cochlea, U_c the rms volume velocity of the stapes, and φ the phase lag of U_c versus P_c function. According to several authors (Tonndorf et al, 1966; Khanna and Tonndorf, 1971; Dancer and Franke, 1980; Lynch et al,

TABLE 7-1 **Stapes Volume Velocities for a Stimulus Level of 94 dB (in $m^3 \cdot Pa^{-1} \cdot s^{-1}$)**

	FREQUENCY		
SPECIES	**2 kHz**	**4 kHz**	**8 kHz**
Cat	$1.9 \cdot 10^{-10}$	$3.3 \cdot 10^{-10}$	$2.0 \cdot 10^{-10}$
Chinchilla	$3.5 \cdot 10^{-10}$	$3.5 \cdot 10^{-10}$	$2.1 \cdot 10^{-10}$
Guinea pig	$2.2–5.5 \cdot 10^{-10}$	$0.9–2.5 \cdot 10^{-10}$	$0.9–2.0 \cdot 10^{-10}$

TABLE 7-2 **Acoustic Power Entering the Cochlea (in $W \cdot Pa^{-1}$)**

	FREQUENCY		
SPECIES	**2 kHz**	**4 kHz**	**8 kHz**
Cat	$3.3 \cdot 10^{-9}$	$7.0 \cdot 10^{-9}$	$2.5 \cdot 10^{-9}$
Chinchilla	$8.4 \cdot 10^{-9}$	$6.3 \cdot 10^{-9}$	$3.5 \cdot 10^{-9}$
Guinea pig	$5.1–12.8 \cdot 10^{-9}$	$1.1–3.2 \cdot 10^{-9}$	$1.0–2.4 \cdot 10^{-9}$

TABLE 7-3 **Acoustic Power Corresponding to the Threshold of Stereocilia Damage (in W)·**

	FREQUENCY		
SPECIES	**2 kHz**	**4 kHz**	**8 kHz**
Cat	$530 \cdot 10^{-8}$	$120 \cdot 10^{-8}$	$20 \cdot 10^{-8}$
Chinchilla	$190 \cdot 10^{-8}$	$17 \cdot 10^{-8}$	$0.7–1.3 \cdot 10^{-8}$
Guinea pig	$80–210 \cdot 10^{-8}$	$7–20 \cdot 10^{-8}$	$0.6–1.5 \cdot 10^{-8}$

1982), in a passive cochlea, the acoustic input impedance is purely resistive in the frequency range under consideration (thus $W_c \approx P_c \cdot U_c$). Having measured P_c it remains to determine U_c in order to calculate W_c. The stapes displacement can be used to calculate its volume velocity:

$$U_c = 2\pi f \cdot A_s \cdot X_s$$

where A_s is the area of the stapes footplate, X_s its displacement, and f the driving frequency. To determine X_s we can use, in the cat, the results of Guinan and Peake (1967); in the chinchilla, the results of Ruggero et al (1990); and in the guinea pig, the results of Wilson and Johnstone (1975), Manley and Johnstone (1974), and Dancer et al (1979). For a sound pressure of 1 Pa (94 dB SPL) at the TM, and for the three frequencies (2, 4, and 8 kHz), we obtain the stapes velocities shown in Table 7-1.

The values shown in Table 7-1 are close from one species to another and from one frequency to another. The value of P_c for a sound pressure of 1 Pa (94 dB) at the TM can be obtained from the results presented in Figure 7-7. Using these results, we can calculate the acoustic power that enters the cochlea. The results of these calculations are shown in Table 7-2.

Taking into account the uncertainties that affect the numerous measures involved in the determination of the acoustic power, these results show that in our experimental conditions, for a given sound pressure level at the TM, the acoustic power entering the cochlea is similar in these three species and at the three exposure frequencies. With the help of these calculations and of our previous results (corresponding to the 20-minute exposures), we can evaluate the acoustic power corresponding to the different damage criteria defined earlier. This evaluation shows that the acoustic power that corresponds to a given damage criterion decreases strongly when the stimulation frequency increases (from $\approx 2 \cdot 10^{-6}$ W at 2 kHz to $\approx 1 \cdot 10^{-8}$ W at 8 kHz in the chinchilla for the threshold of stereocilia damage).

For each stimulation frequency and for the various criteria, the values of acoustic power are close between the chinchilla and the guinea pig, whereas they are much larger in the cat. Tables 7-3 and 7-4 show the values of the acoustic power entering the cochlea corresponding to the threshold of stereocilia

TABLE 7-4 **Acoustic Power Corresponding to Isocellular Injury (in W)**

SPECIES	FREQUENCY 2 kHz	4 kHz	8 kHz
Cat	$210 \cdot 10^{-6}$	$180 \cdot 10^{-6}$	$20 \cdot 10^{-6}$
Chinchilla	$60 \cdot 10^{-6}$	$18 \cdot 10^{-6}$	$2.6–5.3 \cdot 10^{-6}$
Guinea pig	$64–164 \cdot 10^{-6}$	$9–26 \cdot 10^{-6}$	$4–10 \cdot 10^{-6}$

TABLE 7-5 **Mean Displacements of the Basilar Membrane Corresponding to an Acoustic Level of 100 dB at the Entrance to the Cochlea**

SPECIES	FREQUENCY 2 kHz	4 kHz	8 kHz
Cat	$0.5 \cdot 10^{-6}$	$0.4 \cdot 10^{-6}$	$0.3 \cdot 10^{-6}$
Chinchilla	$0.7 \cdot 10^{-6}$	$0.8 \cdot 10^{-6}$	$0.15–0.3 \cdot 10^{-6}$
Guinea pig	$1.3–3.2 \cdot 10^{-6}$	$0.7–2.0 \cdot 10^{-6}$	$0.6–1.4 \cdot 10^{-6}$

damage and to isocellular injury, respectively, for a 20-minute exposure.

In evaluating these tables, we reach the same conclusion that had been reached in the evaluation of damage as a function of the acoustic level at the entrance to the cochlea: for a given acoustic power, the cochleas of the chinchilla and the guinea pig seem to have about the same susceptibility, whereas the cochlea of the cat is more resistant (this difference corresponds to about 6 dB in stimulation level).

This phenomenon seems to have a cochlear origin. As a matter of fact the influence of the acoustic reflex of the middle ear can probably be ruled out: all our animals were deeply anesthetized, and Møller (1965, 1974) has shown that this reflex is ineffective beyond 1.5 kHz in the cat. The same observation was made by Lataye (1989) in the guinea pig. Our stimulation frequencies are well beyond these values.

The measurement of the TFME was not sufficient to explain the origin of the interspecies differences in auditory susceptibility. If the transfer function of the peripheral mechanical system (external and middle ear) seems to be responsible for a large part of these differences (especially in the guinea pig and in the chinchilla), there are certainly cochlear factors of some importance.

Cochlear Factors

Efferent Feedback

According to Liberman (1988) and Warren and Liberman (1989a,b), the activity of efferent feedback controlling the OHCs could explain some of the individual differences in susceptibility to noise. The results of these authors were obtained in the cat. But recently Liberman (1990) demonstrated that the olivocochlear efferent bundle was not able to significantly modify the TS induced by a 6-kHz pure tone presented at 100 dB for 10 minutes (deep anesthesia also decreases the activity of the efferent system, especially with the thiopental (Pentothal) used in the cat in our experiments). Without ruling out completely this or many other possibilities, such as vascular, metabolic, or biochemical phenomena, we chose to study the mechanical events that could explain the interspecies differences in susceptibility to noise.

Cochlear Mechanics

For a given input to the cochlea, we have attempted to uncover which cochlear mechanisms might be responsible for acoustic injury and whether these mechanisms differ from one species to another. We have limited our study to the first part of the transduction process—i.e., to the mechanical processes induced by the acoustic stimulus at the level of the cochlear structures and especially of the stereocilia (Décory et al, 1989c).

Average Displacements of the Basilar Membrane. For the stimulation frequencies used in this study, a given volume displacement of the stapes corresponds to an identical average volume displacement of the basilar membrane. This volume displacement affects all of the area corresponding to the traveling wave. For a given acoustic level at the input to the cochlea (100 dB, for example), and taking

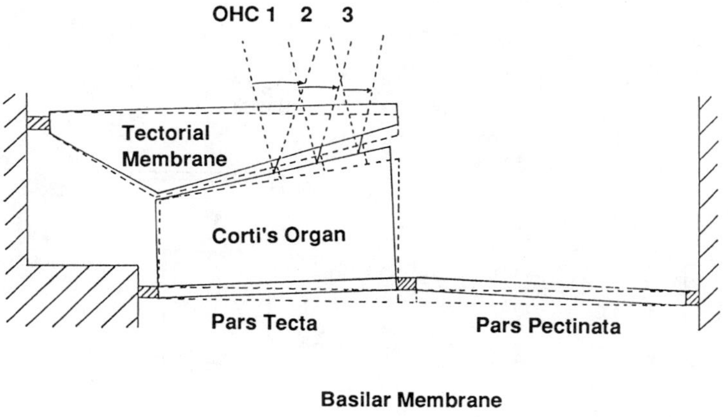

Figure 7-8 Schematic representation of the organ of Corti.

into account the respective dimensions of the cochlear elements, we can calculate the mean displacement of the basilar membrane perpendicular to its surface at 2, 4, and 8 kHz (Table 7-5.) This mean displacement is lower than the maximum displacement because it takes into account neither the shape of the traveling wave nor the fact that the basilar membrane is attached on one side to the spiral lamina and on the other side to the spiral ligament (Décory et al, 1989b,c).

The mean displacements tend to decrease when the stimulation frequency increases. This does not explain the increase in damage as the stimulation frequency increases. On the other hand, the mean displacements cannot explain by themselves the specific resistance of the cochlea of the cat (the largest displacements are observed in the guinea pig). However, this conclusion may not be accurate because we do not know, from these crude estimates, the amplitudes of the relative displacements of the other cochlear structures (e.g., reticular lamina, stereocilia, tectorial membrane) along the organ of Corti in each species.

Cochlear Micromechanics. From a mechanical point of view the displacements of the stereocilia are the basis of the auditory injuries to be seen following exposure to an acoustic stimulus (Saunders and Flock, 1986). According to Liberman (1988), Robertson and Johnstone (1980), and Cody and Robertson (1983), the main anatomic feature that correlates with hearing loss is the rupture of the roots of the stereocilia. Therefore we examined more closely the differences and similarities of the stereocilia of the different hair cell rows in the three species. For this purpose we used anatomical measurements performed by Rhode and Geisler (1966) in the cat; by Spoendlin (1970), Strelioff and Flock (1984), and Wright (1984) in the guinea pig; and by Lim (1980, 1986) in the chinchilla. In each species, the main results of these measurements are that the length of the stereocilia decreases from the apex to the base and from the third to the first rows of the OHCs. Moreover, for a location corresponding to a given CF, the length of the stereocilia decreases from the cat to the guinea pig and from the guinea pig to the chinchilla.

We designed a schematic model of the organ of Corti in each species (Décory et al, 1989c) and evaluated the angular displacements of the stereocilia as a function of the displacements of the basilar membrane. Figure 7-8 shows for example that in our model the shorter stereocilia of the OHC 1 undergo the largest angular displacements. This could explain the high susceptibility of the OHC 1 to acoustic injury. Schematic representations of the organ of Corti in the cat, the chinchilla, and the guinea pig are shown in Figure 7-9. In this figure, the angular displacement of the OHC 1 stereocilia has been determined for a displacement of 1 μm of the basilar membrane and for three locations corresponding to CFs of 1, 4, and 16 kHz. Observe that for a given species and a given displacement of the basilar membrane, the amplitude of the angular deflection seems relatively constant from the base to the apex. Also, note that the angular displacement in the chinchilla is almost three times larger than in the two other species.

If the observations concerning cochlear micromechanics are combined with those concerning the mean basilar membrane displacements (Table 7-5), it is seen that, for a given input to the cochlea, the angular displacements of the stereocilia are comparable in the chinchilla and in the guinea pig but about two times smaller in the cat. Thus, it can be hypothesized that the smaller suscepti-

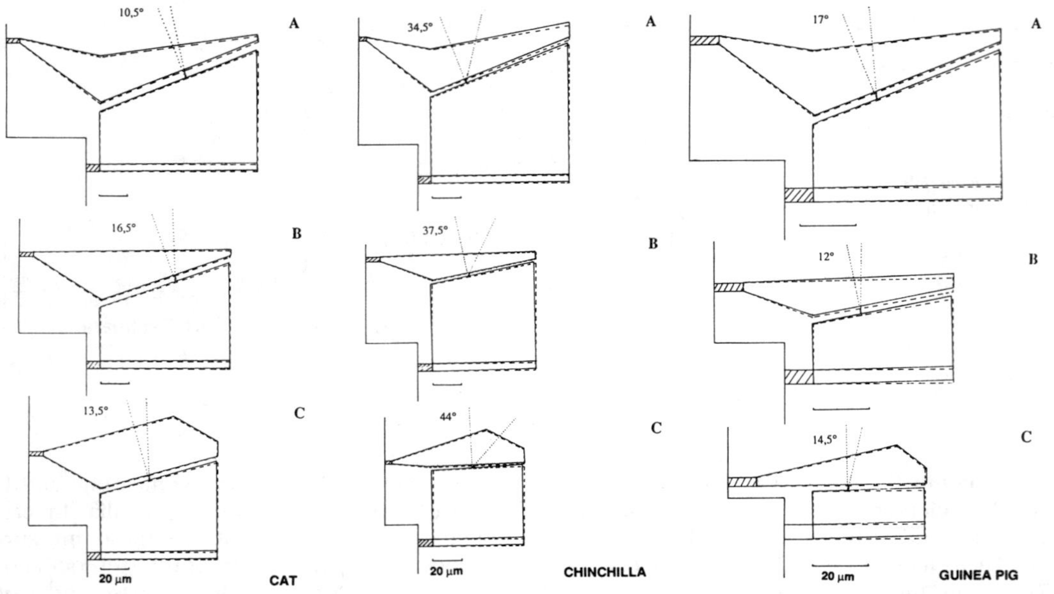

Figure 7-9 Schematic representation of the angular displacements of the outer hair cell 1 stereocilia for a 1-μm displacement of the basilar membrane at three different characteristic frequency locations (*A,* 1 kHz; *B,* 4 kHz; *C,* 16 kHz) in the cat, the chinchilla, and the guinea pig.

bility of the cat's cochlea could be due to the smaller angular displacement of its OHC stereocilia. Furthermore, if the stereocilia damage can be considered to occur as a result of a fatigue failure process (nonlinear phenomenon), then the amplitude *and* the number of cycles undergone by a stereocilium would be of importance.

Differences in Auditory Susceptibility as a Function of Exposure Frequency. In the three species, close to the base of the cochlea (for a given input to the inner ear), the higher the stimulation frequency, the greater the damage. If we consider a location corresponding to a CF of 16 kHz, for the same acoustic level at the input to the cochlea and for all frequencies lower than 16 kHz, the displacement of the basilar membrane (and the angular displacement of the stereocilia) is the same (Dancer et al, 1979) in a given species. Under these conditions the amplitude of the differential cochlear microphonic potential is constant (in its linear range) for all frequencies below the CF of the recording place.

We observed earlier that for a given input to the cochlea the auditory damage observed close to the base (at a CF of 16 kHz, for example) decreases as the stimulation frequency decreases—i.e., to maintain a given amount of damage, the acoustic input to the cochlea has to be increased by 10 to 15 dB each time the stimulation frequency is halved (Décory et al, 1989c).

This observation could be explained by the stress sustained by the stereocilia. This stress depends on numerous physical parameters (e.g., angular displacement, stiffness—see Flock and Strelioff, 1984), but for a given stereocilium and a given exposure condition, it also depends (in a nonlinear way) on the number of cycles (fatigue failure phenomenon). The damage occurring at the level of the stereocilia would then depend on the amplitude of the angular displacement *and* on the number of cycles (i.e., the duration of the exposure in the case of a pure tone).

Conclusion

This study was deliberately conducted with a purely mechanical approach. It was found that that for a given input to the cochlea the interspecies differences in auditory susceptibility are not large between the chinchilla and the guinea pig. However, the cochlea of the cat seems to be more resistant than those of the two other species, by about 6 dB.

The transmission of the acoustic stimulus from the free field to the inner ear seems to be responsible for the largest part of the interspecies differences in auditory susceptibility. Nevertheless, within the limits of our narrow mechanistic approach, it appears that some cochlear factors (such as the angular displacements of the stereocilia) could contribute to the higher resistance of the cat's cochlea to noise trauma.

Différences Interspécifiques de Susceptibilité au Bruit et Mechanismes Lésionnels

La susceptibilité du système auditif vis-à-vis de l'exposition au bruit montre des différences importantes d'une espèce animale à l'autre. Ceci rend difficile l'extrapolation quantitative de données de l'animal à l'homme.

Le but de cette étude était de déterminer si les différences interspécifiques de susceptibilité au bruit sont dues à la fonction de transfert de l'oreille externe et de l'oreille moyenne de chaque espèce, à la susceptibilité proprement dite de la cochlée, ou à la combinaison de ces deux facteurs.

Deux types de résultats quantitatifs d'atteintes auditives induites par des surstimulations constituées par des sons purs de 2, 4 et 8 kHz (80 à 132 dB SPL au niveau du tympan) sont décrits chez le cobaye, le chinchilla et le chat:

- les déplacements du seuil obtenu par électrocochléographie,
- les altérations des cellules ciliées mesurées par microscopie électronique à balayage.

La fonction de transfert de l'oreille moyenne de chaque espèce a été déterminé grâce à la mesure de la pression acoustique dans le premier tour de la rampe vestibulaire. Connaissant ainsi le niveau acoustique à l'entrée de la cochlée pour un niveau donné de pression devant le tympan, la susceptibilité cochléaire peut être comparée d'une espèce à l'autre.

Dans les conditions expérimentales utilisées par les auteurs, le chat est le moins sensible.

Les auteurs montrent que les différences de susceptibilité interspécifiques existant entre le chinchilla et le cobaye sont essentiellement dues à la fonction de transfert de l'oreille externe et de l'oreille moyenne.

Finalement, le rôle éventuel de la micromécanique des stéréocils dans les différences interspécifiques de susceptibilité est discuté.

References

Cody AR, Robertson D, Bredberg G, Johnstone BM. Electrophysiological and morphological changes in the guinea pig cochlea following mechanical trauma to the organ of Corti. Acta Otolaryngol 1980; 89:440-452.

Cody AR, Robertson D. Variability of noise-induced damage in the guinea pig cochlea: electrophysiological and morphological correlates after strictly controlled exposures. Hear Res 1983; 9:55-70.

Dancer A. Possibilités d'application à l'homme des résultats des études des effets des bruits sur l'audition réalisées chez l'animal. Acustica 1981; 48:239-246.

Dancer A, Franke R, Buck K, Evrard G. Etude de la transmision du stimulus acoustique au niveau du récepteur auditif chez le cobaye. Rapport ISL 1979; 113.

Dancer A, Franke R. Intracochlear sound pressure measurements in guinea pigs. Hear Res 1980; 2:191-205.

Dancer A, Franke R. Pression acoustique intracochléaire: Mesures directes et modèles. Acustica 1982; 51:18-28.

Dancer A, Franke R. Mécanique cochléaire: Onde propagée ou résonance? Rev Acoust 1987; 81:3-9.

Dancer A, Franke R. Mechanics in a "passive" cochlea: Travelling wave or resonance? I1 Valsalva, 1989; 54 (suppl 1):1-5.

Davis H. An active process in cochlear mechanics. Hear Res 1983; 9:79-90.

Décory L, Guilhaume A, Dancer A, Aran J-M, Buck K. Origine des différences interspécifiques de susceptibilité au bruit. Etude électrophysiologique et histologique. ISL-R 1989; 112.

Décory L, Franke R, Dancer A, Evrard G. Mesure de la fonction de transfert de l'oreille moyenne chez le chat, le chinchilla et le cobaye. Application à l'étude des différences interspécifiques de susceptibilité au bruit. ISL-R 1989b; 115.

Décory L, Dancer A. Etude des mécanismes cochléaires responsables des atteintes auditives. ISL-R 1989c; 116.

Décory L, Franke R, Dancer A. Measurement of the middle ear transfer function in cat, chinchilla and guinea pig. Presented at the Meeting on Cochlear Mechanics, Madison, WI, preprints, June 1990, 213-220.

Eldredge DH, Miller JD, Bohne BA. A frequency-position map for the chinchilla cochlea. J Acoust Soc Am 1981; 69:1091-1095.

Flock Å, Strelioff D. Studies on hair cells in isolated coils from the guinea pig cochlea. Stiffness of sensory-cell hair bundles in the isolated guinea pig cochlea. Hear Res 1984; 15:11-28.

Franke R, Dancer A, Lenoir M, et al. Etude des phénomènes hydromécaniques cochléaires aux basses et très basses fréquences chez le cobaye. ISL-R 1982; 121.

Guinan J, Peake WT. Middle ear characteristics of anesthetized cats. J Acoust Soc Am 1967; 41:1237-1261.

Hunter-Duvar IM, Bredberg G. Effects of intense auditory stimulation: Hearing losses and inner ear changes in the chinchilla. J Acoust Soc Am 1974; 55:795-801.

Johnstone JR. Properties of ganglion cells from the extreme basal region of guinea pig cochlea. In: Evans EF, Wilson JP, eds. Psychophysics and physiology of hearing. New York: Academic Press, 1977:89.

Khanna SM, Tonndorf J. The vibratory pattern of the round window in cats. J Acoust Soc Am 1971; 50:1475-1483.

Lataye R. Nocivités comparées de bruits continus d'une durée inférieure ou egale á 8 heures et de bruits intermittents—Etude electrocochléographique chez le cobaye. Thèse de l'Université de Strasbourg, 1989.

Liberman MC. The cochlear frequency map for the cat: labeling auditory-nerve fibers of known characteristic frequency. J Acoust Soc Am 1982; 72:1441-1449.

Liberman MC. Single-neuron labeling and chronic cochlear pathology. I. Threshold shift and characteristic-frequency shift. Hear Res 1984; 16:33-42.

Liberman MC, Dodds LW. Single-neuron labeling and chronic cochlear pathology. II. Stereocilia damage and alterations of spontaneous discharge rate. Hear Res 1984a; 16:43-54.

Liberman MC, Dodds LW. Single-neuron labeling and chronic cochlear pathology. III. Stereocilia damage and alterations of threshold tuning curves. Hear Res 1984b; 16:55-74.

Liberman MC, Dodds LW. Acute ultrastructural changes in acoustic trauma: serial-section reconstruction of stereocilia and cuticular plates. Hear Res 1987; 26:45-64.

Liberman MC. Structural basis for noise-induced threshold shift. Proceedings of the Noise '88 Meeting, Stockholm, August 1988.

Liberman MC. Sound-evoked olivocochlear feedback and the susceptibility to acoustic injury. Proceedings of the 13th ARO Midwinter Research Meeting, February 1990:323-324.

Lim DJ. Cochlear anatomy related to cochlear micromechanics. A review. J Acoust Soc Am 1980; 67:1686-1695.

Lim DJ. Functional structure of the organ of Corti: A review. Hear Res 1986; 22:117-146.

Lynch TJ, Nedzelnitsky V, Peake WT. Input impedance of the cochlea in cat. J Acoust Soc Am 1982; 72:108-130.

Manley GA, Johnstone BM. Middle ear function in the guinea pig. J Acoust Soc Am 1974; 56:571-576.

Møller AR. An experimental study of the acoustic impedance of the middle ear and its transmission properties. Acta Otolaryngol 1965; 60:129-149.

Møller AR. The acoustic middle ear muscle reflex. In: Keidel WD, Neff WD, eds. Handbook of sensory physiology. Berlin, Springer-Verlag, 1974.

Nedzelnitsky V. Sound pressures in the basal turn of the cat cochlea. J Acoust Soc Am 1980; 68:1676-1689.

Rhode WS, Geisler CD. Model of the displacement between opposing points on the tectorial membrane and reticular lamina. J Acoust Soc Am 1966; 42:185-190.

Robertson D. Functional significance of dendritic swelling after loud sounds in the guinea pig cochlea. Hear Res 1983; 9:263-278.

Robertson D, Johnstone BM. Acoustic trauma in the guinea pig cochlea: Early changes in ultrastructure and neural threshold. Hear Res 1980; 3:167-179.

Robertson D, Johnstone BM, McGill TJ. Effects of loud tones on the inner ear: a combined electrophysiological and ultrastructural study. Hear Res 1980; 2:39-54.

Ruggero MA, Rich NC, Robles L, et al. Middle ear response in the chinchilla and its relationship to mechanics at the base of the cochlea. J Acoust Soc Am 1990; 87:1612-1625.

Saunders JC, Flock Å. Recovery of threshold shift in hair-cell stereocilia following exposure to intense stimulation. Hear Res 1986; 23:233-244.

Spoendlin H. Structural basis of peripheral frequency analysis. In: Plomp R, Smoorenburg GG, eds. Frequency analysis and periodicity detection in hearing. Leiden, The Netherlands, Sijthoff, 1970:2.

Strelioff D, Flock Å. Stiffness of sensory-cell hair bundles in the isolated guinea pig cochlea. Hear Res 1984; 15:19-28.

Tonndorf J, Khanna SM, Fingerhood BJ. The input impedance of the inner ear in cat. Ann Otol Rhinol Laryngol 1966; 75:752-763.

Warren EH III, Liberman MC. Effects of contralateral sound on auditory-nerve responses. I. Contributions of cochlear efferents. Hear Res 1989a; 37:89-104.

Warren EH III, Liberman MC. Effects of contralateral sound on auditory-nerve responses. II. Dependence on stimulus variables. Hear Res 1989b; 37:105-122.

Wilson JP, Johnstone JR. Basilar membrane and middle-ear vibration in guinea pig measured by capacitive probe. J Acoust Soc Am 1975; 57:705-723.

Wright A. Dimensions of the cochlear stereocilia in man and the guinea pig. Hear Res 1984; 13:89-98.

CHAPTER 8

Otoacoustic Emissions and Noise-Induced Hearing Loss

J. PATRICK WILSON

Otoacoustic emissions (OAEs) are an indication of mechanically-active mechanisms in the inner ear. The purpose of these mechanisms is to counteract the high level of mechanical damping provided by the structure and composition of the cochlea, thereby providing higher sensitivity and much greater frequency selectivity than would be possible in a purely passive system (Gold, 1948). It might be hypothesized from this that any of the influences that decrease hearing sensitivity or frequency selectivity do so by reducing the involvement of this active process, and thereby lead to a relative reduction of otoacoustic emissions. Such influences may be (1) simultaneous, i.e., occurring during, and not necessarily outlasting, the disturbing influence; (2) temporary, in which a certain period following the cessation of the disturbance is required for hearing to return to normal; or (3) permanent, in which hearing has been irreversibly impaired.

Because the literature on the effects of noise-induced hearing loss on otoacoustic emissions is rather limited, and on its own hard to interpret, all three types of influence will be considered in this chapter.

Simultaneous Influences

There are several ways in which otoacoustic emissions show susceptibilities that would not be expected in a linear system. These properties include (1) a nonlinear input-output function; (2) suppression of the response to one component by the presence of another; or (3) the generation of harmonics and intermodulation products, or "distortion products." In addition to these three major types of nonlinearity, there are some less readily explicable effects such as (4) frequency shifting and (5) remote suppression.

Nonlinear Input-Output Function

The nonlinear properties of otoacoustic emissions were recognized from the earliest report (Kemp, 1978); this property is so ubiquitous that it is used as a criterion for identifying an OAE and distinguishing it from a prolonged middle-ear response. This feature has, for example, been utilized in the IL088 Otodynamic Analyser, in which the linear component is automatically subtracted, leaving only the nonlinear component as the response. Various studies have shown slopes ranging from linearity (1 dB per decibel) to a nearly fully-saturated response (less than 0.1 dB per decibel). At intermediate levels (20 to 60 dB SPL), slopes of 0.3 to 0.7 dB per decibel are frequently found in man (Kemp, 1978; Rutten, 1980; Rutten and Buisman, 1983; Johnsen and Elberling, 1982; Norton and Neely, 1987). In studies that have extended below 20 dB SPL, a tendency towards a linear response can be observed (Wit and Ritsma, 1979; Wilson, 1980a; Grandori, 1983; Dallmayr, 1987). Comparison of different temporal parts of the response shows that the later part has a lower input-output slope and saturates more completely at a lower output level (Rutten, 1980; Wilson, 1980a; Grandori, 1985). Norton and Neely (1987) found no significant difference of slope for frequencies between 0.5 and 2 kHz, whereas Grandori (1985) stated that higher-frequency emissions are more linear. Grandori's statement is consistent with a more linear, early response if high-frequency components of the response occur first (Wilson, 1980a).

By combining two studies on a single ear at the same frequency it is possible to extend linearity measurements over a range of 130 dB. From the interference pattern produced by continuous tonal stimulation (Wilson, 1980c), it is calculated that the OAE remains at 2 to 4 dB below the stimulus from −46 dB to −26 dB using tone-burst stimulation (Wilson, 1980a). The response remained within ± 2 dB of the stimulus from −16 dB to +14 dB SPL, an overall near-linear range of 60 dB. From 24 to 84 dB SPL the response saturated at 20 ± 3 dB SPL.

A similar two-part curve was also observed in the guinea pig (Zwicker and Manley, 1981); in the the bat, *Pteronotus parnellii* (Kössl and Vater, 1985), with the break point shifted upwards by about 20 to 70 dB SPL; and in the starling (Manley et al, 1987), with the break point at 10 dB SPL. In the frog (Wilson et al, 1989) a slope of 0.5 dB per decibel was found with a tendency towards, but no clear region of, linearity or saturation.

Two significant comments can be made concerning the nonlinear input-output characteristics. First, they ensure that when spontaneous OAEs (SOAEs) occur they will be limited to a modest maximum level. The SOAE is viewed as an inevitable but undesirable property of system in which positive feedback is used to enhance sensitivity and selectivity. Unless the system is operated close to instability, however, little benefit will be obtained from it. By having significant deviations from linearity occur as low as 20 dB SPL, SOAEs will normally be limited to about this level. In practice, most SOAEs are below this level and inaudible to the subjects concerned. Conversely, the approach to linearity as level decreases also implies that SOAEs are unlikely to occur substantially below this level, because there would be no automatic self-limiting within a linear region.

Second, the role of the active mechanism in producing enhanced sensitivity and selectivity must be considered. If the saturated level of OAEs represents the maximum available energy output of the active mechanism, or cochlear amplifier, this would imply that it would have negligible influence at normal listening levels. To work effectively as a sharpening mechanism at any particular sound level, the cochlear amplifier would have to have a supply of energy comparable with that of the stimulus. It is known from a variety of studies that even though tuning may broaden somewhat at high stimulus levels, it is still sharper than the passive basilar membrane response. There would appear to be two ways of circumventing this objection: either the saturation of the OAE is not representative of saturation of the active process, or there must be some form of level normalization or automatic gain control preceding the active filter mechanism.

Wilson (1980b) and Sutton and Wilson (1983) suggested that OAEs arose from the incomplete cancellation of components summed from the whole cochlea when the cochlear array has some irregularity of place-frequency mapping or of sensitivity. In such a model, if the degree of irregularity becomes less marked at higher stimulus levels, the cancellation would become greater and the OAE would not increase at the same rate as the stimulus. This could account for the observed low saturation level without implying saturation of the cochlear amplifier at that level. If, however, the OAE level and hearing level are closely related as is described later, this would imply that the amplitude of OAEs is proportional to the involvement of the active process.

The alternative explanation of sharpening over a wide dynamic range is some form of automatic gain control in each channel preceding the active filter. This might take the form of a variable coupling element, perhaps provided by the interface between stereocilia and tectorial membrane. The attraction of this hypothesis is that if this were the physiologically vulnerable element in hearing, changes of sensitivity could occur without necessarily altering the tuning properties. If the active process itself were vulnerable, changes of sensitivity and selectivity would be intimately linked, so that a 6-dB loss of threshold would give rise to a halving of the Q-factor and a doubling of filter bandwidths. With variable coupling, the active mechanism would only be required to match the saturated level of input energy and would be protected from damage until the attenuated signal became excessive. Damage would be manifested as loss of tight coupling at low levels. The question arises as to whether such a variable coupling element would be bidirectional—apparently the simplest implementation. If the OAE has to pass through it in both directions, clearly any effects that this introduces will be doubled compared with direct measures of hearing. In the studies discussed more extensively later, Kemp (1982) found that temporary threshold shift (TTS) was about twice OAE changes (as measured in decibels); Zwicker (1983) found equal TTS and OAE changes; Zwicker and Scherer (1987) found that psychophysical changes were about 1.5 times OAE changes in a masking period paradigm; and Long and

Tubis (1988) found that OAE changes due to aspirin were about 1.5 times the psychophysical changes. The evidence, therefore, does not support a doubled effect on OAEs.

Suppression

The second type of simultaneous influence on the generation of OAEs is suppression of the response to a stimulus by another signal. Again, in a linear system this suppression would not occur. The most readily observed form of suppression is by a frequency component close to that of the response. By setting a certain criterion for suppression (e.g., by 3 dB), it becomes possible to define an isosuppression contour in the level-frequency domain. A number of studies have illustrated such curves (Kemp, 1979; Kemp and Chum, 1980; Wilson, 1980a; Schloth, 1981; Strack et al, 1981; Wilson and Sutton, 1981; Zurek and Clark, 1981; Rabinowitz and Widin, 1984; Baker et al, 1989; Bargones and Burns, 1988), which show similar bandwidths to auditory tuning curves obtained either psychoacoustically or physiologically. In general, however, maximal suppression is obtained for a tone slightly higher than the OAE frequency, the opposite to what would be anticipated from upward spread of masking. Although the effect is small, no explanation has yet been offered for it.

Studies of the growth of suppression with stimulus level (Kemp and Chum, 1980; Zurek, 1981; Rabinowitz and Widin, 1984) have shown that the effect is considerably more steep for frequencies below the OAE, or can be complex (Sutton, 1985). In general, the suppressive behaviors of click, tone-evoked, and spontaneous OAEs are similar. In the case of SOAEs, however, the situation is somewhat more complicated because a comparatively small reduction in the active process may be sufficient in some cases to stop oscillation, and because, when the stimulus is close to the SOAE frequency, it can lock it to the same frequency (Wilson and Sutton, 1981). Two further effects, remote suppression and frequency shifting, will be discussed separately later.

The fact that frequencies close to the OAE frequency are effective suppressors implies that suppression would also occur at the OAE frequency. This is an alternative way of looking at the nonlinear input-output function, because both effects depend on the same process. This is apparent in the similar low levels at which these effects occur.

Distortion Products

Distortion products (DPs) in hearing have long remained a fertile area for research in view of their unusual behavior. Two features have been of particular interest: (1) their level-independent behavior and existence down to low sound levels, and (2) their frequency-specific behavior, indicating an intimate connection with the process of frequency analysis. These properties are particularly apparent with the cubic difference tone (CDT), $2f_1 - f_2$, which has been most extensively researched (Wilson, 1980d). This component has also been extensively investigated in OAEs (CDTOAEs) and indicates that it has useful properties in the present context as a potential objective indicator of temporary or permanent hearing loss.

Attempts to confirm that audible DPs correspond with CDTOAEs have met with variable results. Wilson (1980d) found that CDTOAEs were strongest at frequencies at which $2f_1 - f_2$ corresponded with a strong single-tone emission frequency and corresponded approximately in level with that predicted from psychophysical cancellation levels attenuated and compressed by the OAE mechanism. Other studies have revealed different properties, indicating a second source for the CDTOAE in which the response appears not to depend on cochlear inhomogeneities, shows little delay (Kemp and Brown 1983a,b) and exhibits much less evidence of saturation (Martin et al, 1987; Lonsbury-Martin et al, 1987). The possible use of CDTOAEs in assessing short-term and permanent losses of hearing will be discussed later.

Frequency Shifting

It has been noticed that in an SOAE-suppression experiment, the effect of the "suppressor" may be to shift the frequency of the SOAE even at levels below that producing amplitude suppression (Wilson and Sutton, 1981; Rabinowitz and Widin, 1984; Kössl and Vater, 1985; Baker et al, 1989). Wilson et al (1988) have related this effect to a slight increase in the latency of individual features of the click-evoked OAE as a function of click level (Kemp and Chum, 1980; Wilson, 1980a; Grandori, 1985) to a decreasing OAE tuning frequency with level, to a decrease in the frequencies of ear-canal sound-pressure interference minima as a function of level, and to psychophysical changes of pitch with intensity (van den Brink, 1979; Verschuure and van Meeteren,

1975). These studies consistently show a decreasing tuning frequency, corresponding with an upward pitch shift, up to 60 dB SPL. Stevens' rule only applies above this level, where pitch then shifts downward for low frequencies and upward for high frequencies. There is not yet a satisfactory explanation for any of these frequency shift effects.

Remote Suppression

As discussed earlier, OAE suppression curves resemble psychoacoustic and neurophysiologic tuning curves. If, however, measurements are extended to regions more remote from the OAE frequency, a further lobe of suppression is sometimes found (Evans et al, 1981; Zurek, 1981; Wilson and Sutton, 1983). Care should be taken to ensure that this is true suppression rather than a byproduct of a frequency shift (Wilson and Sutton, 1983). An alternative method to investigate suppression is that adopted by Sutton (1985). Using FFTs of click responses with and without a suppressing tone, he observed that certain frequency regions were particularly susceptible to suppression even by a remote masking tone. He also found that curves sometimes crossed, indicating a decrease in OAE amplitude with stimulus level, probably implying cancellation from two different sites of generation. Remote suppression is interesting because it appears to indicate mechanical interaction over long distances, but again no explanation can yet be offered.

Temporary Influences

A number of influences are known to affect hearing; the ear normally recovers from them on a time scale that depends on the nature and strength of the disturbance. The corresponding changes to OAEs will be considered under the headings of the effects to which they appear to relate: (1) masking period patterns, (2) temporal suppression, (3) temporary threshold shift, (4) hypoxia, and (5) drug-induced changes. This is an area of study that shows the close link between OAEs and conventional measures of hearing.

Masking Period Patterns

The masking period pattern (MPP) technique measures the psychophysical threshold for a short test tone at various phases of a very low-frequency masker (Zwicker, 1977). The idea behind the technique is that the low-frequency masker produces quasistatic displacements to the basilar membrane, thereby biasing the operating point of the transduction process. In the corresponding measures on OAEs, the evoking stimulus is placed at various phases of the low-frequency suppressor to produce a suppression period pattern (SPP) (Zwicker and Manley, 1981) that corresponds with the MPP (Zwicker, 1981). Using three different masking or suppressing pressure functions based on a Gaussian impulse, Zwicker and Scherer (1987) were able to show excellent agreement between MPPs and SPPs. Maximum disturbance appeared to occur at the maximum positive value of the second derivative of the pressure waveform. Although the changes in MPP were slightly larger than SPP changes (3:2), this could be accounted for by the nonlinear behavior of OAEs. As the changes to MPP and SPP appear simultaneous with the changes in pressure waveform, it could be argued that these results should be considered simultaneous influences.

Temporal Suppression

In a click-evoked OAE, the response typically extends from 5 to 15 milliseconds after the stimulus. By adding a second click at various times before or after the stimulus it is possible to localize the time when maximum suppression occurs. Kemp and Chum (1980) used this technique with an alternating polarity for the suppressor so that neither this nor any response that it evokes would appear in the averaged response. The maximum suppressive effects of about 20 dB occurred when stimulus and suppressor coincided, dropping to 3 dB at about 6 milliseconds before or 3 milliseconds after the stimulus. These properties show strong similarities with forward and backward masking (Duifhuis, 1973).

Temporary Threshold Shift

A number of studies have shown that acoustic overstimulation that would normally give rise to temporary threshold shift (TTS) also reduces OAEs. Anderson and Kemp (1979) showed that OAEs in monkeys exposed to wideband noise for 20 minutes at 115 dBA were virtually abolished. Kim (1980) showed that exposure to 2,000 Hz at 90 dB SPL for 2 minutes in cats reduced the CDTOAE by about 7 dB, with partial recovery after 15 seconds. Following overstimulation, a period of enhancement and periodic frequency changes in an SOAE, in addition to the expected loss, were noted by Kemp (1981). Kemp (1982) found that tone overstimulation produced its greatest effect on OAEs at a frequency 0.6 octaves above the stimulus. Comparisons of OAE changes and TTS showed parallel courses, with the effect on OAEs generally being about 0.25 to 0.35 of the TTS, resulting in an exact agreement if allowance is made for an input-output slope of 0.3 dB per decibel for OAEs. Wilson and Evans (1983) measured an OAE at 2.33 kHz in a cat and found that white noise at 57 dB SPL per Hz for ½ minute produced a 4-dB loss that was recovered in 3 minutes. A 1.8-kHz tone at 103 dB SPL for 1 minute reduced the OAE by 18 dB, with substantial recovery over 10 minutes, whereas a 5-kHz tone at 110 dB SPL for 1 minute had little effect.

Zwicker (1983) compared the TTS at 1350 Hz produced by 20-minute exposure to a 40-Hz 112-dB SPL tone with the effects on OAEs and on the cancellation levels of CDTs. All three functions showed similar maximum shifts of 10 to 15 dB at 2 to 3 minutes and similar recoveries to the pre-exposure level after 10 minutes. Schmiedt (1986) compared the effects of half-octave bands of noise centered on 3.1 kHz on CDTOAEs and whole-nerve action potentials in cats and gerbils. Although absolute levels were different, the relative changes were similar, showing peak loss at 4 to 8 kHz. There were, however, discrepancies at some frequencies and between some of the rates of recovery. Lonsbury-Martin et al (1987) looked at the effects of tone overstimulation (2.83 kHz, 90 dB SPL, 45 minutes) on a number of distortion products in the rabbit. The CDT ($2f_1 - f_2$) showed consistent loss and recovery properties (apart from some overshoot at high frequencies); the maximal loss occurred at a frequency (2 to 3 kHz) that implicated the primary tone place, when allowance was made for the half-octave shift. The other distortion products ($2f_2 - f_1$ and $3f_2 - 2f_1$) behaved much less consistently, frequently showing an increase after stimulation. CDTOAEs were no different between the awake and anesthetized animals, and TTSs and recoveries were observed up to an hour postmortem. Martin et al (1987), in the same series of experiments, showed that suppression, an interfering tone, and tone overstimulation produced their maximal effects in the region of the primary tones, not at the CDT. Again, results for $2f_2 - f_1$ were much more variable, but pointed towards greatest sensitivity basal to the $2f_2 - f_1$ place.

Hypoxia

The effects of hypoxia in cats were noted by Kim (1980); a reversible reduction in CDTOAE was produced from about 1.25 minutes after clamping the trachea. Evans et al (1981) found that, 2 minutes after reducing the oxygen concentration to 5 percent, an SOAE and its electrical correlate in a guinea pig rapidly ceased and, about 2 minutes after restoration of oxygen level, suddenly recommenced with a 1- to 2-dB overshoot. Zwicker and Manley (1981), also in a guinea pig, found that an OAE at 2 kHz decreased at 30 to 60 seconds after induction of hypoxia, disappeared at 100 seconds, and started to return about 100 seconds after offset of hypoxia. Substantial recovery had occurred by 300 seconds, but was not complete even at 800 seconds. Although no direct comparisons were made these results correspond with single cochlear fiber properties.

Drug-Induced Changes

The first class of agents to consider is anesthetics. It is generally considered that normal anesthetic levels have no influence on cochlear function; this view is supported by a number of OAE studies. In practice, most human subjects are awake for measurements whereas, for purposes of restraint at least, most animal measurements are done under anesthetic. Lonsbury-Martin et al (1987) compared input-output curves in the rabbit for OAEs at $3f_1 - 2f_2$, $2f_1 - f_2$, and $2f_2 - f_1$ with and without anesthetic and found identical results under all conditions. On the other hand, in the bat, *Pteronotus parnellii,* Kössl and Vater (1985) found that Nembutal and halothane both decreased the amplitude and frequency of an OAE. Furthermore, during awakening, the amplitude of the OAE varied consistently with the behaviorally observed and evoked levels of arousal. There is, however, a considerable amount of evidence that in bats, the cochlea is sensitive to anesthesia, with even the cochlear microphonic showing differences (Pollak et al, 1972). In the starling, Manley et al (1987) also found that anesthetics (halothane, Nembutal, and Ketanest) reduced OAEs, but in the case of halothane, OAE recovery (50 percent in 200 seconds) was slower than the behavioral recovery of the birds (15 seconds). Undoubtedly, there are species differences in the effects of anesthetic. In the case of frogs, Whitehead et al (1986) used various anesthetics purely for restraint and continued recording SOAEs until the frog moved away from the recording microphone, often many minutes after regaining consciousness. In every case, when corrected for temperature, the SOAEs did not vary in amplitude or frequency with anesthetic or arousal level.

A large number of studies have shown changes in OAE corresponding with their known or measured effects on hearing of ototoxic drugs. Anderson and Kemp (1979) found in monkeys that ethacrynic acid (55 mg per kilogram IV) reduced the OAE by 15 dB to background noise level 16 minutes after injection; recovery started at 45 minutes and was complete by 19 hours. Furosemide (40 mg per kilogram IV) caused a substantial reduction after 2 minutes, maximal effect at 4 minutes, and considerable recovery by 30 minutes. Wilson and Evans (1983) found that in the cat furosemide (37 mg per kilogram IV) abolished the OAE after 1 minute; considerable recovery occurred by 23 minutes, but with a somewhat different response pattern. On the other hand, Flaxedil (30 mg per kilogram IV) a muscle relaxant, had no effect. Aspirin has been tested in several studies. Johnsen and Elberling (1982), testing a human subject (10 g every 24 hours, oral), found that the psychophysical threshold to clicks and the pseudothreshold for OAEs were each raised by 15 dB, with full recovery for both after 2 days. McFadden and Plattsmier (1984), also testing human subjects, gave a total dose of 15.6 g distributed over 3.75 days and observed its influence on SOAEs. Small emissions went within 14 to 20 hours of the start of aspirin intake, whereas large emissions sometimes took several days. Recovery was more erratic, taking from one to several days independent of the initial emission size. These authors seemed surprised that their lower dose rate should completely abolish all SOAEs, whereas the click-evoked OAEs of Johnsen and Elberling were merely "diminished." This, of course, is not surprising in a feedback oscillator in which, with marginal gain, a small loss could cause the system to cease to oscillate. Conversely, if the system has excessive gain and a strongly saturating nonlinearity, stable oscillation could be maintained with considerable decreases in the gain factor. Both of these effects were seen in the study of Long and Tubis (1988), who used the same dose rate, although clearly from their results the situation is more complicated. In many cases, aspirin appeared to enhance hearing before threshold elevation occurred, with a corresponding enhancement phase during recovery. In some subjects, at some frequencies, a consistent enhancement was found. Long and Tubis interpret this as being due to the release from the masking produced by an SOAE after it is abolished; they model this effect with a Van der Pol oscillator. Taking these factors into account, there appears to be consistent agreement between hearing and the degree of involvement of the active mechanism.

Permanent Hearing Loss

Kemp (1978) investigated 25 cases of sensorineural hearing loss with normal middle-ear function and found that the OAE was reduced and became unmeasurable when the hearing loss exceeded 30 dB. Four subjects with immobile middle ears also failed to exhibit the phenomenon. Rutten (1980) found that the hearing loss at a specific frequency had to be less than 15 dB for an OAE to be found at that frequency. Bonfils et al (1988) reported that OAEs could not be observed in patients with senorineural hearing loss when subjective click threshold exceeded 30 dB HL. Although two studies (Kollmeier and Uppenkamp, 1989; Tanaka, 1988) have implied that OAEs were present for losses considerably exceeding 30 dB, neither study gives any indication that strict criteria were applied to exclude late, low-level components of the middle-ear response.

In many cases, SOAEs have been found at frequencies associated with irregularities in the audiogram. Wilson and Sutton (1981) reported several cases in which SOAEs were found in a region of normal hearing adjacent to a region with elevated threshold, and suggested that the active mechanism might be enhanced by such an edge effect. This idea was further developed by Ruggero et al (1983) when they suggested that a normally active region of the basilar membrane damps the neighboring regions and fails to do so when the active mechanism breaks down. In fact, not all data fit this picture because sometimes the SOAEs appear to originate from the pathologic region. There are, however, two ways in which this might occur. Firstly, the frequency of an SOAE actually from the intact region may be modified by the adjacent pathologic region; secondly, the elevation of threshold might represent psychophysical masking by the SOAE.

Glanville et al (1971) investigated three members of a family emitting whistles from their ears. These whistles proved to have an enormous number of frequency components, but significantly, in three ears, the strongest component (5.6 to 8 kHz) corresponded with an audiographic notch of 50 to 60 dB SPL. Wilson and Sutton (1983) reinvestigated two of these subjects and were able to confirm that their emissions behaved like SOAEs, although their amplitudes had decreased from 55 to 60 dB SPL to 40 to 45 dB SPL. Although masking by the SOAEs appeared plausible as an explanation for the audiogram notches, the spectra and their predicted masking patterns did not exactly agree with the audiograms. Huizing and Spoor (1973) reported a subject with an emission at 3.5 kHz, now presumed to be an SOAE, adjacent to an audiogram dip at 4 kHz.

In a study on chinchillas, Zurek and Clark (1981) found that none of 22 ears of 15 animals raised in a sound-shielded colony had an SOAE, whereas after sustained exposure to loud sound, two ears produced SOAEs. The first animal's emission was sensitive to suppression and occurred either between 4.6 and 4.73 kHz or between 5.68 and 5.88 kHz. In the other animal, the SOAE frequency would suddenly jump within the range 6.47 to 6.68 kHz. A behavioral audiogram showed a permanent threshold shift for every frequency *except* 6.7 kHz, and histology later revealed a punctate region of hair-cell loss at 7 kHz. Lesions were, however, also found at another point near the center of the cochlea and in the apical region. Furthermore, the three other exposed ears also exhibited punctate basal lesions; thus, their existance is not a sufficient condition for generation of SOAEs.

Ruggero et al (1983) found an SOAE at 7.53 kHz in a region of elevated threshold extending from 4 kHz and becoming particularly prominent at a frequency just below it, at 7 kHz. Ruggero et al (1984) investigated a dog with a strong SOAE of 59 dB SPL at 9.1 kHz in one ear and a four-component SOAE in the other ear (9.4 to 10.9 kHz). Brain-stem audiometry indicated a sudden transition from presumed normal to abnormal hearing between 7 and 8 kHz and a further loss to 10 kHz. In this case, as in the human case of Glanville et al (1971) and Wilson and Sutton (1983), the SOAE lies in the pathologic region, although this again may merely represent masking by the SOAE. Suppression of the SOAE was greatest for lower frequencies, contrary to most of the cases discussed earlier.

Finally, a different approach to the relation between hearing level and OAEs is provided by mutant mice. Horner et al (1985) investigated two types of mice with normal hearing and four types of hearing-impaired mutants. In the normal mice, the CDTOAE was 20 to 25 dB below the primaries (f_1 and f_2) at 60 to 100 dB SPL. In hearing-impaired mutants, the results depended on the type of dysfunction. In *deafness* and *viable dominant spotting* mutants, in which the cochlea is severely disrupted, no CDTOAEs could be detected. The *quivering* mutant, however, in which the dysfunction is central, showed normal CDTOAEs. The *Bronx Waltzer* mutant, in which the outer hair cells appear normal but the inner hair cells are reduced in number, showed detectable but reduced CDTOAEs.

From all the results considered in this chapter it is clear that there is a close, if not exact, correspondence between hearing level and otoacoustic emission. Both stimulus frequency and CDT emissions can provide sensitive monitors of changes in hearing, even though absolute levels may not be reliable indicators of absolute hearing level. OAE data also provide informative constraints to modeling cochlear function, and appear to suggest that the active process might not be the primary site of physiological vulnerability. Clearly this is an important matter to be resolved.

Oto-Emissions Acoustiques et Déficits Audities

Un processus d'amplification mécanique existe dans la cochlée afin de maîtriser son amortissement mécanique. Il en résulte une sensibilité augmentée et une analyse spectrale fine. Dans un système simple ces mesures seraient directement reliées. Il existe, cependant, une dissociation évidente entre les seuils auditifs et la largeur de bande du filtre. Néanmoins il apparaît qu'une perte de sensibilité auditive est due à une réduction du processus d'amplification. Le phénomène d'oto-émission acoustique (OAE) est un sous-produit de l'amplification mécanique. Cette hypothèse est basée sur le fait que plusieurs manipulations connues pour avoir une influence sur le seuil auditif, influencent les oto-émissions acoustiques de la même façon. Cela inclut les pertes auditives neurosensorielles de tous types qui ont été étudiées, la fatigue auditive, le masquage simultané ou anticipé, la courbe de masquage périodique et les effets de l'hypoxie et des drogues ototoxiques. Ces effets ont été observés largement dans les études sur l'homme et sur l'animal. De telles recherches ont utilisé comme critère une réduction des oto-émissions provoquées par des clics ou sons brefs, les oto-émissions par produit de distorsion, une réduction ou une suppression des oto-émissions spontanées. Il existe cependant des phénomènes qui apparaissent pour compliquer le problème tels que le développement des oto-émissions spontanées apres la surstimulation sonore, et des observations fréquentes d'oto-émissions acoustiques à la limite entre une zone normale et une zone pathologique de la gamme auditive. Ces découvertes ne sont pas toutefois en contradiction avec certains types de modèles concernant les mécanismes des oto-émissions. Il est suggéré que l'allure des changements des oto-émissions acoustiques, pourrait constituer un indicateur sensible et objectif des tous premiers stades des déficits auditifs induits par le bruit.

References

Anderson SD, Kemp DT. The evoked cochlear mechanical response in laboratory primates. Arch Otolaryngol 1979; 224:47-54.

Baker RJ, Wilson JP, Whitehead ML. Otoacoustic evidence for nonlinear behaviour in frogs' hearing: suppression but no distortion products. In: Wilson JP, Kemp DT, eds. Cochlear mechanisms: Structure, function, and models. New York: Plenum, 1989:349.

Bargones JY, Burns EM. Suppression tuning curves for spontaneous otoacoustic emissions in infants and adults. J Acoust Soc Am 1988; 83:1809-1816.

Bonfils P, Bertrand Y, Uziel A. Evoked otoacoustic emissions: Normative data and presbycusis. Audiology 1988; 27:27-35.

van den Brink G. Intensity and pitch. Acustica 1979; 41:271-273.

Dallmayr C. Stationary and dynamical properties of simultaneous evoked otoacoustic emissions (SEOAE). Acustica 1987; 63:243-255.

Duifhuis H. Consequences of peripheral frequency selectivity for non-simultaneous masking. J Acoust Soc Am 1973; 54:1471-1488.

Evans EF, Wilson JP, Borerwe TA. Animal models of tinnitus. In: Evered D, Lawrenson G, eds. Tinnitus. London: Pitman, 1981:108.

Glanville JD, Coles RRA, Sullivan BM. A family with high-tonal objective tinnitus. J Laryngol Otol 1971; 85:1-10.

Gold T. Hearing. II. The physical basis of the action of the cochlea. Proc R Soc [B] 1948; 135:492-498.

Grandori F. Evoked oto-acoustic emissions stimulus-response relationships. Rev Laryngol 1983; 104:153-155.

Grandori F. Nonlinear phenomena in click- and tone-burst-evoked otoacoustic emissions from human ears. Audiology 1985; 24:71-80.

Horner KC, Lenoir M, Bock GR. Distortion product otoacoustic emissions in hearing-impaired mutant mice. J Acoust Soc Am 1985; 78:1603-1611.

Huizing EH, Spoor A. An unusual type of tinnitus. Production of a high tone by the ear. Arch Otolaryngol 1973; 98:134-136.

Johnsen NJ, Elberling C. Evoked acoustic emissions from the human ear. I. Equipment and response parameters. Scand Audiol 1982; 11:3-12.

Kemp DT. Stimulated acoustic emissions from within the human auditory system. J Acoust Soc Am 1978; 64:1386-1391.

Kemp DT. Evidence of mechanical nonlinearity and frequency selective wave amplification in the cochlea. Arch Otorhinolaryngol 1979; 224:37-45.

Kemp DT. Physiologically active cochlear micromechanics—one source of tinnitus. In: Evered D, Lawrenson G, eds. Tinnitus. London: Pitman, 1981:54.

Kemp DT. Cochlear echoes: implications for noise-induced hearing loss. In: Hamernik RP, Henderson D, Salvi RJ, eds. New perspectives on noise-induced hearing loss. New York: Raven Press, 1982:189.

Kemp DT, Brown AM. A comparison of mechanical nonlinearities in the cochlea of man and gerbil from ear canal measurements. In: Klinke R, Hartmann R, eds. Hearing—physiological bases and psychophysics. Berlin, Springer, 1983a:82.

Kemp DT, Brown AM. An integrated view of cochlear mechanical nonlinearities observable from the ear canal. In: de Boer E, Viergever MA, eds. Mechanics of hearing. Delft, The Netherlands: Delft University Press, 1983b.

Kemp DT, Chum R. Properties of the generator of stimulated acoustic emissions. Hear Res 1980; 2:213-232.

Kim DO. Cochlear mechanics: Implications of electrophysiological and acoustical observations. Hear Res 1980; 2:297-317.

Kollmeier B, Uppenkamp S. Analysis and influence of lidocaine on evoked otoacoustic emissions from tinnitus sufferers. In: Wilson JP, Kemp DT, eds. Cochlear mechanisms—structure, function, and models. New York: Plenum, 1989:331.

Kossl M, Vater M. Evoked acoustic emissions and cochlear microphonics in the mustache bat, Pteronotus parnellii. Hear Res 1985; 19:157-170.

Long GR, Tubis A. Modification of spontaneous and evoked otoacoustic emissions and associated psychoacoustic microstructure by aspirin consumption. J Acoust Soc Am 1988; 84:1343-1353.

Lonsbury-Martin BL, Martin GK, Probst R, Coats AC. Acoustic distortion products in rabbit ear canal. I. Basic features and physiological vulnerability. Hear Res 1987; 28:173-189.

Manley GA, Schulze M, Oekinghaus H. Otoacoustic emissions in a song bird. Hear Res 1987; 26:257-266.

Martin GK, Lonsbury-Martin BL, Probst R, Scheinin SA, Coats AC. Acoustic distortion products in rabbit ear canal. I. Sites of origin revealed by suppression contours and pure-tone exposures. Hear Res 1987; 28:191-208.

McFadden D, Plattsmier HS. Aspirin abolishes spontaneous oto-acoustic emissions. J Acoust Soc Am 1984; 76:443-448.

Norton SJ, Neely ST. Tone-burst-evoked otoacoustic emissions from normal-hearing subjects. J Acoust Soc Am 1987; 81:1860-1872.

Pollak G, Henson OW Jr, Novick A. Cochlear microphonic audiograms in the "pure tone" bat, Chilonycteris parnellii parnellii. Science 1972; 176: 66-68.

Rabinowitz WM, Widin GP. Interaction of spontaneous oto-acoustic emissions and external sounds. J Acoust Soc Am 1984; 76:1713-1720.

Ruggero MA, Kramek B, Rich NC. Spontaneous oto-acoustic emissions in a dog. Hear Res 1984; 13:293-296.

Ruggero MA, Rich NC, Freyman R. Spontaneous and impulsively evoked otoacoustic emissions: Indicators of cochlear pathology? Hear Res 1983; 10:283-300.

Rutten WLC. Evoked acoustic emissions from within normal and abnormal human ears: comparison with audiometric and electrophysiological findings. Hear Res 1980; 2:263-271.

Rutten WLC, Buisman HP. Critical behaviour of auditory oscillators near feedback phase transitions. In: de Boer E, Viergever MA, eds. Mechanics of hearing. Delft, The Netherlands: Delft University Press, 1983:91.

Schloth E. Relation between spectral composition of spontaneous oto-acoustic emissions and fine structure of threshold in quiet. Acustica 1983; 53:250-256.

Schmiedt RA. Acoustic distortion in the ear canal. I. Cubic difference tones: effects of acute noise injury. J Acoust Soc Am 1986; 79:1481-1490.

Strack G, Klinke R, Wilson JP. Evoked cochlear response in caiman crocodilus. Pflug Arch Suppl 1981; 391:R43.

Sutton GJ. Suppression effects in the spectrum of evoked oto-acoustic emissions. Acustica 1985; 58:57-63.

Sutton GJ, Wilson JP. Modelling cochlear echoes: The influence of irregularities in frequency mapping on summed cochlear activity. In: de Boer E, Viergever MA, eds. Mechanics of hearing. Delft, The Netherlands: Delft University Press, 1983:83.

Tanaka Y. Stimulated otoacoustic emissions from ears with sensorineural hearing loss. Proc Jap Acad 1988; 648:201-204.

Veschuure J, van Meeteren A. The effects of intensity on pitch. Acustica 1975; 32:33-43.

Whitehead ML, Wilson JP, Baker RJ. The effects of temperature on otoacoustic emission tuning properties. In: Moore BCJ, Patterson RD, eds. Auditory frequency selectivity. New York: Plenum, 1986:39.

Wilson JP. Evidence for a cochlear origin for acoustic re-emissions, threshold fine-structure and tonal tinnitus. Hear Res 1980a; 2:233-252.

Wilson JP. Model for cochlear echoes and tinnitus based on an observed electrical correlate. Hear Res 1980b; 2:527-532.

Wilson JP. Subthreshold mechanical activity within the cochlea. J Physiol 1980c; 298:32-33P.

Wilson JP. The combination tone, 2f1-f2, in psychophysics and ear-canal recording. In: van den Brink G, Bilsen FA, eds. Psychophysical, physiological and behavioural studies in hearing. Delft, The Netherlands, Delft University Press, 1980d:43.

Wilson JP, Baker RJ, Whitehead ML. Level dependence of frequency tuning in human ears. In: Duifhuis H, Horst JW, Wit HP, eds. Basic issues in hearing. London: Academic, 1988:80.

Wilson JP, Baker RJ, Whitehead ML. Otoacoustic emissions in frogs. Adv Audiol 1990; 7:47-56.

Wilson JP, Evans EF. Effects of furosemide, Flaxedil, noise and tone over-stimulation on the evoked otoacoustic emission in cat. Proc Int Union Physiol Sci 1983; 15:100.

Wilson JP, Sutton GJ. Acoustic correlates of tonal tinnitus. In: Evered D, Lawrenson G, eds. Tinnitus. London: Pitman Medical, 1981:82.

Wilson JP, Sutton GJ. "A family with high-tonal objective tinnitus"—an update. In: Klinke R, Hartmann R, eds. Hearing—physiological bases and psychophysics. Berlin, Springer, 1983:97.

Wit HP, Ritsma RJ. Stimulated acoustic emissions from the human ear. J Acoust Soc Am 1979; 66:911-913.

Zurek PM. Spontaneous narrowband acoustic signals emitted by the human ear. J Acoust Soc Am 1981; 69:514-523.

Zurek PM, Clark WW. Narrow-band acoustic signals emitted by chinchilla ears after noise exposure. J Acoust Soc Am 1981; 70:446-450.

Zwicker E. Masking-period patterns produced by very-low-frequency maskers and their possible relation to basilar-membrane displacement. J Acoust Soc Am 1977; 61:1031-1040.

Zwicker E. Masking-period patterns and cochlear acoustical responses. Hear Res 1981; 4:195-202.

Zwicker E. On peripheral processing in human hearing. In: Klinke R, Hartmann R, eds. Hearing—physiological bases and psychophysics. Berlin, Springer, 1983:104.

Zwicker E, Manley G. Acoustical responses and suppression-period patterns in guinea pigs. Hear Res 1981; 4:43-52.

Zwicker E, Scherer A. Correlation between time functions of sound pressure, masking, and OAE suppression. J Acoust Soc Am 1987; 81:1043-1049.

CHAPTER 9

Otoacoustic Emissions and Noise-Induced Hearing Loss: Human Studies

D.O. KIM
GERALD LEONARD
JACEK SMURZYNSKI
MARJORIE D. JUNG

Theories about cochlear mechanics have undergone major revisions during the 1970s and 1980s. The issues of the linearity versus nonlinearity and the tuning sharpness of cochlear-partition motion were often debated (Rhode, 1971; Wilson and Johnstone, 1975; Evans and Wilson, 1973; Kim et al, 1973; Kim and Molnar, 1975). The discovery of click-evoked otoacoustic emissions (CEOAEs) by Kemp (1978) occurred during this period. In the subsequent few years, other forms of otoacoustic emissions (OAEs) were also found: distortion-product otoacoustic emissions (DPOAEs) with two-tone stimulation (Kemp, 1979; Kim, 1980), stimulus-frequency otoacoustic emissions (SFOAEs) with continuous pure-tone stimulation (Kemp and Chum, 1980), and spontaneous otoacoustic emissions (SOAEs) (Kemp, 1979; Wilson, 1980; Zurek, 1981). These observations of the OAEs played an important role in supporting nonlinear cochlear theories because the OAEs demonstrated prominent nonlinear behavior. Soon thereafter, by using improved measurement methods, Rhode (1978), Sellick et al (1982), Khanna and Leonard (1982), and Robles et al (1986) demonstrated sharp tuning and nonlinear behavior in the motion of the cochlear partition.

Gold proposed an active cochlear hypothesis in 1948. The observation of prominent SOAEs three decades later provided a major support for active cochlear models that contains internal energy sources (Kim et al, 1980; Neely and Kim, 1983, 1986; Davis, 1983; Zwicker, 1986a,b; Geisler, 1986; Tubis et al, 1989). The active cochlear models postulate that cochlear-partition damping is reduced by an internal energy source. These active models demonstrated an amplification of cochlear mechanical response and a sharpening of frequency tuning. An emerging current concept is that the cochlear mechanical system is both active and nonlinear, reflecting saturation of an active positive feedback (Zwicker, 1986a,b; Neely, 1988).

According to several lines of reasoning, the outer hair cells (OHCs) are believed to be the source of both active and nonlinear behavior of the cochlea (Kim, 1984). Evidence in support of the possible active-nonlinear *mechanical* role of OHCs was provided by the observation that activation of the crossed olivocochlear efferent fibers affected ear-canal acoustic signals (Mountain, 1980; Siegel and Kim, 1982; Guinan, 1986; Kemp and Souter, 1988). These observations implicated a biomechanical role for OHCs, because the efferent fibers make large synaptic contacts directly with the soma of OHCs and not with the soma of IHCs. OHC motility was discovered in the mid-1980s by direct observation of isolated OHCs in vitro under electrical or chemical stimulation (Brownell et al, 1985; Zenner et al, 1985). Subsequent studies have provided further information about OHC motility (Flock et al, 1986; Ashmore, 1987; Santos-Sacchi, 1989; Brundin et al, 1989).

The experimental and theoretical studies cited above suggest the following hypothesis about cochlear mechanism: the active-nonlinear motile mechanism of OHCs amplifies cochlear partition motion 100 to 1,000 times (40 to 60 dB) and, as a byproduct, produces various forms of OAEs. This hypothesis predicts that damage of OHCs in a region of the cochlea should lead to (1) an elevation of hearing threshold (up to 40 to 60 dB) for frequencies corresponding to the damaged region; and (2) a reduction or elimination of nonlinear response such as DPOAEs for stimulus frequencies falling in the damaged region. Observations of SOAEs suggest the following related hypothesis: the generation of SOAEs requires two conditions: (1) the presence of an intact active-nonlinear OHC mechanism in certain regions of the cochlea; and (2) a spatial irregularity of the distribution of the OHC active-nonlinear mechanism. The goal of this chapter is to review studies of the effects of noise-induced and other sensorineural hearing loss on DPOAEs, CEOAEs, and SOAEs, and to evaluate the above hypotheses with observations. This chapter also presents some new OAE data from subjects with noise-induced hearing loss and compares them with results from subjects with normal hearing.

Studies of OAEs as a Test of Human Cochlear Function

In recent years, a number of studies of OAEs have been conducted toward the goal of developing a clinically useful, objective, and noninvasive test of human cochlear function (Cianfrone and Grandori, 1986; Grandori et al, 1990). In general, these studies demonstrated that CEOAEs and DPOAEs were reduced or eliminated in ears that had significant sensorineural hearing loss. We discuss details about the DPOAEs and CEOAEs in the following.

Distortion-Product Otoacoustic Emissions (DPOAEs)

When two tones at frequencies f_1 and f_2 (f_1 is less than f_2) are applied to a normal ear, distortion products at one or more frequencies are observed in the ear canal, with the $2f_1 - f_2$ component being the strongest in general. Thus, our use of the term DPOAE generally refers to the $2f_1 - f_2$ distortion product. Several recent studies have described DPOAE behavior in human ears with normal hearing or sensorineural hearing loss (Kemp et al, 1986; Furst et al, 1988; Harris et al, 1989; Leonard et al, 1990; Lonsbury-Martin et al, 1990; Smurzynski et al, 1990; Kimberley and Nelson, 1990).

Figure 9-1A shows conventional pure-tone audiograms of the two ears of a subject (No. 35) with bilateral noise-induced hearing loss. Figure 9-1B illustrates DPOAE behavior from these two ears in comparison with the normal range. These are previously unpublished data of our study. Details about our experimental methods were described in Smurzynski et al (1990). The triangles in Figure 9-1B show the $2f_1 - f_2$ DPOAE level versus geometric mean of f_1 and f_2, where f_1 and f_2 were varied together while maintaining the $f_2 : f_1$ ratio constant at 1:2. Such a measure is called the "DPOE audiogram." Data in part B were obtained with an ER-10B (Etymotic Research) acoustic probe. In part B, a solid line with two surrounding dotted lines represent the mean ± one standard deviation of the DPOAE level among a group of normally-hearing adults; details about the normally-hearing group are given in the caption of Figure 9-1. The dashed line near the bottom of part B, which corresponds to the mean plus one standard deviation of multiple measurements of DPOAE level in a test cavity, represents the lower limit of DPOAE level detectable by the measurement system. The DPOAE audiograms of the two ears (see Fig. 9-1B) resemble the conventional pure-tone audiograms (see Fig. 9-1A), with both sets exhibiting notches in the 4- to 6-kHz region. These results support our view that the DPOAE method is able to provide frequency-specific information about cochlear function. In a region below approximately 1200 Hz, the DPOAE levels of these two ears are slightly higher than are the DPOAE levels of the normal range; we do not have an explanation for this.

The DPOAEs in subjects with noise-induced hearing loss were also investigated by Martin et al (1990a). Their observations, consistent with our data in Figure 9-1, also demonstrated frequency-specific reduction of DPOAE for stimulus frequencies corresponding to hearing impairment. Further observations of input-output functions of DPOAEs (i.e., DPOAE level versus stimulus level) in a subject with noise-induced hearing loss were reported by Smurzynski et al (1990, Fig. 2, subject No. 13). They showed that, when the stimulus frequencies fell in an impaired region, detection of DPOAEs required higher stimulus levels than were required for a normal ear. When the hearing impairment was severe, DPOAEs could not be elicited at the

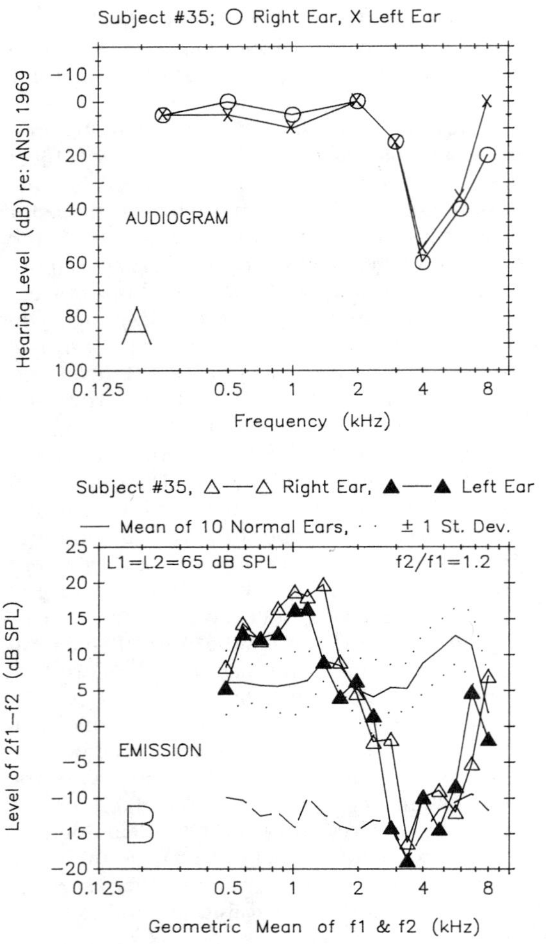

Figure 9-1 *A*, Conventional pure-tone audiograms for the two ears of a human adult with bilateral noise-induced hearing loss; Subject No. 35: male, age 31 years, recreational shooter. *B*, DPOAE audiogram showing $2f_1 - f_2$ DPOAE level versus geometric mean of f_1 and f_2 where f_1 and f_2 were varied with $f_2/f_1 = 1.2$. The data were obtained with an ER-10B probe. The solid line and two surrounding dotted lines represent the normal range as the mean ± one standard deviation among a group of 10 normal human adult ears aged 22 to 29 years who had hearing thresholds of 10 dB hearing level (HL) or better at all standard audiometric frequencies.

highest stimulus levels tested (80 dB SPL re 20 μPa).

Lonsbury-Martin et al (1990) observed that DPOE detection thresholds for stimulus frequencies in the 6- to 8-kHz region were correlated with age among normally hearing young adults; DPOAE detection thresholds were increased for older subjects by about 20 dB in the 18- to 30-year age range. Because the behavioral pure-tone audiometric thresholds of these subjects were all normal (10 dB HL or better), this finding suggests that DPOAEs may be a more sensitive indicator of dysfunction of OHC biomechanical mechanism than the pure-tone audiogram.

The OHC active-nonlinear biomechanical hypothesis predicts that, if OHC mechanisms are impaired in various diseases (such as acoustic trauma, Meniere's disease, hereditary disorders, infections of the ear, and ototoxic effects), these pathologic conditions should all exhibit reduced (or eliminated) DPOAEs. The existing observations are consistent with this hypothesis in that a number of subjects who had sensorineural hearing loss of various etiologies showed a similar characteristic of reduction in DPOAE level for stimulus frequencies falling in the hearing impairment region (Kemp et al, 1986; Leonard et al, 1990; Lonsbury-Martin and Martin, 1990).

A general picture emerges from these studies of DPOAEs: (1) the DPOAE signal can be reliably measured in human ears, although the DPOAE level is considerably lower in human subjects than in laboratory animals; the reason for this human versus animal difference in DPOE level is not well understood now; (2) intersubject and intrasubject variabilities of DPOAEs among human ears appear to be sufficiently small to allow the development of a clinically useful test of cochlear function based on DPOAEs; (3) in ears afflicted with noise-induced hearing loss, DPOAEs are reduced (or eliminated) when two-tone stimulus frequencies fall within a hearing-impairment region, thus providing sensitive and frequency-specific information about cochlear dysfunction; and (4) DPOAEs are similarly reduced (or eliminated) in ears with sensorineural hearing loss of various etiologies that affect cochlear function.

Click-Evoked Otoacoustic Emissions (CEOAEs)

Among various forms of OAEs, the CEOAEs have been the most widely investigated; references can be found in the conference proceedings cited above. Figure 9-2A illustrates the CEOAE of a normally hearing human adult ear measured with an ILO-88 system developed by Kemp (Kemp et al, 1990). This is a typical CEOAE pattern, exhibiting a damped oscillatory "cochlear echo" response waveform lasting for about 10 to 15 msec following a click stimulation. The spectrum of the cochlear response (upper-right inset in Fig. 9-2A) has a complex pattern, exhibiting peaks and notches. The complex CEOAE spectrum is idiosyncratic, like a fingerprint, with the spectral notches occurring even in frequency regions of normal hearing. Possible interpretations of the idiosyncratic CEOAE patterns have been discussed in the literature (Kemp, 1986), but quantitative modeling of the complex spectral patterns of CEOAEs is not available yet.

Figure 9-2B and C show CEOAEs in the same two ears affected with noise-induced hearing loss represented in Figure 9-1. The CEOAEs of these ears exhibited spectral contents only at low frequencies below 2.0 or 2.5 kHz as seen in the spectrum at the upper-right insets of Figure 2B and C. These CEOAE patterns roughly resemble the pure-tone audiograms of these ears (severe hearing loss in the 4- to 6-kHz region, Fig. 9-1A) in the sense that spectral components of the CEOAE are absent above 2.5 kHz. However, the CEOAE data did not provide information about the hearing function for the 6- to 8-kHz region. These examples of CEOAEs illustrate that it is difficult to predict the pure-tone audiometric patterns entirely from the CEOAE data.

The CEOAE spectral components in the 1-kHz region of these two ears (Fig. 9-2B and C) are slightly higher than normal (Fig. 9-2A). This behavior appears to be correlated with the same ears' higher-than-normal DPOAE level in the 1-kHz region (Fig. 9-1B). We postulate that in the 1-kHz region of these ears, the OHC biomechanical mechanism might be hyperactive. It is not known whether these ears had SOAEs in the 1-kHz region, because the SOAEs were not tested in these ears.

A number of studies were reported in the literature for CEOAEs in subjects with normal hearing or sensorineural hearing loss, including subjects with noise-induced hearing loss (Bonfils et al, 1988; Bonfils and Uziel, 1989; Kemp et al, 1990). The findings of these studies are consistent with the results shown in Figure 9-2. In addition, it was found that ears with mean audiometric thresholds higher than about 25 to 35 dB HL did not exhibit detectable CEOAEs (Kemp et al, 1986; Probst et al, 1987; Bonfils et al, 1988).

From observations described in Figures 9-1 and 9-2 as well as other observations in the literature, it appears that the DPOAE method can provide information about human cochlear function with greater frequency specificity. The CEOAE measurement, however, should also be useful for quick screening of cochlear function, e.g., for infants and young children (Johnsen et al, 1983; Norton and Widen, 1990; Stevens et al, 1990), because it can be accomplished more quickly than the DPOAE measurement.

Spontaneous Otoacoustic Emissions (SOEs)

Among normally hearing human ears, SOAEs are commonly observed in 30 to 50 percent (Kemp, 1979; Wilson, 1980; Zurek, 1981, 1985; Wier et al, 1984; Martin et al, 1990b). Among nonhuman primates (presumably with normal hearing), 3 of 122 ears (2.5 percent) exhibited SOAEs (Martin et al, 1985). Among nonprimate laboratory animals such as chinchillas, the occurrence of SOAEs is rare; none of 28 normal ears of chinchillas exhibited SOAEs, but 2 of these 28 ears did exhibit SOAEs after exposure to noise (Zurek and Clark, 1981; Clark et al, 1984). Histologic examinations of these chinchilla ears exhibiting SOAEs revealed a punctate lesion of the organ of Corti located at a place closely corresponding to an SOAE frequency (Clark et al, 1984). Another study suggested that a sharp border between intact and damaged regions of the organ of Corti may have given rise to an SOAE in a dog's ear (Ruggero et al, 1984). These studies lead to the hypothesis that generation of SOAEs in nonprimate animals requires the following conditions: (1) functional disruption of a normally present control for the OHC biomechanical mechanism in a region of the cochlea; and (2) the presence of

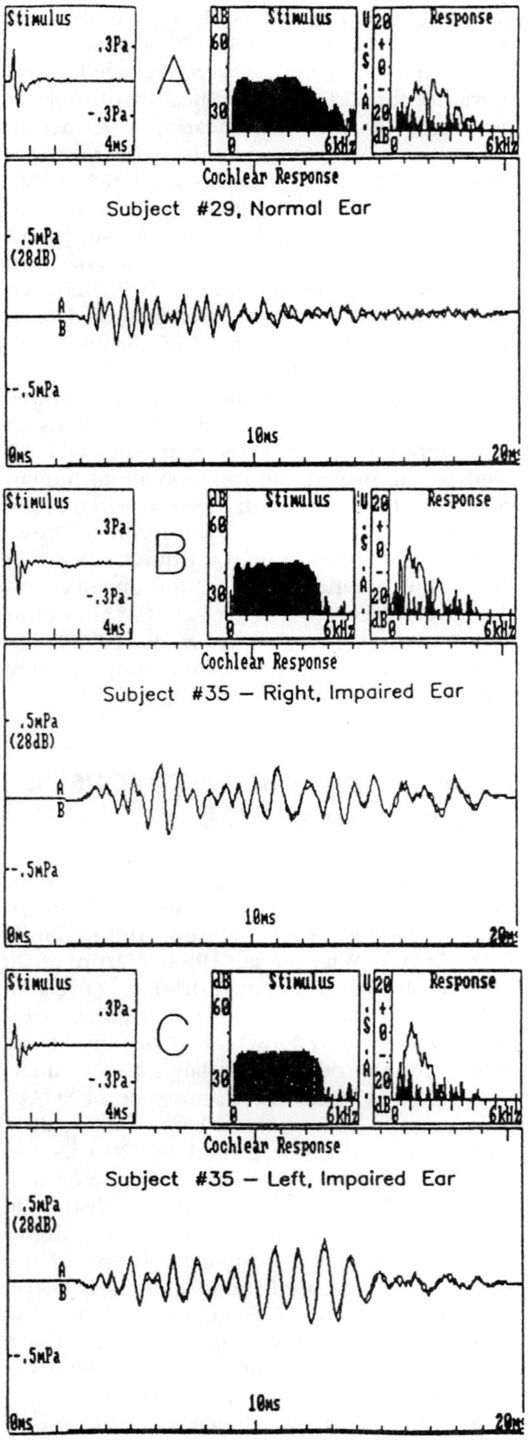

Figure 9-2 Click-evoked otoacoustic emissions (CEOAEs) in three human adult ears, one with normal hearing *(A)* and two with noise-induced hearing loss *(B* and *C)*. Subject No. 29, female, age 25 years, with hearing threshold of 10 dB HL or better at all standard audiometric frequencies. The hearing-impaired subject No. 35 is the 31-year-old male represented in Figure 9-1.

an intact OHC active-nonlinear biomechanical mechanism adjacent to the disrupted region.

The fact that SOAEs are common in normally hearing human ears, particularly those of infants (Strickland et al, 1985), is contrary to the disruption or lesion hypothesis. Histologic examinations of two rhesus monkey ears exhibiting SOAEs (Lonsbury-Martin et al, 1988) also found no circumscribed lesions of the organ of Corti at locations corresponding to the SOAE frequencies. Thus, conditions underlying SOAE generation in human and nonhuman primates in frequency regions of normal hearing may be different from those for nonprimate animals. Observations of SOAEs in human and nonhuman primates suggest the hypothesis that SOAEs in these species arise from irregularities in the normal organ of Corti (such as an extra row of OHCs) rather than lesions (Zwicker, 1986b; Kemp, 1986; Lonsbury-Martin et al, 1988).

Conclusion

Various types of OAEs, such as DPOAEs and CEOAEs, provide noninvasive objective information about cochlear function that can be particularly useful for infants, young children, and the retarded. It appears that the DPOAE method offers advantages by providing greater frequency specificity and more quantitative information about the degree of hearing impairment than the CEOAE method. The OAE methods are promising objective sensitive indicators of early signs and the progression of hearing impairments, including cases of noise-induced hearing loss.

Relations Entre les Oto-Émissions Acoustiques et les Déficits Auditifs: Étude chez l'Homme

Des études récentes sur la cochlée suggèrent l'hypothèse que des mécanismes de motilité actifs et non linéaires des cellules ciliées externes donnent naissance à une amplification de la réponse mécanique cochléaire d'un facteur 100 à 300 (40-50 dB).

Les oto-émissions acoustiques (OAEs) sont supposées être un épiphénomène du mécanisme d'amplification biomécanique cochléaire. Les OAEs comprennent des produits de distorsion et des OAEs évoquées par des clics. Quand une oreille est soumise à un bruit intense ou à des agents tels que des drogues ototoxiques, les cellules ciliées externes sont endommagées et le mécanisme d'amplification biomécanique de la cochlée est interrompu.

Selon la théorie de la biomécanique cochléaire non linéaire, les OAEs devraient être réduites ou éliminées quand les cellules ciliées externes sont endommagées. En effet des mesures effectives d'OAEs sur des sujets présentant des pertes auditives dues au bruit, montrent une telle réduction des OAEs, voire leur élimination. Cet article passera en revue la littérature concernant les oto-émissions sur des sujets humains ayant soit une audition normale, soit des pertes auditives dues au bruit, et les effets des pertes auditives sur les oto-émissions seront discutés.

ACKNOWLEDGMENTS

This work was supported by grants from the Deafness Research Foundation, from the Department of Surgery, from the Division of Otolaryngology, from the Clinical Research Center, and from the Health Center Research Advisory Committee at the University of Connecticut Health Center.

References

Ashmore JF. A fast motile response in guinea-pig outer hair cells: The cellular basis of the cochlear amplifier. J Physiol 1987; 388:323-347.

Bonfils P, Piron JP, Uziel A, Pujol R. A correlative study of evoked otoacoustic emission properties and audiometric thresholds. Arch Otorhinolaryngol 1988; 245:53-56.

Bonfils P, Uziel A. Clinical applications of evoked acoustic emissions: Results in normally hearing and hearing-impaired subjects. Ann Otol Rhinol Laryngol 1989; 98:326-331.

Brownell WE, Bader CR, Bertrand D, de Ribaupierre Y. Evoked mechanical responses of isolated cochlear outer hair cells. Science 1985; 227:194-196.

Brundin L, Flock Å, Canlon B. Sound-induced motility of isolated cochlear outer hair cells is frequency-specific. Nature 1989; 342:814-816.

Cianfrone C, Grandori F, eds. Cochlear mechanics and otoacoustic emissions. Scand Audiol 1986; Suppl 25.

Clark WW, Kim DO, Zurek PM, Bohne BA. Spontaneous otoacoustic emissions in chinchilla ear canals: Correlation with histopathology and suppression by external tones. Hear Res 1984; 16:299-314.

Davis H. An active process in cochlear mechanics. Hear Res 1983; 9:79-90.

Evans EF, Wilson JP. The frequency selectivity of the cochlea. In: Moller AR, ed. Basic mechanisms in hearing. New York: Academic Press, 1973:519.

Flock Å, Flock B, Ulfendahl M. Mechanisms of movement in outer hair cells and a possible structural basis. Arch Otorhinolaryngol 1986; 243:83-90.

Furst M, Rabinowitz WM, Zurek PM. Ear canal acoustic distortion at 2f1−f2 from human ears: Relation to other emissions and perceived combination tones. J Acoust Soc Am 1988; 84:215-221.

Geisler CD. A model of the effect of outer hair cell motility on cochlear vibrations. Hear Res 1986; 24:125-131.

Gold T. Hearing. II. The physical basis of the action of the cochlea. Proc Roy Soc [B] 1948; 135:492-498.

Grandori F, Cianfrone G, Kemp DT, eds. Cochlear mechanisms and otoacoustic emissions. Adv Audiol 1990; 7.

Guinan JJ. Effect of efferent neural activity on cochlear mechanics. Scand Audiol Suppl 1986; 25:53-62.

Harris FP, Lonsbury-Martin BL, Stagner BB, et al. Acoustic distortion products in humans: Systematic changes in amplitude as a function of f_2/f_1 ratio. J Acoust Soc Am 1989; 85:220-229.

Johnsen NJ, Bagi P, Elberling C. Evoked otoacoustic emissions from the human ear. III. Findings in neonates. Scand Audiol 1983; 12:17-24.

Kemp DT. Stimulated acoustic emissions from within the human auditory system. J Acoust Soc Am 1978; 64:1386-1391.

Kemp DT. Evidence of mechanical nonlinearity and frequency selective wave amplification in the cochlea. Arch Otorhinolaryngol 1979; 224:37-45.

Kemp DT, Chum RA. Observations on the generation mechanism of stimulus frequency acoustic emissions—Two tone suppression. In: van den Brink G, Bilsen FA, eds. Psychophysical, physiological, and behavior studies in hearing. Delft, The Netherlands: Delft University Press, 1980:34.

Kemp DT. Otoacoustic emissions, travelling waves, and cochlear mechanisms. Hear Res 1986; 22:95-104.

Kemp DT, Bray P, Alexander L, Brown AM. Acoustic emission cochleography—Practical aspects. Scand Audiol Suppl 1986; 25:71-95.

Kemp DT, Souter M. A new rapid component in the cochlear response to brief electrical efferent stimulation: CM and otoacoustic observations. Hear Res 1988; 34:49-62.

Kemp DT, Ryan S, Bray P. A guide to the effective use of otoacoustic emissions. Ear Hear 1990; 11:93-105.

Khanna SM, Leonard DGB. Basilar membrane tuning in the cat cochlea. Science 1982; 215:305-306.

Kim DO, Molnar CE, Pfeiffer RR. A system of nonlinear differential equations modeling basilar-membrane motion. J Acoust Soc Am 1973; 54:1517-1529.

Kim DO, Molnar CE. Cochlear mechanics: measurements and models. In: Tower DB, ed. The nervous system. Vol. 3. Human communication disorder. New York: Raven Press, 1975:57.

Kim DO. Cochlear mechanics: Implications of electrophysiological and acoustical observations. Hear Res 1980; 2:297-317.

Kim DO, Neely ST, Molnar CE, Matthews JW. An active cochlear model with negative damping in the partition: Comparison with Rhode's ante- and postmortem observations. In: van den Brink G, Bilsen FA, eds. Psychophysical, physiological and behavioral studies in hearing. Delft, The Netherlands: Delft University Press, 1980:7.

Kim DO. Functional roles of the inner- and outer-hair-cell subsystems in the cochlea and brainstem. In: Berlin CI, ed. Hearing science. New York: College-Hill Press, 1984:241.

Kimberley BP, Nelson DA. Time-averaged distortion product emissions. Assoc Res Otolaryngol 1990; 13:240.

Leonard G, Smurzynski J, Jung MD, Kim DO. Evaluation of distortion product otoacoustic emissions as a basis for the objective clinical assessment of cochlear function. Adv Audiol 1990; 7:139-148.

Lonsbury-Martin BL, Martin GK, Probst R, Coats AC. Spontaneous otoacoustic emissions in a nonhuman primate. II. Cochlear anatomy. Hear Res 1988; 33:69-93.

Lonsbury-Martin BL, Harris FP, Stagner BB, et al. Distortion-product emissions in humans: I. Basic properties in normally hearing subjects. Ann Otol Rhinol Laryngol 1990; 99:3-14.

Martin GK, Lonsbury-Martin BL, Probst R, Coats AC. Spontaneous otoacoustic emissions in the nonhuman primate: A survey. Hear Res 1985; 20:91-95.

Martin GK, Lonsbury-Martin BL, Probst R, Coats AC. Spontaneous otoacoustic emissions in a nonhuman primate. I. Basic features and relations to other emissions. Hear Res 1988; 33:49-68.

Martin GK, Ohlms LA, Franklin D, Harris FP, Lonsbury-Martin BL. Distortion product emissions in humans. III. Influence of sensorineural hearing loss. Ann Otol Rhinol Laryngol 1990a; 99:30-42.

Martin GK, Probst R, Lonsbury-Martin BL. Otoacoustic emissions in human ears: Normative findings. Ear Hear 1990b; 11:106-120.

Mountain DC. Changes in endolymphatic potential and crossed olivocochlear bundle stimulation alter cochlear mechanics. Science 1980; 210:71-72.

Neely ST. Transient responses in an active, nonlinear model of cochlear mechanics. In: Duifhuis H, Horst JW, Wit HP, eds. Basic issues in hearing. New York: Academic Press, 1988:106.

Neely ST, Kim DO. An active cochlear model showing sharp tuning and high sensitivity. Hear Res 1983; 9:123-130.

Neely ST, Kim DO. A model for active elements in cochlear biomechanics. J Acoust Soc Am 1986; 79:1472-1480.

Norton S, Widen JE. Evoked otoacoustic emissions in normal-hearing infants and children: emerging data and issues. Ear Hear 1990; 11:121-127.

Probst R, Lonsbury-Martin BL, Martin GK, Coats AC. Otoacoustic emissions in ears with hearing loss. Am J Otolaryngol 1987; 8:73-81.

Rhode WS. Observations of the vibration of the basilar membrane in squirrel monkeys using the Mossbauer technique. J Acoust Soc Am 1971; 49:1218-1231.

Rhode WS. Some observations on cochlear mechanics. J Acoust Soc Am 1978; 64:158-176.

Robles L, Ruggero MA, Rich NC. Basilar membrane mechanics at the base of the chinchilla cochlea. I. Input-output functions, tuning curves, and response phases. J Acoust Soc Am 1986; 80:1364-1374.

Ruggero MA, Kramek B, Rich NC. Spontaneous otoacoustic emissions in a dog. Hear Res 1984; 13:293-296.

Santos-Sacchi J. Asymmetry in voltage-dependent movements of isolated outer hair cells from the organ of Corti. J Neurosci 1989; 9:2954-2962.

Sellick PM, Patuzzi R, Johnstone BM. Measurement of basilar membrane motion in the guinea pig using the Mossbauer technique. J Acoust Soc Am 1982; 72:131-141.

Siegel JH, Kim DO. Efferent neural control of cochlear mechanics? Olivocochlear bundle stimulation affects cochlear biomechanical nonlinearity. Hear Res 1982; 6:171-182.

Smurzynski J, Leonard G, Kim DO, Lafreniere DC, Jung MD. Distortion product otoacoustic emissions in normal and impaired adult ears. Arch Otolaryngol Head Neck Surg. 1990; 116:1309-1316.

Stevens JC, Webb HD, Hutchinson J, Connell J, Smith MF, Buffin JT. Click evoked otoacoustic emissions in neonatal screening. Ear Hear 1990; 11:128-133.

Strickland EA, Burns EM, Tubis A. Incidence of spontaneous otoacoustic emissions in children and infants.

J Acoust Soc Am 1985; 78:931-935.

Tubis A, Long GR, Sivaramakrishnan S, Jones KL. Tracking and interpretive models of the active-nonlinear cochlear response during reversible changes induced by aspirin consumption. In: Wilson JP, Kemp DT, eds. Cochlear mechanisms: structure, function, and models. New York: Plenum Press, 1989:323.

Wier CC, Norton SJ, Kincaid GE. Spontaneous narrowband otoacoustic signals emitted by human ears: A replication. J Acoust Soc Am 1984; 76:1248-1250.

Wilson JP, Johnstone JR. Basilar membrane and middle-ear vibration in guinea pig measured by capacitive probe. J Acoust Soc Am 1975; 57:705-723.

Wilson JP. Evidence for a cochlear origin for acoustic re-emissions, threshold fine-structure and tonal tinnitus. Hear Res 1980; 2:233-252.

Zenner HP, Zimmerman U, Schmitt U. Reversible contraction of isolated mammalian cochlear hair cells. Hear Res 1985; 18:127-133.

Zurek PM. Spontaneous narrowband acoustic signals emitted by human ears. J Acoust Soc Am 1981; 69:514-523.

Zurek PM, Clark WW. Narrow-band acoustic signals emitted by chinchilla ears after noise exposure. J Acoust Soc Am 1981; 70:446-450.

Zurek PM. Acoustic emissions from the ear: A summary of results from humans and animals. J Acoust Soc Am 1985; 78:340-344.

Zwicker E. A hardware cochlear nonlinear preprocessing model with active feedback. J Acoust Soc Am 1986a; 86:146-153.

Zwicker E. "Otoacoustic" emissions in a nonlinear cochlear hardware model with feedback. J Acoust Soc Am 1986b; 80:154-162.

CHAPTER 10

Hysteresis in Cochlear Mechanics and a Model for Variability in Noise-Induced Hearing Loss

ERIC L. LePAGE

An outstanding feature of the many studies of noise on the auditory system is the variability of the hearing loss that results from identical exposures administered to a group of individuals (Salvi et al, 1983; Salvi et al, 1986). Moreover, attempts to predict the degree of permanent threshold shift (PTS) from temporary threshold shift (TTS) have been only partially successful (Mills et al, 1981). The specific reasons for this lack of predictability in individuals are not known. There may be one or more unknown physiologic factors that are varying beyond the control of the experiments, which nevertheless play a major role in determining individual variability in the degree of TTS and susceptibility to PTS.

The problem of dealing with this inherent variability may be partly conceptual. Historically, there has been the expectation that moderate to substantial noise exposures in humans should have produced changes in audiometric thresholds that are statistically significant. The sound energy levels for the lowest thresholds are remarkably low, and the mammalian ear is an exquisitely sensitive mechanoreceptor, so at face value, the human audiogram should be sufficiently sensitive to register very small levels of degradation of cochlear performance for a sample population large enough to lessen the effects of test-retest variability (Burns and Robinson, 1970; Kryter, 1970; Carter et al, 1982).

Numerous studies of damage to the cochlear structures have shown a rise in the threshold of tuning curves of single primary auditory fibers (Liberman and Kiang, 1978; Robertson, 1982). In cases of damage to the organ of Corti, it is nearly always possible to find single units with aberrant tuning properties. An economical hypothesis, therefore, has been to suspect that loss of OHC function leads directly to loss of sensitivity of primary auditory fibers. This should be manifested as changes in the neural tuning curve as well as changes in the microaudiogram, which exhibits fine structure in thresholds associated with areas affected by lesions.

Conversely, it is possible that audiometric sensitivity is not an accurate measure of damage to the cochlea. As a result of otoacoustic emission studies in humans (Kemp et al, 1986, 1989; Kemp, 1989), there appears to be some merit in pursuing *cochlear mechanical loss* as a concept distinct from the concept of hearing loss. Because of multiple sources of redundancy, hearing threshold may be the last parameter to reflect ongoing damage. There is huge redundancy in the numbers of primary afferent fibers and the apparent variability in the dynamic range of these fibers. As the cochlea ages, central reorganization may occur so as to give added weight to the activity of the lowest threshold fibers. There is also considerable redundancy in the outer hair cell (OHC) population. Audiometric thresholds, therefore, may not rise at any one frequency until the threshold of the most sensitive single unit has risen. In these terms, therefore, no signs of hearing loss may be perceived until damage is extensive.

The dominant interest in tuning curves stems from the fact that only the threshold of the sharpest curves correlates best with behavioral and human thresholds. Because of this relationship, the single-unit tuning curve, and more recently, the mechanical tuning curve, have been equated with normal behavior only when the thresholds are lowest and the tuning sharpest. Because the characteristic shape of the tuning curve (LePage, 1987c) is largely preserved irrespective of the method of obtaining it, the prevailing view is that the shape of the traveling-wave excitation pattern remains fixed irrespective of frequency and level. However, threshold mechanical tuning curves describe essentially a "keyhole" view of the spatially distributed excitation pattern, which is most likely varying in some systematic way with tone level in the process of tracking threshold with frequency (LePage, 1987c). The only way to determine whether this is the case is to carry out complete frequency response and intensity functions, making sufficient allowance for active behavior, which has a temporal behavior independent of that for the traveling wave. This is difficult to achieve with any technique, such as the Mössbauer technique, which is slow and which may require limiting assumptions about the nature of the response (e.g., linearity). The data presented here were obtained with two techniques of rapid response and wide dynamic range: a capacitive probe for AC displacement and a fiberoptic lever for the DC displacement responses.

When tuning curves are obtained in this way, in guinea pigs, the description becomes much more complex. A salient feature of the capacitive probe data is that the method of data collection is rapid and reveals frequency responses that are dynamically variable. Yet because the ear is fundamentally a mechanoreceptor, we are obliged to deal with this level of complexity. This chapter is concerned with the nature of the variability and the possibility that its source may be an important component of the variability in the characteristics of noise-induced hearing loss.

Methods

The methods for the capacitive probe technique are described in detail elsewhere (LePage, 1987a), as are those for the fiberoptic lever (LePage, 1989).

Data

LePage and Johnstone (1980) showed that in the vibratory response of the basilar membrane, a decrease of the nonlinear compression (output/input slopes of less than unity, decibel per decibel) was accompanied by a loss of neural sensitivity as determined by the compound action potential. Expansive behavior (slopes greater than unity) also occurred and became more prominent as the compression ceased, partly because the variability decreased (LePage, 1981). With the capacitive probe technique, the most strongly compressive behavior was in fact not at the tuning peak, but some one-fifth of an octave above it, in the region of a notch. Figure 10-1A shows a family of tuning curves obtained as previously described (LePage and Johnstone, 1980; LePage, 1987a,b). Because of the overlap of the curves in this region, the lower-intensity curves are only shown as far as one point above the frequency of the notch. A remarkable feature is that one obtains similar tuning curves whether one uses repetitive clicks, signal averaging and frequency transformation, or fixed-level pure tones presented in steps of 1 kHz and a lock-in amplifier (LePage, 1981). Partially down the high-frequency cutoff is a notch phenomenon that depends on both frequency and level. In Figure 10-1A, the notch occurs in the top trace at 19.5 kHz. This notch is apparently related to OHC contractility (LePage, 1989) and may be much more pronounced. As the stimulus level is increased, the frequency of the notch rises monotonically. In the examples with pure tones, for a level change of 20 dB, the frequency of the notch would rise typically by 1/15 of an octave. In reciprocal terms, this shift describes a slope of 300 dB per octave, coincidentally equaling the high-frequency slope of the threshold tuning curve for the same range of sound pressure levels.

The differential slope of the input-output function (decibel per decibel) may be computed as a function of frequency (Fig. 10-1B). Fresh guinea pig preparations showed strong nonlinear compression for frequencies less than the characteristic frequency (CF), whereas all records showed nonlinear expansive behavior above the CF. This was never revealed by the Mössbauer technique because the expansion rates were high, beyond the limited dynamic range of the technique. In Figure 10-1B the curve with the circles is obtained by dividing the difference between the top two curves of Figure 10-1A by the intensity step (6 dB), and smoothing with a three-point average. Likewise, the curve with the squares represents the slope between the second two curves, and so on. The curves show that the degree of nonlinear compression is higher for the top pair of curves and lowest for the bottom pair. Moreover, the frequency at which the transition toward expansive behavior occurs decreases with stimulus level.

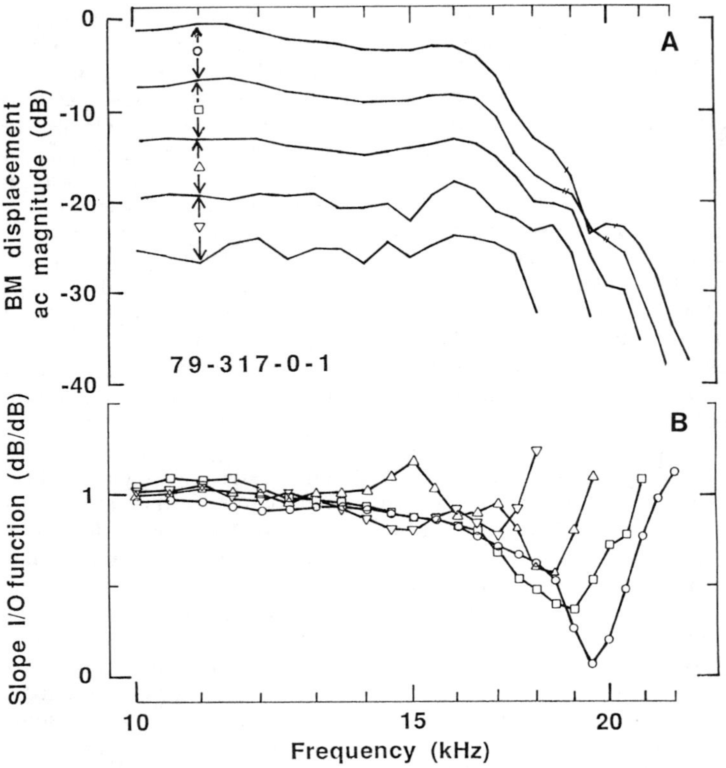

Figure 10-1 Guinea pig tuning curves for a place in the basal turn *(A)*, obtained quasi-simultaneously for repetitive clicks in steps of stimulus level of 6 dB. Each curve represents a response for constant stimulus, not constant basilar membrane response. The curves show a highly reproducible general pattern in which the intensity response functions show greatest nonlinear compression between records for the highest stimulus levels. This pattern of response can be explained if, in addition to the vibratory response of the basilar membrane, the measurement is influenced by a length change of the outer hair cell (OHC), which moves toward scala vestibuli for short delays, leading to apparent compression. *B*, The symbols in the lower panel represent the input/output slopes derived from the differences between adjacent pairs of curves as indicated in the upper panel *(A)*. The circles are for the highest pair of stimulus intensities while the inverted triangles are for the lowest pair. Slopes of unity indicate linear response. Conversely, OHC, which moves the basilar membrane toward ST for longer delays, can account for the swing to expansion. The apparent complexity of the behavior is increased still further by the shift in place of the traveling wave envelope toward the apex, with an increase in level.

The conditions for observing the notch showed considerable variability because the data also strongly depended on the history of the experiment (Fig. 10-2). The level of nonlinear compression could typically decrease over just 1 minute of the stimulus.

In input-output (or intensity) functions, the same notch phenomenon seen in Figure 10-1 is manifested between 50 and 80 dB sound pressure levels (SPL) in the input-output functions (Fig. 10-3A, B). Examination of the phase curves reveals a sharp discontinuity or jump at the frequency of the notch. The tone level at which the notch and phase shift are observed changes with the history of the experiment. Figure 10-3 shows the notch occurring at 74 dB SPL for ascending sound pressure levels. The SPL rises to 99 dB and then descends. The SPL is above 90 dB SPL for 20 to 30 seconds, during which time a slight TTS will have occurred. On descent, the notch has shifted to 63 dB SPL. Figure 10-4 shows a similar history-dependent behavior, which is repeated for a second cycle up and down.

In a series of experiments using the fiberoptic lever, intense tones of 100 to 110 dB SPL are delivered to live guinea pigs using a sealed sound system (voltage to the driver is constant, not the SPL at the tympanum). This results in displacements of the basilar membrane of several micrometers. After an intense sequence of tone bursts (Fig. 10-5A), first increasing frequency and then decreasing frequency, there is a shift of the best frequency of the response pattern to lower frequencies. Two subsequent records at slightly less inten-

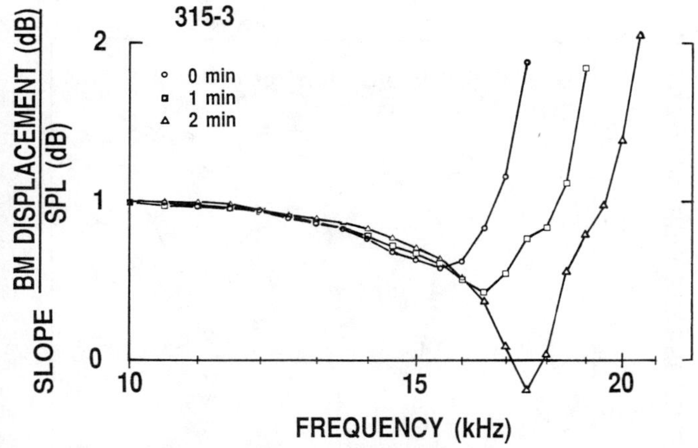

Figure 10-2 Dependence of the slope of the mechanical intensity function on duration of the repetitive click stimulus. The curves are obtained using the method described in Figure 10-1, and are presented at 1-minute intervals. They show pronounced nonlinear compression (slopes < 1 equal to that for the Mössbauer method) that is due directly to the development of a "DC shift" toward scala vestibuli. Greatest compression (triangles) occurs for least exposure. After one minute exposure (squares) the compression is halved. After two minutes exposure the maximum compression is reduced still further (closer to 1). The compression is accompanied by nonlinear expanion (slopes greater than 1) as the basliar membrane moves toward the scala tympani and the traveling-wave envelope slides toward the base with continuation of the expo sure. This leads to a spatial misalignment of the envelope with the position of greatest sensitivity and a decreasing motile response.

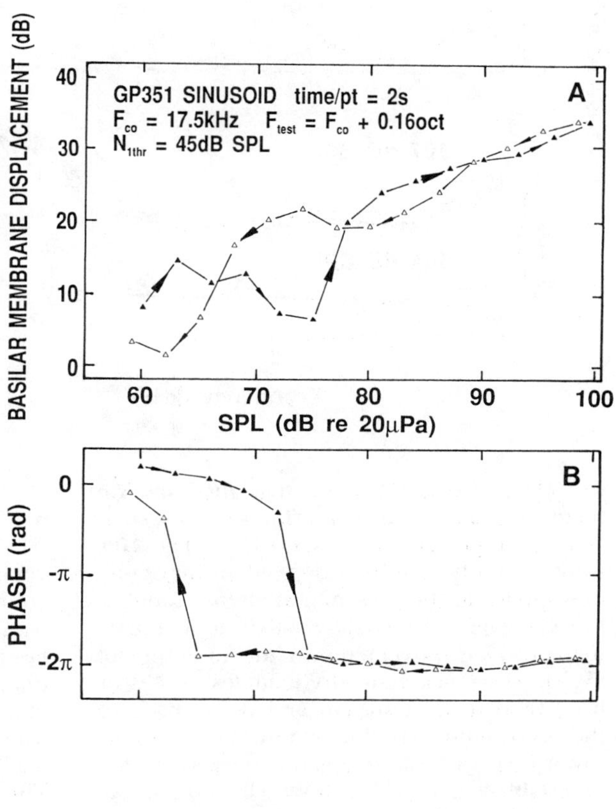

Figure 10-3 History-dependent behavior of basilar membrane vibratory displacement in response to a pure tone ⅙ octave above the best frequency. The sound level of the stimulus tone is increased along the arrows from 60 dB to 100 dB (solid triangles) then decreased back to 59 dB (open triangles). *A,* There is a notch in the vibratory response at 73 dB ascending, due to a rapid transition from a transient "DC" displacement toward the scala vestibuli to a longer-lasting DC displacement toward the scala tympani). *B,* The notch is accompanied by a rapid change in phase. As the sinusoid intensity is raised, the (precorrected) level remains above 90 dB SPL for approximately 1 minute. As the level is reduced on descent, the position of the notch has shifted, as if the place were now responding with a lower best frequency. F_{CO} refers to the 3-dB cutoff frequency on the highest-intensity trace.

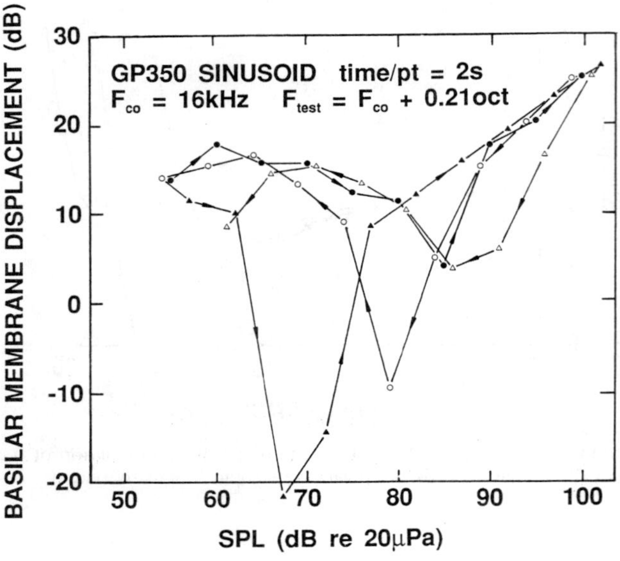

Figure 10-4 Magnitude response function for a sequence similar to that seen in Figure 10-3 but repeated for two cycles instead of one. The lock-in amplifier provides a signal of at least 30 dB to noise improvement. The curves represent the highly compressive behavior of basilar membrane displacement above the cut-off frequency. They also show a generally monotonic decrease in the level for the notch as with exposure to the stimulus at the high levels. The sequence begins with increasing levels (open circles, notch at 79 dB), followed by decreasing levels (open circles, notch at 79 dB), then increasing levels again (filled triangles, notch at 68 dB), followed by decreasing levels (open triangles, a second minor notch at 85 dB).

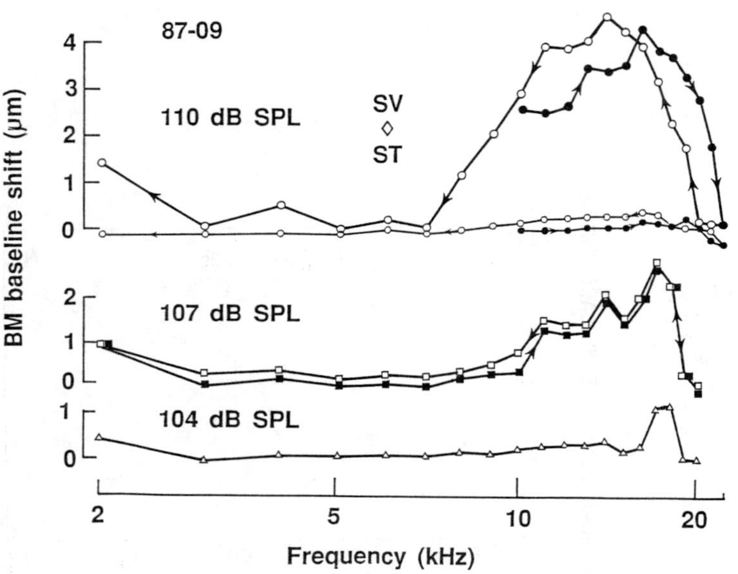

Figure 10-5 History dependence in the DC-displacement response to high-level pure tone bursts using the fiberoptic lever. Each point represents a transient shift toward the scala vestibuli (SV), which returns to a baseline value represented by the small circles. The notable feature is that for tones at 110 dB SPL beginning at 10 kHz, the rapid DC swing behavior (large filled circles) has shifted to lower frequencies by about ⅙ octave (large open circles). Repetition of the curves at lower levels suggests that the new lower "cutoff frequency" lasts longer after the residual swing toward the scala tympani (ST). The reference baseline (0 μm) is not the same for each curve but is subject to the cumulative effects of the residual offsets (small circles).

sity (Fig. 10-5B, C) show that the new CF seems to remain. Expanded time records, such as those reported by LePage (1989, Fig. 10), show a variety of history-dependent behaviors in response to the presence of intense tones at the CF. Figure 10-6 shows that tone bursts that produce movements in the direction of SV, or scala vestibuli (frequencies at CF or less) tend to be transient and decay back to the prestimulus baseline, whereas movements toward ST, or scala tympani (above CF) tend to establish a new baseline. The polarity of these shifts is shown in the insets.

Discussion

These data are difficult to explain by conventional models, which seek primarily to account for behavior at threshold. Instead the data are consistent with the interpretation that nonlinear compression is due to a perturbation of the vibratory response by an influence that is moving the basilar membrane away from the probe tip for short delays, and moving it towards the probe tip sometime later. The velocity of the baseline movement is higher for higher sound levels; this effec-

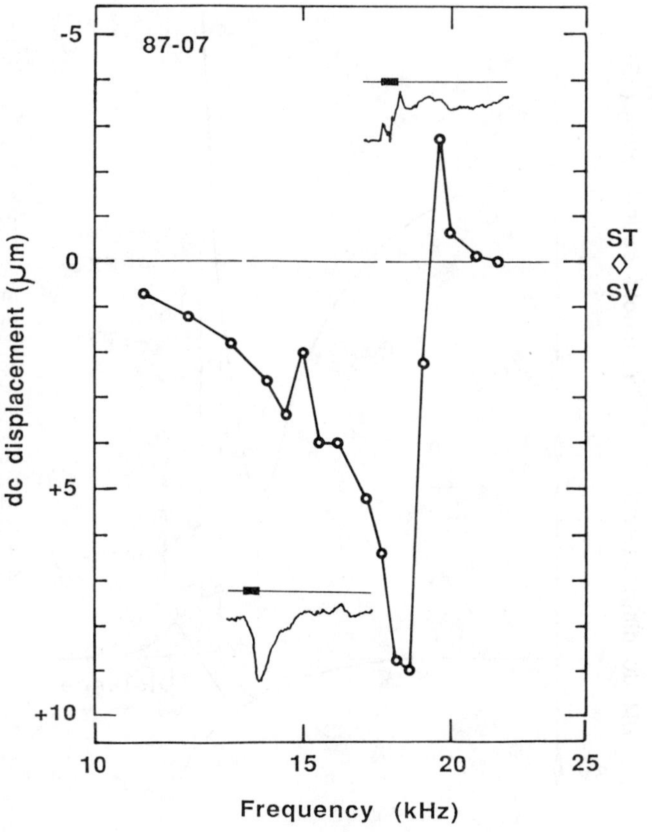

Figure 10-6 Similar experiment as depicted in Figure 10-5, using intense pure tones. However, this shows a clear-cut reversal of the polarity of the basilar membrane DC response. Again, each point represents a transient shift toward the scala vestibuli (SV) for frequencies less than 18 kHz, whereas the swing toward the scala tympani (ST) at 19 kHz and above is more permanent and produces a residual baseline shift. Insets depict shift polarity.

tively reduces probe sensitivity. Conversely, movement towards the scala tympani effectively increases probe sensitivity, accentuating the vibration amplitude and leading to apparent expansion. The velocity is greater for higher levels, so that the apparent nonlinear compression seen in this way is greatest as the level is increased.

The notch constitutes either an antiresonance or, more likely, a cancellation phenomenon in capacitive probe data. The reason that such a notch appears in the intensity functions, but not in the threshold tuning curves, is now apparent. These data suggest that the frequency of the notch shifts with level. In spatial terms, the shift of the notch is similar to what might be expected if the displacement detector had been shifted along the basilar membrane; i.e., the data suggest that the recording position was behaving effectively, as if it were at a more apical place.

It would seem, therefore, that these direct mechanical data describe the behavior of the notch in a manner qualitatively similar to the half-octave shift phenomenon (McFadden, 1986). That is, it represents a transition that *slides along* the cochlear partition toward the base, delimiting the apical extent of the excitation region (Fig. 10-7). An analogy might be the motion of a hard object, such as a pen, between the blades of a pair of scissors as they close. The transverse motion (OHC length change) gives rise to longitudinal motion (the traveling-wave envelope—TWE—or excitation pattern). This "scissors concept" has a plausible physical basis (LePage, 1990; Table10-1) and explains why a notch never actually appears in the threshold tuning curve. Although the complete overview of AC and DC has yet to be obtained, it is evident that the notch and the rapid phase transition are due to the rapid polarity reversal in the DC response from the SV toward the ST, which occurs above the CF. DC displacements toward the SV are excitatory, whereas toward the ST they are inhibitory. Intense tones, in particular those toward the ST, may cause a long-lasting or possibly nonreversible change in OHC turgor; this gives rise to an effective shift in the tonotopy, which in turn gives rise to a TTS. Evidently, in the impulse train experiments, the stimulus was at a high-enough level to produce the mechanical equivalent of a TTS, or a net bias toward the ST adding to the bias ef-

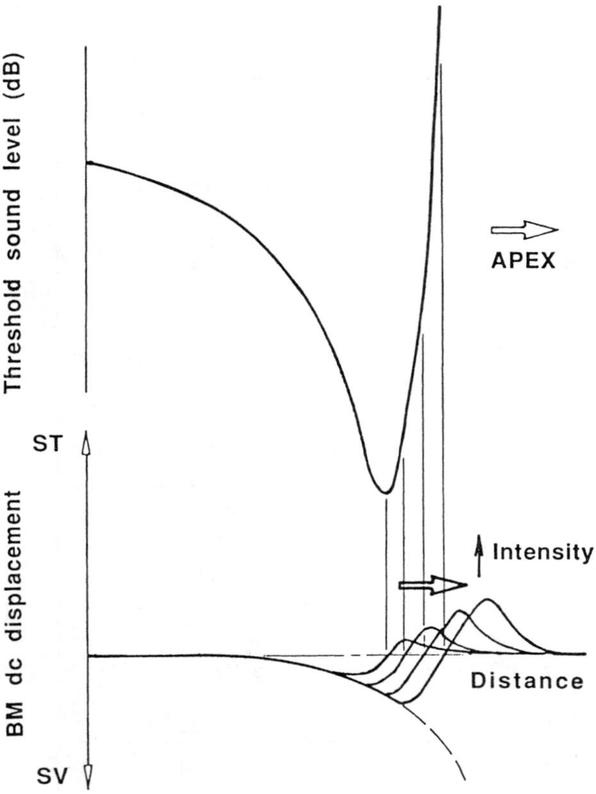

Figure 10-7 Original prediction (LePage, 1981) of the polarity and shape of the "DC-shift phenomenon" from the vibratory motion of the basilar membrane (BM), plus the prediction of its functional significance. The notch in the constant input vibratory tuning curves is now appreciated as a cancellation phenomenon due to the rapid length change of the OHC. The notch in the tuning curves and intensity functions (Figs. 10-1 through 10-4) does not appear in neural or mechanical threshold tuning curves, because it represents a sharp contrast in the excitation pattern, which slides along the basilar membrane, with change in level delimiting the end of the excitation of the inner hair cells. SV, scala vestibuli; ST, scala tympani.

fect of draining the ST for those experiments.

In Figures 10-3 and 10-4 there is systematic behavior in what at first appear to be very badly-behaved intensity and frequency response functions. Again, these data can be explained if the position of the sensor had been shifted along the basilar membrane or, alternately, if the tonotopic map had become permanently distorted. Long-term mechanical recordings were not practical, so a TTS-type of recovery of the shift phenomenon was never seen. Figure 10-5 suggests a shift in the tonotopy with exposure to a very intense tone; this change remained for the two lower sound levels. In response to a train of intense tone bursts, the basilar membrane baseline was seen to be reset to a new value with each new tone burst (LePage, 1989, Fig. 10). The erratic nature of those responses is difficult to explain, unless the presence of each intense burst produces a new distortion of the frequency-place map, which may result in excitation or suppression according to some basic DC-excitation pattern (LePage, 1989). In a series of mechanical experiments in which acetylcholine was perfused into the ST, the notch was apparently inhibited or moved to a higher frequency by the perfusate (LePage, 1989). The notch appears to be correlated with the high-frequency DC reversal seen in Figure 10-7, so that the notch's change of place corresponds to a longitudinal shift of the zero-crossing point, with a general change in OHC tonus caused by the acetylcholine.

In 1990 I suggested that the net turgor of the OHC may have a role in establishing the place (delimiting the apical extent) of the TWE for a fixed tone frequency (LePage, 1990; Table 10-1). The basis of the suggestion is that the slow motility may act to set the resonant frequency in the strings of the "Helmholtz harp," which was originally assumed to be fixed. OHC turgor may not just influence cochlear sensitivity through a conventional bias effect, but may also effectively amplify the change by the development of a spatial disparity. That is, the excitation pattern moves away from the point of maximal effectiveness. It follows that history-dependent variations in OHC turgor, and resulting residual changes in basilar membrane displacement, may influence the susceptibility of OHC to further high-level exposure. Hysteresis may therefore account for variable responses to subsequent exposures—e.g., in Figure 10-6, the subsequent TTS may depend on the starting value of the DC bias.

TABLE 10-1 Basis of the "Modified Helmholtz," or Variable Place Model

1. The primary determinants of tuning along the cochlear partition are a resonance of the radial fiber bundles of the basilar membrane—more specifically, the bundles of the pectinate zone.
2. These strings of "Helmholtz's harp" have a passive resonance, which may extend to high frequencies, and are driven into resonance by the OHCs.
3. The resonance frequency of these strings may not be fixed, as was assumed by Helmholtz; they are fine-tuned by the OHCs. An estimate of the turgor of the OHCs (LePage, 1990) is more than sufficient to apply the required tension to the strings. Regulation of that tension is a prime consideration.
4. There is now ample evidence, both in vitro and in vivo, that the OHCs respond to electric and acoustic stimuli with length changes.
5. Small variations in isometric tension of the OHCs can powerfully influence the resonance frequency. A doubling will produce a half-octave shift.
6. Direct measurements of the baseline position of the basilar membrane in fresh guinea pig preparations exhibit a marked swing towards the ST—more than one-sixth octave above the CF. This suggests that the OHCs have undergone an increase in length.
7. This length change indicates an OHC force-generation pattern, which is regarded as being applied to the tuning of the basilar membrane, controlling the local gradient and degree of dispersion of the traveling wave.
8. It is assumed that OHC shortenings result in a local increase in frequency, whereas lengthenings produce a decrease in frequency.

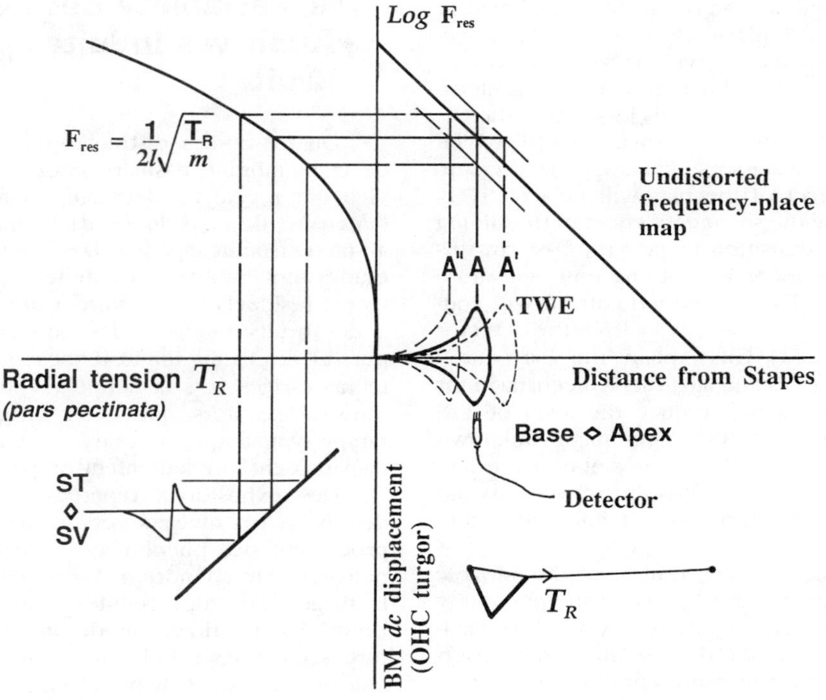

Figure 10-8 General schematic diagram for the cause of the distortions in the frequency-place map caused by the outer hair cell (OHC) length changes. Changes in "place" (positive x-axis) result from variations in resonant frequency (positive y-axis) that are in turn due to changes in radial tension of the basilar membrane fibers (negative x-axis), which in turn are due to changes in outer hair cell turgor (negative y-axis). The reader considers each quadrant in turn, working clockwise from the lower left quadrant. The large "DC shifts" represent the effects of the tension generated by the OHC in the basilar membrane, which fixes its resonance frequency for a given place (A). As the basilar membrane moves toward the scala vestibuli (SV), the tension is increased so that the resonance frequency increases. The effect of this change on a fixed frequency stimulus is that the excitation pattern moves toward the apex (A′). Conversely, a longer-lasting movement toward the scala tympani (ST) will produce a longer-lasting contraction of the traveling wave excitation pattern toward the base (A″). The higher the level, the less the overlap with the detector; thus, increasing intensity will not cause it to depolarize, but inhibit its response still further. For intense tones, therefore, the map will remain permanently distorted until the residual change in OHC tonus subsides. Individual response to loud sounds thus will depend on the viability of the OHC.

The model for variability is schematized in Figure 10-8. The lower-left quadrant shows the hypothetical relationship of basilar membrane DC shift to radial tension in the fiber bundles of the pars pectinata (strings). The upper-left quadrant shows how the resonance frequency of the strings depends on the tension of the strings (Mersenne's first law for a free undamped string). Finally, the upper-right corner shows the standard frequency-place map for the mammalian cochlea. The most pronounced change in basilar membrane baseline is from the SV toward the ST above the CF of the place. Unperturbed from its "rest" position, the TWE will map to a position, *A*. If the basilar membrane moves toward the SV according to the model (LePage, 1990; Appendix 10-1), the lever action of the arch will produce an increase in tension of the fiber bundles of the basilar membrane, raising their resonant frequency. A fixed tone mapping into a small neighborhood of this place will map to a more apical place, *A′*. Conversely, movement toward the ST will slacken the strings, and a fixed tone will map to a more basal location, *A″*. As the frequency is raised past the CF, the DC transition moves toward the ST, which gives rise to a scissors effect. That is, the suppressive effect of the bias will be effectively amplified by the secondary effect of the sliding shift of the transition toward the base. In this scheme, the more intense the tone, the more strongly the TWE excitation pattern will contract towards the base, away from the detector (inner hair cell). This explains the sharp cutoff of tuning curves and suggests a mechanism for priming effects that reduce the level of TTS (Canlon et al, 1988). The major unknown variable in the model is the slope of the line representing the relationship between basilar membrane DC displacement and radial tension.

An important implication of the variable place model is that it opens up the possibility of permanent remapping of the cochlear partition in the case of OHC loss, thereby transferring the frequency representation away from regions in which there is OHC loss to regions in which OHCs remain. This would tend to support the notion of a "fail-safe" mechanism for the cochlea, in which audiometric loss is the last parameter to reflect ongoing damage.

Conclusion

The data suggest that hysteresis occurs in the mechanical displacement of the basilar membrane. The recovery phase takes much longer than the initial changes due to exposure. It is suggested that high-intensity tones produce a slackening of the fibers of the pars pectinata, presumably due to a change of OHC turgor. This then results in a residual bias toward the ST and a loss of sensitivity. Secondly, these tones produce a residual tonotopic shift or spatial misalignment. The TWE moves basalward from the best place, so it is necessary to lower the stimulus frequency to regain the maximal response from the detector. The result is a temporary threshold shift and the observed history-dependent mechanical responses. Permanent loss of OHC may result in varying degrees of remapping of the cochlea and highly unpredictable behavioral losses.

Hystérésis en Mécanique Cochléaire et Modèle de la Variabilité des Pertes Auditives Induites par le Bruit

Quatre études distinctes du mouvement de la membrane basilaire chez le cobaye in vivo ont révélé un décalage, en fonction de l'intensité, de l'enveloppe de l'onde propagée à son extrémité apicale. Deuxièmement, ces études ont montré l'existence de déplacements résiduels faisant suite à une exposition à des bruits intenses, des bouffées de sons purs et des bruits impulsionnels. Les déplacements dirigés vers la rampe vestibulaire sont transitoires, alors que ceux dirigés vers la rampe tympanique sont de longue durée et ne disparaissent que lentement ou pas du tout.

Des expositions répétées ou cycliques depuis les bas niveaux vers les hauts niveaux produisent des phénomènes d'hystérésis qui peuvent correspondre à des modifications de la turgescence des cellules ciliées externes. Un modèle relatif au rôle des modifications de turgescence des cellules sur la mécanique cochléaire est décrit. Il prend en compte l'idée que la motilité des cellules ciliées externes produit des distorsions localisées de la carte fréquencielle cochléaire. En particulier, l'hystérésis qui survient à la suite de sons intenses semble être dû aux variations de turgescence. Le schéma d'excitation continu conduit à l'apparition de régions spatialement adjacentes de contraste élevé. Normalement elles se déplacent vers l'apex quand le niveau croît, mais vont vers la base lorsque le temps d'exposition augmente. Avec le changement de niveau, de petits changements de turgescence seront amplifiés par le décalage le long de la cloison cochléaire et ils pourraient avoir un effet puissant sur la force et la polarité de la motilité des cellules. Une voie est par conséquent ouverte pour expliquer de nombreux phénomènes cochléaires.

ACKNOWLEDGMENTS

This work was carried out as part of a research program into individual susceptibility to noise-induced hearing loss (NIHL) at the National Acoustic Laboratories, Central Laboratory, Sydney, Australia. I thank B.M. Johnstone for assistance in collecting the data and N.M. Murray for assistance with its preparation.

References

Burns W, Robinson DW. Hearing and noise in industry. London: HMSO, 1970, Appendix 10.

Canlon B, Borg E, Flock Å. Protection against noise trauma by pre-exposure to a low level acoustic stimulus. Hear Res 1988; 34:197-200.

Carter NL, Waugh RL, Keen K, et al. Amplified music and young people's hearing. Med J Aust 1982; 2:125-128.

Kemp DT, Bray P, Alexander L, Brown AM. Acoustic emission cochleography—practical aspects. Scand Audiol Suppl 1986; 25:71-89.

Kemp DT. Otoacoustic emissions. Philips Audiol Pract 1989; 6:1-3.

Kemp DT, Slobhan R, Bray P. A guide to the effective use of otoacoustic emissions. Ear Hear 1989; 11:93-105.

Kryter KD. The effects of noise on man. New York: Academic Press, 1970.

LePage EL. The role of nonlinear mechanical processes in the mammalian cochlea. Ph.D. Thesis, The University of Western Australia, 1981.

LePage EL. The application of a capacitive probe technique for direct observation of electromechanical processes in the guinea pig cochlea. J Acoust Soc Am 1987a; 82:126-138.

LePage EL. Frequency-dependent self-induced bias of the basilar membrane and its potential for controlling sensitivity and tuning in the mammalian cochlea. J Acoust Soc Am 1987b; 82:139-154.

LePage EL. A spatial template for the shape of tuning curves in the mammalian cochlea. J Acoust Soc Am 1987c; 82:155-164.

LePage EL. Functional role of the crossed olivo-cochlear bundle: A motor unit control system in the mammalian cochlea. Hear Res 1989; 38:177-198.

LePage EL. Helmholtz revisited: Direct mechanical data suggest a physical model for dynamic control of mapping frequency to place along the cochlear partition. In: Dallos P, Geisler CD, Matthews JW, et al. The mechanics and biophysics of hearing. Lecture notes in biomathematics. New York: Springer-Verlag 1990; 87:278.

LePage EL, Johnstone BM. Nonlinear mechanical behaviour of the basilar membrane in the basal turn of the guinea pig cochlea. Hear Res 1980; 2:183-189.

Liberman MC, Kiang NYS. Acoustic trauma in cats. Acta Otolaryngol Suppl 1978; 358:1-63.

McFadden D. The curious half-octave shift evidence for a basalward migration of the traveling-wave envelope with increasing intensity. In: Salvi R, Henderson D, Hamernik R, Colletti V, eds. Basic and applied aspects of noise-induced hearing loss. New York: Plenum Press, 1986:295.

Mills JH, Adkins WY, Gilbert RM. Temporary threshold shifts produced by wideband noise. J Acoust Soc Am 1981; 70:390-396.

Robertson D. Effects of acoustic trauma on stereocilia structure and spiral ganglion cell tuning properties in the guinea pig cochlea. Hear Res 1982; 7:55-74.

Salvi R, Henderson D, Hamernik R. Physiological basis of sensorineural hearing loss. In: Tobias JV, Schubert ED, eds. Hearing research and theory. Vol 2. New York: Academic Press, 1983:179.

Salvi R, Henderson D, Colletti V (eds). Basic and applied aspects of noise-induced hearing loss. New York: Plenum Press, 1986:173.

SECTION TWO

Central Changes

CHAPTER 11

Effect of Frequency-Specific Losses in Cochlear Neural Sensitivity on the Processing and Representation of Frequency in Primary Auditory Cortex

RAMESH RAJAN
DEXTER R.F. IRVINE
MICHAEL B. CALFORD
LISA Z. WISE

The damaging effects of loud sound exposure on a variety of cochlear responses have been studied extensively. Much is known about the changes in receptor and neural sensitivity, and about the biochemical, morphologic, and physiologic processes that underlie a reduction in neural output from the cochlea due to loud sound exposure. However, only a few studies have examined the effects of this reduction in outflow from the cochlea on the characteristics of neurons in central auditory structures. Such neglect would be justified if the changes in central auditory processing were totally explicable in terms of the cochlear changes. However, the extant studies on the effects of loud sounds on processing in central auditory structures suggest that this simple model cannot fully explain the changes in central auditory processing. For example, many studies have reported that, after exposure to loud noise, threshold losses of neurons in central auditory nuclei are greater than cochlear threshold losses, with different central structures being affected to differing extents (Babighian et al, 1975; Biedermann et al, 1987; Gerken et al, 1986; Lonsbury-Martin and Martin, 1981; Salvi, 1976; Salvi et al, 1975; Starr and Livingston, 1963; Syka and Popelár, 1982). It has also been reported that noise-induced hearing losses can produce an increase in the excitability of central auditory neurons (Gerken et al, 1986; Willot and Lu, 1981). These results suggest that loud noise can produce changes in central auditory structures that are not simply predicted by the cochlear effects. We have been examining the effects of a frequency-specific loss or decrease in neural outflow from the cochlea on processing in the primary auditory cortex (AI) of the cat. In one series of experiments we examined the effects of such a reduction in cochlear outflow on the frequency selectivity of AI neurons. In a second series, we examined the changes in the representation of the cochlea in the AI in animals with restricted cochlear lesions.

Effects of Losses in Cochlear Neural Sensitivity on Frequency Selectivity of AI Neurons

Much of the processing in the auditory system appears to occur in frequency-specific channels (Blauert, 1969/1970; Jenkins and Merzenich, 1984; Viermiester, 1988). Presumably, the substrate for such streaming is provided by the sharp frequency selectivity of neurons along the "core" auditory pathway. Thus, an understanding of the effects of noise exposures on the frequency selectivity of neurons in the core auditory pathway would ap-

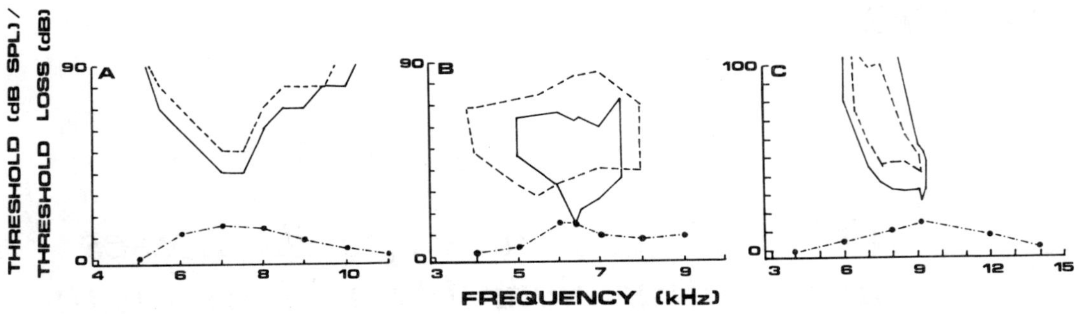

Figure 11-1 Effect of temporary threshold shifts (TTSs) in cochlear sensitivity over restricted frequency regions on the tuning properties of AI neurons. The black dots at the bottom of each panel are the compound action potential (CAP) threshold losses caused by a loud pure-tone exposure (see text), measured after CAP losses had stabilized. Above this are the excitatory response areas of the AI neurons determined before and after TTS. Full lines are pre-TTS tuning curves; dashed lines are post-TTS tuning curves, measured when CAP losses had stabilized. *A*, "Primary-like" effects (see text) on AI tuning curves. *B*, "Disinhibition" effects. *C*, "Increased inhibition" effects. The ordinate is read as threshold (dB SPL) for the tuning curves and as Threshold Loss (dB) for the CAP losses.

pear to be critical for understanding how loud sounds affect human psychophysical performance. In a few studies, the effects of loud sound exposures have been examined on the frequency selectivity of auditory brain stem and midbrain neurons. In essence, these studies found that the effects of loud sound exposures on the excitatory tuning curves of neurons in these parts of the central nervous system mirrored the effects seen at the level of the VIIIth nerve, i.e., there was a loss in threshold sensitivity at and around the characteristic frequency (CF—frequency at which the neuron had the lowest threshold), with little change at more distal frequencies (Henderson and Møller, 1975; Syka and Popelář, 1982; Willott and Lu, 1981). Thus, the general nature of the loss in frequency selectivity in these neurons was attributed to cochlear changes, though the full extent of the central threshold losses was not accounted for in these terms (Salvi, 1976; Salvi et al, 1975; Syka and Popelář, 1982; Willott and Lu, 1981).

We have examined the effects on the frequency selectivity of single neurons in the middle layers (layers III and IV) of the AI, of losses in cochlear neural sensitivity caused by brief loud pure-tone exposures. In each case, the excitatory response area of the single neuron was first defined. A brief (1 to 10 minutes), loud (100 to 115 dB SPL), pure tone was presented to the cochlea at a frequency ½ octave below the CF of the neuron, to produce temporary threshold shifts (TTS) in cochlear neural sensitivity at frequencies in a restricted range about the CF of the neuron. The losses at the cochlea were monitored in the compound action potential (CAP) audiogram (Dallos et al, 1978; Johnstone et al, 1979; Price, 1978). When these losses had stabilized, the frequency response area of the cortical neuron was redetermined using the same method as applied initially.

Three basic types of change in the frequency response areas occurred after loud sound-induced TTS in cochlear sensitivity. The first type, seen in approximately 22 percent of the neurons, basically involved a loss of sensitivity reflecting losses at the periphery (Fig. 11-1A). The second type, seen in approximately 44 percent of the neurons, was more complex, involving a loss in sensitivity around the CF of the tuning curve as well as an expansion of the response area (Fig. 11-1B). The pre-TTS frequency response area of this neuron was bounded both laterally and at higher intensities. Such circumscribed response areas in AI are believed to be shaped by inhibition both from the lateral frequencies and from frequencies from within the response area at high intensities (Calford et al, 1989; Phillips and Cynader, 1985). After the TTS, there was a loss of sensitivity around the CF region of the neuron, corresponding to the cochlear regions in which there were significant CAP threshold losses. Additionally, the neuron's response area expanded to include both frequencies at which it had previously not responded and higher intensities at frequencies within the former response area. The third type of change, seen in approximately 33 percent of the neurons, is illustrated in Figure 11-1C. The initial frequency response area of this neuron was also circumscribed. After the peripheral TTS, there was a loss in sensitivity around the CF, and the response area became more circumscribed in both frequency and intensity.

The first type of TTS-induced change in cortical neural frequency selectivity (Fig. 11-1A) appears to mirror the losses at the periphery, and is fairly similar to the changes seen in VIIIth nerve tuning curves (Cody and Johnstone, 1980; Lonsbury-Martin and Meikle, 1978). Similar effects on tuning curves in neurons in the inferior colliculus have been observed (Popelár and Syka, 1982). In contrast, the other two types of changes observed in AI neurons do not appear to solely mirror the effects at the cochlea. Although both types of change involved a loss in sensitivity at and around the CF, there were also complex changes in the frequency selectivity at off-CF frequencies.

Some of these results are explicable in terms of a mechanism that has been invoked to explain the expansions in the extent of the receptive fields of somatosensory cortical neurons occurring immediately after damage to restricted parts of the peripheral receptor array (analogous to the current experiments). In these studies, the maximal extent of the peripheral receptive field (RF) of a somatosensory cortical neuron was first mapped. When the input from the RF to the neuron was removed by denervation or local anesthesia, the cortical neuron immediately acquired a "new" RF located on body parts immediately adjacent to the former RF—parts that prior to the experimental manipulation had not been able to drive the neuron (Byrne and Calford, 1989; Calford and Tweedale, 1990; Metzlar and Marks, 1979; Nakahima et al, 1966). These results have been explained by invoking an hypothesis of "disinhibition" to explain this immediate expansion of the RF of the cortical neuron.

This hypothesis is predicated on the fact that central somatosensory neurons receive excitatory synaptic input originating from skin regions outside the area defined by the excitatory RF of the neurons (Juliano and Whitsel, 1987; Landry and Deschenes, 1981; Snow et al, 1988; Wall and Werman, 1976; Wilson and Snow, 1990). The disinhibition hypothesis supposes that the extra-RF synapses are functional, but are normally tonically suppressed by input from the dominant RF area (Calford and Tweedale, 1988, 1990; Nakahima et al, 1966). Removal of some or all of the maximal excitatory RF area would remove the tonic inhibition from these regions onto the inputs from the extra-RF regions, thereby "unmasking" the excitatory drive from the extra-RF regions. Thus, as has been observed in recent studies (Byrne and Calford, 1989; Calford and Tweedale, 1988, 1990; Nakahima et al, 1966), removal of some or all of the initial maximal excitatory RF area of a central somatosensory neuron should result in an immediate expansion of the RF area to its maximal excitatory extent.

The basic predictions of the disinhibition hypothesis as applied to our experiments are illustrated in Figure 11-2. As a simplification, it is assumed that the frequency response areas of auditory neurons are equivalent to the RFs of somatosensory neurons. The hypothesis suggests that lateral inhibitory areas (Fig. 11-2A) surrounding the excitatory region (i.e., the excitatory frequency response areas) for auditory cortical neurons can also provide excitatory input to the cortical neuron, but this excitation is suppressed by inhibitory input from the RF center (i.e., from the CF region). Eliminating or reducing the input from the CF region then should also reduce the inhibitory input from the CF region onto the excitatory input from the sidebands, unmasking the excitatory drive from these regions and producing an expansion of the lateral boundaries of the excitatory threshold tuning curve (Fig. 11-2B). In contrast, if disinhibition is not involved in auditory cortical plasticity of the type just described, the loss of input from a restricted region about the CF may only produce changes in the tuning curve that mirror the changes at the periphery (Fig. 11-2C).

The predictions of the disinhibition hypothesis can be applied to the two complex post-TTS changes seen in the frequency response areas of cortical neurons. The pattern of effects seen in the second type of post-TTS change (Fig. 11-1B) is consistent with a loss or reduction in the inhibitory inputs to the neuron contingent on a reduction in the excitatory drive from the CF region. Thus, this type of post-TTS change in cortical frequency selectivity is compatible with disinhibitory effects produced by the peripheral loss in sensitivity. It has been reported that sideband inhibition is reduced in cochlear nucleus neurons in noise-exposed rats (Henderson and Møller, 1975), suggesting that the inhibitory processes might have been more affected by the reduction in cochlear outflow. However, in the third type of change seen following TTS (Fig. 11-1C), the results appear to be the converse of the predictions of the disinhibition hypothesis. Instead, such effects can only be explained by assuming that there was both a loss in sensitivity contingent on the peripheral loss and an increase in the inhibitory inputs to cells of this type.

These results show that the effects of loud sound exposures on the central auditory sys-

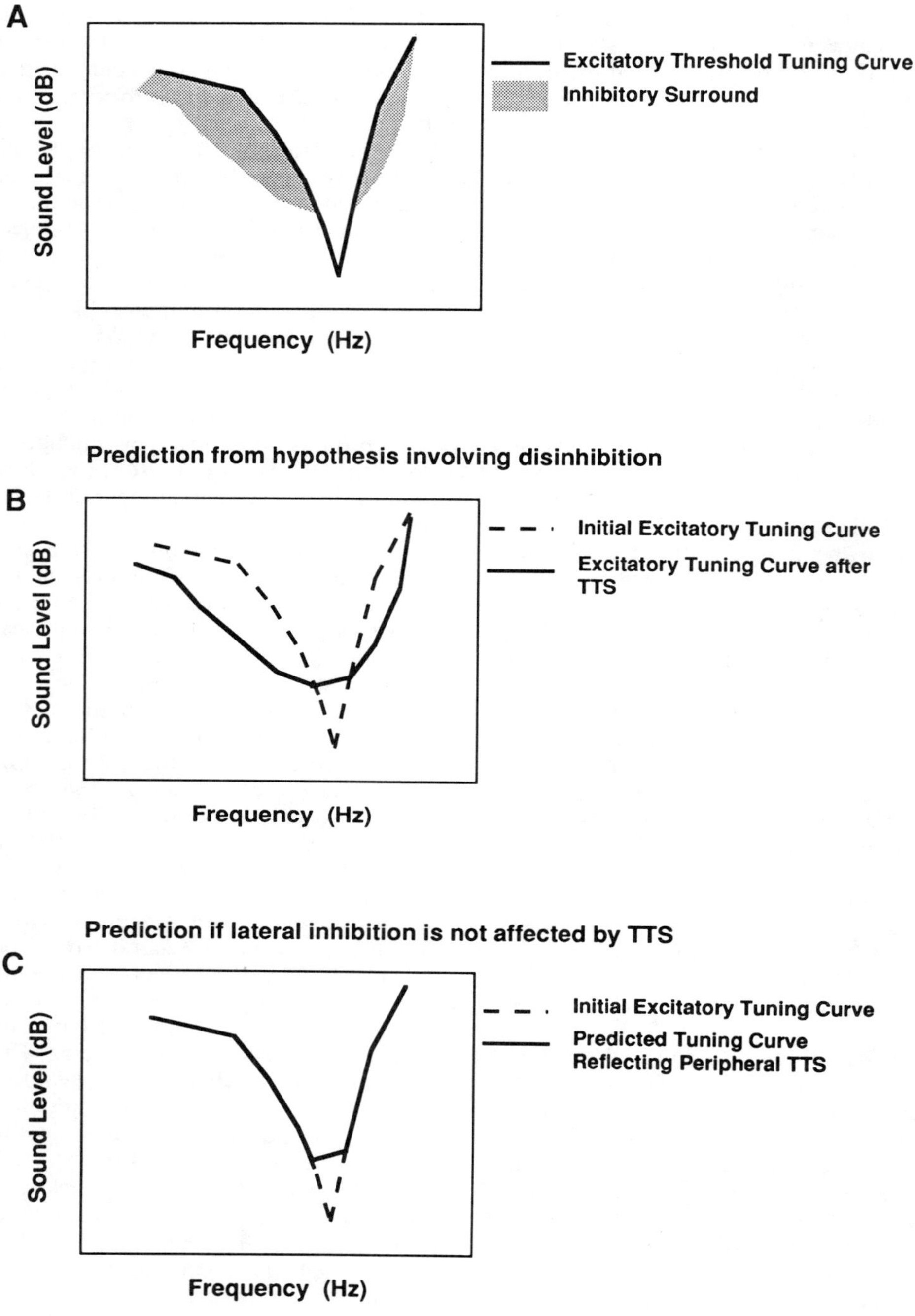

Figure 11-2 Illustration of the hypothesis on the role of inhibition in determining the effects of temporary threshold shift (TTS) on the excitatory tuning curve of primary auditory cortex (AI) neurons. *A*, Generalized example of the excitatory tuning curve of AI neurons flanked by inhibitory surrounds. *B*, Predictions of the disinhibition hypothesis on the effect of a loss in excitatory drive from around the characteristic frequency (CF) region (e.g., after a TTS in cochlear neural sensitivity at frequencies about the AI neuron's CF) on the overall shape of the excitatory tuning curve. *C*, Effect on AI tuning curves if the TTS has no effect on any inhibition shaping the AI neuronal tuning curve.

tem cannot be discussed in terms of only a reduction in the excitation of neurons in central auditory structures. The complex changes that we have observed in the AI, involving changes in the relative levels of both excitatory and inhibitory inputs to AI neurons, suggest that more complex phenomena of this sort must be considered integral to the damaging consequences of loud sounds on the auditory system. The presence of such complex phenomena makes it difficult to predict the effects of a sound-induced loss in peripheral sensitivity on information processing in the auditory cortex. The relatively small numbers of neurons examined prevents us from drawing any conclusions about the predominance of one type of effect as opposed to the others. The complexity of the effects observed does, however, make it imperative that more studies of this sort be done to clarify the central neurophysiologic effects of sound-induced losses in peripheral sensitivity before we begin postulating mechanisms to explain the effects of damaging loud sounds on human psychophysical performance.

Effects of Permanent Losses in Cochlear Neural Sensitivity on the Tonotopic Organization in Primary Auditory Cortex

A second type of change in central structures, produced by losses in peripheral sensitivity, has been shown in recent studies on the effects of restricted damage to the peripheral receptor array on cortical "maps." The term "maps" is used here to denote the ordered representation of the peripheral receptor array that is found in central nervous system structures of the major sensory systems.

In the auditory system, the ordered representation of the peripheral receptor array of the cochlea produces a tonotopic organization of central auditory structures reflecting the basic organization of the cochlea. The cochleotopic organization of the normal cat AI, as determined by microelectrode mapping techniques, is illustrated in Figure 11-3. As has been shown in other studies (Merzenich et al, 1975; Reale and Imig, 1980), high frequencies are represented by neurons at the rostral end of the AI, and low frequencies are represented by neurons at the caudal end, with a systematic representation of intermediate frequencies in between. In each line of caudal-to-rostral penetrations, the CFs of neuron clusters progressively increased. Beyond the rostral AI regions at which the very high frequencies (about 30 to 40 kHz) were represented, the tonotopic sequence reversed, consistent with the electrode having crossed into the anterior auditory field. Along the dorsoventral axis of the AI, points of similar CF can be joined together to form isofrequency lines. In Figure 11-3, such lines have been drawn to separate points with CFs above and below the frequency specified on the line.

Recent studies in the somatosensory and auditory systems have shown that the topographic representation of the receptor surface in the primary sensory cortex is modifiable in the adult following removal of input from restricted regions of the receptor surface (Kelahan and Doetsch, 1984; Merzenich and Kaas, 1982; Merzenich et al, 1983a,b, 1984; Rasmusson, 1982; Robertson and Irvine, 1989; Wall and Cusick, 1984). In the studies of such plasticity of the somatosensory system, removal of input from restricted regions of the body surface by a variety of manipulations results in substantial reorganization of the cortical somatotopic map. In brief, the cortical regions that normally represented the skin surfaces from which input was eliminated did not fall silent after the experimental manipulation. Instead, these cortical regions were occupied by the representation of other, unaffected skin surfaces adjacent to the affected areas. A consequence of this plasticity of the cortical somatotopic representation was that the skin surfaces adjacent to the areas affected by the experimental manipulation now had a much greater area of cortical representation (Kelahan and Doetsch, 1984; Merzenich et al, 1983a,b, 1984; Rasmusson, 1982; Wall and Cusick, 1984).

In an analogous study in the auditory system, Robertson and Irvine (1989) showed that restricted unilateral mechanical lesions of the cochlea in adult guinea pigs, producing permanent losses of cochlear neural sensitivity over a restricted frequency range, result in plasticity of the frequency organization in the cortex contralateral to the lesioned cochlea. The basic features of the results obtained by Robertson and Irvine (1989) are illustrated in Figure 11-4. The mechanical lesion made about 2 months prior to the recording session resulted in a loss in CAP thresholds at frequencies greater than 10 kHz (Fig. 11-4A). When the auditory cortex contralateral to the lesioned cochlea was mapped to determine its

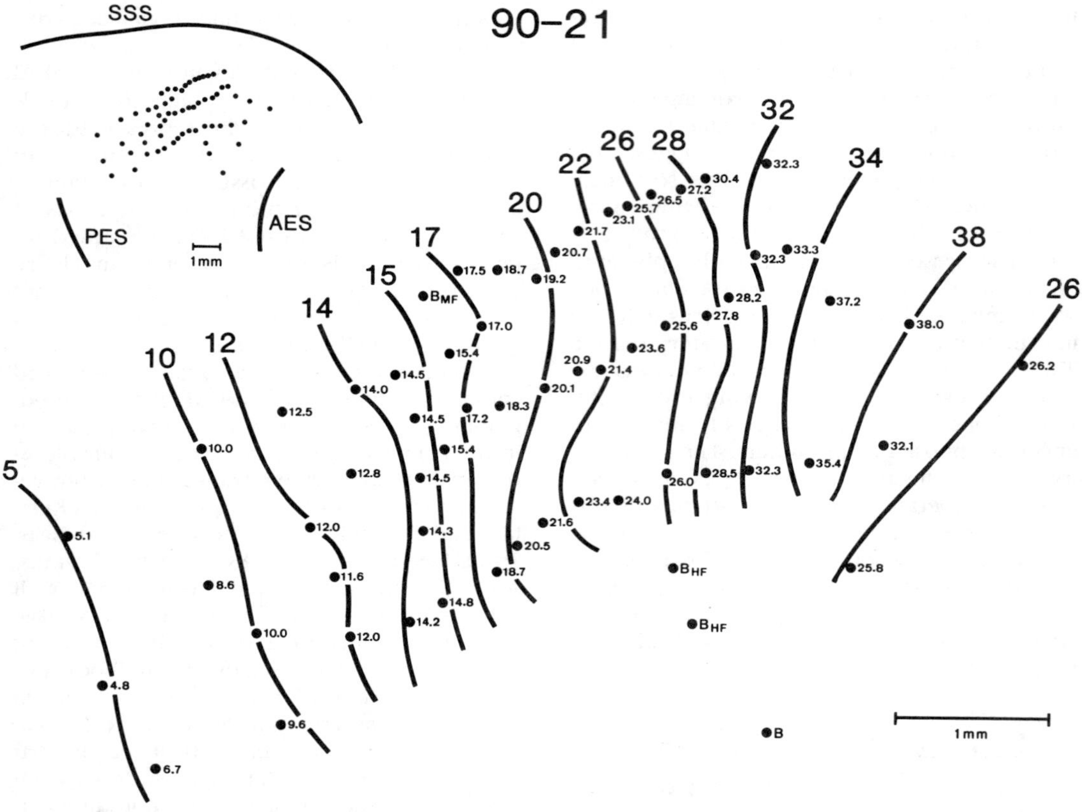

Figure 11-3 Tonotopic organization of the normal cat primary auditory cortex (AI) to contralateral stimulation. The inset shows the location of the recording sites in the AI on the middle ectosylvian gyrus (MEG). Each dot in the figure represents the location of a microelectrode penetration made normal to the cortical surface. Numbers beside each dot represent the characteristic frequency (CF) of a cluster of neurons recorded in that penetration. In penetrations marked "B" neuronal clusters were broadly tuned. Isofrequency lines have been drawn to separate points with CFs above and below the frequency denoted at the top of the line. The frequency reversal at the rostral end of the AI indicates placement of the electrode in the anterior auditory field.

organization to input from the lesioned cochlea (Fig. 11-4B), the representation of the low frequencies in the rostral auditory field, which was mapped in greater detail by these experimenters, appeared to be normal. A normal tonotopic progression of increasing CF from 1.5 kHz to about 9 kHz was observed with caudal displacement of the electrode in this field. In more caudal regions, the organization of the rostral field was distinctly abnormal. There was an expanded representation of the frequency band from 9.1 to 10.6 kHz, and a very large region of cortex that would normally have been devoted to the representation of higher frequencies (Robertson and Irvine, 1989) now contained neuronal clusters with CFs in this restricted range of frequencies, corresponding to the edge of the region at which cochlear losses occurred. Further caudal to this region of cortex was a strip of cortex in which neuronal clusters were either unresponsive or were only weakly responsive to auditory input. Finally, caudal to this strip of cortex, a limited amount of mapping suggested that there had also been an expansion of the representation of the same restricted frequency band in the caudal field, which has a tonotopic organization that is the reverse of the rostral field (Robertson and Irvine, 1989). Thus, the results of this study showed that, some time after a permanent loss in cochlear neural sensitivity, there was a reorganization of the frequency selectivity in the auditory cortex such that neurons deprived of their CF input by the peripheral lesion now acquired a new CF at a frequency at the edge of the region of cochlear losses. Significantly, neuronal responses in the reorganized areas were vigorous, and thresholds of clusters of cortical neurons in these regions were not significantly different from normal thresholds at those frequencies.

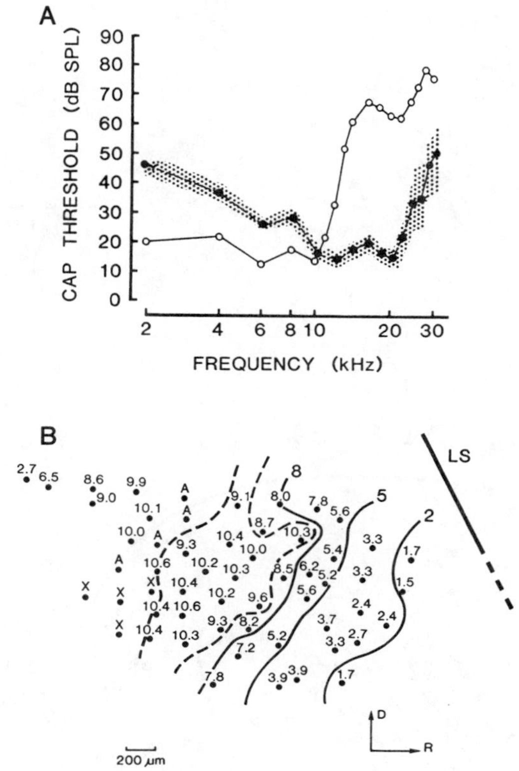

Figure 11-4 Effect of permanent losses in cochlear neural sensitivity over a restricted frequency range on the tonotopic organization of auditory cortex in the guinea pig. *A,* Open circles represent the compound action potential (CAP) audiogram for this animal, measured at the time of the cortical recording session. The black dots and the stippled region represent the mean normal audiogram for normal animals (± 1 S.D.). *B,* Organization of characteristic frequencies (CF) in the cortex contralateral to the lesioned cochlea, to stimulation of the lesioned cochlea. Mapping was done with microelectrode penetrations made normal to the cortical surface. Penetrations marked "A" show neuronal clusters that responded only weakly to auditory input in general, and for which no CF could be determined. The rostral auditory field in the guinea pig, mapped in greater detail here, normally contains a tonotopic progression with low-CF neurons at the rostral edge of the field and high-CF neurons at the caudal edge of the field, which abuts the caudal auditory field. The caudal field has a tonotopic organization that is the reverse of that of the rostral field, such that the high-frequency representations of the two fields abut each other. In penetrations marked "X" neuronal clusters were not responsive to the auditory stimuli used. "LS" indicates the position of the lateral sulcus. From Robertson D, Irvine DRF. Plasticity of frequency organization in auditory cortex of guinea pigs with partial unilateral deafness. J Comp Neurol 1989; 282:456-471.

We have examined the occurrence of effects in the cat, reported by Robertson and Irvine (1989), to determine the generality of their finding of plasticity of the frequency organization in the adult auditory cortex. We employed similar techniques to create mechanical lesions on a restricted region of the basilar membrane (BM) in the left cochlea of adult cats. After a recovery period of a few months, CAP audiograms were measured, and the tonotopic organization of the right AI was determined, under barbiturate anesthesia.

The mechanical lesions to the BM typically produced high-frequency losses at the cochlea. An example of such a loss in cochlear neural sensitivity is illustrated in Figure 11-5A. In this animal, small losses in the CAP occurred at 20 kHz, becoming significant by 22 kHz and larger at all higher frequencies. The effects of these losses on the cochleotopic organization of AI contralateral to the lesioned cochlea are illustrated in Figure 11-5B. In this animal, the low frequencies below about 8 kHz were located in the bank of the posterior ectosylvian sulcus (PES), and two penetrations made along the bank of PES recorded a progressive decrease in CFs with increasing distance down the bank. CFs higher than about 8 kHz were represented on the surface of the middle ectosylvian gyrus. Moving from the caudal end of the gyrus there was a progressive increase in the CFs of neuron clusters, and isofrequency lines progressively shifted rostrally with increasing CF until about 19 kHz, as in normal animals. However, beyond the 19-kHz isofrequency line, the tonotopic organization was distinctly abnormal (see Fig. 11-3). All further rostral penetrations yielded neurons with CFs between 19 and about 21 kHz (except for one point with a CF of 18.2 kHz). The region of cortex with CFs in this restricted range spanned a distance of about 1.5 to 2 mm and, given that all of the most rostral points still had CFs within this range, may have extended even further.

The presence of a much larger than normal (i.e., expanded) region of cortex in which all neurons have a limited range of CF does not in itself mean that a plastic reorganization of the tonotopic map has occurred. As noted by Robertson and Irvine (1989), if cortical neurons have tuning curves that extend to a range of frequencies below CF, the larger-than-normal representation of a frequency at the edge of a cochlear lesion may simply represent residual drive in the high-CF neurons deprived of CF input by the peripheral lesion. That is, a cortical neuron deprived of its CF in-

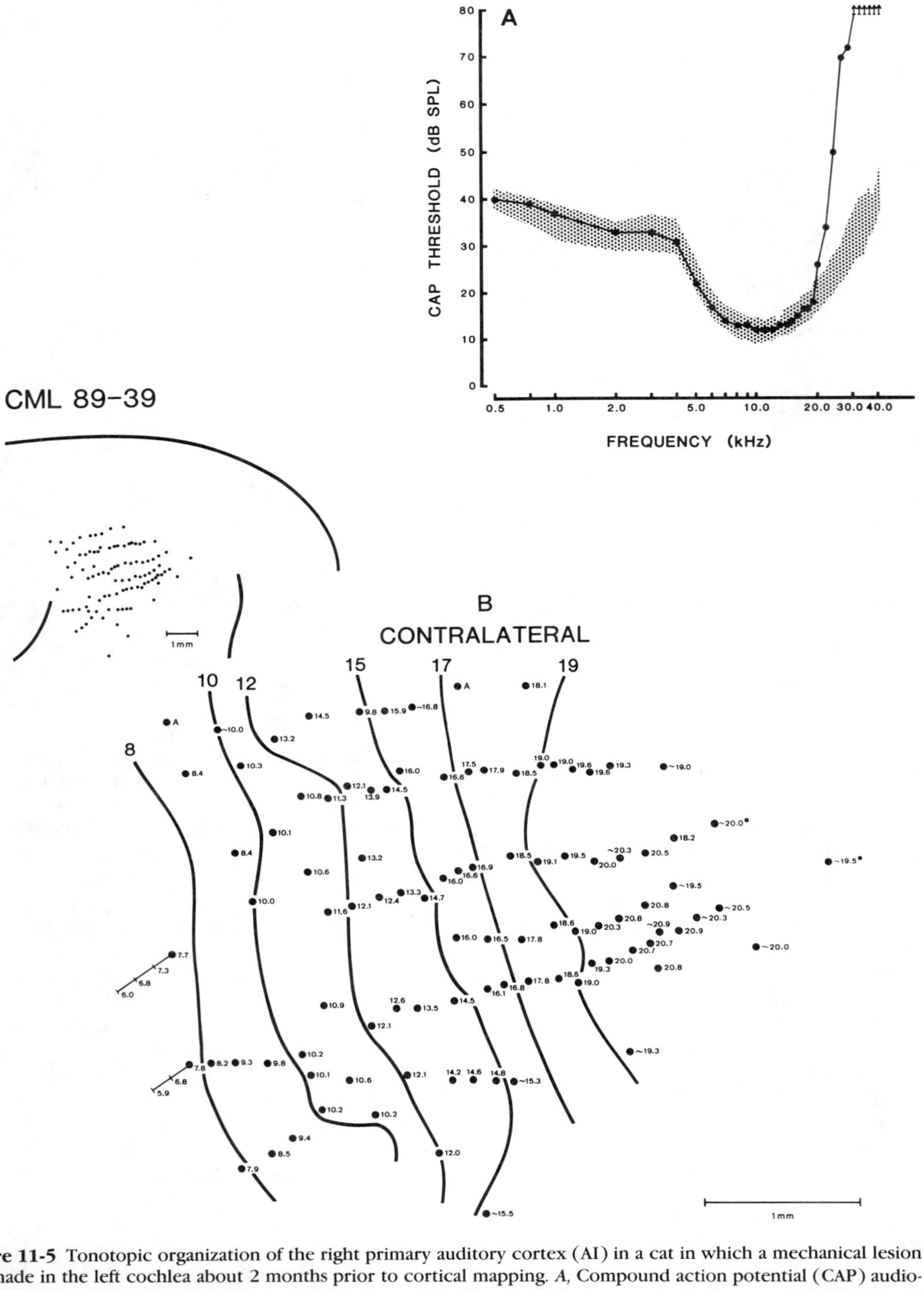

Figure 11-5 Tonotopic organization of the right primary auditory cortex (AI) in a cat in which a mechanical lesion was made in the left cochlea about 2 months prior to cortical mapping. *A,* Compound action potential (CAP) audiogram from the left cochlea at the time of cortical mapping. The stippled area represents the range ±1 S.D. around the mean audiogram from normal animals. In the test animal, the CAP audiogram lay within this range until about 20 kHz, at which there was a loss of about 6 dB compared to normal mean CAP thresholds. Thereafter, CAP losses in this animal were considerably greater. *B,* Tonotopic organization of the AI contralateral to the lesioned cochlea to stimulation of that cochlea. Tildes indicate that the assigned CF was the midpoint of a narrow range of frequencies (no more than 3 kHz wide) to which the neuronal clusters were equally sensitive. Note the rostral region containing an expanded representation of the frequency range 19 to 20.9 kHz. Two rostral points are marked with an asterisk to indicate that they had very high thresholds (about 50 dB SPL).

put would still be able to respond to the lower frequencies that fell within its response area and would thus exhibit a "new" CF at a frequency at the edge of the lesion. However, given the sharp frequency tuning of most AI neurons (Phillips and Irvine, 1981), residual responses of this sort would have higher-than-normal thresholds. Thus, assessing whether the expanded representation is a manifestation of plasticity depends critically on whether the CF thresholds in the region of expanded representation are comparable to normal thresholds.

We therefore compared the CF thresholds in the expanded region to the CF thresholds in normal cortical regions immediately adjacent to the region of nominal expansion, selecting all points within the 2-kHz band of frequencies just caudal to the start of the region of expansion as the "normal" band for comparison. The adjacent 2-kHz band was chosen because this band of frequencies was sufficiently close so as to be unaffected by the confounding factor of differences in normal cochlear sensitivity. In the case illustrated in Figure 11-5, the "control" points were the 12 points lying between the 17- and the 19-kHz isofrequency lines. The mean threshold for these points was about 7 dB lower than the mean threshold in the region of expansion. Although this difference was statistically significant, it can be acounted for by the loss of 6 dB in the CAP threshold at the frequencies of expansion, compared to normal CAP thresholds at these frequencies.

In all cases with lesions made to restricted regions of the BM, we have observed the basic phenomenon of an expansion of the cortical representation of a restricted band of frequencies represented at BM loci at the edge of the region affected by the lesion. This confirms the results obtained by Robertson and Irvine (1989) in the guinea pig and extends the generality of the result to another mammalian species. As illustrated by the consideration of thresholds in the regions of reorganization, the expanded cortical representation of a frequency band at the edge of a peripheral lesion appears to represent a genuine plastic reorganization of the frequency map rather than just the result of residual drive from the edge frequencies.

These results reveal a large degree of plasticity in a cortical map of the adult auditory system, similar to the plasticity observed in maps of adult central nervous system structures in other sensory systems (Byrne and Calford, 1989; Calford and Tweedale, 1988, 1990; Devor and Wall, 1978, 1981; Dostrovsky et al, 1976; Kelahan and Doetsch, 1984; Merrill and Wall, 1978; Merzenich and Kaas, 1982; Merzenich et al, 1983a,b, 1984; Rasmusson, 1982; Wall and Cusick, 1984; Wilson and Snow, 1990). This suggests that this phenomenon is common among sensory representations in the adult central nervous system. How such plasticity of frequency selectivity and auditory cortical maps after damage to the peripheral receptor array affects perceptual function is still a matter of speculation. Nevertheless, the reorganization of the tonotopic map and the expanded representation of frequency regions adjacent to the regions of cochlear losses may result in abnormal patterns of processing in an auditory cortex showing such effects.

Effets des Deficits Auditifs sur la Sélectivité en Fréquence et sur l'Organisation Tonotopique du Cortex Auditif

Les aires corticales primaires de l'audition, de la somesthésie et de la vision contiennent une représentation ordonnée du champ récepteur périphérique. Dans la somesthésie et la vision, cette topographie correspond à des "cartes" respectives de l'espace corporel et de l'espace visuel. Dans le système auditif, la représentation ordonnée de l'organe récepteur périphérique correspond à une organisation tonotopique du cortex auditif primaire (AI). Les hautes fréquences sont représentées à un bout du champ cortical et les basses fréquences à l'autre, avec les fréquences intermédiaires entre les deux. Beaucoup d'études récentes, principalement du système somesthésique, ont montré que la représentation topographique corticale est malléable non seulement chez un organisme en cours de développement mais aussi chez l'adulte suite à l'élimination d'informations en provenance de régions spécifiques et restreintes de la surface du récepteur périphérique. Dans le système auditif périphérique, Robertson et Irvine (1989) ont montré que chez le cobaye adulte, des lésions cochléaires unilatérales et restreintes provoquant des pertes permanentes de la sensibilité neuro-cochléaire sur une étendue restreinte de fréquences, entraînaient une plasticité de l'organisation en fréquence dans le cortex auditif contralatéral à la cochlée lésée. De 35 à 81 jours après la lésion, l'analyse de la sensibilité des groupements de neurones dans le cortex auditif contralatéral, révéle que l'aire corticale où le domaine fréquentiel lésé aurait normalement été représenté est partiellement occupé par une expansion des domaines fréquentiels adjacents au domaine fréquentiel endommagé par la lésion. Les réponses des neurones de l'aire réorganisée sont vigoureuses et les seuils des groupements de neurones corticaux ne sont pas différents des seuils normaux à ces fréquences. Ces effets n'ont pas été observés quand le cortex contralatéral était examiné quelques heures après la réalisation des lésions.

Chez le chat, en utilisant des lésions cochléaires induites mécaniquement ou par du bruit, nous avons tenté de reproduire les résultats de Robertson et Irvine et de déterminer s'il est possible de généraliser leur découverte relative à la plasticité de l'organisation fréquentielle du cerveau adulte. La robustesse du chat en tant qu'animal expérimental, nous a permis d'examiner d'autres aspects de la plasticité, telle que l'arrivée d'informations binaurales dans la région de réorganisation fréquentielle. Dans l'étude de Robertson et Irvine, la carte en fréquence du cortex auditif contralatéral à l'oreille lésée, a été examinée en utilisant des stimulations monaurales de l'oreille lésée car la grande majorité des neurones auditifs corticaux d'un hémisphère reçoivent des afférences excitatrices en provenance de l'oreille contralatérale. Cependant, la plupart de ces neurones rçoivent aussi des informations en provenance de l'oreille ipsilatérale. Nous avons essayé de déterminer si les afférences d'origine ipsilatérale des neurones de la région d'expansion et de réorganisation maintiennent un registre normal entre les cartes fréquentielles ipsilatérales et contralatérales. Finalement, afin de tenter d'élucider les mécanismes qui pourraient contribuer à cette plasticité, nous avons examiné les effets, induits par le bruit, de réaménagements temporaires des seuils de sensibilité neuro-cochléaire sur la sélectivité en fréquence des neurones du cortex auditif.

References

Babighian G, Moushegian G, Rupert AL. Central auditory fatigue. Audiology 1975; 14:72-83.

Biedermann M, Emmerich E, Kaschowitz H, Richter F. Cochlear potentials and responses from structures of auditory pathway influenced by high-intensive noise. In: Syka J, Masterson RB, eds. Auditory pathway: structure and function. New York: Plenum Press, 1987:217.

Blauert J. Sound localization in the median plane. Acustica 1969/1970; 22:205-213.

Byrne J, Calford, MB. Acute plasticity of primary somatosensory cortex (SI) in adult rats. Proc Aust Neurosci Soc Neurosci Letts Suppl 1989; 34:S67.

Calford MB, Rajan R, Irvine DRF. Effect of pure-tone induced temporary threshold shift on the response areas of auditory cortical neurons in the cat. Proc Aust Neurosci Soc Neurosci Letts Suppl 1989; 34:S68.

Calford MB, Tweedale R. Immediate and chronic changes in responses of somatosensory cortex in adult flying-fox after digit amputation. Nature 1988; 332:446-448.

Calford MB, Tweedale R. The capacity for reorganization in adult somatosensory cortex. In: Rowe M, Aikin LM, eds. Information processing in mammalian auditory and tactile systems. New York: Wiley-Liss, 1990:221.

Cody AR, Johnstone BM. Single auditory neuron response during acute acoustic trauma. Hear Res 1980; 3:3-16.

Dallos P, Ozdamar O, Ryan A. Behavioral, compound action potential, and single unit thresholds: relationship in normal and abnormal ears. J Acoust Soc Am 1978; 64:151-157.

Devor M, Wall PD. Reorganization of spinal cord sensory map after peripheral nerve injury. Nature 1978; 276:75-76.

Devor M, Wall PD. Plasticity in the spinal cord sensory map following peripheral nerve injury in rats. J Neurosci 1981; 1:679-684.

Dostrovsky JO, Millar J, Wall PD. The immediate shift of afferent drive of dorsal column nucleus cells following deafferentation: A comparison of acute and chronic deafferentation in gracile nucleus and spinal cord. Exp Neurol 1976; 52:480-495.

Gerken GM, Simhadri-Sumithra R, Bhat KHV. Increase in central auditory responsiveness during continuous tone stimulation or following hearing loss. In: Salvi RJ, Henderson D, Hamernik RP, Colletti V, eds. Basic and applied aspects of noise-induced hearing loss. New York: Plenum Press, 1982:195.

Henderson D, Møller A. Effects of asymptotic threshold shift in the neural firing patterns of the rat cochlear nucleus. J Acoust Soc Am 1975; 57:S53.

Jenkins WM, Merzenich MM. Role of cat primary auditory cortex for sound-localization behaviour. J Neurophysiol 1984; 52:819-847.

Johnstone JR, Alder VA, Johnstone BM, et al. Cochlear action potential threshold and single unit thresholds. J Acoust Soc Am 1979; 65:254-257.

Juliano SL, Whitsel BL. A combined 2-deoxyglucose and neurophysiological study of primate somatosensory cortex. J Comp Neurol 1987; 263:514-525.

Kelahan AM, Doetsch GS. Time-dependent changes in the functional organization of somatosensory cerebral cortex following digit amputation in adult racoon. Somatosens Res 1984; 2:49-81.

Landry P, Deschenes M. Intracortical arborizations and receptive fields of identified ventrobasal thalamocortical afferents to the primary somatic sensory cortex in the cat. J Comp Neurol 1981; 199:345-371.

Lonsbury-Martin BL, Martin GK. Effects of moderately intense sound on auditory sensitivity in rhesus monkeys: Behavioral and neural observations. J Neurophysiol 1981; 46:563-586.

Lonsbury-Martin BL, Meikle MB. Neural correlates of auditory fatigue: Frequency-dependent changes in activity of single cochlear nerve fibers. J Neurophysiol 1978; 41:987-1005.

Merrill EG, Wall PD. Plasticity of connection in the adult nervous system. In: Cotman CW, ed. Neuronal Plasticity. New York: Raven Press, 1978:97.

Merzenich MM, Kaas JH. Organization of mammalian somatosensory cortex following peripheral nerve injury. Trends Neurosci 1982; 5:434-436.

Merzenich MM, Kaas JH, Wall JT, et al. Topographic reorganization of somatosensory cortical areas 3b and 1 in adult monkeys following restricted deafferentation. Neuroscience 1983a; 8:33-55.

Merzenich MM, Kaas JH, Wall JT, et al. Progression of change following median nerve section in the cortical representation of the hand in areas 3b and 1 in adult owl and squirrel monkeys. Neuroscience 1983b; 10:639-665.

Merzenich MM, Knight PL, Roth GL. Representation of the cochlea within primary auditory cortex in the cat. J Neurophysiol 1975; 38:231-249.

Merzenich MM, Nelson RJ, Stryker MP, et al. Somatosensory cortical map changes following digit amputation in adult monkey. J Comp Neurol 1984; 224:591-605.

Metzlar J, Marks PS. Functional changes in cat somatic sensory-motor cortex during short-term reversible epidermal blocks. Brain Res 1979; 177:379-383.

Nakahima H, Nishioka S, Otsuka T. Excitation and inhibition in ventrobasal thalamic neurons before and after cutaneous input deprivation. Prog Brain Res 1966; 21:180-196.

Phillips DP, Cynader MS. Some neural mechanisms in the cat's auditory cortex underlying sensitivity to combined tone and wide-spectrum noise stimuli. Hear Res 1985; 18:87-102.

Phillips DP, Irvine DRF. Responses of single neurons in physiologically defined primary auditory cortex (AI) of the cat: frequency tuning and responses to intensity. J Neurophysiol 1981; 45:48-58.

Popelár J, Syka J. Noise impairment. II. Changes of single unit responses in the inferior colliculus. Hear Res 1982; 8:273-283.

Price GR. Action potentials in the cat at low sound intensities: thresholds, latencies and rates of change. J Acoust Soc Am 1978; 64:1400-1405.

Rasmusson DD. Reorganization of racoon somatosensory cortex following removal of the fifth digit. J Comp Neurol 1982; 205:313-326.

Reale RA, Imig TJ. Tonotopic organization in auditory cortex of the cat. J Comp Neurol 1980; 192:265-291.

Robertson D, Irvine DRF. Plasticity of frequency organization in auditory cortex of guinea pigs with partial unilateral deafness. J Comp Neurol 1989; 282: 456-471.

Salvi R. Central components of the temporary threshold shift. In: Henderson D, Hamernik RP, Dorsanjh DS, Mills JH, eds. Effects of noise on hearing. New York: Raven Press, 1976:247.

Salvi R, Henderson D, Hamernik R. Auditory fatigue: retrocochlear components. Science 1975; 190:486-487.

Snow PJ, Nudo RJ, Rivers W, et al. Somatotopically inappropriate projections from thalamocortical neurons to the SI cortex of the cat demonstrated by the use of intracortical microstimulation. Somatosens Res 1988; 5:349-372.

Starr A, Livingston RB. Long-lasting nervous system responses to prolonged sound stimulation in waking cats. J Neurophysiol 1963; 26:416-431.

Syka J, Popelár J. Noise impairment in the guinea pig. I. Changes in electrical evoked activity along the auditory pathway. Hear Res 1982; 8:263-272.

Viermiester N. Intensity coding and the dynamic range problem. Hear Res 1988; 34:267-274.

Wall JT, Cusick CG. Cutaneous responsiveness in primary somatosensory (S-I) hindpaw cortex before and after partial hindpaw deafferentation in adult rats. J Neurosci 1984; 4:1499-1515.

Wall PD, Werman R. The physiology and anatomy of long ranging afferent fibers within the spinal cord. J Physiol (Lond) 1976; 225:321-334.

Willott JF, Lu S-M. Noise-induced hearing loss can alter neural coding and increase excitability in the central nervous system. Science 1981; 216:1331-1332.

Wilson P, Snow PJ. The capacity for reorganization within spinal somatosensory systems. In: Rowe M, Aitkin LM, eds. Information processing in mammalian auditory and tactile systems. New York: Wiley-Liss, 1990:205.

CHAPTER 12

Deafness-Induced Changes in the Central Nervous System: Reversibility and Prevention

JOSEF M. MILLER
RICHARD A. ALTSCHULER
JOHN K. NIPARKO
DUANE O. HARTSHORN
ROBERT H. HELFERT
JEAN K. MOORE

As our understanding of the peripheral effects of noise on inner-ear structures and the mechanisms underlying these effects increases, so does concern about the central consequences of noise-induced pathology as well as the effects of deafness on the central auditory system. From studies dating to the last century, we know that normal structure and function of the central pathways of sensory systems depend on the integrity and activity of the receptor (Coleman and Buell, 1985). In aging, as well as in development, anatomic studies suggest that afferent input strongly influences axonal and dendritic characteristics, synapse morphology and, to a lesser degree, cell size. It is apparent that the "hard-wired" concept of brain circuitry is not correct. Rather, the capacity for neural reorganization in response to the presence or absence of afferent input is now well established. In the auditory system, the dependency of auditory nerve and central auditory structures on normal cochlear function has been well described in both neonatal and mature animals. Although the effects tend to be more dramatic in the neonate, they certainly are evident in the mature auditory system.

In the auditory system, such studies have taken on a special emphasis with the development of clinical procedures to bypass the pathologic receptor and directly activate central auditory paths in an attempt to rehabilitate the profoundly deaf. It seems intuitive that the development and application of cochlear and central nervous system (CNS) prostheses depend on the condition of the auditory nerve and the rest of the central auditory pathways. Increasingly, data indicate that the benefits of a prosthesis depend on the integrity of the auditory nerve and secondary central auditory structures. Direct observations supporting this contention include animal studies that illustrate a relationship between the threshold, dynamic range of hearing and discrimination performance, and the density of surviving spiral ganglion cells (SGCs) (Pfingst et al, 1981, 1983, 1985, 1988). Indirect observations are based on findings in human beings of an inverse relationship between perceptual benefits and length of deafness before implantation, and between perceptional benefits and interaction of signals across stimulation electrodes ("channel interaction"), both presumably reflecting a decreased density of nerve fibers (Kileny and Zimmerman-Phillips, 1988).

Most recently, observations have indicated that under some conditions, the central degenerative consequences of inner-ear deafness may be reduced. Together these observations raise three questions: (1) What is the state of our current knowledge of the consequences of deafness on central auditory structures? (2) What are the mechanisms that may underlie these changes? (3) To what extent are they preventable or reversible?

Current Knowledge on Central Consequences of Deafness

Deprivation of sensory input can have profound effects on the structure and function of an afferent neural network. Most dramatic are the changes that take place in the developing organism. These effects have been particularly well described in the visual system; Hubel and Wiesel have made hallmark contributions (Hubel and Wiesel, 1965; Wiesel and Hubel, 1965; Hubel et al, 1976, 1977). Unilateral visual deprivation during development permanently eliminated representation of the deprived eye in binocular cells within visual cortex. It is interesting that if the monocular deprivation is reversed within a critical period of development, the physiologic changes can also be reversed (Wiesel and Hubel, 1965). Thus, not only can reduced afferent input decrease the functional projections of the system, but stimulation can increase functional connectivity. Moreover, in rats with monocular deprivation, there is an extensive hemispheric ingrowth of callosal fibers, which invade and make functional connections on binocularly deprived cells within the contralateral hemisphere (Lund et al, 1984). Many of these fibers would be gradually lost in the normal preparation, reflecting routine programmed cell death that occurs widely throughout the nervous system. Thus, activity may permanently eliminate the development of functional afferent connections and may reduce programmed cell death by promoting growth of neuronal processes in the visual system. In general, these findings are consistent with observations in the somatosensory (Harris and Woolsey, 1981), olfactory (Meisami, 1976; Meisami and Manoochehri, 1977), and auditory systems.

In the auditory system, previous studies on both neonatal and mature mammalian models indicate that deafening can produce significant morphologic changes in the central pathways. These changes are most obvious when the deafening occurs during development. In neonatally sound-deprived mice, Webster and Webster (1977) found that both globular cells of the ventral cochlear nucleus (CN) and principal cells of the medial nucleus of the trapezoid body were reduced in size, and that the dorsal CN was reduced in volume. These findings, although of a lesser extent, were similar to those observed in the brain of a 9-year-old child with profound congenital sensorineural hearing loss (Webster and Webster, 1977). Following cochlear ablation in neonate mice, Trune (1982) found fewer and smaller neurons in the octopus cell and multipolar cell regions, as well as in the ipsilateral cochlear nucleus in the deep layer of the dorsal cochlear nucleus. Additionally, he observed fewer normal-sized spherical and globular cells. In cats with fully-developed auditory systems, cochlear ablation results in a significant reduction in volume of the CN and nuclei of the superior olivary complex, primarily due to a reduction of cell size, with no obvious decrease in cell number (McGee and Olszewski, 1962; Powell and Erulkar, 1962; Kane, 1974). Similar findings were observed in the adult guinea pig cochlear nucleus by Webster and Webster (1978) and gerbil CN (Hashisaki and Rubel, 1989).

Human Investigations

The questions and challenges in this area of research can be defined on the basis of the examination of human material. Figure 12-1 illustrates the results of an analysis of auditory nerve survival and cochlear pathology in the temporal bones of a 62-year-old male who was bilaterally profoundly deaf. He had lost hearing in his right ear following a mastoidectomy 40 years prior to death. Deafness in his left ear occurred as a result of a slowly progressive hearing loss from 1952 onward. In 1987 he was implanted with a nucleus cochlear prosthesis, which he used regularly during the last 9 months of his life. The principal finding of this temporal bone analysis is that there is a close relationship between SGC survival and damage to structures of the organ of Corti.

The central auditory structures in the patient described above were also examined. Figure 12-2 illustrates a comparison between the ventral CN in a normal subject (Fig. 12-2A) and the bilaterally deaf patient (Fig. 12-2B). In the deaf subject, the CN shows a markedly increased packing density of neurons and glia and a much more diffuse staining of cellular elements. The greater density of cells in the ventral nucleus is highly suggestive of regression of auditory nerve axons and their collateral branches. Diffuse neuronal staining was also observed in higher auditory nuclei, and was particularly obvious in cells of the medial superior olive (Fig. 12-3A). The change in staining characteristics was restricted to auditory structures and was not present in other brain-stem structures in the deaf patient, as evidenced by the normal ap-

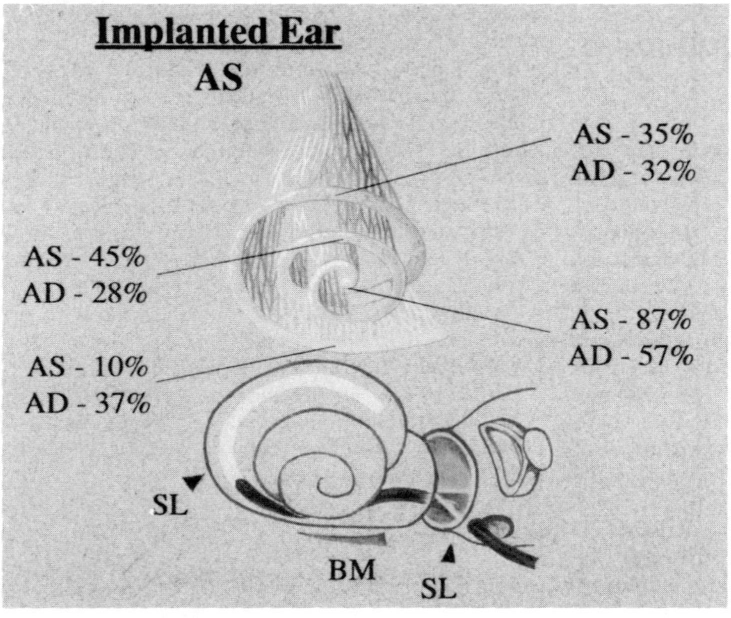

Figure 12-1 Reconstruction of surviving spiral ganglion cells in the right (RD) and left (AS) ears of a profoundly deaf human. The left ear was implanted with a cochlear prosthesis. Initial placement of the prosthesis is indicated by the white line in the figure of the cochlea; it was subsequently moved to the position indicated by the dark line in the cochlea drawing. Damage to the spiral ligament (SL) and basilar membrane (BM) occurred at sites indicated. Essentially, all sensory elements were eliminated from the first half of the basal turn in the implanted ear. In both ears it was a gradual increase in sensory element survival from base to apex. A close correlation was found between surviving sensory elements and surviving neural fibers.

pearance of cells in the facial nucleus (Fig. 12-3B).

Our observations in this patient lend support to the suggestion that auditory nerve survival depends on the survival of supporting elements of the organ of Corti (Ghorayer et al, 1980). On the other hand, from this work, as well as from material published by others, it does not seem possible to separate extensive inner hair cell loss from loss of supporting elements as causative factors in producing auditory nerve degeneration. It seems obvious from our observations, in addition to the literature on human subjects, that a wide variety of factors contribute to auditory nerve and secondary pathway degeneration. Indeed, there are even observations of auditory nerve degeneration and concomitant hearing loss in the presence of normal hair cells and organ of Corti following aminoglycoside treatment (Hinojosa and Lerner, 1987). In general, in the literature on human subjects, a wide spectrum of eighth-nerve survival has been reported with inner-ear pathology (Otte et al, 1978; Hinojosa and Marion, 1983), which to a limited extent appears to depend on the etiology of deafness (Bergstrom, 1975; Hinojosa and Marion, 1983). These data indicate that a number of factors involved with normal inner-ear function may contribute to maintenance of a normal auditory nerve; also, as demonstrated in controlled animal investigations, a number of peripheral mechanisms underlie auditory nerve survival. We suggest that controlled animal studies in parallel with the investigation of human material are necessary to clearly define the factors that contribute to CNS changes with deafness.

Animal Investigations

To pursue these questions under controlled conditions, we have studied degeneration in the ototoxically-deafened guinea pig. The combination of kanamycin and ethacrynic acid in a single systemic injection as described by West et al (1973) has been used throughout these studies. This drug produces a profound deafness with a typically complete elimination of all hair cells except a few scattered outer hair cells remaining at the apex of the cochlea. With such broad destruction of hair cells of the organ of Corti, widespread degeneration of auditory nerve and SGCs begins 1 to 2 weeks following drug administration. By 9 weeks the density of SGCs has been reduced to approximately 50 percent of normal; by 16 weeks it is reduced to 20 to 25 percent of normal (Fig. 12-4). Although there is significant variability across animals within this group, as Figure 12-4 shows, a reliable and consistently progressive change in cell survival was observed. In animals with a sparing of hair cells in the apical region of the cochlea (approximately one in ten, with the drug dose used) significant survival of SGCs in the apex of the cochlea was observed. As opposed to

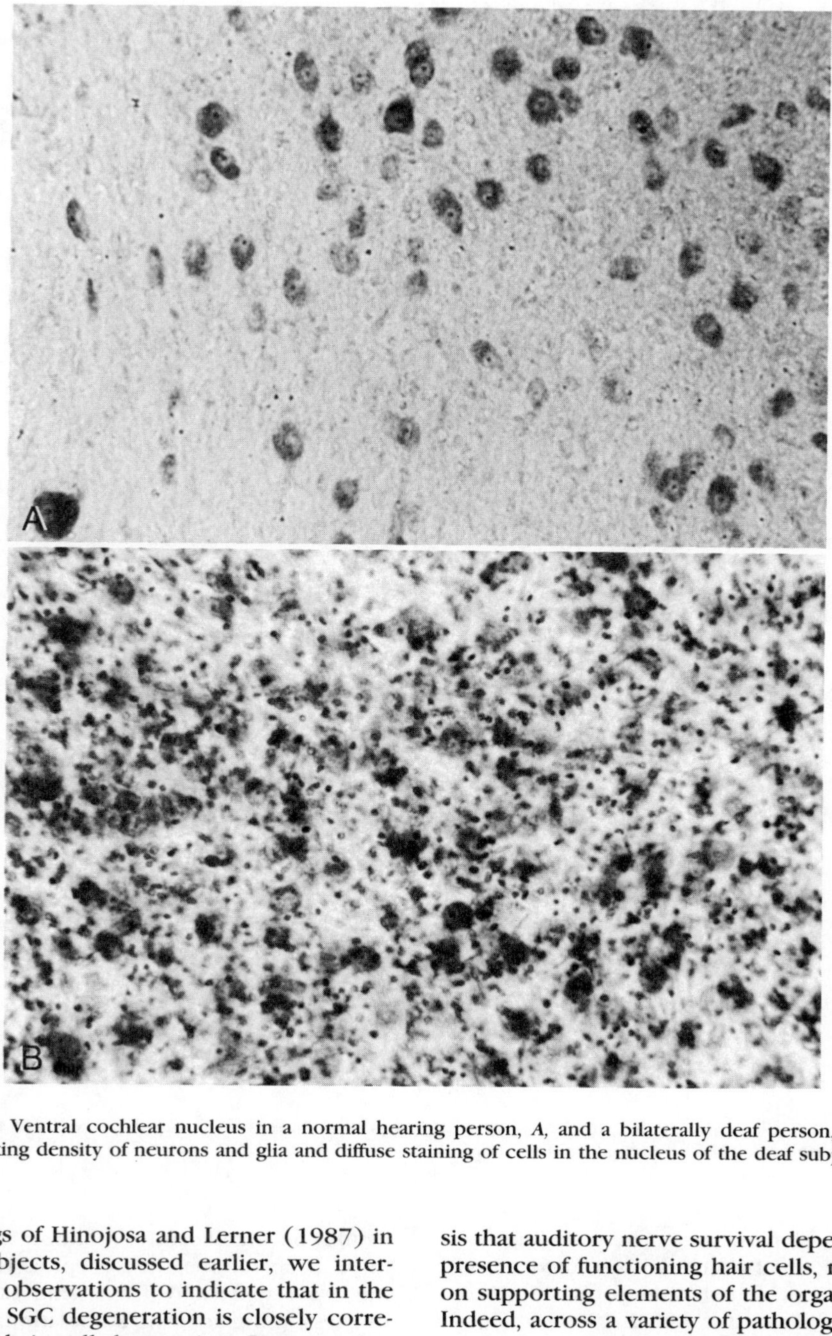

Figure 12-2 Ventral cochlear nucleus in a normal hearing person, *A*, and a bilaterally deaf person, *B*. Note increased packing density of neurons and glia and diffuse staining of cells in the nucleus of the deaf subject.

the findings of Hinojosa and Lerner (1987) in human subjects, discussed earlier, we interpret these observations to indicate that in the guinea pig SGC degeneration is closely correlated with hair cell destruction. Degeneration does not appear to be a direct effect of the ototoxic drug on distal processes of the auditory nerve fibers in this preparation. Moreover, the observation that initial SGC degeneration could be seen in less than 2 weeks following drug administration, as well as in preparations in which a relatively normal supporting structure of the organ of Corti could yet be observed, supports the hypothesis that auditory nerve survival depends on the presence of functioning hair cells, rather than on supporting elements of the organ of Corti. Indeed, across a variety of pathologic material in the guinea pig, our observations support this view.

These data have recently been extended to examine the effects of deafening on cells of the CN. In a preliminary study, we measured the areas of nucleolus-containing somatic profiles in the rostral anteroventral cochlear nucleus (AVCN) in guinea pigs 12 months after ototoxic drug administration. Figure 12-5 shows that we observed a 15 to 20 percent

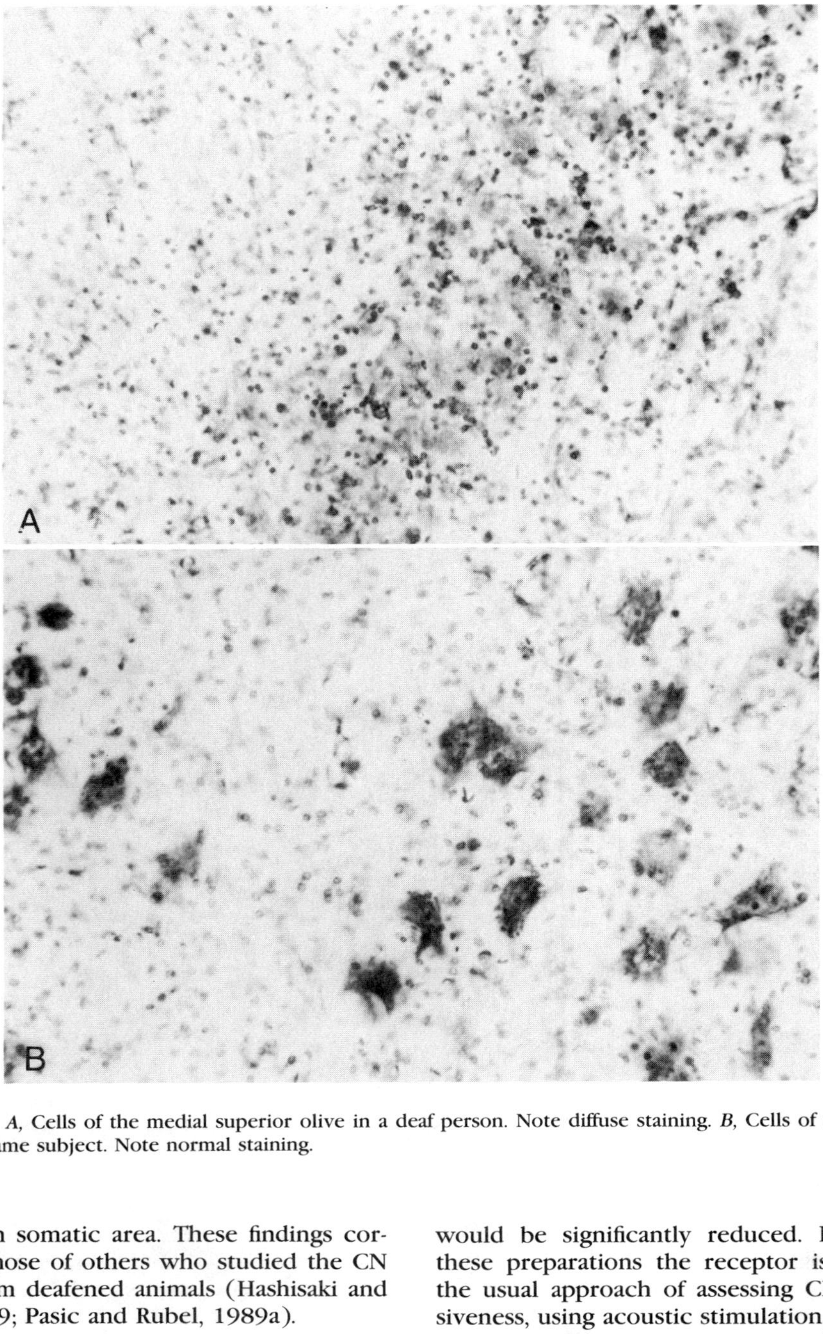

Figure 12-3 *A,* Cells of the medial superior olive in a deaf person. Note diffuse staining. *B,* Cells of the facial nucleus from same subject. Note normal staining.

decrease in somatic area. These findings corroborate those of others who studied the CN of long-term deafened animals (Hashisaki and Rubel, 1989; Pasic and Rubel, 1989a).

Functional Implications of CNS Changes

It would seem obvious that with degeneration of auditory nerve and changes in cells of the auditory brain stem the responsiveness of the central auditory pathways to excitation would be significantly reduced. Because in these preparations the receptor is damaged, the usual approach of assessing CNS responsiveness, using acoustic stimulation, cannot be employed. One alternative approach is the use of electrical stimulation that can bypass the auditory receptor. Smith and Simmons (1983) demonstrated that the slope of the amplitude input/output function for the electrically evoked auditory brain-stem response (EABR) was reduced with a reduction in density of SGCs in pathologic cat preparations. Hall (1990) demonstrated that various measures of the EABR amplitude strongly correlate with

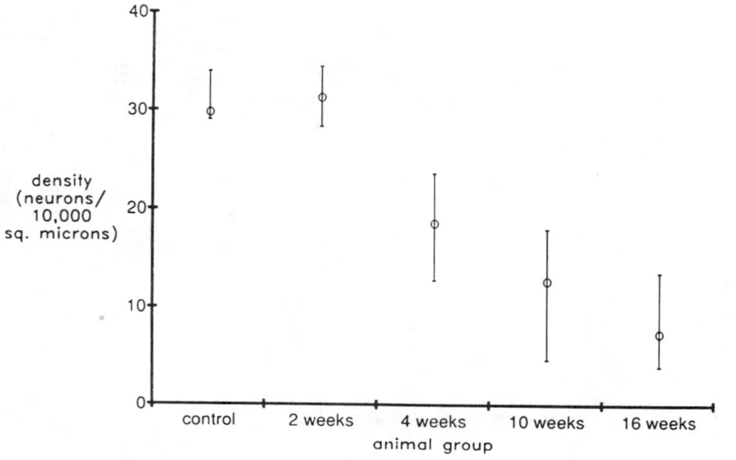

Figure 12-4 Density of surviving spiral ganglion cells in guinea pigs following administration of ototoxic drugs. From Jyung RW, Miller JM, Cannon SC. Evaluation of eighth nerve integrity using the electrically evoked middle latency response. Otolaryngol Head Neck Surg 1989; 101(6):670-682.

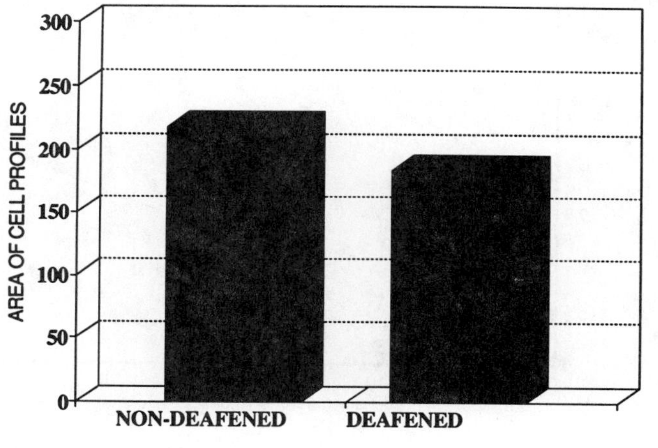

Figure 12-5 Spherical cell size in the anteroventral cochlear nucleus of guinea pigs 12 months following ototoxic drug treatment and of age-matched, normal-hearing subjects.

SGC populations in pathologic rat preparations. Stypulkowski et al (1986) indicated that for individual animals the variability was sufficiently great that at best only a tenuous relationship existed between decreased responsiveness as measured by the EABR and SGC density. We have suggested that this variability may, in part, reflect a susceptibility of the EABR measure to electrical artifact contamination, due to its short latency. We have evaluated the utility of the electrically evoked middle latency response (EMLR) to assess changes in electrical evoked responsiveness of the auditory pathways. We demonstrated that the measure was less sensitive to electrical artifact than the EABR and exhibited equal threshold sensitivity and sensitivity to changes in the site of peripheral stimulation (Burton et al, 1989a,b). Following treatment with ototoxic drugs the slope of the amplitude input/output function of the EMLR in guinea pigs decreases with time following treatment both across animals and within individual subjects (Jyung et al, 1989; Hartshorn et al, 1989). This effect is demonstrated in Figure 12-6, which shows, for an individual animal, the change in amplitude input/output function of the EABR during a 9-week period following treatment with ethacrynic acid and kanamycin. Figure 12-7 demonstrates the correlation coefficient observed between the slope of the input/output function of the EMLR and density of surviving SGCs in drug-treated subjects with survival times from 2 to 16 weeks following ototoxic administration. These findings indicated that significant changes in excitability of the central auditory pathways occur with reduction of SGCs.

Most recently these findings have been extended to the study of evoked metabolic activity in ototoxically-deafened animals using 2-deoxyglucose (2DG) measures. Figure 12-8 illustrates the density of 2DG in the inferior colliculus (IC) of normal and deafened subjects. These data demonstrate that, 4 weeks following deafness from ototoxic drug admin-

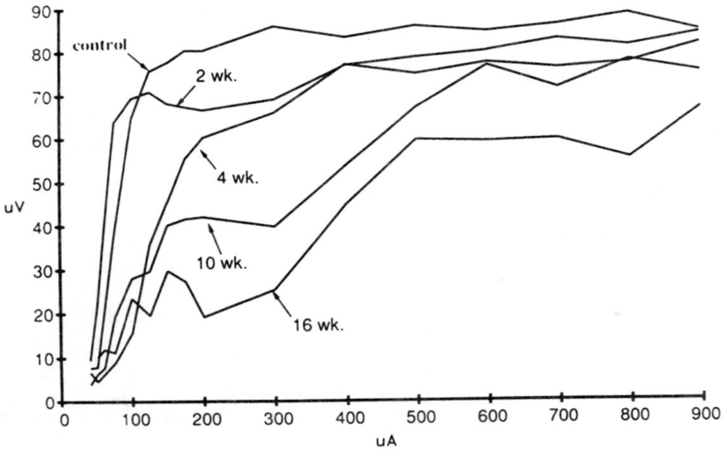

Figure 12-6 Amplitude input/output functions of the electrically evoked middle latency response (EMLR) in a guinea pig prior to (control) and following ototoxic drug administration. From Jyung RW, Miller JM, Cannon SC. Evaluation of eighth nerve integrity using the electrically evoked middle latency response. Otolaryngol Head Neck Surg 1989; 101(6):670-682.

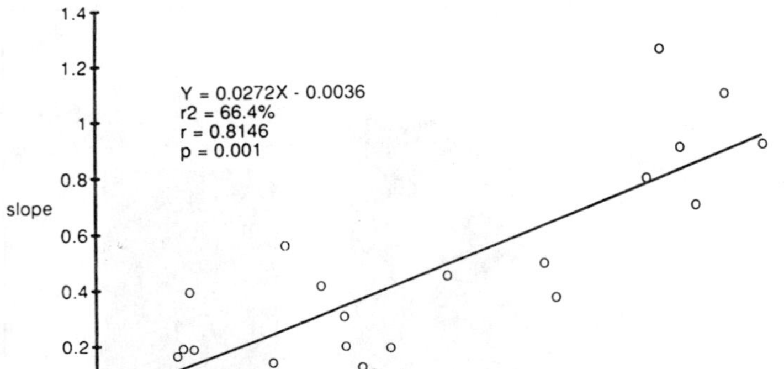

Figure 12-7 Correlation coefficient observed between the slope of the input/output function of the electrically evoked middle latency response (EMLR) and density of surviving spiral ganglion cells in ototoxic drug–treated guinea pigs with varying survival times following drug administration. From Jyung RW, Miller JM, Cannon SC. Evaluation of eighth nerve integrity using the electrically evoked middle latency response. Otolaryngol Head Neck Surg 1989; 101(6):670-682.

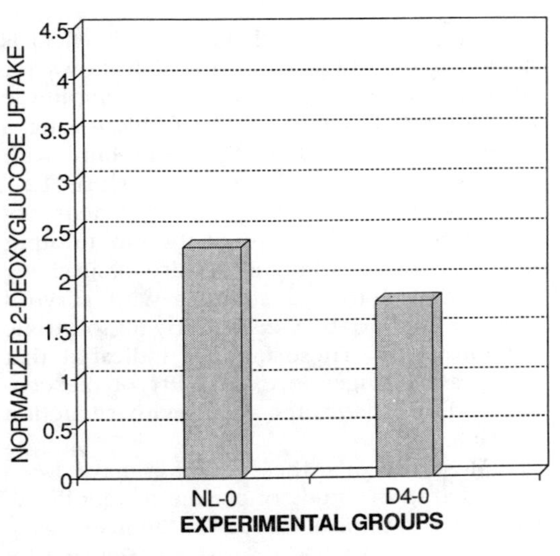

Figure 12-8 A comparison of the level of 2-deoxyglucose uptake (without electrical or auditory stimulation) in the inferior colliculus of a normal (NL-0) guinea pig and a guinea pig 4 weeks after deafening from kanamycin and ethacrynic acid (D4-0).

istration, there is a marked reduction in metabolic activity in the IC in comparison to that observed in the normal subject. Significant changes in electrically evoked metabolic responsiveness in the central auditory pathways were observed in the ipsilateral CN complex, contralateral nuclei of the lateral lemniscus, and contralateral IC after 4 weeks of deafness. These data strongly support the hypothesis that deafness produces significant physiologic changes in the responsiveness of central auditory pathways as well as in resting and evoked metabolic activity. Important, then, is the question of whether these changes are subject to regulation by activation of afferent fibers via prosthetic electrical stimulation.

Effects of Electrical Stimulation

A few studies have addressed the effect of electrical stimulation on the maintenance of the central auditory system in deafened animals. Intracochlear electrical stimulation preserved the neuronal activity in the brain-stem auditory nuclei of unilaterally deafened cats and kittens (Wong-Riley et al, 1981; Leake et al, 1989). Chouard et al (1983) found that chronic prosthetic stimulation prevents, at least partially, atrophy in the guinea pig lower auditory brain stem resulting from drug-induced deafening. The latter study provides some interesting observations; however, from the standpoint of experimental design, it suffers because of uncontrolled stimulus parameters (i.e., the use of a hearing aid in a "normal" sound environment), the lack of adequately-defined statistical measures, and a small sample size (17 experimental and control groups from a pool of 22 animals). Recent studies suggest that prosthetic stimulation may enhance the survival of SGCs. Lousteau (1987) examined the effects of electrical stimulation on SGC degeneration induced by ototoxicity. Guinea pigs were implanted with scala tympani electrodes and then deafened by injection of kanamycin and ethacrynic acid. In comparison to implanted and unstimulated deafened animals, animals receiving electrical stimulation maintained higher SGC densities. In chemically-deafened kittens and in genetically-deaf white cats, electrical stimulation with a scala tympani electrode was associated with higher SGC survival when compared to unimplanted, deafened controls (Leake et al, 1989, 1990). We have also shown that in the chemically-deafened guinea pig, stimulation with a cochlear implant reduces loss of SGCs (Hartshorn et al, 1989).

Using our ototoxically-deafened guinea pig model, we examined the effects of unilateral electrical stimulation at various levels over a 9-week survival period following drug administration. Immediately after ototoxic drug administration, subjects were stimulated for 2 hours per day, 5 days per week with electrical sinusoidal stimulation at 1,000 Hz, 50 percent duty cycle at intensities of 100, 200, 300, and 400 μA. EMLR growth functions were measured weekly from these subjects over 9 weeks of survival, and SGC densities were evaluated. Figure 12-9 illustrates the input/output EMLR functions recorded in one subject stimulated with 100 μA. As opposed to previous investigations and findings in nonstimulated animals in this study, a smaller reduction in the slope of the input/output functions was observed. In these chronically stimulated animals, significant across-subject variability in slope changes was found. However, the reduction in EMLR slope in subjects stimulated at 100 μA was statistically less than that observed in control animals, and although slope changes in animals stimulated at 200, 300, and 400 μA were not significantly different from those of control animals, all of them demonstrated a tendency toward less slope change than in stimulated animals. Moreover, the mean slope of all stimulated animals at all intensity levels showed a statistically significant smaller slope change than that observed in the control, unstimulated subjects.

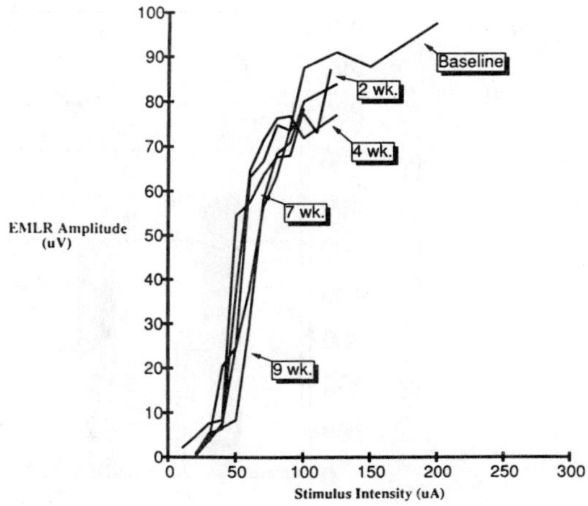

Figure 12-9 Amplitude input/output electrically evoked middle latency response (EMLR) functions recorded from one subject, following ototoxic drug administration, who received daily exposure to electrical stimulation at 100 μA, 2 hours per day. Unlike unstimulated subjects this subject's slope of the input/output function did not decrease with time following drug administration.

Figure 12-10 illustrates the density of SGCs in segments of the guinea pig cochlea from the basal 2½ turns of the cochlea in stimulated versus nonstimulated ears in each group of subjects. The observed differences in SGC density between stimulated and unstimulated ears were statistically significant in each of these groups. Figure 12-11 illustrates the survival of SGCs in the implanted versus the unimplanted ear of control, unstimulated subjects. Clearly, in most basal regions of the cochlea, the presence of the electrode itself appears to have reduced SGC degeneration. This observation is similar to that of Lousteau (1983). Figure 12-12 illustrates the mean difference in density of surviving SGCs in the stimulated ear versus the nonstimulated ear of all stimulated subjects, minus the difference in survival of SGCs in the implanted versus the unimplanted ears of control animals. This figure indicates that electrical stimulation influences survival of SGCs in the lower portions of the cochlea. We suggest that the lack of

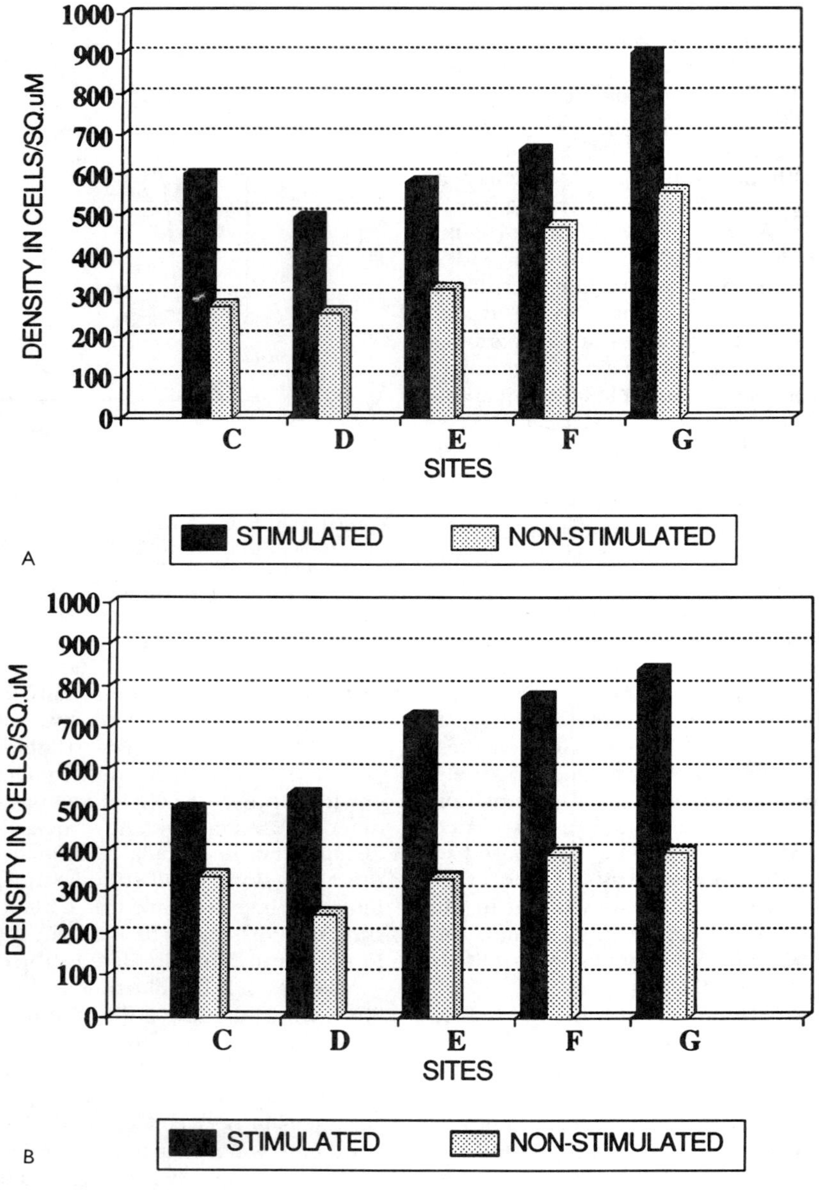

Figure 12-10 Spiral ganglion cell survival 9 weeks following ototoxic drug administration in the guinea pig from unstimulated ears and ears receiving electrical stimulation at various intensity levels: *A*, 400 μA; *B*, 300 μA.

ototoxic injury in the extreme base of the cochlea reflects the presence of the electrode that alone reduced ototoxically-induced SGC loss.

Figure 12-13 illustrates that chronic electrical stimulation also affects metabolic responsiveness of the central auditory pathways. This figure demonstrates the effects of 5 weeks of low-level electrical stimulation on responsiveness of the IC to electrical stimulation. Following 5 weeks of stimulation via an intrascalar cochlear implant, the evoked metabolic activity is higher than in an animal that received no stimulation during the 5-week period and is, in fact, comparable to that observed in the nondeafened subject.

Mechanisms of Pathology and Electrically-Elicited Survival

A variety of mechanisms have been proposed to account for the effects of "deafferentation" on normal development (including

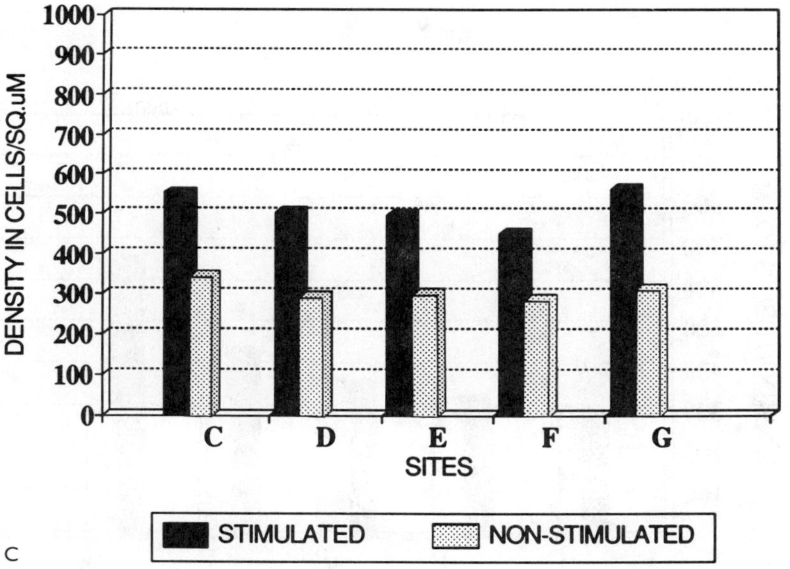

C

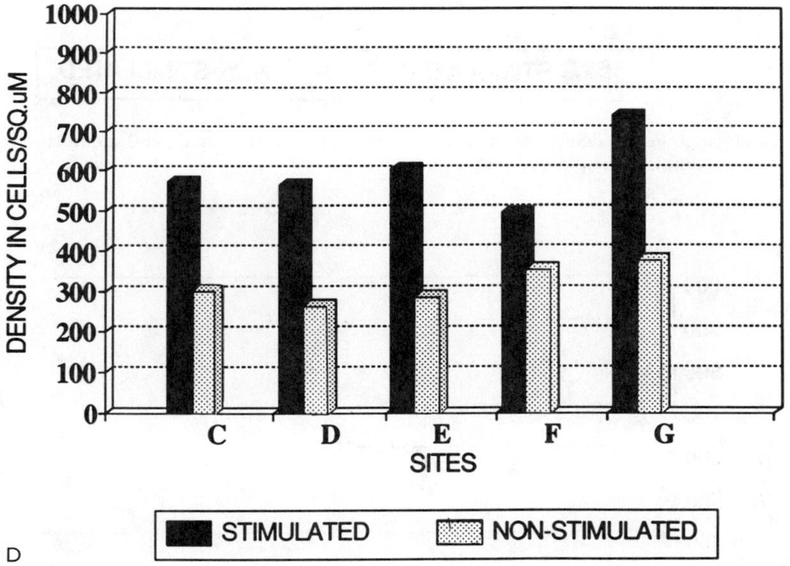

D

Figure 12-10 *Continued C,* 200 μA; *D,* 100 μA.

programmed cell death) and activity of postsynaptic neural elements (Greenough and Juraska, 1986; Cowan et al, 1984; Ding et al, 1983). Deitch and Rubel (1989a,b) have reported rapid atrophy of dendrites of auditory brain-stem cells in the chick following deafferentation. Atrophy was specific to the portion of the dendritic tree of individual cells receiving the blocked input and occurred within 96 hours of deafferentation. The authors speculated that the denervation atrophy might reflect "(1) disruption of the physical contact between presynaptic and postsynaptic elements; (2) the elimination of a specific 'trophic substance' released from the presynaptic element; or (3) the elimination of local depolarizations of the postsynaptic membrane by afferent activity." More recently, Sie and Rubel (1989) demonstrated in the gerbil a rapid reduction in spherical cell size and metabolism in the CN following pharmacologic blockade of cochlear nerve with tetrodotoxin. The decrease in spherical cell metabolism was observed 1 hour after blockade; the reduction

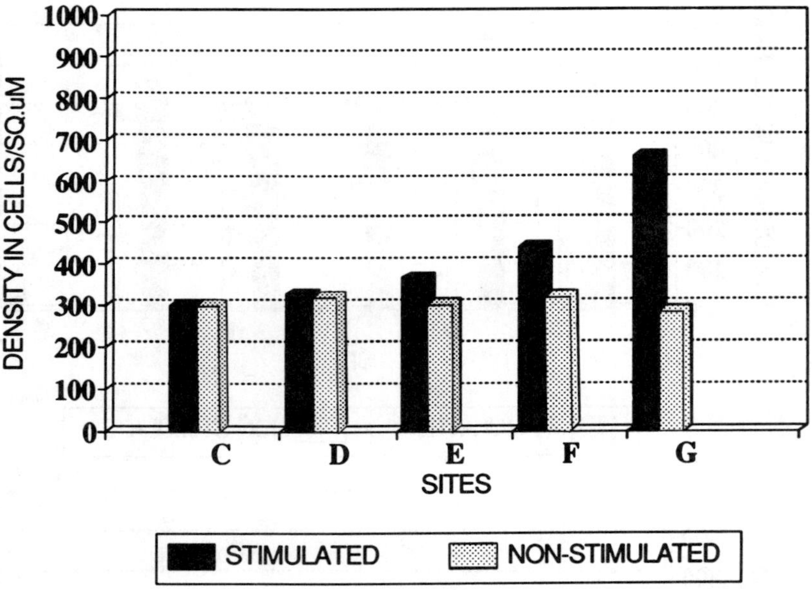

Figure 12-11 Spiral ganglion cell density in drug-treated animals in unstimulated and unimplanted temporal bones versus contralateral unstimulated implanted temporal bones.

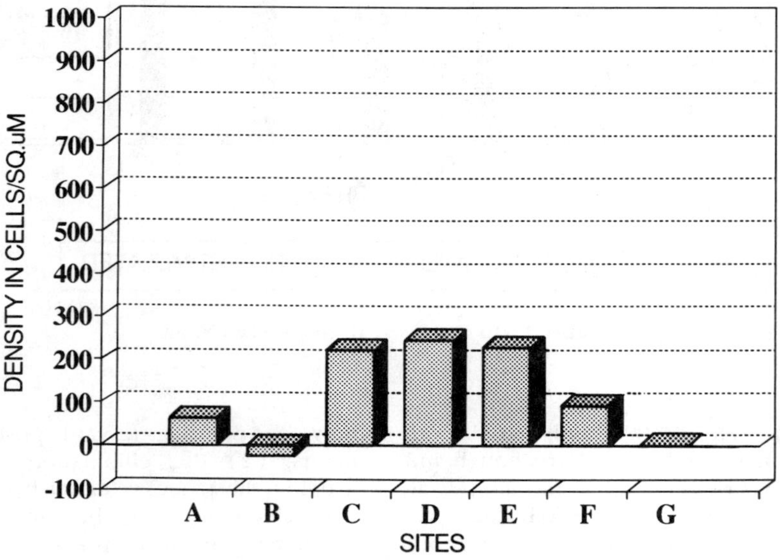

Figure 12-12 Mean difference in density of surviving spiral ganglion cells in implanted subjects stimulated at various intensity levels, compared to the temporal bone of subjects implanted but unstimulated following drug treatment.

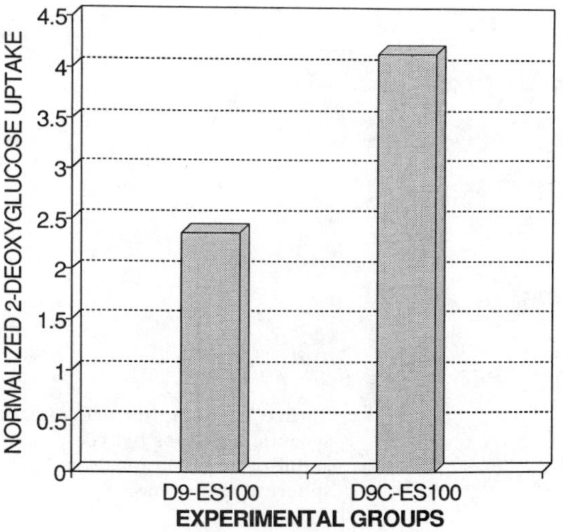

Figure 12-13 A comparison of the levels of electrically-evoked (by an intrascalar cochlear implant) 2-deoxyglucose uptake in the inferior colliculus 9 weeks after deafening by kanamycin and ethacrynic acid. The level of uptake is higher in the guinea pig that received 5 weeks of chronic stimulation via the cochlear implant (D9C-ES100) than in the guinea pig that didn't receive stimulation (D9-ES100).

in cell size was evident 17 hours later. The effect was found to be reversible in subjects allowed to recover for 7 days following a 24- to 48-hour episode of eighth-nerve blockade (Pasic and Rubel, 1989b). Rubel and his colleagues concluded that electrical activity of the eighth nerve was responsible for the regulation of cell size of central auditory neurons.

In general, most authors emphasize the role of specific neural activity at the synapse in maintenance of cell function and structure. Thus, the maintenance of a simple "physical contact" between presynaptic and postsynaptic elements would seem inadequate to account for the majority of findings in this field. Our observations of a maintenance of electrical and metabolic responsiveness of auditory pathways and a reduction in degeneration of SGC with low-level electrical stimulation would seem to support the importance of neural activity following deafness. Electrical stimulation may cause the generation and propagation of action potentials along the auditory nerve and, thus, account for their survival. If so, one might hypothesize that changes in characteristics of synapses of afferent fibers terminating on cells of the CN, observed with deafness, might be reduced with electrical stimulation. Indeed, we have examined this question and recently found that auditory nerve synapses tend to maintain both the normal concave appearance of their active zone and a rich vesicularization in guinea pigs deafened and stimulated at low levels on a daily basis for 9 weeks, as compared to deafened, unstimulated controls, in which active zones are flattened. Figure 12-14 shows electron micrographs of normal- and abnormal-appearing afferent terminals on the spherical cells of the CN. In Figure 12-14A, normal concave active zones are shown in auditory nerve synapses. Following 9 weeks of deafness, all synaptic terminals were flattened, as typified in Figure 12-14B. Figure 12-14C shows the effects of low-level chronic stimulation in the deafened subject. In these subjects almost two-thirds of the active zones of auditory nerve terminals remained concave.

It is important to define the mechanism responsible for this action, both for our basic understanding of system function and to increase our potential for modifying the consequences of peripheral deafness, which may significantly help the profoundly deaf who receive a cochlear implant. If electrically evoked activity does promote survival, deafened adults and deafened children should undergo implantation earlier. Obviously, there are other potential contributing factors, such as electrically-induced changes in the homeostasis of the inner ear. For example, enhanced blood flow may play a role (Sillman et al, 1988, 1989a,b; Miller et al, in press). The contribution of such factors may modify the requirements of electrical stimulation that can be used to maintain cell survival in the deafened patient. Obviously, the need for discrete and specifically-patterned electrical stimulation to maintain auditory nerve survival would require an implant with very different approaches in terms of invasiveness and sophistication than those designed to provide low-level general activation of inner-ear structures.

In the auditory system, study of the effects of modification of normal receptor activity contributes to our understanding of the mechanism of central neural processing of sound and the structural features of the CNS on which these mechanisms are based. The elucidation of the CNS changes that follow modification of receptor function, including deafness, is fundamental to our analysis of mechanisms underlying development, maintenance of normal function in the mature system, and changes that occur with aging. Moreover, these studies are basic to our ability to relate physiologic and structural characteristics to perception, and to changes in function during the life span of the organism.

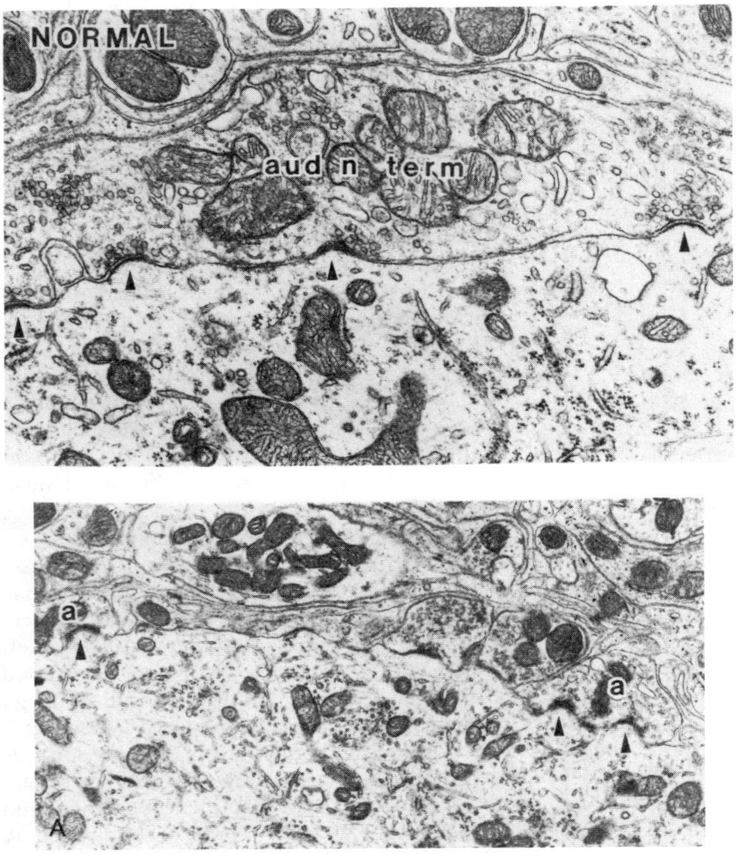

Figure 12-14 *A*, Normal concave synaptic junctions between auditory nerve terminals and spherical cell somas.

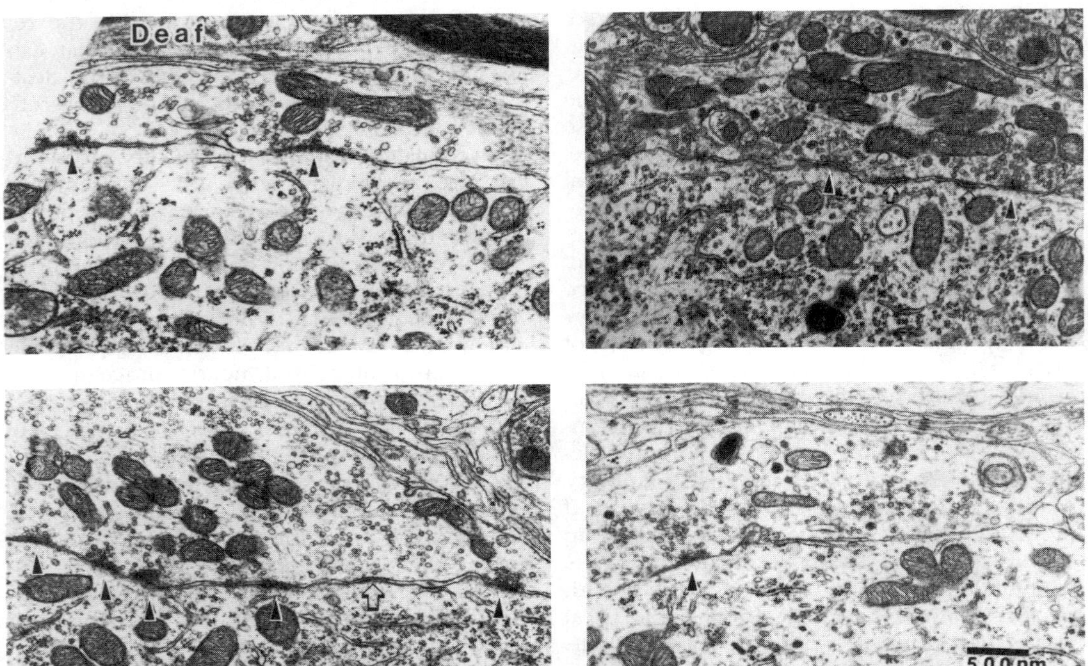

Figure 12-14 *Continued B*, Examples of flattened synaptic terminals observed between afferent auditory nerve fibers and spherical cell somas following 9 weeks of ototoxically-induced deafness.

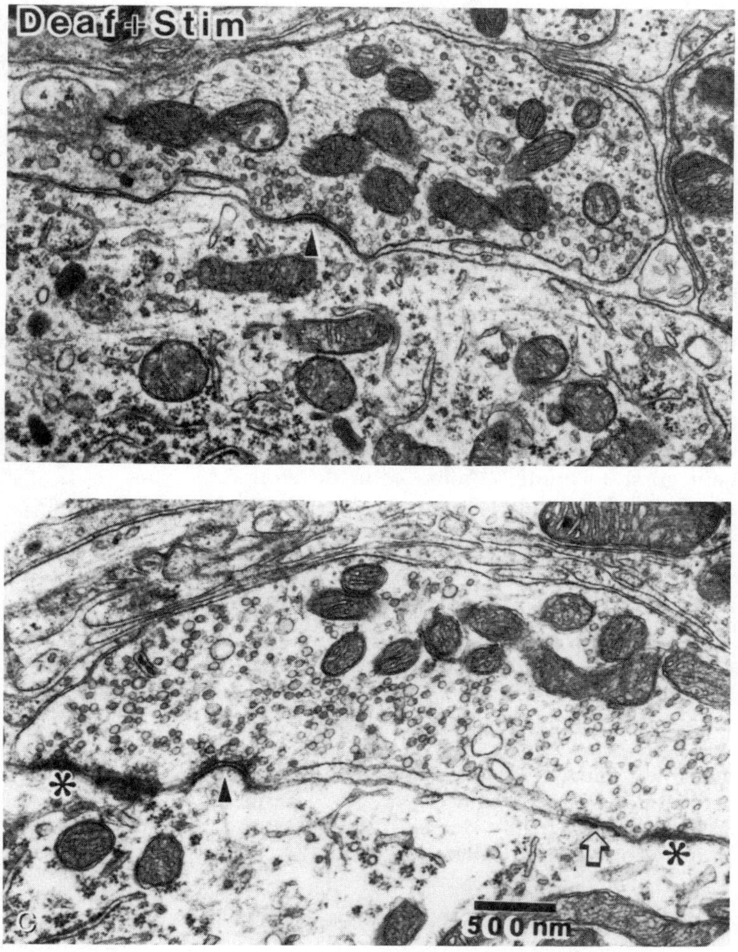

Figure 12-14 *Continued C,* Examples of concave synapses between auditory nerve terminals and spherical cell somas 9 weeks following drug-induced deafness in subjects receiving daily electrical stimulation.

Modifications Centrales Induites par la Surdité leur Reversibilite, leur Prevention

Les pathologies cochléaires associées au trauma acoustique ou à l'ototoxicité sont maintenant bien connues. Les efforts doivent à présent se porter sur les effets secondaires de ces pathologies dans les centres nerveux auditifs. Ces effets sont-ils les mêmes ou varient-ils avec le type de pathologie périphérique? Y a-t-il des effets primaires de certains traumatismes? Les changements dans le CNS sont-ils en partie réversibles et peuvent-ils être prévenus (par les implants cochléaires par exemple)?

On examine ici les atteintes au niveau du nerf cochléaire et du tronc cérébral dans différents modèles de surdité périphérique chez l'animal: ototoxicité chez le cobaye et surdité génétique chez le chien dalmatien. Un sujet humain atteint de surdité neuro-sensorielle acquise et porteur d'un implant cochléaire est aussi inclus dans cette étude.

Dans la plupart des cas, la perte de cellules ganglionnaires est secondaire et parfaitement corrélée à celle des cellules ciliées. Sur les cobayes soumis à une destruction massive des cellules ciliées (induite chimiquement par des aminoglycosides ou de l'acide éthacrynique), les lésions ganglionnaires sont évidentes après 4 semaines et progressent rapidement pour atteindre 90% de pertes 16 semaines après le traitement ototoxique. Ces pertes sont atténuées lorsque les cobayes reçoivent une stimulation électrique: un implant cochléaire étant mis en place après la destruction chimique de la cochlée. Au niveau des noyaux cochléaires on note une diminution de volume des synapses entre le nerf auditif et les deutoneurones. Dans les noyaux auditifs du tronc cérébral on observe une diminution de l'activité métabolique (évaluée par la méthode du désoxyglucose); cette activité métabolique est restaurée, sans atteindre les valeurs normales, sur les animaux porteurs d'implants. Cela est similaire à ce qui a dû se passer sur le sujet humain implanté: la taille et le nombre de neurones des noyaux auditifs du tronc cérébral sont intermédiaires entre les valeurs normales et celles de sujets sourds non implantés.

Sur le modèle du chien dalmatien, la perte de neurones ganglionnaires n'est significative que 8 mois après la dégénérescence des cellules ciliées. L'évaluation des dégâts au niveau du tronc cérébral est en cours sur des animaux implantés ou non. D'autres modèles sont aussi à l'étude, comme celui développé récemment par Rubel et son équipe (instillation locale de TTX).

ACKNOWLEDGMENTS

This work was supported in part by NIH Grant T32DC00024, CIDA DC00037, and NIH Grant P01DC000274. We would like to thank Jeffrey Horn, Donald Schwartz, Elizabeth Plattner, M.D., and Michael Myers, M.D. for their valuable contributions to many of the studies reported in this manuscript. The authors would like to thank Denise Dyson for the preparation of the manuscript.

References

Bergstrom L. Some pathologies of sensory and neural hearing loss. Can J Otolaryngol Suppl 1975; 4(2):1-28.

Burton MJ, Miller JM, Kileny PR. Middle latency responses. I. Electrical and acoustic excitation. Arch Otolaryngol Head Neck Surg 1989a; 115(1):59-62.

Burton MJ, Miller JM, Kileny PR. Middle latency responses. II. Variation among stimulation sites. Arch Otolaryngol Head Neck Surg 1989b; 115(4):458-461.

Cowan WM, Fawcett JW, O'Leary DD, Stanfield BB. Regressive events in neurogenesis. Science 1984; 225(4668):1258-1265.

Chouard CH, Meyer B, Josset P, Buche JF. The effect of the acoustic nerve chronic electric stimulation upon the guinea pig cochlear nucleus development. Acta Otolaryngol 1983; 95(5-6):639-645.

Coleman P, Buell S. Regulations of dendritic extent in developing and aging brain. In: Cotman C, ed. Synaptic plasticity. New York: Guilford Press, 1985:311.

Deitch JS, Rubel EW. Rapid changes in ultrastructure during deafferentation-induced dendritic atrophy. J Comp Neurol 1989a; 281(2):234-258.

Deitch JS, Rubel EW. Changes in neuronal cell bodies in N. laminaris during deafferentation-induced dendritic atrophy. J Comp Neurol 1989b; 281(2):259-268.

Ding RJ, Jansen KS, Laing NG, Tjnnesen H. The innervation of skeletal muscles in chickens curarized during early development. J Neurocytol 1983; 12:887-919.

Ghorayer B, Sarwat A, Linthicum FH Jr. Viable spiral ganglion cells in congenital and acquired profound hearing loss. J Laryngol Otol 1980; 94(4):367-376.

Greenough WT, Juraska JM. Developmental neuropsychobiology. New York: Academic Press, 1986:271.

Hall RD. Estimation of surviving spiral ganglion cells in the deaf rat using the electrically evoked auditory brainstem response. Hear Res 1990; 45:123-136.

Harris RM, Woolsey TA. Dendritic plasticity in mouse barrel cortex following postnatal vibrissa follicle damage. J Comp Neurol 1981; 196(3):357-376.

Hartshorn DO, Miller JM, Altschuler RA. Protective effect of electrical stimulation on the deafened guinea pig cochlea. Otolaryngol Head Neck Surg 1991; 104.

Hashisaki GT, Rubel EW. Effects of unilateral cochlea removal on anteroventral cochlear nucleus neurons in developing gerbils. J Comp Neurol 1989; 283(4):5-73.

Hinojosa R, Lerner SA. Cochlear neural degeneration without hair cell loss in two patients with aminoglycoside ototoxicity. J Infect Dis 1987; 156(3): 449-455.

Hinojosa R, Marion M. Histopathology of profound deafness. Ann N Y Acad Sci 1983; 405:459-484.

Hubel DH, Wiesel TN, LeVay S. Functional architecture of area 17 in normal and monocularly deprived macaque monkeys. Cold Spring Harb Symp Biol 1976; 40:581-589.

Hubel DH, Wiesel TN, LeVay S. Plasticity of ocular dominance columns in monkey striate cortex. Philos Trans R Soc Lond 1977; 278(961):377-409.

Hubel DH, Wiesel TN. Binocular interaction in striate cortex of kittens reared with artificial squint. J Neurophysiol 1965; 28(6):1041-1059.

Jyung RW, Miller JM, Cannon SC. Evaluation of eighth nerve integrity using the electrically evoked middle latency response. Otolaryngol Head Neck Surg 1989; 101(6):670-682.

Kane EC. Patterns of degeneration in the caudal cochlear nucleus of the cat after cochlear ablation. Anat Rec 1974; 179(1):67-91.

Kileny PR, Zimmerman-Phillips S. Effective auditory deprivation on performance with multichannel implants. ASHA 1988; 30:10.

Leake PA, Hultcrantz M, Snyder RL, Hradek GT, Rebscher SJ. Effects of chronic electrical stimulation in neonatally deafened cats. Abstr Midwinter Res Meeting Assoc Res Otolaryngol, St. Petersburg, FL, 1990; 13:328.

Leake PA, Snyder RL, Chambers PL, Hradek GT, Rebscher SJ, Bates GJ, Marks DR. Consequences of chronic electrical stimulation in an animal model of congenital profound hearing loss. Abstr Midwinter Res Meeting Assoc Res Otolaryngol, St. Petersburg, FL, 1989; 12:268.

Lousteau RJ. Increased spiral ganglion cell survival in electrically stimulated, deafened guinea pig cochleae. Laryngoscope 1987; 7:836-842.

Lund RD, Chang FLF, Land PW. The development of callosal projections in normal and one-eyed rats. Brain Res 1984; 316(1):139-142.

McGee TM, Olszewski J. Streptomycin sulfate and dihydrostreptomycin toxicity: Behavioral and histopathologic studies. Arch Otolaryngol 1962; 75:295-311.

Meisami E, Manoochehri S. Effects of early bilateral chemical destruction of olfactory receptors on postnatal growth, Mg-ATPase and Na-K-ATPase activity of olfactory and non-olfactory structures of the rat brain. Brain Res 1977; 128(1):170-175.

Meisami E. Effects of olfactory deprivation on postnatal growth of the rat olfactory bulb utilizing a new method for production of neonatal unilateral anosmia. Brain Res 1976; 107(2):437-444.

Miller JM, Bredberg G, Grenman R, Suonpää J, Lindström B, Didier A. Measurement of human cochlear blood flow. Ann Orl 1991; 100:44-53.

Otte J, Schuknecht H, Kerr A. Ganglion cell populations in normal and pathological human cochleae. Implications for cochlear implantation. Laryngoscope 1978; 88:1231-1246.

Pasic TR, Rubel EW. Rapid changes in cochlear nucleus cell size following blockade of auditory nerve electrical activity in gerbils. J Comp Neurol 1989a; 283(4):474-480.

Pasic TR, Rubel EW. Gerbil anteroventral cochlear nucleus cell size following reversal of electrical activity blockade. Abstr Midwinter Res Meeting Assoc Res Otolaryngol, St. Petersburg, FL, 1989b; 12:10.

Pfingst BE, Glass I, Spelman FA, Sutton D. Psychophysical studies of cochlear implants in monkeys: Clinical implications. In: Schindler RA, Merzenich MM, eds. Cochlear implants. New York: Raven Press, 1985:305.

Pfingst BE, Rai DT, Tumacder RS. Effects of level on temporally based frequency discrimination. Abstr 11th Midwinter Meeting Assoc Res Otolaryngol 205.

Pfingst BE, Sutton D, Miller JM, Bohne BA. Relation of psychophysical data to histopathology in monkeys with cochlear implants. Acta Otolaryngol 1981; 92(1-2):1-13.

Pfingst BE, Sutton D. Relation of cochlear implant function to histopathology in monkeys. Ann N Y Acad Sci 1983; 405:224-239.

Powell TPS, Erulkar SD. Transneuronal cell degeneration in the auditory relay nuclei of the cat. J Anat 1962; 96:249-268.

Sie K, Rubel EW. The early effects of eighth nerve blockade on protein synthesis and cell size in the anteroventral cochlear nucleus of the young gerbil. Abstr Midwinter Res Meeting Assoc Res Otolaryngol, St. Petersburg, FL, 1989; 12:9.

Sillman JS, LaRouere MJ, Nuttall AL, Lawrence M, Miller JM. Recent advances in cochlear blood flow measurements. Ann Otol Rhinol Laryngol 1988; 97(1):1-8.

Sillman JS, LaRouere MJ, Masta RI, Miller JM, Nuttall AL. Electrically stimulated increases in cochlear blood flow: I. Frequency and intensity effects. Otolaryngol Head Neck Surg 1989a; 100(4):308-316.

Sillman JS, Masta RI, LaRouere MJ, Nuttall AL, Miller JM. Electrically stimulated increases in cochlear blood flow: II. Evidence of neural mediation. Otolaryngol Head Neck Surg 1989b; 101(3):362-374.

Smith L, Simmons FB. Estimating eighth nerve survival by electrical stimulation. Ann Otol Rhinol Laryngol 1983; 92:19-23.

Stypulkowski PH, van den Honert C, Kvistad SD. Electrophysiologic evaluation of the cochlear implant patient. Otolaryngol Clin N Am 1986; 19:249-257.

Trune DR. Influence of neonatal cochlear removal on the development of mouse cochlear nucleus: I. Number, size and density of its neurons. J Comp Neurol 1982; 209(4):409-424.

Webster DB, Webster M. Neonatal sound deprivation affects brainstem auditory nuclei. Arch Otolaryngol 1977; 103(7):392-396.

Webster DB, Webster M. Long-term effects of cochlear nerve destruction on the cochlear nuclei. Anat Rec 1978; 190:578-579.

West BA, Brummett RE, Himes DL. Interaction of kanamycin and ethacrynic acid: Severe cochlear damage in guinea pigs. Arch Otolaryngol 1973; 98(1):32-37.

Wiesel TN, Hubel DH. Extent of recovery from the effects of visual deprivation in kittens. J Neurophysiol 1965; 28(6):1060-1072.

Wong-Riley MTT, Walsh SM, Leake-Jones PA, Merzenick MM. Maintenance of neuronal activity by electrical stimulation of unilaterally deafened cats demonstrable with cytochrome oxidase technique. Ann Otol Rhinol Laryngol Suppl 1981; 90:30-32.

CHAPTER 13

Central Auditory Temporal Processing: Alterations Produced by Factors Involving the Cochlea

GEORGE M. GERKEN

It is well established that cochlear pathology, such as loss of hair cells, reduces the amount of input to the central auditory system. The issue addressed in this chapter is whether cochlear factors, such as pathology, are also accompanied by an alteration in the way the central auditory system operates. In addressing this issue, one aspect of temporal processing is emphasized: temporal integration. Temporal integration is useful as an index of central processing because the time scale on which it occurs is much too long to be supported by events at the peripheral level (Zwislocki, 1960).

The first section below describes the basic approach that was used in assessing acoustic and electrical temporal integration functions. Acoustic stimuli that consisted of multiple, brief tone bursts were particularly important. Not only do these stimuli uncouple the dimensions of duration and power, but the repetitious nature of the stimulus resembles the trains of pulses that should be used with central electrical stimulation. In later sections, the effects of cochlear pathology on temporal integration are discussed, as are the effects of sustained acoustic stimuli of moderate intensity.

Description of Temporal Integration

Many studies have demonstrated that in normal-hearing human subjects, auditory detection threshold is decreased as the duration of the acoustic stimulus is increased. The relation between detection threshold in decibels and the logarithm of stimulus duration plots as a straight line on log-log coordinates. This is a power function of the form:

$$I_T \cdot t^m = C$$

where I_T is the stimulus intensity at threshold, t is the duration of the stimulus, m is the power function exponent, and C is a constant. Data sets that plot in this manner may be found in Algom and Babkoff (1984), Penner (1978), and Florentine et al (1988). Because power functions plot as straight lines in log-log coordinates, these data sets may be characterized by the exponent, m, or, equivalently, by 10 times m, which is the slope expressed in decibels per decade of duration (Gerken et al, 1990). Because the plots are linear, it is proper to average data sets across subjects to obtain grand-mean data. It is convenient, therefore, to succinctly summarize the experimental findings in terms of the slope of the temporal integration function based on grand-mean data. This slope, in turn, serves as an index of the central integration process.

Multiple-burst acoustic stimuli are of intrinsic interest in the study of temporal integration (Carlyon et al, 1990; Plomp, 1961), and they provide a link with the electrical stimuli used to study central auditory mechanisms. Data are available for two sets of acoustic multiple-burst stimuli that provide contrasting views of the temporal integration process: the first stimulus set employed a variable number of bursts with a fixed interburst interval; the second, a fixed number of bursts with a range of interburst intervals (Gerken et al, 1990). For the first stimulus set, thresholds were measured for 1, 2, 4, 8, and 16 brief tone

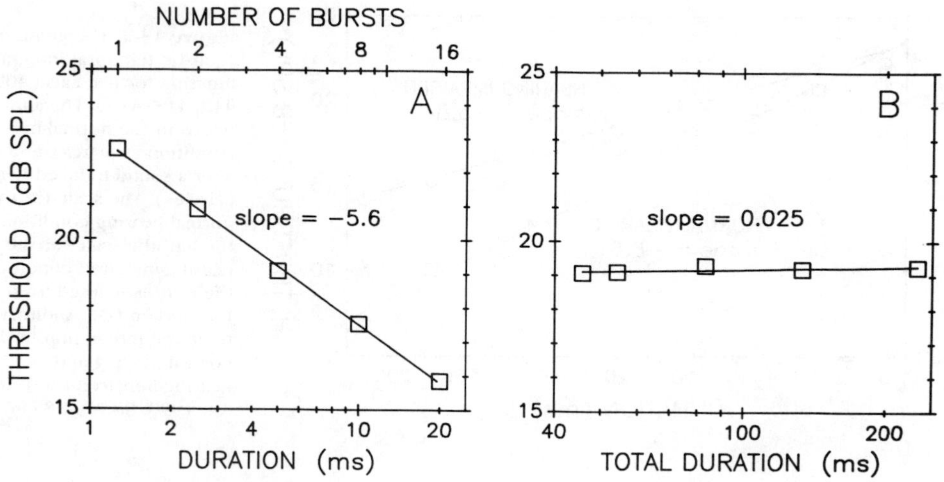

Figure 13-1 *A,* The grand-mean temporal integration function for multiple-burst stimuli obtained from normal-hearing human subjects. Thresholds can be plotted against duration (bottom axis) or against the number of bursts (top axis). *B,* Grand-mean thresholds for multiple burst stimuli with four equally-spaced tone bursts. (Both data sets are from Gerken GM, Bhat VKH, Hutchison-Clutter M. Auditory temporal integration and the power function model. J Acoust Soc Am 1990; 767-778.

bursts (3.125 kHz) with the interburst interval held at 4.16 ms. The grand-mean temporal integration function is shown in Figure 13-1A. Note that the abscissa can be either duration (the sum of the durations of the individual bursts) or simply the number of bursts. The slope that characterizes the integration function, −5.6, is the same whether it is expressed in decibels per factor of 10 bursts or in decibels per decade of duration. Note that no matter what the duration is for one burst, two bursts will have exactly twice that duration and likewise for N bursts. Since all bursts are scaled in duration by the same factor, the slope of the temporal integration function does not depend on the duration of the single burst. Thus the slope of the temporal integration function for multiple-burst stimuli is an excellent means of characterizing the central integrator. Because of the similarity of electrical pulse trains and the multiple acoustic bursts (Gerken, 1984), electrical stimuli provide an equally good characterization.

Stimuli in the second set each contained four brief tone bursts with interburst intervals that varied from 4.16 ms to 66.56 ms (Gerken et al, 1990). It can be seen from the grand-mean data in Figure 13-1B that threshold was almost independent of interburst interval, at least within the 200+ ms total duration used. Thus, the results obtained with multiple-burst stimuli provide the basis for treating the number of pulses in the electrical stimulus as an index of duration. It must be stated, however, that equating the number of electrical pulses and pulse train duration is a working hypothesis that will need additional study to confirm or reject it. All such relations need interpretation and restriction. For example, variation in pulse duration would be expected to affect threshold in the same way as would the duration of a multiple burst. Another obvious restriction is that electrical pulses that are very closely spaced will fall into the relative or absolute refractory period of the stimulated neurons and this will be ineffective. At the other extreme the linear temporal integration function will presumably become asymptotic for long pulse trains. With acoustic stimulation, however, Florentine et al (1988) did not find a break in the function at 500 ms, and Penner (1978) did not report one at 1,000 ms. The extent to which the power function can describe temporal integration has yet to be established. These considerations must be kept in mind when the electrical stimulation work is discussed.

Temporal Integration and Hearing Impairment

Decreased temporal integration associated with hearing loss has been reported numerous times in human beings (Florentine et al, 1988; Watson and Gengel, 1969; Wright, 1968). Much less work has been done with animals, with which the number of hearing-impaired subjects is only slightly larger than

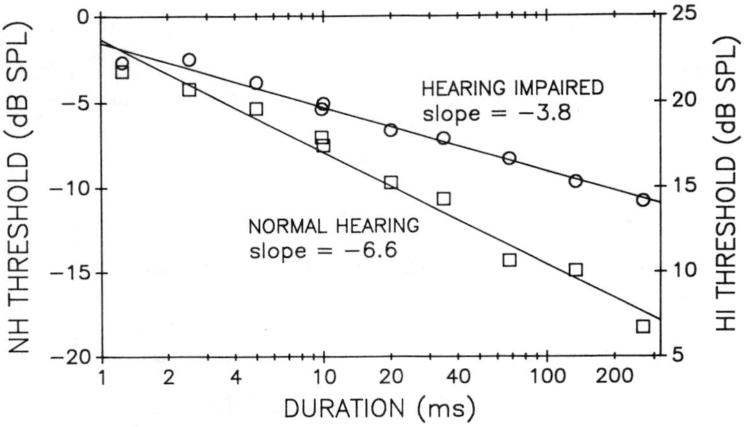

Figure 13-2 The grand-mean acoustic temporal integration function for five cats (409, 410, 412, 413, 414). The animals were tested in the normal-hearing condition (squares), and again after a sound-induced hearing loss (circles). The scale for the normal-hearing condition is on the left; the scale for the hearing-impaired condition is on the right. (Adapted from Solecki JM, Gerken GM. Auditory temporal integration in the normal-hearing and hearing-impaired cat. J Acoust Soc Am 1990; 88:779-785.)

the number of studies (Clark and Bohne, 1986; Henderson, 1969).

A recent study using cats contrasted the temporal integration functions for normal-hearing and hearing-impaired conditions in the same animals (Solecki and Gerken, 1990). Figure 13-2 illustrates a summary of these findings. In both hearing conditions the stimuli were 6.25 kHz. Note that the scales for the two temporal integration functions are displaced by 25 dB. The slope of the normal-hearing function was −6.6 dB per decade of duration; the slope decreased to −3.8 dB per decade in the same animals following a moderate sound-induced hearing loss. The same stimulus set was used with both hearing conditions, and several of the stimuli in the set were multiple-burst stimuli. If, as suggested by Zwislocki (1960), temporal integration is a central process, then the question is raised as to why sound-induced cochlear damage can alter the temporal integration function. It would seem that the reduced input from the damaged cochlea would still be integrated in the same manner as before; hence, pre- and post-exposure slopes should be equal. Clearly, pre- and post-exposure slopes are not equal.

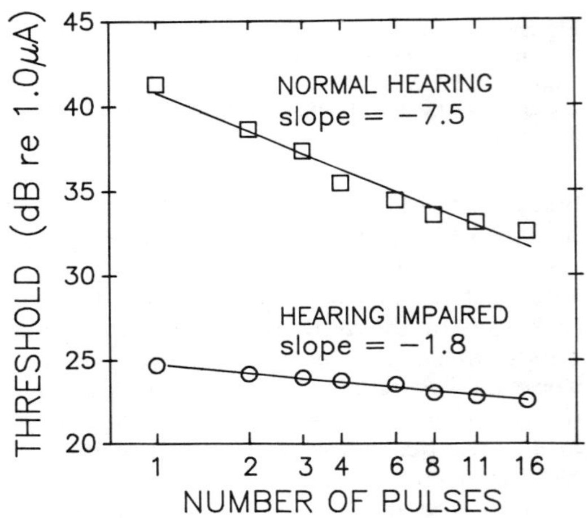

Figure 13-3 The grand-mean electrical temporal integration function for four cats (401, 402, 403, 408). One electrode in the inferior colliculus was tested extensively in each animal. After completion of testing in the normal-hearing condition (squares), a mean permanent threshold shift of 48 dB was produced by exposure to intense sound. The animals were retested in the hearing-impaired condition (circles), starting 1 month after the sound exposure. Note that detection thresholds are given in decibels re 1.0 μA.

Temporal Integration of Central Electrical Stimulation

It has been amply demonstrated in cochlear prosthesis work that electrical stimulation is effective in conveying information (Gray, 1985; Schindler and Merzenich, 1985). Stimulation of different regions of the cochlea or stimulation at different rates often yields discriminably different sensations, whereas reduction of the amplitude of the electrical stimulus reduces the magnitude of the sensation (Miller and Spelman, 1989; Shannon, 1983). In animals, behavioral responses have been obtained for electrical stimuli applied to sensory areas of the central nervous system including the visual cortex (Doty, 1965) or the brainstem auditory nuclei (Nieder and Neff, 1961).

For the determination of a temporal integration function based on electrical stimulation of the central nervous system, the parameters of the stimuli used must be chosen on

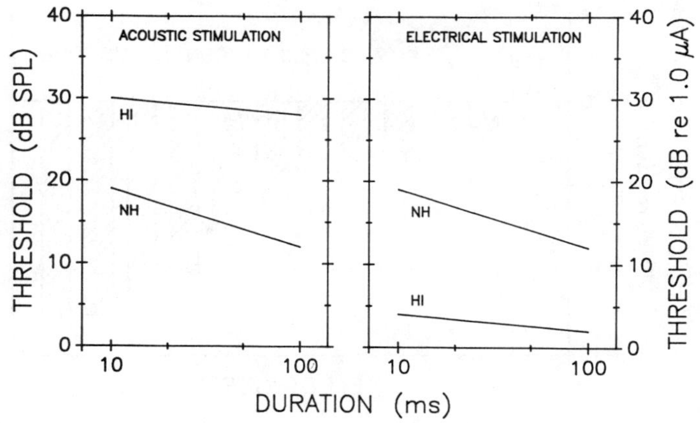

Figure 13-4 Schematic summary of the threshold changes and temporal integration effects obtained with acoustic and electrical stimuli in normal-hearing (NH) and hearing-impaired (HI) subjects.

the basis of neural effectiveness, and consequently will differ significantly from the parameters of the acoustic stimuli used in the corresponding auditory task. Brief (shorter than 1 ms) monophasic cathodal stimuli simplify interpretation of the results and can be used without concern for polarization or tissue damage so long as presentation rates are low and charge transfer is small. A stimulus of long duration cannot be obtained by increasing the duration of a pulse because a long pulse is not an efficient neural stimulus and could cause cell damage. To increase stimulus duration, it is necessary to repeat the brief electrical pulse to produce a train of pulses. A train is described, therefore, by specifying the duration of the basic pulse and by giving the number of pulses in the train as well as the interpulse interval. The number of electrical pulses in the train is taken, as discussed above, as an index of duration.

It was possible to study the process of temporal integration by using direct electrical stimulation of the central auditory system because absolute thresholds can be measured for electrical stimulation in the same manner used for acoustic stimuli (Gerken et al, 1989). The grand-mean temporal integration function for electrical stimulation, based on data for four normal-hearing cats, is shown in the top portion of Figure 13-3. The electrodes were located in the central nucleus of the inferior colliculus. One electrode in each animal was tested extensively in order to obtain the data shown. The same animals were tested after exposure to an intense sound, which produced a mean permanent threshold shift of 48 dB. The resulting grand-mean, postexposure temporal integration function is shown in the bottom portion of Figure 13-3.

In the normal-hearing animals, the slope of the temporal integration function for electrical stimulation of inferior colliculus was −7.5 dB per factor of 10 pulses. This slope was slightly steeper than the −6.6 dB per decade of duration obtained for cat with acoustic stimuli (Solecki and Gerken, 1990). In the hearing-impaired animals, the slope of the temporal integration function obtained from the same electrodes decreased to −1.8 dB per factor of 10 pulses. This was less steep than the −3.8 dB per decade of duration obtained with acoustic stimuli in hearing-impaired cats (Solecki and Gerken, 1990). The decrease in slope for the electrical temporal integration function from the normal-hearing to hearing-impaired condition was a critical finding. In no way did the electrical signal that was detected by the animal directly involve the cochlea. The decrease in slope must have been produced by a change in the central auditory system, one that had its origin in the pathologic cochleas.

The temporal integration functions in Figure 13-3 were plotted on a common ordinate that encompassed the entire range of pre- and postexposure thresholds. This was done to emphasize that in the hearing-impaired animals, the detection thresholds for electrical stimulation were *decreased.* A supersensitivity to electrical stimulation was a second major consequence of the hearing impairment (Gerken et al, 1984). As with the change in slope, the supersensitivity did not directly involve the cochlea, but must have had its origin in a factor related to the cochlea.

A schematic summary is given in Figure 13-4 of the effects on the temporal integration functions for acoustic and electrical stimuli. For acoustic stimuli, detection thresholds increased following hearing loss, whereas for electrical stimulation, detection thresholds decreased. For both types of stimuli, the temporal integration functions in the hearing-impaired condition are less steep than in the normal-hearing condition.

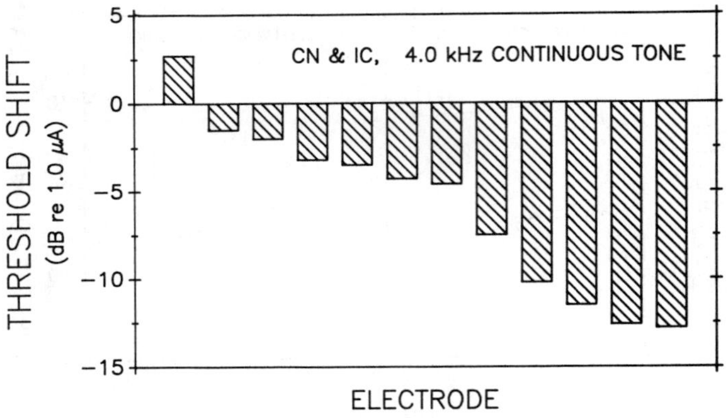

Figure 13-5 Comparison of electrical stimulation thresholds for six electrodes in the cochlear nucleus (CN) and six electrodes in the inferior colliculus (IC). A negative threshold shift indicates a lower electrical stimulation threshold in the presence of the 4.0-kHz, 80-dB SPL continuous tone than in quiet conditions. The threshold shifts are shown in order of increasing magnitude. The histogram is not labeled with respect to anatomic loci of the electrodes because both loci showed large and small shifts.

Continuous Tone and Stimulation Supersensitivity

Acoustic stimulation can also produce a central supersensitivity for electrical stimulation of the central auditory system (Gerken et al, 1985). Whether the central mechanism activated by the continuous tone is the same as the mechanism affected by cochlear pathology is not known. The effects, however, were of the same magnitude. Figure 13-5 shows the threshold shifts obtained for electrical stimulation in quiet conditions versus the presence of 4.0-kHz tones of 80 dB SPL. A negative decibel value (threshold decrease) indicates supersensitivity in brain-stem auditory nuclei in the presence of the continuous tone. Note that for one of the electrodes, the tone produced several decibels of masking. For the other 11 electrodes, however, varying amounts of supersensitivity occurred.

In Figure 13-5, half the placements were electrodes in cochlear nucleus and half were electrodes in the inferior colliculus. There was no apparent difference in the amount of threshold shift obtained: large and small shifts occurred in both loci. The local anatomy and the neural connections are different in the two nuclei and, logically, the consequences of electrical stimulation should also differ. It is surprising, therefore, that the results are so similar. The auditory nerve projects to the three major subdivisions of the cochlear nucleus, which in turn give rise to three distinct striae (Osen, 1970). Presumably, the striae are not redundant and thus carry information concerning different aspects of the acoustic signal. An electrical stimulus applied to the cochlear nucleus could activate one, two, or all three pathways. An electrode positioned in the inferior colliculus almost certainly produces a different pattern of neural activation within the auditory system. The implication is that the electrical stimulus may not actually be detected at the locus of stimulation, but rather at a higher level in the system at which the several pathways may again converge. Supersensitivity in the several portions of the subcortical auditory system may reflect a change in a rostrally located detector (e.g., in cortex). The obvious next step is to measure electrical temporal integration functions in the absence and in the presence of continuous tone, but this has not been done. It can only be speculated, therefore, that continuous tone would mimic hearing loss in flattening the slope of the electrical temporal integration function.

Continuous Tone and Human Auditory Temporal Integration

In regard to the decrease in temporal integration that is associated with sensorineural hearing loss, the question has been raised as to whether the decrease is due to the cochlear pathology or to the elevated sound pressure levels that were needed to test hearing-impaired subjects. To answer this question, temporal integration has been measured in persons with conductive loss and in persons with a sensorineural loss. In addition, temporal integration was measured in normal-hearing subjects in the presence of masking noise. The general conclusion was that cochlear pathology did affect temporal integration, whereas conductive loss or masking noise did not (Florentine et al, 1988; Garner and Miller, 1947;

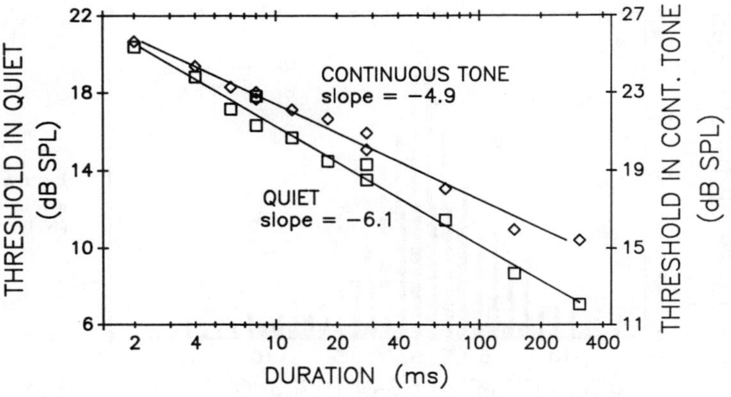

Figure 13-6 Temporal integration functions for 2.0-kHz stimuli in quiet conditions (squares; left scale) and with a 2.52-kHz, 60-dB SPL continuous tone (diamonds; right scale) presented to the same ear as the stimulus. (Grand-mean data for eight subjects from Bhat VKH. Human auditory temporal summation in the presence of ipsilateral and contralateral continuous tones. Unpublished PhD dissertation, The University of Texas at Dallas, Richardson, TX, 1988.)

Gengel, 1972; Green et al, 1957; Sheeley and Bilger, 1964; Wright, 1968; Wright and Cannella, 1969; Zwicker and Wright, 1963).

Given that conductive loss and masking noise do not alter the amount of temporal integration, it is surprising that continuous tone produces a different effect. Human auditory temporal integration functions were measured by Bhat (1988) in quiet conditions and in the presence of a continuous tone. Grand-mean data for eight subjects, for which the test signal was 2.0 kHz and the continuous tone was ⅓ octave higher (2.52 kHz), are shown in Figure 13-6. The continuous tone acted to raise detection threshold (note the difference in the left and right scales in Fig. 13-6) and to decrease the slope of the temporal integration function to −4.9 dB per decade of duration from −6.1 dB per decade of duration. This pattern of results is identical to that shown in Figure 13-2 for hearing-impaired cats, although the effects produced by the continuous tone are less pronounced than those produced by the hearing impairment. It is possible that if a more-intense (but not injurious) continuous tone had been employed—80 dB SPL, for example—stronger effects would have been obtained.

Variability of Thresholds

There is variability in any series of threshold measurements. It seemed that variability across thresholds was reduced both with hearing loss and in the presence of a continuous tone. In this section, this reduction in variability is evaluated.

If thresholds were repeatedly measured for only one stimulus, variability across thresholds would be simply expressed as the standard deviation of the thresholds. The data available, however, were not for a single stimulus but for a set of stimuli that were repeated exactly in two contrasting conditions: normal-hearing versus hearing-impaired, or quiet conditions versus continuous tone (Bhat, 1988; Gerken et al, 1990; Solecki and Gerken, 1990). In these data sets, there were 10 or 12 threshold measurements for each subject, stimulus, and condition. Deviations from the means for subject, stimulus, and condition were converted to deviation histograms as a display of threshold variability. The histograms for normal-hearing and hearing-impaired cats are shown in Figure 13-7 (unpublished data from Solecki and Gerken, 1990). The distribution of thresholds for the hearing-impaired animals is significantly narrower at the 0.002 level ($F = 1.97$, $N = 595$ per condition).

Electrical stimulation thresholds are also less variable in the hearing-impaired animal. The same procedure used to obtain the data displayed in Figure 13-7 was used with the electrical stimulation thresholds obtained from inferior colliculus (Gerken et al, 1989). These histograms are shown in Figure 13-8. It is clear without statistical analysis that the distribution for the hearing-impaired animals is narrower. Finally, the variability of the data sets summarized in Figure 13-6 was calculated. The variability of the thresholds obtained in the presence of the 60-dB SPL continuous tone was less than it was in quiet conditions ($F = 1.65$, $N = 96$ per condition, $p = 0.02$).

Conclusion

It was hypothesized that factors involving the cochlea, apart from amount of input per se, affect the manner in which the central au-

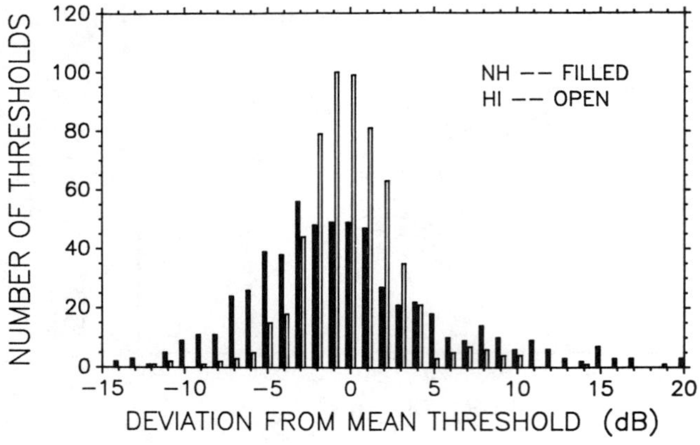

Figure 13-7 Distribution of normalized acoustic thresholds for normal-hearing (NH) and hearing-impaired (HI) cats.

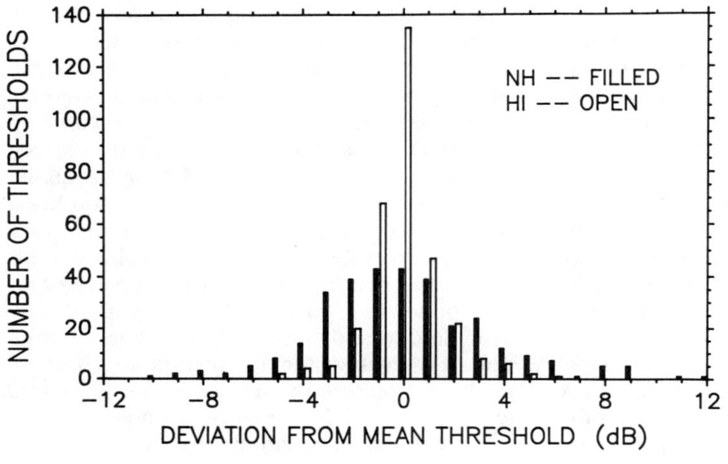

Figure 13-8 Distribution of normalized electrical thresholds for normal-hearing (NH) and hearing-impaired (HI) cats.

ditory mechanisms operate. Note the following:

1. Auditory temporal integration, an assumed central process, was reduced in the hearing-impaired animal
2. Temporal integration with electrical stimulation of inferior colliculus was reduced in the hearing-impaired animal
3. Auditory temporal integration was reduced in human subjects in the presence of a background of continuous tone of moderate intensity
4. In the hearing-impaired animal, a central supersensitivity to electrical stimulation occurred
5. In the normal-hearing animal, continuous tone also produced a central supersensitivity for electrical stimulation
6. Variability in auditory detection thresholds was reduced in hearing-impaired cats
7. Variability in detection thresholds for electrical stimulation of the inferior colliculus was reduced in hearing-impaired cats
8. Variability was reduced in auditory detection thresholds in human subjects in the presence of a continuous tone
9. In comparison with the results obtained with continuous tone, noise was relatively ineffective in altering the state of the central auditory system

These results support the hypothesis that factors involving the cochlea affect the operation of the central auditory system. Central effects were obtained whether the cochlea was permanently altered, as in sound-induced hearing loss, (see items 1, 2, and 4 in the above list), or was simply used to transmit a non–information bearing signal such as a continuous tone (see items 3, 5, and 8 in the above list).

A further conclusion relates to the apparent symmetry of the effects produced by hearing loss and the presence of continuous tone. The symmetry was seen in effects on temporal integration (items 1 and 3 above), the production of stimulation supersensitivity (items 4 and 5 above), and in the reduction of the variability of detection thresholds (items 6, 7, and 8 above). The symmetry of effects for hearing loss and continuous tone suggests that these two factors affect the central auditory system in a similar manner. It may be that supersensitivity is associated with an auditory mechanism used for discrimination of one sound in the presence of another. In a normal-hearing listener, such a mechanism would presumably be activated in a limited manner related to the spectrum of the nontarget signal (e.g., in this simplest case, the frequency of the continuous tone). In the hearing-impaired listener, however, it seems that the mechanism would be more globally activated. The global supersensitivity would thus serve as a means of partially offsetting the peripheral loss. There must be a cost in this maneuver to increase sensitivity, however, or else the system would normally be in the supersensitive state. Possibly, the central auditory system has increased its ability to detect at the expense of its ability to discriminate.

One aspect of auditory processing known to be affected by hearing loss is temporal integration. Compare, for example, the acoustic and electric temporal integration functions. With acoustic stimuli (see Figs. 13-2 and 13-4), the thresholds for long stimuli are apparently elevated more than the thresholds for short stimuli. With electrical stimuli, however, the reverse was observed (see Figs. 13-3 and 13-4): the thresholds for short stimuli decreased more than the thresholds for long stimuli. It is in the electrical stimulation data that the basis for the acoustic result may be seen. Specifically, the greater increase in central sensitivity to brief electrical stimuli may result in less apparent loss for the brief acoustic stimuli.

In summary, although the traditional role of the cochlea is the transduction of acoustic input, it was argued that the cochlea is also involved in concomitant processes that influence the state of the central auditory system—influences that go beyond the basic metric of quantity of input and perhaps relate to the control of the processing.

Bruit, Son Continu et Déficits Auditifs: Effets Centraux sur l'Analyse Temporelle

La cochlée et le système auditif central peuvent être affectés par les mêmes facteurs ou conditions dont les effets sur le traitement temporel de stimulus auditifs présentent un intérêt particulier. Parmi les facteurs et les conditions qui affectent la cochlée, figurent la pathologie cochléaire ainsi que certaines combinaisons de stimulus acoustiques. La différenciation en ce qui concerne la cochlée et les effets sur le système auditif central est un problème difficile en raison de la relation séquentielle entre la périphérie et le système central. Il est certain que des lésions périphériques réduiront l'envoi d'informations vers le système central; cependant, si l'hypothèse de l'altération des processus de traitement est confirmée, les opérations centrales doivent être affectées qualitativement et pas seulement quantitativement.

La réduction de la pente de la fonction d'intégration temporelle, qui intervient après une perte auditive, est un exemple d'altération des processus de traitement temporel. Des explications en termes de mécanismes centraux ou périphériques pourraient tout aussi bien rendre compte de ce phénomène.

Des travaux récents ont montré qu'après stimulation électrique au niveau central la pente de la fonction d'intégration temporelle était aussi réduite de manière similaire (Gerken, Solecki et Boettcher, 1989). En cas de stimulation centrale, le signal qui doit être détecté ne passe pas par la cochlée et le traitement central est ainsi mesuré directement. Il découle de ce qui précède que la pathologie cochléaire devrait ainsi induire des changements centraux qui eux produiraient alors la réduction de la pente.

Si certaines combinaisons de stimulus font aussi partie des facteurs et des conditions qui affectent la cochlée, alors une altération des processus centraux de traitement auditif devrait aussi se produire chez des sujets avec des cochlées intactes. Dans une thèse récente, Bhat (1988) a montré que chez des sujets possédant une audition normale, les pentes des fonctions d'intégration auditive temporelle étaient réduites en présence d'un son continu d'intensité modérée. Le travail de Bhat suggère que certaines combinaisons de stimulus acoustiques altèrent le traitement auditif central, mais en eux-mêmes, ils ne démontrent pas un changement des opérations de traitement central.

D'autres données en provenance d'études électrophysiologiques et comportementales chez l'animal ayant une cochlée saine, supportent la conclusion selon laquelle les processus centraux sont altérés par certaines combinaisons de stimulus acoustiques. A titre d'exemple, des stimulus acoustiques brefs induisent des potentiels thalamiques ou corticaux de plus forte amplitude en cas de présentation avec un son continu que sans ce dernier. D'autres exemples qui mettent en relation des résultats électrophysiologiques et psychophysiologiques auraient pû être cités.

Le bruit, les sons continus et les déficits auditifs constituent tous des facteurs ou des conditions qui affectent directement la périphérie. Cependant, il existe des données indiquant que dans certains cas, une altération peut aussi se produire au niveau du fonctionnement auditif central.

ACKNOWLEDGMENTS

This work was supported in part by NIH grant RO1 NS9512. I am grateful to Dr. Vishwa K.H. Bhat for the data analysis used to construct Figure 13-6, and to Janet M. Solecki for the data analysis used to construct Figures 13-2 and 13-7.

References

Algom D, Babkoff H. Auditory temporal integration at threshold: Theories and some implications of current research. In: Neff WD, ed. Contributions to sensory physiology. New York: Academic Press, 1984:131.

Bhat VKH. Human auditory temporal summation in the presence of ipsilateral and contralateral continuous tones. Unpublished PhD dissertation, The University of Texas at Dallas, Richardson, TX, 1988.

Carlyon RP, Buss S, Florentine M. Temporal integration of trains of tone pulses by normal and by cochlearly impaired listeners. J Acoust Soc Am 1990; 87:260-268.

Clark WW, Bohne BA. Cochlear damage: Audiometric correlates? In: Collins MJ, Glattke TJ, Harper LA, eds. Sensorineural hearing loss. Iowa City: University of Iowa Press, 1986:59.

Doty RW. Conditioned reflexes elicited by electrical stimulation of the brain in macaques. J Neurophysiol 1965; 28:623-640.

Florentine M, Fastl H, Buss S. Temporal integration in normal hearing, cochlear impairment, and impairment simulated by masking. J Acoust Soc Am 1988; 84:195-203.

Garner WR, Miller GA. The masked threshold of pure tones as a function of duration. J Exp Psychol 1947; 37:293-303.

Gengel RW. Auditory temporal integration at relatively high masked-threshold levels. J Acoust Soc Am 1972; 51:1849-1851.

Gerken GM. A systems approach to the relationship between the ear and central auditory mechanisms. In: Keidel WD, Finkenzeller P, eds. Advances in audiology: Artificial auditory stimulation theories. Vol 1. Basel, Karger, 1984:30.

Gerken GM, Bhat VKH, Hutchison-Clutter M. Auditory temporal integration and the power function model. J Acoust Soc Am 1990; 88:767-778.

Gerken GM, Saunders SS, Paul RE. Hypersensitivity to electrical stimulation of auditory nuclei follows hearing loss in cats. Hear Res 1984; 13:249-259.

Gerken GM, Saunders SS, Simhadri-Sumithra R, Bhat KHV. Behavioral thresholds for electrical stimulation applied to auditory brainstem nuclei in cat are altered by injurious and noninjurious sound. Hear Res 1985; 20:221-231.

Gerken GM, Solecki JM, Boettcher FA. Temporal integration functions measured using electrical stimulation of subcortical auditory nuclei in normal-hearing and hearing-impaired cat. Paper presented at the Assoc Res Otolaryngol 12th Midwinter Meeting, St. Petersburg, FL.

Gray RF. Cochlear implants. San Diego: College-Hill Press, 1985.

Green DM, Birdsall TG, Tanner WP Jr. Signal detection as a function of signal intensity and duration. J Acoust Soc Am 1957; 29:523-531.

Henderson D. Temporal summation of acoustic signals by the chinchilla. J Acoust Soc Am 1969; 46:474-475.

Nieder PC, Neff WD. Auditory information from subcortical electrical stimulation in cats. Science 1961; 133:1010-1011.

Miller JM, Spelman FA. Cochlear implants: Models of the electrically stimulated ear. New York: Springer-Verlag, 1989.

Osen KK. Course and termination of the primary afferents in the cochlear nuclei of the cat. An experimental anatomical study. Arch Ital Biol 1970; 108:21-51.

Penner MJ. A power law transformation resulting in a class of short-term integrators that produce time-intensity trades for noise bursts. J Acoust Soc Am 1978; 57:431-436.

Plomp R. Hearing threshold for periodic tone pulses. J Acoust Soc Am 1961; 33:1561-1569.

Schindler RA, Merzenich MM. Cochlear implants. New York: Raven Press, 1985.

Shannon RV. Multichannel electrical stimulation of the auditory nerve in man. I. Basic psychophysics. Hear Res 1983; 11:157-189.

Sheeley EC, Bilger RC. Temporal integration as a function of frequency. J Acoust Soc Am 1964; 36:1850-1857.

Solecki JM, Gerken GM. Auditory temporal integration in the normal-hearing and hearing-impaired cat. J Acoust Soc Am 1990; 88:779-785.

Watson CS, Gengel RW. Signal duration and signal frequency in relation to auditory sensitivity. J Acoust Soc Am 1969; 46:989-997.

Wright HN. The effect of sensori-neural hearing loss on threshold-duration functions. J Speech Hear Res 1968; 11:842-852.

Wright HN, Cannella F. Differential effect of conductive hearing loss on the threshold-duration function. J Speech Hear Res 1969; 12:607-615.

Zwicker E, Wright HN. Temporal summation for tones in narrow-band noise. J Acoust Soc Am 1963; 35:691-699.

Zwislocki J. Theory of temporal auditory summation. J Acoust Soc Am 1960; 32:1046-1060.

CHAPTER 14

Enhancement of Evoked Response Amplitude and Single Unit Activity After Noise Exposure

RICHARD J. SALVI
NICHOLAS L. POWERS
SAMUEL S. SAUNDERS
FLINT A. BOETTCHER
ANN E. CLOCK

Noise-induced hearing loss has traditionally been viewed as a peripheral disorder in which the pathophysiologic changes originating in the cochlea are simply relayed up the central nervous system (Salvi et al, 1982a; Siegel and Kim, 1982; Liberman and Kiang, 1978; Schmiedt et al, 1980). Although the altered pattern of neural activity flowing out of the cochlea into the central nervous system may underlie some of the distortions in hearing that accompany sensorineural hearing loss, a full understanding of the phenomenon must ultimately take into account the anatomic and neurophysiologic changes in the central auditory pathway. A number of subtle histopathologies have been observed in several regions of the central auditory pathway following acoustic trauma (Liden et al, 1973; Theopold, 1975; Hall, 1976; Morest, 1982). However, the physiologic consequences of these anatomic changes are not yet fully understood. In fact, there are relatively few reports describing the pathophysiologic changes that occur in the central auditory pathway following acoustic trauma (Starr, 1965; Salvi, 1976; Salvi et al, 1978; Lonsbury-Martin and Meikle, 1978; Lonsbury-Martin and Martin, 1981; Willott and Lu, 1982). Most of the reported effects (e.g., elevated thresholds, poor neural tuning, and compression of spontaneous discharge rates; loss of suppression and distortion product responses) simply mirror the effects seen in the cochlea. For example, acoustic overstimulation leads to loss of sensitivity and tuning in the evoked potentials recorded from the central auditory pathway (Klein and Mills, 1981; Salvi et al, 1976; Saunders and Rhyne, 1970). However, several investigators have observed abnormally large amplitude (enhanced) evoked potentials in the central auditory pathway in subjects with cochlear pathologies arising from a diverse range of factors, including acoustic trauma (Saunders et al, 1972a,b; Gerken et al, 1984, 1986). Because of the preliminary nature of this research, there are still many important but unanswered questions related to the enhancement phenomenon. Specifically, does the magnitude of the enhancement phenomenon vary with the type of noise exposure or the pattern or degree of hearing loss? Is the enhancement phenomenon related to the pattern of hair cell loss along the cochlear partition? Over what time frame does the enhancement phenomenon develop, and what physiologic mechanisms underlie the enhancement phenomenon? The purpose of the present study was to explore some of these issues.

Methods

Evoked Potentials

Adult chinchillas (400 to 800 g) were prepared for chronic evoked response recordings using procedures outlined previously (Henderson et al, 1973; Salvi et al, 1982b). Briefly, the animals were anesthetized (35 mg per kilogram of ketamine, 0.5 mg per kilogram of acepromazine, 0.1 mg per kilogram of xylazine) and monauralized by surgical destruction of the left cochlea, and chronic recording electrodes were implanted into one or more recording locations: round window, cochlear nucleus (CN), inferior colliculus The animals were then allowed to recover for approximately 2 weeks. The awake animal was placed in a yoke-like restraint that fixed the head position within the calibrated sound field. Each evoked response waveform was based on the average of 100 to 250 sweeps to a probe tone (20 ms duration, 5 ms rise/fall time) presented at a rate of 10 per second.

Histology

Each animal was anesthetized with sodium pentobarbital and decapitated. The bulla was quickly removed, perfused with cold glutaraldehyde (2.5 percent), postfixed in 1 percent osmium tetroxide, and dehydrated to 70 percent ETOH. The organ of Corti was dissected out, mounted in glycerin as a flat surface preparation, and viewed at ×400 using a differential interference contrast microscope. Hair cell counts were made over 0.24-mm intervals and plotted in the form of a cochleogram (Salvi et al, 1983a,b).

Single Unit Recording

Each animal was anesthetized (ketamine, 35 mg per kilogram; xylazine, 1 mg per kilogram), tracheotomized, and prepared for single unit recording from the CN as described previously (Salvi et al, 1978). Recordings were made using glass microelectrodes (3 M NaCl and fast green, 5 to 14 MΩ).

Results

Enhancement and Permanent Threshold Shift (PTS)

Evoked response amplitude-level functions were obtained from the inferior colliculus of 10 chinchillas before and 30 to 40 days after exposure to a 2-kHz pure tone (105 dB SPL re 20 μPa; 5 days). This exposure consistently produced 20 to 30 dB of PTS between 2 and 8 kHz, as illustrated by the data for one animal shown in Figure 14-1. The cochleogram for this animal showed a 40 to 50 percent loss of outer hair cells in the 2- to 3-kHz region of the cochlea, roughly a 10 percent loss in the 4- to 10-kHz region, and a 30- to 40 percent loss in the 0.6-kHz region. In this case, there was only a weak-to-moderate correlation between the region of hearing loss and the pattern of hair cell loss.

Figure 14-2 shows the evoked response amplitude-level functions obtained at 0.5 and 4 kHz for the animal shown in Figure 14-1. After the exposure, higher sound levels were required to elicit the evoked response at 4 kHz because of the hearing loss; however, once threshold was exceeded, the amplitude increased rapidly and saturated at a maximum amplitude that was close to the maximum pre-exposure amplitude. At intermediate sound levels, the amplitude exceeded the pre-exposure values. By contrast, there was no PTS at 0.5 kHz. However, the postexposure amplitude-level function increased rapidly and saturated at a level that was almost three times greater than the maximum pre-exposure amplitude. Despite the change in amplitude, there was little or no change in the morphology of the evoked response waveform (Fig. 14-2, bottom).

All 10 chinchillas exposed to the 2-kHz tone developed a hearing loss between 2 and 8 kHz, and eight of the animals had postexposure amplitude-level functions that were larger than their pre-exposure amplitude-level functions at one or more frequencies. In most cases, abnormally large amplitude responses were seen at test frequencies at or below the low-frequency edge of the hearing loss. To provide a comprehensive view of the change in maximum amplitude, the postexposure amplitude-level function was normalized by dividing each of the postexposure amplitudes by the maximum pre-exposure amplitude at a particular frequency. Thus, a normalized amplitude of 1.5 would mean that the postexposure amplitude was 50 percent larger than the largest pre-exposure value. Figure 14-3 shows the 10 normalized amplitude-level functions at the four test frequencies. After the exposure, the maximum amplitude of the evoked response was typically depressed (maximum normalized amplitude less than 1) at 4 and 8 kHz. Only two cases of enhancement were seen at 4 and 8 kHz out of 20 cases. By contrast, the maximum amplitude of the evoked response was typically much larger than normal at 0.5 kHz and 2 kHz. For example, at 0.5 kHz, the maximum amplitude was enhanced by 20 percent or more in 8 of 10 subjects. To put the amplitude changes into perspective, the average PTS and average cochleogram for the 10 animals are shown in Figure 14-4. The results indicate that the enhancement phenomenon is associated with the low-frequency edge of the hearing loss. Although the average hair cell loss was greatest in the 2- to 8-kHz

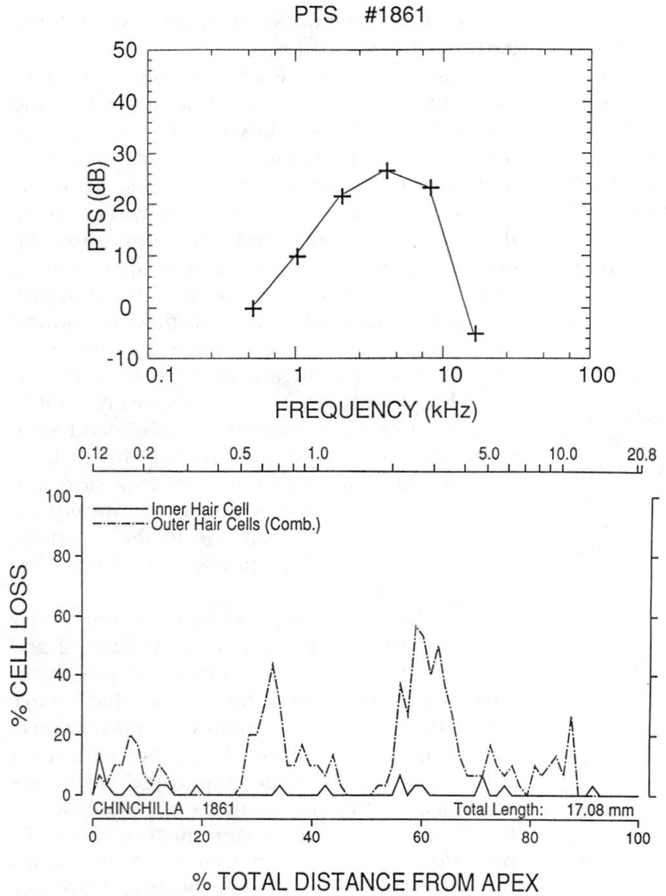

Figure 14-1 Chinchilla #1861. *A,* Permanent threshold shift as a function of frequency. *B,* Percentage of inner and combined outer hair cell loss as a function of percentage total distance from the apex and as a function of frequency. (Eldredge et al, 1981.)

region, the lesions were relatively small and showed only a weak-to-moderate correlation with the hearing loss and the enhancement phenomenon.

Temporary Threshold Shift (TTS)

Does the enhancement phenomenon only occur with PTS or can it occur during TTS? To address this issue, we exposed 10 chinchillas for 5 to 8 days to a 2-kHz tone of 85 dB SPL. This exposure produced virtually no PTS. Testing was carried out by removing the animals from the exposure for approximately 1 hour each day. During the exposure, the average TTS ranged from 25 to 35 dB between 2 and 8 kHz. Little or no TTS was observed at higher or lower frequencies. Figure 14-5 shows the normalized amplitude-level functions measured at 0.5, 2, 4, and 8 kHz. During TTS, the maximum evoked response amplitude was generally depressed (normalized amplitudes less than 1) at 4 and 8 kHz. By contrast, the maximum evoked response amplitude was typically larger than normal at 0.5 and 2 kHz. These results suggest that the enhancement phenomenon can occur with sound exposures that produce virtually no PTS.

Origins of the Enhancement Phenomenon

One important issue related to the enhancement phenomenon concerns its physiologic origins. To address this issue, we implanted chronic electrodes stereotaxically in the cochlear nucleus and inferior colliculus and on the round window. Afterwards, the animals were exposed for 2 hours to a 2.8-kHz tone at 105 dB SPL. Figure 14-6 shows the 1-kHz amplitude-level functions from three different recording locations in the same ani-

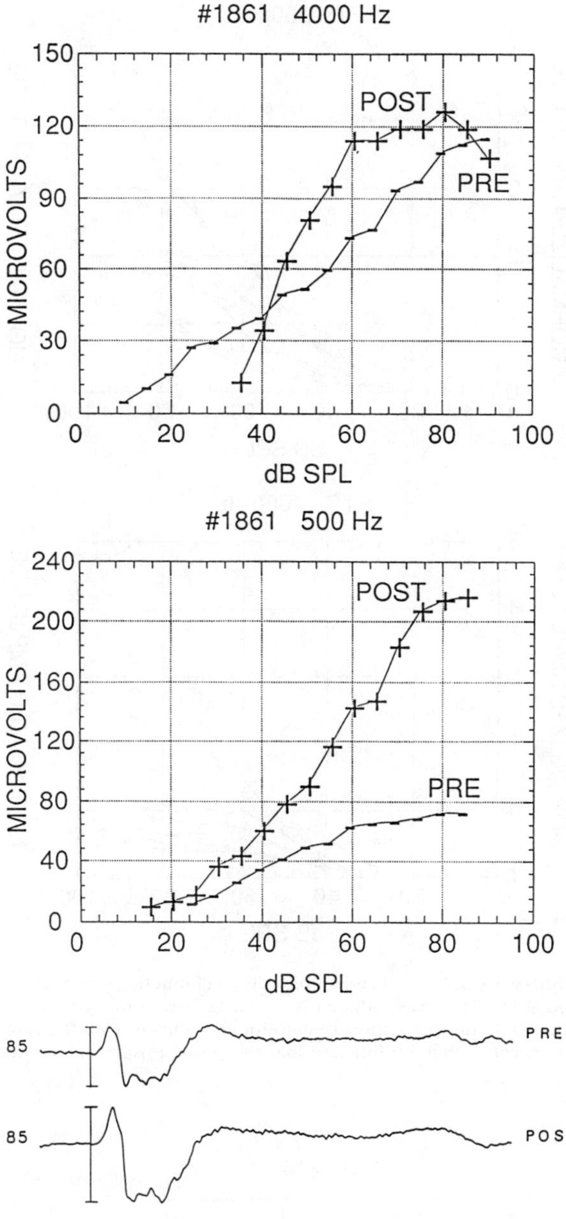

Figure 14-2 Chinchilla #1861. Inferior colliculus, evoked response amplitude (trough-to-peak) as a function of sound pressure level for tone bursts presented at 4 kHz *(middle)* and 0.5 kHz. Evoked response waveforms obtained before and after exposure at 0.5 kHz. Negative polarity is downward. Vertical bar indicates trough-to-peak amplitude. *C,* The waveforms are not plotted to the same scale.

mal. The amplitude-level function for the compound action potential (CAP) showed a loss in sensitivity and a significant reduction in amplitude 24 hours after the exposure. After a recovery period of 30 days, the amplitude-level function was almost identical to the pre-exposure data. The amplitude-level function from the cochlear nucleus also showed a loss in sensitivity and a significant drop in amplitude 24 hours after the exposure. The amplitude-level functions showed a substantial amount of recovery by 30 days after exposure, but the amplitudes were still significantly depressed at high sound levels. The amplitude-level function from the inferior colliculus also showed a loss in sensitivity at 24 hours after exposure. However, the amplitude-level functions measured 24 hours and 30 days after exposure increased steeply once threshold was exceeded and reached maximum amplitudes that were substantially larger than those seen before exposure. It should be noted that these abnor-

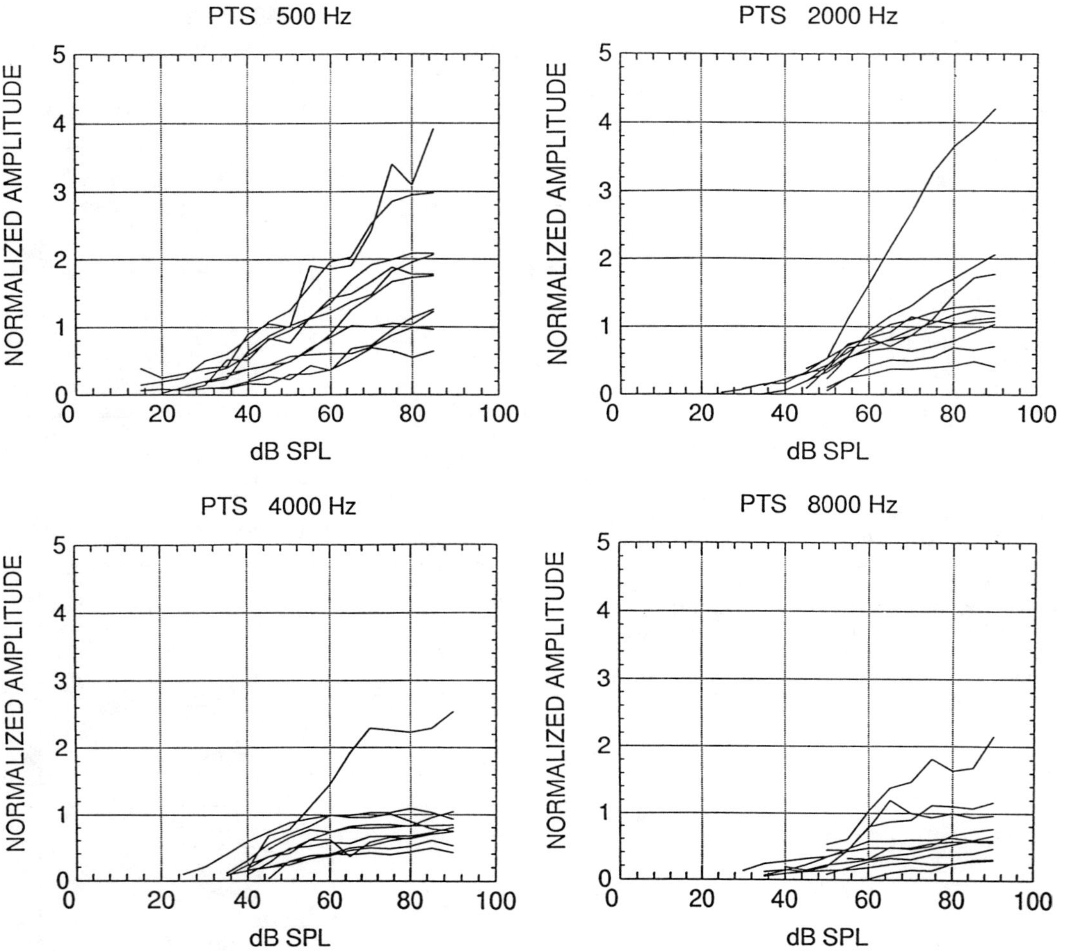

Figure 14-3 Normalized amplitude-level functions from the inferior colliculus of 10 chinchillas. Permanent threshold shift (PTS) was induced by a 2-kHz pure tone. Each postexposure amplitude-level function was normalized to the maximum pre-exposure amplitude obtained from the same animal at that particular frequency. Normalized values greater than 1.0 indicate that the postexposure value exceeded the maximum pre-exposure amplitude.

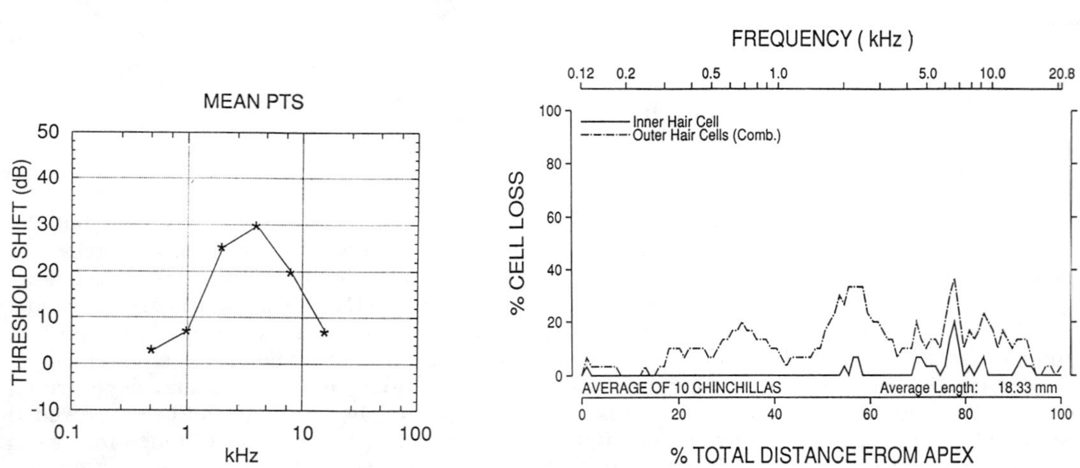

Figure 14-4 *A*, Mean (n = 10) hearing loss as a function of frequency. *B*, Mean (n = 10) inner and combined outer hair cell loss as a function of percentage distance from the apex and as a function of frequency. Average values computed over 1 percent intervals.

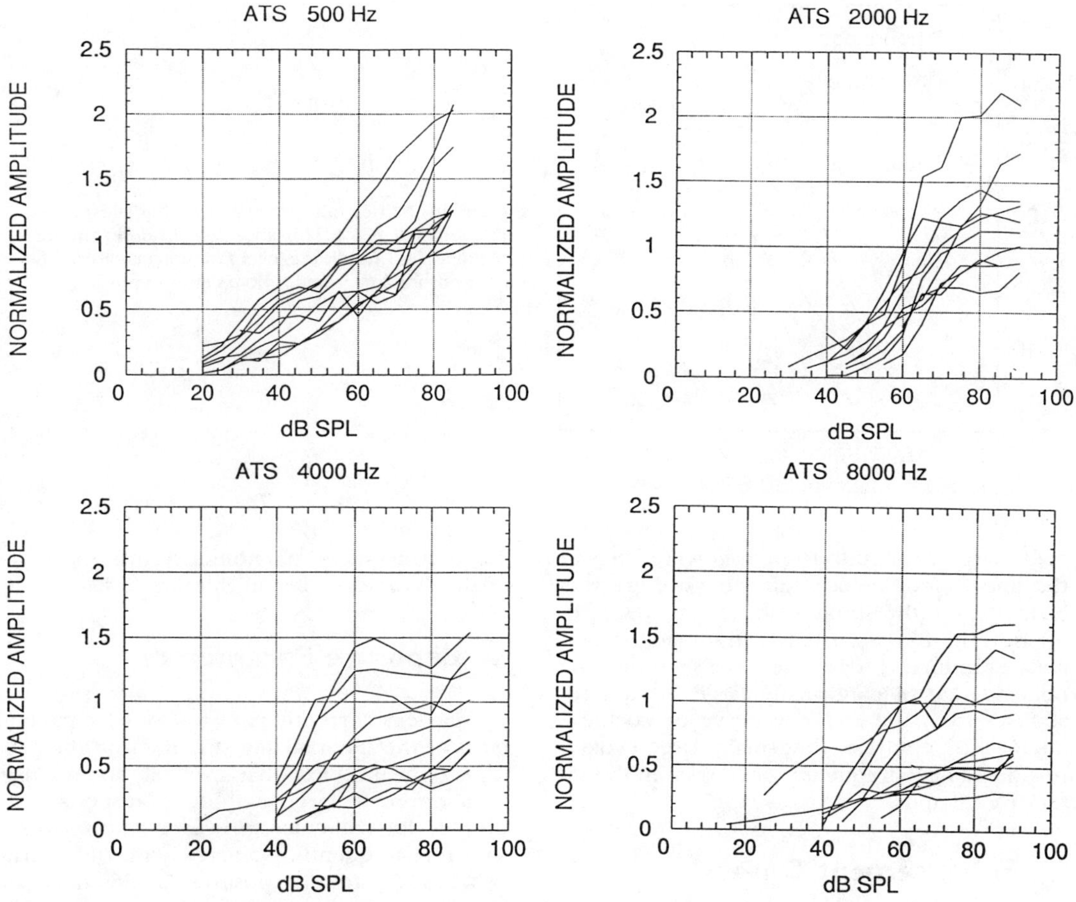

Figure 14-5 Normalized amplitude-level functions from the inferior colliculus of 10 chinchillas. Asymptotic threshold shift (ATS) was induced with a 2-kHz tone. Each postexposure amplitude-level function was normalized to the maximum pre-exposure amplitude obtained from the same animal at that particular frequency. Normalized values greater than 1.0 indicate that the postexposure value exceeded the maximum pre-exposure amplitude.

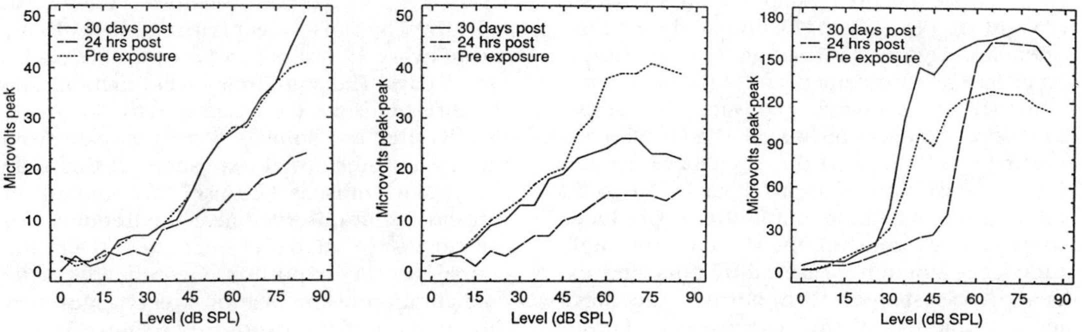

Figure 14-6 Chinchilla #2751. Evoked response amplitude-level functions obtained at *A,* 1 kHz from electrodes on the round window, *B,* in the cochlear nucleus and *C,* in the inferior colliculus. Amplitude-level functions measured before exposure, and 24 hours and 30 days after exposure.

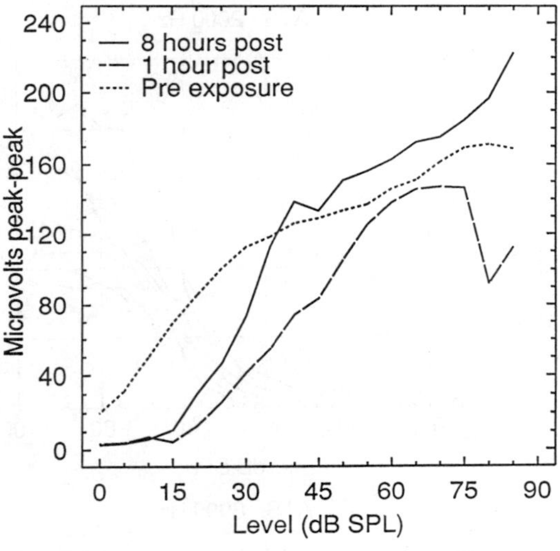

Figure 14-7 Chinchilla #3119. Amplitude-level functions obtained at 1 kHz from an electrode in the inferior colliculus. Amplitude-level functions measured before exposure, and 1 and 8 hours after exposure.

mally large amplitude responses were seen in the inferior colliculus even though there was little or no threshold shift at the test frequency. In the acoustically traumatized animals examined to date, we have seen little or no evidence of abnormally large evoked responses from the auditory nerve or cochlear nucleus. By contrast, abnormally large evoked responses have frequently been seen in the inferior colliculus.

Enhancement Onset

How long does it take for the enhancement phenomenon to develop after acoustic trauma? To examine this issue, we obtained amplitude-level functions (three to five measurements) from each animal prior to exposure. The animals were then exposed for 2 hours to a 2.8-kHz tone presented at 105 dB SPL. Amplitude-level functions were then remeasured at various times following the exposure. The exposure resulted in a significant amount of TTS (60 to 75 dB) at the mid-frequencies. Figure 14-7 shows the amplitude-level functions obtained at 1 kHz between 1 and 8 hours following exposure. The amplitude-level function measured 1 hour after exposure was shifted to the right because of a loss in sensitivity of approximately 15 to 20 dB, and the maximum amplitude was reduced somewhat. By contrast, the slope of the amplitude-level function measured 8 hours after exposure was steeper than normal; the maximum amplitude of the response was consistently larger than the pre-exposure values at high sound levels. These results indicate that the enhancement phenomenon can develop relatively quickly, i.e., in 8 hours or less.

Exposure Parameters

Little is currently known about the parameters of the traumatizing stimulus and the patterns of hearing loss that are likely to give rise to abnormally large amplitude responses in the inferior colliculus. However, one relationship that frequently occurred with our 2-kHz and 2.8-kHz tone exposures is illustrated in Figure 14-8. Abnormally large amplitude evoked responses from the inferior colliculus were generally seen at frequencies below or on the low-frequency edge of the hearing loss (i.e., at or below the frequency of the exposure), whereas response amplitudes were generally depressed at frequencies above the exposure (i.e., in the region of greatest hearing loss). In addition to these results, data are available from a few animals exposed to a 95-dB SPL, octave band of noise centered at 0.5 kHz. The noise was presented for 3 hours out of every 12 hours (25 percent duty cycle) for 15 days. The amplitude-level functions and the thresholds were measured each day immediately after the animals were removed from the noise. Interrupted exposures of this type are rather unusual because the amount of threshold shift observed near the frequency of the exposure actually decreases over the course of the exposure. Consequently, the configuration of the hearing loss changes over the duration of the exposure as shown in Figure 14-9. For example, at 4 kHz, the threshold shift increased from 22 to 32 dB between the

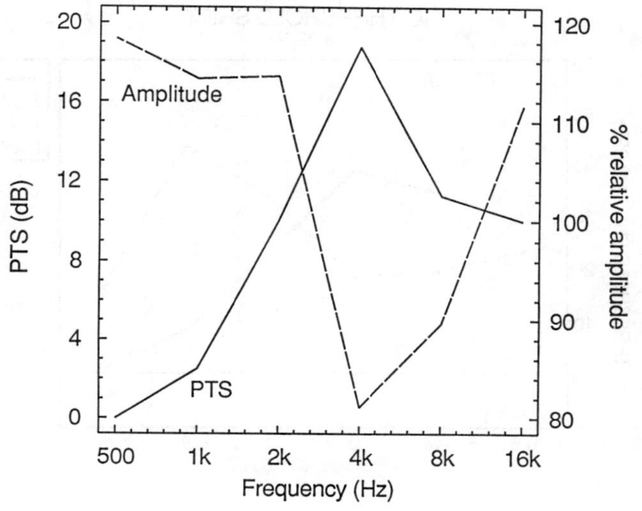

Figure 14-8 Chinchilla #3119. Permanent threshold shift and enhancement as a function of frequency following exposure to a 2.8-kHz tone at 105 dB SPL for 2 hours. Percentage of enhancement is the ratio of the maximum postexposure amplitude to the maximum pre-exposure amplitude at the same frequency in the same animal.

first and fifteenth days of exposure; during this period, there was a corresponding decrease in the amplitude of the evoked response. By contrast, the amount of threshold shift at 1 kHz decreased from 35 to 25 dB between the first and fifteenth days of the exposure, and during this period there was a corresponding increase in the amplitude of the response and a slight enhancement (9 percent) in the maximum amplitude at 1 kHz (and at 0.5 kHz). Although the enhancement effect was relatively small in this case, perhaps due to the residual hearing loss, it was located on the low-frequency edge of the hearing loss.

Single Unit Data

One mechanism that could contribute to the abnormally large amplitude evoked potentials is the selective loss of the inhibitory sidebands that surround the excitatory response area of many units in the central auditory pathway (Evans and Nelson, 1973; Young and Brownell, 1976; Ryan and Miller, 1978). One method for selectively eliminating the inhibitory input to a cell would be to present the traumatizing stimulus in the inhibitory region located on the high-frequency side of the excitatory response area. The reduction or loss of inhibitory inputs on the high-frequency edge of the response area could lead to an expansion of the excitatory response area towards the high frequencies, or to higher-than-normal firing rates to tones presented in the excitatory response area, or to both.

Preliminary data related to this hypothesis have been obtained from a sample of units in the anteroventral cochlear nucleus (AVCN). The response areas of units in the AVCN may be excitatory, or excitatory with inhibitory sidebands (Young, 1984). The excitatory response area was established for each unit. Discharge rate-level functions and post-stimulus time (PST) histograms were then collected in response to frequencies located below, above, and at the characteristic frequency (CF). Measurements were obtained from each unit before and after exposure to a high-level tone presented a half-octave above CF. Figure 14-10A shows the PST histograms collected at CF from a primary-like notch unit with a CF of 8,992 Hz and a threshold of 10 dB SPL. Prior to presenting the traumatizing stimulus, the PST histogram (Fig. 14-10B) to a 50-dB SPL tone presented a half-octave (12,717 Hz) above CF showed almost complete suppression of spontaneous activity followed by a slight rebound in the firing rate at the end of the tone burst. Figure 14-10C and D show the PST histograms after presentation of a 105-dB SPL traumatizing tone of 12,717 Hz for 5 minutes. The shape of the PST histogram obtained at CF was unaffected by the exposure. In contrast, the PST histogram obtained a half-octave above CF (12,717 Hz) showed a loss of single-tone suppression of spontaneous activity after the exposure. The exposure also produced significant changes in the rate level functions (Fig. 14-11). After the exposure, the firing rate at CF was essentially unchanged at low sound levels; however, the maximum firing rate observed at high sound levels showed a significant increase (enhancement). This was reflected as an increase in the peak of the PST histogram near the onset of the stimulus, and

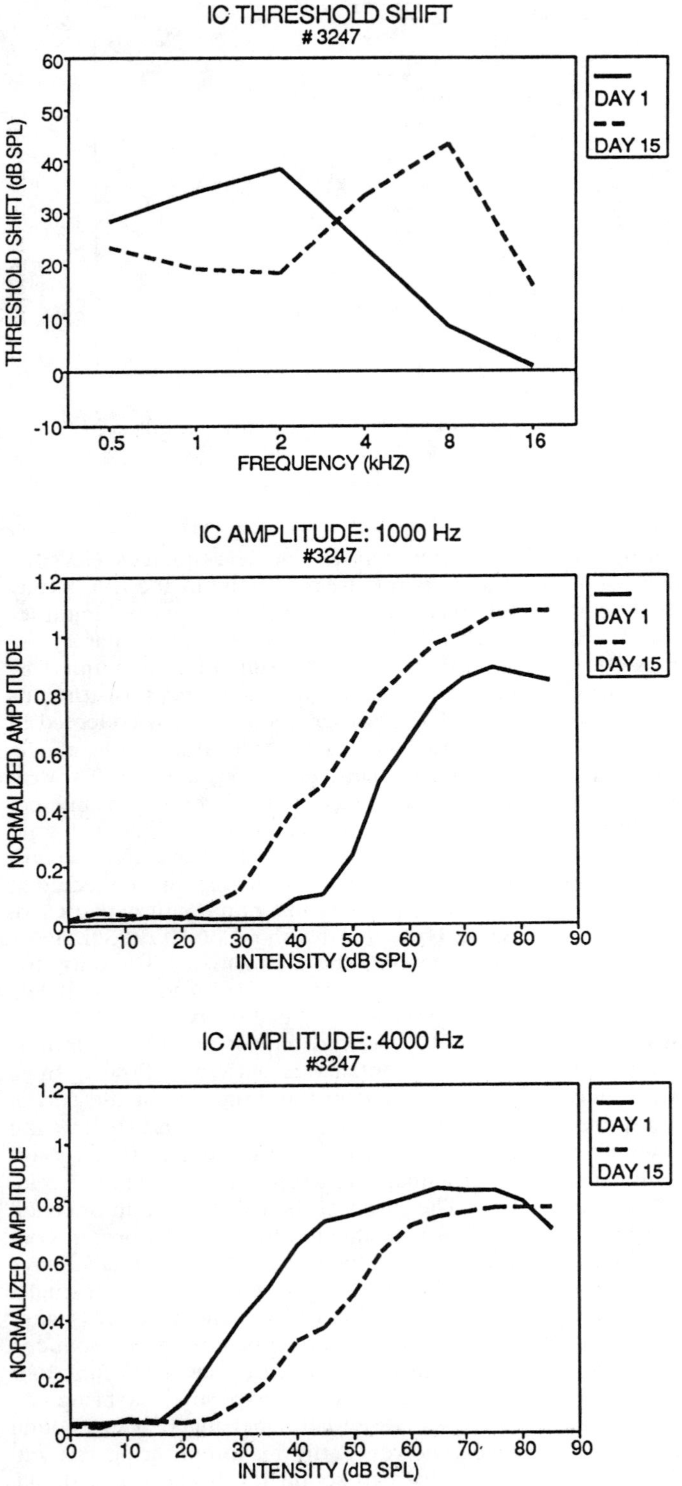

Figure 14-9 Chinchilla #3247. *A*, Threshold shift following 1 day and 15 days of exposure to an interrupted noise with a 25 percent duty cycle (3 hours on, 9 hours off). Octave band noise centered at 0.5 kHz. Exposure level was 95 dB SPL. Each postexposure amplitude-level function was normalized to the maximum pre-exposure amplitude obtained from the same animal at that particular frequency. Normalized values greater than 1.0 indicate that the postexposure value exceeded the maximum pre-exposure amplitude. *B* and *C*, Inferior colliculus amplitude-level functions were measured at 1 kHz and 4 kHz at 1 and 15 days after exposure.

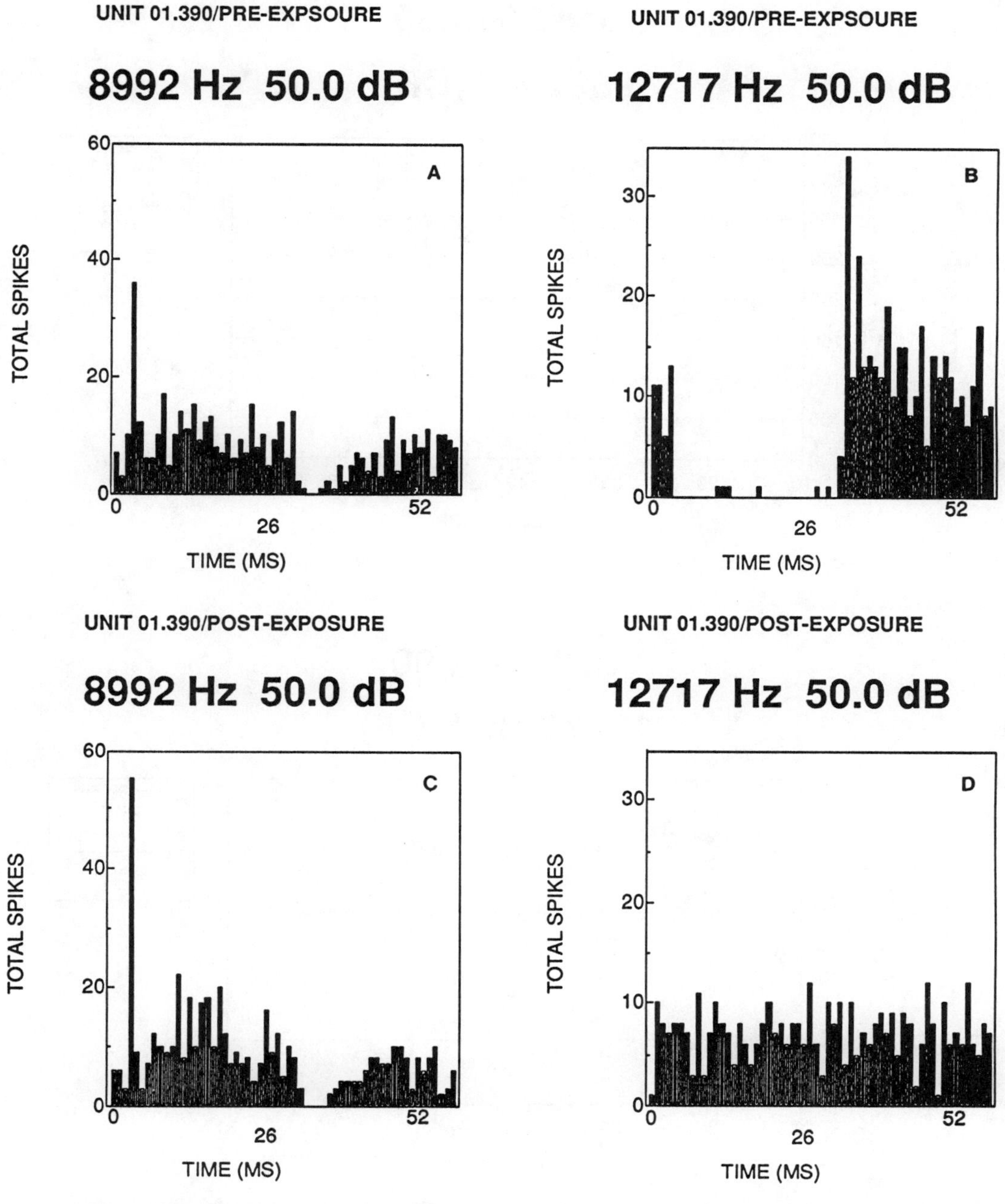

Figure 14-10 Post–stimulus time histograms from a primary-like notch unit. Measurements obtained with 30-ms tone bursts presented at characteristic frequency (CF) and a half-octave above CF. Measurements were obtained before (top two panels) and after (bottom two panels) a 5-minute exposure to a 105-dB SPL tone located a half-octave above CF.

an overall increase in the number of spikes recorded over the duration of the stimulus (Fig. 14-10A versus 14-10C). Examination of the rate-level function obtained a half-octave above CF indicates that the traumatizing exposure virtually abolished any single-tone suppression above CF.

Figure 14-12 shows the results from a Chopper unit (CF 6,221 Hz, threshold 22 dB SPL) with inhibitory sidebands above and below CF. The traumatizing stimulus was a 105-dB SPL tone presented for 5 minutes at a frequency a half-octave above CF. Before the exposure, the rate-level function measured a

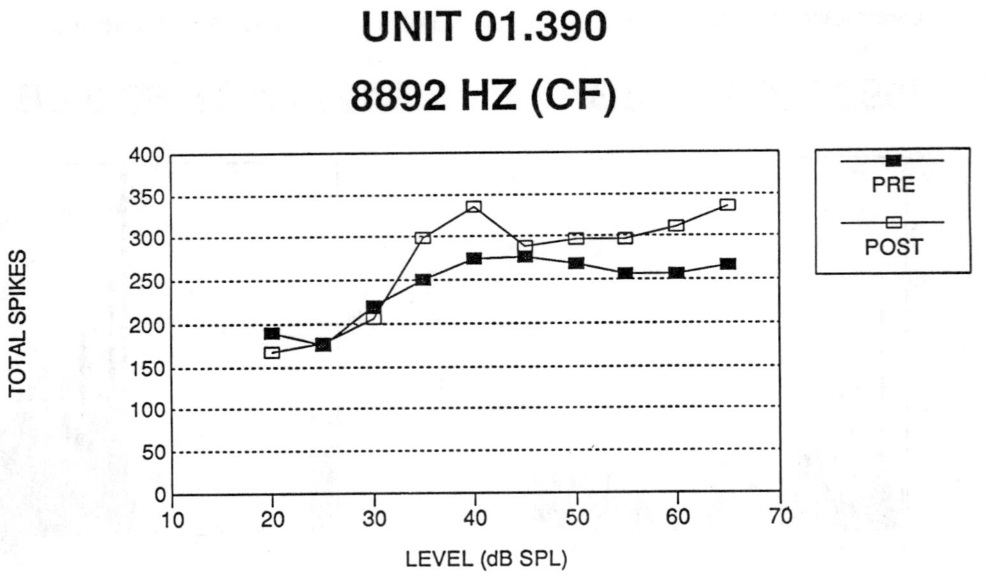

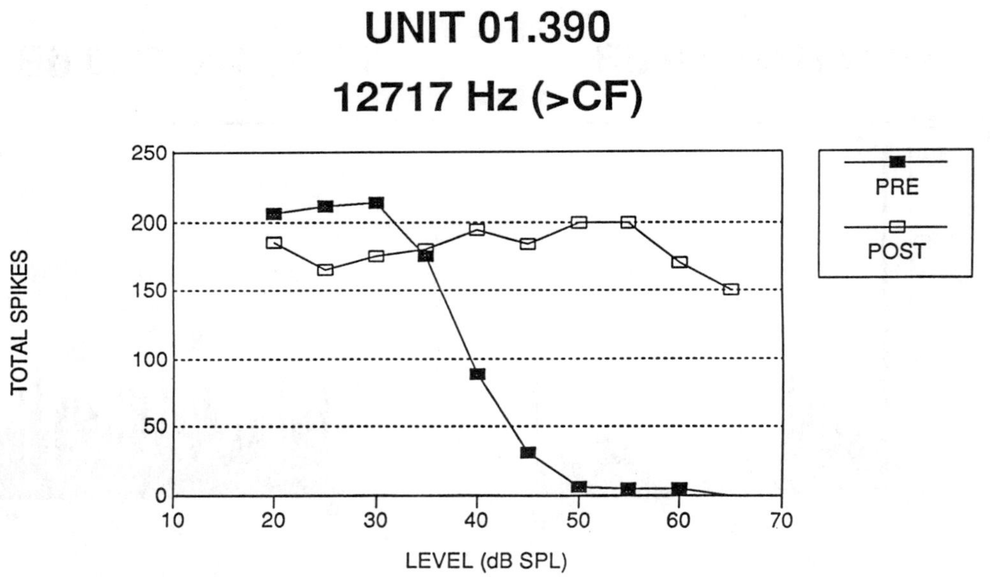

Figure 14-11 Discharge rate-level functions from the primary-like notch unit shown in Figure 14-10. Measurements were obtained before (filled symbols) and after (open symbols) a 5-minute exposure to a 105-dB SPL tone located a half-octave above CF. *A,* Note the increase in the number of spikes to the tone at characteristic frequency (CF) after the exposure. *B,* Note the loss of suppression to the tone presented a half-octave above CF after the exposure.

half-octave above CF (8,799 Hz) decreased as stimulus level increased. However, after the exposure, the firing rate initially increased and remained well above the pre-exposure firing rate until the stimulus level exceeded 63 dB SPL. The traumatizing stimulus also had no effect on the threshold at CF. Nevertheless, it resulted in roughly a 20 percent increase in the maximum firing rate at CF. To summarize, AVCN units with inhibitory sidebands often had elevated discharge rates at CF after presentation of a traumatizing tone a half-octave above CF. However, units that lacked inhibitory sidebands showed little or no change in

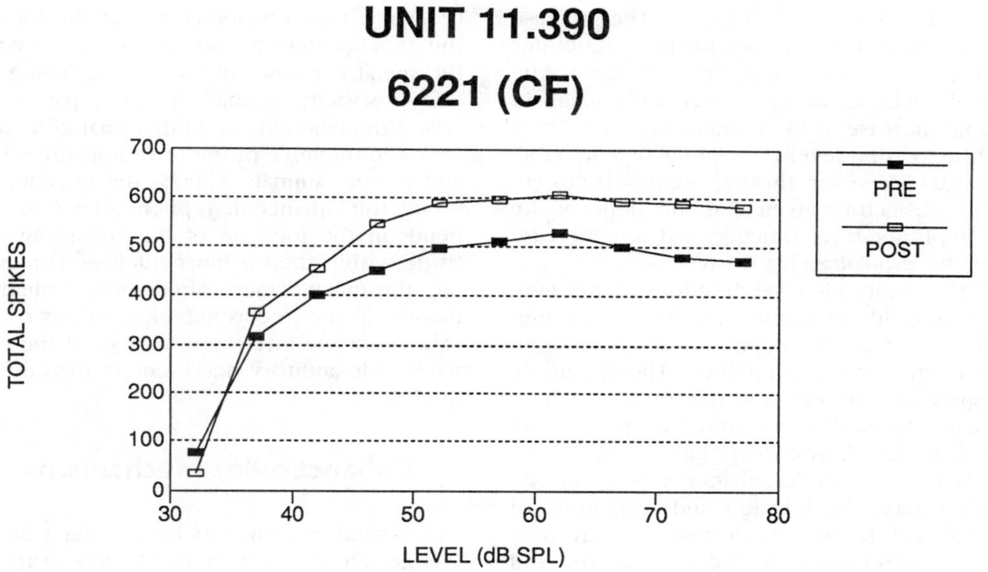

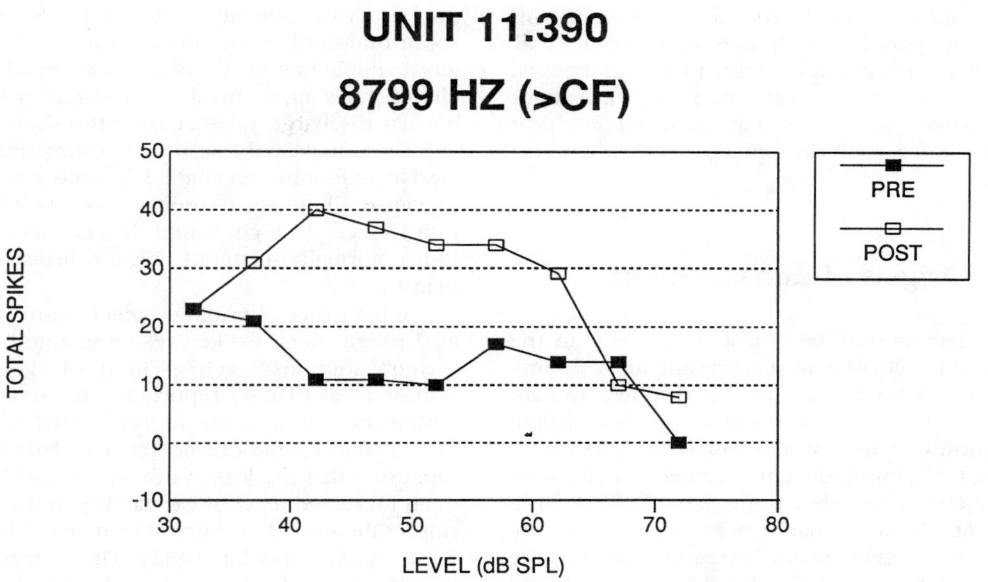

Figure 14-12 Discharge rate-level functions from a Chopper with inhibitory sidebands located above and at characteristic frequency (CF). Measurements were obtained before (filled symbols) and after (open symbols) a 5-minute exposure to a 105-dB SPL tone located a half-octave above CF.

their maximum firing rates after presentation of a traumatizing tone a half-octave above CF.

Discussion

High-level sound exposures that give rise to TTS and PTS produced consistent changes in the evoked response amplitude-level functions from the inferior colliculus. In the region of maximum hearing loss, the amplitude-level functions often increased rapidly, but the maximum response amplitude was generally reduced. This amplitude reduction is consistent with previous results from the auditory nerve as well as the AP data in Figure 14-6 (Eldredge et al, 1973; Salvi et al, 1983a,b). The increase in the slope of the amplitude-level functions from the inferior colliculus may be due to the loss of cochlear tuning, which could result in a rapid increase in the number of active fibers with increasing level (Evans, 1976; Salvi et al, 1983a,b). However, this explanation is not entirely satisfactory given that the slope of the AP amplitude-level function did not increase after the exposure (Fig. 14-6).

The amplitude-level functions on the low-frequency side of the hearing loss also exhibited an increase in slope and an increase in maximum response amplitude. The amplitude enhancement observed at the inferior colliculus cannot easily be accounted for in terms of cochlear pathophysiology, particularly given the lack of amplitude enhancement in the AP. Furthermore, the location and magnitude of the hair cell lesions in our material were only weakly correlated with the hearing loss and enhancement phenomenon. The lack of correlation between structure and function may be due to subtle histopathologies (e.g., stereocilia clumping, fracture of stereocilia rootlets) that cannot be detected with the conventional surface preparation technique (Liberman et al, 1986). Future studies with plastic embedded specimens would clearly be more suitable for studying the relationship between cochlear pathologies and the enhancement phenomenon.

Origins of Enhancement

The amplitude enhancement seen in the inferior colliculus in the present study is similar to that reported in the deafness mutant mouse, in which the onset of cochlear degeneration during development is covariant with onset of amplitude enhancement in the inferior colliculus (Henry and Saleh, 1973). Similar amplitude enhancements have been observed in mice prone to audiogenic seizure (Saunders et al, 1972a,b). After the mice are primed for audiogenic seizures using intense sounds, there is a significant reduction in cochlear microphonic and AP amplitude, whereas the amplitudes of the evoked responses from the CN and inferior colliculus are enhanced. These results would seem to suggest that the enhancement phenomenon originates in the CN. However, we, along with others, have so far not seen evidence of amplitude enhancement in the CN (Powers and Salvi, 1989; Gerken et al, 1984, 1986). There are a number of possible reasons for this discrepancy. One possibility is that the locus of the enhancement phenomenon may vary with the age at the onset of the hearing loss. A second possibility is that the discrepancy may arise from anatomic and functional differences between the mice prone to audiogenic seizure and normal animals. Finally, the likelihood of seeing the enhancement phenomenon may depend on the location of the recording electrode within the cochlear nucleus. For example, the enhancement phenomenon might be missed if the recording electrode were located near the interstitial nucleus at the point where the auditory nerve enters the cochlear nucleus.

Enhancement Mechanisms

Several investigators have studied the discharge rate-level functions of units in the CN and inferior colliculus after acoustic trauma. Lonsbury-Martin and Martin (1981) exposed animals to an intense tone either a half-octave below or at CF. Most units showed a reduction in firing rate after exposure. However, about one-third of the units in the CN and inferior colliculus had lower-than-normal discharge rates near threshold and higher-than-normal discharge rates at suprathreshold levels. They suggested that the exposure affected basilar membrane mechanics in such a way as to cause CF tones to behave like below-CF tones—i.e., at high sound levels, below-CF tones normally generate higher firing rates than CF tones.

What other physiologic mechanism could lead to enhanced evoked response amplitudes at high stimulus levels? Willott (1984) and Willott et al (1984) reported a reduction of inhibition among units in the dorsal CN of mice prone to audiogenic seizure (DBA) and suggested that the loss of inhibition could lead to an increased level of excitability in the inferior colliculus (Lonsbury-Martin and Martin, 1981; Willott and Lu, 1982). They suggested that the lack of inhibition in the DBA strain might be due to the loss of inhibitory interneurons, alterations in inhibitory neurotransmitters, or abnormal dendritic morphology. Our preliminary finding from units in the AVCN are consistent with the preceding hypothesis. After overstimulation with a tone in the high-frequency inhibitory region, there was a reduction in the inhibitory drive to the cell from tones above CF, which in turn was correlated with an increase in the maximum discharge rate to tones near CF. This increase in the maximum discharge rate due to the loss of inhibition could contribute to the enhancement phenomenon if there was an increase in the discharge rate at stimulus onset, such as that seen in Figure 14-10. One problem with this explanation is that the evoked potentials we measure are presumably a response to the onset of the stimulus, whereas the rate level functions reflect the driven level over the duration of the stimulus. Another problem is that we have not observed evoked potential amplitude enhancement in the CN, although there is evidence for such changes in the CN (Saunders et al, 1972a,b). Despite this discrepancy, the proposed mechanism could still provide a satisfactory explanation if the loss of inhibition were to occur proximal to the CN. A third problem relates to the time course of the enhancement mechanism. Enhanced evoked response amplitudes were first observed 8 hours after exposure, whereas single-unit discharge rates showed enhancement within a matter of minutes. Since the duration of the exposure used in the single-unit experiments was much shorter than that used in the chronic experiments, it is difficult to make direct comparisons of the time course of the effect. Also, we have not made detailed evoked response measurements across frequency and time, therefore we do not know if evoked potential enhancement can develop within a matter of minutes.

Studies of the somatosensory cortex have shown that the selective removal of the afferent input from a segment of the receptor surface can result in a change in the topographic organization of the somatosensory cortex such that deprived areas of the cortex become responsive to stimulation of adjacent regions of the skin (Frank, 1980; Rasmusson, 1982; Merzenich and Kaas, 1982; Jenkins and Merzenich, 1987). The expansion of the receptive field boundaries in the somatosensory system has been attributed to unmasking or disinhibition (Metzlar and Marks, 1979; Calford and Tweedale, 1988). Changes in the tonotopic organization of the central nucleus of the inferior colliculus (ICC) have been observed in aging C57BL/6 mice (Willott, 1984). These mice rapidly develop a high-frequency hearing loss as a function of age. Best frequencies of units in the high-frequency regions of the ICC shift to lower frequencies, and as a result there is an over-representation of frequencies at the low-frequency edge of the hearing loss. One mechanism proposed by Willott (1984) to account for these changes is a loss of inhibition from the high-frequency regions of the ICC. More recently, Robertson and Irvine (1989) demonstrated that discrete mechanical lesions of the cochlea resulted in an expanded representation on the auditory cortex of sound frequencies adjacent to the damaged region of the cochlear partition. After a recovery period of 35 to 81 days, the thresholds of units at their "new" characteristic frequencies were close to normal, whereas the thresholds were greatly elevated after a recovery period of only a few hours. They suggested that the pre-existing anatomic receptive fields were actually much wider than those measured physiologically. Thus, when the dominant excitatory inputs to a region are lost because of a peripheral lesion, the pre-existing inputs from adjacent CFs may be expressed. However, the authors did not rule out the possibility that the tonotopic expansion was due to the formation of new synapses. Thus, the enhanced evoked response amplitudes observed on the low-frequency boundary of the hearing loss in the present study (Fig. 14-3) could be due to the over-representation of units with CFs adjacent to the hearing loss.

What functional significance do the enhanced evoked potentials have for auditory processing? One possibility is that the rapid growth and abnormally large amplitudes could be related to loudness recruitment and uncomfortable loudness levels seen in patients with sensorineural hearing loss (Gerken et al, 1986). Alternatively, Rajan (1989) recently reported that electrical stimulation of the contralateral or ipsilateral inferior colliculus during exposure to loud sounds significantly reduced the amount of temporary threshold shift caused by the exposure. The protective effect of stimulating the inferior colliculus was blocked by intracochlear perfusion of hexamethonium. Because this drug also blocks the protective effects due to stimulation of the olivocochlear fibers, it was suggested that the inferior colliculus might modulate the excitability of the olivocochlear neurons that synapse on outer hair cells, thereby altering the response of the basilar membrane (Warr and Guinan, 1979; Rajan, 1989). Thus, an intriguing possibility is that the abnormally large evoked potentials from the inferior colliculus feed back onto the efferent system that innervates the outer hair cells, thereby protecting the cochlea from subsequent exposures to loud sound. Indeed, we have recently found that the second exposure to a traumatizing acoustic stimulus 3 to 4 weeks after the first exposure may produce substantially less elevation in threshold.

Regardless of the mechanism or mechanisms involved, it is clear that the evoked potentials from the central auditory pathway do not simply mirror the changes that occur in the cochlea. Our results, plus those of others, suggest that the pattern of neural activity flowing out of the cochlea and into the central auditory pathway may undergo substantial reorganization.

Amplification des Réponses Evoquées Auditives après Exposition au Bruit

Les pertes auditives induites par le bruit sont traditionnellement considérées comme le résultat d'un dysfonctionnement périphérique impliquant des dommages anatomiques et physiologiques de la cochlée. Cependant, des études récentes indiquent que des changements pathophysiologiques peuvent apparaître au niveau du système auditif central. De tels changements ont été étudiés après avoir implanté des électrodes chroniques à différents emplacements des voies nerveuses auditives pour enregistrer les fonctions amplitude-intensité des réponses évoquées par un "tone-burst" avant et après des expositions sonores à des niveaux capables d'engendrer fatigue et pertes auditives.

Après des expositions sonores de forte intensité, les seuils des réponses évoquées au niveau du nerf auditif, du noyau cochléaire et du colliculus inférieur, étaient élevés. Cependant, alors que le niveau sonore augmentait, l'amplitude des réponses évoquées provenant du colliculus inférieur augmentait à un taux anormalement rapide de telle sorte que, à différentes fréquences, l'amplitude maximale de la réponse était nettement plus grande que la normale. Par contre, les amplitudes maximales des réponses évoquées provenant du noyau cochléaire et du nerf auditif étaient, soit égales, soit plus petites que la normale. Pour les animaux présentant des pertes auditives, les amplitudes des réponses évoquées provenant du colliculus inférieur montraient une augmentation maximale d'amplitude aux limites "basses fréquences" de la zone de fréquences endommagée, tandis que l'amplitude maximale était égale ou plus petite que la normale au centre ou à la limite "hautes fréquences" de cette même zone. Les fréquences présentant une augmentation d'amplitude des réponses évoquées, étaient faiblement corrélées avec le modèle des pertes des cellules ciliées. Une augmentation d'amplitude des réponses évoquées a également été constatée chez les animaux présentant une fatigue auditive. Dans ce cas, les amplitudes ont retrouvé au bout de quelques mois une valeur identique à celle avant exposition. Ces résultats indiquent que les pertes induites par le bruit peuvent être le résultat de changements physiologiques inattendus dans le système auditif central. Les bases physiologiques et la signification de ces changements sont discutées dans cet article.

ACKNOWLEDGMENTS

This work was supported by research grants NS16761 and DC00368, and by the Deafness Research Foundation.

References

Calford MB, Tweedale R. Immediate and chronic changes in responses of somatosensory cortex in adult flying-fox after digit amputation. Nature 1988; 332:446-448.

Eldredge DH, Mills JH, Bohne BA. Anatomical, behavioral, and electrophysiological observations on chinchillas after long exposures to noise. Adv Otorhinolaryngol 1973; 20:64-81.

Eldredge DH, Miller JD, Bohne BA. A frequency-position map for the chinchilla cochlea. J Acoust Soc Am 1981; 69:1091-1095.

Evans EF. Temporary sensorineural hearing loss and VIIIth nerve changes. In: Henderson D, Hamernik RP, Dosanjh DS, Mills J, eds. Effects of noise on hearing. New York: Raven Press, 1976:199.

Evans EF, Nelson PG. The response of single neurones in the cochlear nucleus of the cat as a function of their location and anesthetic state. Exp Brain Res 1973; 17:402-427.

Frank JI. Functional reorganization of cat somatic sensory-motor cortex (SmI) after selective dorsal root rhizotomies. Brain Res 1980; 186:458-462.

Gerken GM, Saunders SS, Paul RE. Hypersensitivity to electrical stimulation of auditory nuclei follows hearing loss in cats. Hear Res 1984; 13:249-259.

Gerken GM, Simhadri-Sumithra R, Bhat KHV. Increase in central auditory responsiveness during continuous tone stimulation or following hearing loss. In: Salvi RJ, Hamernik RP, Henderson D, Colletti V, eds. Basic and applied aspects of noise-induced hearing loss. New York: Plenum Press, 1986:195.

Hall JG. The cochlear nuclei in monkeys after dihydrostreptomycin or noise exposure. Acta Otolaryngol 1976; 81:344-352.

Henderson D, Hamernik RP, Woodford C, Sitler RW, Salvi R. Evoked response audibility curve of the chinchilla. J Acoust Soc Am 1973; 54:1099-1101.

Henry KR, Saleh M. Recruitment deafness: functional effect of priming-induced audiogenic seizures in mice. J Comp Physiol 1973; 84:430.

Jenkins WM, Merzenich MM. Reorganization of neocortical representations after brain injury: A neurophysiological model of the bases of recovery from stroke. Prog Brain Res 1987; 71:249-266.

Klein AJ, Mills HJ. Physiological (waves I and V) and

psychophysical tuning curves in human subjects. J Acoust Soc Am 1981; 69:760-768.

Liberman MC, Kiang NYS. Acoustic trauma in cats. Acta Otolaryngol Suppl (Stockh) 1978; 358:1-63.

Liberman MC, Dodds LW, Learson DA. Structure-function correlation in noise-damaged ears: A light and electron microscopic study. In: Salvi RJ, Hamernik RP, Henderson D, Colletti V, eds. Basic and applied aspects of noise-induced hearing loss. New York: Plenum Press, 1986:163.

Liden G, Engstrom H, Hall JG. Audiological and morphological assessment of effect of noise on cochlea and brain stem in cat. Acta Otolaryngol (Stockh) 1973; 75:325-328.

Lonsbury-Martin BL, Meikle MB. Neural correlates of auditory fatigue: Frequency-dependent changes in activity of single cochlear nerve fibers. J Neurophysiol 1978; 41:987-1006.

Lonsbury-Martin B, Martin GK. Effects of moderately-intense sound on auditory sensitivity in Rhesus monkeys: Behavioral and neural observations. J Neurophysiol 1981; 46:563-586.

Merzenich MM, Kaas JH. Organization of mammalian somatosensory cortex following peripheral nerve injury. Trends Neurosci 1982; 5:428-436.

Metzlar J, Marks PS. Functional changes in cat somatic sensory motor cortex during short-term reversible epidermal blocks. Brain Res 1979; 177:379-383.

Morest K. Degeneration in the brain following exposure to noise. In: Hamernik RP, Henderson D, Salvi RJ, eds. New perspectives on noise-induced hearing loss. New York: Raven Press, 1982:87.

Powers NL, Salvi RJ. Noise induced enhancement and depression of auditory evoked potentials. Abstract. 12th Midwinter Research Meeting, Assn Res Otolaryngol, St. Petersburg, FL, 1989:223-224.

Rajan R. Electrical stimulation of the inferior colliculus at low rates protects the cochlea from auditory desensitization. Abstr Soc Neurosci 1989; 15:1114.

Rasmusson DD. Reorganization of raccoon somatosensory cortex following removal of the fifth digit. J Comp Neurol 1982; 205:313-326.

Robertson D, Irvine DRF. Plasticity of frequency organization in auditory cortex of guinea pigs with partial unilateral deafness. J Comp Neurol 1989; 282:456-471.

Ryan A, Miller J. Single unit responses in the inferior colliculus of the awake and performing rhesus monkey. Exp Brain Res 1978; 32:389-407.

Salvi RJ. Central components of temporary threshold shift. In: Henderson D, Hamernik RP, Dosanjh D, Mills J, eds. Effects of noise on hearing. New York: Raven Press, 1976:247.

Salvi RJ, Hamernik RP, Henderson D. Discharge patterns in the cochlear nucleus of the chinchilla following noise induced asymptotic threshold shift. Exp Brain Res 1978; 32:301-320.

Salvi RJ, Perry J, Hamernik RP, Henderson D. Relationships between cochlear pathologies and auditory nerve and behavioral responses. In: Hamernik RP, Henderson D, Salvi RJ, eds. New perspectives on noise-induced hearing loss. New York: Raven Press, 1982a:165.

Salvi RJ, Ahroon WA, Perry JW, Gunnarson MS, Henderson D. Comparison of psychophysical and evoked-potential tuning curves in the chinchilla. Am J Otolaryngol 1982b; 3:408-416.

Salvi RJ, Hamernik RP, Henderson D. Response patterns of auditory nerve fibers during temporary threshold shift. Hear Res 1983a; 10:37-67.

Salvi RJ, Henderson D, Hamernik RP. Physiological bases of sensorineural hearing loss. In: Tobias J, Schubert E, eds. Hearing research and theory. Vol 2. New York: Academic Press, 1983b:173.

Saunders JC, Rhyne RL. Cochlear nucleus activity and threshold shift in cat. Brain Res 1970; 24:339-342.

Saunders JC, Bock GR, Chen CS, Gates GR. The effects of priming for audiogenic seizures on cochlear and behavioral responses in BALB/c mice. Exp Neurol 1972a; 36:426-436.

Saunders JC, Bock G, James R, Chen CS. Effects of priming for audiogenic seizure on auditory evoked responses in the cochlear nucleus and inferior colliculus of BALB/c mice. Exp Neurol 1972b; 37:388-394.

Schmiedt RA, Zwislocki JJ, Hamernik RP. Effects of hair-cell lesions on responses of cochlear-nerve fibers. I. Lesions, tuning curves, two-tone inhibition and responses to trapezoidal-wave patterns. J Neurophysiol 1980; 43:1367-1389.

Siegel JH, Kim DO. Cochlear biomechanics: Vulnerability to acoustic trauma and other alterations seen in neural responses and ear-canal sound pressure. In: Hamernik RP, Henderson D, Salvi RJ, eds. New perspectives on noise-induced hearing loss. New York: Raven Press, 1982:137.

Starr A. Suppression of single neuron activity in the cochlear nucleus of the cat following sound stimulation. J Neurophysiol 1965; 26:416-431.

Theopold HM. Degenerative alterations in the ventral cochlear nucleus of the guinea pig after impulse noise exposure. Arch Otolaryngol 1975; 209:247-262.

Warr WB, Guinan JG. Efferent innervation of the organ of Corti: Two separate systems. Brain Res 1979; 173:152-155.

Willott JF. Changes in frequency representation in the auditory system of mice with age-related hearing impairment. Brain Res 1984; 309:159-162.

Willott JF, Lu S-M. Noise-induced hearing loss can alter neural coding and increase excitability in the central nervous system. Science 1982; 216:1331-1332.

Willott JF, Demuth RM, Lu S-M. Excitability of auditory neurons in the dorsal and ventral cochlear nuclei of DBA/2 and C57BL/6 mice. Exp Neurol 1984; 83:495-506.

Young ED, Brownell WE. Responses to tones and noise of single cells in dorsal cochlear nucleus of unanesthetized cats. J Neurophysiol 1976; 39:282-300.

Young ED. Response characteristics of neurons of the cochlear nuclei. In: Berlin C, ed. Hearing science. San Diego: College Hill Press, 1984:423.

SECTION THREE

Co-Factors in Development and Aging

CHAPTER 15

Interaction of Noise and Other Agents: Recent Advances

FLINT A. BOETTCHER
MICHAEL ANNE GRATTON
BRIAN R. BANCROFT
VLASTA SPONGR

Noise exposure is the most common cause of acquired hearing loss in industrial societies, and is rated by the United States National Institute for Occupation Safety and Health as a major problem in industrial safety and health. It is estimated that over 10 million civilians in the United States are routinely exposed to hazardous industrial noises (von Gierke, 1990). Despite the prevalence of noise-induced hearing loss, it has proven difficult to predict hearing loss simply given the noise-exposure history of a person. Intersubject variability in the degree of hearing loss is common in demographic studies of noise-induced hearing loss; for example, Passchier-Vermeer (1983) reported a wide variability of hearing loss among factory workers with similar exposure history. Such variability may be a result of one or more factors, such as differences in recreational noise history, health factors, or exposure to ototoxic drugs or environmental toxins.

The major focus of this chapter will be on the interaction of noise with cisplatin and noise with salicylates, because new data are available on these interactions. We will also discuss recent data from other investigators on the interaction of noise with carbon monoxide, toluene, and carbon disulfide. This review of noise-drug and noise–environmental agent interaction is not intended to be exhaustive; studies performed before 1987 were reviewed previously (Boettcher et al, 1987). Furthermore, Aran et al describe the interaction between noise and aminoglycoside antibiotics in detail in Chapter 16.

Interaction of Noise and Cisplatin

Cisplatin (cis-diamminedichloro-platinum) and its derivatives are promising chemotherapeutic agents that act against squamous cell carcinomas of the head and neck and genitourinary systems. Cisplatin is an inorganic heavy metal complex that putatively inhibits DNA synthesis through creation of intrastrand crosslinks between guanine bases (Borch, 1987). Cisplatin is not selectively incorporated only by tumor cells; in addition, it has been shown to have an affinity for the liver, kidney, and cochlea (Schweitzer et al, 1984). Elimination of cisplatin is incomplete, and the drug may bind irreversibly to tissue (Sharma and Edwards, 1983; Safirstein et al, 1986).

Cisplatin administration may result in side effects such as nephrotoxicity, myelosuppression, gastrointestinal disturbance, and ototoxicity. Cisplatin ototoxicity presents as a bilateral, symmetrical sensorineural hearing loss. It is typically permanent, although several investigators have reported recovery in some subjects (Fausti et al, 1984; Aguilar-Markulis et al, 1981). Onset of hearing loss can be detected initially in the ultrahigh frequencies, often after the first or second course of chemotherapy (Fausti et al, 1984). The degree of loss and the frequency range of affected hearing increase as the dose or duration of cisplatin administration increases (Aguilar-Markulis et al, 1981).

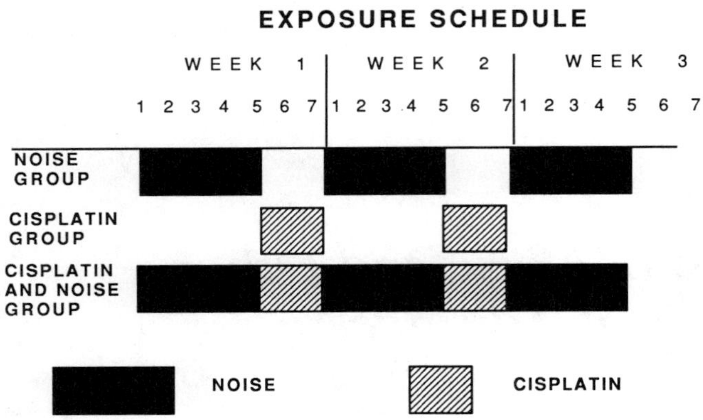

Figure 15-1 Exposure schedule for noise-cisplatin interaction experiments. (From Gratton MA, Salvi RJ, Kamen B, Saunders SS. Interaction of cisplatin and noise on the peripheral auditory system. Hear Res 1990; 50:211-224.)

Mechanism of Cisplatin Ototoxicity

Morphologic studies following cisplatin administration show that the concentration of cisplatin is three times higher in the stria vascularis than in auditory or vestibular neuroepithelial tissue, which would suggest that ototoxic effects of cisplatin may be due to strial damage (Schweitzer et al, 1984; Kohn et al, 1988). However, there is no evidence of decreased $Na^{+}K^{+}$ ATPase after cisplatin administration (Barron and Daigneault, 1987). Instead, it appears that the critical damage caused by cisplatin is at the level of the hair cell. Initially, cisplatin causes damage to outer hair cell (OHC) stereocilia, followed by hair cell degeneration starting at the basal turn of the cochlea and progressing apicalward. Inner hair cells (IHCs) are affected after all three rows of OHCs have degenerated (Fleischman et al, 1975; Wright and Schaefer, 1982; Marco-Algarra et al, 1985; Comis et al, 1986; Barron and Daigneault, 1987). It has been postulated that aminoglycoside antibiotics damage the auditory system via a series of processes, including disruption of hair cells (Schacht, 1986; Williams et al, 1987). It is possible that cisplatin has similar effects, but the mechanisms have not yet been elucidated.

Cisplatin ototoxicity may be exacerbated by concurrent administration of aminoglycoside antibiotics (Schweitzer et al, 1984) or loop-inhibiting diuretics (Brummett, 1981; Kommune and Snow, 1981) as well as by prior cranial irradiation (Granowetter et al, 1985; Baranak et al, 1988). One study suggested that guinea pigs exposed to broadband noise, followed 10 days later by cisplatin administration, did not have greater hearing loss than animals only given the drug (Laurell and Borg, 1986). However, we are aware of no studies that have utilized concurrent administration of cisplatin and exposure to noise.

Methods

Adult chinchillas weighing 450 to 650 g were used as subjects. Status of the auditory system was monitored by the auditory evoked response recorded from the inferior colliculus. Each animal was anesthetized, and a chronic electrode was implanted stereotaxically into the left inferior colliculus. At the same time, the left cochlea was surgically destroyed. Threshold testing occurred in a sound-treated room with the animal awake and lightly restrained. Testing was performed using tone bursts (20 ms duration, 5 ms rise/fall, 10 per second) at octave intervals from 0.5 to 16 kHz and at 11.2 kHz. Baseline audiograms were derived from five complete tests prior to exposure, and permanent threshold shift (PTS) audiograms were derived from five complete tests performed 30 days or more after termination of exposure. Data are also presented that were collected during the noise/drug exposure (termed "asymptotic threshold shift," or ATS).

Animals were assigned to one of seven groups: noise alone (OBN centered at 0.5 kHz, intensities of 70, 85, or 100 dB SPL), drug alone (2.75 mg per kilogram cisplatin IP), or both noise and cisplatin. The exposure schedule is shown in Figure 15-1. The experiment was designed so that each animal received a total of 15 days of noise exposure, four injections of cisplatin, or both. Animals receiving cisplatin were hydrated with lactated Ringer's solution (6 percent body weight) for 80 hours surrounding the injections.

After PTS testing was completed, animals were anesthetized and decapitated. Each bulla was removed and opened, and 2.5 percent glutaraldehyde in veronal acetate buffer (pH 7.3) was perfused through a perforation in the round window. Following overnight refrigeration, the cochlea was again perfused, then later postfixed and stained for 30 minutes via a slow perfusion of cold osmium tetroxide. The cochlea was dehydrated to 70 percent ETOH, then placed in 50 percent EDTA solution. The decalcified cochlea was microdissected and the organ of Corti was mounted in glycerin for light-microscopic study. The sensory epithelium was viewed at ×400 using light microscopy to quantify the number of missing IHCs and OHCs, averaged over 0.24-mm intervals along the basilar membrane. Sensory cells were considered present if the cell body and cuticular plate were intact. Data were plotted as a function of percentage of distance from the apex in order to obtain a cochleogram. Group cochleograms were obtained by averaging data over 1 percent intervals.

Results and Discussion

Figure 15-2 shows cytocochleograms and PTS data for animals exposed to 70 dB noise, cisplatin, or both agents. Cisplatin alone (Fig. 15-2A) caused little PTS and minor OHC loss at the basal region of the cochlea. The noise at 70 dB SPL (Fig. 15-2B) caused minimal PTS and hair cell loss. Animals that received both agents (Fig. 15-2C) had no more PTS or cell loss than those exposed only to cisplatin.

Figure 15-3A shows threshold shifts for animals exposed to 100 dB noise, cisplatin, or both agents, measured 1 hour after the final experimental condition. Cisplatin caused little ATS, whereas animals exposed to either the noise alone or the combination had 40 to 55 dB of ATS. Although the combination group showed a trend toward greater hearing loss, the differences between the groups were not significant. However, the combination group had significantly greater PTS than the noise-alone group (Multiple ANOVA [analysis of variance] p less than 0.001), especially at the high frequencies (Fig. 15-3B).

Figure 15-4 shows average cochleograms of chinchillas exposed to cisplatin, noise (100 dB), or both agents. Those exposed to cisplatin had small losses of OHCs in the basal turn of the cochlea. Animals exposed to noise had scattered IHC and OHC loss, with a peak of 40 percent OHC loss in the region between 0.5 and 2 kHz. Animals exposed to both agents had scattered IHC loss of 20 percent and losses of OHC as great as 70 percent in the basal (hook) region.

Because interaction between noise and cisplatin was observed for intense (100 dB) but not for mild (70 dB) noise exposures, a moderate noise exposure was used (85 dB SPL). When the moderate level of noise exposure was used, animals in the combination group (85 dB plus cisplatin) had significantly more ATS, PTS, and hair cell loss ($p < 0.001$) than those exposed only to the noise.

The results of the experiments are summarized in Figure 15-5. Data are presented for each of the seven groups in terms of PTS and hair cell loss. It is apparent that the combination groups with the moderate (85 dB) and high (100 dB) noise levels had more PTS and hair cell loss than the groups exposed to either the noise or drug alone. The 70-dB combination group did not have greater damage than the noise-alone group. In summary, results of these experiments suggest that concurrent administration of cisplatin and moderate to intense continuous noise can result in greater hearing loss and hair cell damage than such loss and damage that occurs from either agent alone. The interaction effect is greatest in the high frequencies. A threshold of interaction appeared to occur, because no interaction was observed at noise levels below 85 dB. The mechanisms of cisplatin ototoxicity and cisplatin/noise interaction are not yet understood, and further experiments are warranted.

Interaction of Noise and Salicylates

Salicylates are the most commonly used drugs in Western societies. Rainsford (1984) reported that in 1980 over 70 million kg of aspirin were produced in the United States. Salicylates produce the ototoxic symptoms of tinnitus and mild-to-moderate hearing loss in some patients (Myers and Bernstein, 1965; McCabe and Dey, 1965). The symptoms typically disappear within 3 days of the final administration of the drug, and there are few confirmed reports of permanent loss due to salicylates. Typically, the serum salicylate level must exceed 12.5 mg% for ototoxic symptoms to be detectable (Myers and Bernstein, 1965; Jardini et al, 1978).

Mechanisms of Salicylate Ototoxicity

The mechanisms of salicylate ototoxicity are not well understood. Douek et al (1983) reported that salicylate administration re-

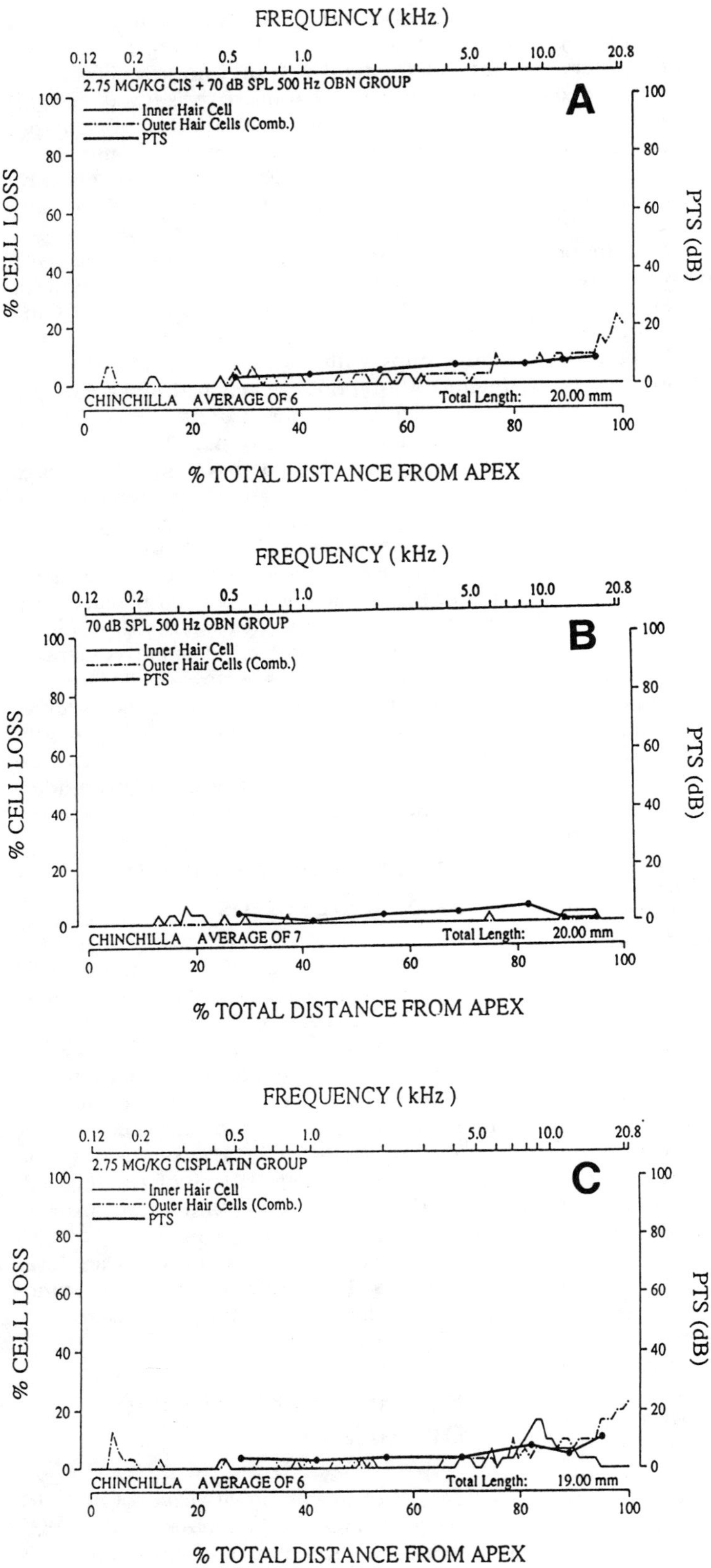

Figure 15-2 Cytocochleograms and permanent threshold shift (PTS) values for animals exposed to *(A)* both cisplatin and noise, *(B)* noise alone—70 dB SPL OBN at 0.5 kHz, and *(C)* cisplatin alone (2.75 mg per kilogram). (From Gratton MA, Salvi RJ, Kamen B, Saunders SS. Interaction of cisplatin and noise on the peripheral auditory system. Hear Res 1990; 50:211-224.)

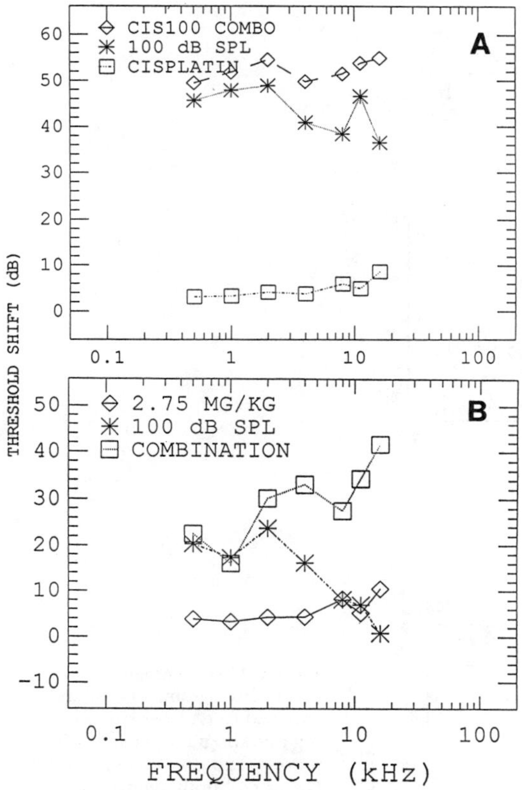

Figure 15-3 Threshold shifts for chinchillas exposed to noise (100 dB SPL, OBN at 0.5 kHz), cisplatin (2.75 mg per kilogram), or both agents. *A*, Threshold shift at termination of exposure. *B*, Permanent threshold shift (average of 5 tests, 30 to 40 days after termination of exposures). (From Gratton MA, Salvi RJ, Kamen B, Saunders SS. Interaction of cisplatin and noise on the peripheral auditory system. Hear Res 1990; 50:211-224.)

sulted in bending of the stereocilia of cochlear hair cells and caused swelling and vacuolization of the smooth endoplasmic reticulum in hair cells. Shehata et al (1990) reported that OHCs lose their turgidity after administration of salicylate and are thus less able to contract. This evidence is consistent with studies that have shown decreased cochlear microphonic potential after salicylate with no concomitant change in the whole-nerve action potential (Mitchell et al, 1973; Stypulkowski, 1989) and with other studies showing decreased otoacoustic emissions after aspirin administration (Long and Tubis, 1988; McFadden and Plattsmier, 1984). Another series of experiments suggested that salicylate causes a decrease in the blood supply to the organ of Corti, possibly through effects on the adrenergic innervation of the vasculature (Cazals et al, 1988) or through decreased prostaglandin synthesis in the cochlea (Escoubet et al, 1985), although this latter observation has been disputed (Puel et al, 1989).

Previous Results of Noise-Salicylate Interaction

Because of the prevalence of exposure to high levels of noise and the common use of aspirin and salicylates, it is critical to understand whether the two agents interact to damage the auditory system. The results of several previous examinations of the question are equivocal. McFadden and Plattsmier (1983) reported that young adult humans received more TTS when exposed to an intense pure tone (2,500 Hz) after administration of 3.9 g of aspirin for 3 days before the exposure than when the exposure occurred in the absence of aspirin. Eddy et al (1976) reported that chinchillas exposed to salicylate (200 mg per cubic centimeter) and noise (85 dBA) received approximately 55 dB of temporary threshold shift at 1 kHz, compared to 35 dB from noise and 30 dB from salicylate. In contrast, Woodford et al (1978) reported that chinchillas exposed to salicylate (400 mg per kilogram IM) and one of three noises (95 dB octave band from 2 to 4 kHz for 1 hour, 80 dB octave band centered at 4 kHz for 96 hours, or 50 impulses of 50 ms overpressure at 158 dB SPL) had no more TTS, PTS, or hair cell loss than control animals exposed to either salicylate or one of the noises alone. Lambert et al (1986) reported no differences in hair cell loss between chicks exposed to noise (115 dB tone at 1,500 Hz for 8 hours) and chicks exposed to noise and salicylate (two or three aspirin per day for 4 days). Lindgren and Axelsson (1986) reported no exacerbation of noise-induced hearing loss by aspirin (1 g per day). Recently, Carson et al (1989) reported that salicylate administration did not increase the noise-induced threshold shift, but did increase noise-induced hair cell loss.

Methods

The experiments recently performed in our lab were designed to answer the following question: Does salicylate administration exacerbate the TTS, PTS, and hair cell loss caused by exposure to noise (octave band centered at 500 Hz) of long duration (15 days)? The experiment differs from some of the earlier studies by using long duration exposure (15 days) and two noise exposures—one that results in

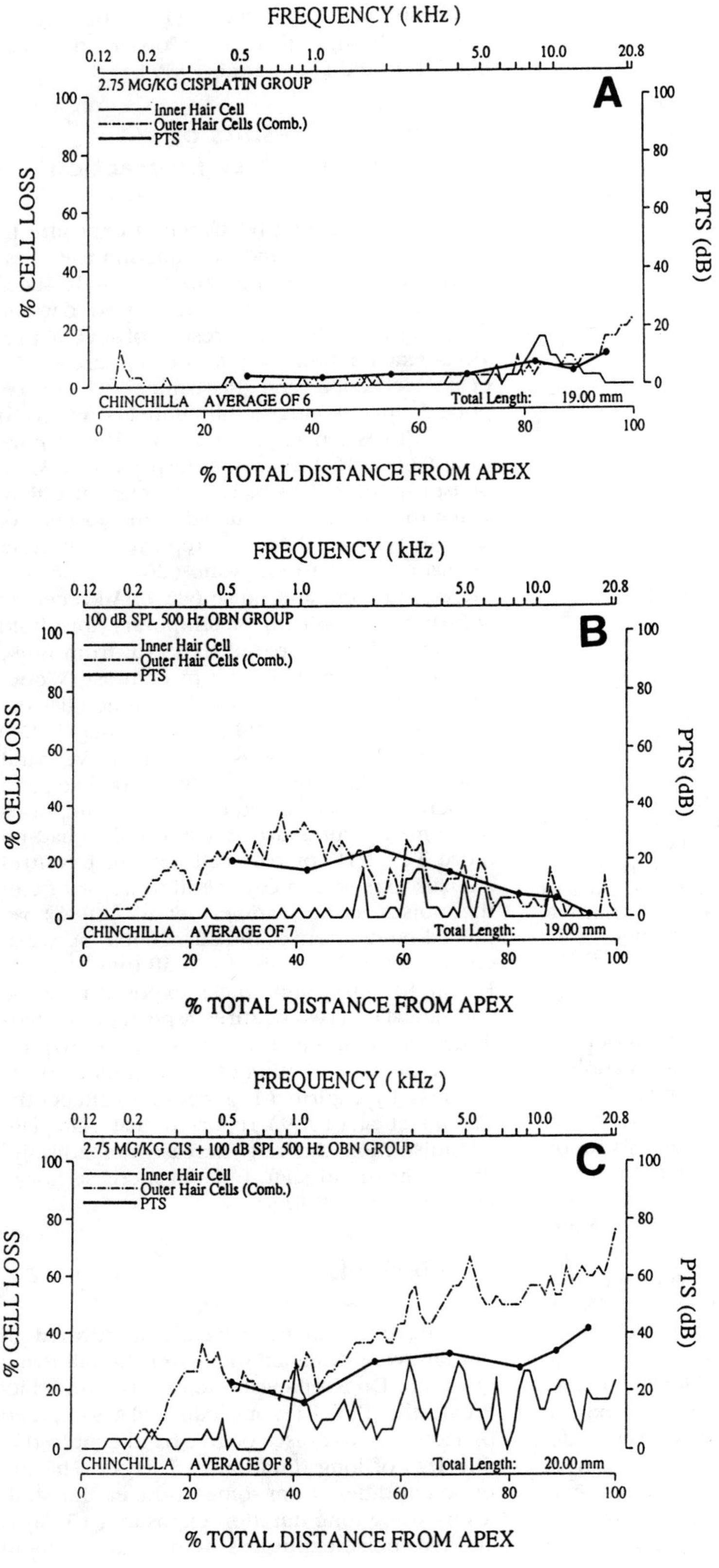

Figure 15-4 Average cytocochleograms of chinchillas exposed to *(A)* cisplatin—2.75 mg per kilogram per day; *(B)* noise—100 dB SPL OBN at 500 Hz; or *(C)* both agents. Key is shown in upper left of each panel. (From Gratton MA, Salvi RJ, Kamen B, Saunders SS. Interaction of cisplatin and noise on the peripheral auditory system. Hear Res 1990; 50:211-224.)

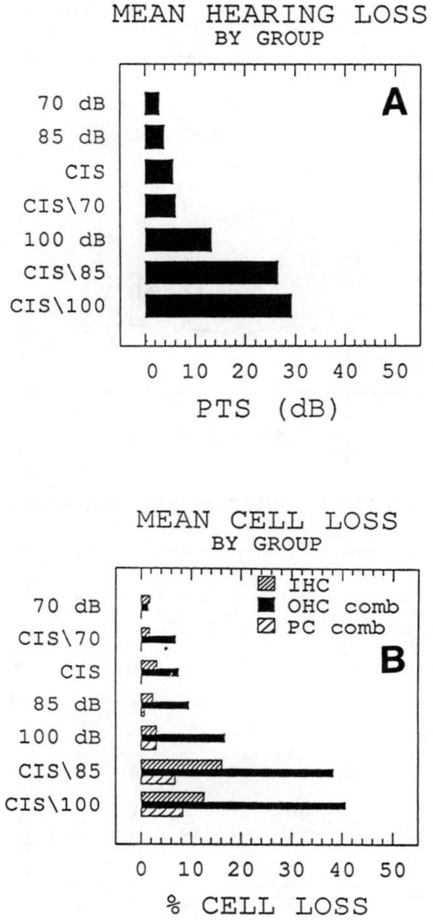

Figure 15-5 Mean hearing loss *(A)* and hair cell loss *(B)* for the seven groups of chinchillas exposed to noise, cisplatin, or both agents. CIS, cisplatin, 2.75 mg per kilogram; CIS/#, cisplatin plus noise exposure in decibels SPL; # dB, noise exposure in decibels SPL, OBN centered at 0.5 kHz.

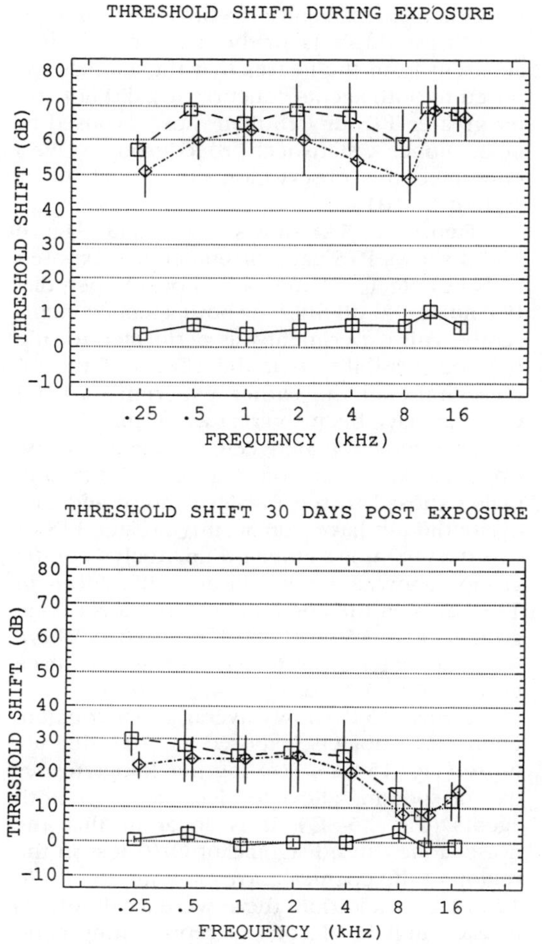

Figure 15-6 Mean threshold shifts of chinchillas exposed to sodium salicylate (300 mg per kilogram per day), noise (105 dB SPL), or both agents. *A,* Threshold shift 50 hours after exposure onset. *B,* Permanent threshold shift measured 30 days after termination of exposure. Open squares and solid line, salicylate; diamonds, noise alone; squares and dashed lines, noise plus salicylate. (From Bancroft BR, Boettcher FA, Salvi RJ, Wu J. Effects of noise and salicylate on auditory evoked response thresholds in the chinchilla. Hear Res 1991 (Accepted for publication).

significant PTS and hair cell loss (105 dB) and one that causes less than 10 dB of PTS and small amounts of hair cell loss (80 dB). A salicylate dose (300 mg per kilogram per day IP) was chosen that results in serum salicylate levels of 20 to 40 mg%, a serum concentration known to result in ototoxic effects in many species (Myers and Bernstein, 1965; Boettcher et al, 1989, 1990).

As in the cisplatin experiments, chinchillas were used in all phases of the experiments. Hearing levels were monitored using the evoked response technique. Cochlear damage was determined as described for the cisplatin experiments, using the surface preparation technique.

Results and Discussion

Figure 15-6A shows temporary threshold shifts for chinchillas exposed to salicylate (300 mg per kilogram), noise (105 dB SPL), or both agents concurrently. The average threshold shift for the drug-alone group was 10 dB or less, whereas that for the noise-alone and combination groups was as great as 70 dB. There were, however, no significant differences in TTS between the noise-alone and combination groups ($F = 4.10$; $df = 1,10$; p

less than 0.01). Figure 15-6B shows permanent threshold shifts for the same animals. It is apparent from the figures that the animals exposed to both agents concurrently did not suffer greater TTS or PTS than those exposed to noise alone. A statistical procedure (ANOVA) confirmed this observation ($F = 0.53$; $df = 1{,}10$; $p > 0.01$).

Figure 15-7A shows TTS, and Figure 15-7B shows PTS data for chinchillas exposed to salicylate (300 mg per kilogram per day IP), noise (80 dB SPL), or both agents concurrently. This experiment was performed to rule out the possibility that the effects of the intense noise in the earlier experiments (105 dB) may have been so great as to "mask" a potential interaction between the agents. However, it is apparent from Figure 15-7 that animals exposed to the low-level noise and salicylate did not have significantly greater TTS or PTS than the noise-alone group. Analysis of the groups showed no significant differences in TTS between the combination and noise-alone groups ($F = 3.57$; $df = 1{,}8$; $p > 0.01$). There were no differences in PTS across the three groups ($F = 0.24$; $df = 2{,}24$; $p > 0.01$).

Figure 15-8 shows average cytocochleograms for subjects exposed to 105 dB SPL noise (Fig. 15-8A), 300 mg per kilogram per day of sodium salicylate (Fig. 15-8), or both agents (Fig. 15-8C). It is apparent that the noise alone caused significant OHC loss in the region of the cochlea corresponding to 300 to 1200 Hz. In addition, there were small lesions in each individual cochlea representing complete IHC and OHC loss. Salicylate alone caused no significant hair cell loss. Cochleograms of the animals exposed to both agents were similar to those of the noise-alone group. There were no significant differences between noise-alone and interaction groups, consistent with the evoked-response data. Results for multiple ANOVA analysis using the combined cochleograms for both experiments (80 and 105 dB SPL noise) were (1) inner hair cells: F ratio = 0.035, $df = 1{,}10$, p less than 0.01; and (2) outer hair cells: F ratio = 0.552, $df = 1{,}10$, p less than 0.01.

In summary, chinchillas exposed to sodium salicylate (300 mg per kilogram) and noise (80 or 105 dB SPL OBN) did not have greater TTS, PTS, or hair cell loss than chinchillas exposed to noise alone. The data are in contrast with those reported by Eddy et al (1976); we suggest that the behavioral tech nique used by Eddy et al may have overestimated the hearing loss caused by salicylate and by the combination of salicylate and noise. It is a common observation that high serum salicylate levels cause lethargy in experimental subjects and thus decrease behavioral responsivity. The data from the present experiment also differ somewhat from those of McFadden and Plattsmier (1983). In the present study, a long-duration noise exposure was used, whereas McFadden and Plattsmier used a 10-second tone to induce acoustic trauma. The combination exposure induced a hearing loss that lasted approximately 30 minutes; it is thus possible that an interaction between noise and salicylate may occur with a short

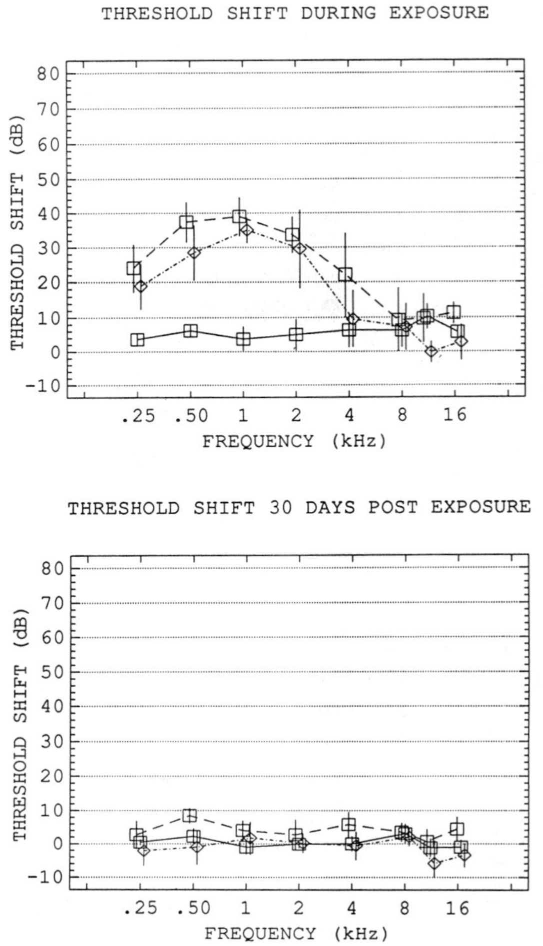

Figure 15-7 Mean threshold shifts of chinchillas exposed to sodium salicylate (300 mg per kilogram per day), noise (80 dB SPL), or both agents. *A,* Threshold shift 50 hours after exposure onset. *B,* Permanent threshold shift measured 30 days after termination of exposure. Open squares and solid line, salicylate; diamonds, noise alone; squares and dashed lines, noise plus salicylate. (From Bancroft BR, Boettcher FA, Salvi RJ, Wu J. Effects of noise and salicylate on auditory evoked response thresholds in the chinchilla. Hear Res 1991 (Accepted for publication).

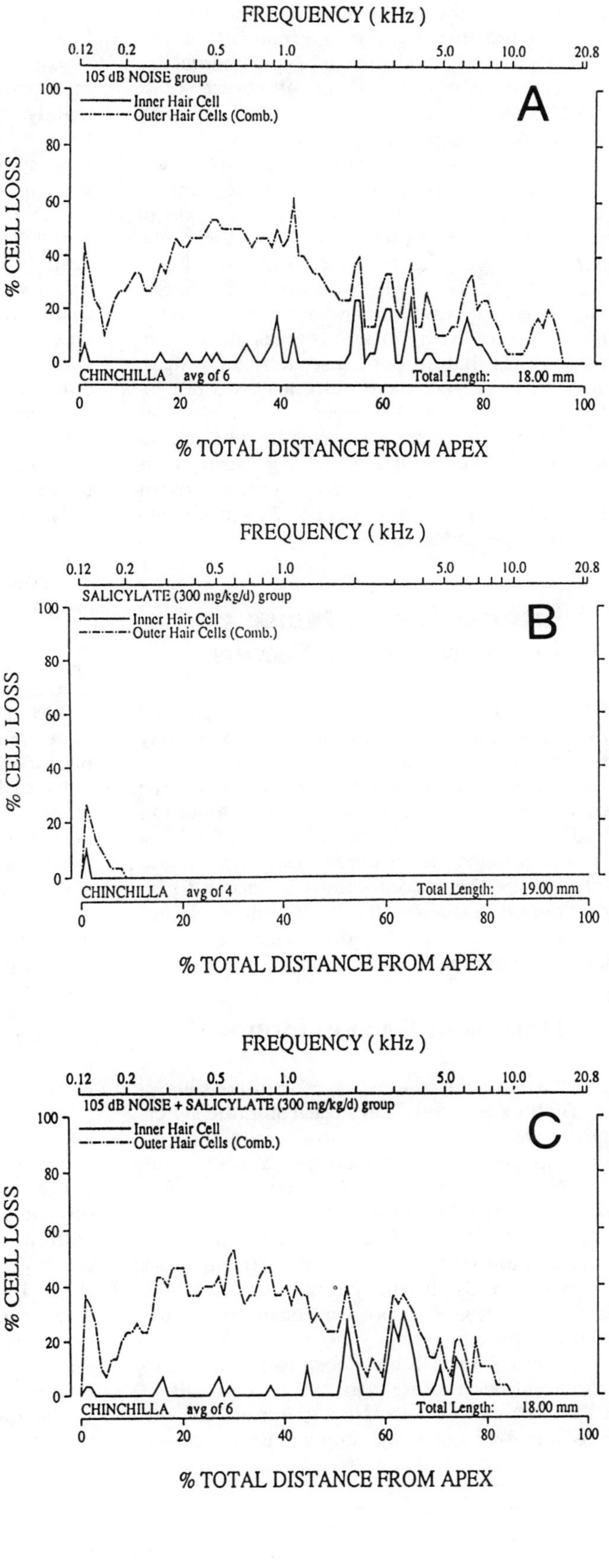

Figure 15-8 Average cytocochleograms of chinchillas exposed to *(A)* noise—105 dB SPL; *(B)* salicylate—300 mg per kilogram; or *(C)* noise plus salicylate. Key is shown in upper left of each panel.

duration, but the data from the present exposure suggest that it is not a permanent effect.

Data from the present experiments are consistent with the data of Woodford et al (1978) and Lambert et al (1986), and with the evoked response data of Carson et al (1989). Because the exact mechanism of salicylate ototoxicity is not completely understood, it is difficult to answer the question of why there is no interaction. Hypothetically, studies suggest that those ototoxic drugs, which themselves cause permanent damage to hair cells (e.g., cisplatin and aminoglycosides), may interact with noise, whereas those ototoxic drugs that do not cause permanent damage (e.g., salicylates and diuretics) will not interact with noise. However, this hypothesis does not provide an answer as to *why* the interactions do or do not occur. Furthermore, as described below, certain environmental toxins that in themselves do not cause PTS may exacerbate noise-induced loss.

Interaction of Noise and Environmental Toxins

Several groups have recently examined the possibility that environmental toxins may exacerbate noise-induced hearing loss. Carbon monoxide, carbon disulfide, and toluene have each been examined for potential interaction with noise and the experiments will be reviewed briefly. Interestingly, only one (toluene) of the three compounds is known to be particularly ototoxic by itself, but each appears to increase noise-induced damage to the auditory system.

Noise and Carbon Monoxide

Two recent studies have been completed by Fechter and colleagues regarding the synergistic effect of noise and carbon monoxide on hearing and cochlear damage (Young et al, 1987; Fechter et al, 1988). They used reflex modulation audiometry to test hearing in rats exposed to noise (110 dBA, 120 minutes), carbon monoxide (1,200 ppm, 210 minutes), or both agents. In the interaction condition, carbon monoxide exposure began before the onset of the noise.

Control animals and those exposed to carbon monoxide alone had −5 to −15 dB of PTS at 10 and 40 kHz. No significant hair cell loss was found in these animals. Rats exposed to noise alone had approximately 25 dB of PTS at 10 and 40 kHz and OHC loss confined to the extreme basal turn of the cochlea. Animals exposed to both agents had approximately 40 dB of PTS at 10 kHz and 60 dB of PTS at 40 kHz. Animals exposed to both agents had significant PTS across the range of hearing and significant hair cell loss throughout the basal half of the cochlea (Young et al, 1987; Fechter et al, 1988). The authors suggested that the interaction is due to decreased oxygen supply to the cochlea, considering that Fechter et al (1987) observed that cochlear vasculature responds to high carbon monoxide levels by increased blood flow, compensating for the decreased oxygen concentration in the blood. However, in the interaction condition, the vasculature cannot compensate by increasing flow because of the putative vasoconstriction in the cochlea that noise produces.

Noise and Carbon Disulfide

Carbon disulfide is a strong lipid solvent used in manufacture of synthetic cloth such as rayon. According to the World Health Organization (1979), carbon disulfide (CS_2) may produce neurotoxicity in the form of peripheral neuropathy, psychological disturbance, or vascular pathology. The ototoxicity of CS_2 is not known. Morata (1989) examined hearing levels of workers in a rayon factory in Brazil. The noise levels in the factory were 86 to 89 dBA and the ventilation was poor, resulting in high air concentration of CS_2 (89.9 mg per cubic meter). The hearing of workers in the factory was compared to the hearing of workers from a factory that had similar noise levels but no CS_2. Approximately 60 percent of workers exposed to both agents had significant hearing loss (hearing level of 30 dB or higher in the better ear at 3,000 Hz or above), whereas 53 percent exposed only to noise had significant loss. Interestingly, 12.7 percent of the workers exposed to both agents had "level IV" loss, which signifies a hearing level greater than 25 dB (average of 500, 1,000, and 2,000 Hz) with no response at 4,000 Hz and greater. Only 3.5 percent of workers exposed to noise alone had level IV loss. To summarize, the data of Morata suggest a possible interaction between noise and CS_2 affecting the auditory system. The location of lesion is not addressed directly in her study, and further examination of the question, using animal studies, is warranted.

Noise and Organic Solvents

Organic solvents, such as toluene, are used in industry and as paint thinners. It is known that inhalation of organic solvents may cause neuropathology in the form of paresthesia and hypesthesia of the peripheral nerves, and that excess exposure may result in motor dysfunction and dementia (Barregard and Axelsson, 1984). Although only a few reports have been presented, it appears that toluene may also damage the peripheral auditory system of young mammals, in the form of IHC and OHC loss (Pryor et al, 1984).

Barregard and Axelsson (1984) presented case reports of audiologic findings from ship painters, who are often exposed to both solvents and high noise levels (from spray painting machines). Each subject had a great deal of hearing loss, more than might be expected from the industrial noise to which they were exposed, but it is not possible to state that an interaction of noise and solvents caused the extreme degree of loss in the painters.

Johnson et al (1988) reported on a series of experiments examining the interaction of noise and toluene on the auditory systems of rats. Rats were exposed to toluene (1,000 ppm, 16 hours a day, 5 days a week, for 2 weeks), noise (maximum 105 dB SPL, 2-kHz band swept from 3 to 30 kHz, 10 hours a day, 7 days a week, for 4 weeks, 50 percent duty cycle), or to toluene followed by noise. Hearing was monitored with far-field evoked potentials. All threshold shifts were determined by comparing postexposure sensitivity with sensitivity in unexposed rats.

Toluene alone resulted in as much as 30 dB of TTS and 10 dB of PTS, primarily at higher frequencies; 12.5 kHz was the most affected frequency. Animals exposed only to noise had as much as 50 dB of TTS at 12.5 kHz; PTS measurements were not made for the noise-alone group. Subjects exposed to both toluene and noise had TTS of greater than 50 dB (thresholds were outside the limits of the acoustic system) and PTS of 25 dB at 3.15 kHz and below and PTS of 45 to 50 dB at 6.3 kHz and greater.

Conclusion

A number of recent studies have expanded our understanding of the interaction of noise and other agents. Data from studies of the chinchilla suggest that cisplatin may make the ear susceptible to noise-induced hearing loss. Recent data with both humans and animals suggest that carbon monoxide, carbon disulfide, and organic solvents may also exacerbate the damage caused by excessive noise exposure. In contrast, data suggest that salicylate does not increase the auditory system's susceptibility to noise. Using the chinchilla, it was shown that animals exposed to noise and salicylate did not have significantly greater TTS, PTS, or hair cell loss than animals exposed to noise.

We do not yet completely understand the mechanisms of the interaction of noise with chemicals, or in fact the mechanisms of the ototoxic effects of most of the chemicals in question. Subjectively, it appears that a synergistic interaction is possible if exposure to the chemical in question may result in permanent damage to the peripheral auditory system. This holds true for the interaction of noise with cisplatin, aminoglycoside antibiotics, and toluene and for the lack of interaction of noise with salicylate and loop-inhibiting diuretics. The exception to the observation is that carbon monoxide does not cause damage in itself, but may increase susceptibility to noise-induced loss. Thus, there appear to be several major issues in noise-chemical synergism that require further investigation. First, the mechanisms of both ototoxicity and noise-chemical interaction need to be addressed, especially at the molecular level. In addition, it is likely that there are chemicals that may increase susceptibility to noise that have not yet been identified, such as trimethyltin and alpha-difluoromethylornithine.

Interactions entre le Bruit et d'autres Agents Ototraumatiques: Résultats Récents

Certains agents ototoxiques tels que les aminoglycosides accentuent les effets traumatisants du bruit. Récemment, plusieurs travaux ont été entrepris au sein de notre laboratoire pour étudier l'interaction d'une part, entre le bruit et le cisplatine et d'autre part, entre le bruit et les salicylates. Les résultats de ces études seront analysés ainsi que ceux provenant d'autres laboratoires ayant étudié les effets combinés du bruit et des agents industriels ou environnementaux tels que le disulfure de carbone, le monoxide de carbone et le toluène.

Le cisplatine est couramment utilisé comme anti-mitotique en dépit de ses effets ototoxiques sévères. Utilisé chez des patients vivant souvent en dehors du milieu hospitalier, une interaction possible de la drogue avec un bruit industriel, ou de tout autre nature, est à redouter. Dans le but d'étudier une éventuelle interaction du bruit avec le cisplatine, une dose de cisplatine (2,75 mg/kg) a été administrée à un premier groupe de chinchillas, trois autres groupes ont été exposés à un bruit de bande centré sur 500 Hz d'un niveau sonore de 70, 85 et 100 dB et, enfin, trois groupes ont été soumis simultanément aux deux agents pour chaque niveau sonore. Le cisplatine, seul, n'a pratiquement pas entraîné de pertes auditives (PTS), tandis que l'exposition à 100 dB a provoqué un PTS d'une amplitude de 20-25 dB dans les basses fréquences. Cependant, lorsque les animaux sont exposés simultanément aux deux agents, un PTS d'une amplitude de 45 dB est obtenu au niveau des hautes fréquences. La combinaison des deux agents est apparue efficace pour les niveaux sonores de 85 et 100 dB mais pas pour l'intensité la plus faible.

L'interaction du bruit et des salicylates a déjà été étudiée chez l'homme et le chinchilla. Les résultats ne sont d'ailleurs pas unanimes. McFadden et Plattsmier (Hear Res 9:295), Eddy et coll. (ISA Trans 15,103) ont suggéré que la fatigue auditive causée par le bruit était accentuée par l'absorption de salicylate, tandis que Woodford et coll. (Ann Otol 87:117) ont trouvé que les salicylates n'augmentaient pas les déficits auditifs causés par le bruit. Dans le but de clarifier et d'approfondir la compréhension des mécanismes régissant les effets combinés du bruit et des salicylates, une dose de salicylate (300 mg/kg/jour/15 jours) a été administrée à un premier groupe de chinchillas, deux autres groupes ont été exposés à un bruit de bande centré sur 500 Hz, à un niveau de 80 dB ou 105 dB et, enfin, deux groupes ont été soumis simultanément aux deux agents pour chaque niveau sonore. Les animaux exposés simultanément au bruit et aux salicylates semblent souffrir de déficits auditifs plus importants bien que la différence avec les autres groupes ne soit pas significative. De plus, les animaux exposés à la fois aux salicylates et au bruit n'ont pas montré d'importantes différences quant aux pertes des cellules ciliées externes par rapport aux animaux exposés uniquement au bruit.

ACKNOWLEDGMENTS

The authors wish to thank Samuel S. Saunders and Nicholas L. Powers for software support and advice on the statistical analyses. Jinghui Wu and Meilin Poon provided excellent technical assistance. Richard Salvi, Donald Henderson, and C.G. Wright provided important advice throughout the projects reviewed here. Our work was supported by grant NIH RO1-23894-03 and the Deafness Research Foundation.

References

Aguilar-Markulis NV, Beckley S, Priore R, Mettlin C. Auditory toxicity effects of long-term cis-dichloro-diammineplatinum II therapy in genitourinary cancer patients. J Surg Oncol 1981; 16:111-123.

Baranak CC, Wetmore RF, Packer RJ. Cis-platinum ototoxicity after radiation treatment: An animal model. J Neurooncol 1988; 6:261-267.

Barregard L, Axelsson A. Is there an ototraumatic interaction between noise and solvents? Scand Audiol 1984; 13:151-155.

Barron SE, Daigneault EA. Effect of cisplatin on hair cell morphology and lateral wall Na,K ATPase activity. Hear Res 1987; 26:131-137.

Boettcher FA, Henderson D, Gratton MA, et al. Synergistic interactions of noise and other ototraumatic agents. Ear Hear 1987; 8:192-212.

Boettcher FA, Bancroft BR, Salvi RJ, Henderson D. Effects of sodium salicylate on evoked-response measures of hearing in the chinchilla. Hear Res 1989; 42:129-142.

Boettcher FA, Bancroft BR, Salvi RJ. Concentration of salicylate in serum and perilymph of the chinchilla. Arch Otolaryngol Head Neck Surg 1990; 116:681-684.

Borch RF. The platinum anti-tumor drugs. In: Powis G, Prough RA, eds. Metabolism and action of anti-cancer drugs. New York: Taylor and Francis, 1987:163.

Brummett RE. Ototoxicity resulting from the combined administration of potent diuretics and other agents. Scand Audiol Suppl 1981; 14:215-224.

Carson SS, Prazma J, Pulver SH, Anderson T. Combined effects of aspirin and noise in causing permanent hearing loss. Arch Otolaryngol Head Neck Surg 1989; 115:1070-1075.

Cazals Y, Li XQ, Aurousseau C, Didier A. Acute effects of noradrenalin related vasoactive agents on the ototoxicity of aspirin: An experimental study in the guinea pig. Hear Res 1988; 36:88-96.

Comis SD, Rhys-Evans PH, Osborne MP, Pickles JO, Jeffreis SJR, Pearse HAC. Early morphological and chemical changes induced by cisplatin in the guinea pig organ of Corti. J Laryngol Otol 1986; 100:1375-1383.

Douek EE, Dodson HC, Bannister LH. The effects of sodium salicylate on the cochlea of guinea pigs. J Laryngol Otol 1983; 93:743-749.

Eddy LB, Morgan RJ, Carney HC. Hearing loss due to combined effects of noise and sodium salicylate. ISA Trans 1976; 15:103-108.

Escoubet B, Amsallem P, Ferray E, Tran Ba Huy P. Prostaglandin synthesis by the cochlea of the guinea pig. Influence of aspirin, genamicin, and acoustic stimulation. Prostaglandins 1985; 29:589-599.

Fausti SA, Schechter MA, Rappaport BZ, et al. Early detection of cisplatin ototoxicity: selected case reports. Cancer 1984; 53:224-231.

Fechter LD, Thorne PR, Nuttall AL. Effects of carbon

monoxide on cochlear electrophysiology and blood flow. Hear Res 1987; 27:37-45.

Fechter LD, Young JS, Carlisle L. Potentiation of noise induced threshold shifts and hair cell loss by carbon monoxide. Hear Res 1988; 34:39-48.

Fleischman RW, Stadnicki SW, Ethier MF, Schaeppi U. Ototoxicity of cis-dichlorodiammine platinum II in the guinea pig. Toxicol Appl Pharmacol 1975; 33:320-332.

Granowetter L, Rosenstock JG, Packer RJ. Enhanced cis-platinum neurotoxicity in pediatric patients with brain tumors. J Neurol Oncol 1985; 1:293-297.

Jardini L, Findlay R, Burgi E, Hinderer K, Agarwal A. Auditory changes associated with moderate blood salicylate levels. Rheumatol Rehab 1978; 17:233-236.

Johnson A-C, Juntunen L, Nylen P, Borg E, Hoglund G. Effect of interaction between noise and toluene on auditory function in the rat. Acta Otolaryngol 1988; 105:56-63.

Kohn S, Fradis M, Pratt H, et al. Cisplatin ototoxicity in guinea pigs with special reference to toxic effects in the stria vascularis. Laryngoscope 1988; 98:865-871.

Kommune S, Snow JB. Potentiating effects of cisplatin and ethacrynic acid in ototoxicity. Arch Otolaryngol 1981; 107:594-597.

Lambert P, Palmer PE, Rubel EW. The interaction of noise and aspirin in the chick basilar papilla. Arch Otolaryngol Head Neck Surg 1986; 112:1043-1049.

Laurell G, Borg E. Cis-platin ototoxicity in previously noise-exposed guinea pigs. Acta Otolaryngol 1986; 101:66-74.

Lindgren F, Axelsson A. Temporary threshold shift induced by noise exposure and moderate salicylate intake. Scand Audiol 1987; 16:41-44.

Long GR, Tubis A. Modification of spontaneous and evoked otoacoustic emissions and associated psychoacoustic microstructure by aspirin consumption. J Acoust Soc Am 1988; 84:1343-1353.

Marco-Algarra J, Basterra J, Marco J. Cis-diamminedichloroplatinum ototoxicity: An experimental study. Acta Otolaryngol 1985; 99:343-347.

McCabe PA, Dey DL. The effect of aspirin upon auditory sensitivity. Ann Otol 1965; 74:312-325.

McFadden D, Plattsmier HS. Aspirin can potentiate the temporary hearing loss induced by intense sounds. Hear Res 1983; 9:295-316.

McFadden D, Plattsmier HS. Aspirin abolishes spontaneous oto-acoustic emissions. J Acoust Soc Am 1984; 76:443-448.

Mitchell C, Brummett R, Vernon J. Interaction between agents which produce temporary hearing threshold shifts: Intense sound and sodium salicylate. J Acoust Soc Am 1974; 55:460.

Morata TC. Study of the effects of simultaneous exposure to noise and carbon disulfide on workers' hearing. Scand Audiol 1989; 18:53-58.

Myers EN, Bernstein JM. Salicylate ototoxicity. Arch Otolaryngol 1965; 82:483-493.

Passchier-Vermeer W. Measurement and rating of impulse noise in relation to noise-induced hearing loss. In: Rossi G, ed. Noise as a public health problem. Milano: Centro Ricerne e Studi Amplifon, 1983:143.

Pryor GT, Dickinson J, Feeney E, Rebert CS. Hearing loss in rats first exposed to toluene as weanlings or as young adults. Neurobehav Toxicol Teratol 1984; 6:111-119.

Puel J-L, Bobbin RP, Fallon M. Salicylate abolishes cochlea potentials through a mechanism that does not involve prostaglandin synthesis and is different than quinine. Otolaryngol Head Neck Surg 1989; 99:154.

Rainsford KD. Aspirin and the salicylates. Boston: Butterworths, 1984.

Safirstein R, Winston J, Goldstein M, et al. Cisplatin nephrotoxicity. Am J Kidney Dis 1986; 8:356-367.

Schacht J. Biochemistry of cochlear function and pathology. Semin Hear 1986; 7:101-114.

Schweitzer VG, Hawkins JE, Lilly DJ, et al. Ototoxic and nephrotoxic effects of combined treatment with cis-diamminedichloro-platinum and kanamycin in the guinea pig. Otolaryngol Head Neck Surg 1984; 92:38-49.

Sharma RP, Edwards IR. Cis-platinum: Subcellular distribution and binding to cytosolic ligands. Biochem Pharmacol 1983; 32:2665-2669.

Shehata WE, Brownell WE, Cousillas H, Imredy JP. Salicylate alters membrane conductance of outer hair cells and diminishes rapid electromotile responses. Abstr 13th Midwinter Meeting Assoc Res Otolaryngol, St. Petersburg, FL, 1990; 13:252.

Stypulkowski PH. The mechanism(s) of salicylate (aspirin) induced hearing loss and tinnitus. Abstr 12th Midwinter Meeting Assoc Res Otolaryngol, St. Petersburg, FL, 1989; 12:189.

Trinder P. Rapid determination of salicylate in biological fluids. Biochem J 1954; 57:301-303.

von Gierke H. The noise-induced hearing problem. Abstr NIH Consensus Conference on Noise and Hearing Loss, 1990: 17-20.

Williams SE, Zenner H-P, Schacht J. Three molecular steps of aminoglycoside ototoxicity demonstrated in outer hair cells. Hear Res 1987; 30:11-18.

Woodford CM, Henderson D, Hamernik RP. Effects of combinations of sodium salicylate and noise on the auditory threshold. Ann Otol 1978; 87:117-127.

World Health Organization, Environmental health criteria 10: Carbon disulphide. Geneva, Switzerland, 1979.

Wright CG, Schaefer SD. Inner ear histopathology in patients treated with cis-platinum. Laryngoscope 1982; 92:1408-1413.

Young JS, Upchurch MB, Kaufmann MJ, Fechter LD. Carbon monoxide exposure potentiates high-frequency auditory threshold shifts induced by noise. Hear Res 1987; 26:37-43.

CHAPTER 16

Noise, Aminoglycosides, and Diuretics

JEAN-MARIE ARAN
H. HIEL
T. HAYASHIDA
J.-P. ERRE
C. AUROUSSEAU
A. GUILHAUME
D. DULON

The overall patterns of functional and morphologic cochlear impairments after exposure to high levels of white noise or after massive aminoglycoside antibiotic treatment are similar. In both cases one usually observes an elevation of thresholds for high frequencies correlated with hair cell destruction at the base of the cochlea, particularly the outer hair cells.*

After combined noise and aminoglycoside treatments, the damage is more extensive than after each treatment applied alone, but the pattern of damage is still the same. Thus, it is difficult to determine which is potentiating the other. It could be that the aminoglycoside treatment increases the damaging effects of noise, for instance, by making the cells metabolically fragile, or vice versa.

However, the pattern of damage, typical also with other causes of cochlear impairments such as in aging, is correlated with the pattern of mechanical excitation of the basilar membrane by noise. Moreover, in the synergistic experiments, damage occurs when the noise levels are close to their traumatic level (greater than 100 dB SPL) (Marques et al, 1975), whereas the drug dosages may be below the ototoxic levels. When the noise level is lower, as in incubators for premature newborns, absence of increased risk of ototoxicity of aminoglycosides has been claimed (Bernard and Pechere, 1984). In these conditions, it has been proposed that the drug enhances the hearing loss and cochlear damage caused by the noise (Boettcher et al, 1987). This is supported by the observation that even with the use of "safe" (low) doses of aminoglycosides, the potentiation of noise damage occurs and may last more than 20 days after cessation of the drug treatment (Gannon et al, 1979).

Conversely, it has been reported on several occasions that when the noise exposure precedes the drug treatment, the damage is larger than when both treatments are presented in an opposite sequence (Darrouzet and De Lima, 1962; Ryan and Bone, 1982; Collins, 1988), suggesting that the damage is due to the toxic action of the drug, potentiated by the sound pre-exposure. Thus, at present, there is no clear description or understanding of the synergistic effects between noise and aminoglycosides.

Although the mechanisms of acoustic impairment to the cochlea are well understood, ranging from direct mechanical injury of hair cells with very high-intensity sounds to meta-

*Only slightly noticeable specific differences have been reported so far in cochlear damage following noise trauma and aminoglycoside ototoxicity. In acoustic trauma the first row of outer hair cells is usually affected first, as with aminoglycosides, although different patterns have been reported (Hawkins et al, 1967). After aminoglycoside treatment inner hair cell loss, with preserved outer hair cells, may occur at the apex of the cochlea, together with outer hair cell destruction at the base. This latter condition has been used to study the function of outer hair cells in the absence of inner hair cells (Dallos et al, 1972).

bolic exhaustion during long-lasting noises of lower levels, such as ambient industrial noises, the mechanisms of aminoglycoside ototoxicity are still not clear.

Other ototoxic agents also work synergistically with noise, aminoglycosides, or both (Boettcher et al, 1987; Humes, 1984; Rybak, 1986). The case of loop diuretics is of particular interest. Loop diuretics such as ethacrynic acid or furosemide, when administered alone, induce profound but totally reversible functional losses due to temporary interference with ionic transport by the stria vascularis. However, when they are administered in association with aminoglycoside antibiotics, a rapid and permanent loss of function and of sensory cells occurs (West et al, 1973), but there is no synergistic effect between noise and loop diuretics (Vernon et al, 1977; Kisiel and Bobbin, 1982).

However, when the three agents (noise, diuretic, and aminoglycoside antibiotic) are used in combination, great synergistic interactions occur, as we have recently observed (Hayashida et al, 1989; Aran, 1990). In particular, the losses usually observed after treatment with ethacrynic acid and gentamicin when the animals are kept in a normal (laboratory or animal's quarters) sound environment, do not develop or are delayed when the animals are kept isolated from sound, in a soundproof room (Hayashida et al, 1989). These results demonstrate the effect of noise, but in the normal, functional, physiologic range of the cochlea, rather than in the damaging range of sound levels.

We will describe experiments using different combination treatments in which we studied the relations between functional or morphologic cochlear changes and the dynamics of aminoglycoside uptake by the hair cells. The results obtained tend to reveal the respective role of each treatment, particularly that of noise, in the development of the pathologic processes.

Experiment I

Guinea pigs equipped with indwelling electrodes on the round window of one ear and on the skull were treated with one intramuscular (IM) injection of gentamicin (GM) (150 mg per kilogram), followed 1.5 hours later by an intracardiac (IC) injection of ethacrynic acid (EA) (30 mg per kilogram). The cochlear function was measured at the beginning and at the end of the experiment by the determination of the thresholds of the auditory nerve compound action potential (CAP) evoked by tone pips (2 ms rise/decay times, no plateau) of different frequencies. It was also regularly monitored every 2 or 5 minutes during the hour following the EA injection by recording the CAP in response to a train of 256 clicks (70 dB peak equivalent sound pressure level [pespl] 10 per second).

In every case we observed, during the first hour, a rapid decrease of the amplitude of the CAP followed by a progressive recovery. But when the animals were kept thereafter in the soundproof room, without any acoustic stimulation, the recovery was complete after 24 hours, i.e., the thresholds were normal (Fig. 16-1, *C*). However, if the animals were placed in the animal quarters, with an ambient sound level with peaks at about 60 dB SPL, then the recovery was not complete and there was, at 24 hours, a definite high frequency threshold elevation (Fig. 16-1, *A*). After 48 hours in silence, some guinea pigs showed a profound loss, whereas others still displayed normal CAP audiograms (Fig. 16-1, *D*). By contrast, all animals maintained in ambient sound had profound losses at all frequencies (Fig. 16-1, *B*).

The uptake of GM was studied using autoradiography or immunohistochemistry (Hayashida et al, 1989). The main observations were (1) GM is specifically, and exclusively, labeled in the hair cells of the cochlea, with inner to outer hair cells and apex to base gradients (Fig. 16-2); (2) GM is preferentially localized at the apex of the hair cells, below the cuticular plate, in the area of dense lysosome accumulation, around the basal body, the hair bundle (Fig. 16-3), and on the nucleus (Hiel et al, in preparation); (3) GM is clearly identified within numerous hair cells in cochleas of guinea pigs that did not show, at time of sacrifice, any threshold elevation, particularly those kept in silence and sacrificed at 24 hours. However, although it was impossible to precisely quantify the amount of GM taken up by the hair cells, GM labeling was apparently more pronounced in the guinea pigs exposed to sound than in those kept in silence.

The results of this first series of experiments confirm the potentiation of aminoglycoside ototoxicity by loop diuretics. But they indicate additionally (1) GM specifically penetrates into hair cells; (2) normal acoustic stimulation (functional depolarization) is essential for GM uptake and toxicity—in other words, silence could prevent the development of ototoxicity; (3) the patterns of GM uptake and of functional loss parallel that of sound activation in the cochlea; (4) GM uptake by the hair

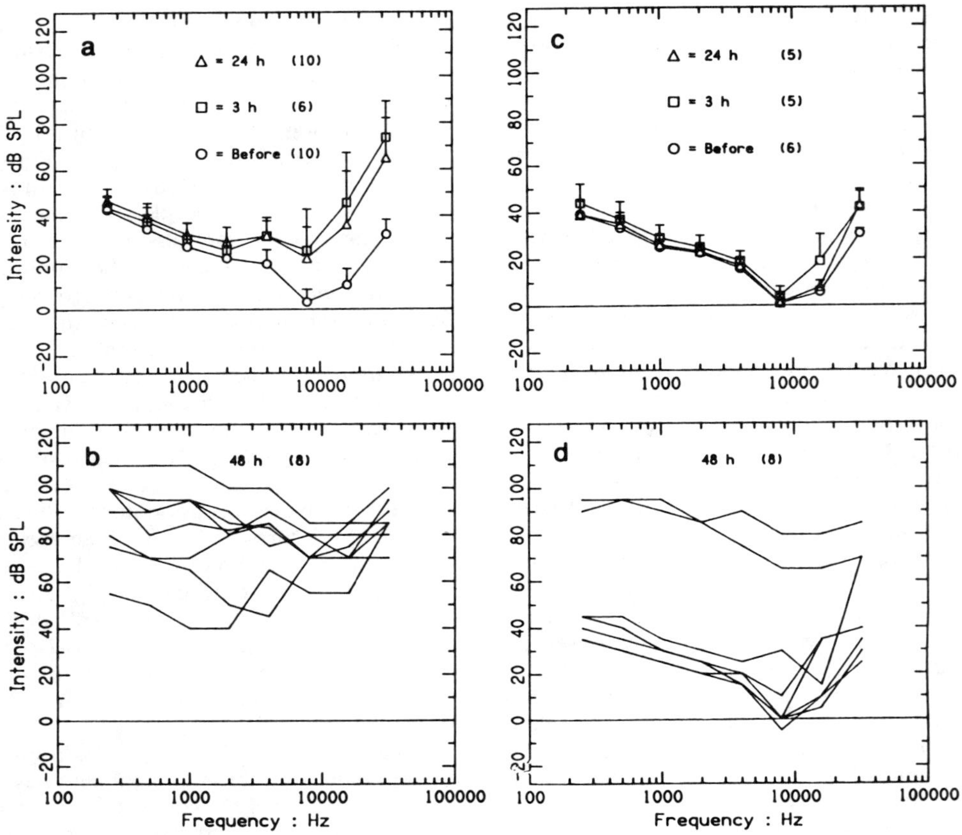

Figure 16-1 Comparison of compound action potential (CAP) frequency threshold curves between two groups of guinea pigs (GPs) having received one IM injection of gentamicin (GM) (150 mg per kilogram) followed, 1.5 hours later, by an IC injection of ethacrynic acid (EA) (30 mg per kilogram). Group I was exposed to sound *(A,B)* and group II was isolated from sound *(C,D)*. Means and standard deviations are represented for GPs before EA injection and 3 and 24 hours after injection, just before sacrifice *(A,C)*. Numbers of GPs are in parentheses. For GPs sacrificed at 48 hours, there is great variability in the results, so that individual curves are presented separately *(B,D)*. (From Hayashida T, Hiel H, Dulon D, Erre J-P, Guilhaume A, Aran J-M. Dynamic changes following combined treatment with gentamicin and ethacrynic acid with and without acoustic stimulation. Acta Otolaryngol (Stockh) 1989; 108:404-413.)

cells precedes the development of ototoxicity, and thus (5) toxicity is an intracellular process that could be also potentiated by sound.

Experiment 2

To separate out the role of EA from that of GM, we have studied the relation between uptake and functional and morphologic impairments in the course of a chronic treatment with GM alone (60 mg per kilogram per day IM). In such a chronic treatment with aminoglycosides alone, it is well known that ototoxicity develops only after several days of treatment (Aran and Darrouzet, 1975). Here threshold elevations did not occur before about the tenth day of treatment. However, we were able to identify, immunohistologically, GM in hair cells as soon as 2 days after the beginning of the treatment—that is, in cochleas with normal threshold curves, 8 days before the development of functional changes (Hiel et al, in preparation). Moreover, the pattern of GM uptake along the cochlea after such a chronic treatment also parallels that of the functional changes across frequency.

The results from this experiment are similar to those obtained after the acute GM/EA treatment; in particular, they confirm that GM uptake precedes the development of ototoxicity. Thus, they indicate also that the changes seen after GM/EA treatment are associated with GM toxicity and that potentiation by EA can be a convenient tool for the study of aminoglycoside ototoxicity.

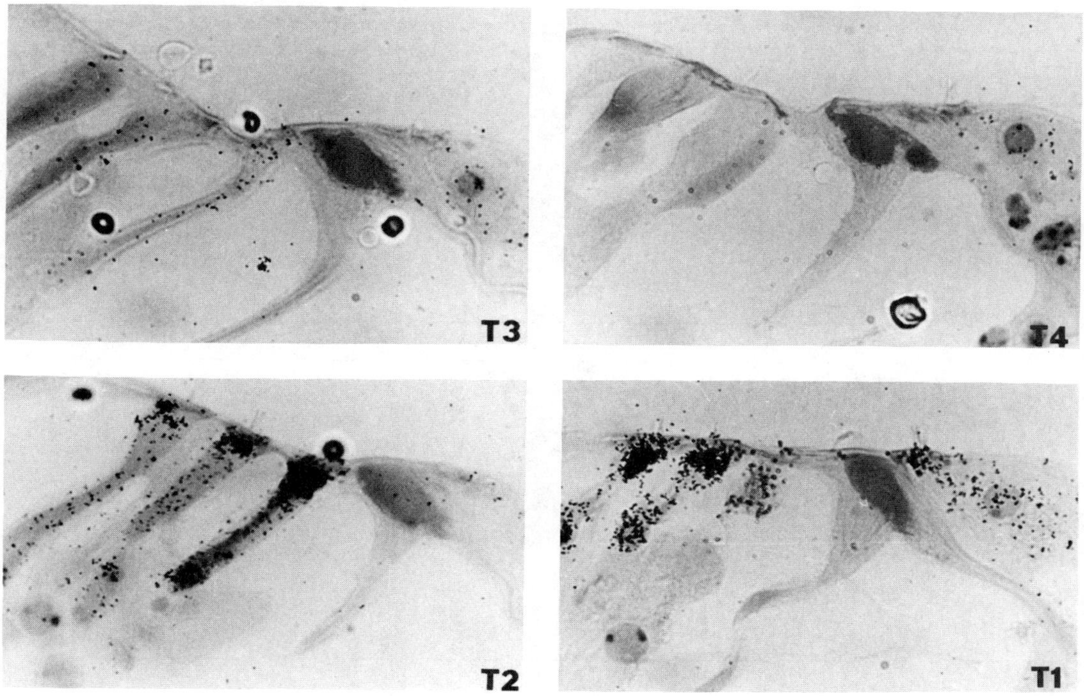

Figure 16-2 Autoradiography of sections of the four turns (T1 through T4) of a guinea pig having received the gentamicin/ethacrynic acid (GM/EA) treatment, kept in normal sound environment and sacrificed 24 hours after the EA injection. Two milligrams of [^{3}H]GM (Amersham, 1 mCi per milligram) were added to the dose of GM. (From Hayashida T, Hiel H, Dulon D, Erre J-P, Guilhaume A, Aran J-M. Dynamic changes following combined treatment with gentamicin and ethacrynic acid with and without acoustic stimulation. Acta Otolaryngol (Stockh) 1989; 108:404-413.)

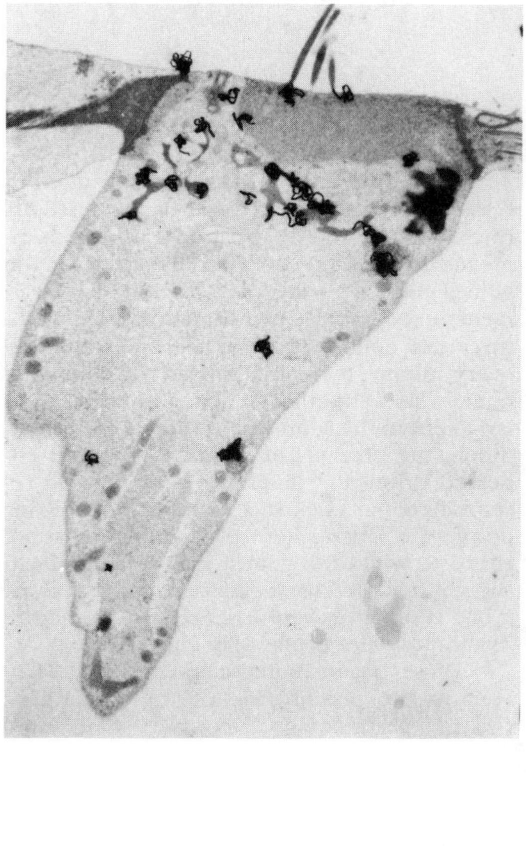

Figure 16-3 Transmission electron microscopic view of a labeled autoradiographic section of the apical part of an outer hair cell of the second turn of the same guinea pig as seen in Figure 16-2.

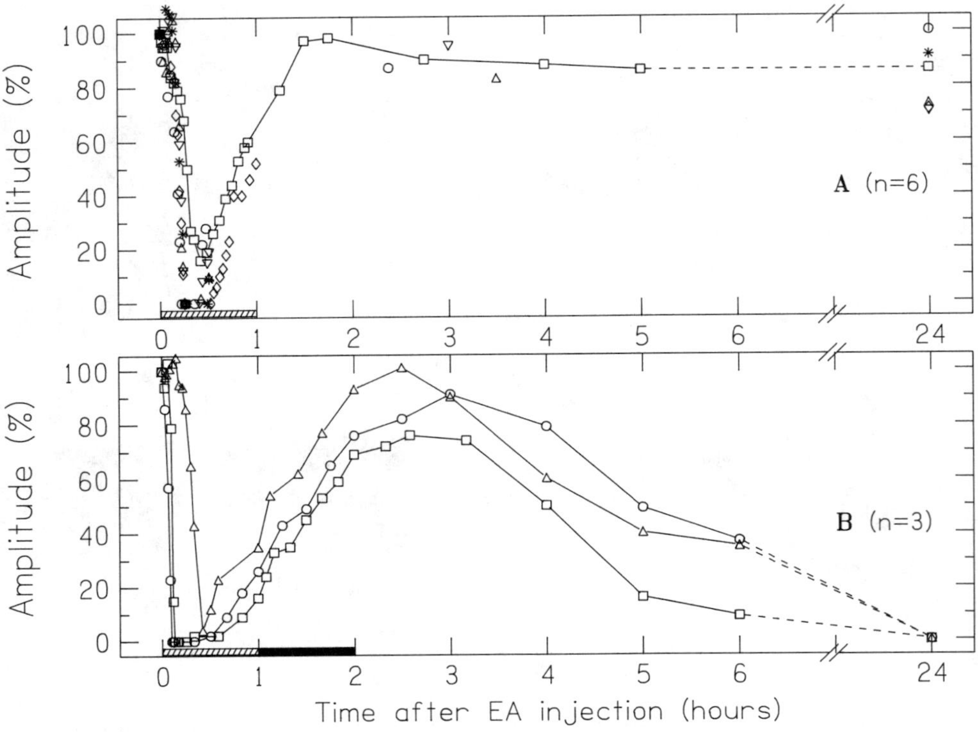

Figure 16-4 Changes in amplitude of the compound action potential (CAP) response to the click over 24 hours after the ethacrynic acid (EA) injection (1.5 hours after the gentamicin (GM) injection). *A*, GPs monitored during the first 30 to 60 minutes (256 clicks, 70 dB pespl, 10 per second, every 2 to 5 minutes), thereafter kept in the soundproof room and only occasionally tested until 24 hours. *B*, GPs exposed during the second hour to the same train of clicks (256 clicks, 70 dB pespl, 10 per second, every minute) and kept similarly in silence thereafter.

Experiment 3

To analyze the role of sound activation in GM uptake and toxicity, we first studied its role after the GM/EA treatment. The experiment was the same as experiment 1, with the guinea pigs receiving the same GM/EA treatment, except that their function was monitored not only during the first hour, but also every minute thereafter during the following hour. Afterward, the guinea pigs were similarly kept in the soundproof room. In this condition, the changes in the CAP response appeared drastically different. Although the response to the click did continue to recover during the second hour of sound stimulation, later on, while the guinea pigs were again in silence, it started to decrease and, at 24 hours, it had completely vanished (Fig. 16-4) and the thresholds were profoundly elevated.

These observations are significant. They confirm the potentiation of the toxicity of GM/EA treatment by acoustic stimulation. They indicate also that this potentiation does not occur at the peak of the EA effect, when the cochlea is completely deprived of activity, but rather when this activity recovers. The delay between the sound activation and the development of the functional losses suggests that these alterations are not directly due to the noise. If that was the case, they would develop instantly, as they do during acoustic trauma. We know that EA facilitates entry of GM into endolymph (Tran Ba Huy et al, 1983), and it is likely that, in turn, sound activation facilitates its entry from endolymph into the hair cells. The intracellular toxicity would then develop without the participation of sound, because by that time the animals are isolated from sound.

Experiment 4

In a fourth experiment, we tried to determine whether silence would also prevent the development of ototoxicity during a chronic treatment with GM alone. Because it is difficult to maintain the animals in a silent environment during a long period because of self-generated noise, they were kept in the animal's quarters, but one ear was protected from ambient sound by surgically disrupting the incudostapedial joint, thereby inducing a mean 30-dB conductive loss. In doing so, we also provided each animal with its own control ear. However, after 21 days of IM injection of GM (60 mg per kilogram per day) and 1 month of delay between the end of the treatment and sacrifice, we did not notice any significant difference in hair cell loss between the protected and unprotected ears.

These observations thus fail to show any difference between a sound-activated and a sound-protected ear with respect to aminoglycoside-induced ototoxicity as in the case of acute GM/EA treatment. Thus, it could be possible that the effect of noise on GM ototoxicity is also potentiated by EA. However, it is well documented that diuretics do not potentiate the damaging effects of noise (Vernon et al, 1977), whereas the interaction of noise and aminoglycosides is well established (Darrouzet and De Lima, 1962; Marques et al, 1975). Moreover, all the other observations about GM and noise interactions with or without EA tend to indicate that the synergistic mechanisms are the same.

These negative results during chronic treatment with GM could be related to the fact that only one ear was (partially) sound protected. Another side effect of aminoglycoside antibiotics is their neuromuscular blocking potency (Paradelis et al, 1980). We have observed that aminoglycosides do not, over the short term, penetrate the hair cells in vitro, but that they concentrate at the basal end, in the synaptic efferent area, which is most probably cholinergic, and that they block the calcium channels (Dulon et al, 1989). Thus, it is possible that the aminoglycoside action at the synaptic area modifies the function of the hair cell, and thus indirectly, its penetration mechanisms. This synaptic area is normally activated during excitation of the efferent system, which occurs bilaterally after afferent sensory excitation. In our chronic experiment in which one ear was unprotected, the efferent system was activated and could exert its influence on the two ears. However, there does not seem to be a correlation between the degree of ototoxicity and of neuromuscular blockade potency of the different aminoglycosides (Rutten et al, 1980; Aran, 1990).

Conclusion

In our GM/EA conditions, it is likely that (1) EA facilitates entry of GM into endolymph (Tran Ba Huy et al, 1983); (2) sound, and possibly EA, facilitate, in turn, entry of GM from endolymph into the hair cells; and (3) GM accumulates inside the hair cells until its concentration reaches a toxic level. These two steps should also occur during the chronic treatment with GM and sound stimulation alone, but with a much slower pace, following the kinetics of GM in the inner ear fluids and tissues. However, evidence of sound interaction with aminoglycosides has been presented only for high sound levels.

These results and interpretations apparently contradict the observation by Hudspeth that dihydrostreptomycin applied to bullfrog isolated saccular hair cells in vitro blocks the transduction channels (Hudspeth and Kroese, 1983; Howard et al, 1988), whereas we observe that functional changes occur only after the aminoglycoside has penetrated the hair cells. However, it is possible that such a blockade of the transduction channels, which is rapidly reversible, remained undetected in our global physiologic measurements, and that it could be a step towards the penetration of the molecule into the cell. Thus, the activation of the transduction channels by sound may effectively facilitate the entry of the aminoglycoside molecule into the cell.

Bruits Antibiotiques Aminóglycosidiques et Diurétiques

La synergie entre bruit et antibiotiques aminoglycosidiques a été découverte très tôt, mais contestée et insuffisamment explorée. Comme les deux agressions affectent principalement les cellules ciliées externes de la base de la cochlée, il est encore difficile de définir précisément le rôle de chacun de ces agents.

Les quelques observations cliniques et expérimentales disponibles spécifiquement sur les interactions bruit/aminoglycosides sont tout d'abord analysées, puis comparées à celles obtenues à propos d'autres synergies, telles que les synergies diurétiques/aminoglycosides, et celles observées plus récemment sur le plan expérimental entre les trois agents: bruit, diurétiques et aminoglycosides.

Les combinaisons bruit/aminoglycosides sont toxiques principalement quand les deux agents sont administrés chacun à des doses proches du niveau traumatique ou toxique. Par contre l'association diurétique/aminoglycoside (dans nos expériences: acide éthacrynique et gentamicine) peut être très toxique, sur les plans fonctionnels et morphologiques, alors que chaque traitement est, individuellement, parfaitement non toxique. A cette occasion nous avons observé que ces effets toxiques pouvaient être retardés, voire annulés, lorsque les animaux ainsi traités étaient gardés dans le silence. Nous démontrions ainsi qu'un environnement sonore normal pouvait être un facteur additionnel dans l'établissment des lésions. De plus nous avons pu démontrer simultanément que, en présence d'acide éthacrynique, la pénétration de la gentamicine spécifiquement dans les cellules ciliées, et vraisemblablement aussi les mécanismes cytotoxiques intracellulaires, étaient potentialisés par un environnement acoustique normal.

Un certain nombre de considérations suggèrent que c'est l'acide éthacrynique qui potentialise la toxicité de la gentamicine, en facilitant sa pénétration dans l'endolymphe, sa clearance étant ensuite très lente. Dans des expériences récentes nous montrons que le délai entre le traitement gentamicine/acide éthacrynique et l'exposition au bruit est déterminant dans l'étendue et la cinétique des modifications fonctionnelles et morphologiques. Il est donc vraisemblable que la stimulation acoustique potentialise l'effet de l'acide éthacrynique vis-à-vis de la pénétration et de la toxicité de l'antibiotique.

La protection contre les traumatismes acoustiques est déjà recommandée lors d'un traitement clinique par aminoglycosides. Nos expériences suggèrent qu'une protection même envers les sons de la vie courante pourrait être nécessaire. Cependant d'autres expériences sont encore nécessaires avant qu'une telle recommandation puisse être faite.

References

Aran J-M. Physiopathology of sensory hair cells: In vivo and in vitro studies on aminoglycoside uptake and toxicity. Adv Audiol 1990; 7:42-46.

Aran J-M, Darrouzet J. Observation of click evoked compound VIII nerve responses before, during and over several months after kanamycin treatment in the guinea pig. Acta Otolaryngol (Stockh) 1975; 79:24-32.

Bernard PA, Pechere JC. Does incubator noise increase risks of aminoglycoside ototoxicity? Audiology 1984; 23:309-320.

Boettcher FA, Henderson D, Gratton MA, Danielson RW, Byrne C. Synergistic interactions of noise and other ototraumatic agents. Ear Hear 1987; 8:192-212.

Collins PWP. Synergistic interactions of gentamicin and pure tones causing cellular hair cell loss in pigmented guinea pigs. Hear Res 1988; 36:249-260.

Dallos P, Billone MC, Durrant JD. Cochlear inner and outer hair cells: Functional differences. Science 1972; 177:356-358.

Darrouzet J, De Lima E. Oreille interne, Kanamycine et traumatisme acoustique. Etude expérimentale. Rev Laryngol Otol Rhinol (Bord) 1962; 83:781-806.

Dulon D, Zajic G, Aran JM, Schacht J. Aminoglycoside antibiotics impair calcium entry but not viability and motility in isolated cochlear outer hair cells. J Neurosci Res 1989; 24:338-346.

Gannon RP, Tso SS, Chung DY. Interaction of kanamycin and noise exposure. J Laryngol Otol 1979; 93:341-347.

Hawkins JE Jr, Beger V, Aran J-M. Antibiotic insults to Corti's organ. In: Graham AB, ed. Sensorineural hearing processes and disorder. Boston: Little, Brown, 1967:411.

Hayashida T, Hiel H, Dulon D, Erre J-P, Guilhaume A, Aran J-M. Dynamic changes following combined treatment with gentamicin and ethacrynic acid with and without acoustic stimulation. Acta Otolaryngol (Stockh) 1989; 108:404-413.

Hiel H, Erre JP, Hayashida T, et al. Autoradiographic cellular and subcellular localization of gentamicin in the cochlea following combined treatment with ethacrynic acid (in preparation).

Howard J, Roberts M, Hudspeth AJ. Mechanoelectrical transduction by hair cells. Ann Rev Biophys Chem 1988; 17:99-124.

Hudspeth AJ, Kroese ABA. Voltage-dependent interaction of dihydrostreptomycin with the transduction channels in bullfrog sensory hair cells. J Physiol (Lond) 1983; 345:66P (Abstract).

Humes LE. Noise-induced hearing loss as influenced by other agents and by some physical characteristics of the individual. J Acoust Soc Am 1984; 76:1318-1329.

Kisiel DL, Bobbin RP. Interaction of aminooxyacetic acid and ethacrynic acid with intense sound at the level of the cochlea. Hear Res 1982; 6:129-140.

Marques DM, Clark CS, Hawkins JE Jr. Potentiation of cochlear injury by noise and ototoxic antibiotics in guinea pigs. J Acoust Soc Am 1975; 57:S1 (Abstract).

Paradelis AG, Triantaphyllidis C, Giala MM. Neuromuscular blocking activity of aminoglycoside antibiotics. Methods Find Exp Clin Pharmacol 1980; 2:45-51.

Rutten JM, Booij LH, Rutten CL, Crul JF. The comparative neuromuscular blocking effects of some aminoglycoside antibiotics. Acta Anaesthesiol Belg 1980; 31:293-306.

Ryan AF, Bone RC. Non-simultaneous interaction of exposure to noise and kanamycin intoxication in the chinchilla. Am J Otolaryngol 1982; 3:264-272.

Rybak LP. Ototoxic mechanisms. In: Altschuler AR, Hoffman DW, eds. Neurobiology of hearing: The cochlea. New York: Raven Press, 1986:441.

Tran Ba Huy P, Manuel C, Meulemans A, et al. Ethacrynic acid facilitates gentamicin entry into endolymph of the rat. Hear Res 1983; 11:191-202.

Vernon J, Brummett R, Brown R. Noise trauma induced in the presence of loop-inhibiting diuretics. Trans Acad Ophthalmol Otolaryngol 1977; 84:407-413.

West BA, Brummett RE, Himes DL. Interaction of kanamycin and ethacrynic acid. Severe cochlear damage in guinea pigs. Acta Otolaryngol (Stockh) 1973; 98:32-37.

CHAPTER 17

Sensitive Developmental Period and Acoustic Trauma: Facts and Hypotheses

RÉMY PUJOL

Sensitive periods have been identified in the developing mammalian cochlea (Uziel, 1985; Pujol and Uziel, 1988). They can be described as developmental periods during which an epigenetic factor has a damaging effect, or an increased damaging effect on cochlear structures and function. Reasonably well-defined sensitive periods exist for thyroid deprivation (Uziel, 1986) and aminoglycoside antibiotics (Pujol, 1986). Similarly, a sensitive period for acoustic trauma has been reported. During this period, juvenile animals show an enhanced susceptibility to noise exposure: i.e., both temporary threshold shifts (TTS) (Bock and Seifter, 1978) and/or permanent threshold shifts (PTS) (Bock and Saunders, 1977) were first reported in the hamster cochlea after a noise exposure that was nontraumatic for an adult of the same species.

This article will not review the experimental data, as little has been added to the literature since the previous report (Lenoir et al, 1986). However, the main results will be briefly summarized and two major questions that were raised at that time will be discussed further. The first question concerned the anatomic correlates that could account for the sensitive period to noise trauma. Some of the most recent findings in cochlear physiology (e.g., active mechanisms and neurochemistry) must presently be considered to complement the hypotheses already proposed. We will particularly discuss: (1) a possible immaturity of the inner hair cell-auditory nerve synapse, resulting in an increased excitotoxicity to amino acids; (2) the fragility of the incompletely developed outer hair cell active mechanism; and (3) the weaker protective effect of efferents at the end of the developmental period as compared with adulthood. The second question concerns the existence of a sensitive period in human babies. Because of the great similarities in cochlear structure and development among most mammalian species, including humans, it is highly probable that a sensitive period for acoustic trauma exists during the last trimester of pregnancy, or in premature babies. Some recent data supporting this assumption will be presented.

Sensitive Period for Noise-Induced Damage: Experimental Data

Experimentally, the first suggestion that developmental factors needed to be considered in evaluating the effect of noise on the auditory system came from studies on the phenomenon of priming for audiogenic seizures (e.g., Henry and Bowman, 1970; Saunders et al, 1972). These studies clearly demonstrate "that an elevated absolute threshold per se is not sufficient to induce seizure susceptibility, but that a prolonged reduction of input during a sensitive period might be a better explanation" (Willott and Henry, 1974).

An age-dependent susceptibility of the cochlear structures to acoustic trauma was first observed in guinea pigs (Falk et al, 1974). Exposure to traumatic noise, when presented during the first week after birth, resulted in more severe cochlear lesions than when presented to adult guinea pigs. Similar findings were then reported by others, using different types of noise exposure or different measurements (physiologic versus anatomic) of the traumatic effect (Lenoir et al, 1986).

However, the first clear demonstration that an enhanced period of susceptibility to acoustic trauma exists in the mammalian cochlea was from observations on young hamsters (Bock and Saunders, 1977; Stanek et al, 1977; Bock and Seifter, 1978). In this animal, which exhibits a delayed cochlear maturation as compared to most of the other experimental models, the following conclusions were reached:

1. Young hamsters pass through a developmental stage during which they show a heightened susceptibility to acoustic trauma.
2. Increased susceptibility to acoustic trauma is evident using both the PTS or TTS criteria.
3. The sensitive period appears to depend on developmental changes within the cochlea, not in the middle ear.
4. The developmental changes remain unidentified, but occur after the completion of the apparent structural and functional maturation of the cochlea.

Experiments performed with rats further confirm the above conclusions (Lenoir et al, 1979). A sensitive period to noise exposure existed in the rat pup between day 16 and day 40 of postnatal age. From anatomic and physiologic data showing that the rat cochlea reaches its adult-like properties at the end of the third week, it was concluded that the increased susceptibility appeared at the end of cochlear maturation. The peak of sensitivity, i.e., the time when the noise exposure causes the maximum PTS, occurred at day 22 when the rat cochlea is considered to be fully mature. Moreover, the sensitive period extends for approximately 1 month after the apparent completion of cochlear maturation. In order to determine the nature of the cochlear damage responsible for the PTS, a histologic study (surface preparation visualized with transmission electron microscopy) was done on the same animals (Lenoir and Pujol, 1980). Although not obviously conclusive, the results indicated that different metabolic impairments in different cochlear structures may account for the traumatic processes. Interestingly, these impairments were first noted not only on the hair cells (especially outer), but also on the nerve endings (especially the efferents to the outer hair cells).

A series of experiments was completed recently on several strains of mice (Henry, 1984a,b). The results largely agree with what has been found in other species. A sensitive period for acoustic trauma was found in both the CBA and C57BL/6 mice during the second month of life (Henry, 1984b), while their cochlea are believed to be mature by the end of the first month (Shnerson and Pujol, 1983). However, in the CBA mouse, it appears that this increased susceptibility does not involve the whole cochlea. The high-frequency portion of the organ of Corti seems to be equally sensitive throughout the mouse's lifespan (Henry, 1984a).

Anatomic Correlates of the Sensitive Period

From the above reported experimental data, the most surprising and general finding is that it is not possible to closely correlate the period of sensitivity to acoustic trauma with a specific maturational event in the cochlea. Cochlear structures and functions appear fully developed when the sensitive period is at its peak. Thus, authors refer to "an unidentified and late developmental change" (Bock and Saunders, 1977), or to "a metabolic stabilization period that would follow the structural maturation" (Lenoir et al, 1979). Our concept of cochlear physiology has drastically changed within the last decade (Santos-Sacchi, 1988; Pujol, 1989); therefore, new hypotheses can now be developed. We will review only three of them involving the synapses between inner hair cells (IHCs) and the auditory nerve, the outer hair cell (OHC) active mechanism, and the regulation of the active mechanism by the medial efferents.

IHC-Auditory Nerve Synapse

The morphology of the synapses between the IHCs and the radial auditory afferent endings of the type I ganglion cells clearly indicates that synaptic transmission is of a neurochemical type (Pujol and Lenoir, 1986). The best candidate for the neurotransmitter is glutamate (Eybalin and Pujol, 1989). This has physiologic as well as pathophysiologic implications.

Glutamate is considered to be an excellent neurotransmitter in the central nervous system when fast excitation is needed, which is the situation one would expect in the cochlea. However, glutamate is also known to have neurotoxic effects when excessively released, and/or incompletely recycled. A glutamatergic synapse, to be safe, should be provided with an efficient mechanism for removing the neurotransmitter from the synaptic cleft. In the cochlea (Eybalin and Pujol, 1983), as generally occurs in the brain, this is achieved by glial recycling of glutamate into glutamine. But when glutamate is released in excess, as may occur during overstimulation, or in pathologic conditions such as ischemia or anoxia, this mechanism is not adequate and neurotoxic processes affect the postsynaptic targets. This neurotoxicity is first characterized by a swelling of nerve endings, followed by degeneration of glutamoceptive neurons (Mayer and Westbrook, 1987). In the cochlea, exposure to kainic acid, a glutamate analog, results in an acute and specific swelling of radial afferent dendrites connected to IHCs (Pujol et al, 1985). Subsequently, a loss of type I spiral ganglion neurons occurs (Juiz et al, 1989). It is striking to compare this acute damage with what occurs in anoxia (Spoendlin, 1970; Billett et al, 1989) or some cases of acoustic trauma (Spoendlin, 1976; Robertson, 1983). In all cases, the same type of immediate swelling (Fig. 17-1), probably linked to glutamate excitotoxicity, is observed (Pujol et al, 1990a).

Glutamate neurotoxicity is now taken into account in the CNS to explain some of the degenerative processes occurring in aging (Meldrum, 1985). This could also be a valuable working hypothesis in some forms of presbycusis (Pujol et al., 1990a). Similarly, it would be interesting to investigate more carefully IHC-afferent auditory synapses after noise exposure during the sensitive period. An increase of the swelling, as compared to similar exposure in adulthood, would indicate that glutamate neurotransmission and/or glutamate recycling is not fully mature, accounting for part of the increased sensitivity of the cochlea. Interestingly, in two of the experimental studies that have characterized the histologic damage that follows acoustic trauma during the sensitive period, the loss of IHCs (Price, 1976) and the degeneration of their afferent supply (Lenoir and Pujol, 1980) were pointed out.

OHC-Active Mechanism

The OHCs are no longer considered to be conventional mechanoreceptors. However, they are excited in the same way as the IHCs (through displacement of their stereocilia and opening of potassium channels), but they react to auditory stimulation in a completely different manner, probably by contracting. The demonstration, in in vitro preparations, that OHCs could contract or elongate depending on changes in the membrane potential, represents one of the major steps in the understanding of cochlear physiology (Brownell, 1984). In fact, an active mechanism enhancing and filtering the vibration of the basilar membrane was strongly suggested when oto-acoustic emissions were discovered (Kemp, 1978). Moreover, the finding that in normal conditions, the basilar membrane (Sellick et al, 1982; Khanna and Leonard, 1982) as well as the IHCs (Russell and Sellick, 1978) are perfectly tuned suggested that this active mechanism must take place before the sensorineural transduction at the IHC level. Even though the exact mechanism occurring in vivo is still not completely understood, OHCs are clearly involved. As the OHCs are firmly coupled to the basilar membrane by means of supporting cells, and to the tectorial membrane by means of their tallest stereocilia, their contraction may result in an enhancement and a tuning of the vibration of the cochlear partition. Thus, the OHC active mechanism is considered to be responsible for the exquisite sensitivity (gain of about 50 dB at threshold) and frequency selectivity of the cochlea.

Possibly relevant to the sensitive period for acoustic trauma are the recent findings on the maturation of the OHC active mechanisms. A developmental study of acoustic distortion products in the rat cochlea (Lenoir and Puel, 1987) points out the relatively late maturation of the active mechanism phenomenon as compared with other indices of the cochlear function (Puel and Uziel, 1987). The $2F_1$-F_2 otoacoustic emissions for midfrequencies (3 to 7 kHz) reach their adult value at the very end of the first postnatal month. The gradient of maturation observed in this study, from the lowest (3 kHz) to the highest (7 kHz) frequencies, suggests that subtle developmental changes may occur in the basal portion of the rat cochlea well after the end of its apparent structural maturation. Thus, it is tempting to correlate both the location (high frequency region) and the timing (peak at the end of the first month) of the sensitive period to acoustic trauma (Lenoir et al, 1979) with the increased sensitivity of the OHC active mechanisms, which are not yet fully stabilized.

Efferent Supply to OHCs

OHCs, especially in the region that is most sensitive to acoustic trauma in the developmental period (i.e., 8 to 20 kHz; Lenoir et al, 1979), are innervated by the medial efferent endings that form huge axosomatic synapses (Lenoir et al, 1980). This so-called medial efferent system (Warr and Guinan, 1979)

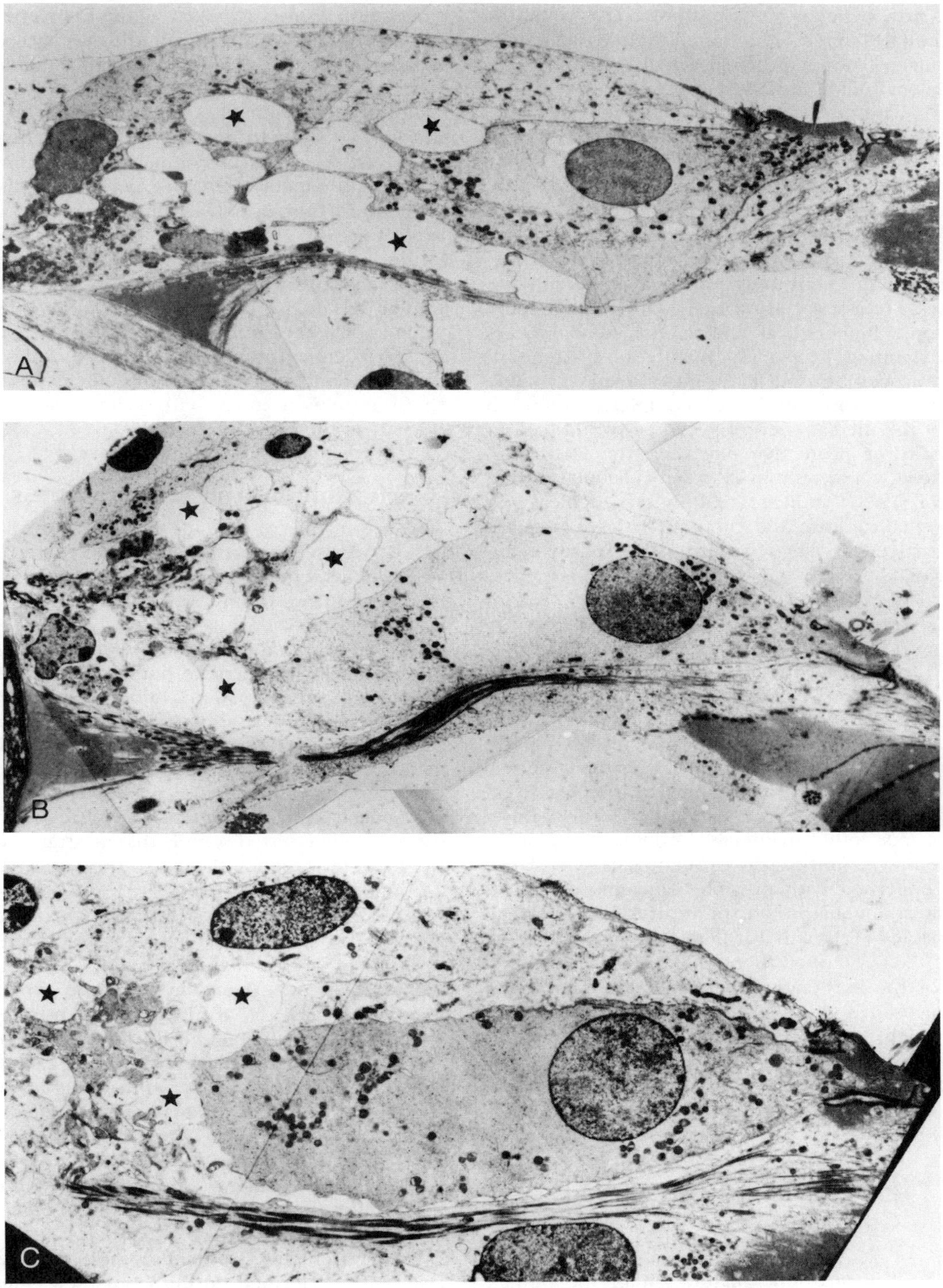

Figure 17-1 Comparison of acute damage affecting the radial afferents below the inner hair cells of the guinea pig after: *A*, kainic acid (glutamate analog) exposure; *B*, acoustic trauma (closed system: 10 kHz, 120 dB, ½ hour); and *C*, anoxia. In all cases, a selective and drastic swelling of radial afferents (some of them indicated by a star) is observed, possibly due to glutamate excitotoxicity.

is now believed to have a protective effect on the OHCs via a reduction of their active mechanisms (Mountain, 1980; Rajan and Johnstone, 1983; Puel et al, 1990).

The maturation of the efferent-OHC synapses is known to be the last event of cochlear synaptogenesis in the rat (Lenoir et al., 1980) as well as in all other mammalian species that have been investigated (Pujol and Sans, 1986). These synapses reach an apparent mature stage just before the sensitive period to acoustic trauma, but only anatomic criteria were used to assess this maturity. One could expect some biochemical and/or molecular process extending the synaptic maturation or stabilization well beyond the point estimated by electron microscopy. Thus, incomplete maturation of the medial efferent synapses would lead to a lower protective effect on the OHCs. Indeed, very preliminary results (Lenoir and Pujol, 1980) indicate that in rat cochleas exposed to noise, the efferent-OHC synapses are particularly affected during the sensitive period.

Human Data

Whatever the anatomic correlates, the existence of a period of increased sensitivity to acoustic trauma in young rodents can no longer be questioned. Because of the remarkable similarities of cochlear anatomy and/or function between mammalian species, it is highly probable that such a period also exists in most other mammals. In humans, the problem was first raised by clinicians who were concerned with possible damaging effects of noisy incubators on the hearing of premature babies (Falk and Farmer, 1973; Douek et al, 1976). Although there is little direct evidence for the existence of a sensitive period in humans, it is worth reviewing some relevant data which provide information about (1) maturation of the human cochlea; (2) the onset of fetal hearing; and (3) the evaluation of risk factors for hearing loss in the fetus and newborns.

Maturation of the Human Cochlea

The anatomic maturation of the human cochlea has been thoroughly investigated in the recent past (Pujol and Uziel, 1988; Lavigne-Rebillard and Pujol, 1990). These studies confirm that the fetal cochlea is structurally ready to function as soon as the eighteenth week of pregnancy, and that complete structural maturation is achieved by the last trimester. By comparing the maturational stages in humans to those reported in experimental mammals, it can be proposed that a 6- or 7-month fetal cochlea could function with a sensitivity close to mature values. Furthermore, on the basis of comparison with rats, one would expect a sensitive period to noise trauma to occur in humans from 5 months in utero to a few months after birth, with a peak within the last trimester of normal pregnancy. Thus, an enhanced risk factor for acoustic trauma has to be estimated in two different populations: the term newborns, who spend most of their sensitive period in utero, and the premature infants, who are directly exposed to a noisy environment within the most critical part of the sensitive period.

Hearing by the Human Fetus

A precise evaluation of the intensity of sound to which the fetus is exposed in utero is a prerequisite to any estimation of the risk of noise trauma during pregnancy. Recently, data have been published concerning the uterine sound environment in human mothers as well as in suitable animal models such the ewe. From these studies it appears that the sensory information reaching the amniotic cavity is far richer than previously expected. Two sets of experiments in pregnant ewes give a clear idea of the intensity and frequency of externally emitted sounds that are transmitted to an intact amniotic sac. In the first study (Armitage et al, 1980), a hydrophone implanted on the fetus neck indicated an attenuation of about 20 dB or less for frequencies lower than 2 kHz; higher frequencies have a higher level of attenuation. Another experiment (Gerhardt et al, 1988) demonstrated that application of a sound source directly on the surface of the maternal abdomen can result in very high sound pressure levels in the uterine cavity. When stimulating with an artificial larynx (frequency spectrum below 1 kHz), something that is done clinically for surveillance of high-risk pregnancies, the sound level recorded at the hydrophone reached 130 to 140 dB!

Measurements in human mothers have also been performed during labor (see Querleu et al, 1989). Most of these measurements are concordant with the animal results: i.e., the attenuation is lower than 20 dB below 1 kHz and increases linearly from 20 to 40 dB when the frequency is increased from 1 to 10 kHz. It is, however, important to note that both the external and middle ears are filled with amniotic fluid in the fetus and the transmission of sounds to the cochlea may be completely different than in the adult. Nevertheless, the feasibility of prenatal testing (see Granier-Deferre et al, 1985) is a good indication that this fluid transmission is really not too bad. In these conditions, during the last trimester of pregnancy, when cochlear thresholds of the fetus have probably dropped close to normal values, one should expect sound stimulation to have both physiologic and pathologic effects limited mainly by the attenuation discussed above and by some frequency distortions.

Noise Trauma in the Human Fetus

The possibility of fetal cochlear damage resulting from noise exposure of the mother during pregnancy has been postulated on the basis of correlations with experimental data (see Lenoir et al, 1986). However, a direct evaluation has also been reported in two clinical studies. In the first investigation (Daniel and Laciak, 1982), 75 children were tested: all were born from mothers who had worked during their pregnancy in a weaving factory (within a 100 dB noise environment). Only 40 of these children had normal hearing for their age! The other 35 presented high frequency losses of 20 to 55 dB. This dramatic result has been confirmed in another study (Lalande et al, 1986) in which 131 children were examined. Their mothers had worked while pregnant in noisy conditions ranging from 65 to 95 dB. Results show that children whose mothers were exposed to noise of 85 to 95 dB had a three-fold increase in the risk of having a high-frequency hearing loss. Moreover, there was a correlation between exposure to low-frequency noise and the risk of hearing loss at 4 kHz.

Noise Trauma in Premature Babies

The results described above clearly suggest that a period of increased sensitivity to the damaging effect of noise also exists in the human cochlea. The demonstration that a noise exposure around 90 dB has a noxious effect on the fetal ear, despite the attenuation provided by the uterine environment, implies that a similar noxious effect should be expected to occur in premature babies at lower levels of exposure. This raises again the problem of a possible traumatic effect of incubator noise. Depending on the incubator model, such noise can reach 60 to 75 dB under normal working conditions. Is this level of noise sufficient to damage the cochleas of premature babies? Experiments done in the rat show that during the sensitive period a noise can have deleterious effect at levels 10 to 20 dB lower than in adulthood (Lenoir et al, 1979). If this is also true in human cochleas, a 1-month exposure to 75 dB could well be damaging.

The last point that must be discussed concerns premature babies. They are sometimes given, when in an incubator, ototoxic drugs such as aminoglycosides. A combination of noise (nontraumatic by itself) and drug (at a dose which is nonototoxic by itself) could produce a potentiating effect (Lenoir et al, 1986), especially during the sensitive period. This is a serious matter even if most of the studies done with infants in intensive care units do not clearly indicate auditory defects with noise and/or drug exposures. Damage could well be small enough or limited to a high-frequency range so as to be overlooked at the time of treatment. Taking into account that all assaults of noise and drugs may accumulate over time (Hawkins, 1973), very early damage could well be significant in the late appearance of a perceptible hearing impairment.

Traumatisme Sonore et Période de Susceptibilité au cours du Développement: Faits et Hypothèses

Au cours du développement cochléaire, plusieurs périodes d'hypersensibilité ont été décrites (voir Uziel, 1985 et Pujol et Uziel, 1989 pour revues). Elles correspondent à des périodes du développement où un facteur épigénétique peut affecter, ou avoir un effet délétère accru sur la structure et la fonction cochléaire. C'est ainsi qu'une période d'hypersensibilité a été mise en évidence pour l'insuffisance thyroïdienne et l'ototoxicité aux antibiotiques aminoglycosides; il en est de même pour le trauma acoustique. Dans ce dernier cas, des animaux en cours de développement, soumis à une exposition bruyante inoffensive chez l'adulte de même espèce, présentent des pertes auditives temporaires ou définitives.

Le présent article n'a pas pour objectif de passer à nouveau en revue les travaux expérimentaux sur le sujet, car très peu de résultats ont été publiés depuis le précédent rapport (Lenoir, Bock et Pujol, 1986). Toutefois les principales données seront résumées avant de prolonger la discussion sur deux points essentiels. Le premier concerne les corrélations anatomiques qui pourraient expliquer la période d'hypersensibilité au trauma acoustique. De fait, il faut à présent tenir compte des développements les plus récents concernant la physiologie cochléaire (mécanismes actifs, neurochimie, . . .) pour compléter ou modifier les hypothèses déjà avancées. Nous nous proposons de discuter particulièrement: (1) une possible immaturité de la synapse entre cellules ciliées internes et fibres auditives, ayant pour conséquence une toxicité accrue aux acides aminés; (2) une fragilité des cellules ciliées externes et des mécanismes actifs avant leur complète maturation; (3) un effet protecteur du système efférent plus faible au cours de cette période que dans l'âge adulte. Le second point concerne la transposition chez l'homme de la période d'hypersensibilité au trauma acoustique. En fait, il existe trop de similarités dans la structure et le développement de la cochlée de la plupart des mammifères, homme y compris, pour que l'on ne puisse pas généraliser la notion de périodes d'hypersensibilité. Dans ces conditions, il doit exister une période de risques accrus pour la cochlée humaine, face au trauma acoustique, au cours du dernier trimestre in utero, ou chez les prématurés. Quelques observations récentes venant à l'appui de cette idée sont discutées.

ACKNOWLEDGMENTS

Thanks are due to W. Lippe and M. Mayat for carefully reviewing the manuscript, to P. Sibleyras for printing the photographs, and to A. Bara for editing.

References

Armitage SE, Baldwin BA, Vince MA. The fetal sound environment of sheep. Science 1980; 208:1173-1174.

Billett TE, Thorne PR, Gavin JB. The nature and progression of injury in the organ of Corti during ischemia. Hear Res 1989; 41:189-198.

Bock GR, Saunders JC. A critical period for acoustic trauma in the hamster and its relation to cochlear development. Science 1977; 197:396-398.

Bock GR, Seifter EJ. Developmental changes in susceptibility to auditory fatigue in young hamsters. Audiology 1978; 17:193-203.

Brownell WE. Microscopic observation of cochlear hair cell motility. Scanning Electr Microsc 1984; 3:1401-1406.

Daniel T, Laciak J. Observations cliniques et expériences concernant l'état de l'appareil cochléo-vestibulaire des sujets exposés au bruit durant la vie foetale. Rev Laryngol 1982; 103:313-318.

Douek E, Dodson HC, Bannister LH, et al. Effects of incubator noise on the cochlea of newborn. Lancet 1976; 20:1110-1113.

Eybalin M Pujol R. A radioautographic study of [^{3}H]L-glutamate and [^{3}H]L-glutamine uptake in the guinea pig cochlea. Neuroscience 1983; 9:863-872.

Eybalin M, Pujol R. Cochlear neuroactive substances. Arch Otorhinolaryngol 1989; 246:228-234.

Falk SA, Cook RO, Haseman JK, Sanders GM. Noise-induced inner ear damage in newborns and adult guinea pigs. Laryngoscope 1974; 84:444-453.

Falk SA, Farmer JC. Incubator noise and possible deafness. Arch Otolaryngol 1973; 97:385-387.

Gerhardt KJ, Abrams RM, Kovaz BM, et al. Intrauterine noise levels produced in pregnant ewes by sound applied to the abdomen. Am J Obstet Gynecol 1988; 159:228-232.

Granier-Deferre C, Lecanuet JP, Cohen H, et al. Feasibility of prenatal hearing test. Acta Otolaryngol (Stockh) Suppl 1985; 421:93-101.

Hawkins JE Jr. Comparative otopathology: Aging, noise, and ototoxic drugs. Adv Otorhinolaryngol 1973; 20:125-141.

Henry K. Cochlear damage resulting from exposure to four different octave bands of noise at three ages. Behav Neurosci 1984a; 98:107-117.

Henry K. Noise and the young mouse: Genotype modifies the sensitive period for effects on cochlear physiology and audiogenic seizures. Behav Neurosci 1984b; 98:1073-1082.

Henry KR, Bowman RE. Acoustic priming of audiogenic seizures. In: Welsch BL, Welch AS, eds. Physiological effects of noise. New York: Plenum Press, 1970:185.

Juiz JM, Rueda J, Merchàn JA, Sala ML. The effects of kainic acid on the cochlear ganglion of the rat. Hear Res 1989; 40:65-74.

Khanna SM, Leonard DGB. Basilar membrane tuning in the cat cochlea. Science 1982; 215:305-306.

Kemp DT. Stimulated acoustic emissions from the human auditory system. J Acoust Soc Am 1978; 64:1386-1391.

Lalande NM, Hétu R, Lambert J. Is occupational noise exposure during pregnancy a risk factor of damage to the auditory system of the fetus? Am J Industr Med 1986; 10:427-435.

Lavigne-Rebillard M, Pujol R. Auditory hair cells in human fetuses: Synaptogenesis and ciliogenesis. J Electron Microsc Techn 1990; 15:115-122.

Lenoir M, Puel J-L. Development of $2F_1$-F_2 otoacoustic emissions in the rat. Hear Res 1987; 29:265-271.

Lenoir M, Pujol R. Sensitive period to acoustic trauma in the rat pup cochlea: Histological findings. Acta Otolaryngol (Stockh) 1980; 89:317-322.

Lenoir M, Bock GR, Pujol R. Supra-normal susceptibility to acoustic trauma in the rat pup cochlea. J Physiol (Paris) 1979; 75:521-524.

Lenoir M, Shnerson A, Pujol R. Cochlear receptor development in the rat with emphasis on synaptogenesis. Anat Embryol 1980; 160:253-262.

Lenoir M, Pujol R, Bock GR. Critical periods of susceptibility to noise-induced hearing loss. In: Salvi RJ, Henderson D, Hamernik RP, Colletti V, eds. Basic and applied aspects of noise-induced hearing loss. New York: Plenum Press, 1986:227.

Mayer ML, Westbrook GL. Cellular mechanisms underlying excitotoxicity. Trends Neurosci 1987; 10:59-61.

Meldrum B. Excitatory amino acids and anoxic/ischaemic brain damage. Trends Neurosci 1985; 8:47-48.

Mountain DC. Changes in endolymphatic potential and crossed olivocochlear bundle stimulation alter cochlear mechanics. Science 1980; 210:71-72.

Price GR. Age as a factor in susceptibility to hearing loss: Young versus adult ears. J Acoust Soc Am 1976; 60:886-892.

Puel J-L, Uziel A. Correlative development of cochlear action potential sensitivity, latency, and frequency selectivity. Dev Brain Res 1987; 37:179-188.

Puel J-L, Rebillard G, Pujol R. Active mechanisms and cochlear efferents. In: Grandori F, Cianfrone G, Hoke M, eds. Advances in Audiology. Basel: Karger, 1990:156-163.

Pujol R. Anatomie et physiologie de la cochlée. Arch Int Physiol Bioch 1989; 97-4, A51-A78.

Pujol R, Lenoir M. The four types of synapses in the organ of Corti. In: Altschuler RA, Bobbin RP, Hoffman DW, eds. Neurobiology of hearing: The cochlea. New York: Raven Press, 1986:161.

Pujol R, Lenoir M, Robertson D, et al. Kainic acid alters auditory dendrites connected with cochlear inner hair cells. Hear Res 1985; 18:145-151.

Pujol R, Rebillard G, Lenoir M, et al. Glutamate neurotoxicity in the cochlea: A possible consequence of ischemic or anoxic conditions occurring in aging. Acta Otolaryngol [Suppl] (Stockh), 1990a; In press.

Pujol R, Lavigne-Rebillard M, Uziel A. Physiological correlates of development of the human cochlea. Semin Perinatol 1990b; 14:275-280.

Pujol R, Sans A. Synaptogenesis in the mammalian inner ear. In: Aslin R, ed. Advances in neural and behavioral development. Norwood, NY: Ablex Press, 1986:18.

Pujol R, Uziel A. Auditory development: Peripheral aspects. In: Timiras PS, Meisami E, eds. Handbook of human growth and development biology. Vol. 1. Boca Raton, FL: CRC Press, 1988:109.

Pujol R. Period of sensitivity to antibiotic treatment in the developing cochlea. Acta Otolaryngol [Suppl] (Stock) 1986; 429:29-33.

Querleu D, Renard X, Boutteville C, Crepin G. Hearing by the fetus? Semin. Perinatol 1989; 13:409-423.

Rajan R, Jonhstone BM. Crossed cochlear influences on monaural temporary threshold shifts. Hear Res 1983; 9:279-294.

Robertson D. Functional significance of dendritic swelling after loud sounds in the guinea pig cochlea. Hear Res 1983; 9:263-278.

Russell IJ, Sellick PM. Intracellular studies of hair cells in the mammalian cochleas. J Physiol (Lond) 1978; 284:261-290.

Santos-Sacchi J. Cochlear physiology. In: Jahn AF, Santos-Sacchi J, eds. Physiology of the ear. New York: Raven Press, 1988:271.

Saunders JC, Bock GR, Chen CS, Gates G. The effects of priming for audiogenic seizures in cochlear and behavioral responses in BALB/c mice. Exp Neurol 1972; 36:426-436.

Sellick PM, Patuzzi R, Johnstone BM. Measurement of basilar membrane motion in guinea pig using the Mössbauer technique. J Acoust Soc Am 1982; 72:131.

Shnerson A, Pujol R. Development: Anatomy, electrophysiology, and behavior. In: Willott JF, ed. The auditory psychobiology of the mouse. Springfield, IL: CC Thomas, 1983:395.

Spoendlin H. Auditory, vestibular, olfactory, and gustatory organs. In: Bischoff A, ed. Ultrastructure of the peripheral nervous system and sense organs. Stuttgart: George Thieme Verlag, 1970:173.

Spoendlin H. Anatomical changes following various noise exposures. In: Henderson D, Hamernik RP, Dosanjh DS, Mills JH, eds. Effects of noise on hearing. New York: Raven Press, 1976:69.

Stanek R, Bock GR, Goran ML, Saunders JC. Age dependent susceptibility to auditory trauma in the hamster: Behavioral and electrophysiologic consequences. Trans Am Acad Ophthalmol Otolaryngol 1977; 84:465-472.

Uziel A. Non-genetic factors affecting hearing development. Acta Otolaryngol [Suppl] (Stockh) 1985; 421:57-61.

Uziel A. Sensitive periods to thyroid hormone in the organ of Corti. Acta Otolaryngol [Suppl] (Stockh) 1986; 429:23-27.

Warr WB, Guinan Jr, JJ. Efferent innervation of the organ of Corti: Two separate systems. Brain Res 1979; 173:152-155.

Willott JF, Henry KR. Auditory evoked potentials: Developmental changes of threshold and amplitude following early acoustic trauma. J Comp Physiol Psychol 1974; 86:1-7.

CHAPTER 18

Regeneration of Hair Cells in the Avian Inner Ear

EDWIN W. RUBEL

Most of this volume deals with parameters affecting noise-induced hearing loss. It is of considerable importance to examine factors such as exposure duration, sound intensity, and age, individually and as they interact. In addition, investigators are providing important new information about the cellular events involved in noise or drug damage to the inner ear. These events seem to involve a constellation of mechanical and chemical events that lead to disruption and phagocytosis of hair cells, as well as varying degrees of support cell disruption and ganglion cell loss. Understanding relationships between the physical parameters of sound and the degree of sensorineural damage may allow prediction and prevention of damage due to noise exposure. Understanding the mechanical and chemical events underlying receptor damage from noise exposure may lead to methods for protection or early treatment that will prevent or retard the deleterious effects.

Conversely, it is safe to assume that damage to the inner ear through exposure to noise, environmental chemical toxins, medications, and disease will continue to cause hearing and balance disorders in millions of people each year. An ultimate objective, therefore, would be to develop methods to replace lost receptor elements through transplantation or regeneration. This chapter deals with recent studies on regeneration of hair cells in the avian inner ear.

The potential for vertebrate hair cells to proliferate and differentiate throughout life has been recognized for over 50 years (Corwin et al., 1989). For example Stone (1933; 1937) studied regeneration of lateral line organs following tail amputation in amphibian embryos. He found that regenerated organs were numerically similar to the previous complement and that they were supplied by migration of precursor cells from the last organ of the proximal tail stump. More recently, a number of groups have investigated both continued production of hair cells in the saccule of rays and fishes as well as regeneration of hair cells in the lateral line of amphibians (Corwin, 1983; Corwin et al., 1989; Presson and Popper, 1990a,b).

Until recently, however, it was generally accepted that postembryonic production of hair cells is limited to cold-blooded vertebrates, as is the ability to restore damaged populations of hair cells. That is, birds and mammals have lost this ability during evolution. In both birds and mammals, the hair cells that will normally populate the inner ear are produced relatively early in embryogenesis (Ruben, 1967). Although some mitotic activity may continue after this time, the new cells were not thought to differentiate into hair cells. Recent studies on birds have suggested that we must re-evaluate these assumptions.

Initial Experiments

Two serendipitous findings suggested that birds were able to restore the population of hair cells following elimination of embryonically produced hair cells due to ototoxic drugs or noise exposure. Raul Cruz (Cruz et al., 1987) performed an experiment intended to examine the time course of aminoglycoside destruction of hair cells in the chick. Cruz gave a large group of neonatal chicks a 50 mg/kg injection of gentamicin each day for 10 days. Experimental and vehicle-injected control animals were allowed to survive varying amounts of time ranging from 1 day to 32 days. Earlier studies in our laboratory (Johns et al., 1980) demonstrated that when animals were given this injection regimen and allowed to survive for 40 days, hair cell loss was evident throughout the basal two-thirds of the cochlea. In the Cruz et al. study, the cochleas were serially sectioned and the number of hair cells was counted at 100 μm intervals from the base to the apex. Hair cell counts revealed that after the ten day aminoglycoside treatment there was a nearly total elimination of hair cells in the basal one-third of the cochlea. A week later the damage had spread to eliminate a majority of the hair cells throughout the basal two-thirds of the cochlea, but counts at the basal pole revealed that the number of hair cells had been partially restored. After another 2 weeks, the number of hair cells throughout the basal two-thirds of the cochlea appeared to be recovering toward normal.

While these data strongly suggested that new hair cells were being produced to replace those destroyed by the aminoglycoside treatment, other interpretations were possible. For example, it was possible that the aminoglycosides caused deterioration or dedifferentiation of hair cells to the extent that they were unrecognizable in the microscopic sections, and then recovery ensued. Even if new hair cells were taking the place of embryonically produced cells that had been destroyed by the drug, we could not conclude that this was due to the production of new cells. Instead, it was possible that the aminoglycosides or the resulting damage induced support cells differentiate into new hair cells. In other receptor organs, such as taste buds, there is continual replacement of receptors by so-called support cells.

While Cruz was counting hair cells following aminoglycoside ototoxicity, Cotanche (1987a) was examining the neonatal chick cochlea by scanning electron microscopy following acoustic trauma. Although the initial purpose of these studies was to examine age differences in the position of damage produced by overstimulation (Rubel and Ryals, 1983; Ryals and Rubel, 1985; Lippe and Rubel, 1983, 1985), Cotanche also noted the repopulation of hair cells a few days following noise damage. Again, this observation is open to several interpretations including both cell regeneration and recovery of stereocilia. Cotanche made two additional important observations: the apical surfaces of the cells that appeared to be repopulating the cochlea bore a striking resemblance to immature hair cells, and the sequence of differentiation paralleled the embryology of stereocilia.

Taken together, these two studies (Cruz et al., 1987; Cotanche, 1987a) suggested that the restoration of hair cells was not due to recovery, but represented newly created hair cells or transformed support cells. Three studies then used tritiated thymidine (^{3}H thymidine) to label mitotically active cells in the inner ear of postnatal birds in order to prove that new hair cells were being produced. This method makes use of the fact that the nucleic acid, thymidine, is incorporated into DNA during the S-phase of mitosis. It then remains in the nucleus throughout the life of the cell. If an abundance of radioactive thymidine is introduced into the environment of mitotically active cells during S-phase, all progeny become radioactively labeled. With successive cell divisions in the absence of radioactive thymidine, the "label" is serially diluted. However, if the radioactive thymidine is present during the final cell division, both daughter cells will be strongly radioactive. This method is commonly used to study the "birth date" of cells, the time that cells leave the mitotic cycle (Sidman, 1970). By following treatments of ^{3}H thymidine with an abundance of nonradioactive ("cold") thymidine, it is possible to label cells that are produced during a restricted period of time. This method is commonly referred to as "pulse labelling." Cells labelled by ^{3}H thymidine can be identified at any subsequent time by histologic tissue processing and autoradiography. Reduced silver grains in the photographic emulsion overlying the nucleus of labelled cells are an indication that the stem cell was undergoing mitosis while the ^{3}H thymidine was available for incorporation.

Using this method, Corwin and Cotanche (1988) and Ryals and Rubel (1988) demonstrated that damage to the avian cochlea causes a population of stem cells to re-enter the mitotic cycle and produce new cells, which subsequently differentiate into new hair cells as well as new support cells. Corwin and Cotanche used intense sound to destroy receptors in the cochlea of neonatal chicks. Tritiated thymidine was infused into the animals for 7 days postexposure by means of an osmotic pump. The cochleas were then processed for autoradiography. Both labelled hair cells and labelled support cells were observed. In a parallel study (Ryals and Rubel, 1988), we exposed young, sexually mature quail (*Coturnix*) to an intense, pure tone (1500 Hz) to destroy hair cells in the middle region of the cochlea. One group of animals was given two daily injections of ^{3}H thymidine over the ensuing 10 days. The remaining animals were

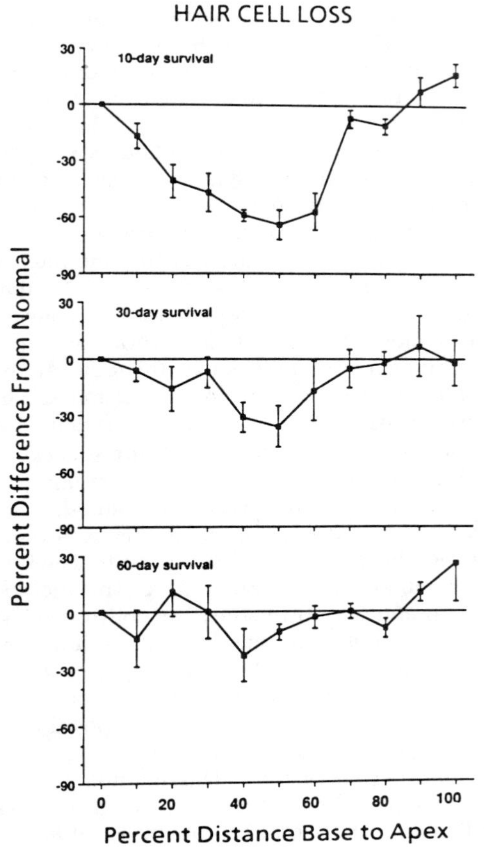

Figure 18-1 Regeneration of quail hair cells. The mean percentage difference in hair cell number as compared to normal controls ($n = 6$), after acoustic trauma for *(A)*, 10-day, *(B)*, 30-day, and *(C)*, 60-day survival times. Normal hair cell number in controls is shown by a straight line at 0 along the cochlea from base to apex. Average percentage difference in hair cells from normal (± 1 SEM) is shown in 10 percent intervals along the cochlea from base to apex at each survival time (n = 6, 5, and 3 for 10-day, 30-day, and 60-day survival, respectively). (From Ryals BM, Rubel EW. Hair cell regeneration after acoustic trauma in adult *Coturnix* quail. Science 1988; 240:1774-1776.)

allowed to survive for either 10, 30, or 60 days. Figure 18-1 shows the percent reduction in hair cell number (compared to control cochleas) as a function of position along the cochlea. Ten days after the noise damage there is a massive reduction in the basal half of the cochlea. During the ensuing 50 days, the population of hair cells is restored to near normal numbers.

The animals treated with tritiated thymidine provide convincing evidence that the repopulation of hair cells is due to the production and differentiation of a new generation of cells. Both support cells and hair cells were labelled by the ^{3}H thymidine (Fig. 18-2). In control animals, which were not exposed to the pure tone but were given the 10 days of thymidine injections, no labelled hair cells or support cells were found.

The studies by Corwin and Cotanche (1988) and Ryals and Rubel (1988) indicate that, in both neonatal and mature precocial birds, damage to the cochlea induces a "quiescent" population of precursor cells to re-enter the mitotic cycle. Newly produced cells can then differentiate into either hair cells or support cells. Jorgensen and Mathiesen (1988) also reported on the production of new hair cells in the postembryonic inner ear of birds. In this case, normal, adult budgerigars were labelled with ^{3}H thymidine, following which the vestibular epithelia were sectioned and processed for autoradiography. Scattered labelled hair cells and support cells were seen in each receptor epithelia. This result, which we have recently replicated in neonatal chicks (Roberson et al, 1989), indicates that there is a low level of continual turnover of vestibular hair cells.

In summary, it has become clear that the *assumption* that birds and mammals cannot restore hair cells lost due to injury is wrong. Both young and adult birds can regenerate new hair cells to repopulate areas damaged by aminoglycosides or noise, and the avian vestibular epithelium appears to slowly replace hair cells throughout life. It appears that this property was lost during evolution of the mammalian inner ear. We have begun to address a number of issues that may lead to further understanding of the process of hair cell regeneration in birds in the hope that the answers will suggest methods to induce this ability in mammals, including man.

Identity of the Precursor Population

One of the foremost questions is the identification of the cellular population or populations that re-enter the mitotic cycle and produce new hair cells. This issue has been elegantly addressed by Corwin et al (1989) in the axolotl lateral line where it was confirmed that support cells lying at the periphery of the receptor organ are the progenitors of new hair cells. This system is advantageous because it lies on the periphery of the organism and therefore can be directly observed. In the inner ear we are not so fortunate. The situation is complicated by the fact that there are a

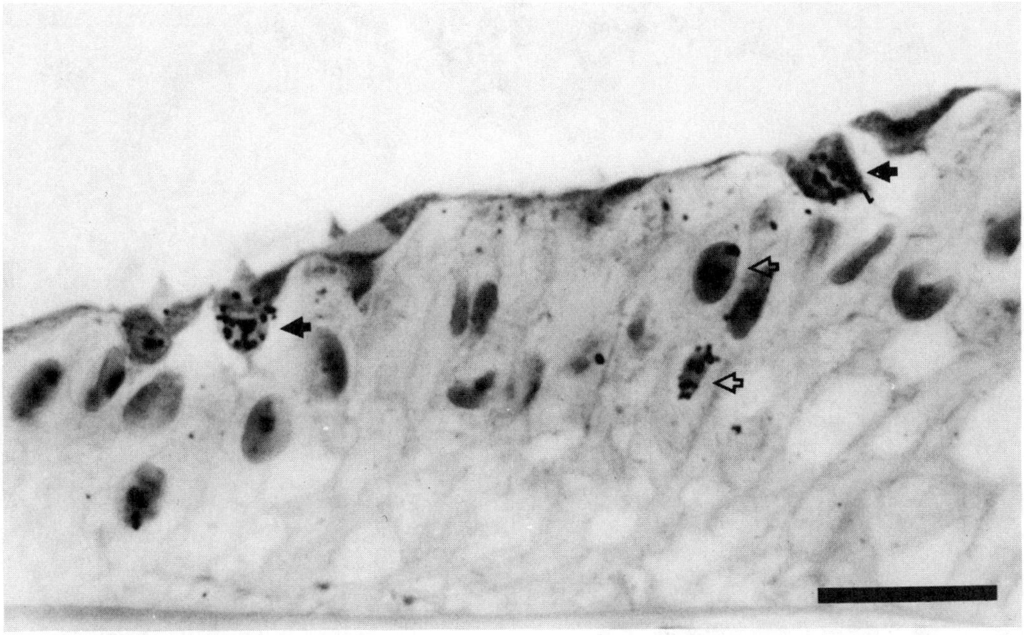

Figure 18-2 ^{3}H thymidine-labelled quail hair cells and support cell 10 days after acoustic trauma. Bar = 20 μm. (From Ryals BM, Rubel EW. Hair cell regeneration after acoustic trauma in adult *Coturnix* quail. Science 1988; 240:1774-1776.)

large number of support cell types in the vicinity of the avian basilar membrane (Takasaka and Smith, 1971).

A tangential section of the avian cochlea is shown in Figure 18-3. Likely precursors are the following:

1. Remaining hair cells that could dedifferentiate and become mitotically active.
2. Support cells whose nuclei lie underneath the hair cells and extend apical processes to the lumen, surrounding the apical surface of each hair cell or other support cells in this area that have not been characterized.
3. Epithelial cell populations that lie either toward the neural or abneural borders of the hair cell populations.
4. An unidentified stem cell population whose progeny migrate into the receptor epithelium.

The first experiment to address this issue (Girod et al., 1989) involved determining the first cells that become mitotically active following damage and attempting to follow the fate of their progeny. The design of this experiment is shown in Figure 18-4. Neonatal chicks were exposed to a 120 dB, 1500 Hz pure tone for 18 hours. Beginning either during the tone exposure (after 12 hours) or immediately after the tone exposure, the animals began receiving injections of ^{3}H thymidine. One group was given an abundance of "cold" thymidine following three days of ^{3}H thymidine. The remaining animals were sacrificed at various times during ^{3}H thymidine treatment, ranging from 6 hours to 3 days following noise exposure. One cochlea from each animal was processed for autoradiography; the other was examined by scanning electron microscopy (SEM).

Figure 18-5 shows the appearance of the receptor epithelium 6 hours following the noise exposure. The epithelium is severely damaged; it has pulled away from the basilar membrane and most of the short hair cells are extruded. At this time, no cells in the vicinity of the receptor epithelium are labelled. An occasional cell in the nerve fiber bundle is labelled and a few nuclei of tympanic border cells, lying under the basilar membrane, are labelled. By 15 or 24 hours after noise exposure, the undifferentiated epithelial cells lying at the inferior edge of the receptor epithelium have spread out and are rapidly proliferating (Fig. 18-6). As these cells continue to proliferate (Fig. 18-7, *A*), the single cell lamina is transformed to two to three cells deep and labelled nuclei are abundant. At this time, a few cells can already be recognized as immature hair cells because their apical tips contact the lumen and are beginning to develop immature

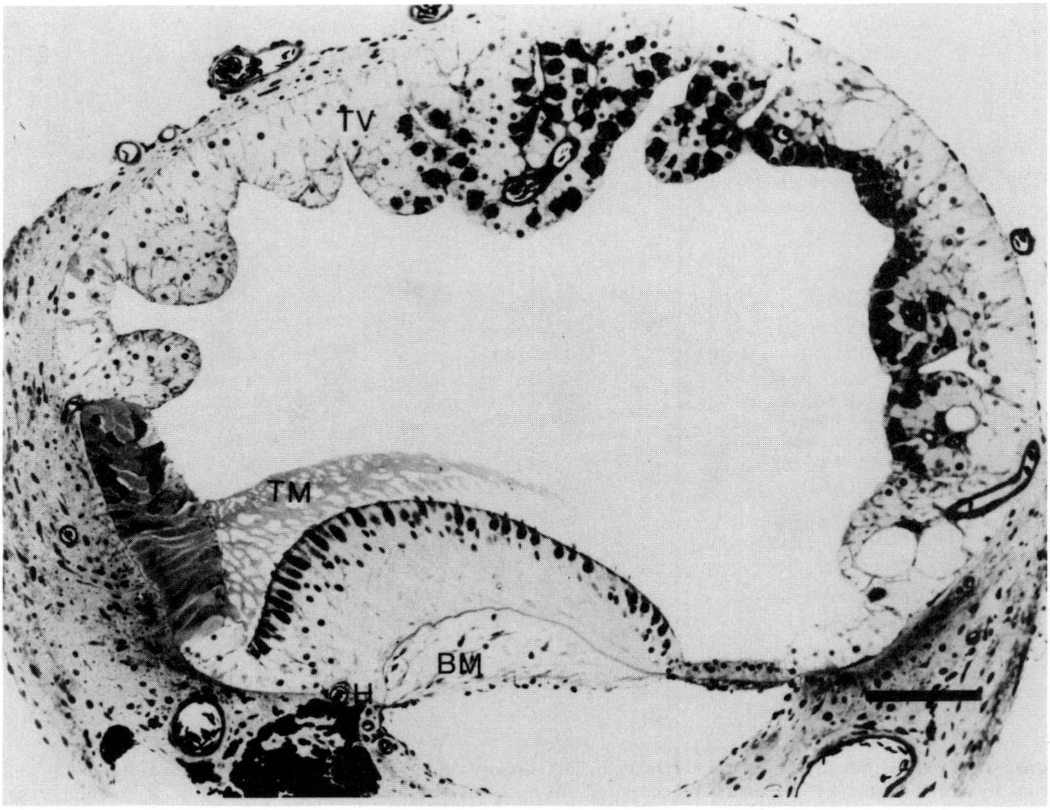

Figure 18-3 Transverse section through basilar papilla (approximately 3.3 mm from proximal tip) in a normal 40-day-old chicken. At this point, tall hair cells predominate the width of the basilar membrane. TV = tegmentum vasculosum, BM = basilar membrane. H = habenula, TM = tectorial membrane. Bar indicates 100 μm. (From Rubel BM, Ryals EW. Patterns of hair cell loss in chick basilar papilla after intense auditory stimulation: Exposure duration and survival time. Acta Otolaryngol 1982; 93:31-41.)

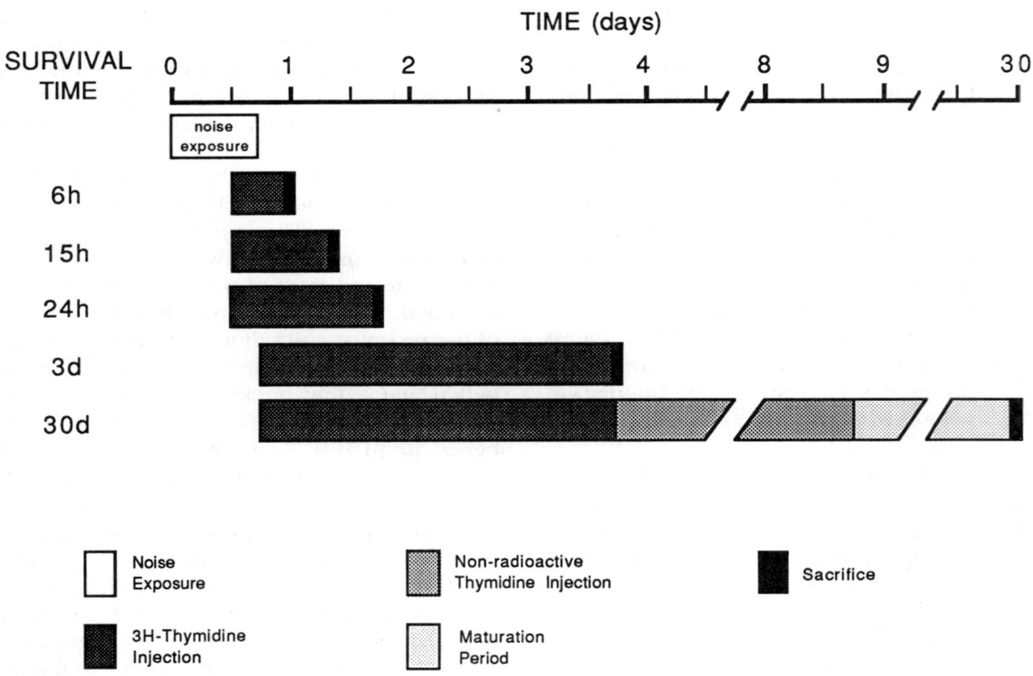

Figure 18-4 Schematic representation of the experimental design for "pulse labelling" experiment. The animals were divided into five subgroups based on survival time following the completion of the noise exposure. Tritiated thymidine labeling was initiated 12 hours into the noise exposure for the early survival groups (≤24 hours) and on completion of the noise exposure for the longer survival groups (≥3 days). N = 4 in each group. (From Girod DA, Duckert LG, Rubel EW. Possible precursors of regenerated hair cells in the avian cochlea following acoustic trauma. Hear Res 1989; 42:175-194.)

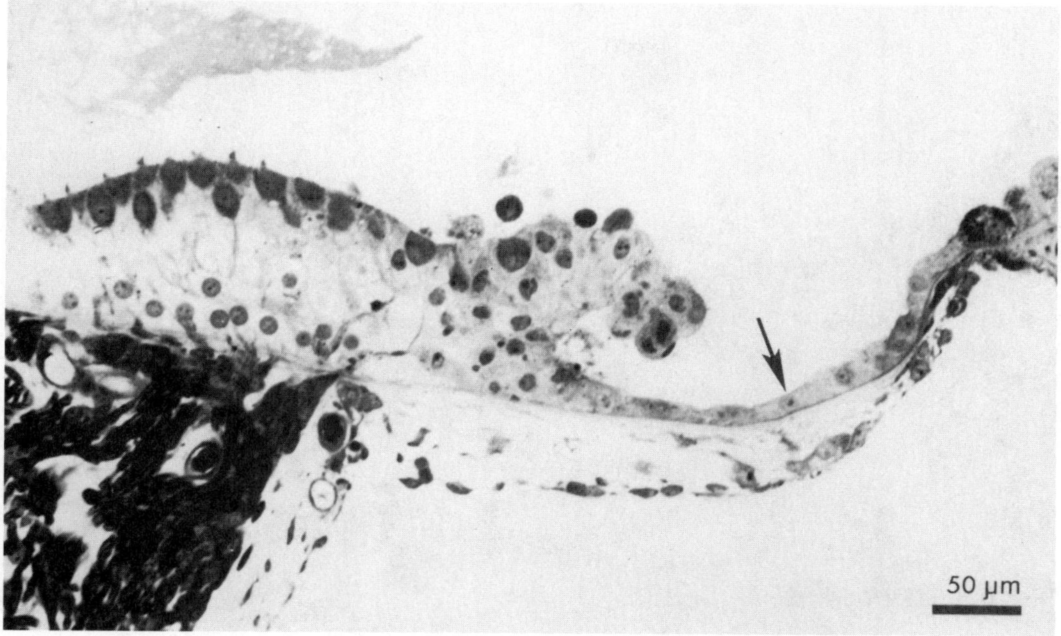

Figure 18-5 Transverse light microscopic sections through the 1500 Hz region of the chick cochlea 6 hours after completion of noise exposure, demonstrating extensive hair cell and supporting cell loss at the inferior edge of the sensory epithelium. Note the thin monolayer of cells spreading to cover the basilar membrane (arrow). (From Girod DA, Duckert LG, Rubel EW. Possible precursors of regenerated hair cells in the avian cochlea following acoustic trauma. Hear Res 1989; 42:175-194.)

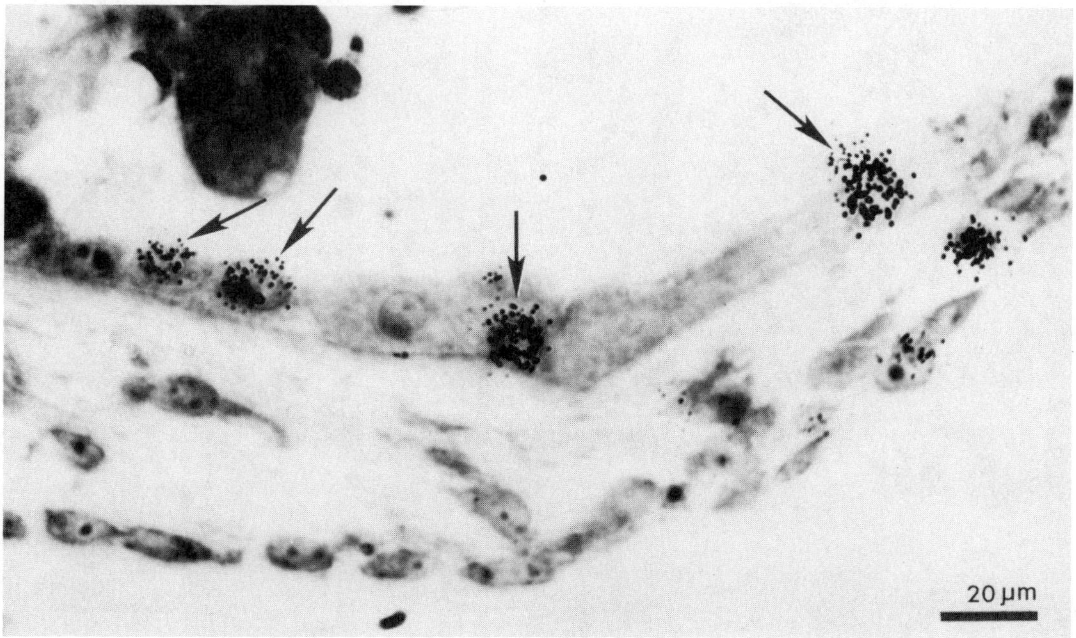

Figure 18-6 Inferior border of the sensory epithelium in the 1500 Hz region of experimental cochleae, 15-hour survival. Labeled nuclei (arrows) indicating mitosis within the cellular monolayer. (From Girod DA, Duckert LG, Rubel EW. Possible precursors of regenerated hair cells in the avian cochlea following acoustic trauma. Hear Res 1989; 42:175-194.)

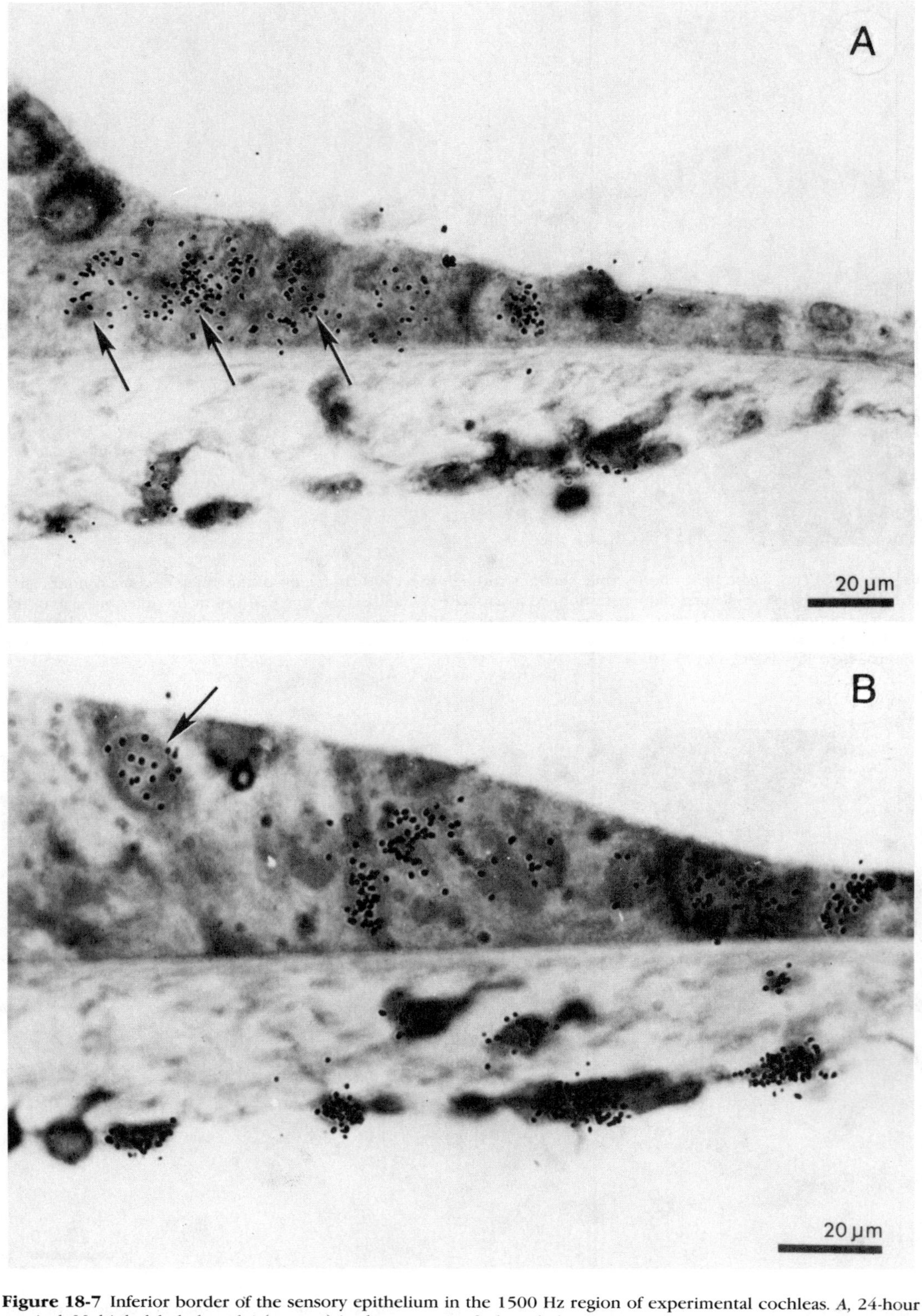

Figure 18-7 Inferior border of the sensory epithelium in the 1500 Hz region of experimental cochleas. *A*, 24-hour survival. Multiple labeled nuclei (arrows) in the now stratified epithelium covering the basilar membrane. *B*, 3-day survival after inferior hair cell loss. Labelled regenerated hair cell (arrow) with lightly staining cytoplasm and a large round nucleus adjacent to the region of active proliferation. Plane of focus is on the overlying silver grains putting the cells partially out of focus. (From Girod DA, Duckert LG, Rubel EW. Possible precursors of regenerated hair cells in the avian cochlea following acoustic trauma. Hear Res 1989; 42:175-194.)

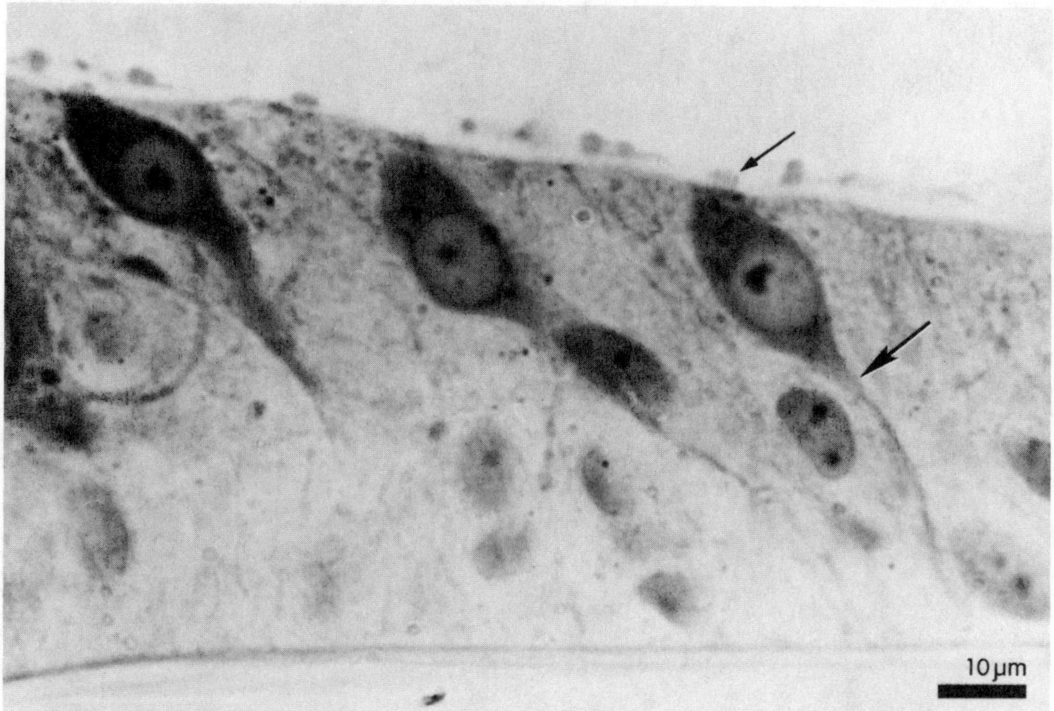

Figure 18-8 Immature regenerated chick hair cells seen 3 days after noise exposure. Plane of focus is now on the cells and not on the overlying silver grains. The regenerated hair cells have a unique appearance including a tall spindle-shaped cell body with lightly stained cytoplasm, a large, round nucleus, and very short stereocilia (small arrow). Processes seen at the cell bases are probably trailing cytoplasmic processes showing the path of migration from the basilar membrane to the lumen (large arrow). (From Girod DA, Duckert LG, Rubel EW. Possible precursors of regenerated hair cells in the avian cochlea following acoustic trauma. Hear Res 1989; 42:175-194.)

stereocilia. Three days following noise exposure (Fig. 18-7, *B*), most of the cellular debris from dying and extruded cells has been cleared. Now many labelled new hair cells as well as support cells can be observed toward the inferior side of the receptor epithelium. The new hair cells are easily recognized by the staining characteristics of their cytoplasm, a thin apical process extending to the lumen already bearing a tuft of immature cilia, and a basal process extending down toward or to the basilar membrane (Figs. 18-7, *B* and 18-8). In scanning electron microscopy (Fig. 18-9), the tips of immature stereocilia are clearly recognized.

The labelled hair cells shown in Figure 18-10 were proliferated during the 3 days following noise damage (30-day group). At the light microscope level they cannot be distinguished from normal hair cells. In addition, when viewed by SEM (Fig. 18-11), the mosaic pattern of hair cells is largely restored. It is not normal, however; persistent defects are observed and the apical surfaces of hair cells in the repopulated area appear larger, suggesting that the total complement of hair cells has not been fully restored. Marsh et al (1990) have measured the packing density and apical surface areas of hair cells in the repopulated area and confirmed these observations.

The picture that emerges from studies of the inferior region after noise damage is summarized in Figure 18-12. Initially, support cells near the inferior margin of the receptor epithelium spread out to cover the area of the basilar membrane that has been damaged. This process seems to involve changes in the shape of the border cells, hyaline cells, and possibly, cuboidal cells. This epithelial covering of the basilar membrane is seen as early as we have examined the tissue, at the end of the 18 hours of sound exposure. We assume that proliferation of epithelial cells is not involved in this process because no ^{3}H thymidine labelling is seen in this region until 15 hours after the sound exposure.

The next phase involves rapid proliferation of this epithelial layer that begins between 6 and 15 hours following exposure. These new cells appear to form a pseudostrat-

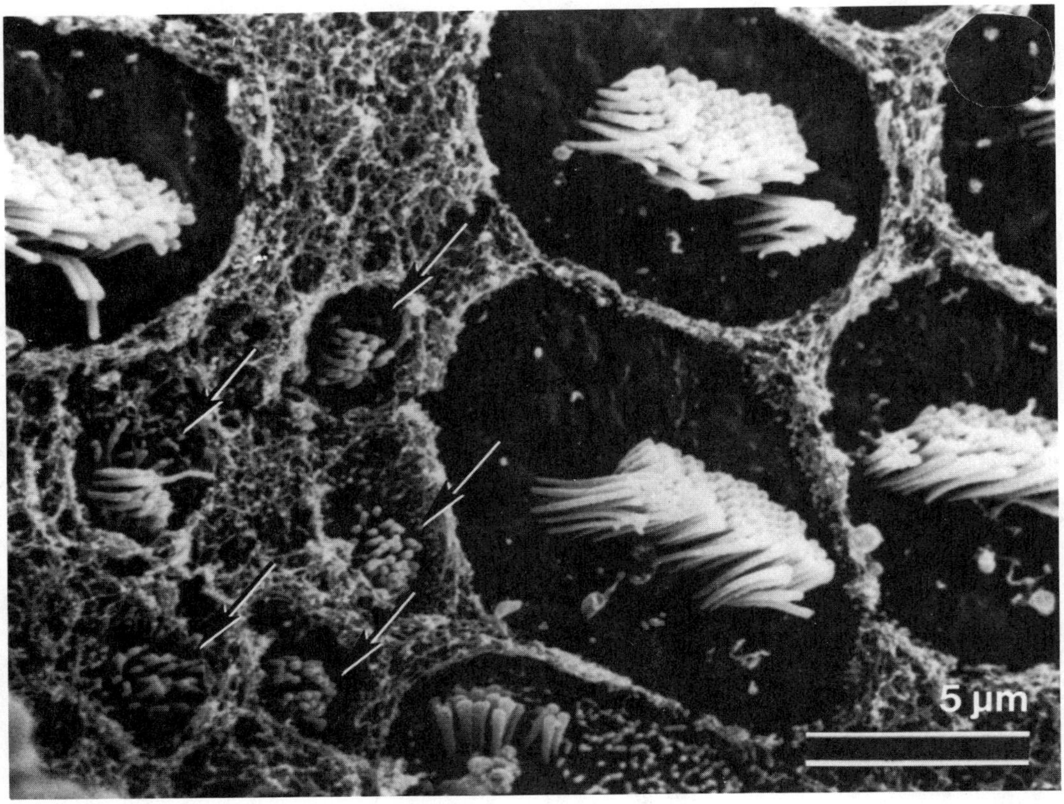

Figure 18-9 Scanning electron micrograph of the sensory epithelium in the 1500 Hz region of the chick cochlea at 3-day survival. Contrast the stereocilia of newly regenerating hair cells (arrows) to the adjacent mature hair cell. (From Girod DA, Duckert LG, Rubel EW. Possible precursors of regenerated hair cells in the avian cochlea following acoustic trauma. Hear Res 1989; 42:175-194.)

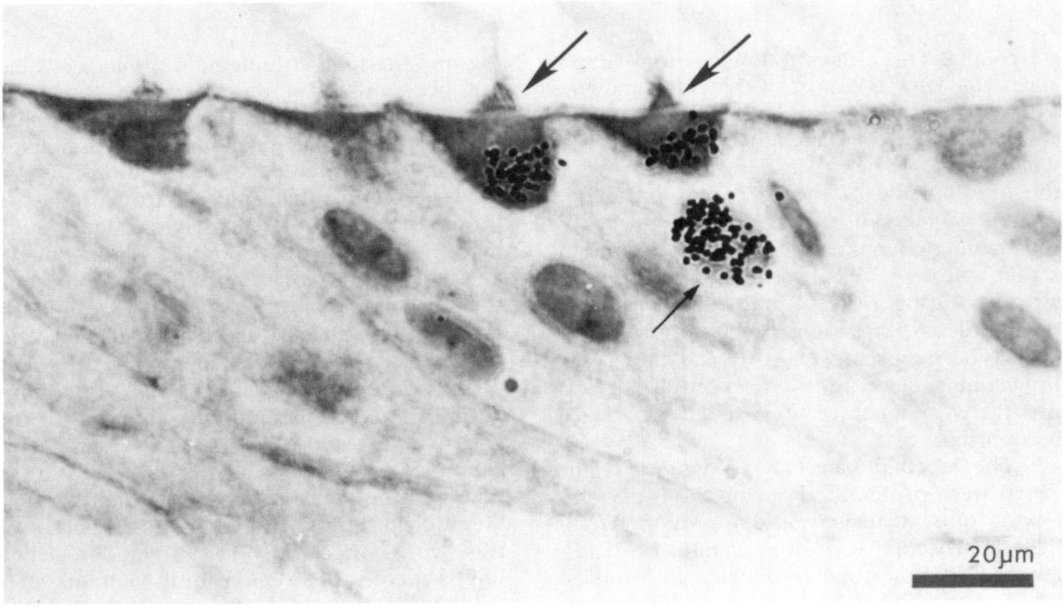

Figure 18-10 Superior portion of the sensory epithelium in the 1500 Hz region of experimental cochleas. 30-day survival. Labelled regenerated short hair cells (small arrows) are indistinguishable from adjacent non-labelled hair cells. Labelled mature supporting cell (large arrow) underneath labelled hair cells. There is no evidence of residual damage. Bar = 10 µm. (From Girod DA, Duckert LG, Rubel EW. Possible precursors of regenerated hair cells in the avian cochlea following acoustic trauma. Hear Res 1989; 42:175-194.)

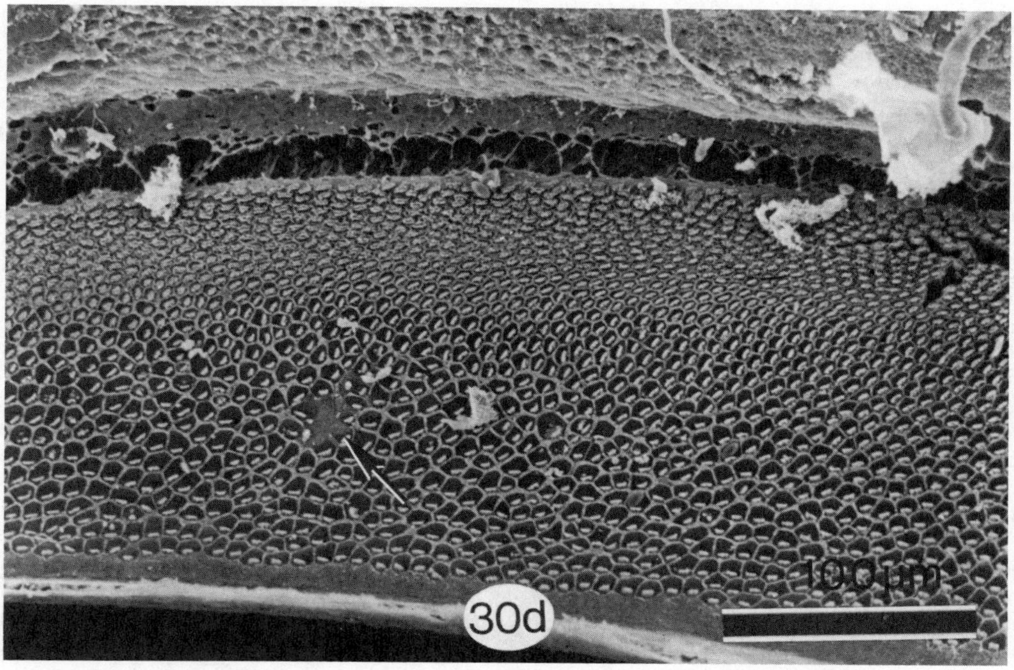

Figure 18-11 Scanning electron micrograph of the sensory epithelium in the 1500 Hz region of the chick cochlea at 30-day survival. Note the mild disorganization of the normal hair cell mosaic pattern and the very small residual scar (arrow). (From Girod DA, Duckert LG, Rubel EW. Possible precursors of regenerated hair cells in the avian cochlea following acoustic trauma. Hear Res 1989; 42:175-194.)

Figure 18-12 Schematic representation of the proposed phases of regeneration of the inferior sensory epithelium following noise exposure. Normal (pre-exposure) border, hyaline, and cuboidal epithelial cells are shown on the inferior basilar membrane at the left. The superior normal sensory epithelium is to the right. Time after noise exposure is on the X axis. Phase I: Migration of border cells or hyaline cells or cuboidal cells to cover basilar membrane exposed by lost hair cells and supporting cells. Phase II: Proliferation of border cells to increase cell number. Phase III: Differentiation of proliferating cells into hair cells and supporting cells. Phase IV: Maturation of the regenerated sensory epithelium. (Modified from Girod DA, Duckert LG, Rubel EW. Possible precursors of regenerated hair cells in the avian cochlea following acoustic trauma. Hear Res 1989; 42:175-194.)

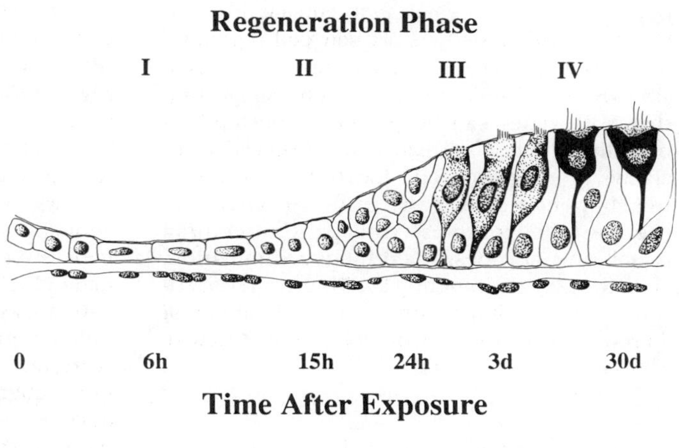

ified epithelium and may show nuclear translocation from the basilar membrane to the lumen during mitosis (Presson and Popper, 1990a). As cells leave the mitotic cycle, the epithelium thickens and a portion of the cells rapidly begin to differentiate into hair cells. The incipient hair cells can be recognized as they migrate toward the lumen by their relatively greater cytoplasmic staining density, which is associated more with organelles than with surrounding support cells. After the apical tip of the differentiating hair cell contacts the luminal surface, specializations begin to appear. These specializations include small microvilli, immature stereocilia, and condensation of actin filaments into a cuticular plate (see later). These and other surface modifications have been described in detail by others (Cotanche, 1987a; Cotanche and Corwin, 1990; Marsh et al., 1990). During the next 30 days, the new hair cells mature to the point that they are indistinguishable (except for ^{3}H thymidine labelling) from normal hair cells in that part of the cochlea. As discussed later in this chapter, even such individualized and specialized features as number and height of stereocilia appear to be replicated in the postembryonically produced hair cells, suggesting that whatever factors regulate these gradients in the embryo persist into adulthood or also emerge from the damaged epithelium.

In a few cases we have observed hair cell loss limited to a strip of cells lying at the junction between short hair cells and long hair cells (Cotanche et al., 1987). In these cases, we have not observed proliferation of the border or hyaline cells, suggesting that another cell population is generating the new hair cells. We have not yet identified this progenitor population; it could be the support cells suggested by Corwin and Cotanche (1988) or a population of stem cells that has heretofore remained unrecognized.

Because most of the damaged animals that have been studied with radioactive thymidine have sustained short hair cell damage, it is not surprising that mostly short hair cell regeneration has been seen. We have, however, occasionally seen labelled tall hair cells, suggesting that both types can be produced postembryonically. The few tall hair cells observed were always at an appropriate location, superior to the short hair cells. Early in the regeneration process following noise damage, the tectorial membrane, also destroyed by overstimulation, is re-formed (Cotanche, 1987b). Its reconstitution may be important for the alignment of stereocilia bundles (Cotanche and Corwin, 1990).

Do Regenerated Hair Cells Restore Hearing?

The ability of regenerated hair cells to restore hearing after sensorineural damage is of obvious importance. This issue has been difficult to evaluate following noise damage for two reasons. First, high intensity noise exposure severely disrupts the integrity of the tectorial membrane (TM) (Cotanche, 1987b). Reconstitution of the TM and its interaction with the surviving hair cells precedes maturation of the regenerated hair cells and appears correlated with evoked response threshold recovery (McFadden and Saunders, 1989). Second, in addition to loss and regeneration of hair cells and TM, there are likely to be a variety of other changes that complicate making direct structure-function correlations. For example, Ryals et al (1990) have shown continuing loss of ganglion cells for several weeks following noise trauma even though hair cells are regenerating. Thus, there is likely to be continual remodeling of synaptic connections in the inner ear during this period. Finally, we have not observed noise damage that ever produces complete loss of hair cells in any part of the cochlea. Although the site of lesion can be made quite specific by using pure tone exposure (Ryals and Rubel, 1982; Rubel and Ryals, 1982), some hair cells always remain in the injured area. Thus, the extent to which the remaining, presumably injured, hair cells are responsible for restoration of hearing, as opposed to new hair cells, is difficult to determine.

To avoid some of these problems we have examined functional recovery primarily in animals treated with aminoglycosides. After 5 days of aminoglycoside treatment at the dosage of gentamicin we typically use (50 mg/kg body wt/day), there is virtually complete loss of both tall and short hair cells in the basal 25 percent of the cochlea. Thus, in this region, recovery of function *must* be due, in part, to regenerated hair cells. Furthermore, as will be apparent below, the protracted time course of hair cell loss and recovery has allowed some structure/function correlations to be made.

We have undertaken two experiments aimed at revealing functional properties of regenerated hair cells. In both experiments neonatal chicks were given 10 days of gentamicin (50 mg/kg/day). Control animals were given either vehicle injection or no injections, but were matched for age. In the first experiment, one subgroup of animals was tested after 5 days of aminoglycoside. The other groups were tested either after 10 days of aminoglycoside injections or were allowed to survive 1 to 24 weeks with no further manipulations.

In the first study (Tucci and Rubel, 1990), evoked potential thresholds were determined by recording from electrodes implanted in the brainstem in a region near the cochlear nuclei. Short tone bursts ranging in frequency from .250 kHz to 5 kHz were used as the stimuli and separate groups of 8 to 16 chickens were

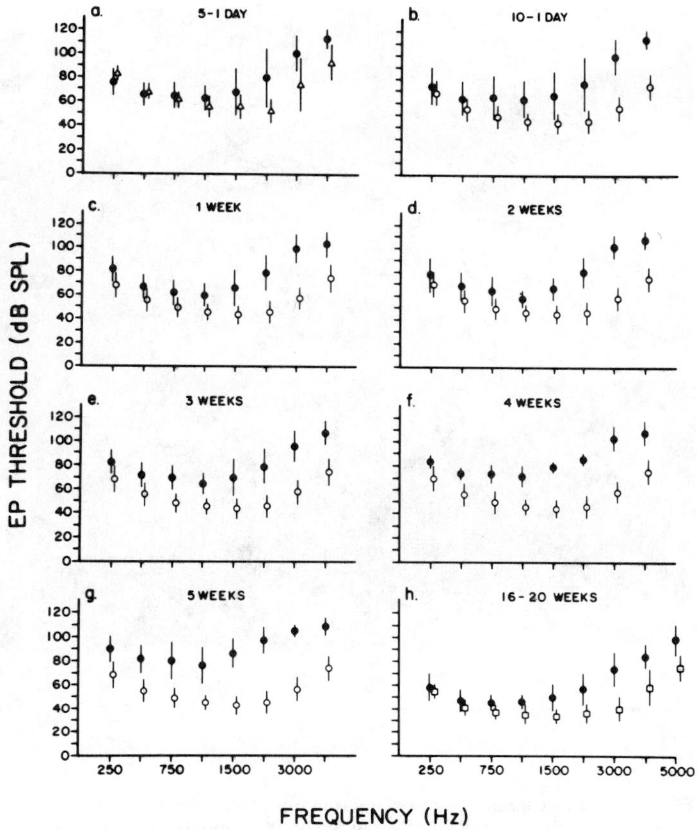

Figure 18-13 Evoked potential thresholds in dB SPL, mean (± one standard deviation), for experimental (filled circles) and control (open symbols) animals at the survival intervals indicated following gentamicin treatment. (From Tucci DL, Rubel EW. Physiological status of regenerated hair cells in the avian inner ear following aminoglycoside ototoxicity. Otolaryngol Head Neck Surg 1990; 103:443-450.)

studied at the following survival times: 5 days of aminoglycoside treatment plus 1 day recovery; 10 days aminoglycoside plus recovery times of 1 day, 1 week, 2 weeks, 3 weeks, 4 weeks, 5 weeks, and 16 to 20 weeks. Gentamicin injections were begun on the day of birth. Thus, separate age-matched control groups (n = 5 per group) were also examined for comparison with each of the experimental groups. In addition to the electrophysiologic experiments, a cohort of animals (three to four) from selected groups was used for morphologic analyses. One ear of these animals was processed for scanning electron microscopy (SEM) and the other ear was studied by transmission electron microscopy (TEM). The SEM studies allow for comparison of the patterns of hair cell loss, and then recovery, with the electrophysiologic results (Girod et al., 1990); the TEM studies (Duckert and Rubel, 1990) allow the study of ultrastructural properties of regenerated hair cells and their associated neural elements.

Figure 18-13 summarizes the results of our electrophysiologic studies. Each panel of this figure shows the mean evoked-potential thresholds as a function of stimulus frequency for gentamicin treated and control chicks at the survival times indicated. Panels a and b show data from animals 1 day after 5 days or 10 days of aminoglycoside treatment, respectively. At these early times, significant hearing loss is restricted to frequencies above 1.5 kHz. The evoked-potential threshold elevation ranges between 10 dB in the mid frequencies to 25 dB at high frequencies. At these times, hair cell loss appears restricted to the basal (proximal) 20 to 30 percent of the cochlea. In fact, the basal 20 percent is nearly entirely devoid of mature hair cells at this time (Fig. 18-14).

The results shown in Figure 18-13, *A* (5 days of gentamicin) are somewhat surprising. At this time there is essentially complete loss of hair cells in the basal 20 percent of the cochlea and the remaining 80 percent *appears* essentially normal in SEM. In contrast, the hearing loss is relatively mild (10 to 15 dB) at the high frequencies and extends down to the mid frequencies (2 kHz). The pattern of hair cell damage seen in SEM might be expected to produce greater threshold shift at high frequencies and a more restricted frequency range of threshold shift. Two explanations appear likely. First, evoked potentials to short

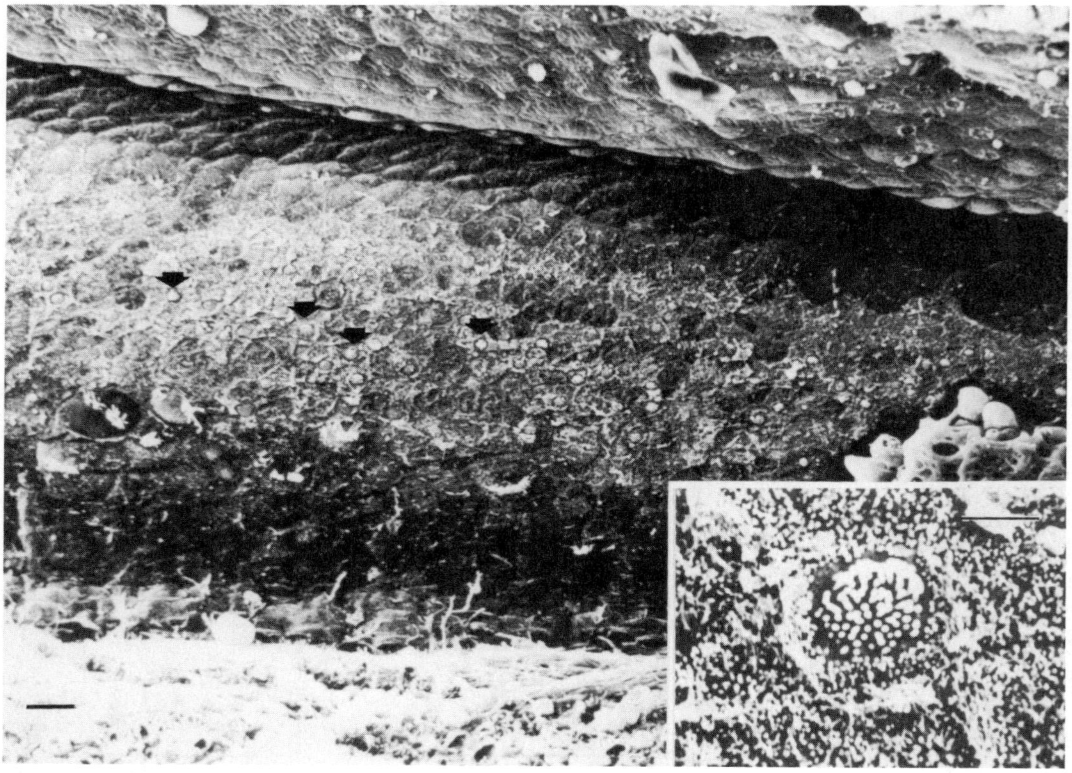

Figure 18-14 Scanning electron micrograph of proximal (basal) portion of the basilar papilla, approximately 400 microns from the tip, 1 day following 5 days of aminoglycoside treatment. Newly erupted hair cells are identified by stereocilia tufts (arrows). Bar = 10 μm. *Insert:* Higher magnification scanning electron photomicrograph of newly regenerated hair cell identified by sensory hair tuft. Bar = 2 μm. (From Duckert LG, Rubel EW. Ultrastructural observations on regenerating hair cells in the chick basilar papilla. Hear Res 1990; 48:161-182.)

tone bursts do not provide particularly "place-specific" information about the site of cochlear damage. Second, the aminoglycoside treatment has probably caused damage to the intact hair cells that is not apparent in our SEM observation. It is important to remember that the presence of hair cells with intact stereocilia cannot be taken as evidence that they are metabolically and functionally normal.

By 4 to 5 weeks after the aminoglycoside treatment (Fig. 18-13, *F* and *G*), significant evoked potential threshold shifts are seen throughout the frequency range examined. The hearing loss at low frequencies (under 1.5 kHz) averages 20 to 25 dB, but at higher frequencies it tends to be greater (35 to 50 dB).

The pattern of hair cell morphology seen by SEM, although complex, is consistent with the functional data. In the basal region of the cochlea, some hair cell regeneration has occurred, but the stereocilia orientation is in disarray. In addition, many hair cells appear damaged and the others appear immature. It is entirely possible that the process of hair cell loss and recovery is still occurring. The damaged region has now spread to include all but the apical pole of the cochlea by this time. Throughout this region large patches devoid of hair cells are observed intermixed with degenerating hair cells immature regenerating hair cells, and normal-appearing hair cells (Fig. 18-15).

In this study, the next time points examined were 16 and 20 weeks after the aminoglycoside treatment (Fig. 18-13, *H*). The results were similar and are combined in the figure, but inspection of the raw data reveals that the recovery process is still occurring; the 20-week animals show slightly, but consistently, lower thresholds than the 16-week animals. In both groups, it is apparent that considerable functional recovery has occurred. Once again, significant hearing loss is restricted to high frequencies. Below 2 kHz, thresholds are either normal or within 10 dB of normal. These results are also consistent

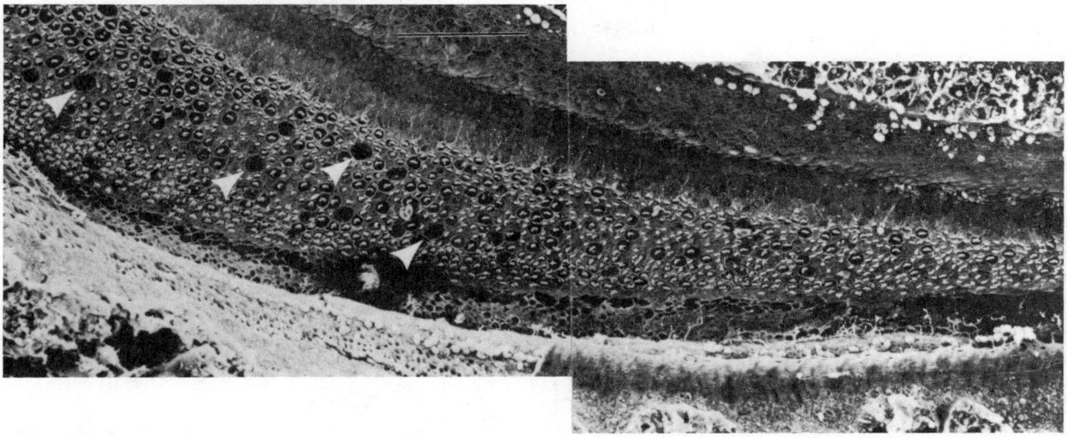

Figure 18-15 Scanning electron micrograph of the proximal one-third of the reticular surface at 28 days following gentamicin treatment. Numerous "giant" hair cells (arrows) are randomly distributed across the surface. Large areas are devoid of normal hair cells and the mosaic pattern is disrupted. Bar = 100 μm. (From Duckert LG, Rubel EW. Ultrastructural observations on regenerating hair cells in the chick basilar papilla. Hear Res 1990; 48:161-182.)

with our SEM observations on the cochleas from these animals. By 20 weeks, most of the cochlea appears almost normal. There are some defects in the packing of hair cells and the cell surfaces appear slightly larger than normal, suggesting that the full complement of hair cells may not have been replaced. At the basal end, however, some disorganization is still apparent, particularly in the alignment of stereocilia bundles, which may be the reason for the hearing loss seen at the high frequencies. The fact that functional improvement is still occurring between 16 and 20 weeks following the drug treatment suggests that with longer survival times, the basal part of the cochlea may show further morphologic and functional recovery.

The protracted time course of recovery following aminoglycoside treatment enticed us to attempt dissociating recovery of hair cell function and eighth nerve function. That is, we wished to ascertain whether recovery of hair cell function was coincident with or preceded recovery of evoked potentials. This information is important in that it can indicate whether formation of the receptor complex is the only barrier to functional recovery or if maturation of mature connections with ganglion cells and the central nervous system imposes further constraints. To address these issues, we have begun studying evoked otoacoustic emissions (Kemp, 1978) in chicks during the course of hair cell regeneration (Norton et al, 1990).

In this study, we again treated newborn chicks with gentamicin (50 mg/kg/day) for 10 days. These animals and age-matched controls were studied from 1 day to 22 weeks following the treatment. In addition to examining tone burst–evoked potentials recorded from brainstem electrodes, acoustic distortion products (ADPs) produced by tones ranging from 0.5 kHz to 5.0 kHz were studied. The acoustic distortion products were produced by simultaneously presenting two tones at a frequency ratio of $F_1/F_2 = 1:1.3$. The levels of the two tones were equal and ranged from 20 dB SPL to 80 dB SPL in 5 dB steps. Cubic difference tones ($2F_1 - F_2$) were recorded with an Etymotic ER 10B probe microphone assembly sealed to the ear canal. The cubic difference tone emission at low stimulus intensities has been shown to be a sensitive indicator of outer hair cell integrity in mammals (Brown et al, 1989) and does not depend on the integrity of the eighth nerve (Horner et al, 1985; Arts et al, 1990).

The changes in evoked potential thresholds generally replicated those of our earlier study, discussed above. Threshold elevations were first observed at high frequencies and then at all frequencies tested. Between 1 and 22 weeks there was a gradual improvement in thresholds, first at low and mid frequencies and later at high frequencies. Figure 18-16, *A* shows the time course of evoked potential threshold shifts and ADP threshold shifts to a 1500 Hz stimulus relative to age-matched control animals. The abrupt evoked potential threshold elevation seen at 10 to 12 weeks was a consistent, unexplained finding. We suspect it is related to synaptic remodeling that occurs because of transneuronal degeneration of some ganglion cells and subsequent rein-

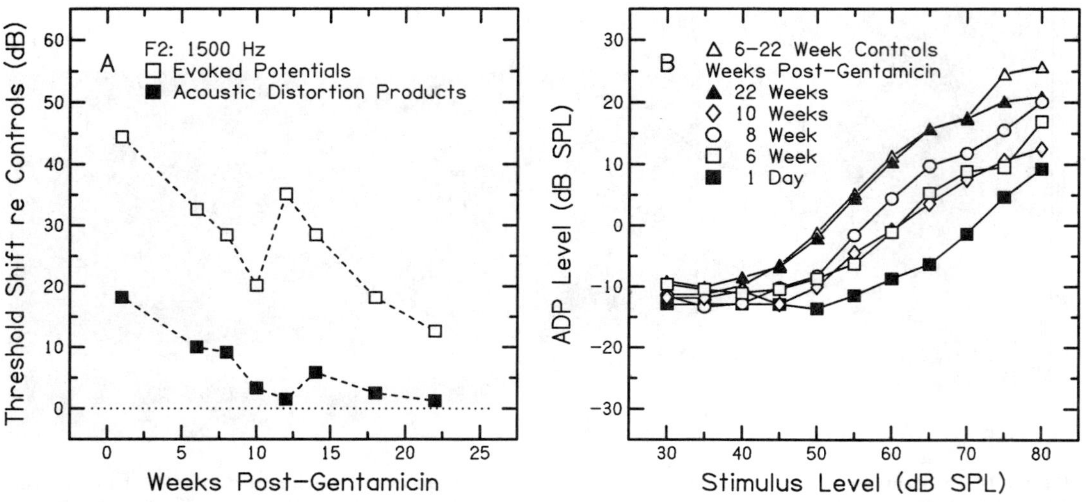

Figure 18-16 *A,* Comparison of evoked potential (EP) threshold and acoustic distortion product (ADP) threshold recovery following 10 day treatment of gentamicin in neonatal chicks. Mean threshold shift (compared to age-matched control animals) as a function of weeks after gentamicin treatment. For EPs, the stimulus was a 1500 Hz tone burst. For ADPs, F_2 equaled 1500 Hz and F_1 equaled 1154 Hz (F_2/F_1 = 1.3). Note that ADP threshold recovered by 10 to 12 weeks. While EP threshold recovered, some residual hearing loss persisted until 22 weeks. *B,* ADP input/output functions during recovery. Mean ADP level is plotted as a function of stimulus level. All data are to F_2 = 1500 Hz stimulus (F_1 = 1154 Hz). The levels of F_1 and F_2 were equal and the frequency ratio was F_2/F_1 = 1.3. Mean input-output function from control animals (open triangles) is compared to mean values obtained at various times (from 1 day to 22 weeks) after the gentamicin treatment.

nervation of regenerating as well as surviving hair cells.

As seen in Figure 18-16, *A,* the time course of ADP recovery is parallel to, but not coincident with, evoked potential recovery. ADP thresholds at F_2 = 1.5 kHz have recovered to within 5 dB of normal by 10 to 12 weeks after the aminoglycoside treatment, whereas evoked potential thresholds approach normal levels at 22 weeks. This difference, which was seen at all frequencies, suggests that hair cell recovery precedes neural recovery by several weeks. The site of this delay will require further investigation.

Figure 18-16, *B* shows averaged input-output functions for ADPs as a function of stimulus intensity. The separate lines represent various times after the termination of gentamicin treatment from 1 day to 22 weeks. In normal mature animals, ADP input-output functions may reflect two components that have different biologic generators or cellular mechanisms. Emissions to low and moderate intensity sounds are extremely vulnerable to anoxia, tend to saturate as intensity is increased, and appear to be ATP dependent. At higher intensities, emissions are less vulnerable to insult and rise linearly with stimulus intensity (Norton and Rubel, 1990). Initially (1 day), the threshold is shifted and only emissions to high level stimuli (>65 dB) are seen. At these relatively high intensities, the ADPs tend to be linearly related to stimulus intensity. Around 8 to 10 weeks, the threshold is reduced and the input-output function begins to show saturation, suggesting that "active" elements are becoming functional. However the ADP dynamic range remains reduced. By 22 weeks, the ADP input-output function (at F_2 = 1.5 kHz) has fully recovered.

In summary, the studies reported above strongly suggest that the regenerated hair cells are functional and relay information to the central nervous system. In addition, regions of the cochlea that appear morphologically normal correspond to the frequencies at which response parameters also show the best recovery. This correlation suggests that the regenerated hair cells develop the frequency specificity characteristics appropriate to their cochlear location. While we have shown results *consistent* with these conclusions, several important avenues of functional research remain to be carried out. At this time little is known about behavioral capacities during regeneration. In addition, single unit recordings from the eighth nerve, coupled with axonal injections of label to determine which fibers connect to regenerated hair cells, are needed to prove their functional capability. Finally, it would be extremely interesting to examine the development of ionic channels and frequency tuning in isolated regenerating hair cells.

Ultrastructural Properties of Regenerated Hair Cells

Along with the functional studies reported above, our group, as well as other groups (e.g., Cotanche, 1987a; Marsh et al, 1990; Cotanche and Corwin, 1990), have begun to study the ultrastructural properties of the regenerated epithelium following noise-induced or drug-induced damage. In this section I will briefly describe ultrastructural observations on the regenerated hair cells following aminoglycoside treatment. More detailed descriptions can be found in Duckert and Rubel (1990).

The two issues to be addressed here are related to the conclusions we have drawn from our functional analyses. First, it is of interest to determine if regenerated hair cells make synaptic connections with the central nervous system and, if so, the time course over which these connections mature. Second, because in normal animals the stereocilia bundle morphology varies precisely as a function of cochlear location, it is important to examine the number, length, and orientation of stereocilia bundles on regenerated hair cells. These stereocilia properties are thought to be related to functional properties of mature hair cells and their coupling to the tectorial membrane.

Synaptic Connections with Regenerated Hair Cells

To study the establishment of synaptic connections with regenerating hair cells, we took advantage of the fact that aminoglycoside treatment with the parameters noted above destroys virtually all mature hair cells in the basal part of the newly hatched chick cochlea. Therefore, by concentrating our TEM analysis on this region, we were assured that synaptic complexes were associated with regenerating, as opposed to "surviving" or degenerating, hair cells. The principal questions we wish to address here are (1) when can afferent and efferent terminals be recognized on the regenerating hair cells; and (2) what is their relative maturity? More detailed analyses involving quantitative studies of synaptology are in progress.

Immature cells destined to become hair cells can be recognized soon after they begin migrating from the basilar membrane toward the luminal surface. In contrast to the supporting cells, the cytoplasm of regenerating hair cells is more electron dense because of an increase in the number of organelles. As the cells approach the luminal surface this difference increases. A good example is shown in Figure 18-17. The three immature hair cells lined up under the luminal surface show progressively decreasing electron density, but all are more dense than the surrounding support cells. Circled elements in Figure 18-17 are nerve fibers in close approximation to an immature hair cell, which has yet to reach the luminal surface or to produce stereocilia.

Figure 18-18 shows afferent synaptic terminals on regenerated hair cells. Afferent synaptic complexes on immature cells are seen as early as we have looked. They are seen 1 day after the termination of gentamicin treatment, but are more numerous at 1 week or 4 weeks. They are found both on cells that have reached the luminal surface (erupted), which are beginning to produce stereocilia, and on unerupted cells. The synaptic complexes appear immature, but have the full complement of specializations including synaptic ball, vesicles, presynaptic density, and postsynaptic density. The terminals are usually boutons and are less densely packed than on normal cells. We have not examined the innervation pattern beyond 4 weeks following the gentamicin treatment.

Vesiculated terminals, which are presumably efferents from the central nervous system, are also seen on both erupted and unerupted immature hair cells (Fig. 18-19). These have not been observed prior to 1 week after aminoglycoside treatment. In both normal and regenerating cochleas, they tend to occur most often on short hair cells. Typically they are packed with synaptic vesicles. Often, but not always, subsynaptic cisterna are seen. At early times, these endings tend to be boutons while at later survival times and in normal animals they form flattened cups around the base of the short hair cells.

Thus, both afferent and efferent terminals can be identified early in the regeneration process. We have observed both types of terminals on erupted and on nonerupted cells, and all the normal components are present. Further analyses will be required to describe the

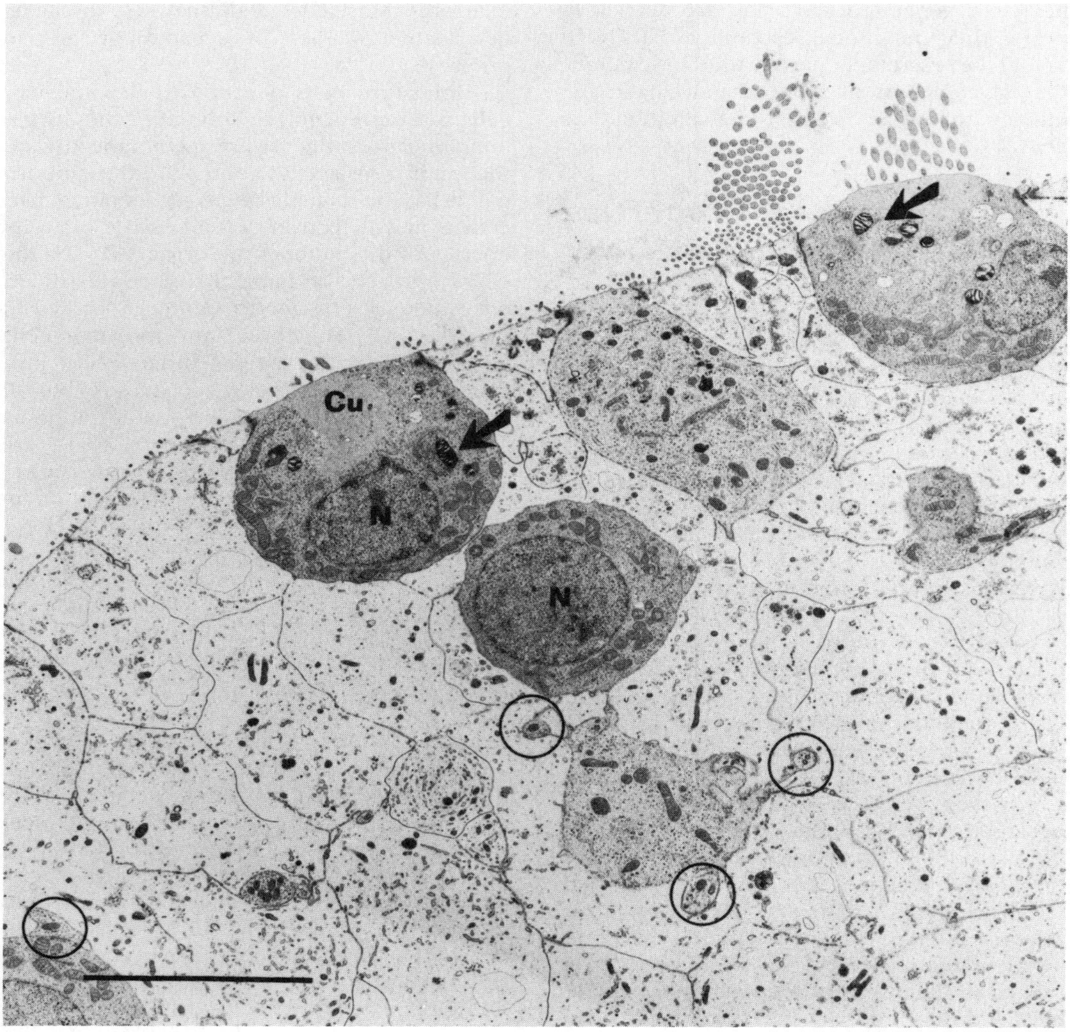

Figure 18-17 Transmission electron photomicrograph showing erupted and unerupted regenerated hair cells 28 days after gentamicin treatment. The cells at the surface are rotund with a basally located nucleus (N). Note increasing electron density as cells migrate toward the surface. Cu = cuticular plate, arrows = myelin figures. Nerve fibers are circled. Bar = 10 μm. (From Duckert LG, Rubel EW. Ultrastructural observations on regenerating hair cells in the chick basilar papilla. Hear Res 1990; 48:161-182.)

maturation of synapses, which may be important for understanding the lag between recovery of hair cell function (emissions) and recovery of evoked potential thresholds.

Stereocilia

The maturation of stereocilia in regenerating hair cells has been described by a number of investigators (Cotanche, 1987a; Henry et al, 1988; Girod et al, 1989; Duckert and Rubel, 1990). Recently, Cotanche and Corwin (1990) have provided quantitative analyses of stereocilia bundle orientation during regeneration following noise trauma. They showed that the orientation of stereocilia bundles initially varies over approximately 100 degrees. Then, over approximately 4 days, the bundles became aligned with those of other regenerating cells and with the orientation of surviving hair cells surrounding the lesion. In their study, this change took place rapidly, between 6 days and 10 days following the sound exposure. Although the reorientation of stereocilia bundles following aminoglycoside ototoxicity has not been quantified, the same general phenomenon has been seen, but with a much

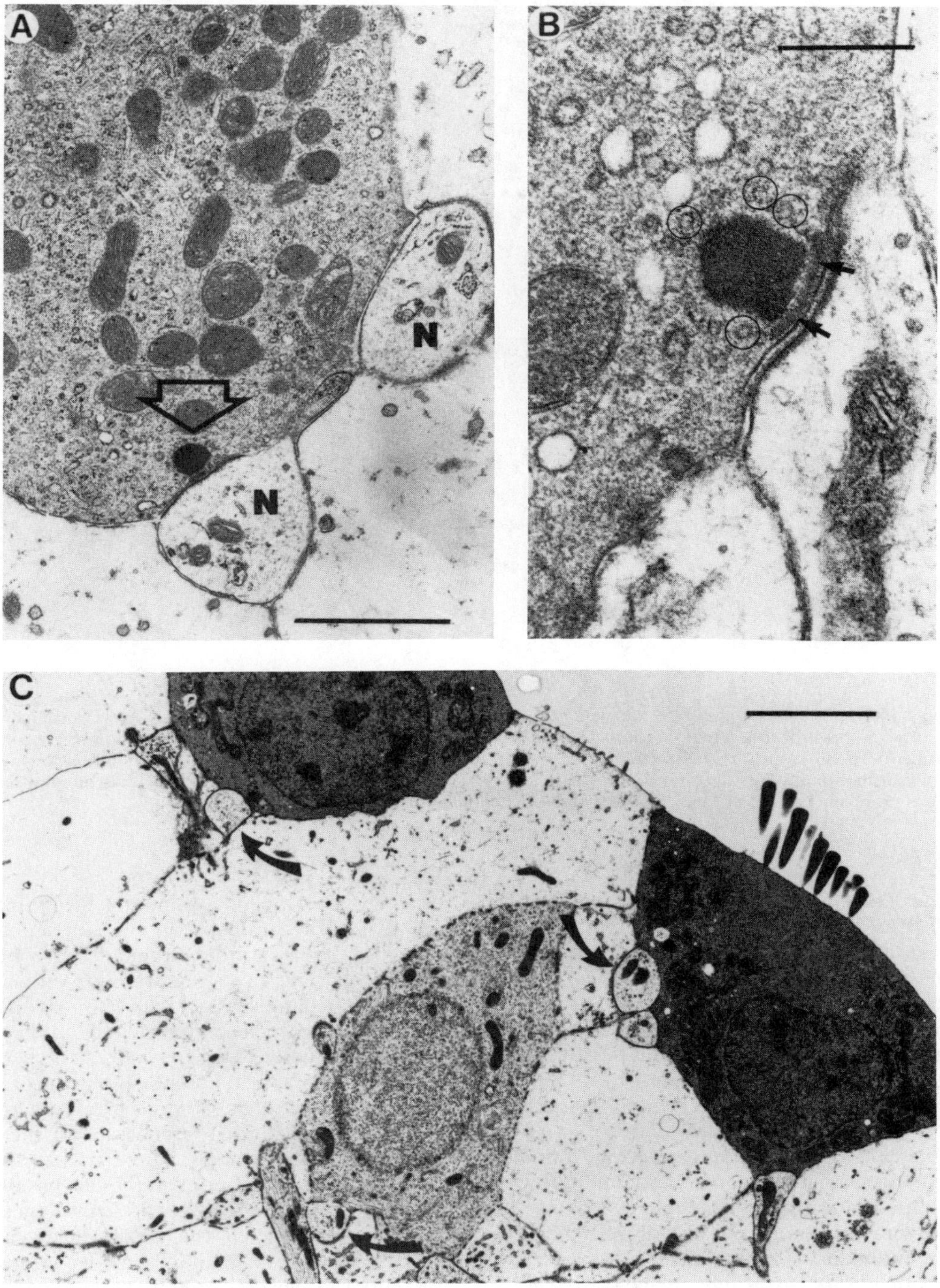

Figure 18-18 *A,* Small bouton afferent nerve endings (N) opposed to basal portion of regenerated sensory hair cell 1 day following termination of gentamicin treatment. Arrow = synaptic complex consisting of synaptic ball and vesicles. Bar = 1 μm. *B,* High magnification of synaptic complex in a regenerated hair cell 1 day following termination of gentamicin treatment. Note row of vesicles surrounding synaptic ball (circles). A granular synaptic membrane (arrows) is found between the ball and the cell membrane. Bar = 0.5 μm. *C,* Transmission electron photomicrograph of primitive regenerated hair cells 7 days following termination of gentamicin treatment. The more mature sensory cells are more densely stained than the unerupted precursor cell below the reticular surface. Numerous afferent nerve terminals (arrows) approximate the basal portion of both erupted and unerupted sensory cells. Bar = 5 μm. (From Duckert LG, Rubel EW. Ultrastructural observations on regenerating hair cells in the chick basilar papilla. Hear Res 1990; 48:161-182.)

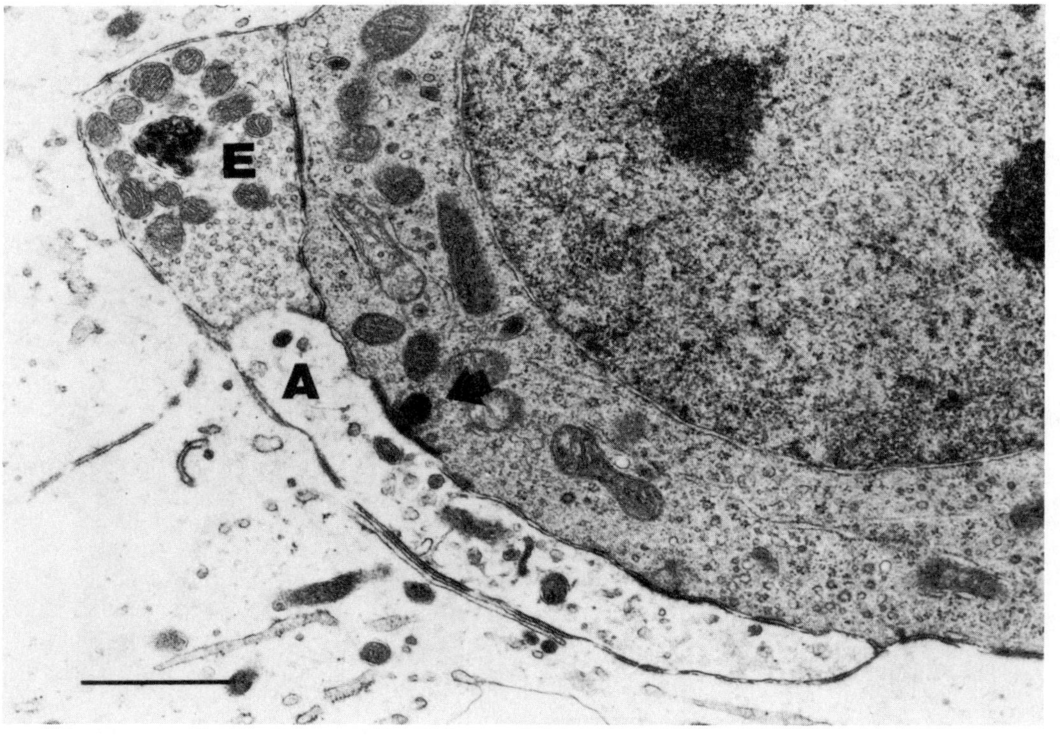

Figure 18-19 Transmission electron micrograph showing both afferent (A) and efferent (E) nerve terminals opposed to the basal portion of an unerupted primitive sensory hair cell 7 days following termination of gentamicin treatment. The efferent terminal contains multiple small, round vesicles in addition to mitochondria. A synaptic complex (arrow) opposes the afferent terminal. Bar = 1 μm. (From Duckert LG, Rubel EW. Ultrastructural observations on regenerating hair cells in the chick basilar papilla. Hear Res 1990; 48:161-182.)

longer time course (Duckert and Rubel, 1990). SEM observations indicate that at 5 weeks after gentamicin treatment, stereocilia bundles throughout the basal two-thirds of the cochlea are disoriented. By 10 to 12 weeks, some reorientation is apparent in the middle region, but in the basal and mid-basal regions high variability still predominates. By 22 weeks, all but the basal region appears to show consistent bundle orientation.

In the chick cochlea, stereocilia bundles vary systematically in length and number of elements (Tilney and Saunders, 1983). At the basal end the bundle consists of many (200 to 300) individual stereocilia and the tallest row extends ~5 μm from the hair cell surface; toward the apical end, the number decreases and the height increases. Development of this gradient has been studied in detail by Tilney et al (1986, 1988). It is of considerable interest to understand the signals underlying the ontogeny of this pattern and it might be expected that these signals are restricted to the embryologic period. To begin addressing this issue we have begun examining the number and height of stereocilia in regenerated hair cells. Although few measurements have been obtained to date, even cursory observation reveals the striking finding that after 20 to 25 weeks, the normal patterns have been restored. The height of stereocilia of regenerated hair cells appears identical to that of the remaining hair cells at any given position along the cochlea, and at the basal end, the entire complement of new hair cells has short stereocilia. The number of stereocilia has been counted on several mature-appearing regenerated hair cells from the basal region in a 4-week survivor. The number was between 150 and 170 per cell, which is comparable to the number reported by Tilney and Saunders (1983). Examples of stereocilia on a regenerated hair cell from the basal region of a gentamicin-treated animal and a normal hair cell from approximately the same region of a control animal are shown in Figures. 18-20, *A* and 18-20, *B*, respectively. Without more extensive measurements of stereocilia height and

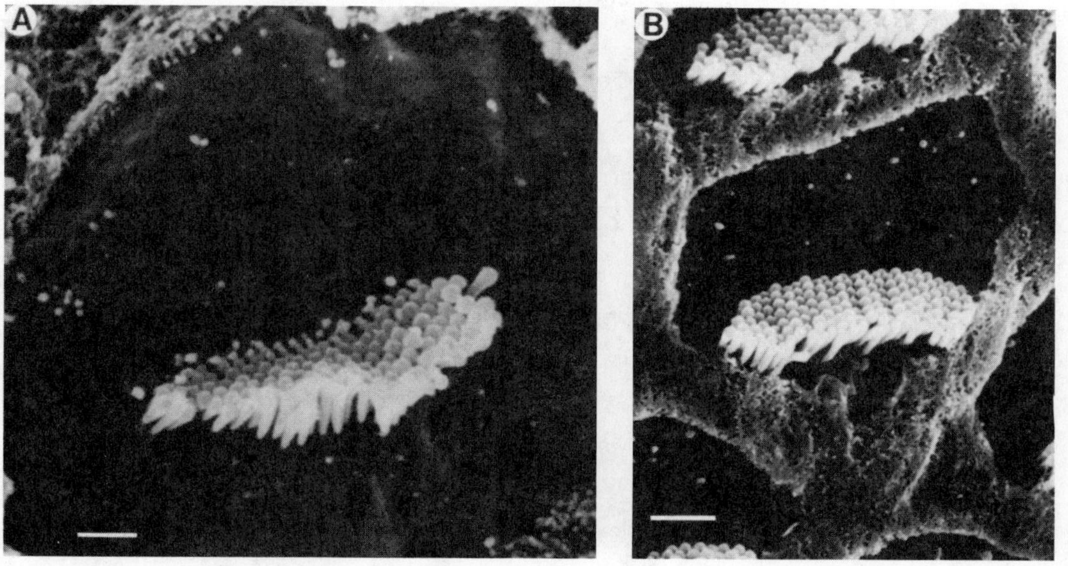

Figure 18-20 Comparison of stereocilia on regenerated and normal basal short hair cells. *A,* At 28 days following termination of gentamicin treatment the stereocilia bundle is centrally located on the apical surface of the regenerated hair cell. The staircase orientation is easily recognized. The stereocilia bundle is better organized than at earlier times, and the tightly packed hexagonal lattice configuration observed in normal control animals is seen. *B,* Apical surface of short sensory hair cell from control animal showing hexagonally packed lattice of stereocilia. Bar = 2 μm.

number throughout the length of the cochlea, the precision of this pattern cannot be evaluated, but our observations to date strongly suggest that the signals regulating this pattern persist in the mature avian cochlea. The site of these signals remains to be determined. They may be expressed by the genome of the stem cell population or be obtained from the local environment of the differentiating hair cells.

Regeneration of Hair Cells in the Vestibular Epithelium

In the cochlear portion of the postnatal avian inner ear, neither we, nor other investigators have observed ongoing proliferation of hair cells. That is, in control animals and in regions outside of an area subjected to noise damage, thymidine incorporation studies have not revealed labeled hair cells. In the vestibular epithelium, on the other hand, Jorgensen and Mathiesen (1987) reported a low rate of hair cell and support cell proliferation in mature budgerigars. We have recently confirmed this observation on posthatch chicks (Roberson et al., 1989). In normal animals, we have successfully labeled type II hair cells and supporting cells in each ampulla, the utricle, the saccula, and the macula lagena with ^{3}H thymidine and with bromodeoxyuridine (BrdU—a thymidine analog) (Fig. 18-21). In addition, recent studies by Pedro Weisleder and the author have shown that the rate of receptor cell production is dynamically regulated. When the vestibular epithelium is damaged by streptomycin injection, the production of receptor cells increases by approximately four-fold (Fig. 18-22).

These findings on postembryonic production of vestibular hair cells are of considerable importance. They show that the ability to restore lost receptor cells is not limited to the cochlear portion of the avian inner ear. Second, they suggest that the proliferation of hair cells is not a binary process; either cell cycle times or the number of stem cells induced to re-enter the mitotic cycle can be regulated by tissue "needs." Finally, the fact that vestibular system structure is highly conserved across virtually all classes of vertebrates, including mammals, suggests that regeneration of hair cells in the mammalian inner ear can eventually be induced.

Conclusion

Postembryonic production of receptor cells in fish and reptiles has been known for

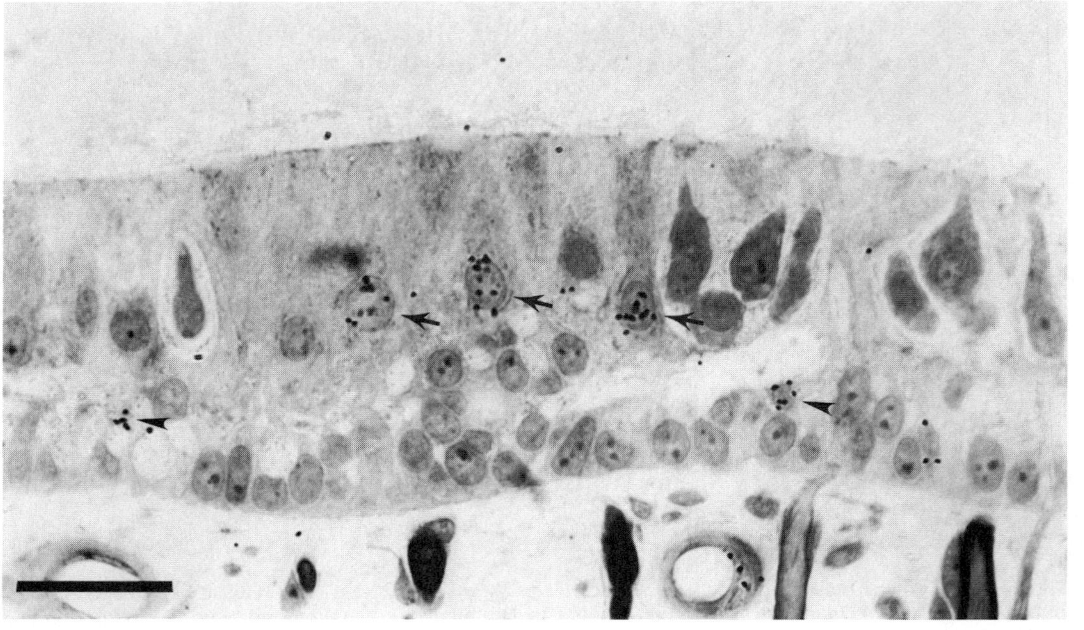

Figure 18-21 Photomicrogragh of normal saccule from a 15-day-old chicken. The animal was given ^3H thymidine for 5 days and was allowed to survive for an additional 2 weeks. Labeled type II hair cells (arrows) and support cells (arrowheads) are seen. Bar = 20 μm.

several decades. Until recently, we assumed that this capacity was absent in the more highly specialized inner ears of birds and mammals. Recent research has shown that birds have the capacity to rebuild a damaged inner ear, and physiologic studies strongly suggest that the restored receptor epithelium can restore hearing. Although advances are being made toward identifying stem cells, examining function, and documenting morphologic changes during regeneration, little is known about the intercellular signals that induce stem cells to re-enter the mitotic cycle. We know that damage to the epithelium by noise or drugs is a sufficient stimulus to trigger these events, but the subsequent chain of cellular events remains to be discovered. The fact that all vertebrate classes, with the exception of mammals, have this capacity suggests to this author that proliferation in mammals is actively suppressed. Discovery of the signals that trigger regeneration in birds and elucidation of the chain of cellular events will provide critical information. It may then be feasible to identify the steps that are blocked in mammals. Such steps may someday lead to the ability to stimulate hair cell regeneration in humans.

Régénération des Cellules Ciliées de l'Oreille Interne chez l'Oiseau

Dans la cochlée des Mammifères, une exposition à un bruit traumatique qui endommage les cellules ciliées cause une perte auditive permanente. Cela est dû à notre incapacité à produire des cellules ciliées en dehors de la période embryonnaire et donc à remplacer celles qui ont été détruites par un facteur environnemental toxique, comme le bruit ou certaines drogues. A l'opposé, les Vertébrés à sang froid, ont une production continue de cellules ciliées et peuvent donc remplacer celles qui ont été endommagées. La papille basilaire des Oiseaux présente un état intermédiaire: normalement, toutes les cellules ciliées sont produites au cours de l'embryogenèse, mais celles qui sont détruites par traumatisme peuvent être remplacées.

Cet exposé concernant ce dernier cas de figure comprendra 3 parties. Dans la première, la preuve que les dégâts causés par le bruit stimulent la production de nouvelles cellules ciliées est apportée.

La seconde partie décrit une série

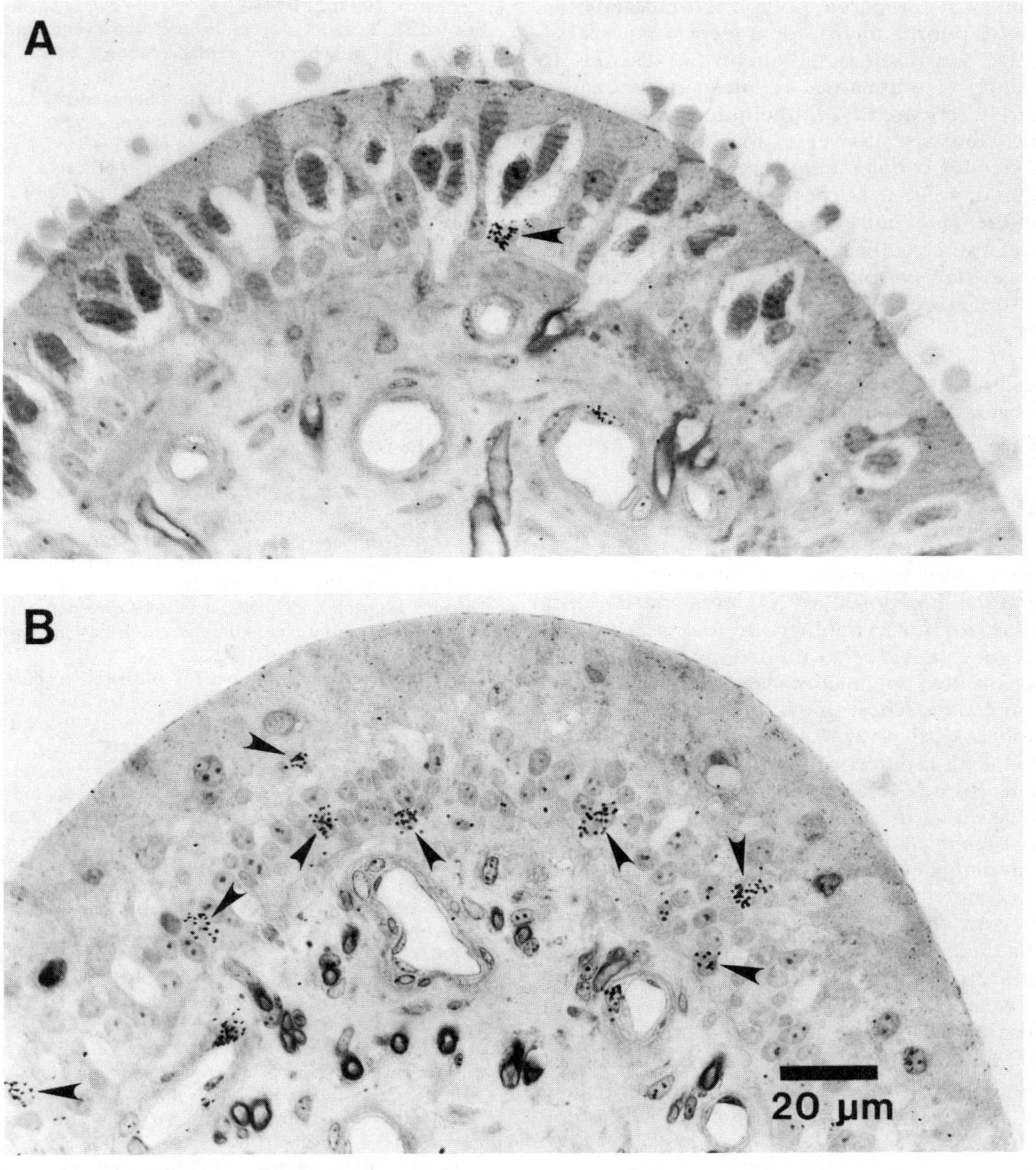

Figure 18-22 Up-regulation of hair cell regeneration in the avian vestibular system. Ampullary tissue from 2-week old animals sacrificed 1 day after a 3-day-course of 20 µCi/g/day tritiated thymidine. Arrowheads point to cells in the sensory epithelium that have incorporated tritiated thymidine. *A,* Ampulla from a control animal. Note the presence and normal complement of type I and type II hair cells, and the single row of supporting cells. Only one labeled cell is seen. *B,* Ampulla from a bird treated with 600 mg/kg/day streptomycin sulfate for 7 days and then given tritiated thymidine. Note the absence of all type I and most type II hair cells, and the presence of several rows of supporting cells. Numerous labeled cells are seen.

d'expériences autoradiographiques destinées à identifier les éléments précurseurs des cellules régénérées. Après une exposition de 18h à un bruit traumatique (1,5 kHz, 120 dB SPL) les animaux (poulets) reçoivent une injection de thymidine tritiée entre 6 et 72 h et sont sacrifiés. Un autre groupe reçoit de la thymidine tritiée jusqu'au troisième jour, puis de la thymidine froide jusqu'au cinquième jour; ils sont sacrifiés à 30 jours. Sur chaque animal une cochlée est préparée pour l'autoradiographie, l'autre pour la microscopie électronique à balayage. Les résultats indiquent que dans les 15 h après le trauma des cellules situées en bordure inférieure de l'épithélium récepteur commencent à se diviser et forment, ensuite, de nouvelles cellules ciliées et de nouvelles cellules de soutien. Les nouvelles cellules ciliées se différencient entre 48 et 72 h; cette différenciation est caractérisée par l'accroissement des organelles cytoplasmiques, une migration vers la surface de l'épithélium et la poussée des stéréocils.

La dernière partie de l'exposé décrit les résultats de la microscopie électronique à balayage concernant les cellules précurseurs et les cellules régénérées.

ACKNOWLEDGMENTS

The studies reported in this chapter were carried out by an outstanding group of collaborators, composed of students, postdoctoral fellows, otolaryngology residents, and colleagues. It is due to their untiring efforts and loyalty that speculations and passing ideas became data. These individuals include Pamela Bohrer, Raul Cruz, Larry Duckert, Douglas Girod, Paul Lambert, Susan Norton, David Roberson, Brenda Ryals, Debara Tucci, and Pedro Weisleder. In addition, outstanding technical assistance and advice was provided by Dale Cunningham and Glen MacDonald. I also appreciate the valuable suggestions of Susan Norton and Douglas Cotanche for improving the manuscript. Expert secretarial assistance was provided by Terry Hogley. The research was supported by PHS grant DC00395, funds from the Deafness Research Foundation, and funds from the Departments of Otolaryngology–Head and Neck Surgery at the University of Virginia and at the University of Washington.

References

Arts HA, Norton SJ, Rubel EW. Influence of perilymphatic tetrodotoxin and calcium concentration on hair cell function. Presented at Midwinter Meeting of the Association for Research in Otolaryngology, St. Petersburg, FL, February, 1990.

Brown AM, McDowell B, Forge A. Acoustic distortion products can be used to monitor the effects of chronic gentamicin treatment. Hear Res 1989; 42:143-156.

Corwin JT. Postembryonic growth of the macula neglecta auditory detector in the ray, *Raja clavata:* Continual increases in hair cell number, neural convergence, and physiological sensitivity. J Comp Neurol 1983; 217:345-356.

Corwin JT, Balak KJ, Borden PC. Cellular events underlying the regenerative replacement of lateral line sensory epithelium in amphibians. In: Coombs S, Görner P, Münz H, eds. The mechanosensory lateral line: neurobiology and evolution. New York: Springer-Verlag, 1989:161-183.

Corwin JT, Cotanche DA. Regeneration of sensory hair cells after acoustic trauma. Science 1988; 240:1772-1774.

Cotanche DA. Regeneration of hair cell stereociliary bundles in the chick cochlea following severe acoustic trauma. Hear Res 1987a; 30:181-194.

Cotanche DA. Regeneration of the tectorial membrane in the chick cochlea following severe acoustic trauma. Hear Res 1987b; 30:197-206.

Cotanche DA, Corwin JT. Stereociliary bundles reorient during hair cell development and regeneration in the chick cochlea. Hear Res 1990, In press.

Cotanche DA, Saunders JC, Tilney LG. Hair cell damage produced by acoustic trauma in the chick cochlea. Hear Res 1987; 25:267-278.

Cruz RM, Lambert PR, Rubel EW. Light microscopic evidence of hair cell regeneration after gentamicin toxicity in chick cochlea. Arch Otolaryngol Head Neck Surg 1987; 113:1058-1062.

Duckert LG, Rubel EW. Ultrastructural observations on regenerating hair cells in the chick basilar papilla. Hear Res, 1990; 48:161-182.

Girod DA, Duckert LG, Rubel EW. Possible precursors of regenerated hair cells in the avian cochlea following acoustic trauma. Hear Res 1989; 42:175-194.

Girod DA, Tucci DL, Rubel EW. Anatomical correlates of functional recovery in the avian inner ear following aminoglycoside ototoxicity. Presented at Midwinter Meeting of the Association for Research in Otolaryngology, St. Petersburg, FL, February, 1990.

Henry WJ, Makaretz M, Saunders JC, et al. Hair cell loss and regeneration after exposure to intense sound in neonatal chicks. Otolaryngol Head Neck Surg 1988; 98:607-611.

Horner KC, Lenoir M, Bock GR. Distortion product otoacoustic emissions in hearing-impaired mutant mice. J Acoust Soc Am 1985; 78:1603-1611.

Johns ME, Ryals BM, Guerry TL. Effects of aminoglycoside antibiotics on hair cells of the chick basilar papilla. Presented at Midwinter Meeting of the Association for Research in Otolaryngology, St. Petersburg, FL, February, 1980.

Jorgensen JM, Mathiesen C. Continuous production of hair cells in vestibular sensory organs, but not in the auditory papilla. Naturwissenschaften 1988; 75:319-320.

Kemp DT. Stimulated acoustic emissions from within the human auditory system. J Acoust Soc Am 1978; 64:1386-1391.

Lippe WR, Rubel EW. Development of the Place Principle: Tonotopic organization. Science 1983; 219:514-516.

Lippe WR, Rubel EW. Ontogeny of tonotopic organization of brain stem auditory nuclei in the chicken: Implications for development of the Place Principle. J Comp Neurol 1985; 237:273-289.

Marsh RR, Xu L, Moy JP, Saunders JC. Recovery of the basilar papilla following intense sound exposure in the chick. Hear Res 1990; 46:229-238.

McFadden EA, Saunders JC. Recovery of auditory function following intense sound exposure in the neonatal chick. Hear Res 1989; 41:205-216.

Norton S, Tucci D, Rubel EW. Comparison of acoustic and neural responses from avian ears following gentamicin. Presented at Midwinter Meeting of the Association for Research in Otolaryngology, St. Petersburg, FL, February, 1990.

Norton SJ, Rubel EW. Active and passive ADP components in mammalian and avian ears. In: Geisler D, Dallos P, Mathews J, Ruggero M, eds. Mechanics and biophysics of hearing. New York: Plenum, 1990, In press.

Presson JC, Popper AN. A ganglionic source of new eighth nerve neurons in a post-embryonic fish. Hear Res 1990a; 46:23-28.

Presson JC, Popper AN. Possible precursors to new hair cells, support cells, and Schwann cells in the ear of a post-embryonic fish. Hear Res 1990b; 46:9-22.

Roberson DW, Bohrer PS, Duckert LG, Rubel EW. Ongoing production of new sensory epithelial cells in the chick vestibular organs. Presented at Midwinter Meeting of the Association for Research in Otolaryngology, St Petersburg, FL, February, 1989.

Rubel EW, Ryals BM. Patterns of hair cell loss in chick basilar papilla after intense auditory stimulation: Exposure duration and survival time. Acta Otolaryngol 1982; 93:31-41.

Rubel EW, Ryals BM. Development of the Place Principle: Acoustic trauma. Science 1983; 219:512-514.

Ruben RJ. Development of the inner ear of the mouse: A radioautographic study of terminal mitoses. Acta Otolaryngol 1967; 220:1-44.

Ryals BM, Rubel EW. Patterns of hair cell loss in chick basilar papilla after intense auditory stimulation: Frequency organization. Acta Otolaryngol, 1982; 93:205-210.

Ryals BM, Rubel EW. Ontogentic changes in the position of hair cell loss after acoustic overstimulation in avian basilar papilla. Hear Res 1985; 19:135-142.

Ryals BM, Rubel EW. Hair cell regeneration after acoustic trauma in adult *Coturnix* quail. Science 1988; 240:1774-1776.

Ryals BM, Ten Eyck B, Westbrook EW. Ganglion cell loss continues during hair cell regeneration. Hear Res 1990; 43:81-90.

Sidman RL. Autoradiographic methods and principles for study of the nervous system with thymidine-H^3. In: Nauta WJH, Ebbesson SOE, eds. Contemporary research methods in neuroanatomy. New York: Springer-Verlag, 1970:252-274.

Stone LS. The development of lateral-line sense organs in amphibians observed in living and vital-stained preparations. J Comp Neurol 1933; 57:507-540.

Stone LS. Further experimental studies of the development of lateral-line sense organs in amphibians observed in living preparations. J Comp Neurol 1937; 68:83-115.

Takasaka T, Smith CA. The structure and innervation of the pigeon's basilar papilla. Ultrastruct. Res 1971; 35:20-65.

Tilney LG, Tilney MS, Cotanche DA. Actin filaments, stereocilia and hair cells of the bird cochlea V. How the staircase pattern of stereociliary lengths is generated. J Cell Biol 1988; 106:335-365.

Tilney LG, Tilney MS, Saunders JC, DeRosier DJ. Actin filaments, stereocilia, and hair cells of the bird cochlea. III. The development and differentiation of hair cells and stereocilia. Dev Biol 1986; 116:100-118.

Tilney LG, Saunders JC. Actin filaments, stereocilia, and hair cells of the bird cochlea: I. The length, number, width, and distribution of stereocilia of each hair cell are related to the position of the hair cell on the cochlea. J Cell Biol 1983; 96:807-821.

Tucci DL, Rubel EW. Physiological status of regenerated hair cells in the avian inner ear following aminoglycoside ototoxicity. Otolaryngol Head Neck Surg 1990; 103:443-450.

CHAPTER 19

Function-Structure Correlation During Recovery from Aminoglycoside Ototoxicity in the Avian Auditory System

ERI HASHINO
MASAHIRO SOKABE
YASUO TANAKA

Some species of fish and amphibians are known to produce hair cells over their entire life span (Corwin, 1981, 1983; Popper and Hoxter, 1984). However, the production of hair cells in the cochlea of birds and mammals occurs during embryogenesis. Thus, the loss of hair cells after birth has been assumed to result in permanent hearing loss. This assumption, however, proved to be incorrect in neonatal chicks, because hair cells have been shown to regenerate after being destroyed by noise exposure (Cotanche, 1987b; Corwin and Cotanche, 1988) and ototoxic drugs (Cruz et al, 1987). In noise-exposed hatchling chicks, scanning electron microscopy (SEM) showed that regions of the basilar papilla devoid of hair cells were replaced with new hair cells 10 to 15 days after exposure (Cotanche, 1987b; Marsh et al, 1990). Autoradiographic studies with tritiated thymidine indicated that regenerated hair cells had proliferated from supporting cells or unidentified stem cells (Corwin and Cotanche, 1988; Girod et al, 1989). McFadden and Saunders (1989) recorded auditory evoked potentials from noise-exposed chicks and found that thresholds from evoked potentials had almost completely recovered by 15 days after treatment, suggesting that functional recovery accompanies hair cell regeneration.

Although hair cell regeneration has been shown to occur in some avian ears, a number of issues need to be clarified. For example, there are little or no data concerning the recovery of structure or function after aminoglycoside ototoxicity. Although hair cell regeneration is known to occur in adult quail after acoustic trauma (Ryals and Rubel, 1988), little or no evidence of hair cell regeneration was seen in adult chickens treated with gentamicin (Seidman et al, 1989). The reasons for these differences are presently unclear; however, they could be related to the mechanism or to amount of cell damage or to species differences.

We have previously shown in adult budgerigars that impulse noise induces an unusual pattern of hearing loss. Immediately following the exposure, a hearing loss of 40 to 60 dB was evidenced at both the low and high frequencies. However, hearing thresholds completely recovered at the high frequencies, whereas a significant permanent threshold shift was present below 1 kHz (Hashino et al, 1988). The propensity of the budgerigar to develop a noise-induced low-frequency hearing loss is exactly the opposite of what is seen in mammals (Henderson and Hamernik, 1982). Because the tonotopic organization of the avian cochlea parallels that of mammals (Manley et al, 1989), the permanent hearing loss at low frequencies implies that there is some structural damage in the apical region of the basilar papilla.

The present study was designed to answer two major questions arising from the preceding studies. The first question was whether the aminoglycoside antibiotics would induce a low-frequency hearing loss in the budgerigar similar to that which occurs with impulse noise, i.e., the low-frequency region especially vulnerable in the budgerigar. If so, what structural changes are associated with this unusual pattern of hearing loss? The second question was whether there is any evidence of hair cell regeneration or recovery of function in the adult budgerigar following aminoglycoside ototoxicity.

Methods

Subjects

Twenty-three adult budgerigars (approximately 5 to 6 months old) were used as subjects. Four birds were used for the behavioral study; the others were used for SEM. The birds received intramuscular injections of kanamycin (KM) at a dose of 200 mg per kilogram per day for 10 successive days. This dose was shown to induce a significant hearing loss in the budgerigars (Hashino and Sokabe, 1989).

Psychophysical Procedures

Each bird was required to bite a response bar during the presentation of a tone lasting 5 seconds. When a bird failed to respond to the tone, the sound of a buzzer served as a conditioned negative reinforcer; in 20 percent of the error trials, a mild electric shock (0.1 mA p-p rectangular pulse lasting 100 ms, 5 Hz) was paired with the buzzer in order to maintain the response behavior. After the bird had mastered the detection task, absolute thresholds were measured using a psychophysical tracking procedure. Six test frequencies between 0.25 and 8 kHz were evaluated, and five threshold estimates were obtained at each frequency.

Histologic Procedures

The birds in the histologic part of the study were allowed to survive for either 1, 7, or 14 days after the last KM injection and then were deeply anesthetized and decapitated. The cochleae were fixed by perfusing 1 percent osmium tetroxide (in 0.1 M phosphate buffer, pH 7.4) through the exposed distal end of the cochlea, and were kept in the fixative at 4° C for 45 minutes. The fixed tissues were dehydrated in ethanol up to 70 percent and dissected out in order to expose the luminal surface of the basilar papilla. Afterwards, the cochleae were dehydrated in a graded series of ethanol, which was then replaced with 100 percent tert-butyl alcohol and dried with an Eiko ID-2 freeze drier. The specimens were sputter-coated with platinum/palladium and viewed on a Jeol JSM-820 scanning electron microscope at an accelerating voltage of 15 kV.

Results

Psychophysical Testing

During KM treatment, the behavioral thresholds initially deteriorated, resulting in threshold shifts of 60 to 80 dB. Figure 19-1 shows the time course of recovery from the kanamycin-induced temporary threshold shift (TTS) at 0.5, 2, and 4 kHz. After KM treatment was terminated, the thresholds improved by approximately 40 dB until about 14 days after treatment, after which the thresholds stabilized. The exact time course of recovery, however, varied across test frequency. At 2 and 4 kHz, the TTS reached a peak 3 to 5 days after treatment rather than 1 day after the final injection of KM. This delayed peak of TTS was followed by a period of rapid recovery (4.5 dB per day), which continued for about 10 days. After 2 weeks following treatment, the TTS at 2 and 4 kHz converged toward a stabilized value of approximately 15 dB. By contrast, the TTS at 0.5 kHz peaked at 1 day after treatment and then gradually decreased (2 dB per day) to a stable value around 2 weeks after treatment.

At least five measurements of threshold were taken at the six frequencies during the last 20 days of recovery in order to determine the amount of permanent threshold shift (PTS). The inset of Figure 19-1 depicts the mean PTS from four birds as a function of frequency. Note that the PTSs below 1 kHz were much greater than those above 1 kHz. Low-frequency threshold shifts remained stable at approximately 40 dB even 40 days after the termination of drug treatment.

Our preliminary results using auditory evoked potentials are consistent with our behavioral data. We successfully recorded far-field auditory evoked potentials from KM-treated budgerigars with a chronic electrode inserted in the skull. Three days after treatment, the evoked response threshold to 4-kHz tone bursts was elevated 60 dB relative to the pretreatment thresholds. However, threshold improved by 40 dB in the next 27 days (Fig. 19-2). The threshold shifts measured with the evoked response agreed with those measured behaviorally.

SEM Study

The basilar papilla of the budgerigar has the same general shape as that of the chick (Gleich and Manley, 1988). The length of the long axis of the papilla is approximately 2 mm. Figure 19-3*A* shows a typical basilar papilla observed 1 day after the cessation of KM administration. Extensive damage was seen over the basal 55 to 75 percent (mean = 67 percent) of the basilar papilla. Both short and tall hair cells were completely lost in this region (Fig. 19-3*B*). Only several clusters of microvilli, which were expected to become stereociliary bundles, could be identified in the most basal end of the cochlea (Fig. 19-3*C*).

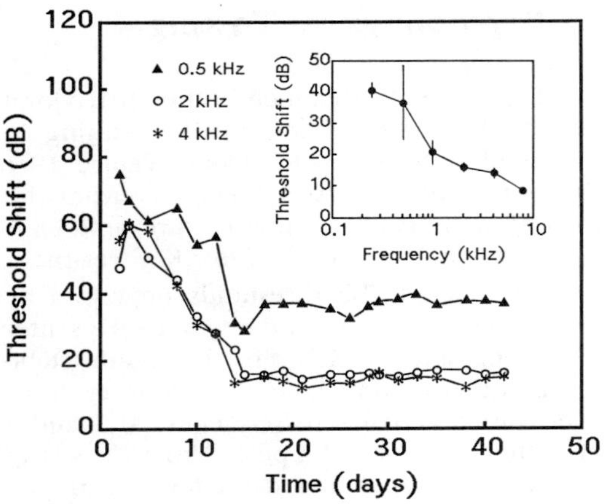

Figure 19-1 Time course of behavioral threshold shifts and permanent threshold shifts (inset) in the kanamycin-treated budgerigars. (Redrawn from Hashino E, Sokabe M. Kanamycin induced low-frequency hearing loss in the budgerigar *(Melopsittacus undulatis)*. J Acoust Soc Am 1989; 85:289-294.)

Seven days following KM intoxication, the basal 20 percent of the papilla was covered with regenerating hair cells (Fig. 19-4*B*). These hair cells were immature, but tip links had already formed between neighboring stereocilia (data not shown). In the adjacent apical region, the number of hair cells had increased to one-third of the normal level. The area at 40 to 60 percent of the distance from the base was still devoid of hair cells (Fig. 19-4*A*).

By 14 days after treatment, regenerated hair cells had appeared over all of the damaged regions of the basilar papilla. In the basal 40 percent, the basilar papilla was completely covered with new hair cells (Fig. 19-5*B*). On the apical surfaces of these cells, there were numerous microvilli similar to those that transiently appear in normally developing hair cells (Cotanche, 1987a). In the remaining areas, except for the undamaged apex, the number of hair cells had increased, but was signifi-

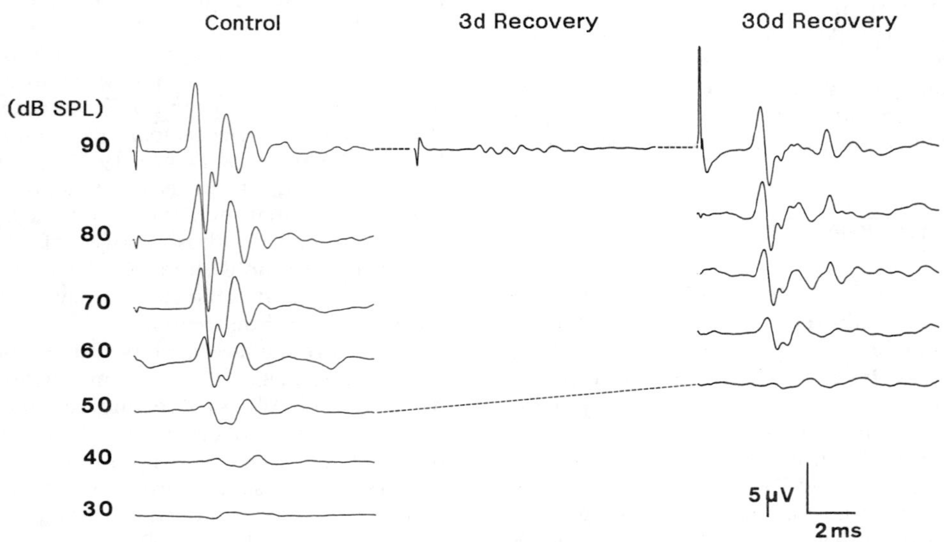

Figure 19-2 Auditory evoked responses (AER) of a budgerigar obtained with a 4-kHz tone burst before (control) and 3 days and 30 days after kanamycin (KM) treatment. The AERs were recorded by a screw electrode implanted in the skull at the vertex; the neck was used as a reference.

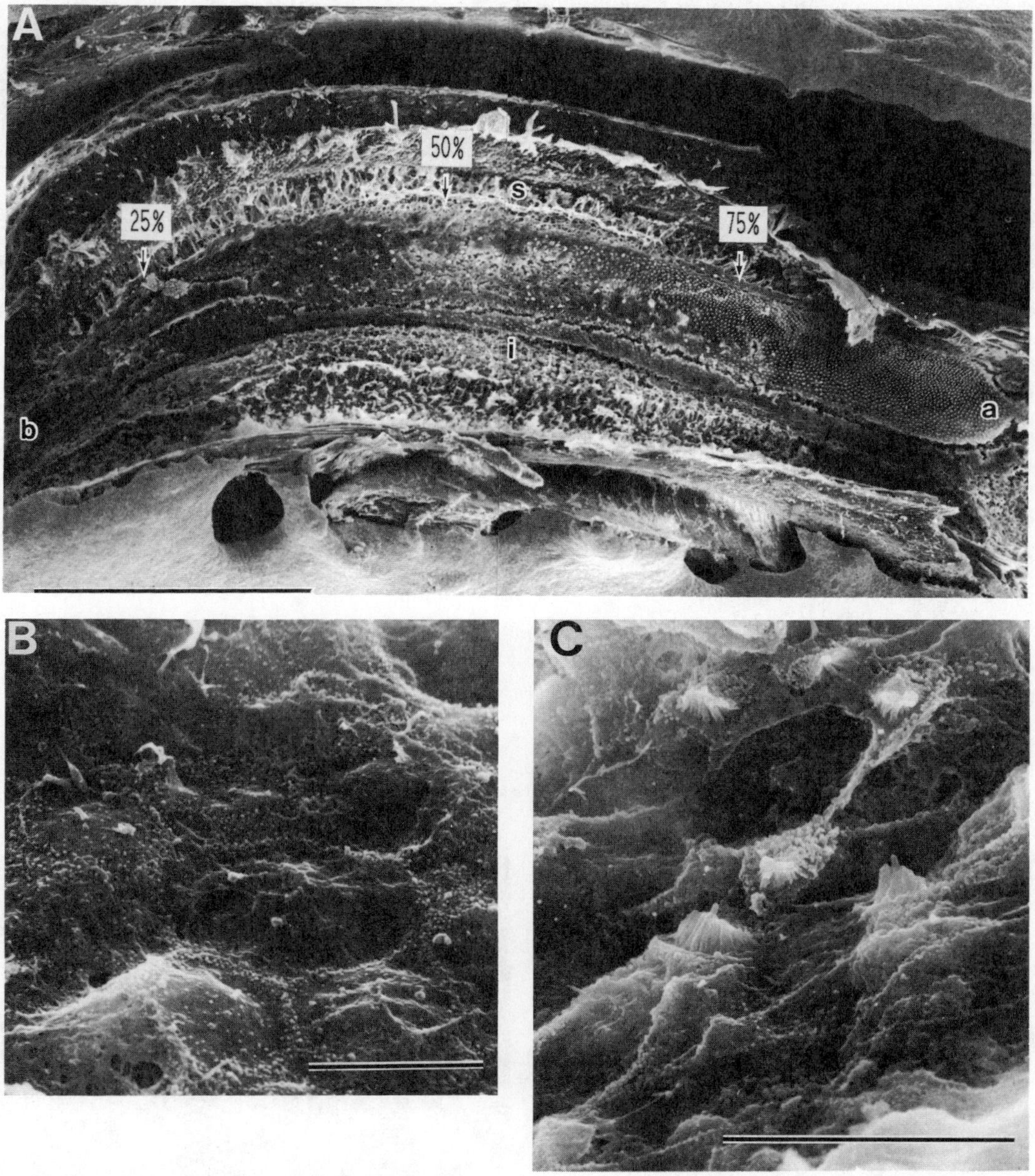

Figure 19-3 Scanning electron micrograph of the budgerigar's cochlea 1 day after treatment. *A,* Basilar papilla: a, apical; b, basal; s, superior; i, inferior. Bar = 500 μm. *B,* Degenerated region located at 50 percent of the distance from the base. *C,* Presumably regenerating hair cells observed at the most basal part of the cochlea. Bars in *B* and *C* = 10 μm.

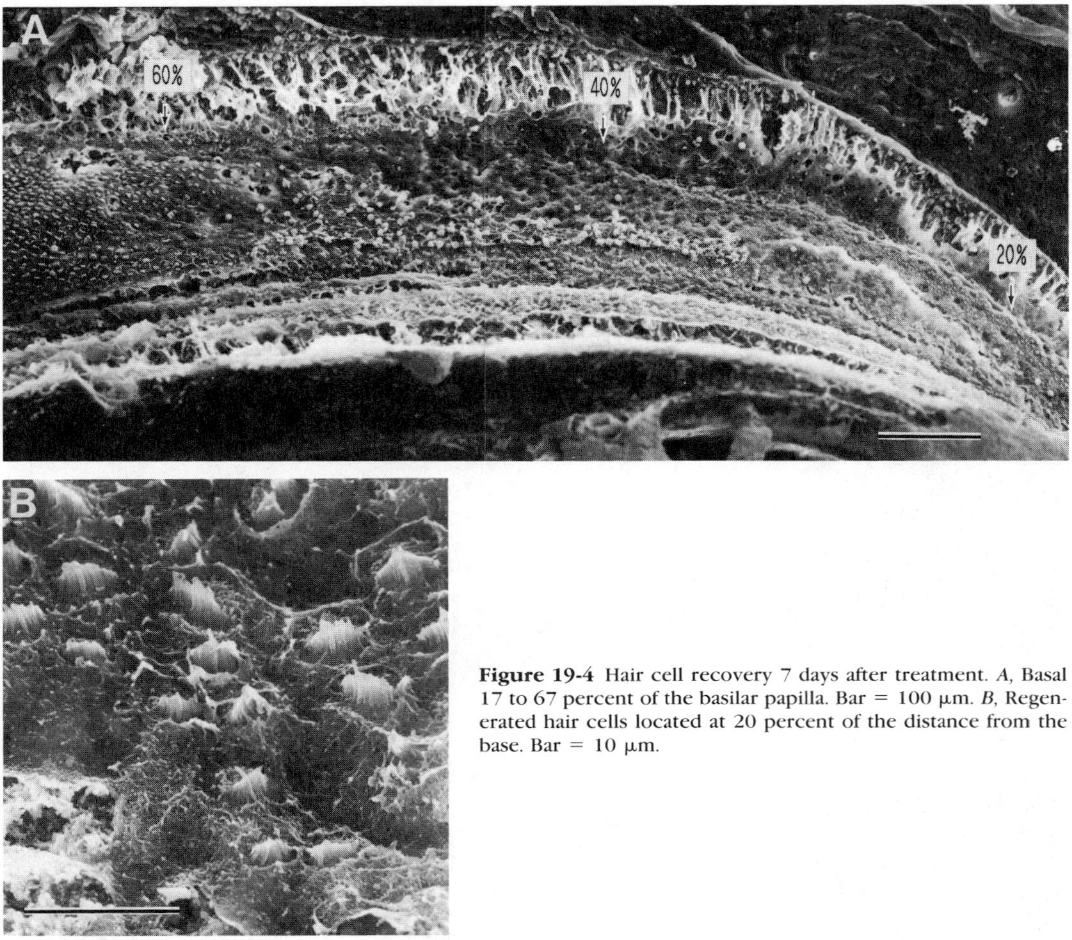

Figure 19-4 Hair cell recovery 7 days after treatment. *A*, Basal 17 to 67 percent of the basilar papilla. Bar = 100 μm. *B*, Regenerated hair cells located at 20 percent of the distance from the base. Bar = 10 μm.

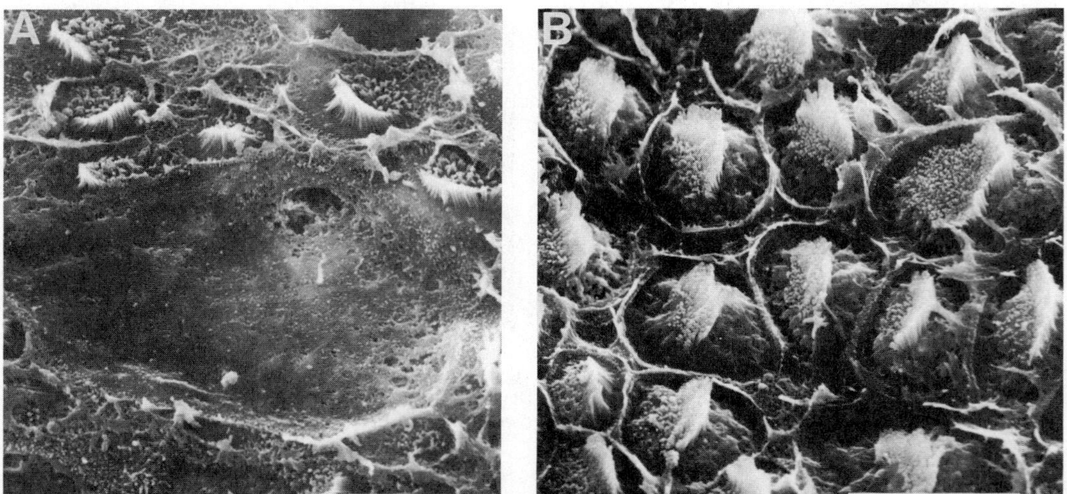

Figure 19-5 Hair cell recovery at 60 percent *(A)* and 20 percent *(B)* from the basal end of the cochlea 14 days after treatment. Bars = 10 μm.

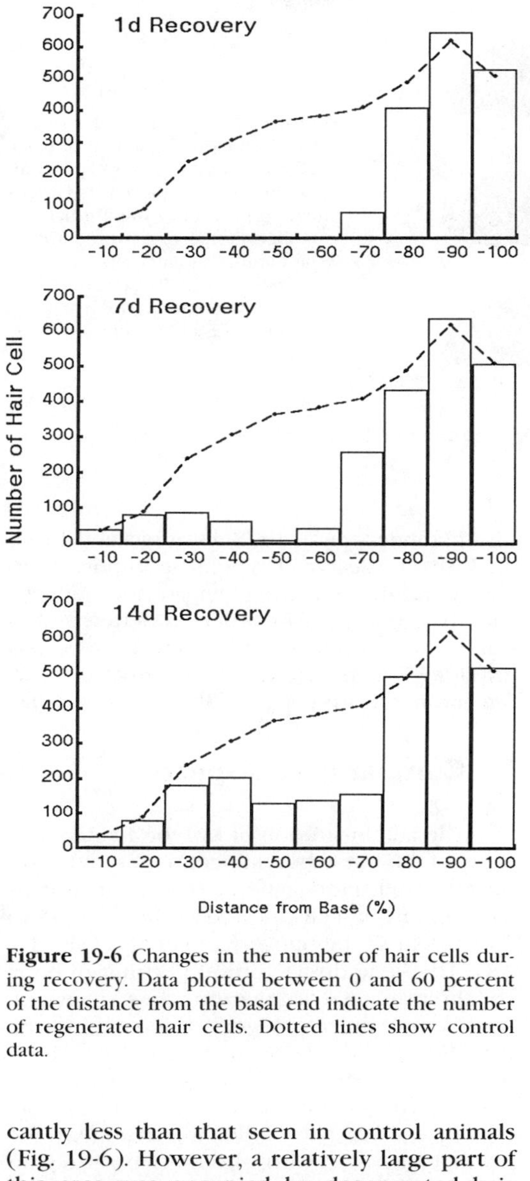

Figure 19-6 Changes in the number of hair cells during recovery. Data plotted between 0 and 60 percent of the distance from the basal end indicate the number of regenerated hair cells. Dotted lines show control data.

cantly less than that seen in control animals (Fig. 19-6). However, a relatively large part of this area was occupied by degenerated hair cells (Fig. 19-5*A*).

Discussion

Correlation Between Hair Cell Regeneration and Functional Recovery

Based on the frequency-place maps derived from single-fiber staining of functionally characterized primary auditory neurons in several avian ears, one would predict that virtually all of the test frequencies used in the present study, including 0.25 kHz, would be transduced in the basal 70 to 75 percent of the basilar papilla (Manley et al, 1987; Gleich, 1989). Behavioral threshold testing at 1 day after treatment showed a hearing loss of 50 to 80 dB at all of the test frequencies. However, given that the basal 70 percent of the basilar papilla was devoid of nearly all short and tall hair cells, it is surprising that the threshold shifts were not higher. Threshold measurements were not obtained below 0.25 kHz because of limitations of the acoustic system; however, it is reasonable to assume that thresholds in this region were normal, given that there was little or no hair cell loss. Thus, in damaged ears, it is likely that the high-frequency stimuli are detected on the basis of spectral splatter into the low-frequency regions.

According to our histologic data, the process of hair cell regeneration had begun as early as 1 day after treatment, at which time several presumptive cilia bundles were identified in the basal tip of the budgerigar's cochlea. Hair cell regeneration was initially greatest in the basal region of the basilar papilla, and then progressed towards the apex. At 14 days after treatment, the basal 40 percent of the papilla was covered with regenerating hair cells, whereas only partial regeneration was seen in more apical regions (Fig. 19-7). The base-to-apex gradient observed in the pattern of hair cell regeneration coincided with the recovery of the behavioral thresholds. The thresholds at frequencies above 1 kHz recovered promptly, whereas recovery of thresholds at frequencies below 1 kHz was delayed.

The number of hair cells in the basal region of the basilar papilla had recovered to normal levels by 14 days after treatment. Additionally, both hair cell surface area and the length of the cilia bundles on the regenerated hair cells were not significantly different from those of normal hair cells at the same position along the cochlea. Despite the fact that hair cell regeneration was nearly complete in the basal region, the behavioral thresholds at the high frequencies remained elevated at approximately 15 dB. There are a number of possible reasons for this discrepancy. First, the orientation of the cilia bundles is rotated by as much as 90 degrees from normal on some regenerated hair cells. A second possibility is that processes proximal to the hair cells may be involved. For example, Ryals et al (1989) showed that ganglion cells began to degenerate well after hair cell regeneration had begun. Furthermore, it is unclear whether the dis-

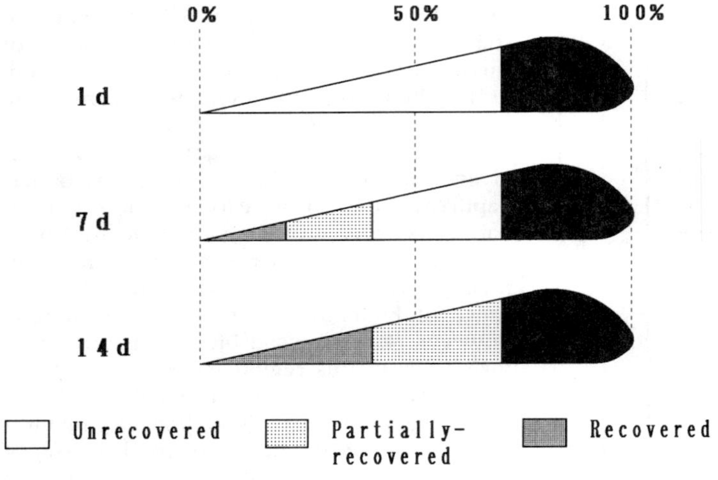

Figure 19-7 Schematic drawing of spatiotemporal gradient in hair cell regeneration. Recovered area: The number of hair cells is larger than 70 percent of the normal number. Partially-recovered area: The number of hair cells is between 10 and 70 percent of the normal number. The black area indicates an undamaged region.

charge patterns of neurons that innervate regenerated hair cells are in fact normal.

Another important facet of our results is the fact that hair cell regeneration in the middle of the basilar papilla was incomplete 14 days after treatment. It is conceivable that more hair cells would have regenerated with longer survival times. However, this possibility seems unlikely given that the behavioral thresholds had stabilized by 2 weeks after treatment. Clearly, it would be important to determine if any additional hair cells regenerate in the budgerigar with longer survival times. Based on these results, plus our previous behavioral data with impulse noise (Hashino et al, 1988), it appears that the hair cells in more-apical regions of the basilar papilla are less likely to regenerate than those in the base. Obviously, it would be important to determine which factors regulate the process of regeneration.

It has been suggested that ciliary length is one factor that may determine the tuning properties of hair cells (Hudspeth, 1989). Thus, it is conceivable that the low-frequency loss might be brought about by a reduction in length of the regenerating stereocilia bundles so that the hair cells are tuned to a higher frequency than one would predict on the basis of position along the basilar papilla. However, this possibility seems unlikely given that the lengths of the stereocilia on fully regenerated hair cells were within normal limits.

The frequency representation on the basilar papilla is known to vary across avian species (Manley et al, 1989; Gleich, 1989). Moreover, the unusual shape of the critical band function in the budgerigar suggests that the tonotopic organization along the basilar papilla may not be logarithmic in this species of bird (Saunders et al, 1978; Okanoya and Dooling, 1987). Clearly, it would be important to determine the frequency map of the budgerigar's basilar papilla in order to better understand the correlation between the various physiologic and behavioral measures of hearing and the morphology of the basilar papilla.

Comparative Aspects

The administration of KM for 10 days at a dose of 200 mg per kilogram per day produced significant degeneration of the hair cells and supporting cells located in the basal 55 to 75 percent of the budgerigar cochlea (Fig. 19-3*A*). The same dosage of KM per unit of body weight produced significantly less degeneration (approximately 35 to 40 percent) in the hatchling chick (Hashino et al, 1991). Moreover, the basilar papilla of the budgerigar required a longer time to recover than it did in the chick. After 1 day following treatment, the number of hair cells in the most basal region of the chick cochlea had reached a normal level. By contrast, there were only several immature kinocilia and cilia bundles in the budgerigar. Fourteen days after treatment, the chick basilar papilla was essentially normal in appearance, whereas the adult budgerigar papilla had obvious pathologies. One possible explanation for these differences is that the basilar papilla of adult birds is more easily damaged by ototoxic drugs than that of young birds. However, this explanation seems unlikely given that adult (52-week-old) chickens appear to be more resistant to aminoglycoside ototoxicity than hatchling chicks (Seidman et al, 1989). Another possibility is that the propensity for hair cell regeneration is reduced in adult animals, as suggested by the recent work of Seidman et al (1989). Finally, it is conceivable that the propensity for hair cell regeneration varies across species; however, little information is currently available on this issue.

It is clear from the present experiment that adult budgerigars have the potential to generate new hair cells even following significant damage to the cochlea by KM. In contrast, Seidman et al (1989) reported little or no hair cell regeneration in adult chickens treated with gentamicin. The reason for these differences is not yet clear; however, it is conceivable that the lack of regeneration in the adult chick may be related to the fact that the ototoxic effects of gentamicin are more prolonged or severe than the ototoxic effects of KM (Hashino et al, 1991).

Récupération du Traumatisme Acoustique et Ototoxicité des Aminoglycosides chez les Oiseaux

Cette étude analyse les effets de bruit intenses ou d'injections d'antibiotiques aminosides sur l'audition et la structure de la papille basilaire des oiseaux.

Après une exposition binaurale à un bruit impulsif de 170 dB SPL, des perroquets sont testés en continu (conditionnement d'évitement) pour leurs capacités auditives entre 0,125 et 8 kHz. On observe des pertes auditives temporaires (TTS) pour les fréquences supérieures à 1,5 kHz et des pertes auditives permanentes (PTS) au dessous de cette fréquence; la structure de ces PTS est tout à fait différente de celle rencontrée chez les Mammifères.

Sur la même espèce, et avec le même type de test, des injections de kanamycine (100 à 200 mg/jour/10 jours) provoquent aussi des TTS et PTS avec des élévations de seuil plus importantes pour les fréquences au dessous de 1 kHz.

Dans les deux cas, on peut donc noter une récupération fonctionnelle pour les fréquences élevées, ce qui est tout à fait différent de ce qui se passe chez les Mammifères.

Les corrélations morphologiques, recherchées sur les animaux traités à la kanamycine, montrent dans un premier temps des dégâts importants au niveau des cellules ciliées de la partie basale (35-40%) de la papille. Une récupération de ces dégâts intervient dans les deux semaines après le traitement, ce qui correspond au délai de récupération fonctionnelle.

En utilisant une autre espèce avienne, le poulet, les résultats après kanamycine sont différents avec des PTS aux fréquences élevées. Les corrélations morphologiques sont en cours pour analyser cette différence spécifique entre les cochlées de perroquet et de poulet. Quoi qu'il en soit, la récupération des dégâts et la structure particulière des PTS observés confèrent au modèle avien une importance particulière pour explorer les mécanismes moléculaires de la régénération des cellules ciliées, ainsi que les relations spatiales entre la morphologie et la physiologie de ces cellules.

ACKNOWLEDGMENTS

We would like to thank Dr. F. Ito for helpful suggestions on photomicrographs, and Dr. R.J. Salvi for critical reading of the manuscript. Our work was supported by grants from the Deafness Research Foundation, Inoue Foundation for Science, Kanehara Ichiro Foundation, and National Science Foundation BNS 9007822.

References

Corwin JT. Postembryonic production and aging of inner ear hair cells in sharks. J Comp Neurol 1981; 201:541-553.

Corwin JT. Postembryonic growth of the macula neglecta auditory detector in the ray, *Raja clavata:* Continual increases in hair cell number, neural convergence, and physiological sensitivity. J Comp Neurol 1983; 217:345-356.

Corwin JT, Cotanche DA. Regeneration of sensory hair cells after acoustic trauma. Science 1988; 240:1772-1774.

Cotanche DA. Development of hair cell cilia in the avian cochlea. Hear Res 1987a; 28:35-44.

Cotanche DA. Regeneration of hair cell ciliary bundles in the chick cochlea following severe acoustic trauma. Hear Res 1987b; 30:181-196.

Cruz RM, Lambert PR, Rubel EW. Light microscopic evidence of hair cell regeneration after gentamicin toxicity in chick cochlea. Arch Otolaryngol Head Neck Surg 1987; 113:1058-1062.

Girod DA, Duckert LG, Rubel EW. Possible precursors of regenerated hair cells in the avian cochlea following acoustic trauma. Hear Res 1989; 42:175-194.

Gleich O, Manley GA. Quantitative morphological analysis of the sensory epithelium of the starling and pigeon basilar papilla. Hear Res 1988; 34:69-87.

Gleich O. Auditory primary afferents in the starling: Correlation of function and morphology. Hear Res 1989; 37:255-267.

Hashino E, Sokabe M, Miyamoto K. Frequency specific susceptibility to acoustic trauma in the budgerigar *(Melopsittacus undulatus)*. J Acoust Soc Am 1988; 83:2450-2453.

Hashino E, Sokabe M. Kanamycin induced low-frequency hearing loss in the budgerigar *(Melopsittacus undulatus).* J Acoust Soc Am 1989; 85:289-294.

Hashino E, Tanaka Y, Sokabe M. Hair cell damage and recovery after chronic application of kanamycin in the chick cochlea. Hear Res 1991; In press.

Henderson D, Hamernik RP. Asymptotic threshold shift from impulse noise. In: Hamernik RP, Henderson D, Salvi R, eds. New perspectives on noise-induced hearing loss. New York: Raven Press, 1982:265-281.

Hudspeth AJ. How the ear's works work. Nature 1989; 341:397-404.

Manley GA, Brix J, Kaiser A. Developmental stability of the tonotopic organization of the chick's basilar papilla. Science 1987; 237:655-656.

Manley GA, Gleich O, Kaiser A, Brix J. Functional differentiation of sensory cells in the avian auditory periphery. J Comp Physiol [A] 1989; 164:289-296.

Marsh RM, Xu L, Moy JP, Saunders JC. Recovery of the basilar papilla following intense sound exposure. Hear Res 1990; 46:229-238.

McFadden EA, Saunders JC. Recovery of auditory function following intense sound exposure in the neonatal chick. Hear Res 1989; 41:205-216.

Okanoya K, Dooling RJ. Hearing in passerine and psittacine birds: A comparative study of absolute and masked auditory thresholds. J Comp Psychol 1987; 101:7-15.

Popper AN, Hoxer B. Growth of fish ear: 1. Quantitative analysis of hair cell and ganglion cell proliferation. Hear Res 1984; 15:133-142.

Ryals BM, Rubel EW. Hair cell regeneration after acoustic trauma in adult Coturnix quail. Science 1988; 240:1774-1776.

Ryals BM, Eyck BT, Westbrook EW. Ganglion cell loss continues during hair cell regeneration. Hear Res 1989; 43:81-90.

Saunders JC, Denny RM, Bock GR. Critical bands in the parakeet *(Melopsittacus undulatus).* J Comp Physiol [A] 1978; 125:359-365.

Seidman DA, Lambert PR, Rigby PL. Absence of hair cell recovery in adult chickens after gentamicin toxicity. Abstr Assoc Res Otolaryngol 1989; 12:135.

CHAPTER 20

Noise-Induced Hearing Loss: Effects of Age and Existing Hearing Loss

JOHN H. MILLS

The most common causes of hearing loss in adults are exposure to noise, the effects of aging, the interaction of noise and aging effects, and the interaction of noise with other variables. Thus, it is not surprising to note that a clinical and research topic of longstanding interest is the interaction of noise effects and aging effects. A related topic and currently one of great interest is the effect of an existing hearing loss (whether age- or noise-induced) on the production of a subsequent hearing loss, such as that induced by exposure to noise. The timeliness of this topic is due, in large part, to recent studies of the effects of the efferent auditory system (Rajan and Johnstone, 1983) and to studies of the sensory cells of the organ of Corti, which attribute a motor (muscle-like) function to the outer hair cells (Brownell et al, 1985; Flock et al, 1986; Zenner, 1986). In this chapter, I will address the issue of the effects of an existing hearing loss (noise-induced) on the production of a subsequent noise-induced hearing loss. I will also examine the interaction between a noise-induced hearing loss and a presbycusic loss.

Susceptibility of the Noise-Damaged Ear to Additional Noise Damage

Which person is at greater risk of noise-induced hearing loss: the person with normal auditory sensitivity or the person with a mild (or moderate or severe) noise-induced hearing loss? Currently, there is no straightforward answer to this question, although the "damaged-ear theory of noise-induced hearing loss" suggests that the already-damaged ear is at greater risk of additional injury from subsequent noise exposures than the undamaged ear. The damaged-ear theory is part of the scientific basis of hearing-conservation programs and the assignment of workers to or away from excessively noisy environments.

The damaged-ear theory has a long history. Davis et al (1950) were perhaps the first to raise the issue of the susceptibility of the acoustically-injured ear. Their results with temporary threshold shift (TTS) in normal and hearing-impaired human subjects equivocally supported the damaged-ear theory. This equivocation was due in part to massive variance. For example, in one subject the first exposure to a 4.0-kHz exposure at 130 dB SPL for 8 minutes produced a temporary hearing loss of 51 dB. When the identical exposure was repeated on a later date, a temporary loss of only 12 dB was observed. Dramatic differences of this magnitude (50 dB) were noted for other subjects as well. Although Davis et al did not speculate about the physiologic bases of such dramatic intraindividual differences, they were certain that the data were not artifactual, and that individual differences were a significant factor in noise-induced hearing loss. These data, gathered at the famous Psychoacoustics Laboratory (PAL) at Harvard during World War II, gave rise to the speculation that ears resistant to noise-induced hearing loss can become susceptible to damage, or the reverse hypothesis, that susceptible ears can be toughened by acoustic experience.

Field studies and epidemiologic data suggest that persons with an existing permanent hearing loss are at greater risk of additional noise-induced hearing loss from occupational sources (Klockhoff et al, 1986; Franks et al, 1989; Elmore, 1989). These data are from hearing-conservation programs involving nearly 40,000 recruits of the Swedish Army (Klockhoff et al, 1986), and more than 100,000 U.S. Air Force personnel who were studied over a 10-year period (Elmore, 1989). These data, impressive by their sheer numbers, can be interpreted to support the damaged-ear theory—i.e., that the person with an acoustic injury of the ear is at greater risk of further noise-induced damage than the person with an uninjured ear. There are, of course, alternative explanations, including the inappropriate use of ear protective devices and the influence of nonoccupational exposures to noise.

Laboratory experiments with human subjects and with experimental animals are inconsistent in their support of the damaged-ear theory. Human TTS data (Harris, 1955) and some animal data (Voldrich, 1979) suggest the impaired ear is at greater risk of damage, whereas a number of other investigations suggest no effect or even a protective effect (Trittipoe, 1958; Miller et al, 1963; Mills et al, 1981; Ward, 1976; Pye, 1974). Mills (1973) showed that in chinchillas with pre-existing hearing losses of 0 to 30 dB, the absolute sound pressure level (SPL) or shifted threshold produced by a given exposure was independent of the pre-exposure hearing level. This result is supported by Humes (1980, 1984).

A recent report by Canlon et al (1988) supports the idea that the ear can be "toughened" by acoustic experience. In this experiment, guinea pigs were pre-exposed to a low-level tone (1.0 kHz at 81 dB SPL) for 24 days, and then to a 1.0-kHz tone at 105 dB SPL for 72 hours. A control group received only the 105-dB tone for 72 hours. The group receiving the low-level tone incurred no permanent effects, whereas the control group had permanent threshold shifts of 14 to 35 dB, depending on frequency. In light of these data, the field data of Elmore (1989) and Klockhoff et al (1986), and data on the efferent auditory system (Rajan and Johnstone, 1983), it was decided to re-examine the damaged-ear theory.

Interaction of Noise-Induced Hearing Loss and Presbycusis

In the preceding section I considered the interaction of an existing noise-induced hearing loss on the production of a subsequent noise-induced hearing loss. Now, I will consider the interaction of age-related hearing loss (presbycusis) and noise-induced hearing loss. Currently, in the quantitative audiologic assessment of occupational hearing loss, a presbycusic component is assumed to be present and is subtracted from the measured hearing levels. Indeed, there is little disagreement about the need for a presbycusic correction factor. Debate arises over the specific details of the "interaction" between noise effects and aging effects, and on the quantitative methods to correct for the effects of aging (see, for example, Corso, 1980). Although there is much literature on the interaction of noise effects and aging effects, most of the data are retrospective analyses of epidemiologic data and field studies of noise-induced hearing loss. Some of the most basic questions have never been addressed experimentally. For example, what are the biologic effects of aging on the inner ear when the inner ear has not been affected by exposure to noise (sociocusis) or disease (nosoacusis)? Do "pure presbycusic effects" differ from other forms of hearing loss? Are there several (four) distinct types of presbycusis? Are there several types of noise-induced hearing loss, such as metabolic loss from long-duration, low-level exposures, and mechanical loss from intense impulses on one occasion (acoustic trauma)? Most of these questions can only be addressed experimentally through the use of an animal model (Mills et al, 1990). Here, I will report some of the results in which hearing losses of gerbils born and reared in a quiet environment were compared with hearing losses of gerbils that spent most of their adult lives in 85-dBA noise.

Procedures

Effects of Existing Noise-Induced Loss

Details of the noise exposure and schedule are described briefly in Table 20-1. The experimental animals, Mongolian gerbils, were born and reared in a quiet vivarium. Auditory sensitivity was assessed by recording brainstem potentials elicited by tone bursts (1.8 ms) with center frequencies from 1 to 16 kHz in octave steps. Details of the audiometric procedure are given elsewhere (Mills et al, 1990). After pre-exposure audiometry was completed and it was assured that the auditory thresholds of each animal were within ±5 dB, animals were assigned randomly to Group I or to Group II. Group I was exposed first to a mon-

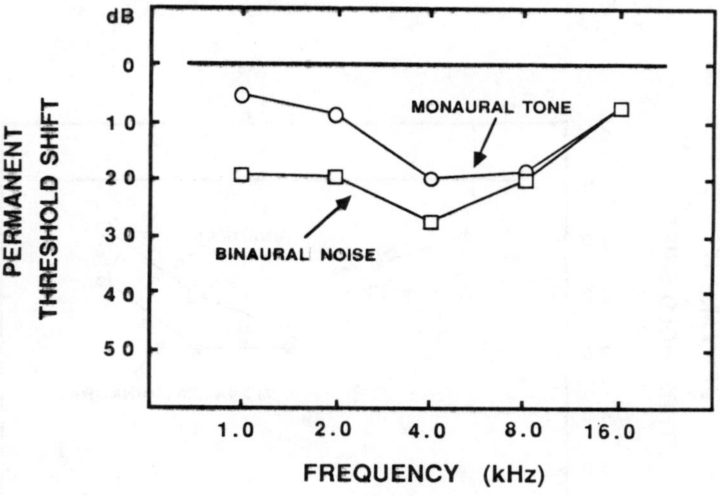

Figure 20-1 Permanent threshold shift produced by a monaural exposure to a 3.5-kHz pure tone for 1 hour at 113 dB SPL. Measurements were made 6 weeks after the exposure. Nine animals were in Group 1, 10 animals were in Group 2. The open squares show permanent threshold shifts produced by a binaural exposure to a wide-band noise for 14 days at 95 dBA.

TABLE 20.1 **Experimental Procedures**

GROUP I: Monaural/Binaural	
A. Monaural exposure:	3.5-kHz pure tone 113 dB SPL for 1 hour
B. 6 weeks recovery, measure hearing loss	
C. Binaural exposure:	Wide-band noise (0.5–4.0 kHz) 95 dBA for 2 weeks
D. 6 weeks recovery, measure permanent threshold shift (PTS)	
E. 14 weeks recovery, final measurement	
GROUP II: Binaural/Monaural	
A. Binaural exposure:	Wide-band noise (0.5–4.0 kHz) 95 dBA for 2 weeks
B. 6 weeks recovery, measure hearing loss	
C. Monaural exposure:	3.5-kHz pure tone 113 dB SPL for 1 hour
D. 6 weeks recovery, measure PTS	
E. 14 weeks recovery, final measurement	

aural tone, then to a binaural noise after 6 weeks of recovery. Group II was first exposed to a binaural noise, then to the monaural pure tone after 6 weeks of recovery. Specific details are given in Table 20-1.

Interaction of Noise and Aging Effects

The experimental procedures and rationale for the use of an animal model is discussed elsewhere (Mills et al, 1990). Briefly, the strategy was to compare hearing losses in a group of Mongolian gerbils raised in quiet quarters with hearing losses in a group that spent most of their lives in a noise chamber in which the A-weighted SPL was 85 dBA. Prior to the exposure, audiograms of 6- to 8-month-old gerbils were obtained using auditory brain-stem response (ABR) methods. Then, animals were placed in a sound field until they were about 34 months of age. At periodic intervals between 6 to 8 months and 34 months, an animal was removed from the noise field and thresholds were measured. At 36 months, a final audiogram was obtained, the animal underwent additional physiologic study, and then the ears and brain were removed for further study.

Results

Effects of Existing Hearing Loss

Permanent threshold shifts (PTSs) produced by the monaural exposure to a 3.5-kHz pure tone for 1 hour are shown in Figure 20-1. PTS was largest at 4 and 8 kHz and decreased at adjacent test frequencies. These results are consistent with earlier results both with gerbils and with other species. The open squares in Figure 20-1 show PTS produced in the right ear by a binaural exposure for 14 days to a wide-band noise (500 to 4,000 Hz) at 95 dBA. PTS was 20 to 25 dB from 1 to 8 kHz, and decreased to less than 10 dB at 16 kHz. These results are unremarkable given the spectrum, level, and duration of the exposure. Although not shown in Figure 20-1, PTS in the left ear for the binaural exposure was virtually identical to PTS in the right ear. The monaural pure-tone exposure in the right ear produced 5 dB or less PTS in the left ear.

Figure 20-2 shows PTS (right ears) in the Group II animals after the binaural exposure and PTS in the Group I animals after both the

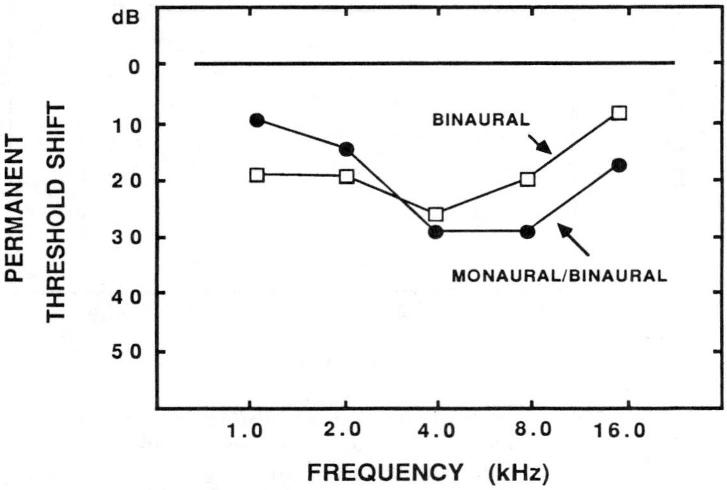

Figure 20-2 Permanent threshold shift produced in the Group II animals after the binaural exposure compared with permanent threshold shift in the Group 1 animals after both the monaural and binaural exposures. Note that at 1 and 2 kHz the monaural/binaural group has about 8 dB and 3 dB less permanent threshold shift, respectively, than the binaural group. At 8 and 16 kHz, on the other hand, the binaural group has about 10 dB less permanent threshold shift. These data thus suggest that an intense pure-tone exposure at 3.5 kHz protected the ear at 1 kHz from a subsequent exposure to a wide-band noise. At 8 and 16 kHz, the first exposure to the 3.5-kHz pure tone did not protect the ear from the effects of a subsequent exposure to a wide-band noise. Indeed, the effects of the first exposure added to the effects of the second. The damaged-ear theory is thus supported by the data at 8 and 16 kHz.

monaural and binaural exposures. In other words, the data in this figure address the question of whether or not the monaural exposure protected the ear from the subsequent binaural exposure. At 1 kHz the monaural/binaural group had about 8 dB less PTS than the binaural group. At 2 kHz this difference was reduced to about 3 dB. On the other hand, at 8 and 16 kHz the binaural group has about 10 dB less PTS than the monaural/binaural group. These data suggest that an intense pure-tone exposure at 3.5 kHz protected the ear at 1 kHz from a subsequent exposure to a wide-band noise. At 8 and 16 kHz the monaural exposure to the 3.5-kHz tone did not protect the ear from the effects of a subsequent exposure to a wide-band noise. The damaged-ear theory is thus supported by the data at 8 and 16 kHz, whereas the protective theory is supported by the data at 1 kHz.

Figure 20-3 compares PTS produced by the monaural/binaural sequence of exposures with PTS produced by the opposite sequence, that is, binaural/monaural. It is obvious that PTS is less in the animals exposed to the monaural/binaural sequence than in the animals exposed to the binaural/monaural sequence. This is particularly the case for test frequencies of 1, 2, and 4 kHz at which the standard error of the mean is about 2 dB. This order effect is not predicted by the either the damaged-ear theory, the protective theory, or any of the methods used to predict the combined effects of different exposures, such as the intensity or pressure rules (Kryter et al, 1966; Ward, 1963).

The present results are not directly comparable to reported data in which the protection was provided by temporary changes (Davis et al, 1950; Miller et al, 1963; Ward, 1963; Mills, 1981; Canlon et al, 1988). Perhaps the present data are most pertinent to field studies, which are consistent in their support of the damaged-ear theory (Franks, 1986; Klockhoff, 1986; Elmore, 1989). In other words, data from well-controlled laboratory experiments with animals, and field studies of noise-induced permanent threshold shift, show that, under some exposure conditions, the ear with an existing noise-induced permanent hearing loss may be at greater risk than the unexposed ear.

We speculate that the monaural/binaural versus binaural/monaural order effect may reflect differences in the nature of the acoustic injury produced by the different exposures. The monaural exposure is an intense, pure-tone exposure of short duration (113 dB for 1 hour), whereas the binaural exposure is a wide-band noise at a moderate level that is of

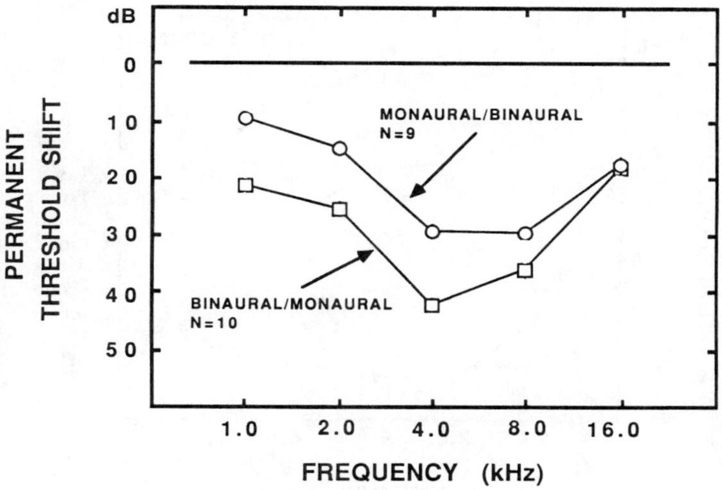

Figure 20-3 Permanent threshold shift produced in the Group I animals after the monaural/binaural sequence of exposures compared with permanent threshold shift in the Group II animals after the binaural/monaural sequence of exposures. Clearly, there is less permanent threshold shift in the monaural/binaural animals, particularly at 1, 2, and 4 kHz. This result is not predicted by the damaged-ear theory or by any other method of predicting the combined effects of noise exposures.

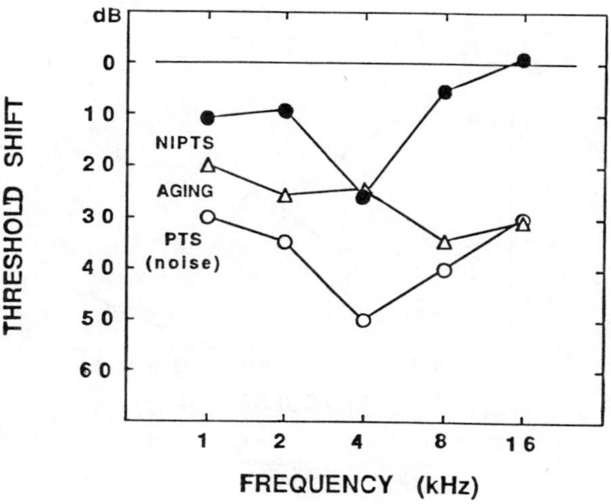

Figure 20-4 Permanent threshold shifts (open circles) measured about 90 days after termination of a 720-day exposure to a wide-band noise at 85 dBA. Aging threshold shift data (triangles) are means from 32 animals (37 ears) that were raised in a quiet vivarium (see Mills et al, 1990). Both the noise-exposed gerbils and the gerbils raised in a quiet environment were 36 months of age when these data were obtained. Noise-induced permanent threshold shift (NIPTS) is defined as noise-induced threshold shifts corrected for the effects of aging. PTS, permanent threshold shift.

long duration (95 dBA for 14 days). It is possible that the acoustic injury produced by these two distinct classes of exposures produces two distinct types of acoustic injury, and therefore complicates interactions, including an order effect.

Interaction of Noise and Aging Effects

Figure 20-4 summarizes normative aging data obtained from 37 ears of 32 Mongolian gerbils that were born and reared in a quiet vivarium for 36 months (Mills et al, 1990). Permanent threshold shift data in Figure 20-4 were measured about 90 days after termination of a 700- to 720-day exposure to a wide-band noise at 85 dBA. Both the noise-exposed animals and the animals reared in a quiet environment were 36 months of age (± 2 wks) when these measurements were made. Noise-induced permanent threshold shift (NIPTS) was defined as noise-induced threshold shifts corrected for the effects of aging. The most commonly used correction factor assumes additivity (in decibels) between noise-induced threshold shifts and "age-induced" threshold shifts. Thus, in Figure 20-4 we have simply subtracted our normative data for aging gerbils from the measured PTS. The result is NIPTS as shown in Figure 20-4.

Is the simple subtraction carried out in Figure 20-4 an appropriate or even valid method? Two factors support the procedure. One is the coincidence between the shape of the NIPTS (age-corrected) audiogram and the asymptotic threshold shift (ATS) audiogram observed after 30 to 60 days of exposure. The other is the coincidence between the spectral shape of the wide-band noise (500 to 4,000 Hz) and the audiometric configuration of

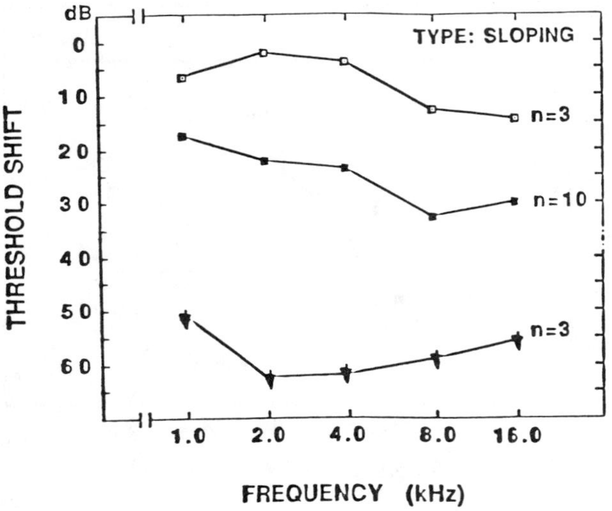

Figure 20-5 Examples of threshold shifts in 36-month-old Mongolian gerbils. Note that the range of threshold shifts is greater than 65 dB. Arrows on the datum points indicate no response at the maximum output of the audiometer.

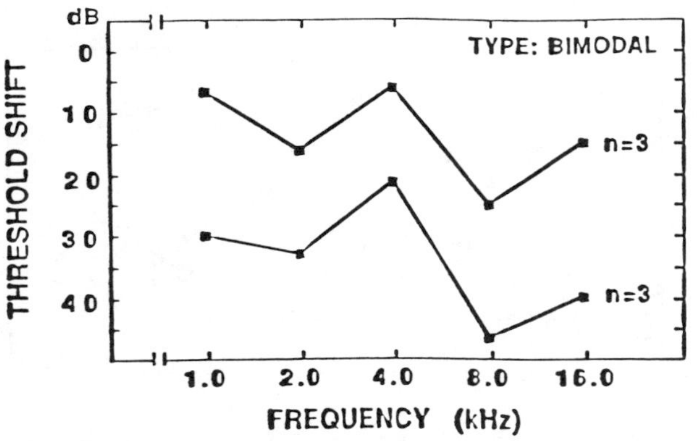

Figure 20-6 A bimodal audiometric configuration observed in some 36-month-old Mongolian gerbils. Bimodal is defined as a peak in the audiogram at 4 kHz with a 10-dB or greater loss at adjacent test frequencies. Note that in Figure 20-4, permanent threshold shifts produced by exposure to noise were greatest at 4 kHz and decreased at adjacent frequencies. In other words, the audiometric configuration associated with noise-induced permanent threshold shift in gerbils is opposite in shape to the audiometric configuration found in some gerbils who have aged in a quiet environment.

NIPTS. That is, NIPTS is present only in the frequency region of the noise. There is 5 dB or less NIPTS at 8 and 16 kHz where the spectrum of the noise contained very little energy. If indeed the subtraction procedure is valid, then the PTS audiogram shown in Figure 20-4 is mainly an aging component at 8 and 16 kHz, and a mixture of noise and aging components at lower frequencies.

Although the simplicity of the additivity notion of PTS and aging effects is appealing and is perhaps supported by coincidental observations, there are other features of the normative gerbil data (and normative human data) that detract from the additivity notion. The most obvious is the variance in the data. Figure 20-5 shows extreme examples of 16 of the 37 normative ears from Figure 20-4. The range of threshold shifts in these normative animals is greater than 65 dB. It is important to recall that these animals were born and reared in an acoustically controlled vivarium where the ambient sound levels rarely exceeded 40 dBA. It is highly unlikely that sound levels of 40 dBA and less produced hearing losses of the magnitude shown in Figure 20-5. In addition, none of the animals had impacted or infected ears, and none had ever received medicinal drugs. Room temperature, diet, and humidity were also under control. Truly, variance of the magnitude shown in Figure 20-5 is remarkable, and makes it virtually impossible to separate noise effects from aging effects in individual animals.

Figure 20-6 shows an unusual audiometric configuration, which we have called bimodal. That is, threshold shift is least at 4 kHz and increases by 10 dB or more at adjacent frequencies. This audiometric configuration was observed in 11 of 37 ears. It is interesting for several reasons. One is that the audiometric configuration noted in Figure 20-6—bimo-

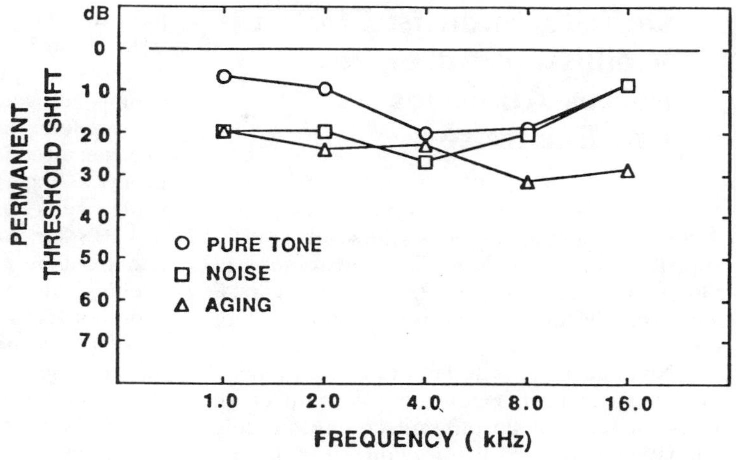

Figure 20-7 Permanent threshold shifts (1) produced by exposure to a monaural pure tone (3.5 kHz, 1 hour, 113 dB SPL); (2) produced by exposure to a wide-band noise (95 dBA, 14 days); and (3) from normative aging data from 37 ears of 32 gerbils, age 36 months, that were reared in a quiet vivarium (see Mills et al, 1990).

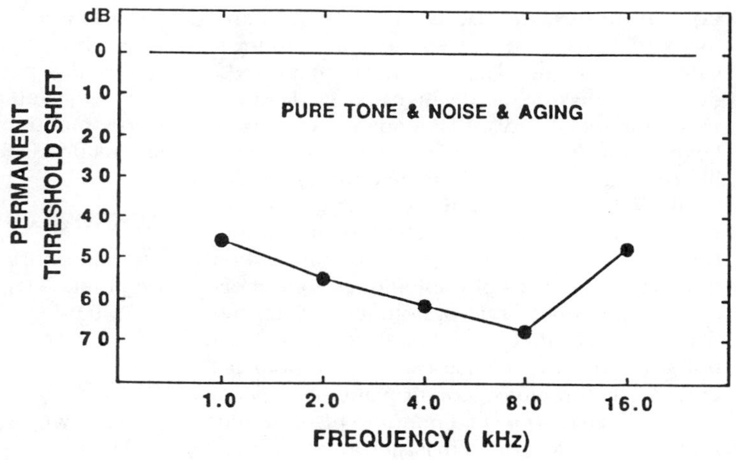

Figure 20-8 Interaction of two separate noise exposures, from Figure 20-7, with the effects of aging in a quiet environment, also from Figure 20-7. Data shown in Figures 20-1 through 20-3 support the proposition that the effects of the two noise exposures are multiplicative (additive in decibels). The data of Figure 20-4 support the assertion that presbycusic threshold shifts add (in decibels) to the threshold shifts produced by exposure to noise. Thus, when the threshold shifts of Figure 20-7 are added (in decibels) as shown here, seemingly minor permanent threshold shifts become serious when considered along with potential interactions.

dal—is opposite in shape to the NIPTS audiometric configuration shown in Figure 20-4. That is, in the bimodal category, threshold shifts are minimal at 4 kHz and increase at adjacent frequencies, whereas in NIPTS, threshold shifts are maximal at 4 kHz and decrease at adjacent frequencies. Additional analyses of bimodal audiograms await analyses of the cochlear anatomy of these animals.

In Figure 20-7 we have replotted the normative aging data from Figure 20-4, the PTS data from Figure 20-1 for a monaural pure-tone exposure, and the PTS data from Figure 20-1 for a binaural noise exposure. Each one of these three events produced a seemingly minor permanent hearing loss. That is, in the medicolegal definition of hearing handicap, the permanent threshold shifts shown in Figure 20-7 produce a minimal, if any, handicap. However, if we combine the effects of these three events in a manner dictated by the results of the experiments reported here, then the permanent threshold shifts produced by the three events are multiplicative. That is, the permanent threshold shifts are additive (as measured in decibels). The result is demonstrated in Figure 20-8 in which threshold shifts are 45 dB at 1 and 16 kHz, and 60 to 70 dB between 2 and 8 kHz. Thus, if we generalize these results from laboratory experiments to the field, seemingly minor noise-induced hearing losses incurred at a young age may very well become major when combined with the deleterious effects of age and other noise exposures as well as the possible effects of other agents including drugs and disease. Indeed, perhaps we should be careful about what we call a seemingly minor noise-induced permanent hearing loss. Of course, many additional data are needed to specify the rules for predicting the combined effects of sequential ototoxic events.

Déficits Auditifs: Effets du Vieillissement et des Pertes Auditives Pré-Existantes

Les causes les plus communes des pertes auditives neurosensorielles chez les adultes sont l'exposition au bruit, le vieillissement, et l'interaction de ces deux facteurs entre eux, ainsi que beaucoup d'autres facteurs exterieurs.

Nous avons abordé l'étude expérimentale des effets du bruit et du vieillissement et de leurs interactions en utilisant comme modèle animal la gerboise de Mongolie. L'approche expérimentale est directe. Les gerboises sont élevées dans un vivarium dont le niveau sonore moyen est de 40 dB (A). Quelques animaux témoins passèrent 36 mois dans un local calme tandis que d'autres étaient exposés à des bruits de durées, de niveaux, et de spectres variables. Avant, pendant et après l'exposition, pour les animaux testés, et régulièrement pour les animaux témoins, les seuils auditifs sont estimés à partir des potentiels évoqués du tronc cérébral. A un âge déterminé, habituellement 36 mois, un certain nombre de mesures physiologiques sont effectuées (potentiel microphonique, potentiel d'action, potentiel endocochléaire, et fibre unitaire), ensuite l'animal est préparé pour les études anatomiques comprenant la microscopie électronique et l'immuno-histochimie. Dans cet article nous envisagerons 2 interactions possibles, le vieillissement et l'exposition au bruit, et les effets d'une perte auditive préexistante due au bruit sur une nouvelle perte auditive due au bruit.

Dans le cadre de l'étude de l'interaction des effets du bruit et des effets du vieillissement, les seuils auditifs d'un groupe d'animaux témoins ont été comparés à ceux d'un groupe d'animaux exposés pendant 700 jours à un bruit large bande de 85 dBA. La moyenne des pertes auditives du groupe exposé au bruit était supérieure à la moyenne du groupe témoin; toutefois quand la moyenne des pertes du groupe témoin était soustraite (en dB) de celle des pertes du groupe exposé au bruit, la courbe représentant la différence avait la même forme que le spectre du bruit. Cette correspondance autorise la pratique courante de la correction des PTS (pertes auditives permanentes) induits par le bruit par soustraction (en dB) d'un facteur de correction lié à l'âge. Bien que cette pratique semble valable pour des données de groupes, elle serait inadéquate pour des données individuelles. Ceci étant, les PTS de plusieurs animaux témoins étaient supérieurs à ceux mesurés sur des animaux soumis au bruit.

Au sujet des pertes auditives dues au bruit préexistantes à d'autres pertes auditives, des groupes de gerboises ont été exposés, sur une seule oreille, à un son intense qui produisait des PTS sur l'oreille exposée. Ensuite les animaux étaient exposés à un bruit sur les deux oreilles. Pour d'autres groupes, l'ordre de présentation était inversé. Les résultats ne confirment pas la notion selon laquelle une perte auditive permanente protège l'oreille en cas d'expositions sonores ultérieures. En fait les PTS produits soit par l'exposition monaurale/binaurale soit par l'exposition binaurale/monaurale étaient prévisibles en additionnant les PTS obtenus (en dB) suite aux expositions séparées. Cet effet multiplicatif (additivité en dB) n'est pas en accord avec les règles courantes des pertes auditives dues au bruit et avec les résultats obtenus dans d'autres laboratoires montrant les effets protecteurs d'expositions préalables.

ACKNOWLEDGMENTS

The work in this chapter was supported by grants NIH-NIDCD P50-DC00422 and R01 ES 1301.

References

Brownell WE, Bader CR, Bertrand D, DeRibaupierre Y. Evoked mechanical responses of isolated cochlear outer hair cells. Science 1985; 227:194-196.

Canlon B, Borg E, Flock A. Protection against noise trauma by pre-exposure to a low level acoustic stimulus. Hear Res 1988; 34:197-200.

Corso JF. Age correction factor in noise-induced hearing loss: A quantitative model. Audiology 1980; 19:221-232.

Davis H, Morgan CT, Hawkins JE, et al. Temporary deafness following exposure to loud tones and noise. Acta Otolaryngol Suppl 1950; 88:1-57.

Elmore J. Employment of hard-of-hearing workers in hazardous noise and the probability of additional hearing loss. Symposium on hazardous exposure to steady state and impulse noise. Presented at the Committee on Hearing, Bioacoustics, and Biomechanics Meeting in Washington, D.C., 1989.

Flock Å, Flock B, Ulfendahl M. Mechanisms of movement in outer hair cells and a possible structural basis. Arch Otorhinolaryngol 1986; 243:83-90.

Franks JR, David RR, Krieg EF. Analysis of a hearing conservation program data base: Factors other than workplace noise. Ear Hear 1989; 10:273-280.

Harris JD. On latent damage to the ear. J Acoust Soc Am 1955; 27:177-179.

Humes LE. Temporary threshold shift for masked pure tones. Audiology 1980; 19:335-345.

Humes LE. Noise-induced hearing loss as influenced by other agents and by some physical characteristics of the individual. J Acoust Soc Am 1984; 76:1318-1329.

Klockhoff I, Lyttkens L, Svedberg A. Hearing damage in military service. Scand Audiol 1986; 15:217-222.

Kryter KD, Ward WD, Miller JD, Eldredge DH. Hazardous exposure to intermittent and steady-state noise. J Acoust Soc Am 1966; 39:451-464.

Miller JD, Watson CS, Covell W. Deafening effects of noise on the cat. Acta Otolaryngol Suppl 1963; 176:1-91.

Mills JH. Threshold shifts produced by exposure to noise in chinchillas with noise-induced hearing losses. J Speech Hear Res 1973; 16:700-708.

Mills JH, Gilbert R, Adkins WY. Temporary threshold shifts produced by wideband noise. J Acoust Soc Am 1981; 70:390-396.

Mills JH, Schmiedt RA, Kulish L. Age-related changes in auditory potentials of Mongolian gerbil. Hear Res 1990; 46:201-210.

Pye A. Acoustic trauma after double exposure in mammals. Audiology 1974; 13:320-325.

Rajan R, Johnstone BM. Residual effects in monaural temporary threshold shifts to pure tones. Hear Res 1983; 12:185-197.

Trittipoe WJ. Residual effects of low noise levels on the temporary threshold shift. J Acoust Soc Am 1958; 30:1017-1019.

Voldrich L. Noise-noise effect upon the spreading of the posttraumatic progressive necrosis in the organ of Corti. Arch Otorhinolaryngol 1979; 222:169-173.

Ward WD. Susceptibility and the damaged-ear theory. In: Hirsh SK, Eldredge DH, Hirsch IJ, Silverman SR, eds. Hearing and Davis. St. Louis: Washington University Press, 1976:127.

Ward WD. Auditory fatigue and masking. In: Jerger J, ed. Modern developments in audiology. New York: Academic Press, 1963.

Zenner HP. Motile responses in outer hair cells. Hear Res 1986; 22:83-90.

CHAPTER 21

Physiologic and Histopathologic Changes in Quiet- and Noise-Aged Gerbil Cochleas

RICHARD A. SCHMIEDT
BRADLEY A. SCHULTE

Presbycusis, the loss of hearing function with age, is still poorly understood, largely owing to the lack of controlled studies on appropriate animal models. We have been using the Mongolian gerbil to explore the interaction of age and exposure to chronic, low-level noise on hearing. The gerbil has some compelling advantages over other animal models. For example, its auditory system is well characterized (Schmiedt and Zwislocki, 1977; Smith, 1977; Ryan and Bone, 1978; Ryan et al, 1982; Schwartz and Ryan, 1983; Keithley et al, 1989; Schmiedt, 1982, 1986, 1989; Schulte and Adams, 1989; Smith et al, 1990). The gerbil is inexpensive to breed and rear, it is relatively free of middle-ear disorders that plague other rodents, it lives for about 3 years, and it has an audibility curve that closely matches that of humans. Finally, the gerbil is also used as an animal model for aging in other organ systems (Cheal, 1986).

This chapter summarizes some of the changes in the gerbil cochlea that occur with age and with chronic exposure to low-level noise. Two experiments attempted to clarify how environment and genetics combine to yield an overall hearing loss with age. The first experiment was simply to age animals in a quiet environment. Our "quiet-aged" gerbils are born and reared in a colony where the mean noise level is approximately 35 dBA, with a statistical distribution such that the levels are below 49 dBA 99 percent of the time. In the second experiment, gerbils were raised in quiet conditions until approximately 8 months of age and then were transferred to a separate enclosure, wherein a band-limited noise was continuously present. The noise level was 85 dBA overall, and the spectral half-power frequencies were 0.5 and 4 kHz. These "noise-aged" animals lived in the noise continuously for between 1 and 2 years. Animals from either group were removed for terminal physiologic studies when (1) they approached 36 months of age; (2) they showed hearing losses in excess of 60 dB as assessed by longitudinal brain-stem recordings; or (3) either ear showed signs of an impending outer-ear impaction. The median life span for gerbils in our colony is about 36 months. A more detailed description of these procedures can be found in Mills et al (1990) and Schmiedt et al (1990).

Quiet-Aged Results

Hearing thresholds were assessed by recording compound action potentials (CAPs) with round-window electrodes during the terminal experiment. Thresholds of six quiet-aged animals along with mean control data from 10 young gerbils are shown in Figure 21-1. There is an essentially parallel shift in thresholds in the older gerbils at frequencies below 4 kHz. Above 4 kHz, the threshold shifts increase, often with substantial variability among animals.

While collecting the CAP data, we noticed that the amplitude of the CAP waveform did not grow normally with increasing stimulus intensity. This lack of growth is a consistent finding in all quiet-aged gerbils. Examples of CAP input/output (I/O) functions from young and old animals are shown in Figure 21-2. Further analysis demonstrates that both the slope

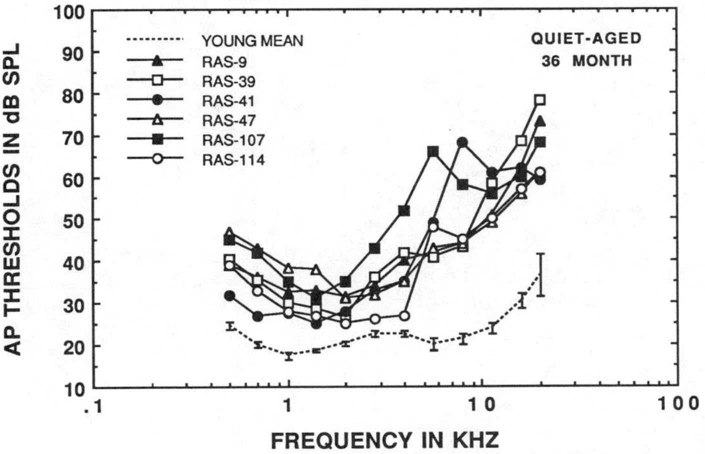

Figure 21-1 Compound action potential (CAP) thresholds obtained with tone pips in six quiet-aged gerbils. Dashed line plots the mean thresholds from 10 young controls, with error bars indicating the standard error of the mean (SEM). Note the parallel shift at low frequencies compared to the control data, and the larger shifts for frequencies above 4 kHz.

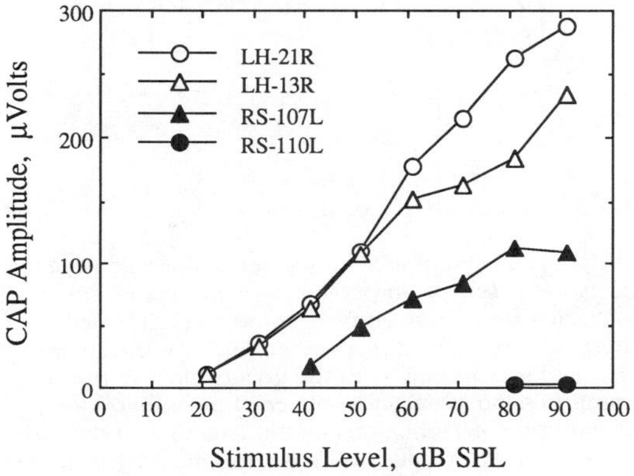

Figure 21-2 Compound action potential input/output (CAP I/O) functions in young (open symbols) and quiet-aged, 36-month-old (closed symbols) gerbils. CAP responses were elicited with a 2-kHz tone pip and recorded at the cochlear round window with a silver-ball electrode. The amplitude was measured from the negative to the positive peak on the CAP waveform after averaging 50 responses. Generally, the CAP I/O function is less steep and saturates at lower maximum values in aged gerbils as compared with young control gerbils.

and the maximum amplitude of the CAP I/O functions in quiet-aged gerbils are significantly less than those found in young animals (Hellstrom and Schmiedt, 1990a). This evoked-response decrement also carried over to the brain-stem evoked response (Mills et al, 1990), but is not present at the level of primary cochlear fibers; i.e., the intensity functions of single fibers are normal in shape and in dynamic range in quiet-aged gerbils (Hellstrom and Schmiedt, 1990b). A possible cause for the decrement in the CAP I/O function may be spiral ganglion cell degeneration (Keithley and Feldman, 1982; Keithley et al, 1989); our preliminary anatomic results tend to support these data.

Hair-cell loss in the quiet-aged animals is variable and is almost entirely accounted for by the loss of outer hair cells (OHCs). The OHC loss is most often greatest in the apex, although scattered losses are always present throughout the cochlea. Figure 21-3 illustrates a typical cochleogram from a quiet-aged gerbil (RAS-39). Respective evoked-potential thresholds, single-fiber tuning curves, and two-tone suppression boundaries are also shown for gerbil RAS-39 in Figure 21-3.

Single-fiber characteristics in these quiet-aged gerbils are, for the most part normal. An exception is that tuning curves (Fig. 21-3) are elevated around their characteristic frequencies (CFs). Tail thresholds are approximately normal, resulting in a decreased tip-to-tail ratio in these old animals. The boundaries of two-tone rate suppression are clearly defined and are approximately normal in threshold, both above and below CF. Suppression is present even when the CF threshold is elevated as much as 40 to 60 dB (Schmiedt et al, 1990).

Despite the relatively normal single-fiber characteristics, the DC endocochlear potential (EP) in the scala media is definitely abnormal in aged gerbils, almost certainly owing to degeneration of the lateral wall and stria vascularis (see Figs. 21-7 and 21-8). Figure 21-4 illustrates some mean EP data with percentage loss of strial function as the parameter. Note that even with a 25 to 75 percent functional loss as estimated subjectively by evaluating the decreased intensity of immunohistochemical staining for Na^+,K^+-ATPase, the EP can still be maintained at about 60 mV over most of the cochlear duct. The stria always degener-

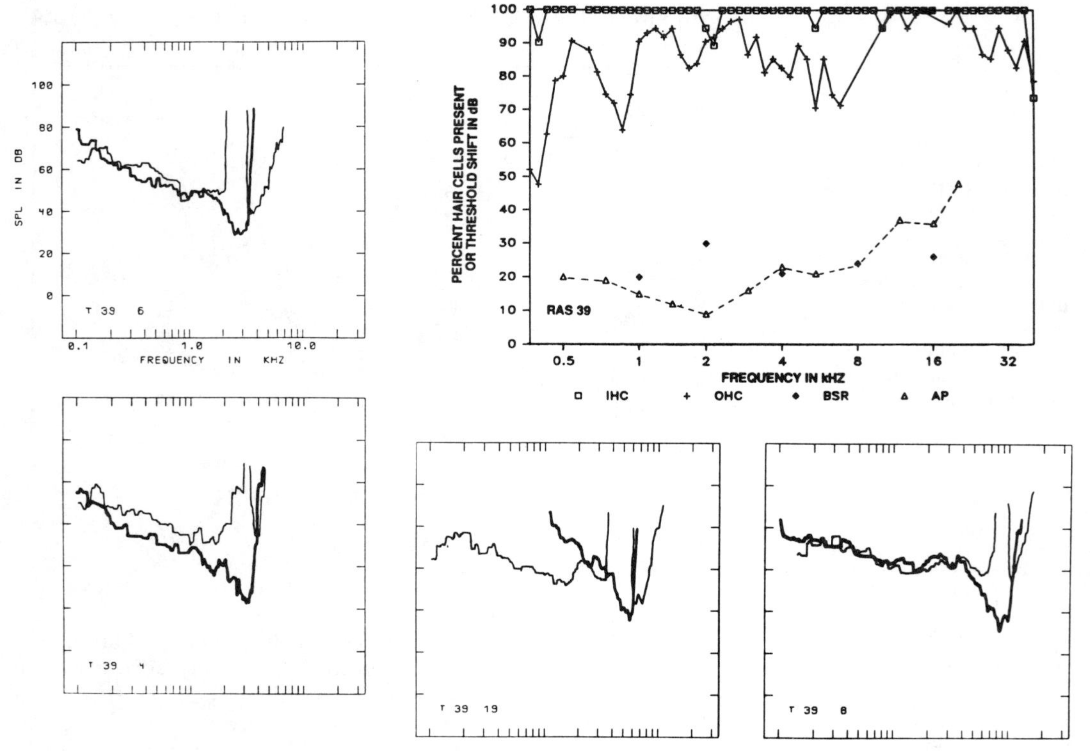

Figure 21-3 Cochleogram, evoked response thresholds (top right) and single-fiber tuning and suppression boundaries from a quiet-aged gerbil (RAS-39). The cochleogram plots the presence, in percent, of inner (open squares) and combined outer hair cells (OHCs) (plus signs). The cochlear map is derived from the data of Schmiedt and Zwislocki (1977). The compound action potential (CAP) thresholds are plotted as a dashed line; the thresholds of the brain-stem response are plotted with filled diamonds. OHC loss is scattered, with the greatest loss in the apex. Tuning curves (thick lines) and boundaries of two-tone rate suppression (thin lines) obtained from four auditory-nerve fibers are also shown. Suppression contours were obtained in the presence of a continuous tone at the characteristic frequency (CF) of the fiber at 15 dB above threshold (see Schmiedt, 1982). All the quiet-aged gerbils showed clear suppression boundaries above and below CF despite 20- to 40-dB shifts in CF threshold as compared to controls. (Adapted from Schmiedt RA, Mills JH, Adams JC. Tuning and suppression in auditory nerve fibers of aged gerbils raised in quiet or noise. Hear Res 1990; 45:221-236.)

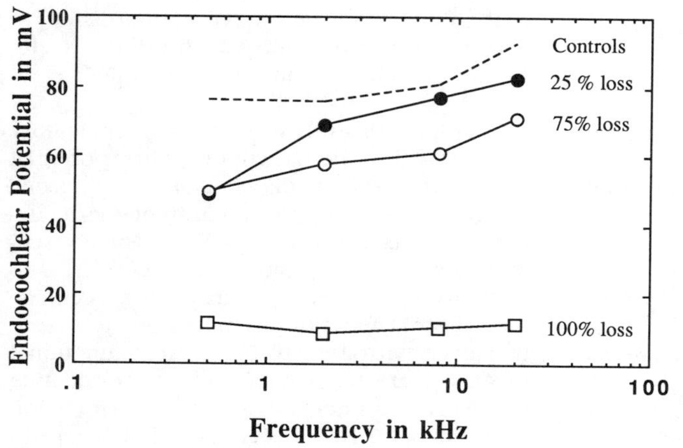

Figure 21-4 Mean endocochlear potentials (EPs) recorded at four places in young and quiet-aged (36-month-old) gerbil cochleas. The cochlear locations correspond to the third, second, and first turns and the round-window region, going from low to high frequency. The upper dashed line plots mean data from seven young controls. Cochleas were grouped according to the amount of strial loss as judged subjectively from the intensity of immunohistochemical staining for Na^+K^+ ATPase in 5-μm paraffin sections taken at 125-μm intervals along the entire cochlear duct. No immunoreactive Na^+K^+ ATPase was present in the apical turn of any of the old cochleas. Later degenerative changes began in the basal turn and progressed toward the middle turn. The 25 percent group had a 0 to 25 percent loss of staining compared to controls over the remaining cochlea; the 75 percent group had a loss of between 25 and 75 percent; and the 100 percent group had a loss of between 75 and 100 percent. The numbers of cochleas in the 25, 75, and 100 percent groups were 5, 5, and 4, respectively.

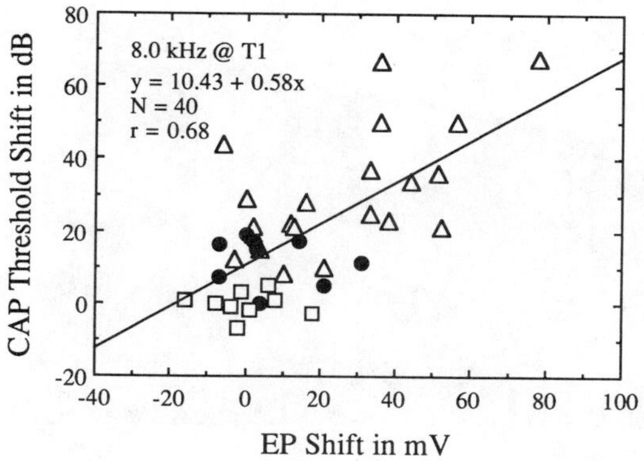

Figure 21-5 Correlations between the compound action potential (CAP) threshold shift at 8 kHz and the endocochlear potential (EP) recorded at the 8-kHz location for young (open squares), 30-month-old (filled circles), and 36-month-old, quiet-aged (open triangles) gerbils. Each point represents a paired measurement of the EP and CAP from one cochlea. The greatest effects of the EP shift on CAP thresholds are seen in the 36-month-old group.

ates first in the apex, then in the basal turn. In this group of cochleas, all 33 months or older, none had any strial function in the apical turn, but most retained at least some normal-appearing regions of striae in the middle turn. When strial loss is 75 to 100 percent throughout the cochlea, the EP essentially disappears, as one would expect.

Sewell (1984) showed a direct relation between CAP thresholds and EP in acute studies of cats using furosemide to modulate the EP. A linear decrement of EP logarithmically shifted the CAP threshold, thus giving rise to a relationship of approximately 1 mV per dB; i.e., a 1-mV decrease in the EP resulted in a 1-dB increase in the CAP threshold. However, the slope constant was variable among cats and among single-fiber thresholds in any given cat. The point is that there is a direct relationship between the EP in millivolts and neural thresholds in decibels in normal, acutely-prepared cats. Thus, it was of interest to analyze our CAP threshold data and relate it to the EP recorded at the appropriate place.

CAP thresholds were correlated with EP in young controls and in 30-month-old and 36-month-old gerbils aged in quiet. EP was recorded at four locations along the cochlear duct corresponding to 0.5, 2, 8, and 20 kHz. The resulting correlation between the CAP thresholds and the value of the EP present in the scala media at the 8-kHz location is shown in Figure 21-5. A correlation coefficient of 0.68 implies that about 46 percent of the variability of the CAP data can be accounted for by the variation in the EP. The data show that there is a correlation between EP values and CAP thresholds only in the 36-month-old group; in the 30-month-old group, there is an EP shift in many animals, but it is not correlated with shifts in CAP thresholds. Obviously, other factors besides the decrement in EP are involved in the neural threshold shifts in these quiet-aged gerbils.

Some morphologic differences between the stria vascularis of young and old gerbils are illustrated in Figures 21-6 and 21-7. Marginal cells show extensive atrophic changes in regions of strial degeneration in old gerbils; thus, it is not surprising that the EP is decreased in these animals. Changes in strial function with age are more clearly demonstrated by a decrease or loss of immunostaining for Na^+,K^+-ATPase, as shown in Figure 21-8. This technique provides a much more accurate and reproducible means of evaluating strial function than does the examination of histologic preparations under the light or electron microscope.

Noise-Aged Results

CAP thresholds from five noise-aged gerbils are shown in Figure 21-9. The midfrequency loss is almost certainly due to the noise exposure and not to aging (compare Fig. 21-1). Moreover, the low-frequency thresholds of these animals vary considerably and are less sensitive than those of the quiet-aged group.

Single-fiber data from two noise-aged animals are shown in Figures 21-10 and 21-11. The data in both figures are arranged as in Figure 21-3. Gerbil RAS-28 (Fig. 21-10) was only aged in the noise for 12 months and was 24 months old at the time of the terminal experiment. This animal was removed from the noise prematurely because of an impending impaction in an outer-ear canal. Even so, scattered hair-cell loss is present throughout the cochlea, but concentrated in the midfrequency region, the region most affected by the noise. The tuning and suppression boundaries of the primary fibers were definitely abnormal: tuning curves were mostly bowl-shaped for CFs below about 10 kHz, and suppression was absent above and below CF. For CFs above 10 kHz, the tuning curves regained their normal tip and tail features, although the CF thresholds were still elevated by 10 to 15 dB over those of young controls. Two-tone suppression reasserted itself in these high-CF fibers as well. Thus, the basal turn of this co-

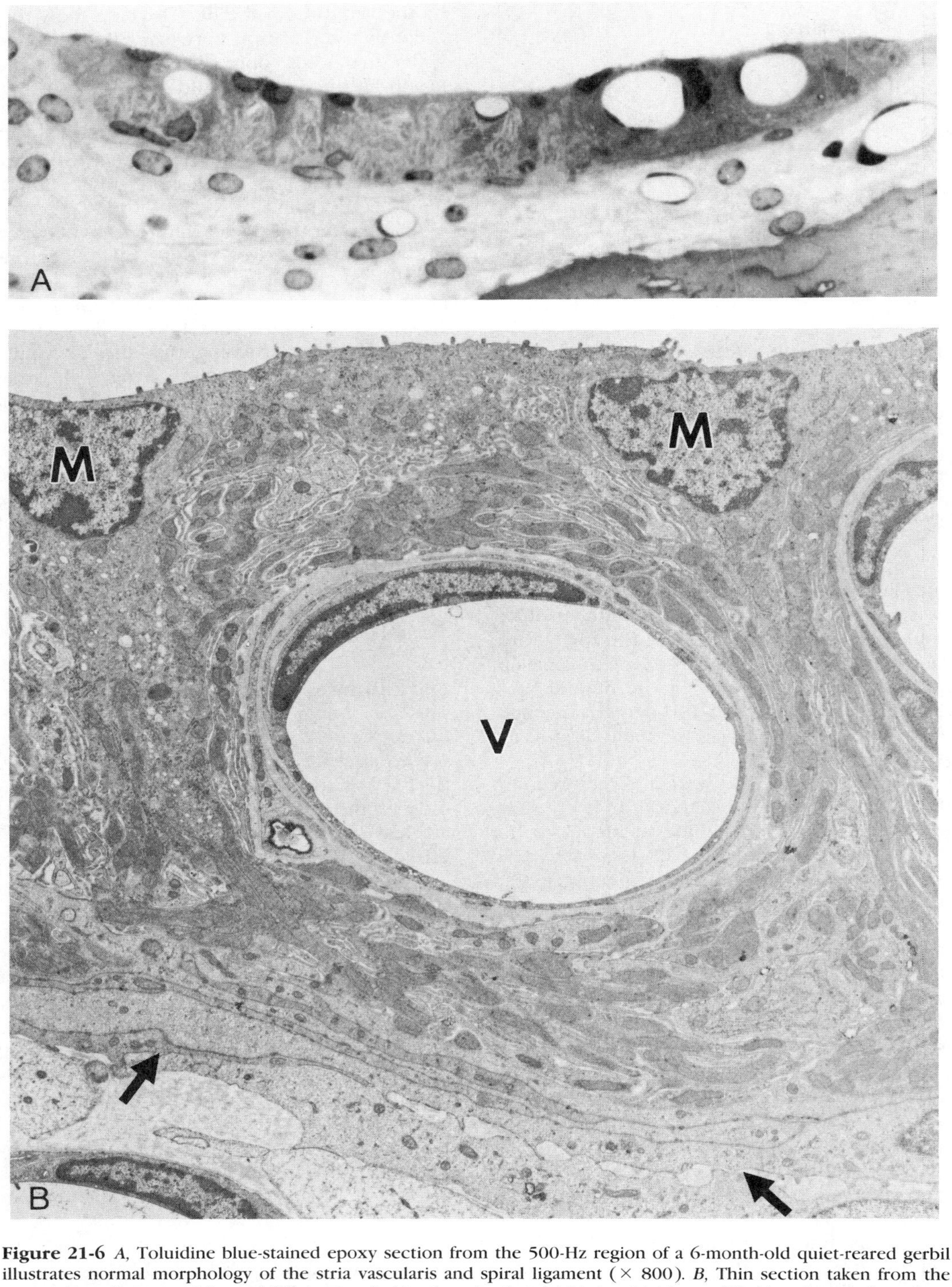

Figure 21-6 *A,* Toluidine blue-stained epoxy section from the 500-Hz region of a 6-month-old quiet-reared gerbil illustrates normal morphology of the stria vascularis and spiral ligament (× 800). *B,* Thin section taken from the same region shows a strial vessel (V) surrounded by the mitochondrial-laden, highly-amplified basolateral plasmalemma of marginal cells (M). Interdigitating processes of basal cells (arrows) form the boundary between the stria vascularis and the underlying spiral ligament (× 13,000).

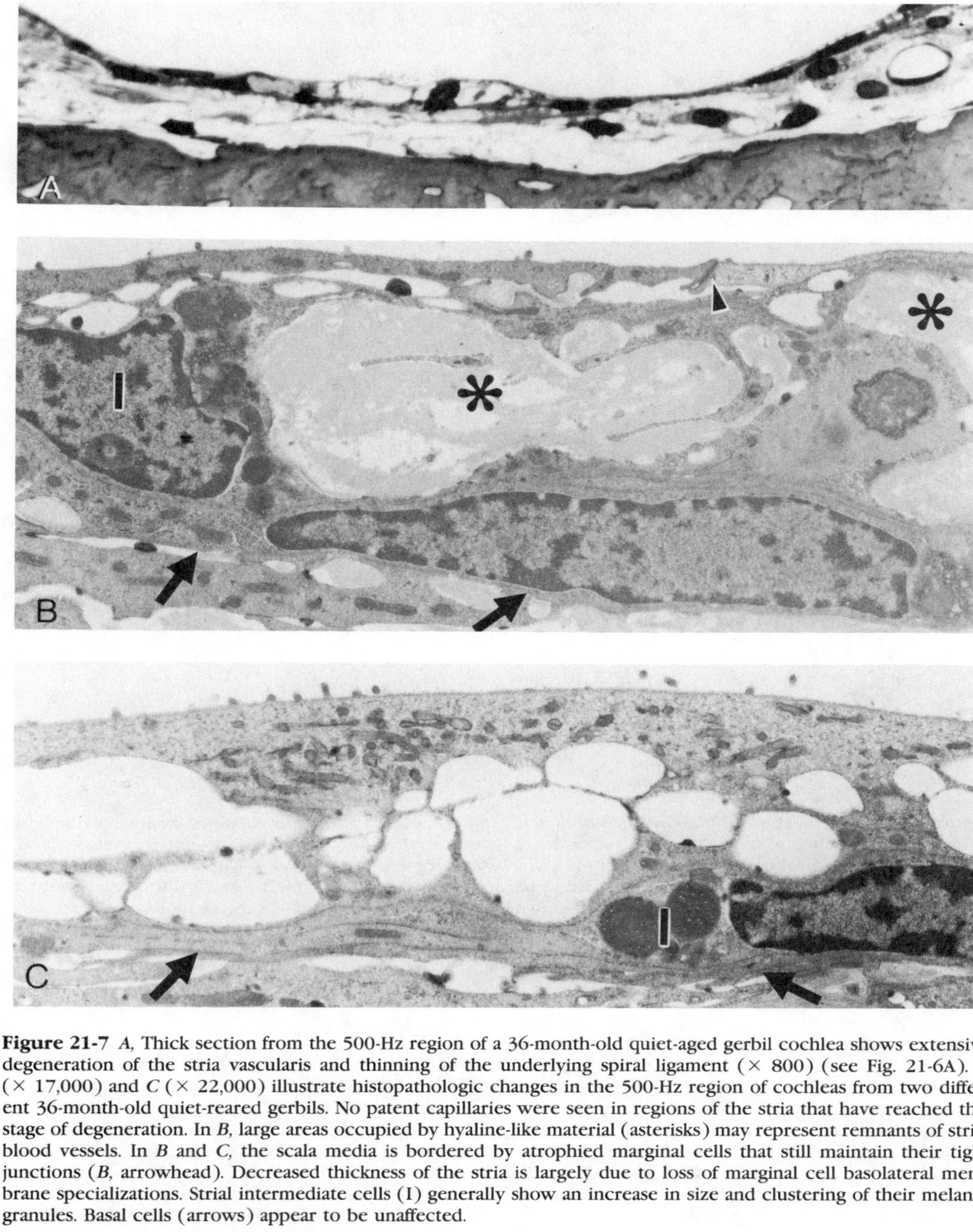

Figure 21-7 *A*, Thick section from the 500-Hz region of a 36-month-old quiet-aged gerbil cochlea shows extensive degeneration of the stria vascularis and thinning of the underlying spiral ligament (× 800) (see Fig. 21-6A). *B* (× 17,000) and *C* (× 22,000) illustrate histopathologic changes in the 500-Hz region of cochleas from two different 36-month-old quiet-reared gerbils. No patent capillaries were seen in regions of the stria that have reached this stage of degeneration. In *B*, large areas occupied by hyaline-like material (asterisks) may represent remnants of strial blood vessels. In *B* and *C*, the scala media is bordered by atrophied marginal cells that still maintain their tight junctions (*B*, arrowhead). Decreased thickness of the stria is largely due to loss of marginal cell basolateral membrane specializations. Strial intermediate cells (I) generally show an increase in size and clustering of their melanin granules. Basal cells (arrows) appear to be unaffected.

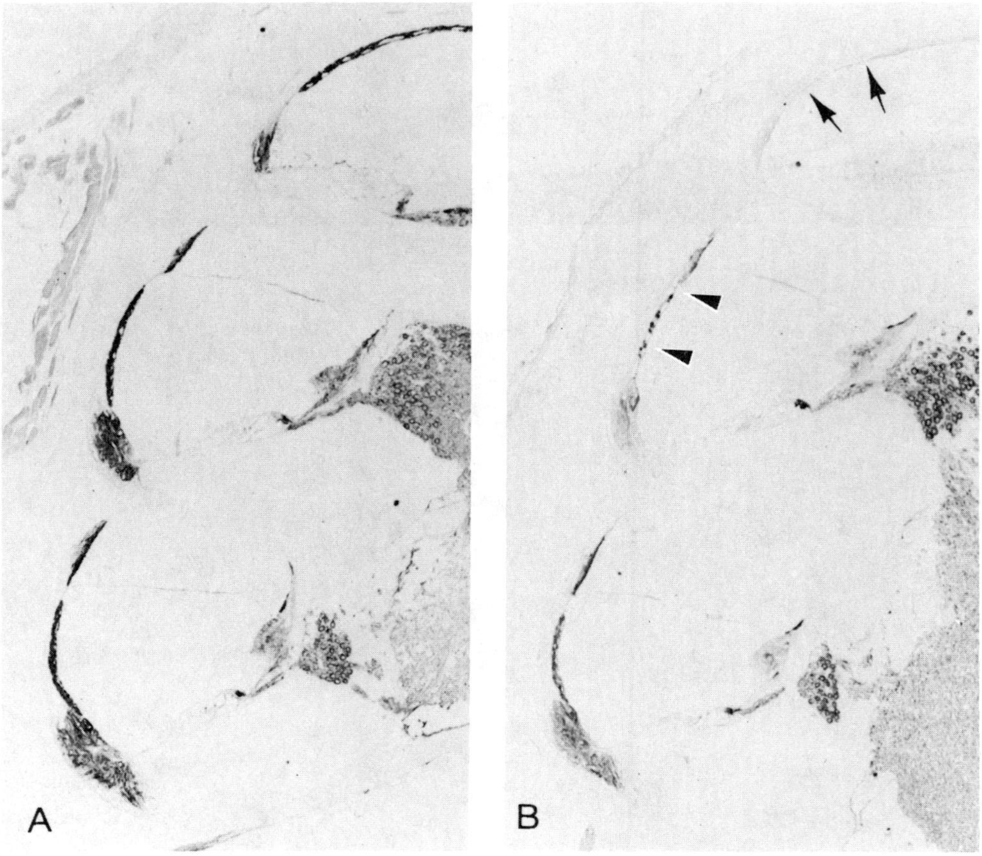

Figure 21-8 Gerbil cochleas immunostained with a 1:2,000 dilution of an antiserum raised against bovine brain cortex Na^+K^+ ATPase. *A*, Cochlea from a 6-month-old quiet-reared animal shows uniform distribution of Na^+K^+ ATPase in strial marginal cells of all three turns (× 60). *B*, Cochlea from a 30-month-old quiet-reared animal shows complete loss of immunoreactive Na^+K^+ ATPase in the stria vascularis of the apical turn (arrows) and greatly diminished immunoreactivity in the middle turn (arrowheads) (× 60). More details of the methods can be found in Schulte and Adams (1989).

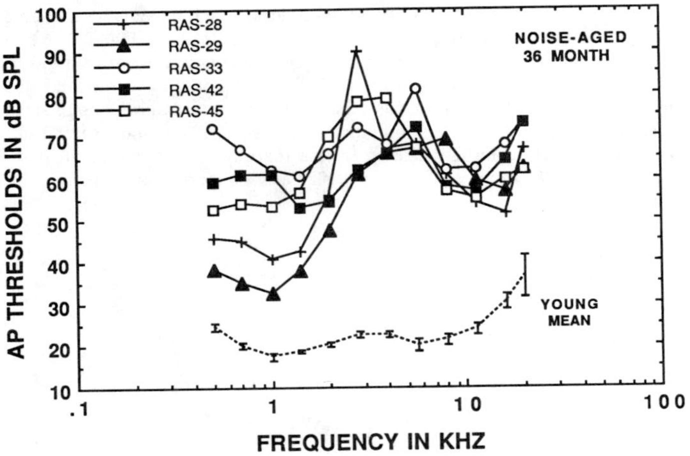

Figure 21-9 Compound action potential (CAP) thresholds obtained with tone pips in five noise-aged gerbils. Otherwise, the figure is the same as Figure 21-1. Note the midfrequency elevation in thresholds caused by the noise exposure (0.5 to 4 kHz, 85 dBA). Also, variability is greatest at low frequencies, opposite to that which is found in quiet-aged animals.

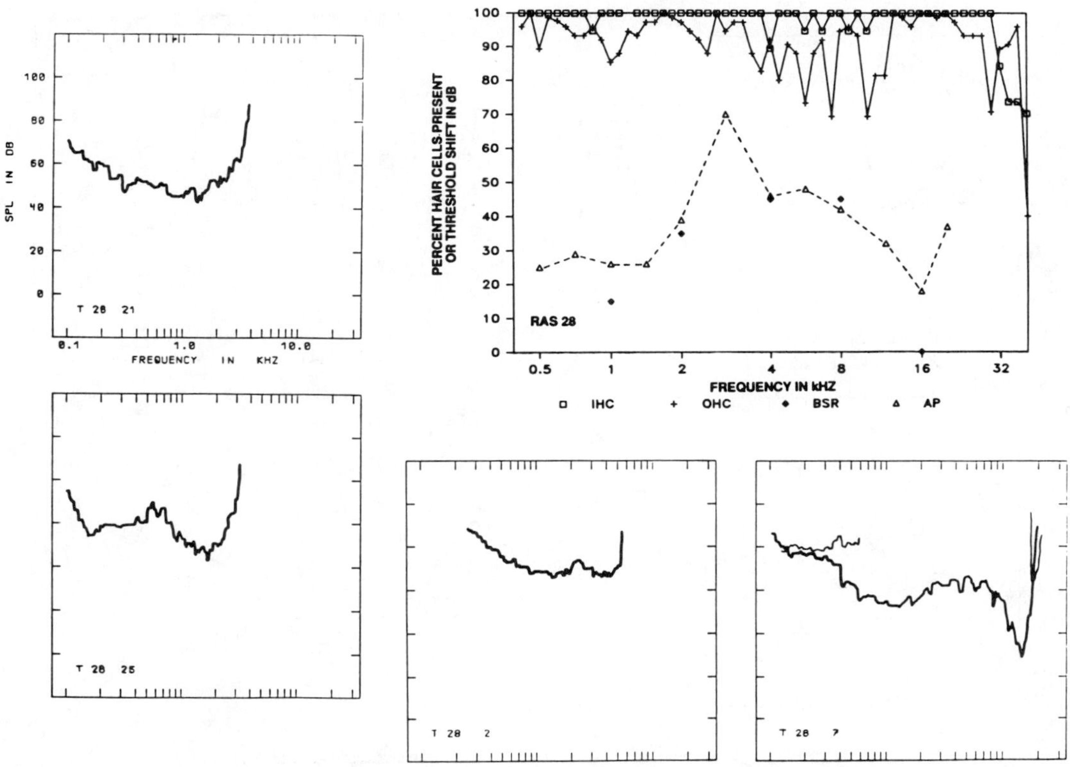

Figure 21-10 Cochleogram, evoked response thresholds (top right) and single-fiber tuning curves and suppression boundaries from a noise-aged gerbil (RAS-28). Otherwise, the data are plotted as in Figure 21-3. The compound action potential (CAP) audibility curve has a notch that does not correspond to any large loss of hair cells or ganglion cells. Single-fiber tuning curves were bowl-shaped, except for fibers of high characteristic frequency (CF). Similarly, two-tone suppression was absent except for high-characteristic frequency fibers. It is hypothesized that the noise exposure destroyed the normal two-tone interactions in this cochlea; however, the basal coil was spared, given the decreasingly small amount of noise energy above 4 kHz. (Adapted from Schmiedt RA, Mills JH, Adams JC. Tuning and suppression in auditory nerve fibers of aged gerbils raised in quiet or noise. Hear Res 1990; 45:221-236.)

chlea was able to "age" normally despite the 1-year exposure to the noise.

Gerbil RAS-45 remained in the noise for 700 days and was 36 months old at the terminal experiment. The hair-cell loss in the mid and apical turns under these conditions was far more pronounced than that for the younger animal, RAS-28 (Fig. 21-10). Yet, even with losses of OHCs approaching 60 percent, two-tone suppression below CF was always present, even for fibers with bowl-shaped tuning curves. Suppression above CF reappeared in fibers with CFs above about 8 kHz. Thus, it seems that a full complement of OHCs is not necessary for suppression below CF, and that suppression above and below CF are independent phenomena (Schmiedt et al, 1990). As in the previous noise-aged animal, the basal-most fibers seemed to escape the effects of the noise exposure.

Perhaps the secret to maintaining suppression below CF is the condition of the inner hair cells (IHCs). The photomicrographs in Figure 21-12 show a view of the mid-cochlea of RAS-45 focused at the plane of the stereocilia (left) and radial fibers (right). OHC loss is certainly evident, yet few IHCs are missing, and the density of radial fibers is apparently normal. Sections of missing radial fibers were rarely seen in either the quiet- or noise-aged gerbils. The ears were not processed in a way to optimize observation of stereocilia; thus stereocilia have not been systematically examined in either the quiet- or noise-aged group. It is probable, however, that stereocilia hold at least part of the explanation of the elevated thresholds seen in the noise-aged animals as compared to the quiet-aged animals. We have seen stereocilia aberrations in both groups, but it is difficult to determine

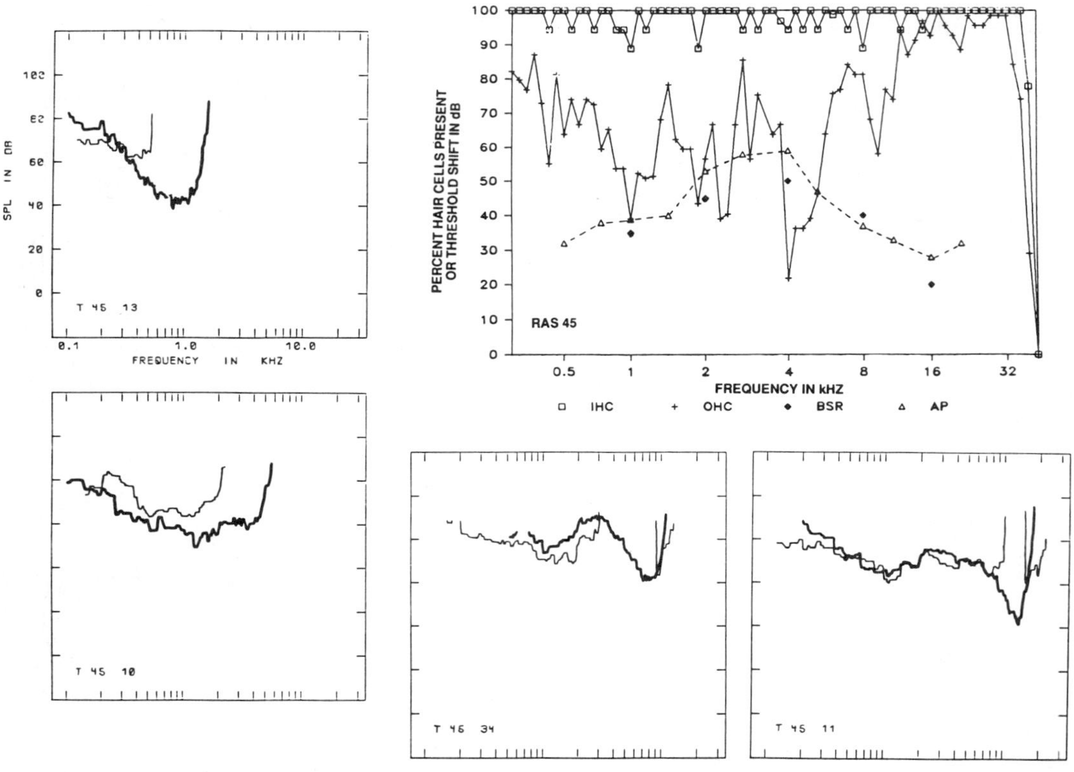

Figure 21-11 Cochleogram, evoked response thresholds (top right) and single-fiber tuning curves and suppression boundaries from a noise-aged gerbil (RAS-45). Otherwise, the data are plotted as in Figure 21-3. This gerbil had extensive hair-cell loss, especially in the region corresponding to the noise spectrum. Unlike the previous noise-aged gerbil (RAS-28), most of the contacted auditory-nerve fibers in this gerbil had well-defined suppression below characteristic frequency (CF), even those fibers having bowl-shaped tuning curves. Those fibers associated with the noise, however, exhibited no suppression above CF. Data such as these suggest that suppression above CF is more vulnerable than suppression below CF to chronic, low-level noise, and that suppression areas above and below CF are more or less independent. (Adapted from Schmiedt RA, Mills JH, Adams JC. Tuning and suppression in auditory nerve fibers of aged gerbils raised in quiet or noise. Hear Res 1990; 45:221-236.)

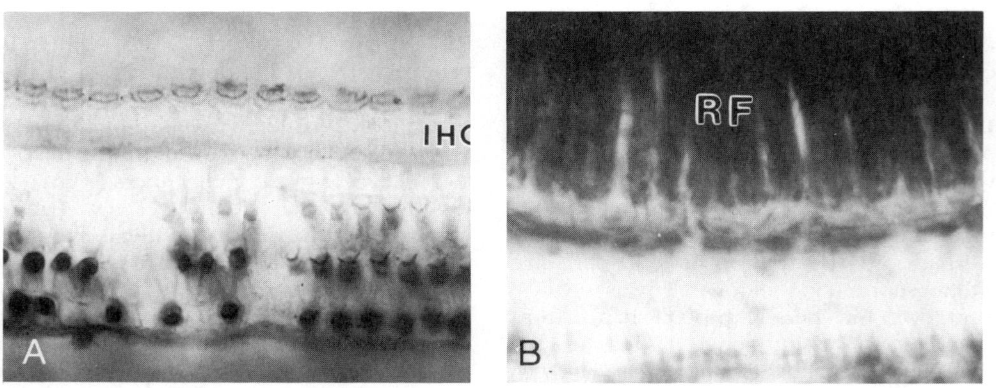

Figure 21-12 Photomicrographs taken from the 4-kHz region of a surface preparation of a 36-month-old gerbil raised in noise (RAS-45R). *A,* More than 50 percent of the outer hair cells (OHC) are missing or damaged, but the inner hair cells (IHC) appear to be in relatively good shape. The condition of the stereocilia could not be judged with certainty in these preparations (× 880). *B,* Despite the large number of missing OHCs *(A)* and a compound action potential threshold elevation of around 60 dB, the density of radial fibers (RF) does not appear to be diminished (× 440). With the exception of the greater number of lost or damaged OHCs in noise-exposed ears, no obvious morphologic differences were seen in surface preparations of age-matched animals raised in quiet or noise.

whether the abnormalities are real or artifactual.

In summary, we find that the effects of chronic, low-level noise are additive to the effects of age in a qualitative and quantitative sense (Mills et al, 1990; Schmiedt et al, 1990). Thus, no matter what the genetic background of the individual, the environmental influence of noise exposure during a lifetime will add to any loss dictated by genetics.

Modifications Physiologiques et Histopathologiques Observées sur des Cochlées de Gerboises Elevées dans un Environnement Calme ou dans le Bruit

Les facteurs génétiques et environnementaux sont les causes principales des pertes auditives chez les personnes âgées. L'interaction du bruit et de l'âge a été explorée sur deux groupes de gerboises de Mongolie qui étaient élevés, l'un dans le calme, l'autre dans un local bruyant (bruit de 85 dB (A), fréquences 0,5 à 4,0 kHz). La durée d'exposition au bruit était comprise entre 365 et 724 jours. Les résultats ont été comparés avec ceux d'un groupe contrôle composé de jeunes sujets élevés dans le calme. A la fin des expérimentations l'âge des sujets variait de 24 à 43 mois, l'âge moyen de notre colonie étant de 36 mois. L'audition était contrôlée au moyen des tests suivants: potentiel d'action global (CAP), potentiel endocochléaire (EP) et réponse de fibres unitaires au niveau du nerf auditif. Les cochlées des groupes de contrôle "sujets jeunes", et des groupes de sujets âgés vivant au calme "âgés-calme" ont été soumis aux mêmes examens morphologiques et immunohistochimiques. Les cochlées des sujets agés soumis au bruit "âgés-bruit" ont été soumis aux examens morphologiques seulement.

Les seuils auditifs montrent une variabilité considérable à l'intérieur des deux groupes de sujets âgés, ceux vivant dans le calme et ceux vivant dans le bruit, mais ils augmentent avec l'âge dans les deux groupes. Dans le groupe "âgés-calme", la moyenne des seuils du CAP à 36 mois montre une variation uniforme de 20 dB de 0,5 à 4 kHz, qui croît jusqu'à 30 dB pour les fréquences plus élevées. Les courbes "fibres-unitaires" montrent également des variations de seuils, mais seulement autour de la fréquence caractéristique (CF), les seuils aux autres fréquences sont normaux. Par conséquent le rapport maxi-mini (tip-to-tail) est réduit chez les sujets "âgés-calme". Les non-linéarités correspondant à la suppression entre deux tons, sont présentes à la fois au-dessus et au-dessous de la fréquence caractéristique dans le groupe "âgés-calme".

Les cochlées du groupe "âgés-calme" montrent des pertes dispersées de cellules ciliées externes (OHCs), principalement à l'apex et à la base, mais presque pas de pertes de cellules ciliées internes (IHCs). L'atrophie de la strie vasculaire dans le groupe "âgés-calme" est une découverte intéressante. La dégénérescence de la strie vasculaire apparait d'abord dans le tour apical et ensuite dans le tour de base quand le sujet avance en âge. Les colorations immunohistochimiques Na,K-ATPase confirment une réduction notable de la fonction de la strie vasculaire avec l'âge, corrélée avec la réduction du potentiel endocochléaire pour certains sujets pris individuellement.

Les sujets "âgés-bruit" ont des variations de seuils plus importantes que les sujets "âgés-calme" pour les fréquences comprises dans la bande de bruit. Comme pour le groupe "âgés-calme" elles sont localisées principalement à la pointe des courbes de fibres unitaires. Contrairement aux sujets "âgés-calme" la suppression entre deux tons est souvent absente dans le groupe "âgés-bruit." On n'a jamais remarqué de suppression au-dessus de la fréquence caractéristique, pour les fibres avec CFs dans la bande de bruit, quoique la suppression a pu quelquefois être démontrée en-dessous de la fréquence caractéristique.

Les sujets "âgés-bruit" montrent une plus grande perte de cellules ciliées externes (OHCs) que les sujets "âgés-calme" sur les emplacements de la cochlée correspondants au bruit. Comme pour les sujets "âgés-calme" on observe peu de pertes de cellules ciliées internes. L'atrophie de la strie vasculaire n'a pas été observée chez les sujets "âgés-bruit".

Ces résultats démontrent que l'exposition au bruit exacerbe les pertes auditives dues à l'âge. Cependant, la nette variabilité dans l'étendue des changements physiologiques, morphologiques et histochimiques observée entre les sujets "âgés-calme", restés dans le même environnement suggère une influence génétique directe sur les pertes auditives dues à l'âge.

ACKNOWLEDGMENTS

We thank J.C. Adams, L.I. Hellstrom, F.S. Lee, J.H. Mills, and S.S. Spicer for their help with data collection and analysis. Support was provided by NIH grants P50 DC00422 and DC00713, and from NSF grant BNS-8607921.

References

Cheal M. The gerbil: A unique model for research on aging. Exp Aging Res 1986; 12:3-21.

Hellstrom LI, Schmiedt RA. Compound action potential input/output functions in young and quiet-aged gerbils. Hear Res 1990; 50:163-174.

Hellstrom LI, Schmiedt RA. Comparisons of compound action potential and single-fiber characteristics in young and quiet-aged gerbils. Abstr Assoc Res Otolaryngol 1990b; 13:149.

Keithley EM, Feldman ML. Hair cell counts in an age-graded series of rat cochleas. Hear Res 1982; 8:249-262.

Keithley EM, Ryan AF, Woolf NK. Spiral ganglion cell density in young and old gerbils. Hear Res 1989; 38:125-134.

Mills JH, Schmiedt RA, Kulish LF. Age-related changes in auditory potentials of Mongolian gerbil. Hear Res 1990; 46:201-210.

Ryan AF, Bone RC. Noise-induced threshold shift and cochlear pathology in the Mongolian gerbil. J Acoust Soc Am 1978; 63:1145-1151.

Ryan AF, Woolf NK, Sharp FR. Tonotopic organization in the central auditory pathway of the Mongolian gerbil: A 2-Deoxyglucose study. J Comp Neurol 1982; 207:369-380.

Schmiedt RA. Boundaries of two-tone rate suppression of cochlear-nerve activity. Hear Res 1982; 7:335-351.

Schmiedt RA. Acoustic distortion in the ear canal. I. Cubic difference tones: Effects of acute noise injury. J Acoust Soc Am 1986; 79:1481-1490.

Schmiedt RA. Spontaneous rates, thresholds, and tuning of auditory-nerve fibers in the gerbil: Comparisons to cat data. Hear Res 1989; 42:23-36.

Schmiedt RA, Zwislocki JJ. Comparison of sound-transmission and cochlear-microphonic characteristics in Mongolian gerbil and guinea pig. J Acoust Soc Am 1977; 61:133-149.

Schmiedt RA, Mills JH, Adams JC. Tuning and suppression in auditory nerve fibers of aged gerbils raised in quiet or noise. Hear Res 1990; 45:221-236.

Schulte BA, Adams JC. Distribution of immunoreactive Na^+,K^+-ATPase in gerbil cochlea. J Histochem Cytochem 1989; 37:127-134.

Schwartz IR, Ryan AF. Differential labeling of sensory cell and neural populations in the organ of Corti following amino-acid incubations. Hear Res 1983; 9:185-200.

Sewell WF. The effects of furosemide on the endocochlear potential and auditory-nerve fiber tuning curves in cats. Hear Res 1984; 14:305-314.

Smith DI, Mills JH, Schmiedt RA. Frequency selectivity of the middle latency response. Hear Res 1990; 43:95-106.

Smith RL. Short-term adaptation in single auditory nerve fibers: Some poststimulatory effects. J Neurophysiol 1977; 40:1098-1112.

SECTION FOUR

Performance Changes

CHAPTER 22

Psychoacoustic Characterization of Two Types of Auditory Fatigue

MARIE-CLAIRE BOTTE
SABINE MÖNIKHEIM

Auditory fatigue generally refers to the temporary loss of auditory sensitivity that takes place after exposing the ear to an intense sound. Auditory fatigue has been measured in many experiments by the increase in absolute threshold, or temporary threshold shift (TTS), and in a few others by the reduction of loudness, or temporary loudness shift (TLS). However, TTS and TLS also appear with exposures to moderate and even low-level sounds, provided that the test level (for TLS measurement) is lower than the exposure level. This second type of auditory fatigue has been known for many years, but its study was never totally completed. Insofar as TTS was very small, few experiments measured TLS from low-level exposures, probably because it was expected to be even weaker than TTS.

This chapter examines the psychoacoustic specifics of these two types of fatigue in the domain of intensity perception. Physiologic data strongly suggest a cochlear origin of the shifts of threshold and loudness (Abbas, 1983; Cody and Johnstone, 1981; Lonsbury-Martin and Meikle, 1978). Focusing on threshold and loudness during auditory fatigue is useful in forming a theory of active cochlear mechanisms, because threshold and loudness are involved in the detection of low-level sounds (Johnstone et al, 1982).

We will present a series of "fatigue patterns" due to different exposure levels and frequencies. Fatigue patterns show the amounts of TTS and TLS as a function of the test frequency in the fatigued range. The patterns for high-level and low-level exposures will be described. In turn, the role of exposure duration, frequency, and level will be examined to the extent that data are available.

TTS and TLS Patterns from High-Level Exposures

According to a number of studies reviewed by Ward (1973), TTS that persists for longer than 2 minutes but shorter than 16 hours after the end of the exposure may be regarded as "physiologic" long-term fatigue that is always completely recovered. This type of fatigue appears once the exposure SPL exceeds a critical value of 70 to 75 dB. Few experiments have compared threshold recovery to loudness recovery extensively. McPherson and Anderson (1970) found the time course of recovery similar for TTS and TLS after a 5-minute exposure; however, for longer exposure durations (30 to 90 minutes), Botte and Chocholle (1979) suggested that TLS at low sensation levels recovers more slowly than TTS.

The frequency pattern of TTS shows a maximum loss for a frequency higher than the exposure frequency, a peculiarity that is commonly designated "the half-octave shift" of TTS. The amount of TTS at the exposure frequency is much smaller and often not measurable.

Role of Exposure Duration

After exposures to continuous octave-band noises in human subjects, TTS increases as a function of exposure duration for 4 to 12 hours and then reaches a plateau or asymptote (Mills et al, 1979), whereas the asymptotic level of TTS appears after only 1 to 2 hours in cases of impact noises (Laroche et al, 1988). Maximum TTS, as well as the rate and duration of its growth, depend on the frequency and level of exposure (Ward et al, 1959; Mills et al, 1970, 1979). Despite the absence of systematic measurements, according to the pioneer work of Davis et al (1950) and the later confirmations of Mills et al (1970) and McPherson and Anderson (1970), the growth of loudness shift is supposed to reproduce that of TTS. However, McFadden and Plattsmier (1982b, 1983) demonstrated TLS without TTS at the exposure frequency. Sebald (1987) also found TLS both at frequencies higher than the exposure frequency and at the exposure frequency itself. These results suggest some discrepancy between the respective growths of TTS and TLS.

Role of Exposure Frequency

Maximum Amount of TTS and TLS

TTS from tones or noise bands with equivalent SPL in different frequency regions have often been measured (Davis et al, 1950; Mills et al, 1979; Thompson and Gales, 1961; Ward, 1962). It has generally been assumed that for constant SPL, "the higher the exposure frequency, at least up to 4,000 or 6,000 Hz, the greater the TTS" (Ward, 1973). Moreover, Botte et al (1990) found no significant differences among maximum TTSs from pure-tone exposures (250 to 6,000 Hz) at equal sensation levels (80 dB above threshold) and suggested, after averaging data of a number of subjects, that a constant power input to the cochlea results in a constant TTS whatever the exposure frequency, at least for levels that are close to the critical value.

A peak of TLS also occurs at the test frequency showing the maximum TTS, but TLS dependence on the exposure frequency has never been investigated in detail. During auditory fatigue, the amount of TLS strongly depends on the test level. At test frequencies showing a noticeable TTS, the loudness function is similar to those observed for a partially masked sound, and to those observed in sensorineural pathologies with typical recruitment. For a fatigued ear, when the level of stimulus increases above an abnormally elevated threshold, the loudness grows more rapidly than for an unfatigued ear; then TLS decreases as a function of the test level. Because of different exposure conditions, the test level at which TLS becomes negligible varies among experiments between 70 dB SLH (Piazza, 1966), 80 dB HL (Young and Harbert, 1975), and 100 dB SPL (Davis et al, 1950). Botte and Scharf (1980) measured loudness functions for a 1500-Hz tone with and without masking by a 700-Hz tone, before and after an exposure to a 1,000-Hz fatiguing tone. They demonstrated that TLS from auditory fatigue accumulates with TLS due to partial masking.

Extension of the Fatigued Range

Few experiments have investigated the TTS frequency pattern as a function of exposure frequency, yet once again Davis et al (1950) set the example. However, instead of plotting TTS for the different tested frequencies as a function of the frequency, level, and duration of the exposure, they calculated an "average hearing loss" covering two octaves. Figure 22-1 shows frequency patterns of TTS as a function of exposure frequency of pure tones at a constant exposure level (80 dB SL).

Differences in the ranges of fatigue are clear: as the exposure frequency increases, not only does the maximum TTS come closer to the exposure frequency, but also the total range of frequencies over which there is TTS diminishes (3.5 octaves for 250-Hz exposure, 2 octaves for 1,000- and 2,000-Hz exposures, 1 octave for 4,000- and 6,000-Hz exposures). When the exposure frequency becomes higher, maximum TTS occurs at frequencies that are closer and closer to the exposure frequency (1.3 octaves for 250-Hz exposure, 0.9 octaves for 500-Hz exposure, 0.6 to 0.5 octaves for 1,000-, 2,000-, and 4,000-Hz exposures, and 0.3 octaves for 6,000-Hz exposure). These results depart from the half-octave rule and show that the frequency pattern of TTS, and probably also that of TLS, strongly depends on the exposure spectra. Figure 22-2 presents similar results for band-limited noise exposures. Four different noise bands having a width of four critical bands (200 to 630 Hz, 630 to 1,270 Hz, 1,270 to 2,300 Hz, and 2,300 to 4,400 Hz) were monaurally presented for 45 minutes at 90 dB SPL. Average TTSs of 10 subjects are plotted as a function of the distance between the test frequency and the central frequency of the exposure sound.

Maximum TTSs occur at test frequencies 0.7 to 0.8 octaves above the central frequency of the exposure for the three noise bands with the highest frequencies, but occur at 1.3 octaves above the central frequency for the band of 200 to 630 Hz. By comparing Figures 5, 6, and 7 from Mills et al (1979), one can see that TTS range extends farther, in octaves, above the spectral components of the exposure

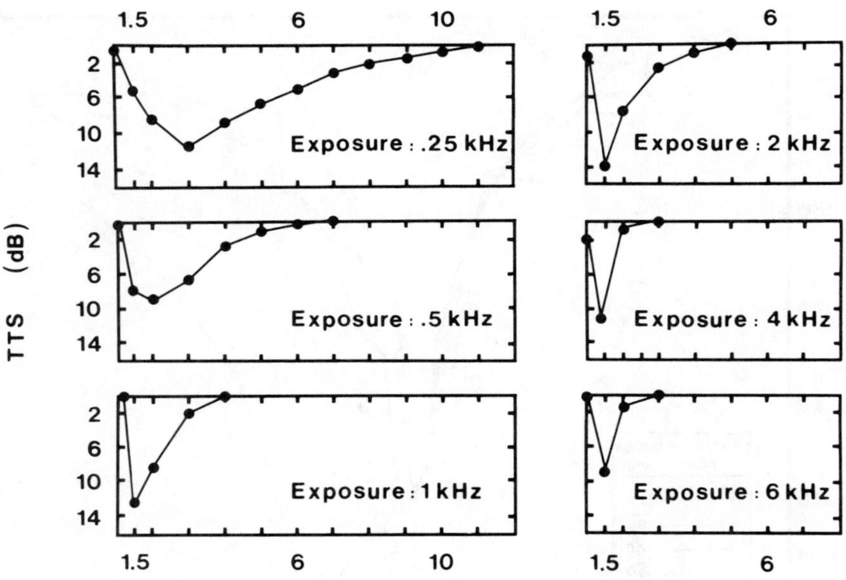

Figure 22-1 For 12 subjects, mean monaural temporary threshold shift (TTS) plotted as a function of the ratio of the test frequency to the ipsilateral exposure frequency (F_{test}/F_{expo}). Each panel is for a different exposure frequency with constant level (80 dB SL) and duration (30, 45, or 60 minutes, depending on the subjects). (From Botte MC, Baruch C, Dancer A. TTS as a function of exposure frequency. J Acoustique 1990; 3:53-57.)

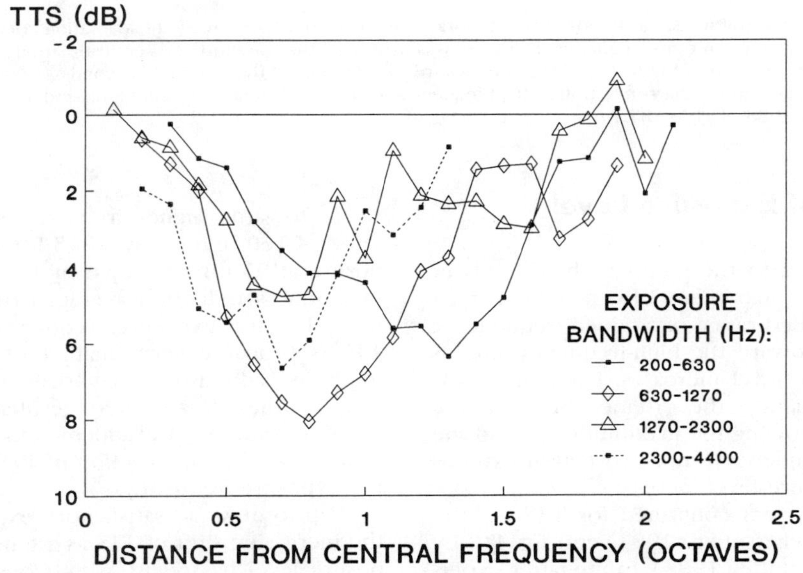

Figure 22-2 For 10 subjects, mean monaural temporary threshold shift (TTS) after a 45-minute ipsilateral exposure to a noise band at 90 dB SPL as a function of the distance between the test frequency and the central frequency of the noise band.

noise band as the exposure spectrum is moved toward lower frequencies.

Frequency patterns for TLS as a function of exposure frequency exhibit the same trends as the TTS patterns, with two differences: (1) TLS is much larger than TTS at the exposure frequency as mentioned earlier, and (2) the higher the exposure frequency, the larger the extension of TLS pattern for a given SPL of exposure (Botte et al, to be published).

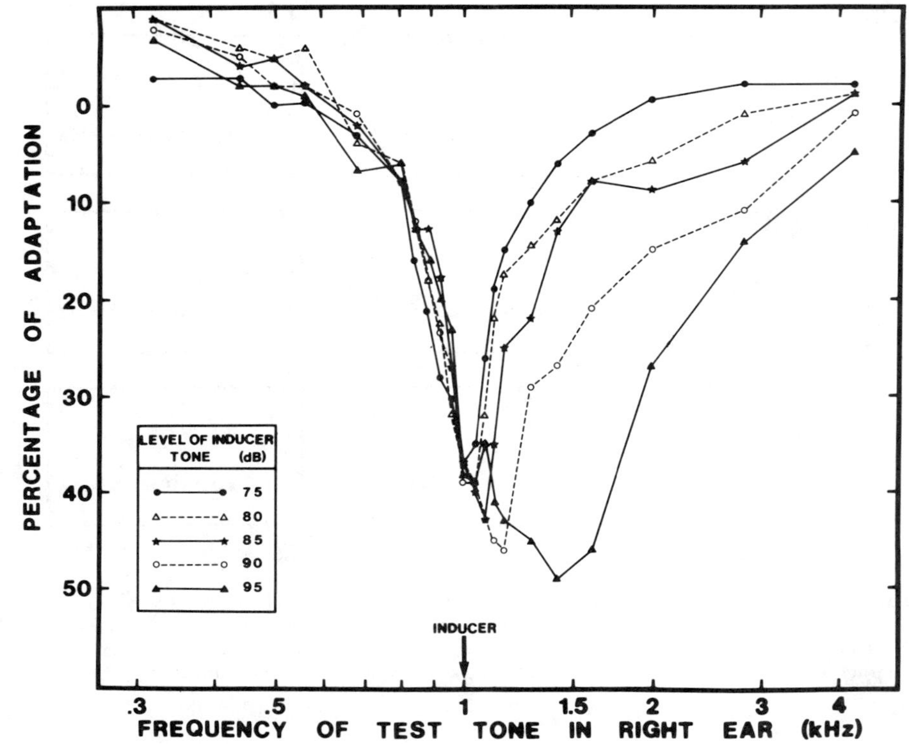

Figure 22-3 For 10 subjects, mean monaural temporary loudness shift (percentage of adaptation) of a 60-phon test tone plotted as a function of its frequency. Loudness was measured by a method of direct estimations before and 34 seconds after cessation of a 1,000-Hz ipsilateral exposure tone (inducer) that lasted 24 seconds. Exposure levels are given in the inset. (From Charron S, Botte MC. Frequency selectivity in loudness adaptation and auditory fatigue. J Acoust Soc Am 1988; 83:178-187.)

Role of Exposure Level

According to the monograph of Davis et al (1950), the maximum TTS and TLS, as well as the extended range of fatigued frequencies, are shifted toward the high-frequency side as the exposure level increases. For a given exposure frequency, the distance between the frequency showing the maximum TTS and the exposure frequency is not constant: it extends as the exposure level increases.

This fact was confirmed for TTS by McFadden and Plattsmier (1983) and for TLS by Charron and Botte (1988). In the latter experiments, TLS was expressed as the percentage of loudness reduction obtained by a method of direct estimation of loudness. Frequency patterns for TLS after a 24-second exposure to a 1,000-Hz tone at different levels are shown in Figure 22-3.

As the level of the exposure increases from 75 to 95 dB, the TLS of a 60-phon test tone remains sizable at the test frequency of 1,000 Hz, but the maximum moves progressively towards higher frequencies: to 1,040, 1,080, 1,160, and finally 1,415 Hz with the exposure at 95 dB, as shown by the percentage of loudness reduction averaged over 10 subjects. For the exposure frequency, at which TTS is probably very small, the 40 percent loudness reduction is remarkable; these data support the already-cited results of Sebald (1987) and of McFadden and Plattsmier (1982b) on the dissociation of TTS and TLS at the exposure frequency.

Up to now, no satisfactory explanation of the increasing shift of TTS as a function of exposure level has been given. Consistent with the cochlear models of Davis (1983) and Kim (1986), the proposal by McFadden and Plattsmier (1982b), argued for by McFadden (1986), is that the shift in the frequency showing the maxium TTS occurs because "the point of maximal displacement (of the basilar membrane) at high intensity is basal to the displacement maximum at low intensity, and thus the region maximally fatigued is one associated with higher frequencies at threshold in-

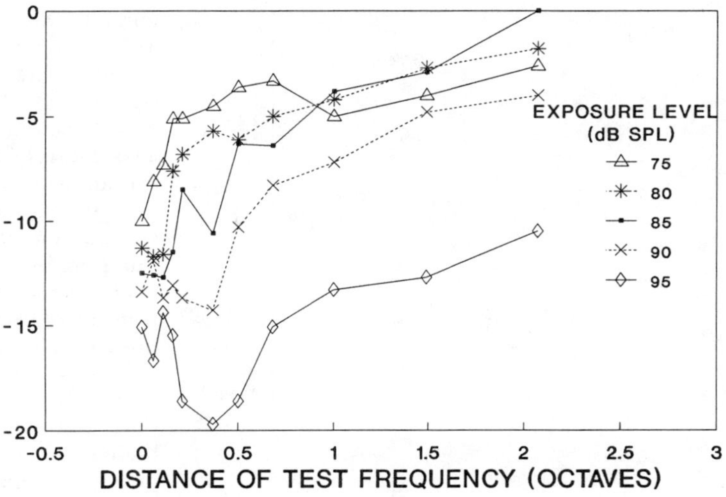

Figure 22-4 For 14 subjects, mean monaural temporary loudness shift (TLS), in decibels, of a 60-dB test tone plotted as a function of its frequency. Loudness was measured by a method of direct estimation before and 15 seconds after cessation of a 1,000-Hz ipsilateral exposure tone that lasted 60 seconds and was set at five different levels.

tensities." When progressively higher levels are tested at the exposure frequency, the activated regions have greater overlap with the fatigued area because of the intense exposure. Therefore, according to this theory, the TLS at the exposure frequency should increase regularly, at least as long as the recruitment mechanism is too limited to reverse that trend. Moreover, McFadden's hypothesis predicts that for a given test level, the amount of TLS should vary nonmonotically over the range of fatigued frequencies, with a single maximum located farther from the exposure frequency as the exposure level is set higher. On the contrary, the results of an experiment by Botte et al (to be published) show more complicated TLS patterns (Fig. 22-4). The experimental conditions for this study were basically the same as the experimental conditions for the data of Figure 22-3, but the total exposure duration was now 60 seconds. TLSs were only measured for test frequencies higher than the exposure frequency, and were converted into equivalent level reduction in decibels, owing to the individual loudness functions of the 14 subjects.

Instead of a curve with a single maximum, the TLS patterns resulting from 85-, 90-, and 95-dB exposure levels clearly show two separate peaks: the frequency of the first maximum almost exactly coincides with the exposure frequency, and its amplitude slowly increases by 5 dB as the exposure level increases from 75 to 95 dB, whereas the second peak, which is located at a higher frequency, varies from 10 to 20 dB for increasing exposure levels from 85 to 95 dB. A similar double-peaked curve is seen in Figure 22-3 for the 95-dB, 24-second exposure tone.

Conclusion

TTSs and TLSs from high-level exposures may stem from two different mechanisms, each with its own frequency selectivity and rules of growth as a function of the level, duration of exposure, or both. The type-I mechanism produces predominant TTSs and TLSs at frequencies higher than the exposure frequency; for these frequencies losses culminate at threshold and decrease as test level is increased. The type-II mechanism mainly causes TLSs to the exposure frequency, eventually without any corresponding TTS at the same frequency.

The temporal persistence of type-I effects is much better known than that of type-II effects, which still have to be measured in an extended range of exposure levels. Even if type-II effects have always been measured shortly after the end of exposure, the two types of fatigue may be concomitant for periods of several seconds or minutes after the end of exposure.

TTS and TLS Patterns from Low-Level Exposures

Most of the environmental sounds to which we are exposed do not exceed 80 dB. Thus, their practical influence on auditory sensitivity is at least as important as that of intense sounds. However, it has long been thought that auditory fatigue due to moderate and low-level sounds is almost negligible: small TTSs were observed (Caussé and Cha-

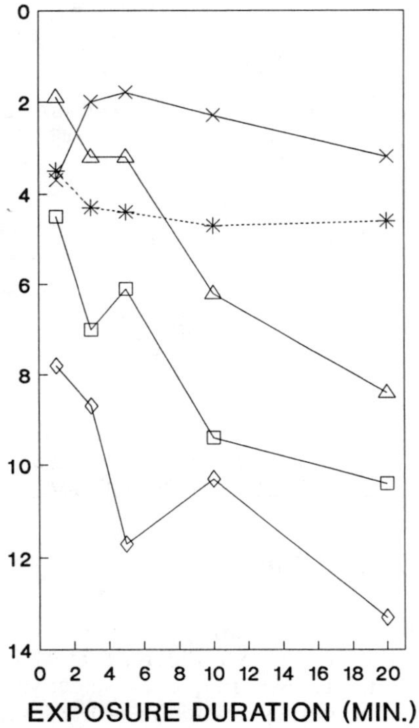

Figure 22-5 For 7 subjects, mean monaural temporary threshold shift (TTS) and temporary loudness shift (TLS) at four test levels, in decibels, of a 1,000-Hz tone as a function of the duration of an ipsilateral exposure to a 1,000-Hz, 75-dB tone. Measurements were made before and within 60 to 80 seconds following cessation of exposure by a method of Békésy tracking for threshold, or direct loudness estimation.

vasse, 1947), which were almost independent of the exposure level (Hirsh and Bilger, 1955). They reached their maximum after a 1-minute exposure, and their recovery was achieved within 2 minutes. Exposures below 85 dB lasting about 1 minute result in this type of short-term auditory fatigue (Ward, 1973). Recent experiments have provided new insight into this type of low-level fatigue. However, because of the lack of extensive data on the role of exposure conditions and tested levels, as well as on recovery, our characterization of low-level fatigue is incomplete and sometimes incoherent. Nevertheless, the frequency pattern of this fatigue is commonly assumed to be symmetric, with a maximum located at the exposure frequency.

Effect of Exposure Duration

As shown in Figure 22-5, the amount of TTS is actually independent of exposure duration. Seven subjects were exposed to a monaural 1,000-Hz tone at 75 dB SPL for 1, 3, 5, 10, or 20 minutes. The mean TTS (about 4 dB 1 minute after cessation of exposure) does not significantly change as a function of the exposure duration. The duration of TTS recovery is also equivalent for the five exposure periods (about 50 seconds).

For the same subjects, the mean TLSs show an increase as a function of the exposure duration for test levels below 70 dB SPL. However, to measure these TLSs, loudness functions were established before and after the exposure by a method of direct estimation with numbers. The different levels were successively presented in increasing order, a procedure that could have reduced the TLSs at the higher test levels because of longer recovery periods compared to those for the lower levels, which were tested first.

A clear result of this experiment is that TLS is greater than TTS, especially at moderate test levels.

Role of Exposure Frequency

The data of Caussé and Chavasse (1947) indicate that for an exposure to a 30-dB tone, there is no TTS for exposure frequencies lower than 800 Hz; the maximal TTS is approximately equivalent for the higher exposure frequencies (3 to 4 dB). Plotted on a logarithmic scale of frequency, the extent of the TTS pattern after a 40-dB exposure tone of 1,000, 3,000, or 8,000 Hz becomes larger as the exposure frequency decreases. In each case, the TTSs become maximal at the exposure frequency and diminish symmetrically as a function of the distance of the test frequency above and below the exposure frequency.

The data of Charron and Botte (1988) show a similar shape of the TLS pattern for a test level close to 60 dB, after a 24-second exposure to tones of 500, 1,000, or 3,000 Hz at 75 dB SPL (Fig. 22-6). However, there is no change of the extent of the TLS pattern as a function of the exposure frequency; this is different from the variation of TTS extent in Caussé and Chavasse's experiments. Thus, there are indications that TTS patterns differ from TLS patterns not only for high-level but also for low-level fatigue.

In a recent experiment, we measured TTS and TLS at three different test levels (20, 40, and 60 phons) after 3-minute exposures to a 65-dB tone of 500, 1,000, or 3,000 Hz. The results for the 3,000-Hz exposure are shown in Figure 22-7. For the TLS measurements, we used a method of alternate binaural loudness

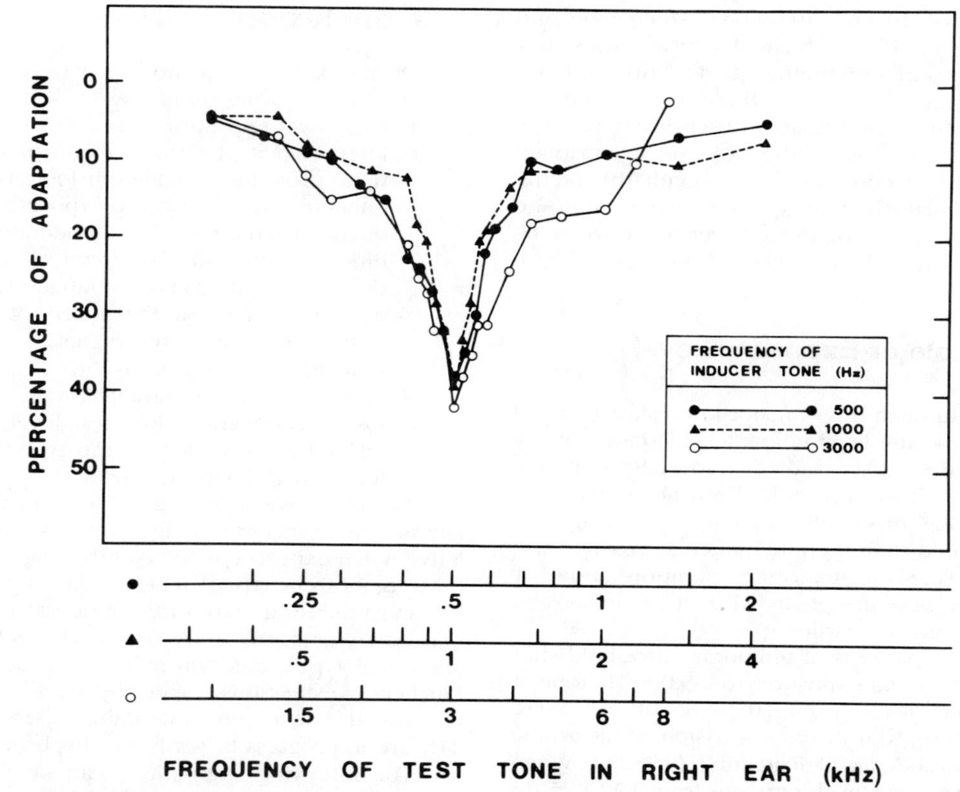

Figure 22-6 For 18 subjects, mean monaural temporary loudness shift, or TLS (percentage of adaptation) for a pure tone as a function of its frequency. Loudness was measured by a method of direct estimation before and 26 or 34 seconds after cessation of a 24-second, 75-dB ipsilateral exposure tone (inducer) of 500, 1,000, or 3,000 Hz. For each exposure tone, all test tones were of the same loudness level (equal to that of the inducer at 60 dB SPL). (From Charron S, Botte MC. Frequency selectivity in loudness adaptation and auditory fatigue. J Acoust Soc Am 1988; 83:178-187.)

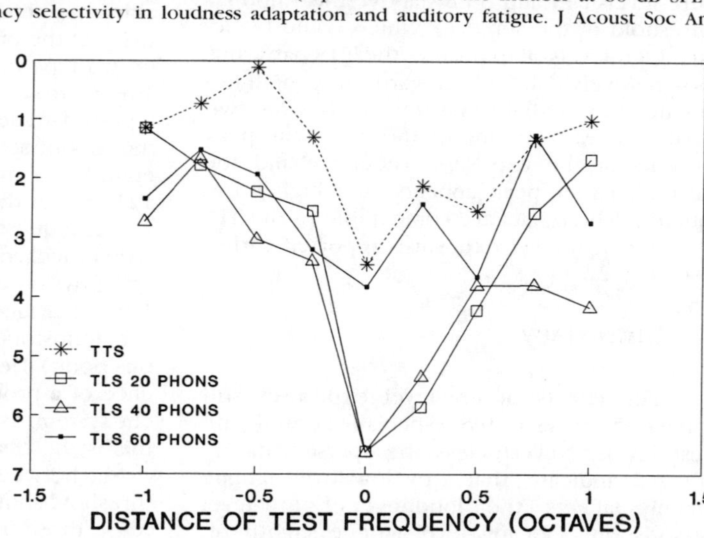

Figure 22-7 For 10 subjects, mean monaural temporary threshold shift (TTS) and temporary loudness shift (TLS) at 20, 40, and 60 phons, in decibels, as a function of test frequency. Measurements were made before and within 30 seconds after a 3-minute ipsilateral exposure to a 3,000-Hz, 65-dB tone by a method of Békésy tracking for threshold, or by binaural loudness comparison.

comparison. The smallest TTS and TLS resulted from the 500-Hz exposure, but these are not negligible, as found by Caussé and Chavasse (1947); this could be due to the higher level of exposure in our present experiment. The extent of the pattern of TTS is similar for the three exposure frequencies and only slightly narrower than the TLS pattern. Moreover, the maximum loss of sensitivity is not found at threshold but at the intermediate levels of 20 and 40 phons. McPherson and Anderson (1970) obtained similar results after an exposure of 5 minutes to a 50-dB, 1,000-Hz tone, but they believed that the observed TLS was actually "not related to sensitivity changes in the ear" but rather to the comparison method. If confirmed, this peculiarity of the loss of sensitivity for low test levels would be a new feature of the difference between fatigues from high-level and low-level exposures.

Role of Exposure Level

Although it is of major interest, the role of the exposure level in low-level fatigue is probably the least studied, especially for test sounds above threshold. Even if the exposure level has practically no effect on temporary threshold shift, it could influence TLS, because increasing the exposure duration above 1 minute provides greater TLS at moderate test levels, as seen earlier.

The patterns of temporary threshold shift for 30-second exposures to a 5,000-Hz tone at different levels from 10 to 65 dB SPL were shown by Kim in the discussion of his article by McFadden and Plattsmier (1982b). When the exposure level increases from 10 to 25 dB SPL, the pattern of TTS remains centered on the exposure frequency, and the maximum TTS grows from 1.5 to 3 dB. For higher exposure levels (45 and 65 dB above the 5,000-Hz threshold of the subject), which could be actual high levels of exposure, the TTS pattern is progressively shifted toward the high-frequency side with a trend toward showing two peaks, at least for one of the ears. One peak appears at the exposure frequency and the second, larger peak appears at a higher frequency. These data are comparable to the TLS data for high-level exposures reported earlier (see Fig. 22-4).

Summary

The effects of low-level exposures still have to be investigated, especially at moderate test levels. Nevertheless the sparse data reviewed indicate that (1) low-level fatigue mainly affects the loudness of low-level sounds, and (2) low-level fatigue slightly affects the threshold. Maximum TLS is found for test tones of the same frequency as the exposure tone. Moreover, the TLS increases with exposure duration and is greater for the highest exposure frequencies.

Conclusion

On the basis of TTS and TLS patterns, we propose the following summary:

1. High-level exposures result in two different types of fatigue: (1) type-I fatigue provides a maximum loss at frequencies higher than the exposure frequency from threshold to moderate audition levels, with maximum effect at threshold; and (2) type-II fatigue has a maximum effect at low levels of test tones at the exposure frequency.
2. Low-level exposures produce a slight increase in threshold and a noticeable loss of loudness at low test levels, an effect that is similar to the type-II effect of high-level exposures.

Therefore, we suggest that there are actually two mechanisms of fatigue that are cumulative when exposure is sufficiently long or intense or both. A type-II mechanism only acts for short-duration exposures, moderate-level exposures, or both; above a critical level, an additional type-I mechanism is set in action. Further investigations, especially on the role of exposure level on concomitant TTS and TLS, are in progress to verify this hypothesis.

The following suggestions can be made about the cochlear processes involved in the two types of sensitivity loss. Because the type-II mechanism leaves threshold almost unaffected, it is logical to suppose that the cochlear amplifier mechanisms linked to the activity of the outer hair cells are also preserved in this type of fatigue. A modulation of the afferents from inner hair cells could explain type-II fatigue. Regarding the type-I effects, the loss of sensitivity from threshold to moderate levels may be more directly assigned to a change in the activity of the outer hair cells.

The question of the protective role of the type-I mechanism is now clearly posed by several physiologic studies (Guinan and Gifford, 1988; LePage, 1989; Puel et al, 1988; Rajan and Johnstone, 1988; also see Chapter 38 of this book). Does TTS simply indicate the existence of a protective mechanism via the efferent system, as suggested by LePage (1989)? If this is the case, an inverse correlation should exist between temporary and permanent threshold shifts in a population of subjects, because those having greater TTS should benefit from better protection against hearing impairment; yet, as far as we know, this has never been noticed in animal or epidemiologic human studies. Moreover, above a certain amount of exposure-induced threshold shift, only a partial or considerably delayed recovery occurs; for that reason, psychophysicists avoid exceeding a maximum TTS of 20 dB—except for those who do so with their own ears. Because actual auditory impairment develops despite this protection, TTS should not be considered solely as evidence of a protective reflex like the stapedius reflex; rather, TTS and TLS probably involve protective loss of sensibility as well as true impairment of the hair cells when the protective mechanisms are overloaded.

Caractérisation Psychoacoustique de deux Types de Fatigue Auditive

La fatigue auditive qui fait suite à une exposition sonore est une diminution temporaire de la sensibilité de l'oreille. Son origine est située essentiellement au niveau cochléaire. Actuellement, la compréhension des processus mécaniques et nerveux dans la cochlée progresse rapidement. Toutefois plusieurs problèmes restent en discussion, en particulier ceux qui concernent les relations entre la fatigue auditive et ce que l'on appelle "l'amplificateur cochléaire". Cet article fait une revue des caractéristiques psychoacoustiques spécifiques de la fatigue auditive dans le domaine de la perception de l'intensité et dégage leurs implications en relation avec la théorie des mécanismes cochléaires.

Depuis longtemps, deux types de fatigue auditive ont été décrits. Ils sont respectivement appelés fatigue "à long terme" ou "à niveau intense" et fatigue "à court terme" ou "à niveau faible" selon la durée de récupération et le niveau d'exposition. Pour le type I (exposition à niveau intense), on sait que la gamme des fréquences fatiguées présente un écart d'une demi-octave entre le TTS maximum et la fréquence d'exposition. Mais, en fait, l'extension de la gamme des fréquences fatiguées, de même que le déplacement du TTS maximum, augmentent à mesure que la fréquence d'exposition diminue. Pour la majorité des fréquences fatiguées, le TLS est inférieur au TTS et décroît régulièrement avec le niveau du son test. En fonction du niveau d'exposition, non seulement le TTS et le TLS augmentent mais, de plus, l'ensemble de la gamme des fréquences fatiguées se déplace vers les fréquences plus élevées. En dépit du manque relatif de données expérimentales, la fatigue auditive de type II (exposition à niveau faible) se produit probablement plus couramment dans les conditions naturelles d'écoute. Elle résulte de l'exposition à des niveaux inférieurs à environ 75 dB SPL. Le pattern de fréquences du TTS, comme celui du TLS, est distribuée symétriquement de part et d'autre de la fréquence d'exposition pour laquelle il atteint son maximum. Au contraire du type I, dans le type II, la perte de sensibilité n'est pas maximale au seuil et ne décroît pas régulièrement avec l'augmentation du niveau du son test: le TLS dépasse un TTS très faible. Le TLS maximum apparaît aux niveaux modérés et diminue pour les niveaux plus intenses. Les montants de TTS et de TLS dépendent peu du niveau et de la durée d'exposition.

A partir de l'ensemble des caractéristiques des types I et II, nous suggérons que la fatigue résultant d'expositions à niveau intense comprend en fait une composante de type II ainsi qu'une composante supplémentaire et dominante, de type I. Puisque les deux types de fatigue sont très variables d'un individu à l'autre et peu corrélés entre eux, leurs bases physiologiques sont probablement différentes. Les caractéristiques de la perception de l'intensité suggèrent aussi que le type II est la manifestation d'une diminution de l'efficacité de l'amplificateur cochléaire sur toute sa gamme dynamique tandis que le type I résulterait d'une augmentation du seuil du même mécanisme à un endroit différent sur la membrane basiliaire.

References

Abbas PJ. Recovering from long-term and short-term adaptation of the whole nerve action potential. J Acoust Soc Am 1983; 75:1541-1547.

Botte MC, Chocholle R. Etude de la fatigue auditive chez l'homme. Comparaison de la récupération au niveau du seuil et aux niveaux supraliminaires. Audiology 1979; 18:125-132.

Botte MC, Baruch C, Dancer A. TTS as a function of exposure frequency. J Acoustique 1990; 3:53-57.

Botte MC, Charron S, Bouayad H. Frequency patterns and correlations for TTS and TLS.

Botte MC, Scharf B. La sonie. Effets simultanés de fatigue et de masque. Acustica 1980; 46:100-106.

Caussé R, Chavasse P. Etudes sur la fatigue auditive. L'Année Psychologique 1947; 43–44:265-298.

Charron S, Botte MC. Frequency selectivity in loudness adaptation and auditory fatigue. J Acoust Soc Am 1988; 83:178-187.

Cody AR, Johnstone BM. Acoustic trauma: Single neuron basis for the "half-octave shift." J Acoust Soc Am 1981; 70:707-711.

Davis H. An active process in cochlear mechanics. Hear Res 1983; 9:79-90.

Davis H, Morgan CT, Hawkins JE Jr, Galambos R, Smith FW. Temporary deafness following exposure to loud tones and noise. Acta Otolaryngol Suppl (Stockh) 1950; 88:1-57.

Guinan JJ Jr, Gifford ML. Effects of electrical stimulation of efferent olivocochlear neurons on cat auditory-nerve fibers. I. Rate-level functions. Hear Res 1988; 33:97-114.

Hirsh IJ, Bilger RC. Auditory-threshold recovery after exposures to pure tones. J Acoust Soc Am 1955; 27:1186-1194.

Johnstone BM, Robertson D, Cody A. Basilar membrane motion and hearing loss. Hear Prophylax Scand Audiol Suppl 1982; 16:89-93.

Kim DO. Active and nonlinear cochlear biomechanics and the role of outer-hair-cell subsystem in the mammalian auditory system. Hear Res 1986; 22:105-114.

Laroche C, Hétu R, Poirier S. The growth and recovery from TTS in human subjects exposed to impact noise. J Acoust Soc Am 1988; 85:1681-1690.

LePage EL. Functional role of the olivo-cochlear bundle: A motor unit control system in the mammalian cochlea. Hear Res 1989; 38:177-198.

Lonsbury-Martin, BL, Meikle MB. Neural correlates of auditory fatigue: Frequency-dependent changes in activity of single cochlear nerve fibers. J Neurophysiol 1978; 41:987-1006.

McFadden DM. The curious half-octave shift: Evidence for a basalward migration of the traveling-wave envelope with increasing intensity. In Salvi RJ, Henderson D, Hamernik RP, Colletti V, eds. Basic and applied aspects of noise-induced hearing loss. New York: Plenum Publishing, 1986:295.

McFadden D, Plattsmier HS. Exposure-induced loudness shifts and threshold shifts. In Hamernik RP, Henderson D, Salvi R, eds. New perspectives on noise-induced hearing loss. New York: Raven Press, 1982b:363.

McFadden D, Plattsmier HS. Frequency pattern of TTS for different exposure intensities. J Acoust Soc Am 1983; 74:1178-1184.

McPherson DF, Anderson CV. Relation of temporary loudness shift to temporary threshold shift. J Acoust Soc Am 1970; 49:1195-1202.

Mills JH, Gengel RW, Watson CS, Miller JD. Temporary changes of the auditory system due to exposure to noise for one or two days. J Acoust Soc Am 1970; 48:524-530.

Mills JH, Gilbert RM, Adkins WY. Temporary threshold shifts in humans exposed to octave-bands of noise for 16 to 24 hours. J Acoust Soc Am 1979; 65:1238-1248.

Piazza RS. The effect of the auditory fatigue upon the loudness and the pitch. Acustica 1966; 17:179-183.

Puel JL, Bobbin RP, Fallon M. An ipsilateral cochlear efferent loop protects the cochlea during intense sound exposure. Hear Res 1988; 37:65-70.

Rajan R, Johnstone BM. Electrical stimulation of cochlear efferents at the round window reduces auditory desensitization in guinea pigs. II. Dependence on level of temporary threshold shifts. Hear Res 1988; 36:75-88.

Sebald A. Temporary loudness shifts scaled by categorical partitioning. In Proceedings of the 3rd Annual Meeting of the International Society for Psychophysics, Durham, NC, 1987:71.

Thompson PO, Gales RS. Temporary threshold shifts from tones and bands of equivalent rms sound-pressure level. J Acoust Soc Am 1961; 33:1593-1597.

Ward WD, Glorig A, Sklar DL. Temporary threshold shift from octave-band noises: Applications to damage risk criteria. J Acoust Soc Am 1959; 31:522-528.

Ward WD. Damage-risk criteria for line spectra. J Acoust Soc Am 1962; 34:1610-1619.

Ward WD. Adaptation and fatigue. In: Jerger J, ed. Modern Developments in Audiology. New York: Academic Press, 1973:301.

Young IM, Harbert F. Types of loudness recruitment in the auditorily fatigued ear. J Auditory Res 1975; 15:162-171.

CHAPTER 23

Tinnitus in Noise-Induced Hearing Loss

ALF AXELSSON
MARIE-LOUISE BARRENÄS

Most reports on the etiology of tinnitus suggest that noise-induced hearing loss (NIHL) is probably the most common cause of tinnitus. Tinnitus caused by noise exposure can be elicited by an acute acoustic trauma or by continuous noise exposure in the work environment or during leisure time activities. Noise-induced permanent tinnitus (NIPT) frequently is combined with presbycusis, particularly in the elderly population. Because of the fairly high incidence of NIPT, the possibilities for effective epidemiologic studies are good. However, a literature survey shows surprisingly few such epidemiologic investigations. This chapter will review the current understanding of the etiology, incidence, treatment, and properties of tinnitus. Three general classes of published work will not be reviewed here. These are (1) the work of authors who have only reviewed the work of others without presenting original material, such as Miller and Jakimetz (1984), Ganz (1986), and Clark and Smith (1981); (2) studies of tinnitus experimentally induced by noise, such as those of Atherly et al (1968) and Hempstock and Atherly (1971); and (3) studies dealing primarily with legal and compensatory issues, which are excluded because such policies vary considerably between countries—for examples, see Coles (1982), Alberti (1987), Dieroff and Meissner (1987), and Coles et al (1988).

Onset

The onset of NIPT is characteristically slow without any specific precipitation (Alberti, 1987). Occasionally, there is a more sudden onset, particularly with acute acoustic trauma caused by exposure to such high-level impulse noises as those from a firecracker, a toy cap gun, a sledge hammer hitting metal, or a gun being fired (Alberti, 1987). There is little information on the characteristics of the onset of tinnitus with NIPT. This is probably due to the fact that many patients do not remember the circumstances in connection with the onset, or report that tinnitus "just appeared one day."

In this context, it is interesting to note the duration of noise exposure before tinnitus appears. McShane et al (1988) found that the incidence of tinnitus was 34 percent in a population exposed to noise for up to 10 years. For those who had worked 11 to 30 years in noise, the incidence of tinnitus was 54 percent; for those who had worked 31 to 50 years in noise, the incidence was 50 percent. Thus, with the exception of those who had worked up to 10 years in noise, the percentage of the population with tinnitus remained reasonably constant.

A common observation is that workers show NIHL long before NIPT appears. This is particularly true of workers in continuous noise. In our own study of 76 industrial workers who had been referred to the Department of Occupational Audiology for assessment of their hearing loss, the average delay between the time of first being employed in a noisy environment and the appearance of tinnitus was 23 years (Table 23-1). We were able to divide the 76 workers into six different occupational groups. As can be seen from Table 23-1, the interval between an individual's first employment in noise and the onset of tinnitus varied considerably. The longest interval was for workshop mechanics (approximately 35 years), and the shortest interval was for mili-

TABLE 23-1 **Interval Between Start of Noisy Job and NIPT, and Laterality of NIPT for Different Professions**

PROFESSION	N	INTERVAL TO NIPT, YEARS	LATERALITY OF NIPT, EAR		
			Left	Right	Both
Rock and stone drillers	8	15	2	1	5
Seamen and fishermen	10	27	3	0	7
Platers	15	26	2	3	10
Workshop mechanics	18	35	7	1	10
Factory and textile workers	14	28	6	3	5
Military personnel	11	11	3	1	7
Total	76	23	23 (30%)	9 (12%)	44 (58%)

tary workers (approximately 11 years). In the latter group there were several subjects whose tinnitus developed immediately as a consequence of acute acoustic trauma. Because tinnitus often has a fairly slow onset and individuals have difficulty remembering the onset of tinnitus, information concerning the duration of tinnitus must be considered with great caution.

Type of Noise

There appears to be a general agreement that NIPT is more common following exposure to impulsive noise than following exposure to continuous noise (Man and Naggan, 1981). Even in individuals with similar hearing thresholds, tinnitus occurred in 63 to 70 percent of a population exposed to impulsive noise, compared to 47 to 57 percent of another population exposed to continuous noise (Alberti, 1987). Only one report has compared the incidence of NIPT in different professions. NIPT was reported in 54 to 58 percent of a population of noise-exposed miners, steel makers, and general manufacturers, and less often in workers in the construction industry (50 percent), automobile manufacturing (46 percent), or paper manufacturing (40 percent) (McShane et al, 1988). Even noisy leisure-time activities such as hunting and target practice could obviously influence hearing and contribute to the onset of tinnitus. Somewhat surprisingly, shooting was not found to be a determinant per se (Coles et al, 1988). Coles et al conclude that gunfire noise appears to be "less damaging than we formerly thought." In a follow-up examination of acoustic trauma in connection with military weapons, where all the cases involved military personnel, tinnitus was clearly related to the degree of hearing loss (Hamberger and Lidén, 1951).

Incidence

The most common subject of studies of tinnitus is the incidence of NIPT in connection with noise exposure. As can be seen in Table 23-2, there is a surprisingly large variability of 5 to 80 percent in the reported incidence of tinnitus. One explanation for the large difference is the heterogeneous composition of the populations that have been reviewed. Further, the method used to determine the incidence of tinnitus may be drastically influenced by the manner of questioning the patient, ranging from only reporting cases in which the patient spontaneously complained of tinnitus to detailed questionnaires concerning the symptoms of tinnitus. Conversely, if we examine populations consisting of patients with tinnitus, 15.5 to 80 percent will show a history of previous damaging noise exposure (Table 23-3).

Age

The question of a relationship between NIPT and age has been addressed by some authors. Because hearing abilities decrease with age, the difference in the incidence of tinnitus in a noise-exposed population versus a corresponding non–noise-exposed control population as a function of age is of interest. Coles (1982) found that in his noise-exposed population younger than age 60 years, tinnitus incidence was fairly constant, at 21 to 22 percent. Of persons older than age 60 years, 33 percent reported tinnitus. In a corresponding control population, Coles found tinnitus in 11

TABLE 23.2 **Prevalence of Tinnitus in Patients with NIHL**

AUTHOR(S)	N	GENDER	AGE, YEARS	POPULATION	% NIPT
Ehman (1965)	1,180	M		Workers in metal industry	4.6 Constant 30.7 Temporary
Harris et al (1983)		F	60	All 60 years old in Malmö	5 Combined with presbycusis
		F	65	" 65 " " " "	5
		M	60	" 60 " " " "	61
		M	65	" 65 " " " "	41
Chung et al (1984)	31,504	M		Noise exposed workers in >85 dBA	6.6
	1,664	F		"	5.6
Prolingheuer (1958)				Miners	6.6 Constant
Coles (1982)	6,804	MF	18–39	Random sample of persons	21.9
			40–60	who reported	21.4
			>60	occupational noise exposure	32.8
Coles et al (1988)		MF		Random sample of population	7.5–20.7, depending on noise level
Arlinger (1983)	224	M		Patient's 1st visit for NIHL	74
		F			17
Chüden (1981)	252			Compensation claimants	35
Weiss (1984)	310	M	Mean 56	Random sample of shipyard workers	43 Right ear 41 Left ear
McShane et al (1988)	3,429	M		Compensation claimants	49.8
	37	F		"	51.3
Alberti (1987)	2,442	M	Mean 56	"	58 (28% Continuous 30% Intermittent)
Man and Naggan (1981)	102		18–35	Patients with acoustic trauma	79.4

TABLE 23.3 **Prevalence of Previous Occupational Noise Exposure in Tinnitus (T-) Patients**

AUTHOR(S)	N	GENDER	POPULATION	% NIPT
Reed (1960)	200		T-patients in ENT clinic	15.5
Axelsson and Barrenäs (1991)	411	M+F	T-clinic patients	33
Meikle and Taylor (1984)	1806	M	T-clinic patients	80
		F	" " " " "	31

percent of persons younger than 40 years of age; in 13 percent of persons between 40 and 60 years of age; and in 18 percent of persons older than 60 years of age. Coles concluded that within each age group, a history of noise exposure almost doubles the risk of tinnitus.

Other authors have also found an increasing incidence of tinnitus with age (Chung et al, 1984; Weiss and Weiss, 1984) but a further analysis showed that the only determinant was the individual's hearing threshold, not his age. A similar conclusion was reached by Coles et al (1988). McShane et al (1988) found a surprisingly small variation (46 to 55 percent) in the occurrence of tinnitus as a function of age in their noise-exposed population.

In summary, previous investigations have shown that the incidence of tinnitus clearly is related to hearing threshold rather than to the age of the patient. With increasing presbycusis and deteriorating hearing thresholds, the incidence of tinnitus can also be expected to increase in noise-exposed as well as non–noise-exposed populations.

Gender

There are comparatively few women working in industrial areas where noise exposure is a problem. Consequently, there are only a few reports available concerning the comparison of NIPT in noise-exposed males and females. The investigations of Chung et al (1984), Coles et al (1988), and McShane et al (1988) did not show any difference in the incidence of tinnitus as a function of gender when comparisons were made on the basis of equivalent hearing thresholds.

Parameters of Tinnitus

Laterality

Previous reports have typically shown that there are no significant differences between the two ears in the occurence of tinnitus (Arlinger, 1983; Alberti, 1987). Most commonly, tinnitus affected both ears with the same intensity (Chung et al, 1984; Axelsson and Sandh, 1985). Only one report (McShane et al, 1988) noted a difference in the intensity of tinnitus between the ears. Bilateral tinnitus was found in 79.6 percent of subjects and unilateral tinnitus was found in 20.4 percent of subjects. Of the unilaterally affected patients, 56 percent had tinnitus in the left and 44 percent in the right ear. This difference between the right and left ears was statistically significant. In our own subject pool of cases with NIHL and NIPT, tinnitus was found in both ears in 58 percent, in the left ear only in 30 percent, and in the right ear only in 12 percent. If the different professions represented in our subjects are divided into two groups, one group exposed to more impulsive types of noise (rock and stone drillers, platers, and military personnel), and the other group exposed to more continuous types of noise (seamen and fishermen, workshop mechanics, factory and textile workers), we see a marked difference in that the latter group had significantly more cases of left-sided tinnitus than the other group (Table 23-1).

Quality

No correlation was found between the subjective description of the tinnitus sound and any diagnosis explaining the tinnitus. Alberti (1987), describing cases of NIHL, found tinnitus to be a ringing sensation in 34 percent, a buzzing in 26 percent, a whistling sound in 12 percent, and a pulsative sound in 9 percent. Most commonly, the tinnitus was tonal and of high pitch (Alberti, 1987). Jakobs and Martin (1978) reported that the tinnitus sound was usually a whistling sound, and seldom a noise or a ringing sound. Axelsson and Sandh (1985) reported pure-tone tinnitus in 42 percent of patients with NIPT, narrow-band tinnitus in 35 percent, and broad-band tinnitus in 7 percent. In another investigation (Chüden, 1981), 60 percent of patients had NIPT of a tonal quality, and 40 percent had NIPT of a noisy quality.

Pitch

When patients with tinnitus are asked to compare their tinnitus sound with an externally presented tone, there generally appears to be a fairly good correlation between the area of hearing loss and the tinnitus pitch. A good correlation between the worst audiometric frequency and the matched tinnitus frequency has been demonstrated (Axelsson and Sandh, 1985), but not consistently (Man and Naggan, 1981). Axelsson and Sandh (1985) found 4 kHz to be the most common pitch for pure-tone tinnitus, followed by approximately equal occurrences for 1.5, 2, 3, 6, and 8 kHz. If pure-tone and narrow-band tinnitus were pooled together, tinnitus most commonly sounded like 4 kHz, followed by 6 and 3 kHz, and less commonly like 1.5, 2, and 8 kHz. Other authors also found that NIHL is often accompanied by NIPT at high frequencies (Man and Naggan, 1981; Cahani et al, 1983). Tinnitus has been found to have a high-frequency pitch in 51 percent of patients with

TABLE 23.4 **Tinnitus Laterality in Patients with Asymmetric NIHL**

AUTHOR(S)	WORST EAR	N	LATERALITY OF NIHL: Both Ears	Right Ear	Left Ear
Cahani et al (1984)	Right	22	3 (14%)	16 (73%)	3 (14%)
	Left	27	7 (96%)	9 (33%)	11 (41%)
Chung et al (1984)	*At 3, 4, 6 kHz:*				
	Right	183		103 (56%)	80 (44%)
	Left	311		150 (48%)	161 (52%)
	At 0.5, 1, 2 kHz:				
	Right	205		139 (68%)	66 (32%)
	Left	231		92 (40%)	39 (60%)
McShane et al (1988)	*At 0.5, 1, 2, 3, 4, kHz:*				
	Right	145		97 (67%)	48 (33%)
	Left	193		50 (26%)	143 (74%)

NIPT, and a low pitch in 49 percent of patients with NIPT (Ehmann, 1965).

Loudness

Tinnitus loudness typically appears to be close to the hearing threshold at the poorest audiometric frequency (Man and Naggan, 1981; Axelsson and Sandh, 1985). The most common tinnitus sensation level, i.e., the difference between the tinnitus audiometric level and the hearing threshold, appears to be 5 dB (Man and Naggan, 1981; Axelsson and Sandh, 1985). Man and Naggan (1981) found a good correlation between the maximum hearing loss and tinnitus intensity in dB HL up to a maximum hearing loss of 84 dB HL. For cases with hearing loss greater than 85 dB HL at the worst test frequency, tinnitus intensity was most commonly at 65 to 84 dB HL.

Severity

Some authors found no correlation between the severity of NIPT and the amount of hearing loss (Weiss and Weiss, 1984; McShane et al, 1988). In 1,727 tinnitus patients with NIHL, McShane et al (1988) demonstrated that tinnitus "did not bother" 9.3 percent of patients, that tinnitus was a minor problem for 61.5 percent of patients, and that tinnitus was a major problem for 29.2 percent of patients. There was no correlation between the severity of tinnitus and the hearing level at the tinnitus frequency either in absolute terms or in sensation level (Axelsson and Sandh, 1985). Alberti (1987) did not find any difference between ears in terms of severity. In patients with bilateral tinnitus, the severity was equal in both ears in 49 percent, worse in the right ear in 23 percent, and worse in the left ear in 22 percent (Alberti, 1987). Comparing problems caused by hearing loss and tinnitus, respectively, it was found that the hearing loss dominated in 90 percent. Tinnitus was considered a minor problem in 39 percent and a major one in 19 percent (Alberti, 1987).

Tinnitus in Relation to Hearing

Generally speaking, the incidence of tinnitus appears to increase with increasing hearing loss (Chung et al, 1984; Weiss and Weiss, 1984; Alberti, 1987; Coles et al, 1988). It has been suggested that the degree of hearing loss, i.e., the hearing threshold, is the most important determinant for tinnitus incidence (Chung et al, 1984; Coles et al, 1988). However, McShane et al (1988) found no such clear correlation with hearing loss at 4 kHz. Only minor variations in the incidence of tinnitus were reported when the threshold was between 10 and 100 dB HL. The incidence of tinnitus varied between 47 and 57 percent.

Tinnitus with Asymmetric Hearing Loss

In cases with asymmetric hearing and tinnitus, one would expect that tinnitus would be more common in the ear with the worst hearing. This is indeed generally the case (Table 23-4) (Cahani et al, 1984; Chung et al, 1984; McShane et al, 1988). Chung et al (1984) considered this finding to be particularly common when low frequencies were affected by the hearing loss. Surprisingly, however, in many cases tinnitus was also heard in the better ear with asymmetric hearing loss, and there was generally a less marked predominance for tinnitus in the worse ear than would be expected.

Effects on Sleep

Difficulties in both falling asleep and being awakened by tinnitus are common sequelae of tinnitus. In cases with NIHL, the proportion of the population who said they had sleeping problems varied between 47 and 50 percent (Axelsson and Sandh, 1985; Alberti, 1987). It has also been demonstrated that there was a correlation between depression and being awakened by tinnitus (Alberti, 1987).

Other Factors

Among other factors that have been considered to influence the incidence of tinnitus are smoking and shooting guns (Chung et al, 1984). However, when hearing levels in smokers and shooters were correlated with tinnitus incidence, the determinant was hearing threshold rather than smoking or shooting per se.

Treatment

Many different treatments have been attempted for tinnitus in general, but only a few treatments are specifically for NIPT. For tinnitus caused by acute acoustic trauma, it was suggested that a combination of pentoxyphyllin and xantinol nicotinate resulted in more improvement than untreated controls. Betahistin produced significantly better therapeutic results compared to a control group and a group treated with pentoxyphyllin and xantinol nicotinate (Jakobs and Martin, 1978). However, because NIHL and consequently NIPT can be prevented by avoiding noise exposure, it seems logical that information on NIPT should be included in occupational prevention programs. This is particularly important because many workers acknowledge that their tinnitus increases severely after a day's work in noise without ear protection. On the other hand, by eliminating the sounds that frequently mask tinnitus, ear protection can increase the discomfort of tinnitus. The issues of tinnitus being worsened by occupational noise exposure, and the increased subjective suffering under ear protectors, are often discussed with patients in the clinic.

Discussion

Because NIHL is the most common cause of tinnitus, it is somewhat surprising that there have been so few epidemiologic investigations. Because the populations with NIHL have many parameters in common, e.g., being almost exclusively males, predominantly in the ages of 20 to 60 years, there are good possibilities for comparative epidemiologic studies that might shed more light on this annoying and more-or-less incurable symptom. The interpretation of epidemiologic studies can be difficult for various reasons. One obvious problem is the selection of cases. In the literature there appears to be a great deal of variability across studies in the choice of patients, ranging from examination of workers in particular industries with noise exposure to clinics for patients suffering from NIHL or clinics for tinnitus sufferers. Others have investigated only cases of individuals who claimed insurance compensation for tinnitus. This variability in the selection of study populations makes it difficult to compare different parameters of NIPT. Furthermore, the method of establishing the incidence of tinnitus varies from recording spontaneous complaints about tinnitus to detailed interrogations concerning the problem.

Another difficulty is that tinnitus in cases with NIHL is not necessarily caused by the noise exposure. It is well known that tinnitus can be induced by a number of factors, e.g., head trauma, surgery, dental treatment, and upper respiratory infections. In addressing the question of tinnitus and NIHL we feel that it is important to put particular emphasis on the onset and first appearance of tinnitus, if possible.

An interesting and difficult question that is rarely examined is the interval between the onset of noise exposure and the onset of hearing loss on the one hand, and the interval between the onset of hearing loss and the onset of tinnitus on the other. In our own study, the interval between the start of employment in noise and tinnitus was approximately 23 years. In contrast, it is a common clinical experience that tinnitus may start acutely after impulsive and blast noise trauma. Indeed, tinnitus may be the only symptom following acute acoustic trauma, in which the audiometric threshold may not be affected despite a permanent severe tinnitus.

An obvious problem with the completely subjective symptom of tinnitus is the evaluation of epidemiologic data in cases of NIHL in which the occurrence of tinnitus and its severity are reported by possible claimants for insurance compensation. If the claim means a higher economic compensation when the patients suffer from severe tinnitus, the reported symptoms may be less trustworthy. Coles et al (1988) introduced the term "auditory honesty," which we feel is appropriate in these matters. If a patient with NIHL, having a compensation claim or not, has given consistent information on his health and working conditions, and additionally appears to be consistent in repeated audiometric measurements, there is reason to more readily believe the information he has given concerning his tinnitus than reports from less consistent patients. However, a confounding variable is the variation in tinnitus symptoms over time.

In terms of insurance compensation, it can be held that in some cases of NIHL the hearing loss can often be rehabilitated, at least to some degree, with hearing aids or other technical aids. The sense of hearing, unlike some cases of tinnitus, is not "switched on" constantly. For many tinnitus sufferers, the symptom of tinnitus is much more incapacitating than the hearing loss, and the tinnitus cannot be switched off at any time. Even if tinnitus is completely subjective, it should be considered in compensation claims, because it frequently increases the total handicap to a considerable extent.

Another reason to focus on tinnitus in cases of NIHL is the possibility of prevention. NIHL is a completely unnecessary condition, except for accidental circumstances, which can be completely prevented by decreasing the noise levels "at the source" and by using ear protection. Because tinnitus is frequently more disabling than the hearing loss itself, we feel that consideration of tinnitus should be incorporated in noise prevention programs much more than it has been. It is well known that it is often of little use to warn comparatively young workers about a possible hearing loss they might incur at an advanced age. They generally have great difficulties in comprehending the consequences of such a hearing loss. Both tinnitus and hearing loss can be acoustically demonstrated to the at-risk population in an attempt to bring about a greater understanding and awareness of the problem and thus to increase the motivation for wearing ear protection in noise.

Conclusion

There is comparatively little information concerning the epidemiology of NIPT. A review of the literature reveals the diversity of findings on tinnitus. The main reason for this diversity are the different methods of investigation. The NIPT population is interesting because of its close association with NIHL, because tinnitus is a serious clinical problem, and because the disorder is preventable. We therefore suggest that relevant information on this condition be collected, in order to better understand its pathophysiology, interactive factors, and possible therapeutic approaches. Such studies should be performed on a random selection of the population, accounting for differences in such areas as age, gender, socioeconomic status, and race. From such a database a more detailed investigation of subjects reporting occupational or leisure-time noise exposure as well as tinnitus could shed more light on problems such as the long interval between the onset of NIHL, the differences in the characteristics of tinnitus, the variations of incidence with different types of noise, the problem with maskability, and the various approaches to the prevention of NIPT.

Tinnitus et Déficits Auditifs

Les examens qui visent à étudier l'étiologie des acouphènes montrent que les pertes auditives induites par le bruit (PAIB) en sont et de loin la cause la plus fréquente. L'incidence la plus typique étant probablement 30-40%. D'autre part, chez les ouvriers qui ont des PAIB, les acouphènes sont retrouvés dans approximativement 30-50% des cas. Cependant il n'est pas facile de savoir pourquoi certains ouvriers travaillant dans le bruit ont des acouphènes alors que d'autres, du même âge et ayant passé le même temps dans le bruit n'en ont pas. Les examens épidémiologiques concernant les acouphènes dans les PAIB sont peu nombreux et sont souvent contradictoires. Si l'on considère que la cause la plus fréquente d'acouphènes est l'exposition au bruit et si l'on considère que les PAIB peuvent être évitées, il est surprenant que si peu d'études épidémiologiques aient été pratiquées. Puisque les PAIB peuvent être évitées, les acouphènes provoqués par le bruit (APB) pourraient l'être également. Beaucoup de questions demandent des études plus approfondies. Nous savons que l'incidence des acouphènes augmente avec l'âge. Nous savons également que les PAIB augmentent en gravité et en fréquence avec la durée d'exposition au bruit. Cependant, il n'a pas pu être établi si les acouphènes pouvaient être attribués à l'âge ou au bruit. Le plus souvent, les acouphènes sont perçus à la dernière bonne fréquence testée et leur intensité est proche du seuil à cette fréquence. En d'autres termes, la sensation d'intensité la plus fréquente, qui correspond à une différence entre le seuil audiométrique et le seuil de l'acouphène, est proche de 0. Dans les PAIB les acouphènes sont en général perçus à des fréquences hautes: entre 3 et 12 kHz. Un autre problème non résolu est la latéralisation inégale des acouphènes. La plupart des investigations ont montré que les acouphènes sont plus fréquents dans l'oreille gauche que dans l'oreille droite mais ce fait n'a pas été confirmé dans tous les travaux. En considérant que les PAIB sont également plus prononcées dans l'oreille gauche que dans l'oreille droite, le fait que les acouphénes soient plus fréquents à gauche n'est pas surprenant. Eu égard au fait que les travailleurs exposés au bruit sont le plus souvent de sexe masculin, on pourrait penser que les hommes devraient présenter des acouphènes plus souvent que les femmes. Entrangement il m'en est pas toujours ainsi. Dans nos propres expériences nous avons trouvé une différence marquée dans le groupe d'âge 50-59 ans où les hommes présentent des acouphènes plus fréquemment que les femmes. Cependant dans le groupe d'âge 60-70 ans, les femmes présentent des acouphènes plus souvent que les hommes. Ceci pourrait être expliqué par la PAIB chez les hommes du groupe d'âge le plus jeune alors que la presbyacousie en serait la PAIB chez les femmes du groupe d'âge le plus élevé.

Il est admis généralement que les acouphènes sont plus facilement provoqués par des bruits impulsionnels aussi bien dans l'environnement professionnel qu'à la suite de l'usage d'armes à feu, de pistolets à amorce, de pétards, etc. Il n'est pas rare qu'un trauma acoustique qui produit une élévation temporaire de seuil sans perte auditive persistante puisse s'accompagner d'acouphènes sévères permanents. Ceci encore démontre l'importance de la prévention contre le bruit non seulement pour l'audition mais également en ce qui concerne les acouphènes.

References

Alberti PW. Tinnitus in occupational hearing loss: Nosological aspects. J Otolaryngol 1987; 16:34-35.

Arlinger S. Tinnitus-epidemiologi i Sverige; en multicenterstudie. 2: A seminariet om tinnitus, Uppsala. Forskningsrådsnämnden och Handikappinstitutet, 1983:40-44.

Atherly GRC, Hempstock TI, Noble WG. Study of tinnitus induced temporarily by noise. J Acoust Soc Am 1968; 44:1503-1506.

Axelsson A, Sandh A. Tinnitus in noise-induced hearing loss. Br J Audiol 1985; 19:271-276.

Cahani M, Paul G, Shahar A. Tinnitus pitch and acoustic trauma. Audiology 1983; 22:357-363.

Cahani M, Paul G, Shahar A. Tinnitus asymmetry. Audiology 1984; 23:127-135.

Chüden HG. Diagnostische Massnahmen bei Tinnitus. HNO 1981; 29:418-421.

Chung DY, Gannon RP, Mason K. Factors affecting the prevalence of tinnitus. Audiology 1984; 23:441-452.

Clark SR, Smith CR. Industrial tinnitus. Hear Aid J 1981; 34:33-37.

Coles RRA. Noise-induced tinnitus. Proceedings of the Institute of Acoustics. Nottingham, U.K. The autumn conference. Bournemouth, 1982:G4.1-G4.5

Coles RRA, Smith PA, Davis AC. The relationship between noise-induced hearing loss and tinnitus and its management. In: Berglund B, Berglund U, Karlsson J, Lindvall T, eds. Noise as a public health problem. Stockholm; Swedish Council for Building Research, 1988:1-26.

Dieroff HG, Meissner W. Prevalence of tinnitus in noise-induced hearing loss. In: Feldman H, ed. Proceedings 3rd International Tinnitus Seminar, Münster. Karlsruhe: Harsch Verlag, 1987:159.

Ehmann G. Problem der Ohrgeräusche bei der Lärmschwerhörigkeit. Diss. Fredrich-Schiller Universität, Jena (cited by Dieroff).

Ganz F-J. Ohrgeräusche: Tinnitus-sprechstunde. Stuttgart-New York: Georg Thieme Verlag, 1986.

Hamberger CA, Lidén G. The prognosis in hearing injuries following acoustic shot traumata. Acta Otolaryngol 1951; 39:160-165.

Harris S, Broms P, Möllerström B. Tinnitus hos 60- och 65-åringar. 2nd seminariet om tinnitus. Uppsala: Forskningsrådsnämnden och Handikappinstitutet, 1983:55.

Hempstock TI, Atherly GRC. Tinnitus and noise-induced tinnitus. In: Robinson DW, ed. Occupational hearing loss. London: Academic Press, 1971:207.

Jakobs P, Martin G. Die Terapie der Tinnitus nach knalltraumatischer Schädigung. HNO 1978; 26:104-106.

Man A, Naggan L. Characteristics of tinnitus in acoustic trauma. Audiology 1981; 20:70-78.

McShane DP, Hyde ML, Alberti PW. Tinnitus prevalence in industrial hearing loss compensation claimants. Clin Otolaryngol 1988; 13:323-330.

Meikle M, Taylor-Walsh E. Characteristics of tinnitus and related observations in over 1800 tinnitus patients. J Laryngol Otol Suppl 1984; 9:17-21.

Miller HM, Jakimetz JR. Noise exposure, hearing loss, speech discrimination and tinnitus. J Laryngol Otol Suppl 1984; 9:74-76.

Prolingheuer KH. Die Geräuschmessung und Untersuchung von Lärmarbeitern in einem Hüttenwerk. Kampf der Lärm 5 (cited by Dieroff).

Reed GF. An audiometric study of two hundred cases of subjective tinnitus. Arch Otolaryngol 1960; 71:84-93.

Weiss AD, Weiss ER. Acoustic trauma: Tinnitus and vertigo. J Laryngol Otol Suppl 1984; 9:82-83.

CHAPTER 24

Objective Evidence of Tinnitus in Auditory Evoked Magnetic Fields

MANFRIED HOKE
CHRISTO PANTEV
BERND LÜTKENHÖNER
KLAUS LEHNERTZ

Tinnitus, an often distressing symptom, can be associated with various diseases of the middle and inner ear (e.g., Ménière's disease, acoustic trauma, sudden hearing loss) or with general diseases (e.g., arteriosclerosis). Tinnitus is a symptom of the aged. Its incidence increases distinctly with age, from approximately 7 percent in the third decade of life to 21 percent in the eighth decade (Axelsson and Ringdahl, 1987). Apart from a minority of cases in which a real (internal) sound source exists ("objective" tinnitus), "subjective" tinnitus consists of purely subjective auditory sensations that can be evaluated so far only by psychoacoustic methods. All attempts to detect the pathophysiologic processes underlying tinnitus in auditory evoked potentials (AEPs) or in the electroencephalogram (EEG) have failed so far, which does not, however, rule out that certain components contributing to the AEP or EEG are affected by tinnitus. In view of the great number of individuals who are unable to lead a normal life and the ineffectiveness of current tinnitus therapy, it is highly desirable that some method be devised to objectively assess the existence of tinnitus and to determine its representation in the central nervous system. Because of the high spatial resolution offered by neuromagnetic measurements, it was natural to study whether the magnetic signals of the brain are affected by tinnitus.

Material and Methods

The auditory evoked magnetic field (AEF) in response to tone bursts (carrier frequency 1,000 Hz, duration 500 ms, rise/decay time 15 ms, interstimulus interval 4 seconds, intensity 60 dB HL) was measured in 25 patients suffering from unilateral tinnitus, and in 40 normal-hearing individuals without tinnitus. Both groups were matched in age (tinnitus group: median age 39 years, quartiles 33 and 56 years; nontinnitus group: median age 36 years, quartiles 26 and 46 years) and hearing loss at the test frequency (tinnitus group: 5 dB—0 dB, 10 dB; nontinnitus group: 0 dB—0 dB, 5 dB). AEFs were measured over the hemisphere contralateral to the side of stimulation at the anterior field maximum. Measurements were taken in an electrically and acoustically, but not magnetically, shielded room (overall noise level 30 to 50 Hz) using a single-channel DC SQUID (Biomagnetic Technologies) equipped with a second-order gradiometer. Average waveforms were computed from 96 stimulus-related magnetoencephalogram (MEG) epochs (sampling frequency 250 Hz, bandwidth 0.1 to 40 Hz) and, in some individuals, from 96 EEG epochs, simultaneously recorded between vertex and contralateral earlobe. Amplitudes and latencies of waves M100 and M200 (AEF) and their electric counterparts N100 and P200 were evaluated off-line (for more details, see Hoke et al, 1989b).

Results

Although the mean amplitudes of waves M100 and M200 do not differ significantly in the nontinnitus group (Fig. 24-1, top), wave M200 is missing or only poorly developed in the tinnitus group (Fig. 24-1, bottom), and the

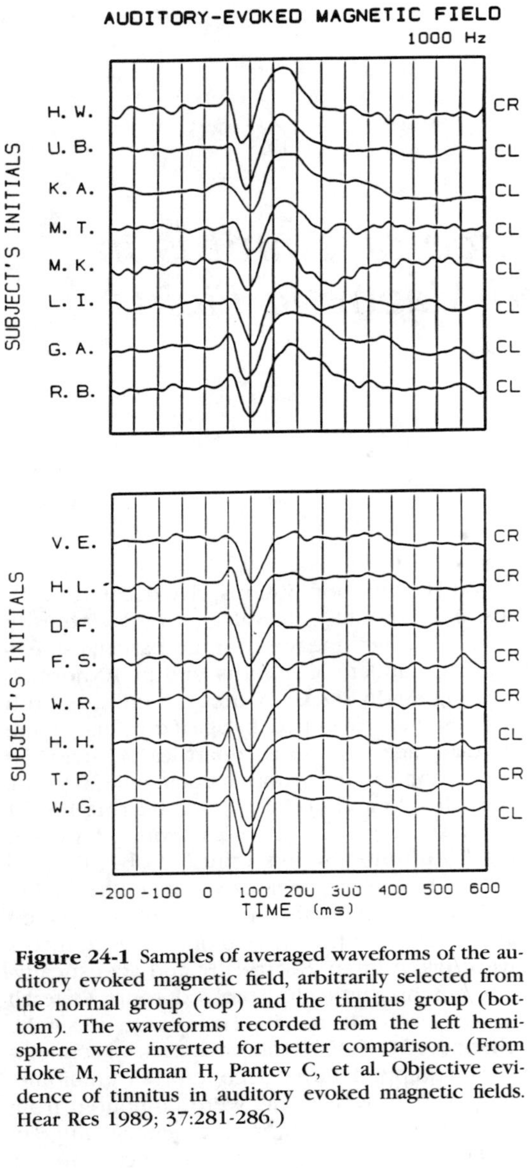

Figure 24-1 Samples of averaged waveforms of the auditory evoked magnetic field, arbitrarily selected from the normal group (top) and the tinnitus group (bottom). The waveforms recorded from the left hemisphere were inverted for better comparison. (From Hoke M, Feldman H, Pantev C, et al. Objective evidence of tinnitus in auditory evoked magnetic fields. Hear Res 1989; 37:281-286.)

amplitude of wave M100 is distinctly larger than the corresponding wave for the normal group. Student t-tests for paired data revealed significant (*p* less than 0.001) differences in both the mean amplitudes of corresponding waves between groups and the mean amplitudes of waves M100 and M200 in the tinnitus group. The mean latencies of wave M100 are not significantly different in the two groups, but the mean latency of wave M200, when developed, is significantly prolonged in the tinnitus group (*p* less than 0.002). Plotting the individual values of the amplitude ratio M200:M100 versus age (Fig. 24-2) shows that the amplitude ratio decreases with increasing age in the normal group, whereas no dependence on age of the amplitude ratio is evident in the tinnitus group. Linear regression analysis revealed that the regression coefficient of the data from subjects with tinnitus is not significantly different from 0, whereas that of the normal subjects differs significantly from 0 (*p* less than 0.05). Simultaneously recorded AEPs showed only a prolonged mean latency of wave P200 with unchanged mean amplitudes of N100 and P200.

We have also been able to trace the process of tinnitus remission in one exemplary case of acute tinnitus secondary to noise trauma (Pantev et al, 1989). During the period of recovery from tinnitus, the waveforms underwent a remarkable reorganization. Initially wave M100 was considerably augmented and wave M200 was totally missing; at the end of the study both waves had normal shapes and amplitudes (Fig. 24-3). As evident from the upper panel of Figure 24-4, the amplitude of wave M100 decreased continuously with time elapsed since the noise trauma from its initial value of 570 fT, asymptotically approaching a value of 180 fT. (Mean and standard deviation for tinnitus patients are, according to Hoke et al [1989b], 436 ± 105 fT, and for nontinnitus individuals, 275 ± 137 fT.) The decrease of the amplitude of wave M100 was accompanied by a recovery of wave M200 from an initial value of 0 (the amplitude of M200 is assumed to be zero if this wave is not detectable) to a final value of 190 fT. (Mean and standard deviation for the tinnitus group is, according to Hoke et al [1989b], 77 ± 69 fT, and for the nontinnitus group, 252 ± 100 fT.) The temporal development of the amplitude ratio M200:M100 is shown in the middle panel of Figure 24-4. The amplitude ratio recovered from 0 to a normal value of 1.1 (1.17 is the normal mean, according to Hoke et al, 1989b).

Conclusion

The results reported here suggest that at least one component of cortical auditory evoked activity with a latency of approximately 200 ms interacts with tinnitus. We explain the diminution or disappearance of wave M200 by pathologically enhanced spontaneous activity in the generator population of that particular component, causing the generator population to be less responsive or completely unresponsive to external stimuli. The enhanced spontaneous activity of the neuronal population that is supposed to depress wave

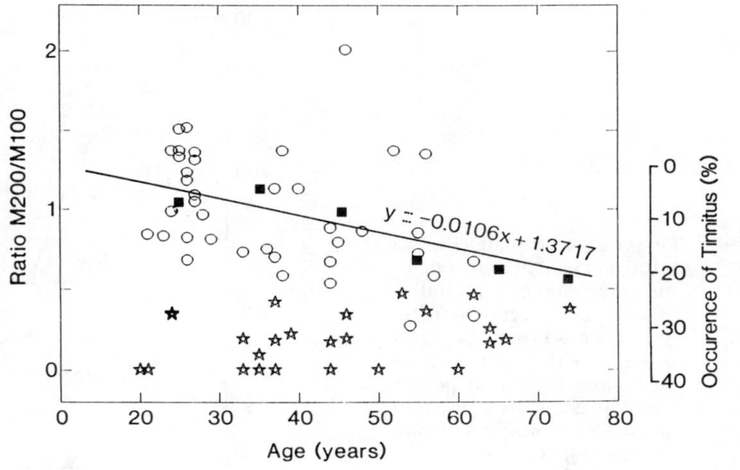

Figure 24-2 Individual amplitude ratios M200:M100 of the normal group (circles) and the tinnitus group (stars) plotted as a function of age. The incidence of tinnitus (squares) is also plotted for comparison. (Amplitude ratios from Hoke B. Incidence of tinnitus plot from Axelsson A, Ringdahl A. The occurrence and severity of tinnitus. A prevalence study. In: Feldmann E, ed. Proc 3rd Int Tinnitus Sem. Karlsruhe, FRG: Hausch, 1987:154.)

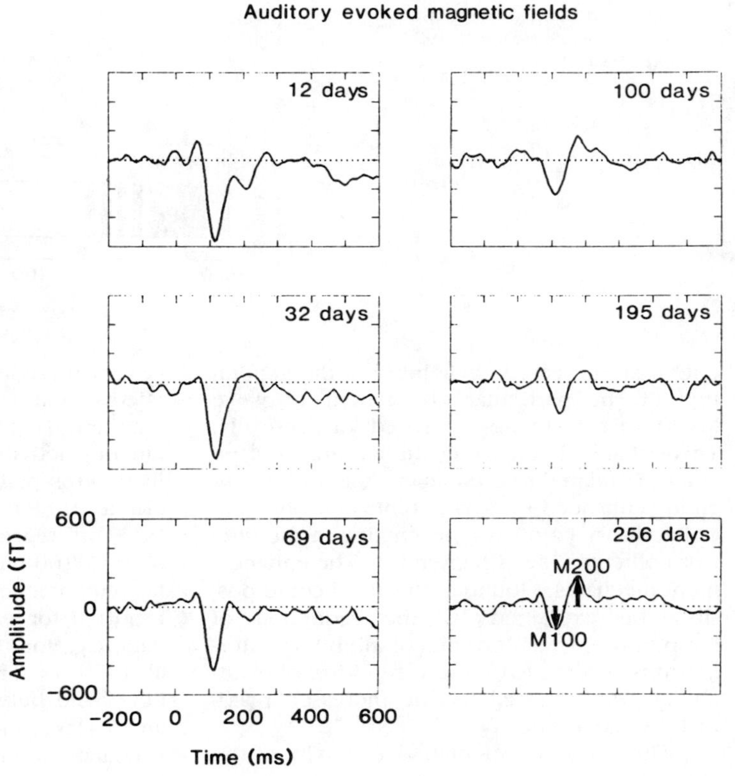

Figure 24-3 Averaged waveforms of the auditory evoked magnetic field recorded over the supralateral surface of the right cerebral hemisphere at the anterior field maximum. The waves M100 and M200 are indicated by arrows in the lower right panel. (From Pantev C, Hoke M, Lütkenhöner B, Lehnertz K, Kumpf W. Tinnitus remission objectified by neuromagnetic measurements. Hear Res 1989; 40:261-264.)

M200 in tinnitus patients has been shown by means of spatiotemporal spectral analysis (Hoke et al, 1989a).

The M100 and M200 components are assumed to reflect different processes. They are assumed to have basically monophasic waveforms of opposite polarity. Wave M200 is assumed to be broader than wave M100, and its deflection is assumed to begin before the maximum of M100, so that both waves partially overlap in healthy subjects. The augmentation of wave M100, however, cannot solely be due to the disappearance of wave M200, as hypothesized in previous publications (Hoke et al, 1989b; Pantev et al, 1989). Recent computer simulations have shown that, under the assumption of a similar shape of wave M100, the increase of its amplitude could also be directly related to tinnitus. The underlying pathologic mechanism is still unclear; it might be

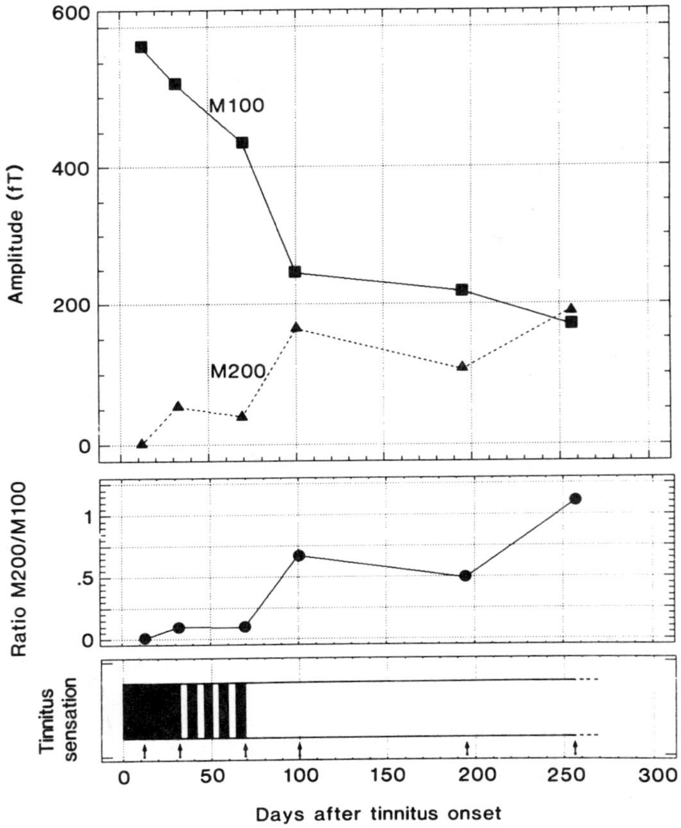

Figure 24-4 Amplitudes of waves M100 and M200 (top) and amplitude ratio M200:M100 (middle) as a function of time since tinnitus onset. The subjective sensation of tinnitus is indicated at the bottom. Black field, permanent tinnitus; vertical bars, intermittent tinnitus; blank field, no tinnitus. (From Pantev C, Hoke M, Lütkenhöner B, Lehnhertz K, Kumpf W. Tinnitus remission objectified by neuromagnetic measurements. Hear Res 1989; 40:261-264.)

due to an increased excitability of the generators of the particular component of wave M100 that is being measured magnetically. This enhanced activity in the auditory cortex could be related to the enhancement phenomenon (enhanced evoked potentials in the central auditory pathway), originating in the inferior colliculus (see Chapter 14). The enhancement mechanism found at this level could possibly be explained by the reduction of inhibition as a result of loss of inhibitory interneurons, leading to an increased level of excitability demonstrated by the increased maximal discharge rate.

The enhanced spontaneous activity of the generator population of one particular component of wave M200, as well as the increased excitability of the generator population of one particular component of wave M100, are supposed to be initiated by (probably multiple) exogenous or endogenous noxious events. If such an event occurs only once or extremely rarely (e.g., acute noise trauma), then these effects may recede, allowing recovery of normal generation of waves M100 and M200, as shown in Figure 24-3. If, however, noxious events happen frequently or are permanent (e.g., with aging), then the pathologic neural effects cannot recede and eventually become manifest. That circumscribed enhanced spontaneous activity in the auditory cortex exists in tinnitus patients has already been asserted (Hoke, 1988).

The regression of the amplitude ratio M200:M100 with age is obviously not a singular phenomenon. Age relationships have been reported for various electroencephalographic data, e.g., for the latency of P300 (Goodin et al, 1978) or for the temporal coherence in the beta band between electrode positions T3T5 and T4T6 (John et al, 1989). It is tempting to speculate whether the same age-related cerebral processes that give rise to those phenomena necessarily pave the way for the occurrence of tinnitus.

The strong correlation between the amplitude ratio M200:M100 and the clinical manifestation of tinnitus points to two important applications: In addition to its usefulness for studying mechanisms of tinnitus pathophysiology, AEF measurements might become an invaluable clinical tool for the objective assessment of tinnitus and an objective measure of the effectiveness of tinnitus therapy.

Mise en Evidence Objective du Tinnitus dans les Champs Magnétiques Evoqués Auditifs

Nous avons pu mettre en évidence un effet objectif des acouphènes dans les champs magnétiques auditifs évoqués par une bouffée tonale (FEA). En comparant les FEA obtenus chez deux groupes de patients, l'un souffrant d'acouphènes et n'ayant que des pertes auditives négligeables à la fréquence test ; l'autre composé d'individus normo-entendants sans acouphène, nous avons trouvé que, bien que l'amplitude moyenne des ondes M100 et M200 du FEA (désignées ainsi en fonction de leurs latences typiques) ne diffèrent pas significativement entre les 2 groupes, l'onde M200 est absente ou très peu développée dans le groupe à acouphènes alors que l'amplitude de l'onde M100 est nettement augmentée dans ce groupe ($p < 0.002$). Le rapport d'amplitude M200/M100 décroît avec l'âge dans le groupe normal, alors qu'aucune relation entre l'âge et le rapport d'amplitude n'existe dans le groupe à acouphènes. Les potentiels évoqués auditifs (PEA) enregistrés simultanément ne présentent qu'un allongement non caractéristique de la latence moyenne de l'onde P200 avec aucun changement des amplitudes moyennes de N100 et P200. Nous avons également pu montrer un processus de rémission dans un cas d'acouphène aigü (trauma acoustique). Dans ce cas le rapport d'amplitude a récupéré de o à sa valeur normale d'environ 1.

Nous expliquons la diminution ou la disparition de l'onde M200 par une augmentation pathologique de l'activité spontanée dans la population nerveuse qui génère cette composante, ce qui rend ces générateurs peu ou pas sensibles à une stimulation extérieure. Les ondes M100 et M200, qui sont probablement générées par des processus différents, sont composées essentiellement d'ondes monophasiques de polarités opposées et qui se superposent partiellement. Donc, si l'onde M200 est significativement plus petite, ou bien absente, l'onde M100 pourra être enregistrée dans sa totalité. On pense que l'augmentation de l'activité spontanée est initiée par des facteurs nocifs exogènes ou endogènes. Cette augmentation localisée de l'activité spontanée dans le cortex auditif existe réellement chez les patients souffrant d'acouphènes comme il l'a déjà été démontré (Hoke, 1988).

ACKNOWLEDGMENT

This text contains parts of already published material (Hoke et al, 1989b; Pantev et al, 1989), which are reproduced with permission.

References

Axelsson A, Ringdahl A. The occurrence and severity of tinnitus. A prevalence study. In: Feldmann E, ed. Proc 3rd Int Tinnitus Sem. Karlsruhe, FRG: Hausch, 1987:154.

Goodin D, Squires K, Starr A. Age-related variations in evoked potentials to auditory stimuli in normal human subjects. Electroencephalogr Clin Neurophysiol 1978; 1101:635-648.

Hoke M. SQUID-based measuring techniques—A challenge for the functional diagnostics in medicine. In: Kramer B, ed. The art of precise measurement in physics and medicine. Weinheim: Verlag Chemie, 1988:287.

Hoke M, Lehnertz K, Pantev C, Lütkenhöner B. Spatiotemporal aspects of synergetic processes in the auditory cortex as revealed by the magnetoencephalogram. In: Başar E, Bullock TH, eds. Springer series in brain dynamics 2. Berlin, Göttingen, Heidelberg: Springer, 1989a.

Hoke M, Feldmann H, Pantev C, et al. Objective evidence of tinnitus in auditory evoked magnetic fields. Hear Res 1989b; 37:281-286.

John ER, Prichep LS, Friedman J, Easton P. Neurometric topographic mapping of EED and evoked potential features: Application to clinical diagnosis and cognitive evaluation. In: Maurer K, ed. Topographic brain mapping of EEG and evoked potentials. Berlin, Heidelberg, New York: Springer, 1989:90.

Pantev C, Hoke M, Lütkenhöner B, et al. Tinnitus remission objectified by neuromagnetic measurements. Hear Res 1989; 40:261-264.

Salvi RJ, Powers NL, Saunders SS, et al. Evoked response enhancement after noise exposure. In: Dancer AL, Henderson D, Salvi RJ, Hamernick RP, eds. Noise-induced hearing loss. Philadelphia: B.C. Decker, 1991.

CHAPTER 25

Choosing Speech Materials to Assess Hearing Impairment

GUIDO F. SMOORENBURG
ARJAN BOSMAN

Hearing impairment, whether or not noise-induced, is primarily assessed in terms of tone audiograms rather than in terms of ability to understand speech. Although in everyday life hearing loss expresses itself in impaired speech perception rather than in a reduced ability to detect pure tones, the speech audiogram is frequently considered secondary information supplementing the tone audiogram. This stepmotherly position of speech audiometry is extreme in the field of noise-induced hearing loss. The presentation of dose-effect relations for noise-induced hearing loss in terms of tone-audiometric losses seems to be a matter of course (e.g., ISO/DIS 1999.2, 1985). Admittedly, tone audiometry possesses outspoken merits. It is very sensitive to small changes in hearing acuity, it is a reliable and efficient method of measurement with small measurement error, it can easily be used to distinguish conductive hearing loss from sensorineural hearing loss, and the shape of the tone audiogram is, to some extent, indicative of the type and origin of the hearing loss. However, tone audiometry does not provide us with direct insight into the handicap that is experienced by the individual with (noise-induced) hearing loss in perceiving speech in everyday life.

In addition to the diagnostic power of tone audiometry, there is another reason why speech audiometry lingers in the shadow of tone audiometry; namely the wide variety of speech materials that can be chosen. Speech audiometry can be based on syllables, either meaningful or meaningless, on multisyllable words including syllable emphasis as a variable (e.g. spondees versus trochees), on sentences (even syntactically correct but meaningless sentences; Nakatani and Dukes, 1973), and on running discourse. For sentences and running discourse, one may choose to assess the receipt of the speech message only, without checking whether the message was understood (by asking the listener to simply repeat the message; this is defined as speech reception), or one may wish to know whether the effort to receive the speech message was sufficiently small to also be able to understand the message (speech understanding). The latter approach is rare in speech audiometry. In measuring speech reception, the score for words can be based on the correct number of individual speech elements (phonemes) in the word or it can be based on the number of words repeated completely correctly. For sentence materials, a similar choice can be made between the syllable or word score and the whole-sentence score. Moreover, the score for sentences may be based on selected key words in the sentence, for example those words carrying the most information and being the least predictable on the basis of syntax (e.g. Fletcher and Steinberg, 1929; Silverman and Hirsh, 1955; and Kalikow et al, 1977). Finally, when assessing the degree of hearing impairment, one has to make choices with respect to the acoustic realization of the speech materials. Should one use a male or a female voice; should one strive for a very precise articulation of the speech material or should the articulation be normal or even sloppy; and, in trying to estimate the everyday life handicap, should one include ambient noise in the measurement because noise is frequently present in practice?

The authors intend to provide some insight regarding the above questions as well as regarding the question of measurement efficiency.

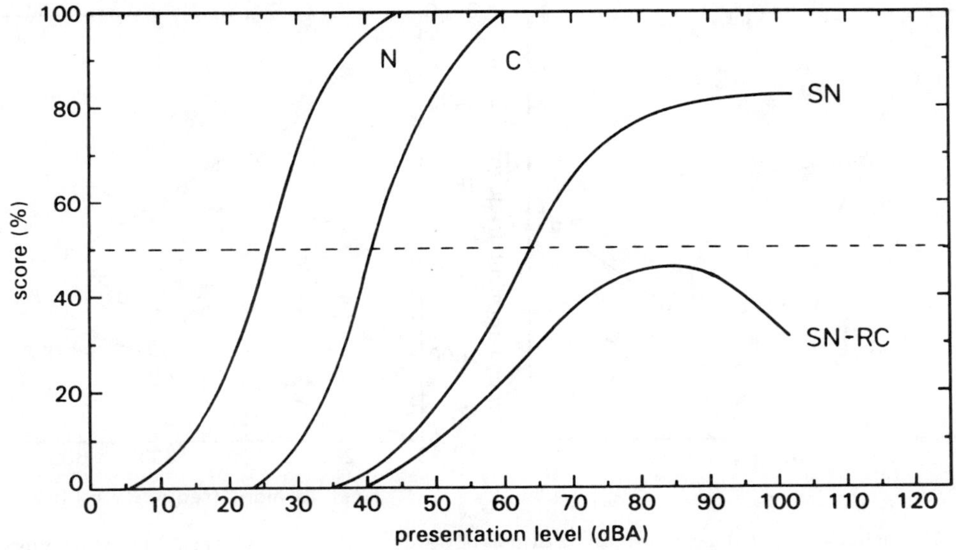

Figure 25-1 Idealized speech audiograms for subjects with normal hearing (N), subjects with a conductive hearing loss (C), subjects with sensorineural hearing loss (SN), and subjects with more severe sensorineural hearing loss, frequently of retrocochlear origin, in which the score decreases at the highest levels tolerated—the so-called rollover phenomenon (SN-RC).

Basic Aspects of the Speech Audiogram

In speech audiometry, the number of speech units (such as phonemes) received correctly is usually plotted as a function of sound level (Fig. 25-1). For normal ears, the speech audiogram appears as an S-shaped curve, running from a score of 0 to 100 percent (curve N). In cases of conductive hearing loss (curve C), and in some cases of (moderate) sensorineural hearing loss, the S-shaped curve may simply shift rightward to higher stimulus levels without changing its shape or slope. Such a shift suggests that the hearing loss simply attenuates the signal; the score curve follows a normal course after amplifying the speech. With more severe sensorineural hearing loss (curve SN), the slope of the curve may become shallower and may not reach the 100 percent level. In some cases of sensorineural hearing loss, in particular those originating with retrocochlear lesions, the score may even decrease at the highest stimulus levels when using words or nonsense syllables as test materials (so-called rollover, curve SN-RC). Except for the scarce cases of rollover, the speech audiogram can be adequately characterized by three parameters: the position of the curve along the abscissa, the slope of the curve, and the maximum score reached at some level. The position of the curve along the abscissa is usually quantified by the sound level at which the curve intercepts the 50 percent score level. This sound level is defined as the speech reception threshold (SRT). However, this definition is limited to moderate hearing impairment for which the maximum score exceeds 50 percent. A general definition can be based on the sound level at which half the maximum score is found (Bosman, 1989). The maximum score reached at some level is defined as the discrimination score (DS).

An interesting aspect of speech audiograms, in comparison with tone audiograms, is that they provide some insight into suprathreshold hearing. Whereas tone audiograms present the level at which a pure tone can just be detected, speech audiograms may indicate that some speech sounds cannot be discriminated from each other, not even at the highest sound levels tolerated. The score may level off below 100 percent. In this respect, it is instructive to note that the S-shaped curve of the speech audiogram has an origin that differs from the origin of the S-shaped detection curve found for pure tones. The detection curve for pure tones represents an increasing probability of detecting speech sounds against, in quiet conditions, an internal (physiologic) noise or against external noise. It is determined by the intensity fluctuations in the noise. The speech audiogram represents a sequence of increasingly weaker speech ele-

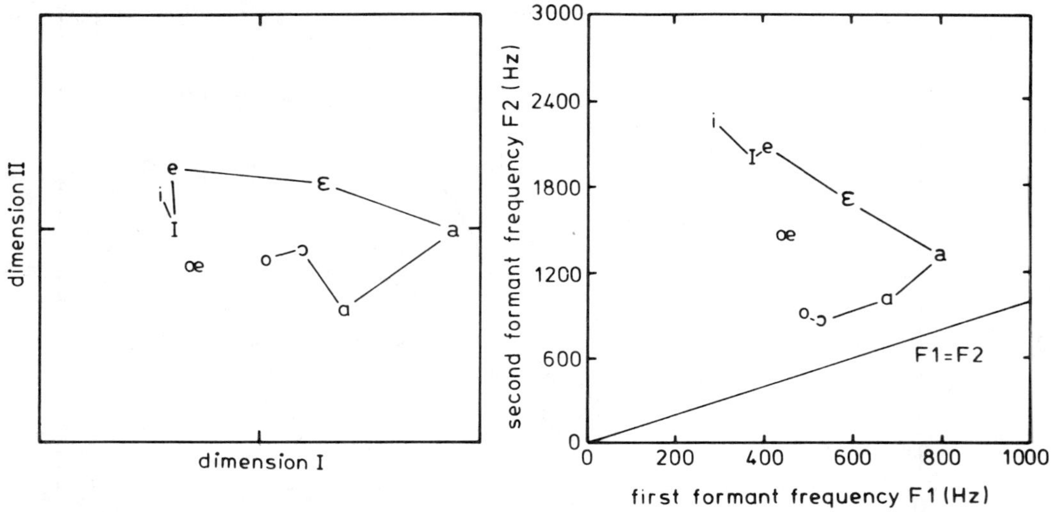

Figure 25-2 Solution of multidimensional scaling analysis of vowel confusions found for subjects with normal hearing *(A)* in relation to the frequencies of the first and second formant *(B)*. The vowels are: /i/ as in bit; /I/ as in see; /e/ as in day (Scottish pronunciation), /ɛ/ as in get, /a/ as in fahren (German), /ɑ/ as in far, /ɔ/ as in hot, /o/ as in no.

ments becoming audible as sound level increases. Hence, it is determined by the distribution of the levels of the speech elements. In addition, it is determined by their mutual discriminability and, depending on the type of materials, by the predictability of nonperceived elements from those elements perceived. While the S-shaped curve for the detection of pure tones may be derived mathematically from the statistical distribution of noise intensity, its counterpart in speech audiometry is primarily based on properties of the speech material itself.

Although speech audiometry is usually restricted to assessment of recognition scores, phoneme confusions may also provide interesting information when the speech materials consist of words or meaningless syllables. The confusions may show which speech features are poorly discriminated. This information can be used in handicap assessment and in hearing aid tuning. Multidimensional scaling techniques (MDS; Kruskal, 1964a, 1964b; Carroll and Chang, 1970) applied to confusion matrices can be very helpful in identifying the speech features used in discrimination. These techniques yield representations of the phonemes in two, three, or more dimensions in which the distance between the phonemes increases with decreasing probability of confusion. The ordering of the phonemes along a certain dimension reveals the speech feature involved. Figure 25-2 (left panel) shows, for example, a result of this technique for vowel perception by subjects with normal hearing. The two dimensions emerging from MDS (according to Kruskal, 1964a,b) applied to the perceptual confusions appear to correspond to the first and second formant frequency of the vowel—measures commonly used to describe the physical (spectral) features of the vowels (see Fig. 25-2, right panel).

Effect of Acoustic Realization of Speech Materials

The effect of articulation is shown in Figure 25-3. Speech reception was measured in 24 individuals with normal hearing (left panel) and in 24 individuals with presbycusis (right panel) using two female speakers: one articulating normally (S1), the other articulating slowly and overprecisely (S2). Speech materials consisted of one- and two-syllable Dutch (meaningful) words. Figure 25-3 shows the phoneme scores separated into those for the vowels and those for the consonants. Emphatic articulation produced higher scores in the subjects with normal hearing, but in presbycusis subjects the scores for the two types of articulation were nearly equal, particularly those for the vowels.

MDS analysis of the vowel confusions showed that with presbycusis the second formant lost its importance in vowel recognition. The orderly arrangement of the vowels, in accordance with the second formant frequency, found for subjects with normal hearing along the second dimension (see Fig. 25-2), disap-

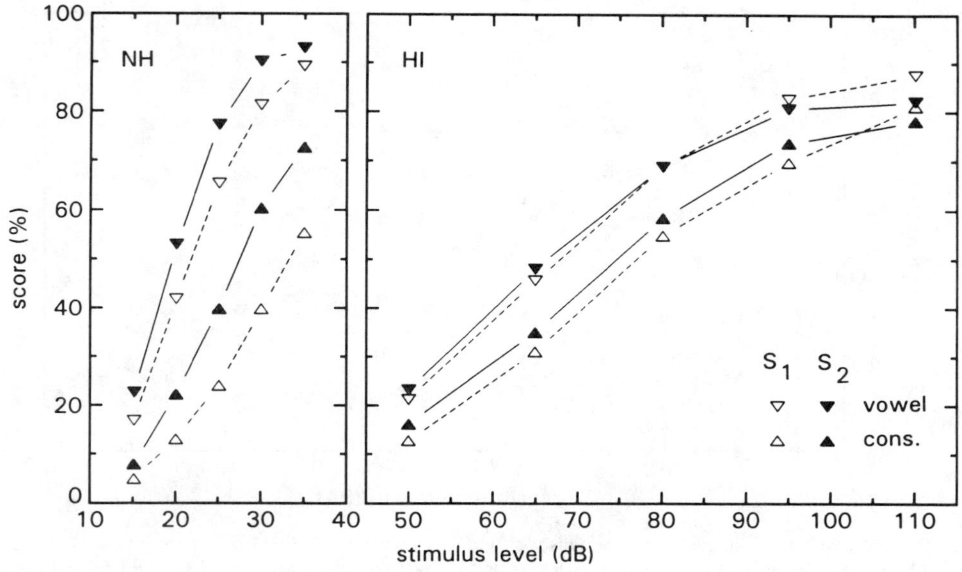

Figure 25-3 The percentage of correctly responded vowels and consonants as a function of stimulus level for normal speech (S1) and for slow and emphatically articulated speech (S2). *A,* Results for normal hearing subjects. *B,* Results for presbycusis subjects.

peared in the result of MDS analysis for the presbycusis subjects (Fig. 25-4; follow the solid line). In contrast, Figure 25-4 shows central clustering of the short vowels (encircled), which implies frequent confusions amongst these short vowels and it shows good discrimination of the long vowels with a certain first formant from their short duration counterparts (/I/ *versus* /i/, /ɛ/ and /ɔ/ *versus* /e/ and /o/, and /ɑ/ *versus* /a/). These results suggest that a third feature, vowel duration, may become the second feature of importance in vowel recognition once the contribution of the second formant disappears. The reduction in importance of the second formant is most likely due to the high-frequency character of the hearing loss.

Further analysis showed that the contribution of the second formant to vowel recognition in normal hearing was important only for the female speaker articulating emphatically, whereas the contribution of the feature "vowel duration" in presbycusis was important only for the female speaker articulating normally. The emphatically articulated speech consisted of unnaturally long vowels with considerable spread in their duration. For the presbycusis subjects, the abnormal vowel durations might have meant that they were less able to use the feature "vowel duration." This would explain why vowel duration was important to the presbycusis subjects for only the speaker articulating normally. The present example suggests that emphatic speech may provide a better basis of discriminating high-frequency hearing loss from normal hearing. When the speaker provides more information that is sensitive to (high-frequency) hearing loss, such as the second formant, and when the speaker provides less, or misleading information in features that become important with hearing loss, such as vowel duration, this may result in larger differences between the

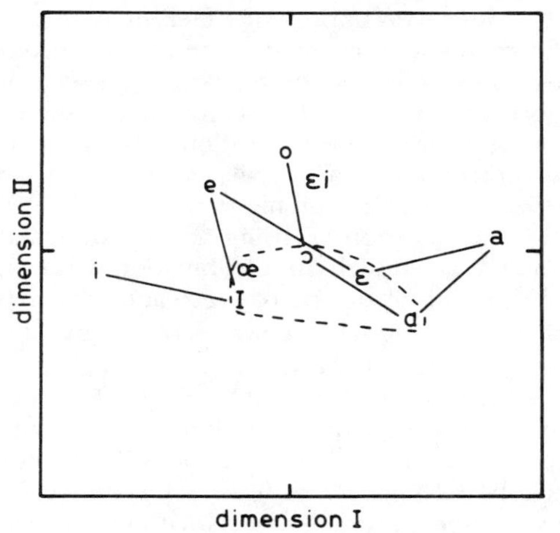

Figure 25-4 Solution of multidimensional scaling analysis of vowel confusions found for listeners with presbycusis. Vowel notation is explained in the legend of Figure 25-2. The short vowels are encircled.

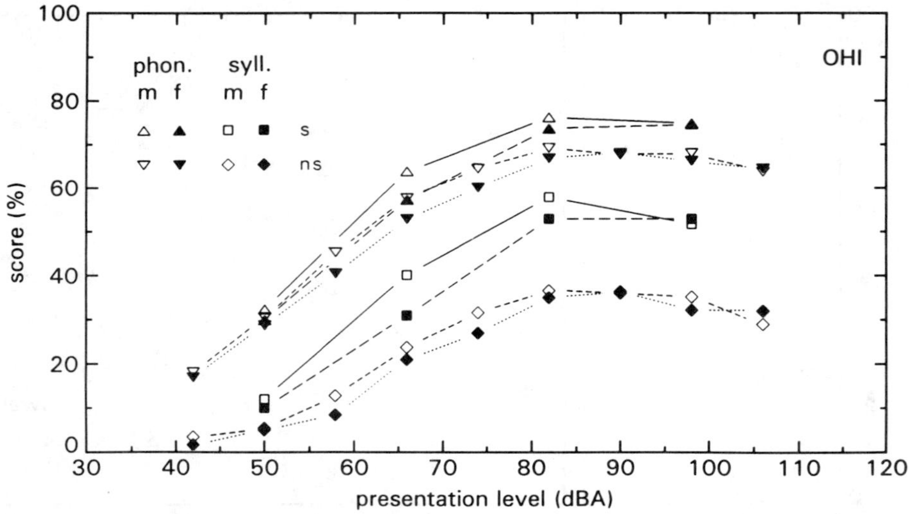

Figure 25-5 Phoneme and syllable scores for sense (s) and nonsense (ns) CVC syllables uttered by a male (m) and a female (f) speaker as a function of stimulus level for presbycusis subjects (OHI). (Adapted from Bosman AJ. Speech perception by the hearing impaired. Dissertation. State University at Utrecht, The Netherlands, 1989.)

scores for normal hearing and those for impaired hearing as was apparent from Figure 25-3. However, improving differential diagnostics in this way means that the results become less representative of everyday speech and more sensitive to unforeseen artifacts, such as the unnatural vowel duration. We therefore recommend normal articulation of speech materials in speech audiometry.

The question of using a male or female voice was studied in combination with the question of what type of score and what type of speech materials are preferable. Figure 25-5 shows scores for meaningful and meaningless syllables (sense and nonsense syllables), consisting of a sequence of an initial consonant, a vowel, and a final consonant (CVC syllables), uttered by either a male or a female speaker and presented to 20 subjects with presbycusis. Two types of scores are given: the count of individual phonemes repeated correctly (the phoneme score), and the count of syllables repeated completely correctly (the syllable score). In this section, we shall address the question of gender.

In Figure 25-5, the difference between the average scores for the male and female speaker appears to be small when either the phoneme scores or the syllable scores are considered, in particular when these differences are compared to the standard deviation of the measurements, which ranges from 4 to 14 percent. For young, normal-hearing subjects, the differences between the two speakers were virtually zero (not shown). For all subjects there was no clear difference between the test-retest error for the male and the female voice. Thus, with respect to scores, this example suggests that the choice of the sex of the speaker is unimportant.

MDS analysis of the confusion matrices, however, revealed an interesting difference (Fig. 25-6). In young, normal-hearing subjects (YNH), we found contributions to vowel recognition from both the first and the second formant for the male speaker (m) but virtually no contribution from the second formant for the female speaker (f). The same difference was found for older subjects with near-normal hearing (ONH) but the contribution from the second formant for the male speaker vanished in the presbycusis subjects (OHI). These results suggest that a male voice may provide more information when one is interested in changes in confusion patterns with high-frequency hearing loss. The difference in the relative contributions from the first and second formant to vowel recognition between the male and female speaker may be due to differences in the level of the second formant above subjective threshold. For the female speaker, this level may have been too low to aid vowel recognition at the sensation levels used. Although these results are limited to one male speaker and to one female speaker, they suggest the choice of a male voice. This conclusion is supported by results found for the consonants. An effect of hearing loss was seen primarily in the feature "voicing" for the male speaker.

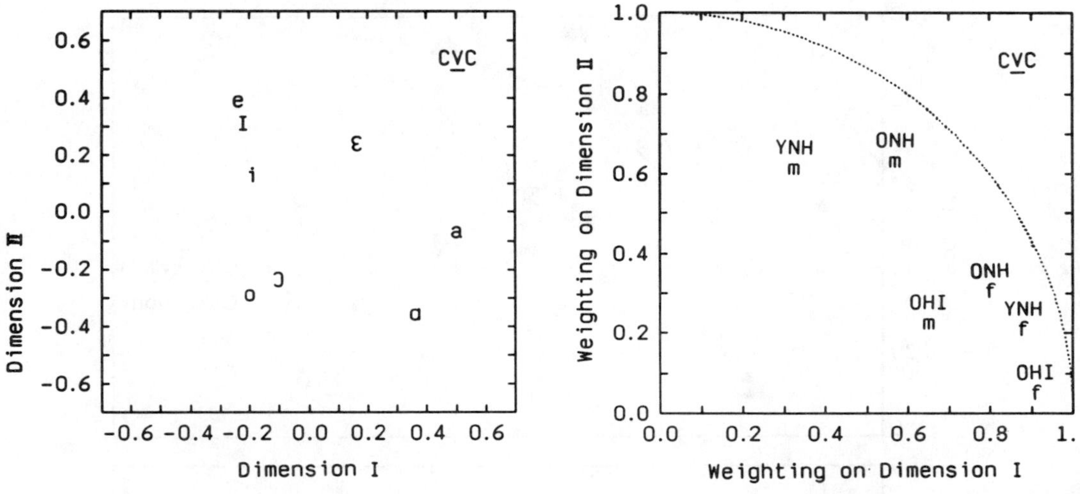

Figure 25-6 Solution of multidimensional scaling analysis of vowel confusions (according to Carroll and Chang, 1970) found for young normal-hearing listeners (YNH), for old individuals with near-normal hearing (ONH), and for old hearing-impaired subjects (OHI). The vowels were uttered in a CVC context by a male (m) and a female (f) speaker. Vowel notation is explained in the legend of Figure 25-2. The short vowels are encircled. (Adapted from Bosman AJ. Speech perception by the hearing impaired. Dissertation. State University at Utrecht, The Netherlands, 1989.)

Effect of Type of Speech Materials and Method of Scoring

The phoneme scores in Figure 25-5 were consistently higher than the syllable scores (both expressed as percentages). This follows straight from the definition. A correct CVC syllable implies three correct phonemes; 0, 1, or 2 correct phonemes imply an incorrect syllable. It is interesting to note that the phoneme scores for the sense and nonsense syllables were almost equal to one another whereas the syllable scores differed considerably. In choosing the method of scoring, this result suggests to prefer phoneme scores above syllable scores. Phoneme scores will be less sensitive to lexical effects.

The syllable score for nonsense syllables closely followed the product of the scores for the three individual phonemes, which agrees with the notion that the recognition of one phoneme in a nonsense syllable should, to a first approximation, and excluding coarticulation effects, not affect the recognition of the other phonemes. For the sense syllables, however, Figure 25-5 shows a higher syllable score at the same phoneme score. Thus, for sense syllables, the syllable score exceeded the product of the individual phoneme scores. This implies that the distribution of responded syllables with 0, 1, 2, and 3 correct phonemes per syllable deviated from the binomial distribution. Subjects tended to respond with a complete syllable or with no syllable at all; they responded with a few incomplete syllables. This result suggests that nonsense syllables are to be preferred. However, untrained subjects tend to respond with meaningful syllables resembling the nonsense syllables presented. This bias is very sensitive to the instruction procedure. Higher reliability is therefore obtained when using sense syllables. We shall show that for Dutch CVC sense syllables, the lexical effects on phoneme scores are limited. With other languages containing few short, meaningful syllables, it may be more difficult to compose lists of meaningful syllables with limited lexical effects.

A comparison between the scores for CVC syllables and those for sentences consisting of eight or nine syllables (Plomp and Mimpen, 1979) is given in Figure 25-7 for YNH subjects (upper panel) and for OHI subjects (lower panel). Again, scores are presented for the male and the female speaker and, again, the CVC syllables are scored in terms of the phoneme count and the syllable count. Similarly, the sentences are scored in terms of the number of individual syllables repeated correctly and the number of sentences repeated completely correctly. For the YNH subjects, the upper panel of Figure 25-7 shows considerably steeper sloping curves for the sentences than for the syllables, irrespective of the type of score. This difference in slope is

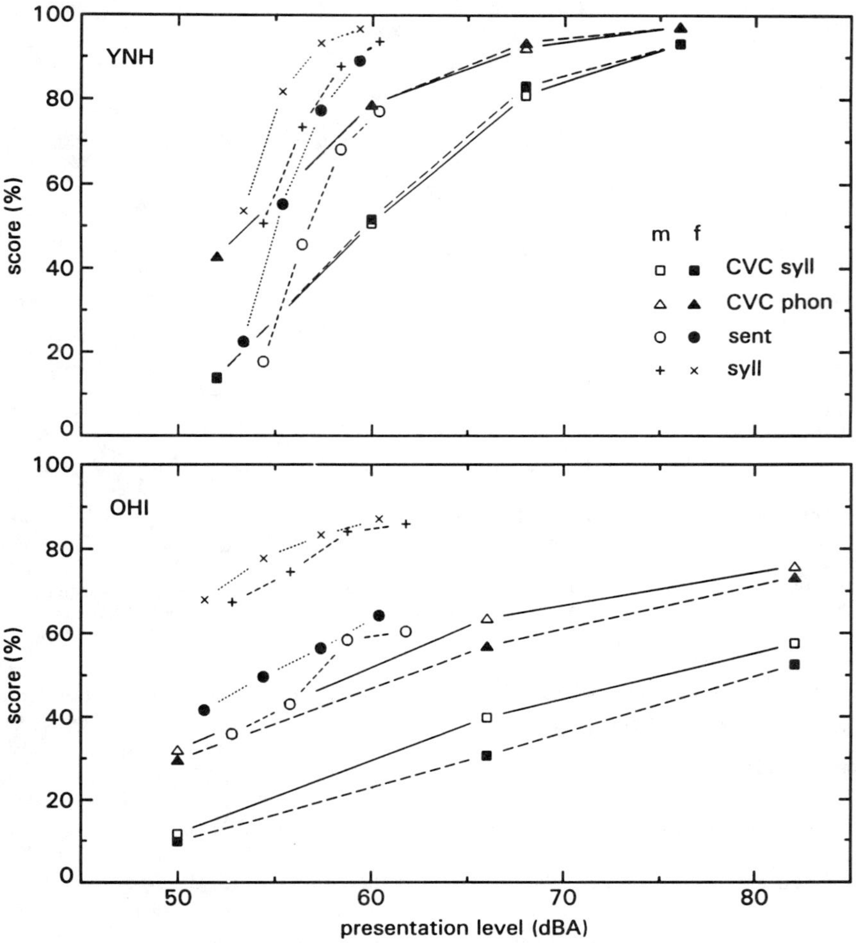

Figure 25-7 Syllable (syll) and whole-sentence (sent) scores for sentences uttered by a male (m) and a female (f) speaker as a function of stimulus level in relation to phoneme and syllable scores for CVC syllables (CVC phon and CVC syll, respectively). Upper panel: Results for young normal-hearing subjects (YNH). Lower panel: Results for old hearing-impaired subjects (OHI). (Adapted from Bosman AJ. Speech perception by the hearing impaired. Dissertation. State University at Utrecht, The Netherlands, 1989.)

less marked for the scores of the OHI subjects in the lower panel of Figure 25-7.

Because the steep slopes found for the sentences were expected, we did not measure the scores at fixed presentation levels. However, the levels were adjusted in relation to the individual SRT for the sentences. Subsequently, the scores averaged across subjects were plotted as a function of the presentation levels averaged across subjects. This procedure guards against a wrong impression of the increase of the score with increasing presentation level. When the individual SRTs cover a large range of presentation levels, data averaging without normalization may result in a reduction of the steepness of the slopes measured individually because of the nonlinear, asymptotic behavior of the score curves at scores of 0 and 100 percent. Thus, for the sentences, the averaged data of Figure 25-7 give a fair impression of the steepness of the individual slopes. Near a score of 50 percent, these slopes are 15 percent per dB for the YNH subjects and 4 percent for the OHI subjects. The averaged data for the CVC syllables were not normalized to individual SRT. They nevertheless give a fair impression of the individual slopes. Estimates of the individual slopes yielded values of 5.5 percent per dB for the YNH subjects and 3.5 percent per dB for the OHI subjects. The large decrease in the slope of the curves for sentences found with hearing loss implies that measurement error in SRT will increase markedly with hearing loss.

The steepness of the score curves for sentences originates with the redundancy of in-

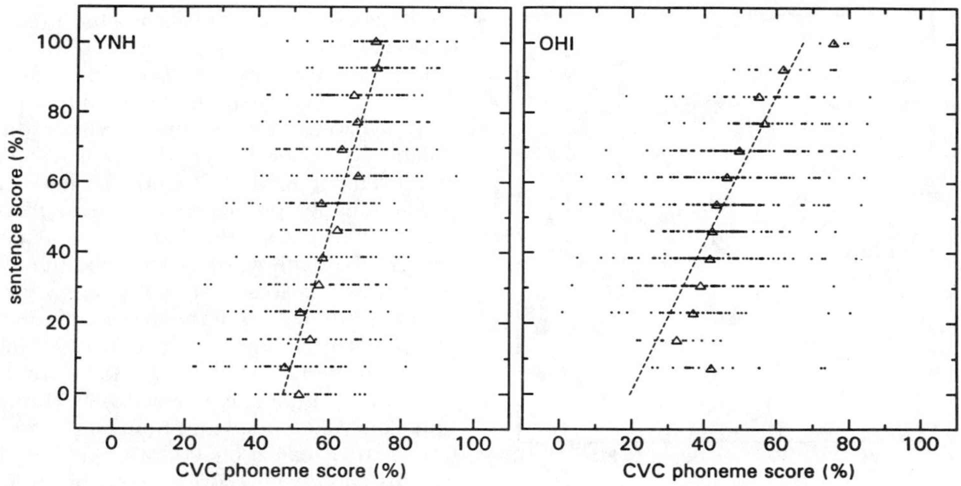

Figure 25-8 Relation between the score for sentences (repeated completely correctly) and the phoneme score for CVC syllables found for young normal-hearing subjects (YNH, left panel) and for old hearing impaired subjects (OHI, right panel). The average phoneme score at a given sentence score is denoted by the triangles. The linear fits are based on principal components (least squares in the direction perpendicular to the line). (Adapted from Bosman AJ. Speech perception by the hearing impaired. Dissertation. State University at Utrecht, The Netherlands, 1989.)

formation in sentences. Once the loud phonemes (the vowels and the loud consonants) are perceived, listeners are able to guess the nonperceived phonemes on the basis of their knowledge of grammar, syntax, and lexicon. This means that negative effects of high-frequency hearing loss on the perception of weak high-frequency consonants, such as fricatives and plosives, may go unnoticed. The choice of sentences as speech material in audiometry has face validity when one is interested in determining the handicap for everyday speech. One should bear in mind, however, that this material does not reveal problems that may arise with high-frequency hearing loss when the hearing impaired has to understand, for example, unfamiliar words.

The relation between the phoneme scores for syllables and the sentence scores shows an interesting aspect of speech perception by the old hearing impaired (Fig. 25-8). Whereas a 100 percent sentence score is reached for both the YNH and the OHI subjects at a phoneme score of about 70 percent, the relation at the low scores shows a difference between the two groups of subjects. For example, a sentence score of 20 percent is reached at an average phoneme score of about 50 percent for the YNH subjects and at only about 30 percent for the OHI subjects. Thus, OHI subjects seem to have better skill in receiving sentences on the basis of fragments of speech information. Figure 25-8 also shows that the correlation between the phoneme scores and the sentence scores is limited. In predicting sentence SRT from the levels at which half the maximum phoneme score for syllables is found, the error is about 5 dB.

Finally, we may consider the use of running discourse in speech audiometry (de Filippo and Scott, 1978). With this material, the score is usually based on the time required to repeat the message completely correctly, including repeated presentations of those parts of the text that were not well received. This method is used in the profoundly hearing impaired because their reception scores for isolated syllables or sentences may be very low. However, the score based on completion time is sensitive to the strategy of the examiner reading the text and deciding when to repeat or spell part of it in response to misreceptions. In view of this limited reliability and the fact that the reception scores for syllables and sentences usually do not fall to very low percentages when dealing with noise-induced hearing loss, the use of isolated syllables or sentences suggests itself for this type of hearing loss.

Measurement Error and Measurement Efficiency

In speech audiometry, measurement error can be predicted on the basis of elementary statistics. We assume that the probability of receiving a speech unit (e.g., a phoneme or a

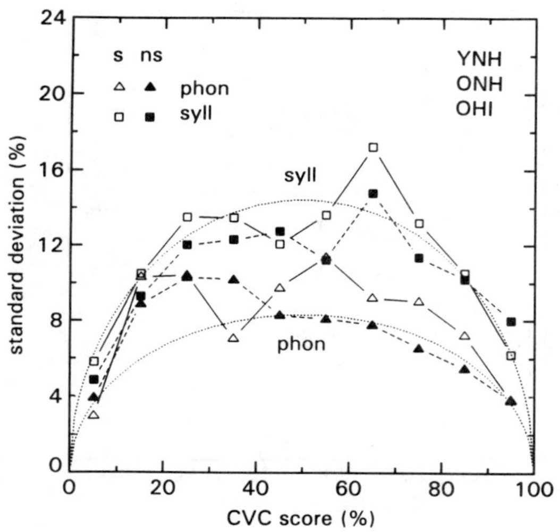

Figure 25-9 Measurement error for phoneme (phon) and syllable (syll) scores with sense (s) and nonsense (ns) CVC syllables at different levels of performance. Performance levels were divided into 10 contiguous classes, each class covering a score interval of 10 percent. Predictions, based on the binomial distribution, are indicated by the dotted lines. The experimental data are derived from test-retest differences. The results are pooled across the three groups of subjects. (Adapted from Bosman AJ. Speech perception by the hearing impaired. Dissertation. State University at Utrecht, The Netherlands, 1989.)

syllable) does not depend on previous failure or success, but that it is an unconditional probability determined by the character of the speech unit and its level. If the probability of a correct response equals p and the number of presentations equals N, we may expect p.N correct responses and, according to the properties of the binomial distribution, a standard deviation of $\sqrt{(p.(1\text{-}p).N)}$. The standard deviation, expressed as a fraction of the number of presentations, becomes $\sqrt{(p.(1\text{-}p)/N)}$. Figure 25-9 shows the calculated standard deviation (in dotted curves) for a list of 12 CVC syllables as a function of p in percent (the score), where N=12 when syllables are scored and N=36 for phonemes. When we compare these calculated values to measurement error, derived from the experimentally determined test-retest reliability, Figure 25-9 shows that the experimental errors for the syllables, either sense or nonsense, closely follow the prediction. Thus, syllable reception can be modeled as the reception of, in this case 12, independent speech units. For the phoneme score, however, measurement error mostly exceeds the calculated standard deviation. With nonsense syllables, it closely follows the prediction when the score exceeds 40 percent, but for lower scores it approaches the prediction for syllables. This suggests that response behavior at these low levels changed from responding phonemes independently (incomplete syllables) to responding either the full syllable or none. With the sense syllables, measurement error is found in between the predictions for phonemes and those for syllables. Hence, the number of independent speech elements was less than the number of phonemes but greater than the number of syllables. A calculation of the effective number of independent elements yielded N=29. This can be interpreted as an average number of 2.4 independent phonemes per syllable. The deviation from 3 independent phonemes is ascribed to primarily lexical effects. We concluded earlier that phoneme scores are to be preferred above syllable scores because they are more resistant to lexical effects. Here, in addition, we conclude that phoneme scores are to be preferred because they carry smaller measurement error.

We applied the same analysis to the results for sentences. Measurement errors for the sentence score, the word score, and the syllable score were all close to the calculated values for the sentence score. This suggests that reception of certain words or syllables in the sentence depends highly on reception of the other syllables. Limited reliability of the measurement error estimates prevented calculation of the number of independent speech units in the sentences. Yet, this could be done on the basis of the relation between the sentence score and the product of the syllable scores. The result was about three independent units. For the design of sentence lists with key words, this result suggests that returns will diminish when the number of key words in one simple sentence (consisting of eight or nine syllables) exceeds a value of three.

We also concluded earlier that, with respect to measurement of speech discrimination abilities, word materials provide more detailed information than sentences. Sentences, however, are frequently advocated to measure the SRT. The steep slope of the score curve for sentences promises small measurement error in the SRT. Calculations of SRT measurement error, where the SRT was based on either interpolation of the score curves around the 50 percent score (or half the maximum score) or on a parametrized fit of the score curve, yielded in YNH subjects an error of about 1.5 dB for the phoneme scores and an error of about 0.9 dB for the sentences. The corresponding values for the OHI subjects were about 4.0 and 3.9 dB. The higher values found for the OHI subjects are in agreement with our previously expressed expectation based on the decrease in the slope of the score curves with hearing loss. Comparing these results in view of measurement efficiency, we should take into account measurement time. The results for syllables were based on three lists of 12 CVC syllables each, the measurement taking about 150 s; the results for sentences were based on two lists of 13 sentences each, taking about 230 s. Assuming an extension of the word lists to 230 s measurement time and a decrease in measurement error with increasing measurement time in accordance with the $\sqrt{N}$-law, estimates of the error for syllables become 1.2 dB in YNH subjects and 3.2 dB in the OHI subjects. These numbers are close to the errors found for the sentences of 0.9 and 3.9 dB, respectively. Thus, the present results, based on carefully developed syllable and sentence materials, suggest that there is no important difference between syllable and sentence materials with respect to the efficiency in determining the SRT. When the measurements are done in a noisy background, the slopes of the score curves (Bosman, 1989) suggest that we may expect to arrive at the same conclusion. Thus it seems justified to restrict the measurements to syllable materials, even when the SRT is the primary measure of concern.

Speech Audiometry in a Noisy Background

So far, the present discussion of speech audiometry was limited to measurements in a quiet condition. However, individuals with noise-induced hearing loss first complain about a hearing handicap when trying to understand speech in a noisy environment (Smoorenburg, 1990). Therefore, we shall conclude this paper with a note on speech reception in noisy conditions. For sentence reception, Figure 25-10 shows that there is little correlation between thresholds measured in a quiet condition and those measured against a background noise (r=0.45). Thus, in order to acquire a good impression of the handicap experienced by an individual with noise-induced hearing loss in a noisy environment, one should include speech audiometry in noise.

With noise-induced hearing loss, speech reception thresholds measured either in quiet or in noise can be predicted to some extent from the tone audiogram. One may wish to consider the accuracy of this prediction against the error in the speech reception measurement itself. In order to gain some insight into this question, the reader is referred to Smoorenburg (1986, 1990, 1991).

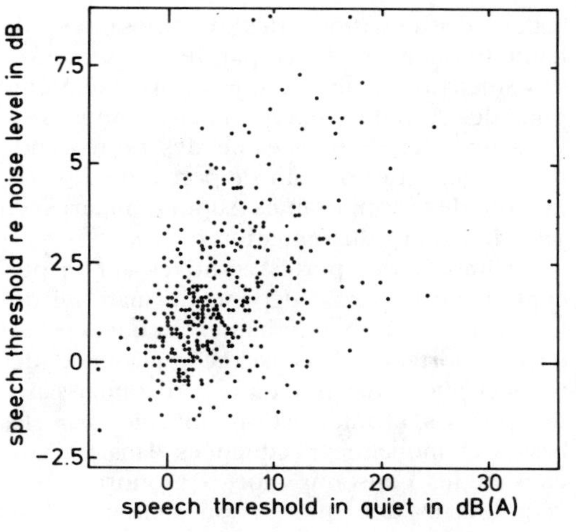

Figure 25-10 Speech reception thresholds measured against a background noise, expressed in the signal-to-noise distance, in relation to the speech reception threshold measured in a quiet condition, expressed in the sound level itself in dB(A) for 400 ears with noise-induced hearing loss (r=0.45). (Adapted from Smoorenburg GF. Hearing handicap assessment for speech perception using pure tone audiometry. In: Noise as a public health problem, new advances in noise research. Part 1, Vol. 4. Stockholm: Swedish Council for Building Research, 1990:245.)

Conclusion

The results presented in this paper suggest that appropriate materials for speech audiometry consist of short (meaningful) words, articulated normally by a male speaker, to be presented in both a quiet condition and against a noisy background, and to be scored in terms of the phoneme count.

Choix des Caractéristiques de la Parole Permettant D'Evaluer les Atteintes Auditives

On soupçonne les pertes auditives induites par le bruit (NIHL) et caractérisées par une augmentation des seuils auditifs dans la région des 4 kHz, d'affecter la perception de la parole par l'atténuation de ses composantes de haute-fréquence. Cependant, l'effet des pertes auditives n'est pas simplement comparable à l'effet d'atténuation des composantes de haute-fréquences de la parole, présentées à des sujets ayant une audition normale. Même pour des stimulus supra-liminaires, nous trouvons un effet dommageable des pertes auditives. Cela peut provenir de pertes de discrimination des composantes supra-liminaires en plus du facteur d'atténuation.

L'impact des pertes auditives sur la perception de la parole dépend du matériel utilisé. L'information des hautes fréquences est plus importante dans la reconnaissance des mots et phonèmes que dans la reconnaissance de phrases. L'information fournie par les basses et moyennes fréquences dans les voyelles et les consonnes fortes (sonores) peuvent fournir une information suffisante pour comprendre les phrases.

Dans cet article nous comparerons les résultats des phonèmes et des mots pour des syllabes significatives et non significatives consistant en des séquences consonne-voyelle-consonne et les scores des syllabes et phrases pour des phrases simples présentées dans un environnement calme ou bruyant sur des sujets présentant des pertes auditives. En plus nous examinerons les confusions de phonèmes, en relation avec les pertes auditives aux hautes fréquences.

References

Bosman AJ. Speech perception by the hearing impaired. Dissertation. State University at Utrecht, The Netherlands, 1989.

Carroll JD, Chang JJ. Analysis of individual differences in multidimensional scaling via an N-way generalization of the "Eckart-Young" decomposition. Psychometrika 1970; 35:283-319.

De Filippo CL, Scott BL. A method for training and evaluation of the reception of ongoing speech. J Acoust Soc Am 1978; 63:1186-1192.

Fletcher H, Steinberg JC. Articulation testing methods. Bell Syst Tech J 1929; 8:806-854.

ISO/DIS 1999.2. (1985) Acoustics—Determination of occupational noise exposure and estimation of noise-induced hearing impairment.

Kalikow DN, Stevens KN, Elliott LL. Development of a test of speech intelligibility in noise using sentences with controlled word predictability, J Acoust Soc Am 1977; 61:1337-1351.

Kruskal JB. Multidimensional scaling by optimizing goodness of fit to a nonmetric hypothesis. Psychometrika 1964a; 29:1-27.

Kruskal JB. Nonmetric multidimensional scaling: A numerical method. Psychometrika 1964b; 29:28-42.

Nakatani LH, Dukes KD. A sensitive test of speech communication quality. J Acoust Soc Am 1973; 53:1083-1092.

Plomp R, Mimpen AM. Improving the reliability of testing the speech reception threshold for sentences. Audiology 1979; 18:43-52.

Silverman SR, Hirsh IJ. Problems related to the use of speech in clinical audiometry. Ann Otol Rhinol Laryngol 1955; 64:1234-1244.

Smoorenburg GF. Speech perception in individuals with noise-induced hearing loss and its implication for hearing loss criteria. In: Salvi RJ, Henderson D, Hamernik RP, Colletti V, eds. Basic and applied aspects of noise-induced hearing loss New York: Plenum Press, 1986:335.

Smoorenburg GF. Hearing handicap assessment for speech perception using pure tone audiometry. In: Noise as a public health problem, new advances in noise research. Part I, Vol. 4. Stockholm: Swedish Council for Building Research, 1990:245.

Smoorenburg GF. Speech reception in quiet and in noisy conditions by individuals with noise-induced hearing loss in relation to their tone audiogram. J Acoust Soc Am 1991, in revision.

CHAPTER 26

Effects of Noise on Binaural Hearing

H. STEVEN COLBURN
CONSTANTINE TRAHIOTIS

During the past decade, there was a great increase in the number of psychophysical investigations of hearing-impaired listeners. The vast majority of those studies were directed toward revealing deficits or discovering mechanisms that mediate the *monaural* processing of sounds. One purpose of this paper is to discuss the relatively few binaural studies of hearing-impaired listeners that were conducted. Additionally, we discuss several recent empirical, theoretical, and practical advances that we believe will stimulate and help shape future studies of binaural processing in hearing-impaired populations. At this time, the discussion cannot focus exclusively, or even principally, on the deleterious effects of acoustic overexposure per se. This is because most published reports do not contain the information necessary to isolate the factor or factors responsible for the subjects' hearing losses.

Studies Prior to 1981

A detailed review of available results from binaural studies of listeners with hearing impairments was presented in 1981 (Durlach et al, 1981); we will not repeat a detailed discussion of the results here. In this part of our presentation, we summarize the studies up to 1981 at a general level, and point out several issues that were raised by that review, either explicitly or implicitly, which remain important in considering binaural studies of hearing-impaired listeners.

As already noted, few studies have specifically addressed the consequences of acoustic exposure for binaural hearing. Therefore we are forced to consider results from subjects in broader categories. Most studies have divided listeners into conductive, cochlear, and retrocochlear categories (with brain-stem and cortical deficits identified as a separate group without audiometric losses), so that a brief summary of the results from subjects with cochlear pathologies may provide insight about patients suffering from noise-induced losses. Individuals with cochlear hearing losses generally can discriminate interaural delays in wide-band signals significantly better than individuals with conductive or retrocochlear impairments. Listeners with cochlear loss appear to have greater difficulties with interaural time discrimination with narrow-band stimuli (see Hawkins and Wightman, 1980, as discussed later), and these deficits may be related to lesions occupying restricted cochlear regions (for some subject categories). The free-field localization tests that have been conducted were primarily of the angle-identification type, and generally revealed that subjects with bilaterally symmetric cochlear losses are better off than subjects with other categories of hearing impairment. Few data on interaural intensity discrimination by subjects with cochlear loss had been obtained prior to 1981. It was already apparent at that time, however, that abilities varied over subjects in a manner that showed little correlation with abilities in interaural time discrimination.

Subjects with cochlear loss also seem to have considerable difficulty in binaural detection of tones in wide-band noise; for example, Quaranta and Cervellera (1974) report abnormally small masking level differences (MLDs) in 86 percent of the cases they studied. These data suggest that patients with bilateral sensorineural losses might have difficulty performing tasks that involve processing of interaural temporal information in narrow frequency bands.

Measurements from subjects who are explicitly identified as having noise-induced losses were almost exclusively from studies of binaural detection (Olsen et al, 1976; Olsen and Noffsinger, 1976). These studies show that most patients with noise-induced hearing losses have MLDs in the normal range for 500-Hz target tones, although a few subjects show very small MLDs. It is interesting to note that the subjects with small MLDs were not necessarily the ones with losses at 500 Hz; therefore, subjects can have abnormal performance at 500 Hz with normal absolute thresholds at 500 Hz. This is one of several examples of the lack of correlation between binaural performance and the monaural audiograms. MLDs with spondee targets are more affected by noise-induced losses; specifically, the average MLD is approximately 2 dB smaller than normal, and a larger percentage of patients show negligible MLDs in this case.

A number of factors interfere with the interpretation and generalization of results of binaural experiments on listeners with hearing impairments. Most of these factors were raised by Durlach et al (1981) or became apparent from their review. First, unless the etiologies of the impairments are known and specified, the subject groups contain relatively heterogeneous types of losses, and characterization of the consequences of the impairments is more difficult. That is, some of the large variability in results may simply be related to the diversity of the subjects' auditory problems. Second, and even more significant, the degree of loss is often unreported and probably contributes to greater variability. For example, Hausler et al (1983) claim that subjects with conductive losses show significant differences in interaural time discrimination tests according to the size of their hearing losses, showing normal performance for losses less than 25 dB HL and significantly abnormal performance (much worse than subjects with sensorineural losses) for losses greater than 35 dB HL. A third issue, which was discussed at some length by Durlach et al (1981), is the lack of consideration of the effective interaural relations in the impaired auditory systems. They note the fact that many data from normal listeners show a decrement in performance when the ears are imbalanced in level and suggest that one component of any abnormalities in binaural performance could be due to an effective shift in the interaural differences in the stimulus. Reports available at that time on the effects of interaurally balancing level were mixed, some studies reporting a big influence and some almost no effect. Fourth, there were few studies that tested several binaural abilities on each subject. Without such studies, performance across experiments could not be compared and the ability to predict performance in some experiments from performance in a subset of experiments could not be investigated. Fifth, there was a lack of sophistication about psychophysical methods, particularly in separating sensitivity from bias in the measurements (e.g., in the many angle identification tests). Sixth, there were few comparisons across stimulus bandwidth or stimulus type for a given test, so that it was difficult to determine whether the conflict noted above, between interaural time discrimination for wide-band and narrow-band stimuli by subjects with cochlear losses, was a conflict between bandwidth effects or stimulus effects (random noise versus deterministic tone) and speech versus tones in other studies. Finally, a general concern is that the normal comparison subjects are often chosen from easily available college students, so that the subject groups are often disparate in ways unrelated to hearing impairments. Optimally, the control subjects would be matched to the population of hearing-impaired subjects in such factors as age, motivation, and education. In the next section, we note that many of these issues have been addressed in the recent studies of binaural performance with hearing-impaired listeners.

Recent Binaural Studies of Hearing-Impaired Listeners

Several important trends separate recent measurements from most of those that were included in the review just discussed. These include the use of modern psychophysical procedures and the design of experiments that address some of the problems just described.

Modern Psychophysical Techniques

One important trend is the use of modern, objective psychophysical techniques with well-practiced hearing-impaired listeners, each of whom is tested over a long period. Such studies reveal that hearing-impaired listeners can provide precise and repeatable data in binaural tasks that are difficult even for normal-hearing listeners. This trend was probably begun when Hawkins and Wightman (1980) studied interaural time discrimination using a constant-stimulus, two-alternative, temporal forced choice (2ATFC) procedure. They tested eight listeners with sensorineural hearing loss and three with normal hearing. Thresholds were estimated by measuring psychometric functions for each condition, and were estimated a number of times at each condition until the data were highly repeatable and no large learning effects were discernible.

There is also an increase in the use of so-called "oddity" procedures that appear to minimize learning, memory, and labeling effects. These procedures appear to have advantages over 2ATFC (sometimes called two-interval, two-alternative forced choice) in some circumstances. In a 2ATFC experiment, the listener must not only discriminate between stimuli but must also recognize and indicate correctly the order of presentation of the stimuli. This additional demand can be avoided if listeners need only indicate which of several intervals (typically three or four) contains the difference of interest. These oddity tasks are also communicated easily both to naive listeners and to listeners with hearing impairments whose auditory perceptions may be very different from those of normal-hearing listeners. It is not unusual to begin testing by providing visual materials indicating that the task is defined by identifying which interval differs from the others. Investigators who wish to retain the formal characteristics of the 2ATFC paradigm may wish to use a 2-cue, two-alternative, temporal forced-choice paradigm (Bernstein and Trahiotis, 1982). This 4-interval procedure utilizes the first and fourth intervals to present the standard (i.e., reference) stimulus and presents the difference to be noted only in either the second or the third interval. This procedure has the virtue of being both an oddity task and mathematically equivalent to the traditional 2ATFC task.

Recently, this procedure was used by Smoski and Trahiotis (1986) in a study of interaural temporal discrimination in listeners with normal hearing, with noise-induced hearing loss, or with hearing loss of viral origin. An important feature of this study is the high degree of consistency of outcomes with those reported earlier by Hawkins and Wightman (1980) in their normal and cochlear-loss subjects. These studies, taken together, indicate that data obtained from hearing-impaired listeners can be highly reliable and repeatable, and that *patterns of results* across frequency for certain types of listeners can be consistently obtained in different laboratories.

Because it is often difficult or impractical to test patients for extended periods, adaptive psychophysical procedures (Levitt, 1971) can be of great benefit. As documented recently by Trahiotis et al (1990), such procedures have been only recently and sparingly applied to studies of binaural hearing that depend on the subjects' use of interaural disparities as cues. This reluctance to use adaptive procedures is an outgrowth of several concerns. One concern is that the listener may not be able to follow changes in the available cue as the independent variable decreases when threshold is approached. For example, in studies of detection utilizing antiphasic (NoSpi) stimuli, large signal-to-noise ratios would foster detectability based on relative power or energy (as in the homophasic [NoSo] case). Then, as the level is decreased following the listener's correct responses, the energy cue becomes unreliable, listeners make errors, and the experimental run may terminate before the listeners discover and use the binaural cues that are available. A related but more general concern is that adaptive procedures may not afford listeners sufficient exposure to near-threshold stimuli, so that they may not learn whatever cues are necessary to reveal their best performance. This would be especially troublesome in some binaural experiments because good performance often depends on the adequate use of small changes in the spatial position, size, and temporal aspects of intracranial images. Even naive normal-hearing listeners often require thousands of trials of practice in fixed conditions in order to learn the subtle, but necessary, cues. (Trahiotis et al [1990] offer a slight modification of the Levitt [1971] procedure that could provide listeners with additional opportunities to gain experience with whatever subjective cues are available while leaving unaltered the statistical aspects of the paradigm.) These concerns notwithstanding, adaptive procedures can be used effectively and efficiently, and Trahiotis et al refer to several successful studies of binaural hearing that used adaptive procedures. That article also includes adaptive MLD data that, happily, indicate great stability over sessions and are, in all respects, consistent with several previous experiments utilizing fixed-increment procedures. Adaptive procedures can also successfully be used in some experiments that require absolute or differential discriminations based on interaural time, interaural intensity, or combinations of both (Trahiotis and Bernstein, 1990). However, adaptive procedures should *never* be used when it is known or suspected that changes in performance are *not* monotonically related to changes in the independent variable.

Recent Empirical Data

Hausler et al (1983) measured performance on a common population of subjects in a number of binaural tasks. Specifically, they measured minimum audible angles and discrimination of interaural time and intensity for a variety of subjects, including 69 with otologic or otoneurologic disease, 32 with neurologic disease (referred to as having central involvement), and 39 in the normal control group. Their angle-discrimination experiments included horizontal angle discrimination at eight reference angles and vertical angle discrimination straight ahead. All the subjects were tested with wide-band noise, and some of them were tested with other stimuli. The authors used an experimenter-controlled, adaptive, 2AFC procedure and showed good correspondence between their normal subjects and previous data. They characterized performance in terms of three aspects of processing that could be separately affected by impairments: interaural time, interaural intensity, and spectral processing. One of the interesting empirical results is that the good performance with a wide-band stimulus did not imply good performance with narrow-band stimuli. It is possible that good performance for a restricted frequency range may be enough to assure good performance for wide-band stimuli. Also, performance as a function of frequency with narrowband stimuli was not predictable from the audiometric data.

Binaural masked detection performance by listeners with impaired hearing has been measured in a number of recent studies (Hall and Fernandes, 1983; Wilson et al, 1985; Hall et al, 1984; Jerger et al, 1984; Hall and Harvey, 1985; Staffel et al, 1990). In general, these studies have measured performance in diotic situations (NoSo) and in dichotic situations allowing a binaural advantage (NoSpi), and have discussed results in terms of MLD. These studies characterize, for cochlear-loss subjects, the dependence of the MLD on several stimulus parameters including masker bandwidth, overall level, interaural level differences, and stimulus frequency. We note that the measured dependence on interaural level difference cannot be separated from the dependence on overall level unless both parameters are varied. Unfortunately, the etiologies of the losses in these subject populations cannot be characterized very precisely, so we do not know how many, if any, of these subjects were affected by acoustic trauma.

Smoski and Trahiotis (1986) provide interaural temporal discrimination data for hearing-impaired listeners, allowing several issues to be addressed. They made measurements at equal sound levels (SLs) and at equal sound pressure levels (SPLs), as did Hawkins and Wightman (1980); they used several types of high-frequency and low-frequency signals (including tones and narrow-band noise at 500 Hz and sinusoidally amplitude-modulated [SAM] tones and narrow-band noise at 4 kHz); and they specified the etiology of their subjects' losses (two diagnosed as noise-induced and two as being of viral origin). When the stimuli were presented at 80 dB SPL to each ear, the hearing-impaired listeners had great difficulty detecting interaural delays with the two high-frequency stimuli. Their thresholds were typically from four to six times larger than those of the normal-hearing listeners and were considerably larger than their own low-frequency thresholds. Interestingly, one subject whose hearing loss was "viral" was totally unable to detect delays with the narrow-band noise stimulus, but could detect as little as 235 μs of interaural delay with SAM tones. When the high-frequency stimuli were presented at 25 dB SL at each ear, that listener discriminated quite well (even better than the normal-hearing listeners) and was now able to detect interaural delays in the narrow-band noise. Another interesting result with the equal-SL stimulus was found with one of the subjects whose loss was noise-induced. This subject, who could detect delays of less than 300 μs with stimuli of equal SPL, was unable to detect delays in either type of high-frequency stimulus when the signals were presented at 25 dB SL. Some of the differences in thresholds between the equal-SL and the equal-SPL conditions could be due to changes in overall level and some may be due to changes in the interaural level per se. In fact, in both cases in which there was a large effect, better performance was obtained with the stimulus at the higher overall level.

Gabriel et al (1990) measured performance in four kinds of experiments for four hearing-impaired subjects. They measured differential discrimination of interaural intensity, differential discrimination of interaural time delays, detection of tonal targets in random noise, and differential discrimination of interaural correlation. Importantly, the binaural abilities of each of four patients were tested as a function of frequency (at octaves from 250 Hz to 4 kHz) in each of the tasks. Based on data collected from normal-hearing listeners and from theoretical formulations, three of the tasks depend, at least in part, on the processing of interaural temporal disparities, and performance across tasks can be compared for consistency. One subject, diagnosed as having multiple sclerosis, could not perform consistently in any task (except for interaural intensity discrimination at 250 and 500 Hz). Another subject, diagnosed as having presbycusis (strial type), showed binaural performance only at 500 Hz for all tasks (except for interaural intensity discrimination at 250 Hz). Two subjects had losses diagnosed as acoustic trauma; both had been pistol shooters and had similar audiograms. Both of these subjects had elevated interaural intensity just-noticeable differences (JNDs), and somewhat elevated NoSo and NoSpi detection thresholds, even though the MLDs were not significantly reduced. One of them had normal interaural time JNDs and slightly elevated interaural correlation JNDs. The other had elevated interaural time JNDs at all frequencies, with very large values at high frequencies, and interaural correlation JNDs that were abnormal at low frequencies, approaching normal values at high frequencies. These results are difficult to interpret with available models of binaural processing and provide clues for improving theories of binaural hearing. In addition, the data may lead to the discovery of underlying general factors or abilities that could successfully characterize the binaural processing abilities of impaired listeners.

Such complexities and difficulties of interpretation should not, in our opinion, lead to pessimism about the quality of data collected from hearing-impaired listeners. Setting aside the fact that relatively few hearing-impaired subjects participate in any typical experiment, one should keep in mind that there can be significant differences between normal-hearing subjects in binaural performance (Koehnke et al, 1986), and that there are low correlations between apparently simple, straightforward tests of monaural hearing in normal-hearing listeners (Seashore, 1919; Karlin, 1942; Elliott et al, 1966; Johnson et al, 1987).

Overall, the data from binaural tests of subjects with noise-induced losses are generally consistent with a disturbance that is limited to the high-frequency regions of the cochlea; however, the data from interaural intensity discrimination (which show abnormal performance at all frequencies) and from interaural correlation discrimination (which show large variability unrelated to the pure-tone audiograms) are not consistent with this simple picture. Also, with regard to the detection data, it is important to consider the threshold signal-to-noise ratios themselves (not only the masking level differences). Recall that the subjects tested by Gabriel et al (1990) had normal MLDs but significantly elevated thresholds.

Another study of the relationships between performances in various binaural tests is under way in Göttingen, although only preliminary results are available at this time (Kinkel et al, 1988). This study includes patients with symmetric and asymmetric sensorineural losses. The binaural tests include MLDs, interaural time and intensity discrimination, and measures of temporal aspects of processing represented in values of time constants.

A survey of binaural performance in impaired listeners is under way at one of our laboratories (Koehnke and Colburn, 1986, 1987; Koehnke et al, 1988, 1989). This survey includes a number of binaural (as well as monaural) tests at 500 Hz and 4 kHz, including the discrimination of interaural differences and binaural detection, and measures the dependence of performance on the interaural reference conditions. This allows us to address the question of whether the effective interaural imbalance in impaired auditory systems affects binaural performance. Results to date indicate that interaural intensity and temporal differences in the reference conditions have relatively small effects on performance, and preliminary conclusions from available data on subjects with asymmetric losses are that level compensation for significant imbalances does not improve performance.

Several of the studies described above indicate that *binaural deficits* can occur even within spectral regions that are considered *audiometrically normal.* This intriguing result may simply indicate that normal listeners performing at their very best utilize a broadly distributed set of nerve fibers. Relatively loud sounds almost certainly stimulate thousands of nerve fibers, many of which reside in portions of the cochlea basal to the region most sensitive to the test frequency. In other words, to the degree that subjects normally use information in the basal turn (i.e., what Kiang and Moxon [1974] would call information in the tails of the high-frequency tuning curves), one would expect that the loss of such neural contribution would result in poorer processing of binaural timing information in the binaural task. This outcome has special import for patients with noise-induced, high-frequency hearing losses defined on the basis of monaural audiograms. These patients are likely to have clinically unnoticed binaural deficits at low frequencies.

Aside from the studies discussed above,

the only other studies (that we are aware of) that included impaired listeners were studies of listeners with conductive losses (Hall and Derlacki, 1986; Magliulo et al, 1990) or essentially monaural studies in which only one ear was usable (Newton, 1983).

Recent Developments That Will Affect Future Studies

At the same time, there have been several developments concerning binaural processing in *normal-hearing* listeners that we believe will have important impact on future studies of hearing-impaired listeners.

Technical Developments

Investigators are now able to use inexpensive computers to generate signals with control over virtually all aspects of binaurally relevant information. For example, one can manipulate separately and in combination interaural delays of the envelope, the carrier, and the phase modulation of complex waveforms (Amenta et al, 1987). Such stimuli could be used in detection, discrimination, and lateralization studies in order to assess how well hearing-impaired listeners utilize interaural information carried by particular features of complex stimuli.

To generate the waveforms of interest, one can multiply two independent low-pass Gaussian random noises by quadrature sinusoids (one sine and one cosine, respectively), and add the product waveforms to obtain narrow-band Gaussian random noise. The envelope and phase modulation of the narrow-band waveform can be computed simply from the two low-pass noises. Specifically, if $N_c(t)$ and $N_s(t)$ are the low-pass noise waveforms, then the envelope A(t) and the phase-modulation phi(t) are given by

$$A(t) = [N_c^2(t) + N_s^2(t)]^{1/2}$$

and

$$\text{phi}(t) = \arctan\,[N_s(t) / N_c(t)]$$

Recently, Hsueh and Hamernik (1990) have shown how one can synthesize random noise waveforms that possess identical (e.g., flat) power spectra and differ in their temporal features. These authors provide algorithms and suggestions for creating and manipulating phase spectra which, in combination with equal-amplitude frequency components, produce several classes of random noise stimuli, including Gaussian and non-Gaussian noises as well as purely impulsive waveforms. This may allow several new lines of inquiry to proceed quickly and inexpensively.

Another type of experiment that has become easy to perform with digitally computed and stored waveforms is masked detection with reproducible noise waveforms (Gilkey et al, 1985; Siegel and Colburn, 1989; Isabelle and Colburn, 1990). Studies of this type allow a "molecular" analysis, and challenge one to explain the dependence of performance on individual waveforms. Results of these studies have allowed detailed evaluations of several models of binaural processing, and may also provide a tool for the study of processing by hearing-impaired listeners.

Empirical Results from Normal-Hearing Subjects

High-Frequency Lateral Position

Several recent studies have reinforced the finding that interaural time differences are discriminable even for waveforms whose spectral content is confined to high-frequency regions of the auditory system. These cues are conveyed via the envelope of the stimulus and, according to the arguments of Colburn and Esquissaud (1976), such temporal information could be essentially equivalent to that provided at lower frequencies by the fine structure of the stimulus. However, it now seems clear that highly detectable interaural delays do not foster appreciable amounts of lateral movement of high-frequency signals (Blauert, 1983; Trahiotis and Bernstein, 1986). Thus, in experiments with normal listeners, there appears to be a divergence between outcomes of "lateralization" experiments utilizing discrimination paradigms and "lateralization" experiments, in which listeners indicate *where* they hear acoustic images.

"Where" listeners hear acoustic images may be measured directly via a rating scale or indirectly via an "acoustic pointer." The latter refers to a procedure by which listeners match the intracranial position of a standard stimulus, the "pointer," to the intracranial position of the stimulus of interest. The rating scale, although a direct estimate of laterality, appears to provide estimates that vary considerably and that can be context-dependent. The acoustic pointer procedure appears to provide rather precise and repeatable data but, of course, only provides a relative measure that must be interpreted carefully across subjects. Bernstein and Trahiotis (1988) (see also Trahiotis and Stern, 1989) discuss how an acoustic pointer can be "calibrated" by having the subjects indicate the position of acoustic images corresponding to various values of the pointer on a representation of a human head.

Discriminability and identification of the external position of sources of sound have been studied with hearing-impaired listeners. However, as pointed out by Durlach et al (1981), both of these types of studies measure resolution of signals occupying differing positions in space and did not assess where the signals were heard. Given the aforementioned ability to generate complex sounds and the vast amounts of new data on extent of laterality of images in normal-hearing listeners, the time seems ripe for studies of *where* sounds are heard by the hearing-impaired. In addition, it will be important and interesting to compare such data with accurate measures of discriminability of binaural cues from the same subjects.

In passing, we note that the acoustic pointing task is known to permit rapid data collection; perhaps adaptive psychophysical procedures will also permit the rapid collection of discrimination data. The efficiency of data collection is an extremely important factor for studies of the hearing-impaired because of the difficulties of scheduling adequate experimental time with such patients.

Spectral Interactions

Although it seems that binaural fusion occurs only for corresponding spectral regions in each ear, it also appears to be true that remote frequency components can interfere with or degrade binaural performance when the critical information is contained only within a narrow spectral portion of a broadband stimulus. Recently, Zurek (1985) and Trahiotis and Bernstein (1990), utilizing normal-hearing listeners, have characterized circumstances under which such interference does and does not occur. As discussed by Trahiotis and Bernstein (1990), the interference is truly binaural and appears to require that the remote frequency components and the target be gated simultaneously.

McFadden and Passanen (1976) were probably the first to show this type of interference when they discovered that the detection of interaural delays of high-frequency complex stimuli were degraded by the presence of a diotic, *low-frequency* band of noise. Interestingly, the converse did not obtain, because the presence of a diotic, high-frequency stimulus did not affect the detection of interaural delays within a low-frequency band of noise. One important question concerning binaural information processing by impaired listeners is the degree to which relatively low-frequency stimuli can interfere with the processing of higher-frequency stimuli. Ironically, such interference, when present, may be even stronger in hearing-impaired listeners who have normal or near-normal low-frequency hearing.

Another interesting phenomenon has been reported by Yost et al (1971) and Yost (1977), who found that normal-hearing listeners detect the presence of interaural delays in nominally high-frequency waveforms by utilizing delays within *low-frequency* information produced by gating the stimuli on and off. These observations and those of Bernstein and Trahiotis (1982) illustrate that great caution must be exercised when attempting to measure binaural performance with high-frequency stimuli. Clearly, normal listeners can utilize interaural disparities within low-level, low-frequency spectral regions even when the energy in such regions is 50 dB or more below the nominal passband of the stimulus! This would be particularly important to preclude when attempting to assess binaural capacities in high-frequency regions for listeners with predominantly high-frequency hearing losses.

Temporal Interactions

Several other recent experiments concerning sensitivity to interaural differences have been conducted. These have focused on the temporal relation between either bursts of noise, which are diotic save for a short segment containing the delay (which could occur at various times within the burst) (Zurek, 1987; Trahiotis and Bernstein, 1990), or transients (pairs or trains of clicks) (Yost, 1976; Hafter et al, 1988; Blauert and Divenyi, 1988). All of these studies illustrate conditions under which sensitivity to interaural delay declines following the first portion of the stimulus.

We believe that these paradigms would be fruitful when used with hearing-impaired listeners, but suggest that interpretation of the data may be somewhat difficult. As Blauert (1983) has clearly discussed, several complex but differentiable phenomena (e.g., summing localization, the law of first wavefront or precedence, and echo suppression) will be factors in such experiments, and it is not clear how pathology will effect these phenomena and their interactions. The interested reader will profit from Blauert's recent discussion (Blauert et al, 1989) of the repeated transient paradigm and its relation to the precedence effect as measured in the sound field.

Theoretical Results

In their model for auditory localization, Searle et al (1976) assumed that the standard deviation of the internal noise increased linearly with the range of angles included within the stimulus set. Although this assumption was consistent with other psychophysical phenomena (e.g., intensity discrimination as modeled by Durlach and Braida, 1969) and the resulting model gave consistent predictions for results from a number of experiments, the assumed dependence could not be verified directly because the data available to Searle et al were gathered from a variety of laboratories using different techniques. The importance of the assumption for the design of experiments and the comparison of results across studies led Koehnke and Durlach (1989) to make direct measurements of this range effect in the identification of interaural time and interaural amplitude differences. Their results demonstrate the validity of the assumption for interaural differences and are completely consistent with a similar range effect in angle identification in a free sound field. This has particular importance for studies of hearing-impaired listeners because studies of angle identification have been and probably will remain a good choice because of the simplicity of the experiment and the direct relation to previous experiences of the subjects. Finally, there are now available models that specify and utilize the shape and location of assumed patterns of neural activity (e.g., Stern and Colburn, 1978; Blauert and Cobben, 1978; Lindemann, 1986; Stern, Zeiberg, and Trahiotis, 1988). These patterns are topographically organized along a two-dimensional surface, and they describe the cross-correlation function of the stimulus as a joint function of the frequency and the delay parameter of the cross-correlation operation. In this fashion, lateralization depends on individual modes of such patterns that are weighted according to their straightness (describing consistency of interaural delay over frequency), centrality (the extent to which interaural delays are small in magnitude), or both. These models have recently been extended to address more complex situations, including precedence, reverberation, and other dynamically changing stimuli.

Effets du Bruit sur l'Audition Binaurale

La dernière décade a vu se multiplier les études psychophysiques sur les handicapés auditifs. Dans leur grande majorité, ces études avaient comme objectif de révéler des déficits ou de découvrir des mécanismes sous-tendant le traitement *monaural* des sons. Un but de ce rapport est de passer en revue les études relativement peu nombreuses qui ont porté sur l'audition binaurale des handicapés auditifs. De plus, nous discuterons de plusieurs avancées récentes, expérimentales, théoriques et pratiques, qui à notre avis stimuleront et aideront à structurer les études futures sur le traitement binaural chez les déficients auditifs. Actuellement, la discussion ne peut pas se focaliser exclusivement, ou même principalement, sur les effets délétères des sur-stimulations acoustiques en elles-mêmes. En effet, la plupart des rapports publiés ne donnent pas les informations nécessaires pour l'isolation du ou des facteur(s) responsable(s) des pertes auditives subies par les sujets.

Malgré le petit nombre d'études sur l'audition binaurale, on peut identifier d'importantes tendances qui sont de bon augure pour l'avenir. L'une est l'usage de tests binauraux multiples, destinés à fournir des données qui permettent de caractériser et délimiter, pour un sujet donné, la nature des déficits sous-jacents. Par exemple, un déficit dans le traitement de l'information temporelle inter-aurale est parfois mesuré (dans des régions spectrales restreintes) avec plusieurs paradigmes: discrimination différentielle de délais inter-auraux, détection de cibles tonales dans du bruit aléatoire, discrimination différentielle de corrélations inter-aurales, etc. . . . Une autre tendance est l'usage de techniques psychophysiques modernes et objectives sur des déficients auditifs bien entraînés et testés chacun sur une longue période. De telles études révèlent que les handicapés auditifs peuvent fournir des données précises et reproductibles dans des tâches binaurales qui sont difficiles même pour des auditeurs normaux. Plusieurs de ces études révèlent que des *déficits binauraux* peuvent être présents même dans des régions spectrales qui seraient ordinairement considérées comme *audiométriquement normales.* Ce résultat a une portée particulière pour les patients chez qui on diagnostique, sur la base d'audiogrammes monauraux, des pertes auditives dans les hautes fréquences et dues au bruit. Il est possible que ces patients aient pour les basses fréquences des déficits binauraux qui passent cliniquement inaperçus.

En même temps, ont été réalisées plusieurs avancées concernant le traitement binaural chez des auditeurs *normaux* et nous pensons que ces avancées auront un impact important sur les études futures sur les handicapés auditifs. Les chercheurs peuvent maintenant utiliser des ordinateurs bon marché pour générer des signaux contrôlés au point de vue de tous les aspects pertinents de l'information binaurale. Par exemple, on peut manipuler séparément et stimultanément les délais inter-auraux de l'enveloppe, du signal porteur, ou de la modulation de phases d'ondes complexes. De plus, on peut exploiter les résultats de plusieurs expériences nouvelles, entre autres, celles qui ont porté sur les interférences d'une région spectrale à l'autre et celles qui ont mesuré les effets de latéralisation produits par diverses caractéristiques des stimulus binauraux. Enfin, sont disponibles maintenant des modèles qui spécifient et utilisent la forme et la position de ce que l'on suppose être des modèles d'activité nerveuse. Ces modèles s'organisent topographiquement sur une surface à deux dimensions et ils décrivent la fonction de corrélation croisée du stimulus comme une fonction conjointe de la fréquence et du paramètre délai de l'opération de corrélation croisée. De cette manière, la latéralisation dépend de modes individuels de tels modèles, modes pondérés d'après leur "rectitude" (cette rectitude représentant le degré de fixité du délai inter-aural quand la fréquence varie) et/ou leur "centralité" (d'autant plus grande que les délais inter-auraux sont petits). Ces modèles ont récemment été élargis afin d'être applicables à des situations plus complexes, entre autres celles où interviennent la réverbération et l'effet d'antériorité, et à d'autres stimulus affectés de changements dynamiques.

ACKNOWLEDGMENTS

This work was supported in part by the following grants from the National Institutes of Health: R01 DC00100 and R01 DC00234.

References

Amenta CA III, Trahiotis C, Bernstein LR, Nuetzel JM. Some physical and psychological effects produced by selective delays of the envelope of narrow bands of noise. Hear Res 1987; 29:147-161.

Bernstein LR, Trahiotis C. Detection of interaural delay in high frequency noise. J Acoust Soc Am 1982; 71:147-152.

Blauert J, Cobben W. Some considerations of binaural cross correlation analysis. Acustica 1978; 39:96-103.

Blauert J. Spatial hearing. Cambridge, MA: MIT Press, 1983.

Blauert J, Divenyi PL. Spectral selectivity in binaural contralateral inhibition. Acustica 1988; 66:267-274.

Blauert J, Canévet G, Voinier T. The precedence effect: No evidence for an "active" release process found. J Acoust Soc Am 1989; 85:2581-2586.

Colburn HS, Esquissaud P. An auditory-nerve model for interaural time discrimination of high-frequency complex stimuli. J Acoust Soc Am 1976; 59(Suppl 1):S23.

Durlach NI, Braida LD. Intensity perception. I. Preliminary theory of intensity resolution. J Acoust Soc Am 1969; 46:372-383.

Durlach NI, Thompson CL, Colburn HS. Binaural interaction in impaired listeners—A review of past research. Audiology 1981; 20:181-211.

Elliott DN, Riach WD, Sheposh JP, Trahiotis C. Discrimination performance of high school sophomores on a battery of auditory tests. Acta Otolaryngol 1966; Suppl 216:1-59.

Gabriel KJ, Koehnke J, Colburn HS. Effects of stimulus frequency on interaural discrimination and binaural detection in listeners with normal and impaired binaural hearing. J Acoust Soc Am

Gilkey RH, Robinson DE, Hanna TE. Effects of masker waveform and signal-to-masker phase relation on diotic and dichotic masking by reproducible noise. J Acoust Soc Am 1985; 78:1207-1219.

Hafter ER, Buell TN, Richards VM. Onset-coding in lateralization: Its form, site, and function. In: Edelman GM, Gall WE, Cowan WM, eds. Auditory function: Neurobiological bases of hearing. New York: Wiley, 1988:647-676.

Hall JW, Derlacki EL. Effect of conductive hearing loss and middle ear surgery on binaural hearing. Ann Otol Rhinol Laryngol 1986; 95:525-530.

Hall JW, Harvey ADG. The binaural masking level difference as a function of frequency, masker level and masking bandwidth in normal-hearing and hearing-impaired listeners. Audiology 1985; 24:25-31.

Hall JW, Fernandes MA. Monaural and binaural intensity discrimination in normal and cochlear-impaired listeners. Audiology 1983; 22:364-371.

Hall JW, Tyler RW, Fernandes MA. Factors influencing the masking level difference in cochlear hearing-impaired and normal-hearing listeners. J Speech Hear Res 1984; 27:145-154.

Hausler R, Colburn HS, Marr E. Sound localization in subjects with impaired hearing. Spatial-discrimination and interaural-discrimination tests. Acta Otolaryngol 1983; Suppl 400:1-62.

Hawkins DB, Wightman FL. Interaural time discrimination ability of listeners with sensorineural hearing loss. Audiology 1980; 19:495-507.

Hsueh KD, Hamernik RP. A generalized approach to random noise synthesis: Theory and computer simulation. J Acoust Soc Am 1990; 87:1207-1217.

Isabelle SK, Colburn HS. Detection of tones in reproducible narrow-band noise. J Acoust Soc Am 1991; 89:352-359.

Jerger J, Brown D, Smith S. Effect of peripheral hearing loss on the masking level difference. Arch Otolaryngol 1984; 110:290-296.

Johnson DM, Watson CS, Jensen JK. Individual differences in auditory capabilities. I. J Acoust Soc Am 1987; 81:427-438.

Karlin JE. A factorial study of auditory function. Psychometrika 1942; 7:251-279.

Kiang NY-S, Moxon EC. Tails of tuning curves of auditory-nerve fibers. J Acoust Soc Am 1974; 55:620-630.

Kinkel M, Holube B, Kollmeier B. Zusammenhang verschiedener parameter binauralen hörens bei schwerhörigen. Forschr Akustik 1988; 629-632.

Koehnke J, Colburn HS. Binaural detection and discrimination: Impaired listeners. J Acoust Soc Am 1986; 79(S1):S22.

Koehnke J, Colburn HS. The dependence of binaural detection and interaural discrimination on interaural time and intensity in normal and impaired listeners. J Acoust Soc Am 1987; 81(S1):527.

Koehnke J, Colburn HS, Durlach NI. Performance in several binaural-interaction experiments. J Acoust Soc Am 1986; 79:1558-1563.

Koehnke J, Colburn HS, Owen GA. Binaural detection and discrimination in listeners with high-frequency sensorineural hearing losses. J Acoust Soc Am 1988; 84(S1):574.

Koehnke J, Colburn HS, Curliss P, Owen GA. Binaural performance in hearing-impaired listeners is not predictable from audiograms. ASHA 1989; 31:69.

Koehnke J, Durlach NI. Range effects in the identification of lateral position. J Acoust Soc Am 1989; 86:1176-1178.

Levitt H. Transformed up-down methods in psychoacoustics. J Acoust Soc Am 1971; 49:467-477.

Lindeman W. Extension of a binaural cross-correlation model by contralateral inhibition. I. Simulation of lateralization for stationary signals. J Acoust Soc Am 1986; 80:1608-1622.

Magliulo G, Gagliardi M, Muscatello M, Natale A. Masking level difference before and after surgery in unilateral otosclerosis. Br J Audiol 1990; 24:117-121.

McFadden D, Pasanen EG. Lateralization at high frequencies based on interaural time differences. J Acoust Soc Am 1976; 59:634-639.

Newton VE. Sound localisation in children with a severe unilateral hearing loss. Audiology 1983; 22:189-198.

Olsen W, Noffsinger D. Masking level differences for cochlear and brain stem lesions. Ann Otol Rhinol Laryngol 1976; 85:820-826.

Olsen WO, Noffsinger D, Carhart R. Masking level differences encountered in clinical populations. Audiology 1976; 15:287-301.

Quaranta A, Cervellera G. Masking level difference in normal and pathological ears. Audiology 1974; 13:428-431.

Searle CL, Braida LD, Davis MF, Colburn HS. Model for auditory localization. J Acoust Soc Am 1976; 60:1164-1175.

Seashore CE. The psychology of musical talent. New York: Silver Burdett, 1919.

Siegel RA, Colburn HS. Binaural processing of noisy stimuli: internal/external noise ratios for diotic and dichotic stimuli. J Acoust Soc Am 1989; 86:2122-2128.

Smoski WJ, Trahiotis C. Discrimination of interaural temporal disparities by normal-hearing listeners and listeners with high-frequency, sensorineural hearing loss. J Acoust Soc Am 1986; 79:1541-1547.

Staffel JG, Hall JW, Grose JH, Pillsbury HC. NoSo and NoSpi detection as a function of masker bandwidth in normal-hearing and cochlear-impaired listeners. J Acoust Soc Am 1990; 87:1720-1727.

Stern RM, Zeilberg AS, Trahiotis C. Lateralization of complex binaural stimuli: A weighted-image model. J Acoust Soc Am 1988; 84:156-165.

Stern RM, Colburn HS. Theory of binaural interaction based on auditory-nerve data. IV. A model for subjective lateral position. J Acoust Soc Am 1978; 64:127-140.

Trahiotis C, Stern RM. Lateralization of bands of noise: Effects of bandwidth and differences of interaural time and phase. J Acoust Soc Am 1989; 86:1285-1293.

Trahiotis C, Bernstein LR. Lateralization of bands of noise and sinusoidally amplitude-modulated tones: Effects of spectral locus and bandwidth. J Acoust Soc Am 1986; 79:1950-1957.

Trahiotis C, Bernstein LR. Detectability of interaural delays over select spectral regions: Effects of flanking noise. J Acoust Soc Am 1990; 87:810-813.

Trahiotis C, Bernstein LR, Buell TN, Spektor Z. On the use of adaptive procedures in binaural experiments. J Acoust Soc Am 1990; 87:1359-1361.

Wilson RH, Civitello BA, Margolis RH. Influence of interaural level differences on the speech recognition masking level difference. Audiology 1985; 24:15-24.

Yost WA, Wightman FL, Green DM. Lateralization of filtered clicks. J Acoust Soc Am 1971; 50:1526-1530.

Yost WA. Lateralization of repeated filtered transients. J Acoust Soc Am 1976; 60:178-181.

Yost WA. Lateralization of pulsed sinusoids based on interaural onset, ongoing, and offset temporal differences. J Acoust Soc Am 1977; 61:190-194.

Zurek PM. Spectral dominance in sensitivity to interaural delay for broadband stimuli. J Acoust Soc Am 1985:78(Suppl 1):S18.

Zurek PM. The precedence effect. In: Yost WA, Gourevitch G, eds. Directional hearing. New York: Springer-Verlag, 1987:85-106.

CHAPTER 27

Cognitive Factors and Selection of Auditory Listening Bands

ERVIN R. HAFTER
ROBERT S. SCHLAUCH

Basic to all work that addresses hearing impairment, including the evaluation of loss, the development of theory, the fitting of prostheses, and the training of new listening habits, is an understanding of the factors that affect the accuracy of perception. When psychoacousticians think of measurement, it is generally in a framework of the rigorous methods of traditional psychophysics. That is not unreasonable for the narrowly defined problems found in the research lab where, for example, such measures as the detectability of single tones in noise have been used to describe filtering properties of the cochlea. However, in the world of everyday listening, the variety of possible signals is almost boundless and competing sounds or maskers can interfere with detection in many complex ways. In these cases, detection may well be affected by factors other than the basic sensory abilities of the listener, factors that can be thought of as cognitive. Among these are signal expectations and the ability to concentrate on specific aspects of a signal, skills in listening and language processing, and the integration of multidimensional information such as visual and auditory. The present paper takes the position that a limitation on the attentional resources employed by the listener can affect all of these abilities and says that we should be aware of these considerations when planning study of or help for the impaired.

Criterion Problem

One might easily argue that the advent of modern psychophysics and perception began with the introduction of the Signal-Detection Theory, often called the Theory of Signal Detectability (TSD) (Green and Swets, 1966). The advantage of TSD is that it gives the psychologist a tool for dealing with subjective factors in detection by viewing the perceiver as a decision maker. The model describes the factors that affect performance with two independent indices. The index of detection, d', quantifies the relation between physical properties of the stimulus and sensory system that determine the sensory "threshold." The index β quantifies the listener's response criterion or willingness to say "yes" to a particular stimulus. β is a function of subjective estimates of the signal probabilities and the costs and values associated with various response contingencies. TSD assumes that d' is a pure measure of signal detectability, leaving factors under control of the listener to be included in β. However, in our laboratory we have found that d' itself can be affected by application of psychological treatments intended to manipulate the subject's attention. If this can be found in a simple psychoacoustical experiment, it suggests that there might be even greater effects in more natural settings such as those faced by an impaired child trying to cope with a busy classroom.

Auditory Attention

Most sounds that we encounter in everyday life are complex, because they are made up of multiple values along one or more acoustic dimensions; there is good reason to believe that discriminable values along those dimensions are represented by separate channels within the auditory nervous system. We commonly think of different frequencies stimulating different cochlear filters (e.g., Greenwood, 1961), although other complex parameters such as amplitude modulation (e.g., Schreiner and Urbus, 1988) and interaural differences (e.g., Yin and Kuwada, 1984) also produce differential activity in separate neural channels. Normal listening thus requires that the listener monitor and integrate multiple channels, a problem further complicated by the need to deal with auditory perception at the same time as demands from the other senses and from ongoing thought processes. In order to understand the constraints in such an environment, psychologists have found it useful to postulate a role for attention, seen as a process whereby the observer applies differential weights to competing perceptual/cognitive tasks (Deutch and Deutch, 1963). In practical terms, attention should allow the listener to concentrate on channels carrying more important features of the environment while rejecting the background or clutter in others (Treisman, 1969). As such, it is akin to processing information through a bandpass filter (Broadbent, 1958). The notion of selective attention has been applied at every level from simple stimulus segregation to higher-order activities such as language perception and comprehension (Norman, 1969). In this paper, however, we will concentrate on the familiar auditory dimensions, frequency, and time. Also, we will not speak separately of the generalized attentional state and the effects of arousal (Kahneman, 1973). Rather, we will assume that all attention is selective, although at times, the competition for it is between observable processes and those that are hidden, which can only be inferred. We will come back to this point later.

A response-criterion view of attention says that quite different values of β in "attended" and "unattended" channels can produce what would seem like differential levels of detection if they were to be considered in a non-TSD framework. This problem is of little concern in the psychoacoustics laboratory, where the effects of sensitivity and response bias can be separated, but it may be important in the clinic, where more rigorous signal detection methods are less accessible and where classes of patients, such as the elderly, may routinely adopt extreme response biases (Rees and Botwinick, 1971; Potash and Jones, 1977). The present discussion will be directed more toward the impact of attention on detectability, and we will argue that attention can, indeed, affect performance, a result with practical implications for the design of hearing aids.

Attention and Stimulus Uncertainty

Kahneman (1973) proposed the idea of attention as a kind of mental effort, both necessary for perceptual processing and limited in quantity. From this view, it follows that when information is presented in multiple channels, the limited attentional capacity of the observer may not allow for optimal processing. Norman and Bobrow (1975) further suggested that the role of attention depends on the nature of the task, with performance being either "data-limited," that is, depending solely on the quality of the data, e.g., the signal-to-noise ratio (S/N), or "resource-limited," that is, improvable by dedication of a greater amount of the attentional resource.

An often given example of a data-limited task is the detection of a weak signal in noise (Norman and Bobrow, 1975). The idea is that for situations in which detectability is determined by an external noise filtered through a fixed sensory filter, the application of extra attention to the task does not improve performance. The belief that masking paradigms are reasonably immune from effects of attention is bolstered by the high reliability of classical data. Indeed, it is the consistency of these results that has allowed theorists to attribute the masking of tones in wideband noise to the amount of that noise falling within fixed auditory filters or "critical bands." However, we have found conditions in which the detectability (d') of a tonal signal in noise is affected by psychological treatments designed to modify attention (Hafter and Kaplan, 1976). Listeners were asked to detect a tone whose frequency changed at random on every trial, a condition of high uncertainty. Under some conditions, the frequency uncertainty was reduced or eliminated by a clearly audible tonal cue presented prior to each trial. The payoff schemes employed to introduce attentional effects ranged from a low-risk condition, in which subjects were paid an hourly wage, to a high-risk condition, in which pay was earned for detections of signals, but a false alarm on one of a few unmarked noise trials meant complete loss. The results showed that when there was no signal uncertainty, payoff had little effect, consistent with the idea of a data-limitation set by the S/N in the various critical bands. In pay-by-the-hour conditions, frequency uncertainty produced a rise in threshold of about 3 dB relative to the condition of minimum uncertainty; this is a common outcome (Green, 1961). The most interesting result appeared in the payoff-by-uncertainty interaction, where the presumably greater attention paid under high risk reduced by half the increase in threshold due to uncertainty.

From the point of view that *fixed* auditory filters determine detectability, the optimal solution under frequency uncertainty is for the listener to monitor all of the potential filters and apply an appropriate decision rule to their combined outputs (Green, 1961). However, Hafter and Kaplan (1976) suggested that the bandwidths used under uncertainty might be *labile*. They argued that only a limited *number* of auditory bands could be monitored in parallel without depleting attentional capacity and reducing the ability to process other ongoing cognitive functions. Thus, the response to high uncertainty about frequency was to diminish the load on attention by pooling the outputs of neighboring filters, even though the use of wider *effective* bands meant lower performance. From their point of view, the reduction of the uncertainty effect reflected the fact that subjects under high risk chose to sacrifice other cognitive functions in order to spend more of a limited attentional resource on processing a larger number of consequently narrower bands. The model is merely speculative, but the important fact remains that increased attention affected performance only under high uncertainty.

Uncertainty, Cueing, and Bandwidth

In order to look more closely at the conclusions of Hafter and Kaplan (1976), we have recently examined several conditions designed to obtain more accurate quantification of the role of attention in masking and to see if uncertainty would lead to wider effective bandwidths (Schlauch and Hafter, 1988). We looked only at frequency uncertainty, although it seems likely that similar constraints might apply if other features of the signal such as envelope timing or spatial location were studied.

In these tasks, the frequency of a brief tonal signal was varied from trial to trial over a range of about 3 octaves. In most cases, each forced-choice trial was preceded by a cue picked to inform the listener about the signal. The exception was the condition of *maximum uncertainty*, which had no cues. In the condition chosen to represent *no uncertainty*, the cues were suprathreshold versions of the signals; because these were images of the signal in the domain of uncertainty, we call them *"iconic"* cues. With a fixed stimulus level (different for each frequency) we obtained 65 percent correct performance under maximum uncertainty and 90 percent correct performance with iconic cues. If converted to thresholds, this represents a loss due to uncertainty of about 5 dB.

To study the bandwidths actually used under uncertainty, one must satisfy two constraints: (1) it is necessary to specify explicitly the number of channels or bands to be monitored; and (2) the bandwidths must be measured directly. Traditionally, the first problem has been solved either by restricting the number of possible signals to a small number whose frequencies are taught through repetition, or by allowing the signal to have many possible values and inferring the number from assumptions based on TSD (Green, 1961). A problem with the former is that there is no way to quantify the amount of experienced-based cueing over the course of an experiment, while the latter requires assumptions about bandwidth, which is the factor being studied. Our solution was to restrict the number of signal possibilities but to vary the actual bands to be monitored from trial to trial. Depending on the condition being tested, each cue consisted of either one, two, or four randomly chosen frequencies, only one of which matched the frequency of the signal. Thus, conditions had an uncertainty of "1", "2", or "4."

For direct measurement of the bandwidths, we used a modified version of the probe-frequency measure of Greenberg and Larkin (1968). They told subjects to listen for a specific *target* frequency that was presented on most trials and then, on occasional *probe* trials, changed the signal to a frequency that differed from the target by one of several fixed amounts. They assumed that subjects listened for signals through a single auditory filter at the frequency of the target and responded to probes only to the extent that the probe fell within the skirts of the monitored filter. Scharf et al (1987) have since shown that the basic results do not change if the subject is told in advance about the probes. In order to be able to change the target frequency on every trial, we modified the way in which probes were selected, setting them to fixed *frequency-ratios* relative to the targets rather than fixed frequency-distances. Then, based on the assumption that the bandwidths of the auditory filters are a fixed proportion of their center

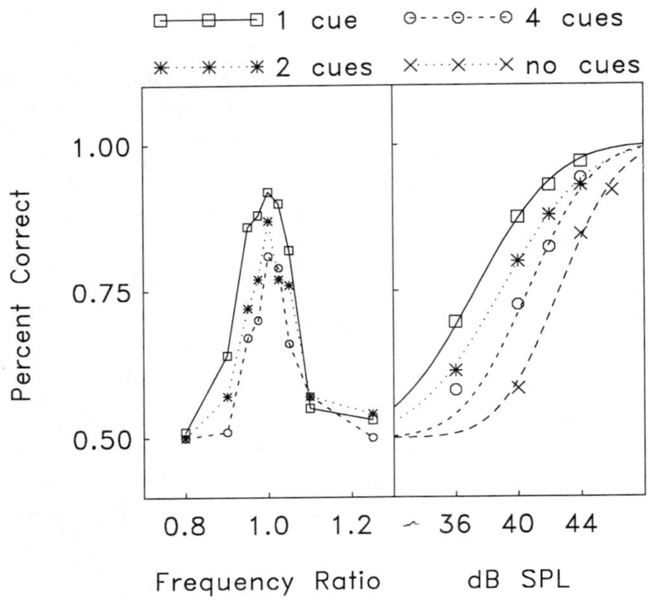

Figure 27-1 *A,* Percent correct performance by one subject, obtained with the modified probe-signal method. The level of frequency uncertainty (1, 2, or 4) was determined by cues. *B,* Psychometric functions for target (correctly cued) signals in each condition of uncertainty as well the condition of complete uncertainty (no cues) from the same subject as in *A.*

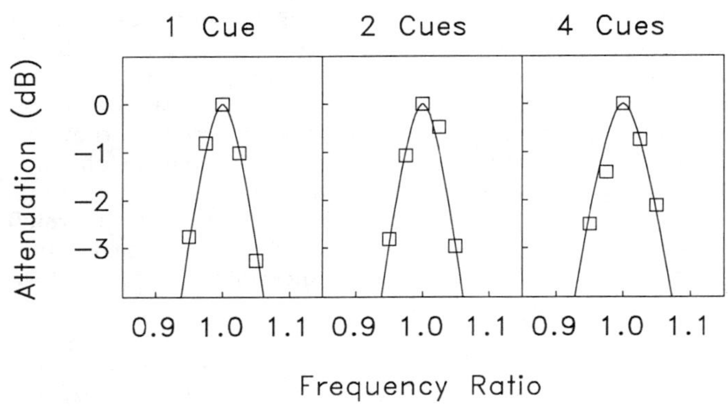

Figure 27-2 Conversions of percent correct to decibels using results of the kind illustrated in Figure 27-1. All points are normalized to performance with the target frequencies. The data are averages across three subjects. The curves are fits from the Patterson et al (1982) model of auditory filters.

frequencies (Moore and Glasberg, 1983), we collapsed data across the entire range of uncertainty, averaging the responses over all probes with the same ratio. Probes were used whether the targets were marked exactly, as in the 1-cue conditions, or marked with uncertainty, as with the 2- or 4-tone cues.

An example of data from one subject in Schlauch and Hafter (1988) is shown in Figure 27-1*A*. Note that best performance for all three conditions of uncertainty (1, 2, or 4 cues) was obtained when the cue matched the signal precisely (probe/target = 1.0), with performance falling off to chance as the match became worse. Clearly, the listener used specific filters, even when required to monitor multiple bands. Because filters are not measured in units of percent correct, we followed the lead of Greenberg (1969) and obtained psychometric functions for the target frequencies in the three conditions of uncertainty. These functions, shown in Figure 27-1*B*, were used to convert the data from Figure 27-1*A* to decibels. Data so converted and normalized to performance with the target are shown in Figure 27-2. In this case, the figure shows averaged results from three subjects. The solid lines represent a fit to the points using the rounded exponential model of the auditory filter proposed by Patterson et al. (1982). Two things are clear. First, the bandwidth of the fit to the 1-cue condition agrees well with an average of Moore and Glasberg's (1983) data across this frequency range, showing that the measurement of bandwidths with trial-by-trial varying signals was successful. Second, as predicted by Hafter and Kaplan (1976), the filters grew wider in response to uncertainty, with the bandwidth for 4-frequency uncertainty being 19 percent wider than that with none, an effect of about .75 dB.

At What Level of Processing is Attention Selected?

When thinking about how results of this kind might relate to realistic problems faced by the hearing impaired, it is important to know how cueing works. How does the listener select the appropriate band or bands to be monitored; what kinds of cues exist in everyday listening; can listeners be trained to use cues for more accurate listening? Without going into detail, we will present further tests of cued detection that address these questions (Hafter and Schlauch, 1989), including results that show that cues need not be a replica of the signal to successfully direct attention. This raises interesting questions about higher-order, more cognitive direction of auditory attention. Collaborators in this work have been Joyce Tang and Lyne Plamondon.

Relative Auditory Cues

First, in a study designed to see if cueing could be invoked with other than an icon of the signal, we presented *relative* cues that differed from the targets to be detected by a fixed (and familiar) ratio, the musical 5th. Again, probe frequencies were used to estimate bandwidths. Not surprisingly, there was a strong learning effect, with initial bandwidths at the 5th being wider than those found with iconic cues. However, performance improved to the point of being nearly as good with the relative cues as with the iconic cues. This showed that stimulation of the filter to be monitored was not necessary.

In a second experiment with non-iconic cues, listeners were asked to use matching *pitches* as cues to the appropriate filters. Cues consisted of harmonic series without the fundamental, while the signal to be detected was the missing fundamental. To discourage relative cueing by the nearest harmonic, the series were varied at random, with half containing harmonic numbers 2 through 6 and half, numbers 3 through 7. Performance with these pitch cues was reduced by 10 percent relative to that with iconic cues, which is still considerably better than with no cue at all. Thus, a shared fundamental pitch was able to guide the listener's attention to the appropriate channel, albeit with some loss.

Visual Cues

Finally, we employed visual cues to direct attention to the appropriate listening bands. Subjects were all chosen on the basis of possessing *absolute pitch,* and the idea was to direct them to the appropriate filters to be monitored by way of auditory memory. The set of signals consisted of sinusoids spaced at semitone intervals ranging from 220 Hz to 1760 Hz. Cueing was done via a visual display that told what the signal would be either by printed text, e.g., "Middle D#," or by musical notation. In the latter case, subjects detected tones as well with the visual cues as with the iconic cues. Thus, higher-order processes used visual information to focus auditory attention.

Attention and Speech

It is interesting to consider some plausible applications of these studies of uncertainty and attention to understanding and dealing with problems of speech in noise. We will discuss two such examples. One concerns the use of place of articulation cues for selection of auditory filters. The second discusses how one should test computerized signal-processing techniques designed to improve speech intelligibility.

Normalization of Vowel Space with Auditory and Visual Cues

Idiosyncratic differences in phoneme production arise from differences in dialect and differences in vocal-tract size. Thus, the formant frequencies for the vowel /a/ of an adult male from San Francisco may differ considerably from those of a child from London. Speaker normalization refers to the listener's correction for these differences. Simple schemes based on ratios or absolute values of formant frequencies have been shown to leave considerable overlap among phonemes.

The point vowels (/i/, /a/, /u/) representing extreme positions in articulation carry information about the vocal tract of a talker. Joos (1948) argued that listeners extract the point vowels from a sample of speech in order to define a talker's vowel space and then use this kind of normalization to help with prediction and analysis of the intermediate vowels. In a sense, one can argue that the listener, so defined, is using relative cues to establish a scheme for detection. In support of Joos' notion is a report from Ladefoged and Broadbent (1959), who found that identification of a vowel depended on both its formant frequencies and the formant frequencies in other vowels pronounced by that same speaker.

It is well known that visual information can make substantial contributions to speech recognition, particularly in hearing-impaired listeners or in noisy backgrounds. For example, Sumby and Pollack (1954) found that observing the face of a talker in white noise was equivalent to increasing S/N by 15 dB. We would like to propose an extension of Joos' (1948) hypothesis that states that listeners may use visual as well as auditory cues to define a speaker's vocal tract. Although studies of phoneme perception in the quiet have led Massaro (1987) to conclude that auditory and visual information in speech are processed independently, our studies of tone detection in noise demonstrate that under some conditions, visual cues can direct attention to the appropriate auditory filters. Hence, it is an unsettled issue whether visual cues can aid in normalization of vowel space and thus improve the auditory processing of speech.

We plan to examine the hypothesis that visual cues can direct auditory attention by measuring the masking patterns for vowels presented with and without visual cues and with special attention paid to performance with new talkers. For conditions of low uncertainty such as with normal listeners in favorable S/N ratios, the practical influence of the visual cues should be minimal. However, in hearing impairment and in noisy backgrounds, the visually obtained knowledge about the locations of formant peaks may make a substantial contribution to discrimination.

Appropriate Testing of Signal-Processing Hearing Aids

It seems certain that the next generation of hearing aids will contain computers that allow for advanced signal processing, just as simple compression aids have already moved toward amelioration of recruitment (Moore and Glasberg, 1988). The primary obstacle still faced by the impaired listeners is that of communication in a noisy environment, and solving that problem will be the goal of a majority of the effort spent on signal processing. Solutions proposed to improve the speech-to-noise ratio range from programs that use speech-like features to identify and enhance the "signal" to programs that mimic features of binaural hearing, using combinations of the inputs from multiple acoustic arrays to cancel the masker. Interestingly, the reports from comparative tests of such schemes are often mixed, with subjects preferring one device over another because the processed speech sounds "clearer" or "easier to listen to," but the speech recognition performance (SRP) showing no difference. Obviously, this is disappointing, implying that the signal processing has not fulfilled the primary goal of improving communication. A common interpretation of this result is that in enhancing some aspects of the speech signal, the processing destroys others.

We will consider a different interpretation of the contradiction implied by "sounds better" with no improvement in SRP. The idea is that selective attention interacts with the use of aided speech in such a way that the results described above may reflect properties of the testing situation more than of the device itself. Imagine tests of a hypothetical speech-processing machine that we will call the "LAP" computer to indicate that it works "like a person." The machine understands vowels and formant frequencies and has clever algorithms that allow it to track sets of harmonics while cancelling the background (a similar technique has been tested by Levitt, 1989.) Further suppose that the LAP fails in the ways described above, creating better sounding speech without improving reception. In considering these results, first note that a mechanical speech processor is an add-on device, intended to help the brain turn auditory information into a representation of speech. Because the LAP algorithm was built to be redundant with processes that the listener can do himself, one might argue that it provides no new information. This would explain why there is no improvement in the SRP but not why the listeners prefer the processed speech. Here we recall a statement made earlier about hidden but active demands on attention. Suppose that doing the same thing as the LAP computer places high demands on attentional resources of the listener. Kahneman (1973) has shown that paying attention is work, requiring mental effort that must come from a limited store. In the typical laboratory setting, where unwanted stimulation is specifically reduced, there are few extraneous demands on attention. There, subjects prefer the computer-processed speech because it demands less attention and thus makes processing easier. But, because the device does nothing that they could not do on their own by supplying full attention, it does not improve performance.

The key words here are "laboratory setting." Suppose instead that testing had taken place in a high-demand environment such as noisy classroom where hearing-impaired children must attend to both the auditory and visual portions of a film or a university lecture where a student tries to process speech and simultaneously understand its content. In natural settings where attention is resource-limited, the information supplied by the LAP computer may no longer be redundant with processes that the listener can do for himself and the device may be of great value. Because these are the very conditions where aided speech processing is most needed, we believe that signal-processing schemes designed for hearing aids should always be tested or compared in situations where there are high levels of competition for attention. Only then can one hope to discover the true value of these algorithms.

Conclusion

Under conditions of stimulus uncertainty, selective attention can be directed to specific stimulus features, thus affecting the detectability of signals in noise. Knowledge of the role of auditory and visual cueing may enhance our understanding of the problems faced by impaired listeners confronted with speech in noise. Finally, the proper evaluation of speech-processing computers designed for hearing-impaired persons requires testing in situations where demands on the attentional capacity of the listener are high.

Facteurs Cognitifs et Sélection Auditive de Bandes de Fréquence

Une compréhension complète des effets des déficits auditifs sur l'écoute quotidienne nécessite une connaissance du rôle de l'attention sélective et d'autres facteurs cognitifs dans la perception des signaux complexes. La Théorie de la Détection du Signal a modifié notre conceptualisation de la détection en distinguant nettement entre éléments du stimulus qui déterminent la détectabilité et les facteurs de réponse qui affectent les décisions. Des fonctions ROC (Receiver Operating Characteristics) furent établies pour montrer que la détectabilité peut rester constante alors même que "l'auditeur idéal" répond de façons très diverses selon les probabilités a priori d'apparition du signal et les coûts relatifs des omissions et fausses alertes; ces observations ont largement convaincu qu'il est une mesure stable de la détectabilité et que les facteurs subjectifs affectent seulement les critères de réponse. Dans le présent rapport, nous proposons que des processus d'ordre supérieur, plus cognitifs, peuvent altérer la détection elle-même. Ceci est spécialement important pour ce qui concerne les sons complexes et peut affecter nos méthodes d'évaluation des données dans les laboratoires où s'élabore la théorie de l'audition, en clinique où il s'agit de déterminer les déficits, et dans la mise au point de prothèses et de programmes d'entraînement pour la récupération de capacités auditives. Nous mettons l'accent ici sur la détermination attentionnelle des positions et les largeurs des bandes fréquentielles d'écoute. Ce faisant, nous distinguons les filtres auditifs fixes qui résultent de la physiologie cochléaire et des bandes d'écoute plus labiles qui peuvent varier avec l'incertitude fréquentielle et d'autres sollicitations de l'attention.

L'hypothèse de l'existence de filtres variables est étayée par des expériences de masque dans lesquelles le sujet a une incertitude sur les fréquences du signal ou du masqueur. Nous avons utilisé des indices variés pour lever l'incertitude, entre autres des sons complexes de même hauteur tonale que le signal et des indices visuels destinés à influencer la sélection de la bande d'écoute en activant la mémoire auditive. Une situation dans laquelle l'attention sélective peut jouer un rôle majeur est la mise à l'épreuve et l'usage subséquent de prothèses auditives destinées à améliorer la perception de la parole dans le bruit. Souvent, lorsque diverses prothèses sont comparées, leurs capacités à augmenter l'intelligibilité s'avèrent égales ou presqu'égales alors que les sujets font état de grandes différences dans la clarté subjective de la parole. Nous pensons que pour être valide, la procédure de test doit inclure des conditions dans lesquelles le sujet est en situation de compétition attentionnelle; si tel n'est pas le cas, l'auditeur peut simplement faire le travail de la prothèse à traitement du signal, rendant ainsi l'instrument superflu. Le test doit également se faire dans des environnements plus naturels, tels que ceux auquels est confronté l'enfant dans une salle de classe active; c'est dans de tels environnements que les bénéfices de la prothèse peuvent être manifestes.

References

Broadbent DE. Perception and communication. London: Pergamon Press, 1958.

Deutch JA, Deutch D. Attention: Some theoretical considerations. Psych Rev 1963; 70:80-90.

Green DM. Detection of sinusoids of uncertain frequency. J Acoust Soc Am 1961; 33:897-903.

Green DM, Swets JA. Signal detection theory and psychophysics. New York: John Wiley & Sons, 1966.

Greenberg GZ. Frequency-selective detection of three signal amplitudes. Perception and Psychophysics 1969; 6:297-301.

Greenberg GZ, Larkin WD. Frequency-response characteristic of auditory observers detecting signals of a single frequency in noise: The probe signal method. J Acoust Soc Am 1968; 44:1513-1523.

Greenwood DD. Critical bandwidth and the frequency coordinates of the basilar membrane. J Acoust Soc Am 1961; 33:1344-1356.

Hafter E, Kaplan R. Unpublished report on attention and flying prepared for NASA Ames Research Center, 1976.

Hafter ER, Schlauch RS. Factors in detection under uncertainty. J Acoust Soc Am 1989; 86:S112.

Joos M. Acoustic phonetics. Language 1948:suppl. 24.

Kahneman D. Attention and effort. Englewood Cliffs, NJ: Prentice-Hall Inc., 1973.

Ladefoged P, Broadbent DE. Information conveyed by vowels. J Acoust Soc Am 1959; 29:98-104.

Levitt H. Personal communication, 1990.

Massaro DW. Speech perception by ear and eye. Hillsdale, NJ: Lawrence Erlbaum, 1987.

Moore BCJ, Glasberg BR. Suggested formulae for calculating auditory filter bandwidths and excitation patterns. J Acoust Soc Am 1983; 74:750-753.

Moore BCJ, Glasberg BR. A comparison of four methods of implementing automatic gain control (AGC) in hearing aids. Br J Audiol 1988; 22:93-104.

Norman DA. Memory and attention. London: John Wiley & Sons, 1969.

Norman DA, Bobrow DG. On data-limited and resource-limited processes. Cogitive Psych 1975; 7:44-64.

Patterson RD, Nimmo-Smith I, Weber DL, Milroy R. The deterioration of hearing with age: Frequency selectivity, the critical ratio, the audiogram, and speech threshold. J Acoust Soc Am 1982; 72:1788-1803.

Potash M, Jones B. Aging and decision criteria for detection of tones in noise. J Gerontol 1977; 32:436-440.

Rees JN, Botwinick J. Detection and decision factors in auditory behavior in the elderly. J Gerontol 1971; 26:33-36.

Schreiner CE, Urbus JV. Representation of amplitude modulation in the auditory cortex of the cat. II. Comparison between cortical fields. Hear Res 1988; 32:49-64.

Scharf B, Quigley S, Aoki C, et al. Focused auditory attention and frequency selectivity. Perception and Psychophysics 1987; 42:215-223.

Schlauch RS, Hafter ER. Attentional filters and frequency uncertainty in the detection of one or more tones. J Acoust Soc Am 1988; 84:S142.

Sumby WH, Pollack I. Visual contribution to speech intelligibility in noise. J Acoust Soc Am 1954; 26:212-215.

Treisman AM. Strategies and models of selective attention. Psych Rev 1969; 76:282-299.

Yin TC, Kuwada S, Sujaku Y. Interaural time sensitivity of the high-frequency neurons in the inferior colliculus. J Acoust Soc Am 1984; 76:1401-1410.

SECTION FIVE

Parameters of Exposure

CHAPTER 28

Damage Risk for Low-Frequency Impulse Noise: The Spectral Factor in Noise-Induced Hearing Loss

GUIDO F. SMOORENBURG

Ten years ago I presented a paper on the damage-risk criterion for impulse noise at a meeting in this series of symposia (Smoorenburg, 1980, 1982). After this presentation, Henning von Gierke stated that impulse-noise standards were being established primarily on the basis of the effects of small-caliber rifle noise whereas, at that time, most of the armies of the world were having problems in defining the hazards associated with artillery noise exposure. He continued that there was reason to believe that the effect of exposure to artillery noise presented a different type of hazard, and subsequently he asked whether or not my damage-risk criterion could be applied to artillery noise. At that time I had to agree with von Gierke that this was a serious point. My proposal for an impulse-noise criterion, based on virtually all data available at that time, did not include the effects of large-caliber weapons. Those data were scarce.

In principle, the proposed damage-risk criterion for impulse noise could have been applied to large-caliber weapons. It presented the maximum peak pressure level that was permitted in view of a certain accepted, small risk of hearing loss as a function of the total duration of the impulses. The total duration was defined as the product of the duration of a single impulse, the D-duration, and the total number of impulses, N, contained in the noise exposure. Exposures to artillery noise with D-durations in the range of 2 to 12 ms and N in the range of 1 to 10, or at most 100, fell well within the range of total durations covered by the damage-risk criterion. However, the range of total durations required to analyze the trade-off between peak pressure level and total duration given in the damage-risk criterion was obtained by combining data sets from (1) small-caliber weapons with D-duration of about 1 ms and N in the range of 1 to 100, (2) small-caliber weapons fired in reverberant environments increasing the D-duration to 70 ms, and (3) industrial impact noises with D-durations in the range of 25 to 85 ms and N exceeding 1,000. The spectral energy distributions of these noises were similar. A-weighting of the noise spectra would have lowered the sound pressure levels of the light-caliber weapons by 1 to 4 dB and those of the industrial impact noises by about the same amounts. The energy spectra of the impulses from large-caliber weapons, however, are characterized by predominantly low-frequency energy. A-weighting would have had a greater effect on these impulses. Because there were insufficient data on the effect of impulses from these large-caliber weapons on hearing, and because the spectral differences between the noises included in my 1980 paper were small, it was, at that time, impossible to evaluate the spectral factor. I had to agree with von Gierke that this question deserved more study.

The need to extend the area of impulse noise research had already been recognized before the 1980 meeting. It was therefore decided to establish an international Research Study Group* on the effects of impulse noise within the framework of the NATO Defense

*Research Study Group 6 on The Effects of Impulse Noise (NATO AC243/Panel 8) consisted of the following members: H.M. Borchgrevink, H. Brinkmann, A. Dancer, M.R. Forrest, S.E. Forshaw, A. Papavasiliou, J.H. Patterson, F. Pfander, Y.Y. Phillips, G.R. Price, and G.F. Smoorenburg (chairman).

Research Group (AC/243, Panel 8/RSG 6). The first meeting of this research study group was held in 1980. As a result of the cooperation within this research study group, the question of the role of low-frequency energy in impulse noise trauma can now be answered in more detail. This chapter primarily addresses this question. Although the analysis presented in this chapter has benefitted substantially from the cooperation within the research study group, I should emphasize that it is solely my responsibility. The conclusions of the research study group were published in a NATO report (1987), which is not classified.

Spectral Factor in Permanent Noise-Induced Hearing Loss Due to Industrial Noise

To solve the question of the spectral weighting function needed to predict noise-induced hearing loss, it is expedient to first consider the dose-effect relations for industrial noise. Data for industrial noise are less scarce than those for impulse noise; moreover, they include permanent, or persistent, threshold shifts (PTSs) in relation to the noise exposure, whereas the data for impulse noise are almost completely restricted to temporary threshold shifts (TTSs) (Smoorenburg, 1982).

The most influential paper of the last decade on the spectral factor in PTS due to industrial noise was published by Robinson (1983). It presented a reanalysis of the Burns and Robinson database (1970), because the first analysis by Burns and Robinson had suggested that B-weighting might yield better predictions. The original database was reduced to a subset containing only stationary noise exposures and sufficient hearing loss to reveal significant effects of spectrum shape. The spectra were divided into classes defined along two dimensions, chosen ad hoc. The first dimension represented spectral slope; the second represented sound level in the mid-frequency range relative to the levels in the low- and high-frequency ranges.

In principle, the question of adequate spectral weighting will be difficult to answer when the shape of the audiogram is related to the spectral energy distribution of the noise. If such a relation exists, the above question cannot be answered without answering the question of how hearing loss should be weighted across the audiometric frequency range. Fortunately, the reanalysis of Robinson showed that there is almost no effect of the spectral distribution of the noise, classified as described above, on the shape of the tone audiogram. Hence, the effects of noises with different spectral distributions could be compared directly, although the analysis could probably be improved by applying principal components and canonic correlation analysis techniques, instead of using the ad hoc classification. The results of Robinson strongly suggest that it is virtually impossible to resolve the optimal spectral weighting function from the industrial PTS data. The data suffered from too much scatter. It was even impossible to choose among either the A-, B- or C-weighting. Because of the lack of counter-evidence, Robinson concluded that his study was "a case for retaining the A-weighting" (Robinson, 1983).

Spectral Factor in Temporary Threshold Shift Due to Exposures to Steady-State Noise

Because Robinson's study (1983) was inconclusive, we now turn to studies on TTS following limited exposures to steady-state, mainly narrow-band noise. These studies are more powerful with respect to the question of the adequate weighting function, because the spectral energy distribution of the noise can be chosen as desired and the exposure is well under control. A disadvantage of TTS studies is, of course, that the relation to PTS is a question in itself.

Although the majority of the TTS studies were carried out decades ago and a discussion of those data would be untimely, there is one aspect of those data, relevant to the theme of this chapter, that received little attention and should be discussed here. The damage-risk contours based on TTS showed an increasing frequency dependence with decreasing exposure duration. This dependence on duration is best illustrated by considering the results of a compilation of TTS studies published by Kryter et al (1966). Figure 28-1 shows the results. The curve for 1.5 minutes or less has considerably steeper skirts than the one for 480 minutes. This effect could be due to the shorter exposure duration, which may have relevance to impulse noise, but it may also be due to the confounding variable, exposure level. Results from Plomp et al (1963), not included in the Kryter et al analysis, shed some light on this question. The curve added in Fig-

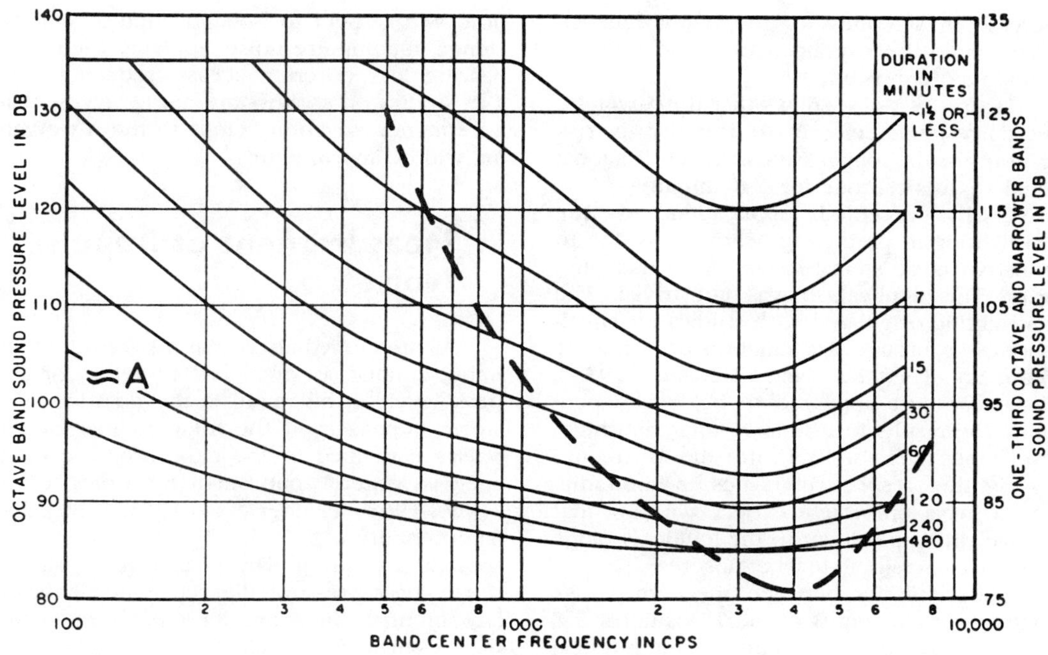

Figure 28-1 Damage-risk contours for steady-state and intermittent noise at different exposure durations. The contours are based on human TTS data. Contours from Kryter KD, Ward DW, Miller JD, Eldredge DH. Hazardous exposure to intermittent and steady-state noise. J Acoust Soc Am 1966; 39:451-464. The broken line indicates a result for a 3-minute human exposure, but a lower TTS criterion. (Adapted from Plomp R, Gravendeel DW, Mimpen AM. Relation of hearing loss to noise spectrum. J Acoust Soc Am 1963; 35:1234-1240.)

ure 28-1 (broken line) shows Plomp et al's result for a 3-minute exposure. The exposure levels are much lower because their criterion was only 5 dB TTS, rather than the 10- to 20-dB figure used in the Kryter et al study. The comparison in Figure 28-1 shows that exposure level by itself does not determine the frequency dependence. Hence, exposure duration may be the principle variable.

The skirts of the curve from Plomp et al, shown in Figure 28-1, are steeper than the contour for 3 minutes from Kryter et al. This difference probably originates with the difference in TTS criterion. The curve of Plomp et al was based on 5 dB TTS at half an octave above stimulus frequency, whereas the contours of Kryter et al were based on maximum TTS at any frequency not exceeding 10 dB up to 1 kHz, 15 dB at 2 kHz, and 20 dB at 3 kHz and above. Although it is frequently stated in the literature that maximum TTS occurs at half an octave above the exposure frequency, this is only valid for a first approximation. The frequency difference tends to be greater at low stimulus frequencies and somewhat smaller at high frequencies (above 3 kHz). Hence, for the low and high stimulus frequencies, measurements at half an octave above the exposure frequency may underestimate maximum TTS. This implies that Plomp et al would have found lower damage-risk levels at these frequencies and, consequently, less-steep skirts, had they used a criterion of 5 dB maximum TTS at any frequency. In addition, the Kryter et al study would have given steeper low-frequency slopes, had the authors used a constant value of TTS across frequency rather than a value increasing with frequency. Together, these two differences may explain the differences in slope.

The dependence of the low-frequency skirt of the damage-risk contours on exposure duration can, at least partly, be explained by the effect of the acoustic middle-ear reflex. The acoustic reflex primarily attenuates the low-frequency components, which will result in an increase of the damage-risk level in this frequency range. The reflex is quickly activated after stimulus onset (within about 30 ms) and relaxes slowly. Although some studies showed that relaxation becomes asymptotic after 2 or 3 minutes, Ward (1962) has found that there is a steady decline of reflex activation for at least 24 minutes. This supports the view that the acoustic reflex contributes to the increase in steepness of the low-frequency skirts of the damage-risk contours in Figure 28-1 at the shorter exposure durations. The increase in steepness of the high-frequency skirts cannot be explained from the acoustic reflex. Its origin is unclear.

Figure 28-1 also shows that the A-weighting corresponds closely to the damage-risk contour for the longer exposures. (It is almost equal to the contour for 240 minutes.) The universally accepted application of the A-weighting in predicting hearing loss due to industrial noise stems, in fact, from this similarity. This application was not trivial. The A-weighting originated with studies on equal-loudness contours as a function of pure-tone frequency (Fletcher and Munson, 1933). These contours appeared to be level-dependent. The results for the low-, mid-, and high-level range were stylized into the A-, B-, and C-weighting, respectively. Thus, in contradiction to what one might expect, we note that the weighting pertinent to the low-level range serves to assess high-level exposures.

The similarity between the damage-risk contours originating with the TTS studies and the A-weighting may point to the physical quantity responsible for hearing damage. The A-weighting is the standardized curve closest to the threshold-of-hearing curve. The low-frequency skirt of this curve is, in fact, somewhat steeper than the A-weighting, which means that a damage-risk contour based on a constant TTS criterion, rather than the frequency-dependent criterion used by Kryter et al, would have been even closer to the threshold-of-hearing curve. The threshold-of-hearing curve represents, as a first approximation, a constant basilar membrane amplitude at the place of resonance as a function of frequency. The B- and C-weightings are flatter, which may be a result of signal processing by the sensorineural system—for example, the result of saturation effects. Thus, risk of a noise lesion (or rather TTS) at some place in the cochlea may be closely related to the magnitude of stimulus-induced basilar membrane movement. This also holds for the shorter exposures, assuming that it is the acoustic middle-ear reflex that alters the frequency dependence of the damage-risk contours (at least up to 3 kHz). The relation between risk of TTS and basilar membrane amplitude suggests that mechanical impact actually causes TTS. This conclusion, however, should be drawn with caution in view of the finding, mentioned earlier, that the site of maximum TTS does not have a fixed relation to exposure frequency. This discrepancy requires further study.

Because the onset time of activation of the acoustic reflex at high intensities is about 30 ms, the reflex will have no protective function with respect to isolated impulse sounds. Hence, for impulse noise, applying a uniform hearing loss criterion across frequency, the TTS studies on steady-state noise suggest that a frequency weighting close to the A-weighting will be appropriate.

Measurement of Impulse Noise

As mentioned already in the introduction, impulse noise is measured in terms of the peak level of the impulse, the duration of a single impulse, and the total number of impulses contained in the exposure. The damage-risk criteria published by Coles et al (1967, 1968), Pfander et al (1975, 1980), and Smoorenburg (1980, 1982) do not include a spectral weighting. The peak level is simply the highest pressure difference occurring at any moment in time. Its measurement requires small acoustoelectric transducers and fast recording apparatus (for details, see NATO, 1987, Appendix 1; Price and Wansack, 1989). Impulse duration is defined in several ways. Lack of agreement on this point arises from lack of knowledge about the relative adequacy of these measures in predicting risk of hearing damage. Figure 28-2 depicts the different definitions (taken from Smoorenburg, 1982). The definition of the A-duration (Coles et al, 1968) is based on the waveform produced by explosive charges in ideal conditions without reflections (the Friedlander wave). In practice, the waveform frequently contains reflections suggesting the use of the B-, C-, or D-duration. The B-duration is based on an idealized, exponentially decaying envelope of the impulse (Coles et al, 1968). In practice, it may often be difficult to fit the recorded impulse with this exponentially decaying envelope, which means limited reliability of reported B-durations. The criterion of −20 dB was based on practical considerations: a simple amplitude criterion (10 percent of the peak level) at a level above possible measurement noise. McRobert and Ward (1973) concluded that 10 dB of decay would be a better criterion than 20 dB, because reflections at 20 dB below peak level do not contribute to hearing loss. The C-duration (Pfander et al, 1975) does not suffer from limited reliability. It is unequivocally defined but it does not represent a simple physical quantity. The D-duration suffers from the same imperfection originating with the supposedly exponentially decaying envelope as the B-duration. It takes

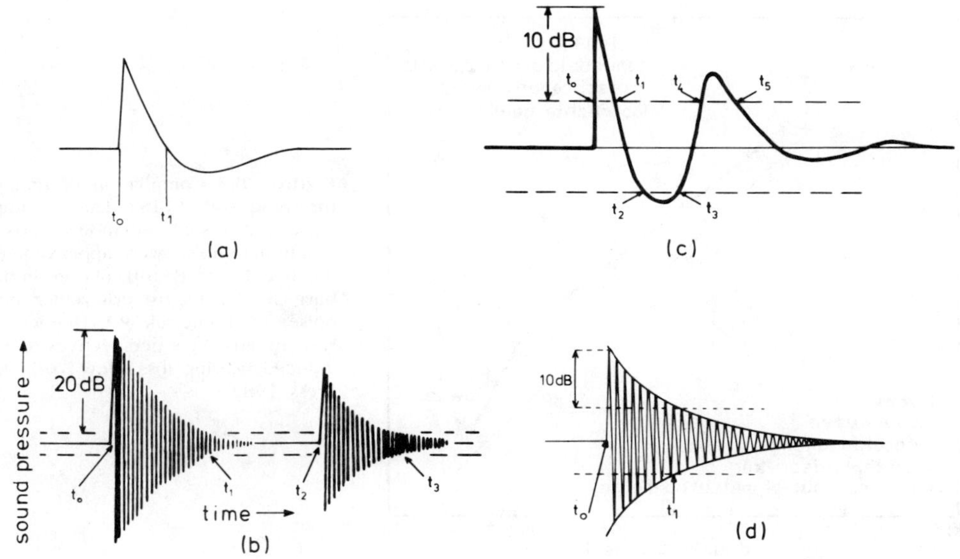

Figure 28-2 Some definitions of impulse duration. *A*, A-duration (t_1-t_0); *B*, B-duration (t_1-t_0) + (t_3-t_2); *C*, C-duration (t_1-t_0) + (t_3-t_2); + (t_5-t_4); *D*, D-duration (t_1-t_0). (From Smoorenburg GF. Damage-risk criteria for impulse noise. In: Hamernik RP, Henderson D, Salvi RJ, eds. New perspectives on noise-induced hearing loss. New York: Raven Press, 1982.)

into account the finding by McRobert and Ward (1973). However, the basis of this measure was mainly the practical purpose of defining a measure as close as possible to the three other measures, which were already in use in order to be able to compile all data available on the basis of a common denominator with the least amount of extrapolation.

Although the physical measures used to assess impulse noise exposure are directly related to typical aspects of the impulses, their application is not the result of a thorough evaluation of all possible measures as to their accuracy in predicting damage risk. Peak level and impulse duration were chosen primarily because of their face validity. When research started in this field, the full pressure-time history of the impulse was recorded simply because there were no fast sound-level meters on the market that could reliably measure relevant aspects of the impulse. Because these sound-level meters have become available and special versions, if needed, can be produced relatively easily using programmable memories, the possibility of a method of measurement simpler than recording the full pressure-time history should be considered. This is even more compelling because the present measures and evaluation schemes to assess damage risk have some serious shortcomings:

1. As mentioned before, A-, B-, and D-duration are based on idealized waveforms which, in practice, do not often occur
2. In contradiction to all current damage-risk criteria, long impulse durations found with large-caliber weapons and characterized by much low-frequency energy do not lead to higher damage risk than short-duration impulses from rifles at equal peak level (to be discussed below)
3. It is not clear how exposures to impulses with different peak levels should be combined
4. Using peak level and impulse duration, attenuation of impulse noise by hearing protectors cannot be calculated from the attenuation figures commonly specified as a function of frequency
5. Acoustic measurements of impulses, using miniature microphones placed in or near the ear canal under ear muffs, show long impulse durations due to low-frequency reverberation, which probably leads to overestimation of damage risk

Items 2 and 5 above suggest that the damage-risk criterion should include some low-frequency attenuation. The damage-risk criteria published by Pfander et al (1975, 1980) and Smoorenburg (1980, 1982) (Fig. 28-3) suggest that damage risk can be assessed, to a fair approximation, on the basis of the total energy

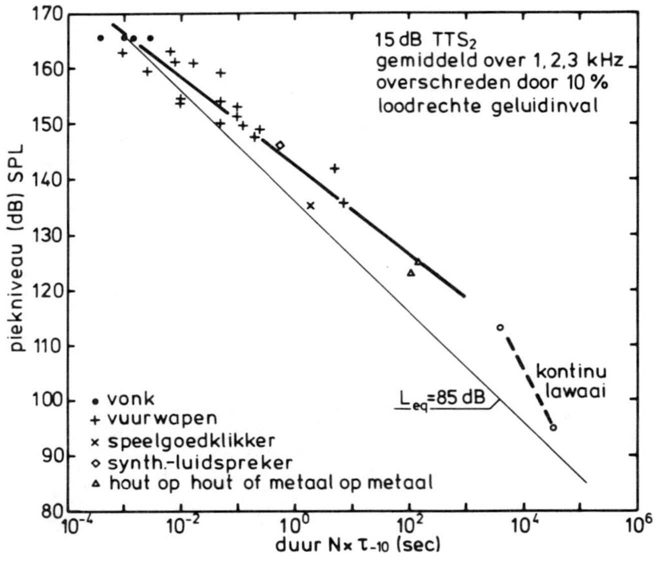

Figure 28-3 Compilation of temporary threshold shift (TTS) data for impulse noise. All results, including those for steady-state noise, were approximated by the line L_{eq} = 85 dB. (From Smoorenburg GF. Damage-risk criteria for impulse noise. In: Hamernik RP, Henderson D, Salvi RJ, eds. New perspectives on noise-induced hearing loss. New York: Raven Press, 1982.)

contained in the impulse exposure. Applying an energy measure would solve items 1, 3, and 4 above. Thus, investigating the applicability of a frequency-weighted total energy measure suggests itself.

Although the application of an energy measure is also supported by a number of other studies (Roberto et al, 1985; Hamernik et al, 1987; Laroche et al, 1989), it is already clear that predicting damage risk from only this measure would be an oversimplification (McRobert and Ward, 1973; Buck et al, 1984; Henderson and Hamernik, 1986; Patterson et al, 1986; Laroche and Hétu, 1990). From Figure 28-3 it is readily clear that somewhat more energy can be tolerated at lower peak levels. Moreover, other variables not yet mentioned, such as impulse rate, also affect damage risk. Nevertheless, the present literature suggests that the energy measure is the best first-order descriptor of damage risk for impulse noise. In the remainder of this chapter I shall focus on the required frequency weighting.

Spectral Factor in Animal Exposures to Impulse Noise

The spectral factor has received little attention in studies on impulse noise, although spectral effects were recognized early on. In the germinal work of Coles et al (1967, 1968), the critical peak level was asymptotic to a constant value with increasing A-duration. This asymptote was related to a spectral factor. When A-duration is increased while peak level is kept constant, all increase in impulse energy is found spectrally in an increase of low-frequency energy; the position of the high-frequency skirt (with the −3 dB per octave slope) is determined solely by the peak level (Fig. 28-4). The increase of low-frequency energy was supposed to have a minor effect on damage risk. Coles et al restricted themselves to this explanation and did not further investigate the spectral effect of impulse noise. Yet, their publication shows that it was clear from the very beginning of research in this field that the spectral energy distribution plays a part in damage risk for impulse noise.

Price should be credited for emphasizing the importance of the spectral distribution of impulse noise for damage-risk estimates. He based his damage-risk contour on threshold shifts measured in the cat immediately after, and 3 hours after, exposures to short tone pips (Price, 1979). For frequencies up to 3 kHz his damage-risk contour bore some resemblance to the A-weighting; above 3 kHz the damage-risk contour showed greater frequency dependence (Price, 1981, 1983a). Results from a similar experiment by Laroche and Hétu (1990), employing human subjects, showed a comparable trend up to 3 kHz. Price interpreted his damage-risk contour in terms of mechanical stress at the level of the basilar membrane in the inner ear (Price, 1979). Mechanical stress was related to the amplitude of basilar membrane movements versus basilar membrane width. Because basilar membrane width changes little with basilar membrane lo-

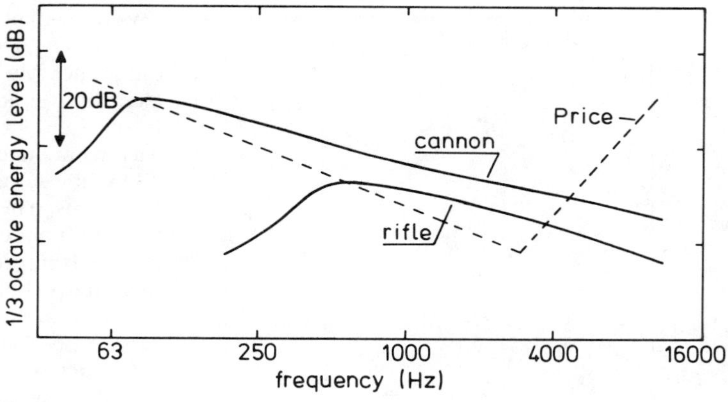

Figure 28-4 Impulse energy measured in ⅓ octaves for a rifle and a howitzer. The damage-risk contour, indicated by a broken line, is from Price GR. Loss of auditory sensitivity following exposure to spectrally narrow impulses. J Acoust Soc Am 1979; 66:456-465.

cation, the criterion is close to the constant basilar-membrane amplitude criterion introduced earlier to describe the TTS results for steady-state noise. Thus, the damage-risk contour proposed by Price must closely follow the threshold-of-hearing curve.

In predicting damage-risk as a function of A-duration, Price (1983a,b) came to the conclusion that impulse noise from cannons with greater A-durations than impulses from rifles would be less hazardous at equal peak levels. In my opinion, this conclusion, although in line with a trend in experimental data, cannot be drawn from the model proposed by Price. As shown before, the spectral energy distribution of weapon noise, measured in ⅓ octaves, has a high-frequency skirt that falls off at a rate of −3 dB per octave (Fig. 28-4). The ordinal position of this skirt depends on peak level only. Doubling A-duration, the peak in the energy distribution shifts downward by one octave while its level increases by 3 dB, in accordance with the −3 dB per octave slope. Following Price, the damage-risk level would be reached when the *peak* of the spectral distribution touches his damage-risk contour. Because his damage-risk contour falls off at a rate of about −6 dB per octave, this would indeed imply that the level of the impulse can be raised when A-duration is increased (about 3 dB doubling A-duration). However, when the peak of the spectral energy distribution touches the damage-risk contour at some frequency below the minimum in this contour at 3 kHz, the energy above the peak will exceed this contour (Fig. 28-4). Hence, damage in the region above the peak in the spectral energy distribution is to be expected. For all peak frequencies below 3 kHz, i.e., A-durations greater than about 0.1 ms, we have to conclude that damage risk will be determined by the energy in the 3-kHz region. This energy is directly related to the peak level. Hence, this would mean that the peak level is independent of A-duration for durations above 0.1 ms. This view was also given in a more recent paper by Price (1986), although in it he did not withdraw his former conclusion (Price, 1983a,b).

In deriving the above conclusion, I have followed Price (1983b, 1986) in comparing the spectral energy distribution of weapon impulses, measured in ⅓ octaves, with his damage-risk contour. However, this comparison is subject to criticism because the damage-risk contour was based on the sound pressure level (SPL) of the tone pips rather than on their energy. The duration of the tone pips was inversely proportional to their frequency. For a first approximation this would reflect the weapon impulses filtered by ⅓ octaves (or by the ear). Consequently, the SPL of the filtered weapon impulses, rather than their energy, should be compared to the damage-risk contour. In terms of SPL, the spectral distribution of weapon noise, measured in ⅓ octaves, is flat where the energy distribution shows the −3 dB per octave slope. Again, the 3-kHz minimum in the damage-risk contour would determine the critical level and, thus, the conclusion that the critical level is independent of A-duration for durations above 0.1 ms remains unaltered when the SPL measure is used instead of the energy measure.

The critical peak levels for rifles and for cannons (howitzers) were studied experimentally by Price in the cat. Threshold shifts, averaged across 2, 4, 8, and 16 kHz and across the two ears, were measured electrophysiologically as a function of peak level for a rifle with the A-duration at 0.3 to 0.4 ms, and for the howitzer at 2 to 3 ms. The results, found 2 months after exposure, are presented in Figure 28-5 (adapted from Price, 1983b). Price calculated the intercept of the regression line with the base line of 0 dB threshold shift that resulted in critical levels of 139 dB for the ri-

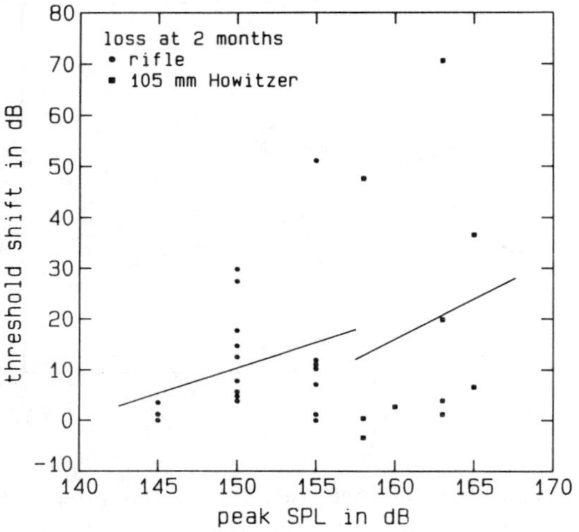

Figure 28-5 Average temporary threshold shift (TTS) across 2, 4, 8, and 16 kHz measured in the cat for rifle and howitzer. The regression lines were presented by Price for the rifle and howitzer separately. (Adapted from Price GR. Relative hazard of weapon impulses. J Acoust Soc Am 1983; 73:556-566.)

fle and of 150 dB for the howitzer. However, Figure 28-5 shows a considerable variability in threshold shifts. The coefficients of correlation between threshold shift and peak level for the rifle and the howitzer were only 0.3 and 0.2, respectively. This high variability is an essential aspect of noise-induced threshold shifts, in particular for impulse noise. It means that the confidence intervals of the critical levels reported by Price are very wide. Therefore, the difference in the peak levels found for the rifle and the howitzer should be accepted with caution. Figure 28-5 suggests, however, that the howitzer is not likely to produce larger threshold shifts than the rifle at the same peak level, although the A-duration is almost 10 times greater for the howitzer than for the rifle.

A later study (Price, 1986) revealed a critical peak level of 147 dB for the howitzer, based on threshold shifts measured at the day of exposure. The data presented in this paper did not permit a direct determination of the critical peak level on the basis of threshold shifts measured 2 months or more after exposure. Yet, the data suggest a value between 142 and 147 dB. Thus, the latter estimates for the howitzer are somewhat lower than the first estimate of 150 dB, but still higher than the estimate of 139 dB for the rifle.

The data published by Price did not allow for a direct comparison of threshold shifts induced by rifle and howitzer impulses at the same peak level and measured at least several days after exposure. In this respect, Dancer et al (1985) published an interesting study. In the guinea pig, they measured threshold shifts electrophysiologically 1 week after exposure. In one series of their experiments, peak level was maintained at a constant level (about 157 dB) while A-duration was varied from 0.05 ms to 1.0 ms. The results suggest that maximum threshold shift occurs at a frequency decreasing with increasing A-duration. Regrettably, thresholds below 2 kHz are not available, which means that maximum threshold shift cannot be assessed for all A-durations. The results suggest, however, that maximum threshold shift at any frequency may be constant across the interval of A-durations investigated or that it may decrease with increasing A-duration. A striking result was the effect of A-duration on the threshold shifts in one frequency region, for example, the 3-kHz region. Although the impulse energy in this frequency region did not change with A-duration, the threshold shift decreased markedly when A-duration was increased up to 1 ms. Thus, an increase of low-frequency energy seems to suppress the threshold shift induced by energy in a higher-frequency region.

In conclusion, the electrophysiologic experiments in animals have shown that damage risk might depend on stimulus frequency. The damage-risk contour may closely follow the threshold-of-hearing curve and bears some resemblance to the A-weighting curve. The damage-risk contour suggests that the critical peak level of impulse noise without reverberations, impulses that can be characterized by the A-duration, is independent of A-duration in the range of durations found for weapon noise. This is in contradiction to the energy concept, even if A-weighted energy is used to predict damage risk. After A-weighting, the howitzer impulse still contains about 5 dB more energy than the rifle impulse at the same peak level. The experimental data on noise exposures suggest that impulses may become even less hazardous when their A-duration is increased. This suggests a nonlinear interaction of the low- and high-frequency components of impulse noise in producing threshold shifts. Low-frequency energy seems to suppress the effect of high-frequency energy. Such a suppression phenomenon was found in studies applying low-frequency biasing stimuli. The response to a probe tone in the mid- or high-frequency range was suppressed at the moment that the basilar membrane was deflected towards scala vestibuli or scala tympani by the low-frequency bias signal of 30 Hz (Klis et al, 1988). The suppression phenomenon may also be re-

TABLE 28-1 **Survey of Important Measures for the 12 Weapons Included in Figure 28-6**

WEAPON	CHARGE	PEAK LEVEL (dB)	D-DUR (ms)	N × D (ms)	A-WEIGHTING (dB)	SB 258 EAR MUFF LIN	SB 258 EAR MUFF A	E.A.R. EAR PLUG LIN	E.A.R. EAR PLUG A	COMFIT EAR PLUG LIN	COMFIT EAR PLUG A
1 LAW 44		181.8	2.0	4.0	2.9	12.3	22.0	—	—	—	—
2 81 mm	3 }	175	3.3	105	(4.0)	(11.3)	(23.3)	—	—	—	—
81 mm	6 }		4.2					—	—	—	—
3 MAW 84		183.5	4.2	16.8	6.6	—	—	22.1	26.4	—	—
4 Viper		183	4.2	8.4	(5.2)	—	—	(22.5)	(26.4)	—	—
5 105 mm	3	172	5.2	312	4.5	—	—	24.2	28.0	19.1	22.1
6 122 mm	3	176.5	4.2	210	4.6	—	—	22.8	26.5	17.6	20.5
7 FH 155-1	7	173	12.2	50	8.0	—	—	21.9	26.3	—	—
8 M 198	7	173.5	9.3	112	(8.7)	—	—	(22.5)	(26.4)	—	—
9 155 mm	3	173	8.8	527	6.3	—	—	22.5	24.6	17.3	18.9
10 FH 70	7 }	178	9.6	115	(8.7)	(10.2)	(24.0)*	—	—	—	—
FH 70	8 }		9.6								
11 M 198	8	177.2	8.4	101	(8.7)	—	—	(22.5)	(26.4)	—	—
12 M 198	8S	180.7	9.5	114	11.7	—	—	(22.5)	(26.4)	—	—

Numbers in parentheses are estimates
*Cosmocord ear muff

lated to middle-ear nonlinearities (Price, 1974).

Spectral Factor in Human Exposures to Impulse Noise

The interaction of low-frequency energy and mid- or high-frequency energy in producing threshold shifts was found already in the early 1970s in a study on human exposures to simulated air-bag noise (Sommer and Nixon, 1973). The noise of air bags, which are used to prevent car drivers from injuries in collisions, consisted of a low-frequency pressure impulse and a mid-frequency (0.3 to 3 kHz) noise burst. After exposures to simulated air-bag noise, the noise burst alone appeared to produce some TTS, but no TTS was found when the low-frequency pressure impulse was added to the noise burst.

I conclude this chapter by evaluating human exposures to large-caliber weapon noise. This evaluation is based on all data that were available within the Research Study Group mentioned earlier. In view of the results from animal experiments, suggesting that damage risk may be independent of A-duration or that it may even decrease with increasing A-duration, I follow a rather conservative approach; I shall test whether inclusion of A-weighting in current damage-risk criteria improves the prediction of threshold shifts, in particular TTS. Applying A-weighting to an energy measure implies that energy, and consequently predicted damage risk, will increase with A-duration, but to a smaller extent than without applying the weighting.

A survey of the weapons, charges, peak levels, D-durations, and total durations (the product of the number of impulses in the exposure, N, and D-duration) used is given in Table 28-1. Impulse durations originally expressed in B- or C-duration were converted to D-duration in accordance with the ratios B:C:D = 4:0.5:1.0. These ratios were experimentally verified for large-caliber weapon impulses.

Because all exposures well exceeded the critical level for unprotected exposure, all subjects wore hearing protectors. This means that the attenuation of the hearing protectors had to be estimated in retrospect. This was done on the basis of the spectral distribution of the weapon impulses and current data on the frequency-dependent attenuation of the hearing protectors worn. In essence, the calculation scheme for continuous noise was followed, assuming no nonlinear effects in protector attenuation for high-level impulse noise. The reduction in total energy was expressed as a corresponding reduction of the peak level, keeping the duration constant. The attenuation data used in this calculation were so-called normal-experimenter-fit values—the values found when placement of the ear plug or ear muff is supervised by the experimenter. It will be clear that the use of hearing protec-

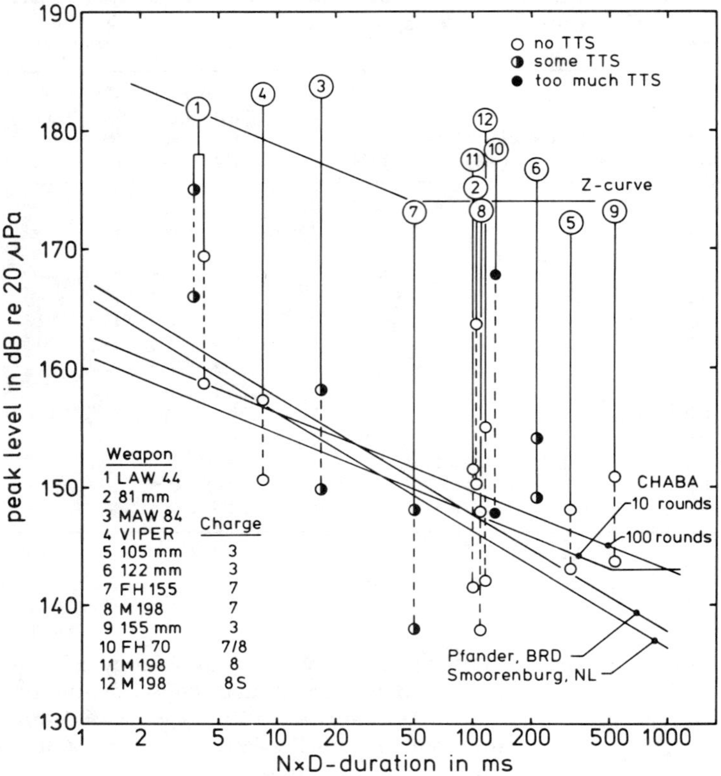

Figure 28-6 Temporary threshold shift (TTS) produced by large-caliber weapon impulses as a function of peak level and total impulse duration (N impulses times D-duration). Encircled digits represent peak levels without hearing protection; upper TTS symbols, connected by solid lines to the encircled digits, represent unweighted exposure levels with hearing protection; lower TTS symbols, connected by broken lines to the upper ones, represent exposure levels with hearing protection including A-weighting. The latter exposure levels are adjusted by +2.5 dB in order to take into account the effect of A-weighting on impulse noise from light-caliber weapons (see text). The Z-curve indicates the highest single exposure, with hearing protection, permitted in the United States. The TTS results for weapon 1 are given for subjects wearing glasses (left-hand set) and for subjects without glasses (right-hand set). (From: NATO Document AC/243, 1987.)

tion may have introduced a source of error in determining the exposure levels. In some of the experiments included in this evaluation, placement of the hearing protector may have been less effective than the normal-experimenter-fit values indicate (see also Smoorenburg and Mimpen, 1982). Consequently, some actual exposure levels may have been higher than calculated. This would lead to overestimation of damage risk. This possible error, however, could not be precluded. The calculated attenuation values, excluding and including A-weighting, are also in Table 28-1, together with the effect of A-weighting on the impulse itself.

In Figure 28-6 the results are compared to existing damage-risk criteria (CHABA, 1968; Coles et al, 1967, 1968; Pfander et al, 1975, 1980; Smoorenburg, 1980, 1982). The digits in circles represent the exposure levels without hearing protection. The Z-curve indicates the highest single exposure, with hearing protection, permitted in the United States. The data points connected by solid lines to the encircled digits represent the exposure levels with hearing protection but without A-weighting. These data points are given in terms of the physical measures on which the damage-risk criteria are based and, thus, can be compared directly to these criteria. Too much TTS (5 percent of subjects selected for highest TTS have more than 25 dB at one or more audiometric frequencies) is expected when the exposure level exceeds the critical level; some TTS (5 percent at more than 10 dB) is expected in a region 10 to 15 dB below the critical level; and no TTS is expected below this region. The results shown in Figure 28-6 for the unweighted levels of all weapons, except number 7, show less TTS than expected from the damage-risk criteria; the result for number 7, some TTS, is in line with expectation. Thus, by and large, damage risk is overestimated on the basis of damage-risk criteria that perform well for light-caliber weapons. This suggested that A-weighting might improve the prediction. In Figure 28-6, the A-weighted exposure levels are indicated by data points connected by broken lines to the data points for the unweighted exposure levels. Because A-weighting would also affect the exposure levels of light-caliber weapons (and the other impulses used in the derivation of Smoorenburg's damage-risk criterion), the criterion itself had to be adjusted. The adjustment would amount to a downward shift of about 2.5 dB (1 to 4 dB; see introduction). However, in order to keep Figure 28-6 simple, we did not add another criterion line, but adjusted the A-weighted exposure levels by +2.5 dB so that they can be compared directly to the damage-risk criterion for unweighted exposure levels. The result shows that for no weapon TTS exceeds the prediction. The results for weapons 7 and 10 are at the borderline of a lower TTS category. We may conclude that present TTS data suggest that current damage-risk criteria for human exposure to impulse noise can be improved by including A-weighting. The trade-off relations between peak level and total impulse duration in the damage-risk criteria by Pfander et al (1975, 1980) and by Smoorenburg (1980, 1982) represent equal energy. Thus, these criteria suggest the application of A-weighted impulse energy to predict damage risk. This method has been chosen by the French army (Dancer, 1982; DTAT, 1983).

Conclusion

Results of animal experiments suggest that some frequency-dependent weighting function should be included in damage-risk criteria for impulse noise. For steady-state and intermittent noise, A-weighting is used. Both human TTS data for steady-state noise and animal data for impulse noise suggest that the damage-risk contours should follow the threshold-of-hearing curve, which corresponds to a first approximation with constant basilar membrane amplitude. A-weighting constitutes a fair approximation of this threshold curve.

Human TTS data suggest that damage risk for impulse noise can be predicted on the basis of the A-weighted energy contained in the impulses. Animal experiments suggest that damage risk for large-caliber weapons may still be overrated after the inclusion of A-weighting in the energy measure. In my opinion, more data on human exposures are required before the criteria are adjusted further. For example, damage risk cannot be based on the peak level alone, irrespective of duration, as the cited animal experiments may suggest. Duration is certainly important in cases of reverberation. In those cases an increase of duration at the same peak level does not imply an increase of only low-frequency energy but it means both more low- and more high-frequency energy. In fact, practice has shown that light-caliber weapon shooting in enclosed (reverberating) shooting ranges and large-caliber shooting from trenches may be relatively hazardous.

The application of A-weighted energy in the damage risk criterion is not based on a general concept. It follows from an analysis of TTS data and it is restricted to exposures that result in small TTS. Only for these exposures, the analysis shows that there is a trading relationship among peak level, impulse duration, and number of impulses in the exposure that corresponds, within reasonable limits, to an energy measure. For higher exposure levels, the relationship may be quite different. TTS increases progressively, once exposure level exceeds the damage risk criterion by more than 5 dB (Smoorenburg, 1982, Fig. 3). This suggests that at higher levels other mechanisms of injury may start to play a role; this may affect the trading relationship.

The restriction discussed above means that regulatory authorities, accepting the A-weighted energy measure, should not set the permitted noise dose at a level in accordance with the level for steady-state and intermittent noise, although the use of the same measure for steady-state noise may suggest such action. My original damage-risk criterion for impulse noise at normal incidence corresponds to an equivalent 8-hour level of continuous noise at 85 dB. After A-weighting this becomes about 82.5 dBA. If this level is increased to 90 dBA, damage risk will be considerably higher than damage risk for continuous noise at 90 dBA.

Critères d'Exposition pour les Bruits Impulsionnels Riches en Basses Fréquences

Actuellement plusieurs critères d'exposition aux bruits impulsionnels en usage dans de nombreux pays sont basés sur le signal pression-temps de l'impulsion acoustique. L'application de ces critères n'est pas facile, car elle nécessite un enregistrement de haute qualité des paramètres de l'impulsion et signifie que l'on ne peut calculer l'effet de protecteurs auditifs à partir de courbes d'atténuation données généralement en fonction de la fréquence. Par conséquent un nouveau critère basé sur l'énergie acoustique totale contenue dans l'impulsion est proposé. Cependant, cette mesure est largement dérivée de données contenues dans le signal pression-temps. Cela signifie que cette mesure n'inclut pas de pondération dépendant de la fréquence, telle que la pondération A, alors qu'au contraire les expositions à un bruit continu ou intermittent sont évaluées à partir de l'énergie pondérée A. L'analyse des déficits auditifs temporaires (TTS) induits par des bruits impulsionnels d'armes lourdes contenant beaucoup d'énergie de basse fréquence, suggère que l'énergie acoustique pondérée A de l'impulsion peut être un meilleur indicateur des pertes auditives induites par les bruits impulsionnels que l'énergie non pondérée. Cette conclusion s'appuie sur les résultats obtenus sur des animaux soumis à des bruits impulsionnels.

La présente analyse est basée sur des données collectées et analysées par le groupe de Recherches N° 6 de l'OTAN (Panel 8) chargé de l'application des Sciences Humaines et Biomédicales à la Défense. La conclusion ci-dessus n'est cependant présentée que sous la seule responsabilité de l'auteur de l'article.

References

Buck K, Dancer A, Franke R. Effect of the temporal pattern of a given noise dose on TTS in guinea pigs. J Acoust Soc Am 1984; 76:1090-1097.

Burns W, Robinson DW. Hearing and noise in industry. London: Her Majesty's Stationery Office, 1970.

Coles RRA, Garinther GR, Hodge DC, Rice CG. Criteria for assessing hearing damage risk from impulse-noise exposure. Technical Memorandum 13-67. Aberdeen Proving Ground, Aberdeen, MD: U.S. Army Human Engineering Laboratories, 1967.

Coles RRA, Garinther GR, Hodge DC, Rice CG. Hazardous exposure to impulse noise. J Acoust Soc Am 1968; 43:336-343.

CHABA, Committee on Hearing, Bioacoustics and Biomechanics, Working Group 57. Proposed damage-risk criterion for impulse noise (gunfire). Washington, DC: National Academy of Sciences, National Research Council, 1968.

Dancer A. Isoenergy principle and A-weighting in the rating of the hazard of noise exposure in the military environment, Scand Audiol 1982; (Suppl 16):49-52.

Dancer A, Buck K, Vassout P. Influence du niveau de crête et de la durée d'ondes de choc (bruit d'armes) sur l'audition du cobaye. Acustica 1985; 59:21-29.

DTAT recommendation on evaluating the possible harmful effect of noise on hearing, May 1983, Saint Cloud, France, AT-83127128.

Fletcher H, Munson WA. Loudness, its definition, measurement, and calculation. J Acoust Soc Am 1933; 5:82.

Hamernik RP, Patterson JH, Salvi RJ. The effect of impulse intensity and the number of impulses on hearing and cochlear pathology in the chinchilla. J Acoust Soc Am 1987; 81:1118-1129.

Henderson D, Hamernik RP. Impulse noise: Critical review. J Acoust Soc Am 1986; 80:569-584.

Klis JFL, Prijs VF, Latour JB, Smoorenburg GF. Modulation of cochlear tuning by low-frequency sound. Hear Res 1988; 36:163-174.

Kryter KD, Ward DW, Miller JD, Eldredge DH. Hazardous exposure to intermittent and steady-state noise. J Acoust Soc Am 1966; 39:451-464.

Laroche C, Hétu R, Poirier S. The growth of and recovery from TTS in human subjects exposed to impact noise. J Acoust Soc Am 1989; 85:1681-1690.

Laroche C, Hétu R. The influence of the spectral content and the decay time of impulse noise on asymptotic threshold shift. Acustica 1990; 70:29-44.

McRobert H, Ward WD. Damage-risk criteria: The trading relation between intensity and the number of nonreverberant impulses. J Acoust Soc Am 1973; 53:1297-1300.

NATO Document AC/243 (Panel 8/RSG.6) D/9. Effects of impulse noise. Brussels, NATO, 1987.

Patterson JH, Lomba-Gautier IM, Curd DL, et al. The role of peak pressure in determining the auditory hazard of impulse noise. In: Salvi RJ, Henderson D, Hamernik RP, Colletti V, eds. Basic and applied aspects of noise-induced hearing loss. New York: Plenum Press, 1986:405.

Pfander F, in collaboration with Bongartz H, Brinkmann H. Das Knalltrauma. Berlin: Springer-Verlag, 1975.

Pfander F, Bongartz H, Brinkmann H, Kietz H. Danger of auditory impairment from impulse noise: A comparative study of the CHABA damage-risk criterion and those of the Federal Republic of Germany. J Acoust Soc Am 1980; 67:628-633.

Plomp R, Gravendeel DW, Mimpen AM. Relation of hearing loss to noise spectrum. J Acoust Soc Am 1963; 35:1234-1240.

Price GR. Upper limit to stapes displacement: Implications for hearing loss. J Acoust Soc Am 1974; 56:195-197.

Price GR. Loss of auditory sensitivity following exposure to spectrally narrow impulses. J Acoust Soc Am 1979; 66:456-465.

Price GR. Implications of a critical level in the ear for assessment of noise hazard at high intensities. J Acoust Soc Am 1981; 69:171-177.

Price GR. Mechanisms of loss for intense sound exposures. In: Fay RR, Gourevitch G, eds. Hearing and other senses: Presentations in honor of E.G. Wever. Groton, CT: Amphora Press, 1983a.

Price GR. Relative hazard of weapon impulses. J Acoust Soc Am 1983b; 73:556-566.

Price GR. Hazard from intense low-frequency acoustic impulses. J Acoust Soc Am 1986; 80:1076-1086.

Price GR, Wansack S. Hazard from an intense midrange impulse. J Acoust Soc Am 1989; 86:2185-2191.

Roberto M, Hamernik RP, Salvi RJ, Henderson D, Milone R. Impact noise and the equal energy hypothesis. J Acoust Soc Am 1985; 77:1514-1520.

Robinson, DW. The spectral factor in noise-induced hearing loss: A case for retaining the A-weighting. J Sound Vibr 1983; 90:103-127.

Smoorenburg GF. Damage-risk criteria for impulse noise. Report IZF 1980-26. Soesterberg, The Netherlands: TNO Institute for Perception, 1980.

Smoorenburg GF. Damage-risk criteria for impulse noise. In: Hamernik RP, Henderson D, Salvi RJ, eds. New perspectives on noise-induced hearing loss. New York: Raven Press, 1982.

Smoorenburg GF, Mimpen AM. Assessment of personal hearing protection in practice. Scand Audiol Suppl 1982; 16:13-22.

Sommer HC, Nixon CW. Primary components of simulated air bag noise and their relative effects on human hearing. AMRL-TR-73-52. Wright-Patterson Air Force Base, Ohio: Aerospace Medical Research Laboratory, 1973.

Ward WD. Studies on the aural reflex. II. Reduction of temporary threshold shift from intermittent noise by reflex activity; Implications for damage-risk criteria. J Acoust Soc Am 1962; 34:234-241.

CHAPTER 29

Parametric Relation Between Impulse Noise and Auditory Damage

ZHI'AN LIANG

Impulse noise from weapons is characterized by an extraordinarily high peak pressure that can cause damage to the auditory system. The potential for permanent hearing loss limits an investigator's ability to make direct observations with human subjects. In the early studies, small arms were primarily used as impulse sources, and temporary threshold shift (TTS) was the chief index for assessing hearing damage. With such constraints, the results of those experiments led to conclusions that were probably on the conservative side (Kryter and Garinther, 1965; Ward, 1968; Coles et al, 1968; Rice and Martin, 1973). With the development of procedures for audiometric measurements in different species of animals, the effect of weapon impulse noise on hearing has become the subject of intensive study (Liang et al, 1983a,b; Liang, 1987; Price, 1986; Henderson and Hamernik, 1986; Patterson et al, 1986; Hamernik et al, 1987).

Unlike the description of steady noises in which a single parameter, decibels (A), may be sufficient for noise control practice, there are a number of impulse noise parameters that must be considered, e.g., the peak pressure, the pulse duration, the waveform, the number of impulses, and the repetition rate. These parameters also interact with each other; therefore, clarification of the parametric relation between impulse noise and auditory damage is only possible by the analysis of vast amounts of experimental data. The results of auditory damage by high-level impulses, especially of heavy-weapon origins, are rarely described in the literature. In this chapter I present the results of an attempt to build such an extensive database. Many of the data are systematically presented for the first time.

Methods in Brief

Impulse Sources

More than 20 different kinds of weapons, discharged on an open proving ground or in a fortification, served as the chief sources of the impulse noises. The weapons' spectrum covered many representative arms, including the heavy weapons such as the 130-mm cannon and the 152-mm gun-howitzer, and the light weapons such as the 12.7-mm machine gun. The sources also included a trinitrotoluene (TNT) explosion, which generated a simple A-type wave, and antitank rockets, which generated impulse noise of the B-type. For supplementary sources, primers, firecrackers, impact sound, and high-level speaker-generating acoustic impulses were also used. The peak pressures (L_{pp}) varied with source and location and included the range 150 to 180 dB (L_{pp}).

Acoustic Measurement

A specially-designed piezoelectric ceramic microphone was used for the high-pressure impulse measurements. The microphone was coupled by a long cable to a B&K precision impulse sound level meter (type 2209). The microphone was fixed at a position corresponding to the location of the animal's head during the exposure. The peak pressure of the impulse was read from the meter set at the linear impulse-hold mode. From the AC output of the sound-level meter the acoustic signal was sent to a high-quality recorder with a looped tape to be displayed later on a memory oscilloscope for measurement of the pulse duration and for plotting of the waveform. Spectral analysis was performed by feeding the recorded signal to a ⅓ octave real-time analyzer. For impulse noise of lower L_{pp} (less than 166 dB), a B&K ¼-inch condenser microphone, type 4138, was used instead of the ceramic gauge. The diaphragm of the measuring microphone was mounted for grazing incidence of the impulse.

Animal and Exposure

More than 2,000 guinea pigs weighing 300 to 500 g with normal hearing were used. The animals were exposed five to a group. The animals' heads were fixed to face the source. The animals were located at the gunner's position or at various distances from the source and at about 1.5 m above the ground.

Audiometric Measurement and Middle-Ear Examination

Audiometry was usually performed 2 days after exposure. Threshold of the pinna reflex to a burst of repetitive clicks (1,000 per second) was measured first; then the animal was anesthetized with nembutal, and thresholds of compound action potential (CAP) and of primary response (PR) from the auditory cortex to click (and, in some experiments, to tone bursts) were determined and taken as the hearing thresholds. The group-averaged values (of 10 ears) were compared with the normal control values, and from the postexposure changes the character, degree, and sites of damage were estimated. Estimates of recruitment and the degree of cochlea damage were made by comparing the reflex and the hearing thresholds. Direct central damage could be ruled out by comparing the CAP and the PR threshold shifts.

After the physiologic tests were completed, the animals were sacrificed for middle-ear inspection. Each auditory bulla was opened, and careful examination of the tympanic membrane, the ossicular chain, and the tympanic cavity was performed under a dissecting microscope. A histologic examination of the organ of Corti was performed in a sampling of animals.

Damage Grading

Damage to the middle ear and to the cochlea was graded separately as safe, marginal, light, moderate, and severe, labeled in succession by 0, I, II, III, and IV. For middle-ear damage, the descriptions were as follows: safe—no damage in all 10 ears of the group or only congestion or faint hemorrhage in not more than two ear drums; marginal—light hemorrhage in some ears, but minute drum perforation only in two ears at most; light—minute perforation, but no medium-sized ones (¼), in more than two ears; moderate—medium-sized perforation, but no large ones (more than ¼), in more than two ears; severe—large perforation, ossicular disruption, or profound tympanic hemorrhage in more than two ears. For cochlear damage, the descriptions were as follows: safe—the group-averaged hearing threshold shift was less than 8 dB (2 days after exposure); marginal—from 8 to 15 dB with no middle-ear damage; light—more than 15 dB with a hearing/reflex threshold difference of from 7 to 20 dB; moderate—from 21 to 30 dB; severe—31 dB or more.

General Features of the Blast Injury

For the wide range of weapons and their diverse levels and spectrum, the damaging effect of the impulse noise was exerted chiefly on the middle-ear structures and on the cochlea. Damage at these two sites did not run parallel. When the peak pressure of the impulse was very high (e.g., above 175 dB) damage was more likely to occur mainly in the middle ear. Middle-ear damage is of minor significance in those studies with small arms in which the effect of much-less-intense impulses was studied (Ward, 1968; Coles et al, 1968; Patterson et al, 1986; Hamernik et al, 1987). A detailed description of blast-induced middle-ear damage under various exposure conditions has been given by Meng et al (1987).

The cochlea seemed more susceptible to impulses of moderate peak pressure with large pulse duration and number of rounds. Histologic examination revealed that the cochlear damage usually started from the second turn and, with increased severity of exposure, the first, third, and fourth turns followed in succession. In mild or moderate damage only receptor cells were affected. In severe conditions, however, the whole organ of Corti might disappear and degeneration of the spiral ganglion and nerve fibers might occur. By contrast, the vestibular organ was usually intact even in cases of extremely severe cochlea damage.

TABLE 29-1 **Damage versus L_{pp} for Single Firing of Cannon 130**

			THRESHOLD SHIFT (dB)		DAMAGE GRADE	
LOCATION	L_{pp} (dB)	T (ms)	Hearing	Reflex	Middle Ear	Cochlea
1	161.7	5	6.1	4.9	0	0
2	166.4	5	6.7	5.6	0	0
3	169.3	4	11.2	7.3	I	0
4	171.2	2	12.1	8.5	II	0
5	171.8	5	19.5	22.6	III	0
6	176.0	5	24.9	22.4	III	0
7	178.5	4	31.7	31.6	IV	0
8	181.7	4	28.8	29.7	IV	0

TABLE 29-2 **Damage versus L_{pp}, Close T, Single Round, Different Sources**

			THRESHOLD SHIFT (dB)		DAMAGE GRADE	
SOURCE	L_{pp} (dB)	T (ms)	Hearing	Reflex	Middle Ear	Cochlea
Antiaircraft 100	168.0	2.6	3.8	0.5	0	0
TNT cylinder 1 Kg	170.0	2	2.2	−1.0	0	0
Machine gun 12.7	172.2	3	6.2	4.7	0	0
TNT cylinder 1 Kg	173.2	2	5.4	−0.1	I	0
Firecracker	175.5	2	12.3	5.1	0	I
TNT sphere 1 Kg	179.4	3	5.9	1.9	II	0
Antiaircraft 100	181.0	2	33.4	21.9	III	II
Primer in free field	182.3	2	21.4	2.3	II	II
Firework A	159.0	20	1.2	1.0	0	0
Rocket 62	169.8	25	3.6	−1.7	0	0
Rocket 82 A	170.0	20	6.5	7.1	0	0
Rocket 82 B	172.2	25	6.5	3.7	0	0
Rocket 82 A	173.0	20	6.6	7.9	I	0
Rocket 82 A	175.0	20	13.3	17.0	III	0
Rocket 82 B	179.0	30	16.8	11.7	III	0
Rocket 82 A	185.5	20	17.5	30.9	IV	0

The CAP and the PR threshold typically shifted to the same degree; thus, there was no sign of immediate central auditory impairment, even when the peak pressure of the impulse was as high as 190 dB. Impediments in central auditory functions occur later and secondary to cochlear damage. Central morphologic changes following acoustic trauma in the periphery have been reported (Morest and Bohne, 1983).

For pure middle-ear blast injury or for mixed trauma of both the middle and the inner ear, hearing loss in guinea pigs is not biased towards high frequencies, as is usually seen in cases of noise-induced deafness in patients wherein the cochlea is often the main site of damage.

Role of Peak Pressure

It is generally agreed that the peak pressure is the first important parameter of an impulse noise. Correlation between the degree of ear damage and L_{pp} in otherwise similar conditions was examined in a series of experiments.

Table 29-1 presents data obtained from firing a single round of cannon 130. The animal groups were located at different distances from the source to vary the received L_{pp}. From the results the following points may be noted: (1) a single blast often damages only the middle ear; (2) there is a general trend for the severity of damage to increase with L_{pp} up to a limit at about 180 dB, where maximum middle-ear destruction is reached.

Results for a single-round exposure to different sources (T = 2 to 3 ms or T = 20 to 30 ms, where T = time) are listed in Table 29-2. They are essentially in agreement with results in Table 29-1 except that marginal or light cochlear damage appears in some high-level exposure groups.

Multiple-round exposures yield a high incidence of cochlear damage as well as middle-

TABLE 29-3 **Damage versus L_{pp} in Multiround Exposure**

				THRESHOLD SHIFT (dB)		DAMAGE GRADE	
SOURCE	**L_{pp} (dB)**	**T (ms)**	**N**	**Hearing**	**Reflex**	**Middle Ear**	**Cochlea**
TNT cylinder 1 Kg	164.9	2	10	5.7	−0.9	0	0
Machine gun 12.7	166.7	3	10	11.4	6.4	0	I
Primer in free field	167.0	2	10	14.6	2.4	0	I
Firecracker	168.4	2	10	13.2	18.1	0	0
Machine gun 12.7	168.9	3	10	7.2	5.9	0	0
Firecracker	170.0	2	10	28.3	9.7	II	II
Primer in free field	173.4	2	10	23.0	14.4	I	II
TNT sphere 1 Kg	174.0	2.5	10	13.6	13.4	II	0
Machine gun 12.7	175.0	3	10	21.9	10.7	0	II
Antiaircraft 100	176.0	2.2	16	47.3	20.5	II	III
Firecracker	177.3	2	10	13.5	11.7	II	0
Antiaircraft 100	182.0	2	16	47.2	28.9	IV	II

TABLE 29-4 **Damage versus T**

				THRESHOLD SHIFT (dB)		DAMAGE GRADE	
SOURCE	**T (ms)**	**L_{pp} (dB)**	**N**	**Hearing**	**Reflex**	**Middle Ear**	**Cochlea**
TNT 200 g	1.2	175.4	I	9.8	4.8	II	0
Double-barreled gun 37	1.4	175.2	I	11.2	0.9	0	I
Firecracker	2.0	175.5	I	12.3	5.1	0	I
Antiaircraft 100	2.2	176.0	I	10.7	7.2	II	0
Gun-howitzer 152	6.0	175.3	I	12.4	16.8	III	0
Rocket 40	7.5	176.0	I	29.6	29.1	III	0
Cannon 130	8.0	176.0	I	24.9	22.4	III	0
Rocket 82 A	20.0	175.0	I	13.3	17.0	III	0
Double-barreled gun 37	1.4	168.0	10	6.6	0.5	0	0
Gun-howitzer 152	>100	167.9	12	47.9	18.7	II	III
TNT cylinder 1 Kg	5	169.9	10	8.2	4.7	I	0
Howitzer 122	40	169.2	12	54.5	19.7	II	III
Machine gun 12.7	3	166.7	60	4.2	1.3	0	0
Rocket 62	25	167.0	60	38.5	17.3	II	III
Howitzer 122	>100	167.0	60	55.5	22.3	II	IV

ear damage. As in the case of single-round exposures, the overall severity of damage also increases with L_{pp}. Examples are given in Table 29-3.

From the data presented in Tables 29-1 through 29-3, it is clear that the peak pressure of weapon impulse noise is an important determinant of the damaging effect. The L_{pp} difference from safe to profound ear injury amounts roughly to 12 to 16 dB, i.e., a 3- to 4-dB L_{pp} increment would raise the damage about one grade. For a single round, and for T not longer than a few milliseconds, an L_{pp} of about 170 dB would begin to cause ear damage.

Because peak pressure is not the sole parameter of an impulse noise, the rules for estimating the damaging effect of exposure to impulse noise must take other parameters into account.

Role of Pulse Duration

The importance of T was examined in several experiments in which L_{pp} and number of rounds (N) are about equal. The data leads to several generalizations: (1) there is a tendency for damage to increase with T; (2) for large-T exposures, cochlear injury may appear and become predominant; (3) when L_{pp} and N are about equal, a 7- to 30-fold T increment would raise the damage two to four grades—i.e., there is a loose correlation of one grade per each three-fold T increment.

Because an increase of L_{pp} or T leads to an increase of the incoming acoustic energy acting on the ear, and because both lead to severe damaging effects, it is reasonable to consider combining these two parameters, as in the case of the equal-energy principle. Several authors had tried to apply the energy princi-

TABLE 29-5 **Damage versus L_{pp} T Product (P)**

					THRESHOLD SHIFT (dB)		DAMAGE GRADE	
SOURCE	P (dB)	L_{pp} (dB)	T (ms)	N	Hearing	Reflex	Middle Ear	Cochlea
TNT 200 g	181.2	180.4	1.2	1	15.6	10.9	III	0
Gun-howitzer 152	181.4	173.5	6.5	1	10.4	16.8	II	0
Rocket 82 B	182.6	169.6	20	1	5.2	3.7	0	0
Machine gun 12.7	178.0	175.0	2	10	36.8	14.5	II	III
Rocket 40	178.0	166.2	15	10	6.2	0.5	0	0
Gun-howitzer 152	177.4	157.4	>100	12	9.4	5.2	0	I
Gun-howitzer 152	181.4	173.5	6.5	30	60.3	28.5	III	IV
Rocket 82 B	181.2	168.2	20	30	13.2	2.2	0	I

TABLE 29-6 **Damage versus N**

				THRESHOLD SHIFT (dB)		DAMAGE GRADE	
SOURCE	N	L_{pp} (dB)	T (ms)	Hearing	Reflex	Middle Ear	Cochlea
Cannon 130	1	166.4	8	6.7	5.6	0	0
	2			13.2	7.2	II	0
	4			14.2	7.6	II	0
	8			24.9	8.5	II	II
	16			30.6	10.4	II	II
	32			45.0	17.6	II	III
Cannon 130	1	171.8	8	19.5	22.6	III	0
	2			28.0	29.4	III	0
	4			28.9	28.2	IV	0
	8			31.2	26.7	IV	0
	16			35.5	28.0	IV	II
	32			47.7	27.2	IV	III
Machine gun 12.7	1	170.9	2	6.2	4.7	0	0
	10			10.0	6.5	0	I
	30			14.5	3.1	II	I
	60			41.5	11.7	II	III
	120			41.3	19.5	II	III
	300			45.3	13.7	II	IV
Rocket 40	1	172.0	20	1.9	−0.3	0	0
	10			12.4	3.7	0	I
	30			16.2	3.5	I	II

ple to predict impulse noise hazard (Atherley and Martin, 1971; Rice and Martin, 1973; Roberto et al, 1985; Henderson and Hamernik, 1986).

Our data provided another perspective to examine this hypothesis under more practical conditions. By simple calculation the $T \cdot L_{pp}$ product for each exposure condition can be easily obtained. For convenience of comparison it is herein expressed in terms of equivalent peak pressure at T equaling 1 ms (denoted by the letter P; $P = L_{pp} + 10 \log T$). Some representative results are listed in Table 29-5. It is obvious for the same P values, damage may vary from safe to moderate or from marginal to severe, indicating that the equal-energy law does not hold for impulse noise hazard, and that the value P cannot be used as a combined parameter for damage prediction.

Damage in Relation to Number of Rounds

Repeated exposure would cause the damaging effect to accumulate and, consequently, the overall hearing impairment would increase with the number of rounds. Such accumulation, however, is different for middle-ear and for cochlear damage. Table 29-6 presents data from a series of experiments designed to demonstrate this difference. With an increase in the number of rounds (N, in one exposure day), the cochlear damage may shift three or four grades (from 0 to IV in the case of exposure to machine-gun firing, or from 0 to III in the case of exposure to cannon 130) whereas the middle-ear damage increases only one or two grades. As a loose estimate, about a three-

TABLE 29-7 **Damage versus Inter-Round Interval**

SOURCE	PAIR NO.	L_{pp} (dB)	N	AVERAGED INTERVAL(S)	THRESHOLD SHIFT (dB) Hearing	Reflex	DAMAGE GRADE Middle Ear	Cochlea
Rocket 82-B	1	165.7	30	232	12.8	4.7	0	I
				44	6.5	1.7	0	0
T = 20 ms	2	167.8	30	232	8.1	6.5	0	I
				44	9.9	3.9	0	I
	3	168.2	30	232	14.8	4.8	0	I
				44	13.2	2.2	0	I
TNT 1 Kg	4	163.0	10	720	5.3	−1.5	0	0
Cylinder				96	3.7	0.1	0	0
T = 3 ms	5	164.9	10	720	9.1	0.1	0	I
				96	5.7	0.9	0	0
	6	169.9	10	720	8.2	4.7	I	0
				96	6.5	−0.4	I	0
	7	177.8	10	720	11.3	2.1	II	0
				96	9.9	3.8	II	0
Impact Noise	8	151.0	30	60	26.0	7.1	0	II
				4	16.3	5.8	0	II
T = 100 ms	9	153.0	30	60	21.4	14.5	0	II
				4	20.6	5.6	0	II
	10	149.0	100	36	14.4	6.1	0	I
				2.4	11.2	6.8	0	I
	11	151.0	100	36	26.6	7.7	0	II
				2.4	23.1	6.0	0	II
	12	153.0	100	36	30.9	12.4	0	II
				2.4	26.2	11.3	0	II
TNT 200 g	13	180.4	4	1350	28.7	15.4	III	II
T = 1.2 ms				450	23.9	25.4	III	0
	14	186.8	4	1350	35.1	30.8	IV	0
				450	27.4	30.4	IV	0
Machine Gun	15	170.9	10	0.1	10.0	6.5	0	I
12.7				10–60	17.0	5.1	0	II
T = 2ms	16	175.0	10	0.1	21.9	10.7	0	II
				10–60	36.8	14.5	II	III
	17	170.9	30	0.1	14.5	3.1	II	I
				10–60	39.9	11.4	II	III
	18	175.0	60	0.1	44.0	23.0	II	III
				10–60	61.7	22.1	II	IV

fold increment in N raises the cochlear damage one grade, comparable to that for increasing T.

Interround Interval

Results for 18 pairs of animal groups, each exposed with different inter-round intervals to the same source, are presented in Table 29-7. For pairs 1 to 14, the shortest interval is only 2.4 seconds, whereas the longest is more than 20 minutes. As shown, in 11 pairs of these 14, the damage grades of both the middle ear and the cochlea are virtually the same for both long and short intervals. Only in pairs 1, 5, and 13 does marginal or light cochlear damage appear in the longer-interval groups, in contrast to the safe grade in the shorter-interval ones. In addition, the hearing threshold shifts seem systematically a little larger in the longer-interval groups. These differences, however, are statistically insignificant. It is likely that the fatiguing factor of hourly exposing the animals of the longer-interval groups to the sun and wind in the open field, rather than the interval parameter itself, may be responsible for the seemingly larger cochlear damage in these groups.

Very long intervals would limit the possible number of rounds within an exposure day, and hence are less interesting. Very short intervals are worth considering. This is demonstrated by the results obtained in the pairs of animal groups exposed to machine-gun firing, in which the damaging effects with short (0.1

TABLE 29-8 **Examples for "Safe" Conditions**

					THRESHOLD SHIFT (dB)	
SOURCE	L_{pp} **(dB)**	**T (ms)**	**N**	**TN**	**Hearing**	**Reflex**
Cannon 130	166.4	8	1	8	6.7	5.6
Antiaircraft 100	168.0	2.6	1	2.6	3.8	0.5
TNT 200 g	170.0	1.8	1	1.8	1.4	2.6
TNT sphere 1 Kg	168.0	5	1	5	2.8	2.1
TNT cylinder 1 Kg	170.0	2	1	2	2.2	−1.0
Rocket 62	169.8	25	1	25	3.6	−1.7
Rocket 82 A	166.0	20	1	20	5.0	3.0
Rocket 82 B	167.0	22	1	22	4.5	2.5
Rocket 40	171.4	16	1	16	1.9	−0.3
Machine gun 12.7	172.2	2	1	2	6.2	4.7
Primer in free field	174.0	2	1	2	−0.8	1.2
Primer in a box	168.4	40	1	40	4.5	0.6
Firecracker	172.0	2	1	1	1.0	2.2
Double-barreled gun 37	168.0	1.4	10	14	6.6	0.5
TNT cylinder 1 Kg	164.9	2	10	20	5.7	−0.9
Firework A salvo	157.0	20	9	180	7.4	3.6
Rocket 82 B	165.7	25	10	250	6.2	4.9
Rocket 40	163.0	18	10	180	6.6	1.8
Machine gun 12.7	168.9	2	10	20	7.2	5.9
Double-barreled gun 37	165.0	11	30	330	−0.1	−0.4
Firework A salvo	154.9	30	75	2250	−0.3	2.4
Rocket 82 A	160.0	20	35	700	4.9	7.5
Rocket 82 B	166.0	25	30	750	4.5	2.4
Rocket 40	158.8	15	30	450	5.7	−0.5
Machine gun 12.7	166.7	2	30	60	5.0	4.7
Firework C	152.7	12	120	1440	1.3	0.7
Machine gun 12.7	162.8	3	300	900	4.7	1.2
Primer in free field	157.2	2	100	200	7.8	−1.7

seconds) and long (10 to 60 seconds) inter-round intervals are compared (pairs 15 to 18 in Table 29-7). As shown, for the short-interval exposures the cochlear damage and hearing loss is less severe than in the long-interval exposures. This may be explained by the protecting mechanism of the acoustic reflex: the 0.1-second interval is short enough for the reflex evoked by the preceding impulse to last and be effective when the succeeding impulse arrives.

Safety Margin for Guinea Pigs

From the experimental data obtained in more than 300 groups of animals exposed to impulse noise of various parameters and under various conditions, we may conclude that the peak pressure, the pulse duration, and the number of rounds are the three essential parameters. In general, injury is aggravated by increasing any of these parameters. There is, however, considerable variability within and across groups. Attention herein is concentrated on the "safe" and "marginal" conditions, which are more important in determining a safety margin. Some representative data are given in Tables 29-8 and 29-9.

By definition, the safety margin should be the demarcation line, or lines, which separate the data points into two populations, holding all the "damaged" points above and leaving only part of the "safe" ones below. This line (or lines) can be drawn in many different ways. After a series of trials we found that L_{pp} versus log (T N) is the simplest. The safety margin of impulse noise for guinea pigs can be expressed as

$$L_{pp} = 172 - 6 \log (T\ N)$$

which is graphically represented by the oblique line in Figure 29-1 in the L_{pp} versus log (T N) format. In this figure the dots represent all the damaged points of marginal or light grades (points of the more severe grades are distributed higher in position and are omitted). The line fits the lower border of the dot distribution strikingly well.

TABLE 29-9 **Examples of Marginal Damage**

SOURCE	L_{pp} (dB)	T (ms)	N	TN	THRESHOLD SHIFT (dB) Hearing	Reflex	DAMAGE GRADE Middle Ear	Cochlea
Cannon 130	169.3	8	1	8	11.2	7.3	1	0
Double-barreled gun 37	172.0	1.4	1	1.4	9.8	2.2	0	1
TNT 200 g	172.6	1.3	1	1.3	11.4	2.0	1	0
TNT 40 g	169.0	3	1	3	8.8	−0.1	1	0
TNT cylinder 1 Kg	171.0	5	1	5	2.9	0.6	1	0
Rocket 82 A	173.0	20	1	20	6.6	7.9	1	0
Rocket 40	174.0	18	1	18	10.9	1.5	0	1
Firecracker	175.5	2	1	2	12.3	5.1	0	1
Double-barreled gun 37	170.8	1.4	10	14	10.1	3.1	0	1
TNT sphere 1 Kg	168.0	5	10	50	5.6	6.1	1	0
TNT cylinder 1 Kg	164.9	2	10	20	9.1	−0.1	0	1
Firework B	159.0	20	9	180	8.6	4.6	0	1
Rocket 82 B	166.0	25	10	250	9.4	2.4	0	1
Rocket 40	172.0	16	10	160	12.4	3.7	0	1
Machine gun 12.7	166.7	2	10	20	11.4	6.4	0	1
Primer in free field	167.0	2	10	20	14.6	2.4	0	1
Firecracker	168.4	2	10	20	13.2	18.1	0	1
Impact impulse	155.0	100	10	1000	9.6	6.3	0	1
Double-barreled gun 37	167.0	1.4	30	42	3.7	0.1	1	0
Firework A salvo	159.5	12	30	360	7.9	2.0	0	1
Rocket 62	160.5	25	60	1500	12.4	3.0	0	1
Rocket 82 A	170.0	20	35	700	10.6	5.7	0	1
Rocket 82 B	165.7	25	30	750	12.8	4.7	0	1
Rocket 40	163.0	18	30	540	9.7	4.2	0	1
Firework A salvo	154.9	30	150	4500	3.7	0.3	1	0
Machine gun 12.7	166.7	2	120	240	8.8	4.1	0	1
Primer in free field	159.0	2	100	200	12.0		0	1
Impact impulse	149.0	100	100	10000	11.2	6.8	0	1

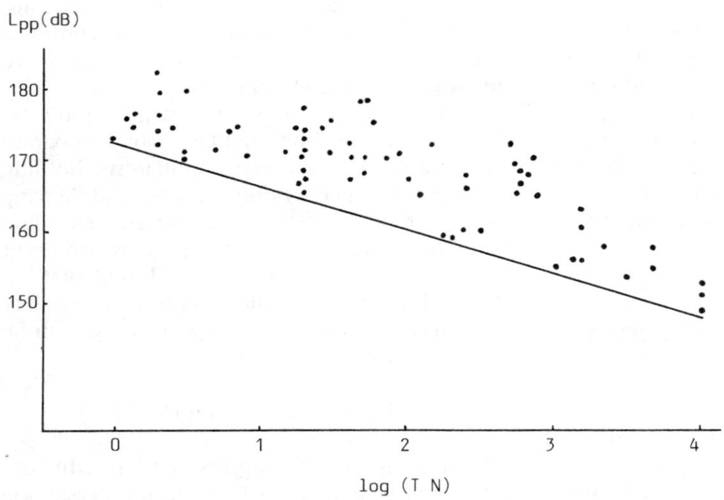

Figure 29-1 Safety margin of impulse noise for guinea pigs. Oblique line represents calculation of $L_{pp} = 172 - 6 \log (T\,N)$ in the L_{pp} versus log (T N) format. Dots represent "damaged" points of marginal or light grades (points of the more severe grades are distributed higher in position and are omitted).

TABLE 29-10 **Percentage of Protection in Exposed Personnel**

dB ABOVE CRITERION	NUMBER OF TESTED SUBJECTS	NUMBER OF "SAFE" SUBJECTS	% OF PROTECTION	EAR PROTECTOR
0.1–9.9	88	80	90.9	Not used
5.0–9.9	81	75	92.6	
11.4–15.1	37	27	73.0	
−3.0–0	138	138	100.0	Earplugs of 20 dB attenuation
0.1–3	263	248	94.3	
3.1–9.9	123	119	96.7	
0.1–9.9	386	367	95.1	

TABLE 29-11 **Examples of Exposure to Different Weapons**

SOURCE	L_{pp} (dB)	T (ms)	N	dB ABOVE CRITERION	TOTAL SUBJECTS	NUMBER OF "SAFE" SUBJECTS	% OF PROTECTION
Machine gun 12.7	175.0	3	2	5.1	45	42	93.3
Gun-howitzer 152*	179.4	>100	4	−12	34	34	100.0
Gun-howitzer 152*	181.0	>100	10	2	31	29	93.5
Cannon 85*	182.4	>100	3	0.3	29	27	93.1

*Firing in fortification; with earplugs of 20 dB attenuation

A Proposed Safety Criterion for Impulse Noise

Taking advantage of some ordinary military practices, a number of contrast experiments between men and guinea pigs were performed with the aim of comparing the damaging effect of weapon impulse noise on the human versus the guinea pig ears. From the results of these experiments it was estimated that the human tolerance to impulse noise is about 8 dB better than the guinea pig's (Liang et al, 1983b). On the basis of the empirical guinea-pig safety margin and the estimated tolerance difference between species, and leaving room to ensure safety, a human safety criterion for grazing incidence of the impulse wave can be proposed to have the form

$$L_{pp} = 177 - 6 \log (T\,N)$$

For simplicity in application, T shorter than 1 ms is taken as 1 ms, so 177 dB is the maximum allowable L_{pp} for the human ear. T longer than 100 ms is taken as 100 ms because the acoustic reflex would then be effective. After proper verification, this criterion was later accepted as the formal Chinese national standard for practical use (Liang et al, 1983b). Part of the verification data is presented in Tables 29-10 and 29-11. As shown, in all tests in which L_{pp} is in the region of the safety criterion, more than 90 percent of the exposed personnel are safe (no middle-ear damage and a complete recovery of hearing threshold shifts within 2 days).

Besides the peak pressure, the pulse duration, the number of rounds, and the inter-round interval quantitatively analyzed, there are still other parameters and factors that may influence the damaging effect of impulse noises; their roles are worthy of detailed study in well-designed and well-controlled experiments.

As a basic acoustic parameter, the spectral composition of the impulse is certainly of importance. The pulse duration or, to be precise, the waveform of the impulse may reflect its spectral properties, but only in a very general way. It is true that most impulse noises of weapon origins possess wide spectra. Significant differences, however, may exist and be effective (Price, 1986). In most of the proposed damage-risk criteria for impulse noises the spectral influence is neglected (Ward, 1968; Coles et al, 1968; Pfander et al, 1980; Liang et al, 1983). This should be understood as a necessary simplification for a military criterion to help ensure regular application.

Frequency of exposure is a factor directly

relevant to the damaging effect of an impulse noise. The proposed safety criterion now being used in the Chinese artillery is suitable when the frequency of exposure is not more than 10 occasions in 1 year with sufficient intervals in between (Liang et al, 1983b). For more-frequent exposures and for repeated exposures on successive days, the maximum allowable peak pressure should be lowered accordingly.

It is not easy to make direct comparisons between the maximum allowable peak pressures in different criteria because of their different forms. On the whole, the maximum allowable peak pressure in the Chinese criterion seems considerably higher than the Western criteria. Doubtlessly, this is not a matter of racial differences in noise tolerance. Rather, the different definitions of the threshold of safety or damage risk and ways of determining damage are responsible for the discrepancy. Take the CHABA criterion (Ward, 1968), for instance. For the same T and N values, the maximum allowable L_{pp} in this criterion is about 10 dB lower than that in the Chinese criterion. CHABA, and some others, took 10 to 20 dB temporary threshold shift (TTS_2) as the threshold of damage risk. With this amount of TTS_2, however, complete recovery of hearing usually takes place within 1 hour (Kylin, 1960; Ward et al, 1961; Loeb and Fletcher, 1968). The CHABA criterion is very conservative and may overestimate the threshold for damage. Judging from the vast amount of animal experimental data presented here, the CHABA criterion seems even too "safe" for guinea pigs, which should be less tolerant to impulse noise than human subjects.

For future consideration, scientists may have to broaden their perspective on what constitutes auditory damage. The reliance on PTS may obscure other significant changes and therefore cause them to go unnoticed. Auditory discrimination that requires the proper functioning of integrating centers may be a measure of central auditory involvement. Prolonged gap detection thresholds in chinchillas after noise exposure have been reported by Salvi et al (1986). Study of systematic changes in difference limens for frequency, for intensity, and for phase in guinea pigs after exposure to impulse noise is now in procession in the Shanghai laboratory. Preliminary results show that these changes as well as the hearing threshold shift do not run parallel, suggesting that the central involvement is by no means simple.

Exposure to steady and impulse noise of appropriate parameters may call forth a phenomenon known as neural facilitation in the brain cortices manifesting as a drastic augmentation of the evoked potentials, marked increase of neuronal discharge rate, and significant lowering of the frequency difference limens (Liang et al, 1982; Gerken et al, 1986; Shao et al, 1988, 1990). This is another interesting aspect of the central involvement in noise hazard.

Relations Paramétriques entre Bruits Impulsionnels et Deficits Auditifs

Pour déterminer l'effet lésionnel des bruits d'armes sur le système auditif, les paramètres essentiels sont la surpression de crête L_p, la durée de l'impulsion T et le nombre de coups N. Sur la base d'études audiométriques portant sur un peu plus de 2000 cobayes exposés dans diverses conditions à des bruits impulsionnels provenant de différents types d'armes, une limite de sécurité valable pour une exposition et pour le cobaye a été formulée comme suit:

$$L_p = 172 - 6 \log(TN)$$

où L_p est exprimé en dB re 0,00002 Pa (incidence rasante), T en ms (les valeurs inférieures à 1 ms étant considérées comme égales à 1 ms), N le nombre de coups sur une journée d'exposition. Lors de l'analyse des données expérimentales, la gravité des lésions est quantifiée selon les classes suivantes: inoffensive, limite, faible, modérée et sévère, en fonction de la variation du seuil d'audition et de la pathologie de l'oreille moyenne. Il apparaît que pour chaque incrément de 3 ou 4 dB de L_p, ou pour toute modification de T ou de N d'un facteur 3 à 5, la gravité lésionnelle augmente d'environ une classe. Ainsi, un dépassement de L_p de 15 dB par rapport à la limite de sécurité, ou un incrément équivalent de NT, risquent d'induire une lésion auditive très sévère.

La destruction de l'oreille moyenne dépend essentiellement de L_p alors que les variations de TN affectent surtout la cochlée. Sous certaines conditions, la destruction du mécanisme de transmission de l'oreille moyenne par quelques premières impulsions peut, d'une manière ou d'une autre, amortir les "coups de fouet" des ondes de choc suivantes au niveau de la cochlée, réduisant ainsi l'effet lésionnel sur cette dernière. Ainsi, il peut arriver dans des cas exceptionnels de tirs répétitifs, qu'un

L_p plus important provoque des lésions auditives globales plus faibles.

La tolérance de l'oreille humaine a été estimée supérieure de 5 dB à celle du cobaye. En élevant la limite de sécurité initiale du cobaye de 172 dB à 177 dB, un critère de sécurité formel pour les bruits d'armes a été proposé pour l'utilisation en milieu militaire en Chine. Des résultats vérifiant la fiabilité de ce critère par la protection de plus de 90% du personnel exposé, seront présentés.

Le spectre de l'impulsion, la polarité du pic principal, l'intervalle entre les salves et la fréquence d'exposition sont également des facteurs significatifs. La réduction de la discrimination auditive consécutive à l'exposition n'est pas en relation directe avec le déplacement du seuil d'audition, ce qui suggère l'existence d'effets induits par le bruit dans les centres auditifs. L'exposition à des impulsions de paramètres appropriés peut provoquer un phénomène connu sous le nom de "facilitation" neurale dans le cortex cérébral qui se traduit par une augmentation importante des potentiels évoqués, une augmentation marquée du rythme des décharges neuronales et une diminution significative de la discrimination fréquencielle.

References

Atherley GRC, Martin AM. Equivalent continuous noise level as a measure of injury from impact and impulse noise. Ann Occup Hyg 1971; 14:11-28.

Coles RRA, Garinther GR, Hodge DC, Rice CG. Hazardous exposure to impulse noise. J Acoust Soc Am 1968; 43:336-343.

Gerken GM, Simhadri-Sumithra R, Bhat KH. Increase in central auditory responsiveness during continuous tone stimulation or following hearing loss. In: Salvi RJ et al, eds. Basic and applied aspects of noise-induced hearing loss. New York: Plenum Press, 1986:159.

Hamernik RP, Patterson JH, Salvi RJ. The effect of impulse intensity and number of impulses on hearing and cochlear pathology in the chinchilla. J Acoust Soc Am 1987; 81:1118-1129.

Henderson D, Hamernik RP. Impulse noise: Critical review. J Acoust Soc Am 1986; 80:569-584.

Kryter KD, Garinther GR. Auditory effect of acoustic impulses from firearms. Acta Otolaryngol Suppl 1965; 221:1-22.

Kylin B. Temporary threshold shift and auditory trauma following steady-state noise. Acta Otolaryngol Suppl 1960; 152:51-56.

Liang Zhi-an, Feng Juming, Qiang Yuhao. Augmentation of evoked potentials from the guinea pig auditory cortex after exposure to intensive noise. Chin J Acoust 1982; 1:190-197.

Liang Zhi-an, Feng Juming, Yang Qionghua. Damaging effect of pressure wave on the auditory organ: I. Sites and features of damage. II. Condition of damage in relation to pressure wave parameters. Acta Physiol Sinica 1983a; 33:369-387.

Liang Zhi-an, Feng Juming, Meng Zhaohui, et al. Safety criterion for pressure waves. Chin J Acoust 1983b; 2:158-164.

Liang Zhi-an. Laws governing the damage of the auditory system by impulse noise of weapon origin. Proc Inter-Noise 1987; 87:1061-1064.

Loeb M, Fletcher JL. Impulse duration and temporary threshold shift. J Acoust Soc Am 1968; 44:1524-1528.

Meng Zhaohui, Cheng Mingkun, Shen Hao. Injury to the middle ear due to high intensity sound. Proc Inter-Noise 1987; 87:925-928.

Morest DK, Bohne BA. Noise-induced degeneration in the brain and representation of the inner and outer hair cells. Hear Res 1983; 9:145-154.

Patterson JH Jr, Lomba-Gautier IM, Curd DL, et al. The role of peak pressure in determining the auditory hazard of impulse noise. In: Salvi RJ et al, eds. Basic and applied aspects of noise-induced hearing loss. New York: Plenum Press, 1986:405.

Pfander F, Bongartz H, Brinkmann H, Kietz H. Danger of auditory impairment from impulse noise: A comparative study of the CHABA damage-risk criteria and those of the Federal Republic of Germany. J Acoust Soc Am 1980; 67:628-633.

Price GR. Impulse noise hazard as a function of level and spectral distribution. In: Salvi RJ et al, eds. Basic and applied aspects of noise-induced hearing loss. New York: Plenum Press, 1986:379.

Rice CG, Martin AM. Impulse noise damage risk criteria. J Sound Vibrat 1973; 28:359-367.

Roberto M, Hamernik RP, Salvi RJ, et al. Impact noise and the equal energy hypothesis. J Acoust Soc Am 1985; 77:1514-1520.

Salvi RJ, Saunders SS, Ahroon WA, et al. Psychological and physiological aspects of auditory temporal processing in listeners with noise-induced sensorineural hearing loss. In: Salvi RJ et al, eds. Basic and applied aspects of noise-induced hearing loss. New York: Plenum Press, 1986:179.

Shao Dianhua, Lin Huaying, Liang Zhi-an. Noise-induced neural facilitation in the brain cortices. Appl Acoust 1988; 25:131-138.

Shao Dianhua, Liang Zhi-an. Noise-induced neuronal activation in the monkey cortex. Chin J Physiol Sci 1990; 6:358-361.

Ward WD. Proposed damage-risk criterion for impulse noise (gunfire). Report of Working Group 57, NAS-NRC CHABA, 1968.

Ward WD, Selter W, Glorig A. Exploratory studies on temporary threshold shift from impulses. J Acoust Soc Am 1961; 33:781-793.

CHAPTER 30

An Experimental Basis for the Estimation of Auditory System Hazard Following Exposure to Impulse Noise

JAMES H. PATTERSON, JR.
ROGER P. HAMERNIK

There are a number of different suggested standards for exposure to impulse/impact noise (Coles et al, 1968; OSHA, Dept of Labor, 1974; Smoorenburg, 1982; Pfander et al, 1980). Although each of these criteria has its proponents, none of them is in complete agreement with existing data (Smoorenburg, 1987). What is needed is a new criterion. Unfortunately, there is an extremely limited empirical database on which a new standard can be built. The difficulties associated with generating such a database are compounded by the extremely broad range of high-intensity noise transients that exist in various industrial and military environments. For example, in industry, impacts with variable peak intensities and a reverberant character often occur. At the other extreme, the diverse military weapon systems produce impulses that originate as the result of a process of shock-wave formation and propagation following an explosive release of energy. These waves, which can have peak levels in excess of 180 dB, can be either reverberant or nonreverberant, depending on the environment in which they are encountered. Trying to develop a single standard to cover this broad range of "acoustic" signals is a formidable task.

Existing or proposed exposure criteria generally lack specific consideration of the frequency domain representation of the impulse. This point has been raised frequently by Price (1979) and others. However, some deference is given to the spectrum in these criteria, in an indirect manner, through the handling of the A and B duration variables.

A more direct spectral approach to the evaluation of impulses and impacts was proposed by Kryter (1970). His suggestions, although based on sound reasoning, never gained acceptance. The Kryter approach was attractive in its ability to predict the amount of temporary threshold shift measured 2 minutes after exposure (TTS_2) to a noise transient. However, this approach was limited to situations in which the TTS_2 was not excessively large or, alternatively, the levels of the transient in any given frequency band were not excessive.

Price (1979, 1983, 1986) has built on and extended the Kryter approach by considering the spectral transmission characteristics of the peripheral auditory system. Price's reasoning led to the following conclusions: (1) There is a species-specific frequency, f_o, at which the cochlea is most vulnerable and that impulses whose spectrum peaks at f_o will be most damaging. This would appear to be true, according to Price, regardless of the distribution of energy above and below f_o. For man, the suggested frequency is 3.0 kHz; and (2) Relative to the threshold for damage at f_o, the threshold for damage should rise at 6 dB per octave when f_p is greater than f_o and at 18 dB per octave when f_p is less than f_o, where f_p is spectral peak of the impulse. Thus, a model for permanent damage was developed that is amenable to experimental testing. In subsequent studies, Price (1983, 1986) has tried to relate, with varying degrees of success, experimental data obtained from the cat to the predictions of this model. More recently, Hamernik et al

(1990) and Patterson et al (1991) have reported on an extensive series of parametric studies in which the spectra of the impulses were varied. A review of the literature indicates that, except for the studies mentioned above, there are few other published results obtained from experiments specifically designed to study the effects of the spectrum of an impulse on hearing trauma.

This chapter presents an analysis of the Patterson et al (1991) data from which a spectral weighting function is derived. This weighting function will then be applied to the blast wave data of Hamernik et al (1990) and to the synthetic impulses from Patterson et al (1986) in order to develop a relation between the permanent threshold shift (PTS) and the sound exposure level (SEL). The intention here is not to present a set of conclusive results, but rather to illustrate a new approach to the analysis of this type of experimental data. It is an approach that develops a direct relation between frequency-specific measures of PTS and the frequency domain representation of the impulse. The results of this approach can be related directly to the Price (1983) model and can be used to estimate the permanent effects of a traumatic impulse noise exposure in a manner similar to that approach proposed by Kryter (1970) for estimating temporary threshold shift (TTS) after an impulse noise exposure.

TABLE 30-1 **Exposure Conditions for the 20 Groups of Animals Used for Series I Exposures**

CF (Hz)	PEAK SPL (dB)	TOTAL SEL (dB)
260	139	132.5
260	146	139.8
775	134	124.8
775	139	129.4
775	144	134.8
1025	129	119.8
1025	134	124.2
1025	139	129.1
1025	144	134.6
1350	129	119.8
1350	134	124.2
1350	139	129.0
2450	129	120.6
2450	134	124.9
2450	139	129.6
2450	144	135.0
3550	124	113.0
3550	129	119.9
3550	134	124.2
3550	139	129.5

Methods

The noise-induced permanent threshold shift (NIPTS) data presented in this report were acquired from 475 chinchillas exposed to high levels of impulse noise. Audiometric data on each animal were obtained using either a shock avoidance procedure (Patterson et al, 1986) or measures of the auditory evoked potential (Henderson et al, 1983). Permanent threshold shifts were computed from the mean of three preexposure audiograms and at least three audiograms taken 30 days after exposure. The behaviorally trained animals were tested at octave intervals from 0.125 kHz through 8 kHz including the half-octave points 1.4, 2.8, and 5.7 kHz. Evoked potential thresholds were measured at octave intervals from 0.5 to 16 kHz and at the 11.2-kHz point. For each animal, measures of compound threshold shift, PTS, and quantitative histology (cochleograms) were obtained. In the analysis that follows, only PTS data will be discussed.

Series I Exposures (N = 118)

Animals were exposed at a normal incidence (i.e., the plane of the external canal was parallel to the speaker exit plane) to 100 impulses presented at the rate of 1 every 3 seconds. This series of exposures consisted of 20 groups of animals, with five to seven animals per group. The stimuli were narrow-band impulses produced by passing a digital impulse through a four-pole Learner-type digital bandpass filter (Gold and Rader, 1969). Following analog conversion, the signal was transduced through an Altex 515 B speaker in a model 815 enclosure. The filter bandwidth was independent of center frequency, with steep attenuation outside the passband permitting the synthesis of equal energy impulses at a variety of center frequencies while assuring minimal spread of energy to other frequencies. The center frequencies of the six sets of impulses varied from 260 to 3,350 Hz. The bandwidth of the impulses was approximately 400 Hz. Impulse peaks were varied from 124 to 146 dB. For each of the exposure conditions listed in Table 30-1 the total SEL was computed as follows (Young, 1970):

$$\mathrm{SEL} = 10 \log_{10} \int_{-\infty}^{\infty} \frac{p^2(t)dt}{p_r^{\,2}\, t_r}$$

where $t_r = 1$ second, $p_r = 20\ \mu\mathrm{Pa}$. Figure 30-1 illustrates an example of the pressure-time his-

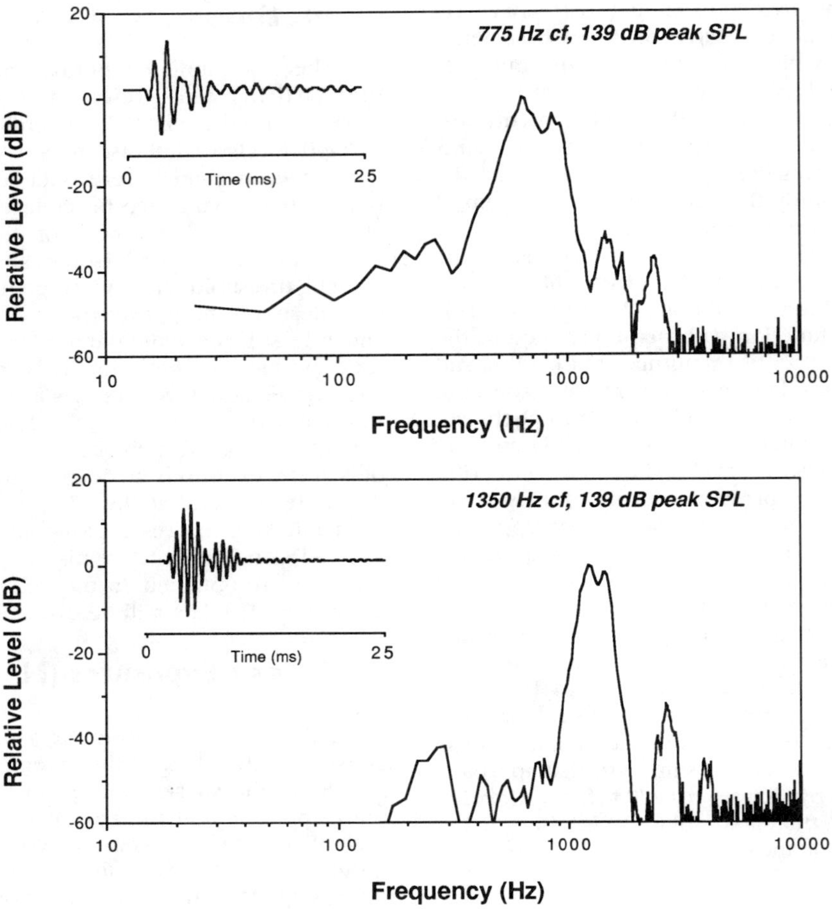

Figure 30-1 Examples of the 775-Hz *(A)* and 1,350-Hz *(B)* center frequency impulses of the Series I exposures along with their respective spectra.

TABLE 30-2 **Exposure Conditions for the Seven Groups Used for Series II Exposures**

WAVE TYPE	PEAK SPL (dB)	TOTAL SEL (dB)	TOTAL P-SEL (dB)	TOTAL P′-SEL (dB)
High Peak	147	130.8	127.6	133.4
Low Peak	139	130.3	127.2	132.9
High Peak	139	123.0	119.9	125.6
Low Peak	131	122.4	119.3	125.0
High Peak	135	119.1	115.8	121.6
Low Peak	127	118.5	115.3	121.0
High Peak	131	115.1	111.9	117.5

tories of the 775-Hz and 1,350-Hz center frequency impulses along with their respective spectra.

Series II Exposures (N = 42)

Animals were exposed at a normal incidence to 100 impulses presented at the rate of 1 every 3 seconds. There were seven different exposure conditions (Table 30-2) to which seven groups of animals were exposed. Each group contained six animals. Two types (low peak and high peak) of relatively broad-band impulses with identically-shaped amplitude spectra were synthesized digitally (Patterson et al, 1986). The peak sound pressure level (SPL) of the impulses was varied from 127 to

147 dB. Hearing threshold data were obtained using the avoidance conditioning procedure. Figure 30-2 illustrates the pressure-time histories of typical high- and low-peak impulses along with their common spectrum.

Series III Exposures (N = 315)

Animals were exposed at a normal incidence to either 1, 10, or 100 impulses, presented at the rate of or 1 every 10 seconds at intensities of 150, 155, or 160 dB peak SPL. All of the above combinations of number, repetition rate, and peak yielded 21 different exposure groups with five animals per group. The impulses were generated by a compressed-air-driven shock tube. This set of 21 exposures was repeated using waves generated by three shock tubes of different diameters that produced blast waves whose spectrum peaked at three different locations of the audible spectrum. The pressure-time traces and spectral analysis of these waveforms are shown in Figure 30-3. In addition, the A-weighted octave band energies are shown in Figure 30-4 so that comparisons could be made for each wave from each source. Because of the high levels of very-low-frequency energy in these blast waves, the resolution at the high frequencies is poor if unweighted energies are plotted. For further details see Hamernik and Hsueh (1990). Table 30-3 summarizes the conditions for the Series III exposures. Only the SELs for the 100-impulse conditions are tabulated. Successive 10-dB adjustments need to be made to obtain the 10-impulse and the 1-impulse SEL values. All animals in this series were tested using the auditory evoked potential procedures.

Results

The results of each series of exposures are presented separately, and the methods used to analyze the NIPTS data from each series are explained.

Series I Exposures

For each of the 20 groups of animals that were exposed to the narrow-band impulses, a mean PTS evaluated at 1, 2, and 4 kHz ($\overline{PTS}_{1,2,4}$) was computed, and the groups were compared on the basis of SEL. This data set is shown in Figure 30-5. The group mean PTS from each set of the two to four groups of animals that make up an intensity series for a specific characteristic frequency (CF) impulse behaves in an orderly manner, with $\overline{PTS}_{1,2,4}$ increasing in an approximately linear fashion with increasing SEL.

The relative susceptibility to NIPTS is seen to be a function of the impulse center frequency, with the lower-frequency impulses producing relatively little NIPTS even at the higher SELs. A relative frequency weighting function can be derived from the data presented in Figure 30-5 by shifting each frequency-specific data set along the SEL axis the amount that is necessary to collapse the data into a single PTS/SEL function using one of the exposures as a "zero" reference.

Such a data-shifting process was carried out "by eye" to produce a best fit using the 1,350-Hz series of data as the reference point. The amounts shifted were 260-Hz CF impulses, −20 dB; 775-Hz CF impulses, −7.2 dB; 1,025-Hz CF impulses, −4 dB; 1,350-Hz CF impulses, 0 dB; 2,450-Hz CF impulses, −4 dB; and 3,550-Hz CF impulses, +4 dB. The realignment of the data that such a shift produces is shown in Figure 30-6, and the weighting function, thus obtained, is shown plotted (solid line with symbols) in Figure 30-7, where it is compared to the conventional A-weighting function (solid line). The new empirical weighting function is referred to as P-weighting in the legends for these figures. A linear regression through the shifted data set showed a correlation coefficient of 0.89 with a slope of 2.6 dB PTS per decibel P-weighted SEL (P-SEL) and a threshold for the onset of $\overline{PTS}_{1,2,4}$ of 116 dB P-SEL. The empirical function derived from the narrow-band impulse data is seen to differ from the A-weighting function by as much as 10 dB at the low frequencies. Also evident in this figure is the anomalous behavior of the data point produced by the exposures to the 2,450-Hz, CF impulses.

Series II Exposures

The detailed histologic and audiometric results of this series of exposures have been published by Patterson et al (1985, 1986). The $\overline{PTS}_{1,2,4}$ data from this series of seven exposures is shown plotted as a function of the SEL and the P-SEL in Figure 30-8. The latter was obtained by applying the empirical weighting function (Fig. 30-7) to consecutive octave bands of the spectrum of the Series II exposures. Also included in this figure are the shifted (or P-weighted) data points from the

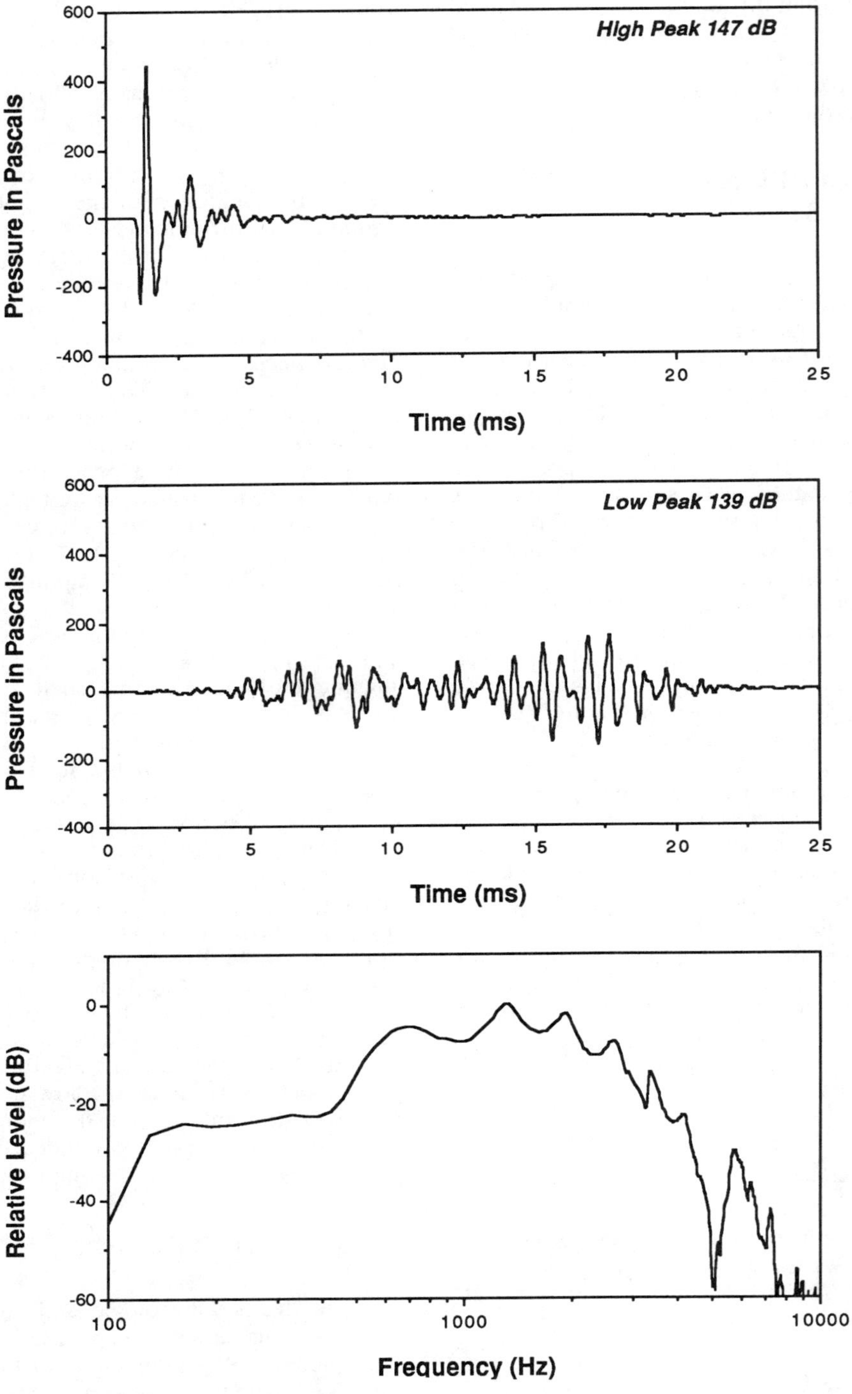

Figure 30-2 Examples of the Series II impulses and their common spectrum. *A,* The high-peaked 147-dB peak SPL impulse. *B,* The low-peaked 139-dB impulse. *C,* The spectrum of each of the above, approximately equal-energy, impulses.

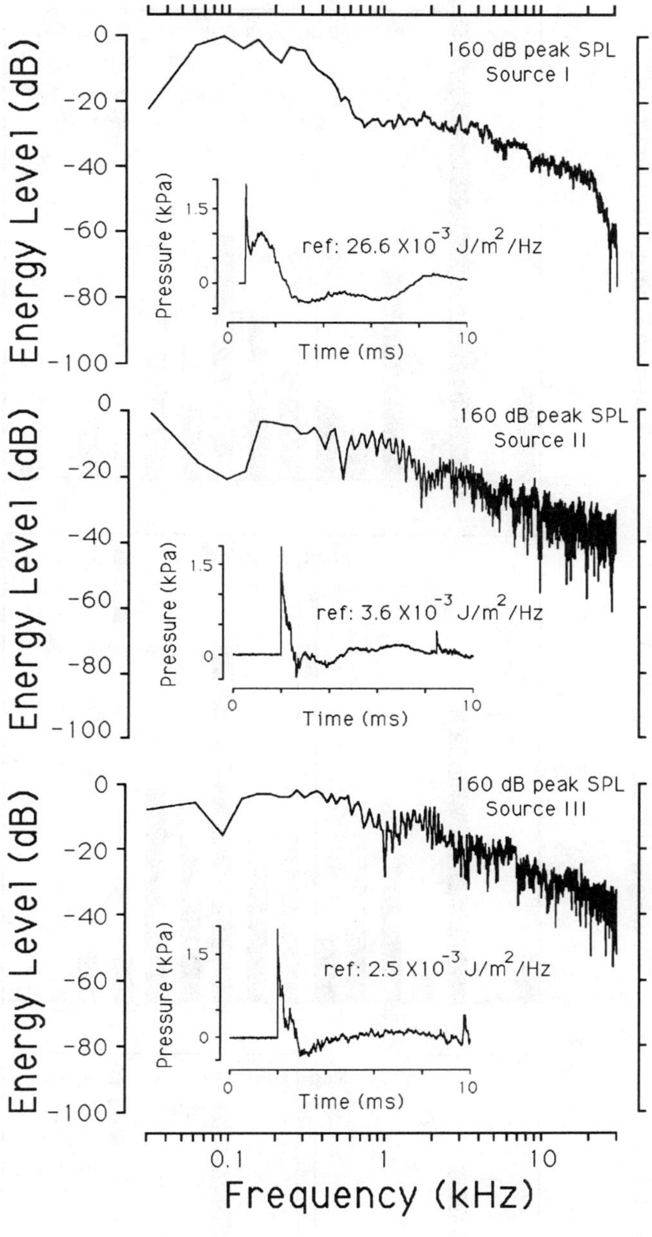

Figure 30-3 Examples of the 160-dB peak SPL impulses produced by the three different shock tubes and their respective spectra. These waves are typical of those used for the Series III exposures.

Series I exposures. It is evident that the P-weighting function does not have the desired effect of increasing the degree of congruence between the Series I and II exposures. Because the Series II exposures had substantial energy in the 2-kHz region of the spectrum, it was apparent that the effect of applying the empirical weighting function to this region of the spectrum would shift the Series II data points in the wrong direction. However, if the empirical P-weighting function is extrapolated as shown by the dotted portion of the function in Figure 30-7, and then used to weight the Series II impulses, the agreement between the Series I and Series II data becomes good, as seen in Figure 30-9. A linear regression analysis (solid line) of the entire data set from the Series I and Series II exposures shows a correlation coefficient of 0.91, a slope of 2.5, and an X-intercept of 116 dB. This modified weighting function is referred to as P′-weighting.

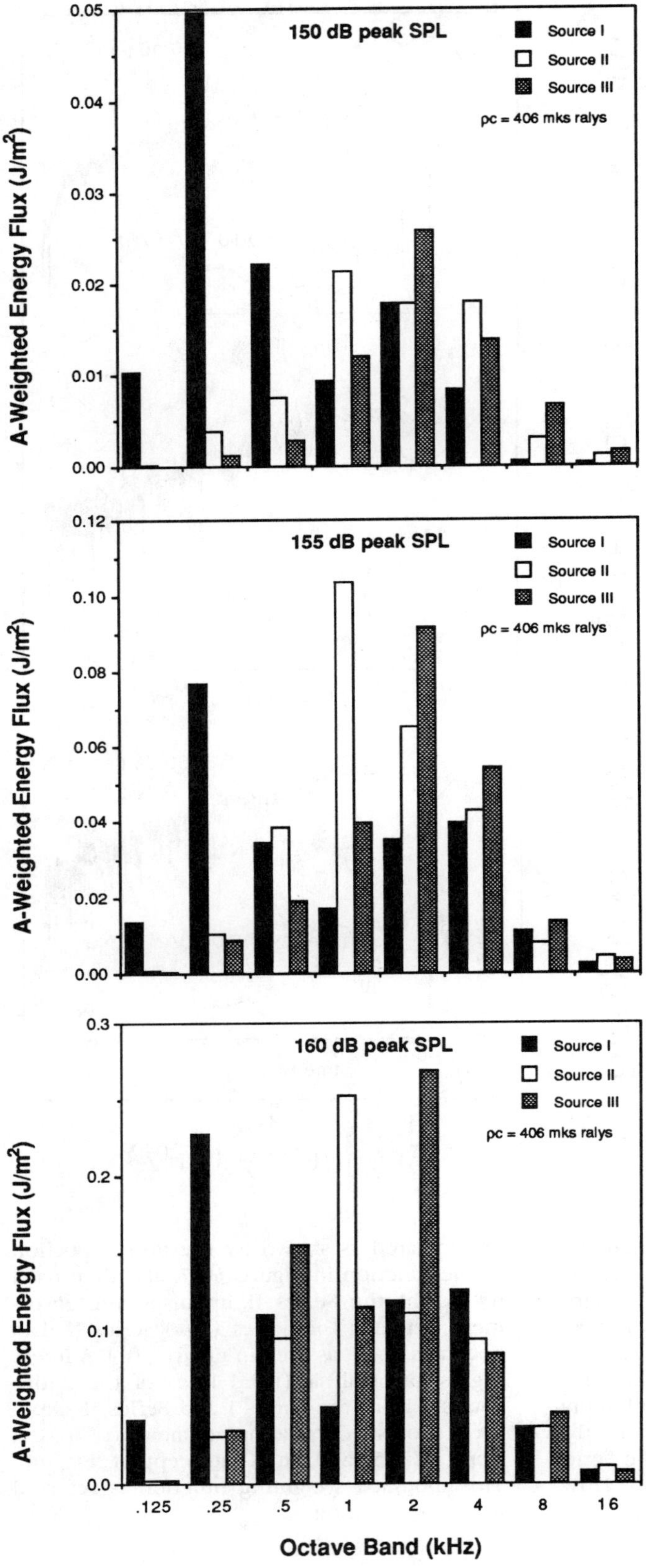

Figure 30-4 A-weighted octave band spectra of each of the waves that were used for the Series III exposures.

TABLE 30-3 **Exposure Conditions for the Nine Groups Used for 100-Impulse Series III Exposures***

SOURCE	PEAK SPL (dB)	TOTAL SEL (dB)	TOTAL P′-SEL (dB)
I	150	140.3	129.2
I	155	141.8	133.6
I	160	146.4	138.8
II	150	131.4	130.3
II	155	136.5	135.3
II	160	140.6	138.6
III	150	129.0	130.8
III	155	135.0	136.2
III	160	139.1	139.9

*Corresponding SEL and P′-SEL values for the 10-impulse and 1-impulse conditions can be obtained by making the appropriate 10-dB adjustments.

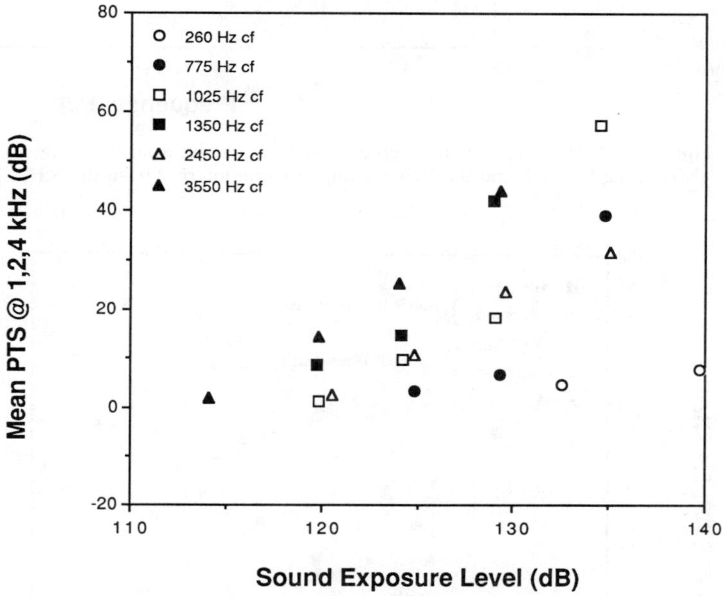

Figure 30-5 The group mean permanent threshold shift (PTS) evaluated at 1, 2, and 4 kHz ($\overline{PTS}_{1,2,4}$) as a function of the total sound exposure level for the six groups exposed to the Series I narrow-band impulses.

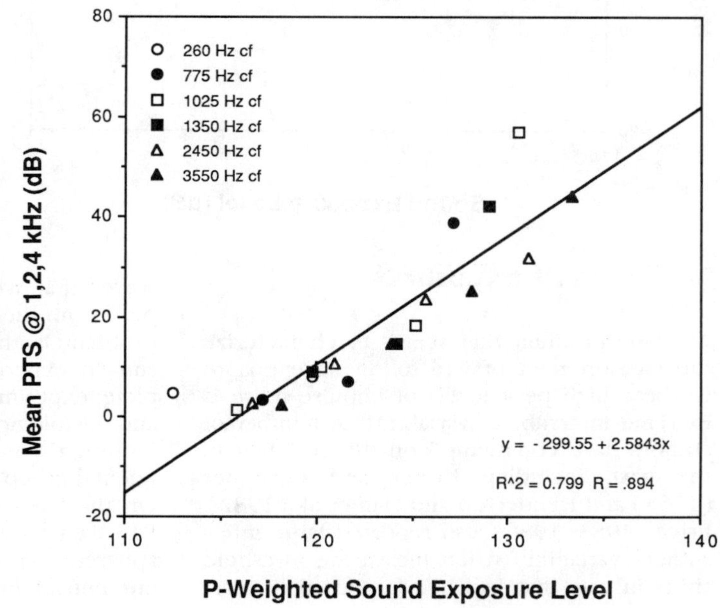

Figure 30-6 The permanent threshold shift at 1, 2, and 4 kHz ($\overline{PTS}_{1,2,4}$) as a function of the empirically-derived P-weighted sound exposure level for all the Series I exposures. The regression line has a slope of 2.6 and an X-intercept of 116 dB.

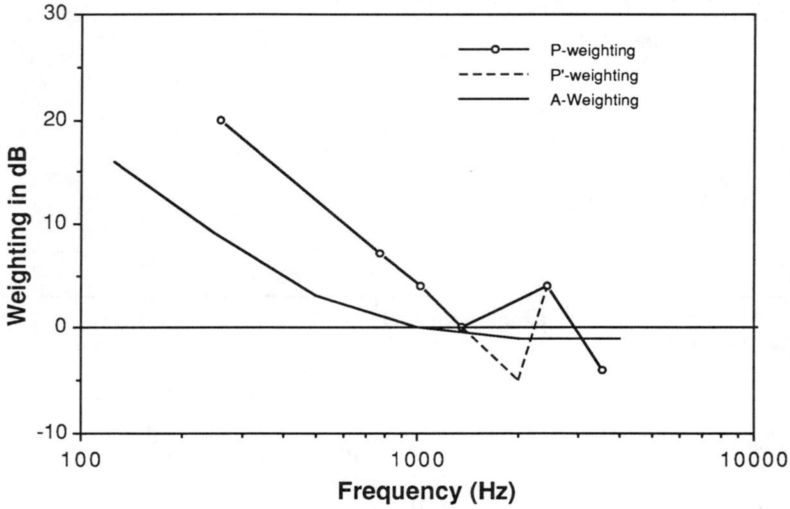

Figure 30-7 The empirical P-weighting function derived from the Series I exposures along with the conventional A-weighting function and the P′-weighting function inferred from the Series II and III experiments.

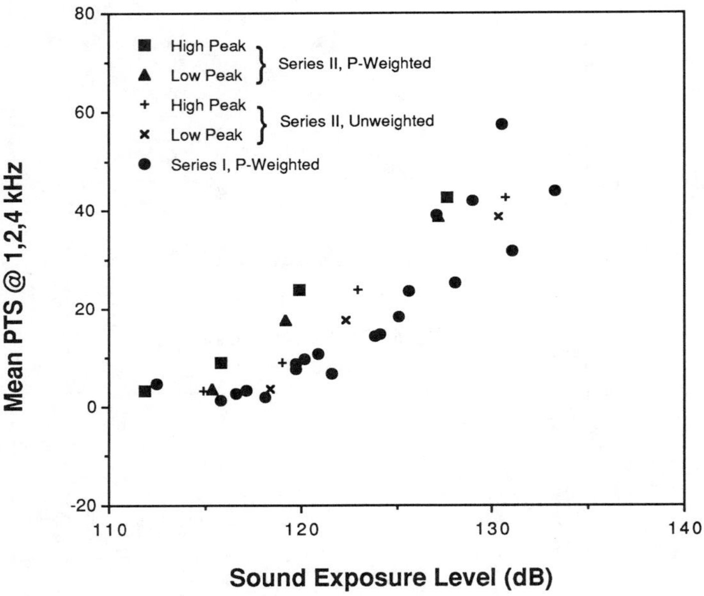

Figure 30-8 The permanent threshold shift at 1, 2, and 4 kHz ($\overline{PTS}_{1,2,4}$) from the Series II exposures shown as a function of unweighted and P-weighted sound exposure level compared to the $\overline{PTS}_{1,2,4}$ versus P-weighted sound exposure level of the Series I exposures.

Series III Exposures

One problem that seems to characterize the measurement of PTS following exposure to these high peak levels of impulse noise is extreme intersubject variability. A number of authors have commented on this problem in the past, including Kryter and Garinther (1965) and Henderson and Hamernik (1982). Price (1983, 1986) also reported large intersubject variability when measuring threshold shifts in cats that had been exposed to blast waves that were similar to some of the impulses in the Series III exposures. Another problem is the excessive time necessary to run an experimental animal through a complete experimental paradigm of audiometric and histologic protocols, thereby effectively limiting the number of animals in each experimental group and hence the statistical power. On the basis of a preliminary analysis of the PTS data (using analysis of variance), it was apparent that the effects on PTS of the different impact presentation rates were, at best,

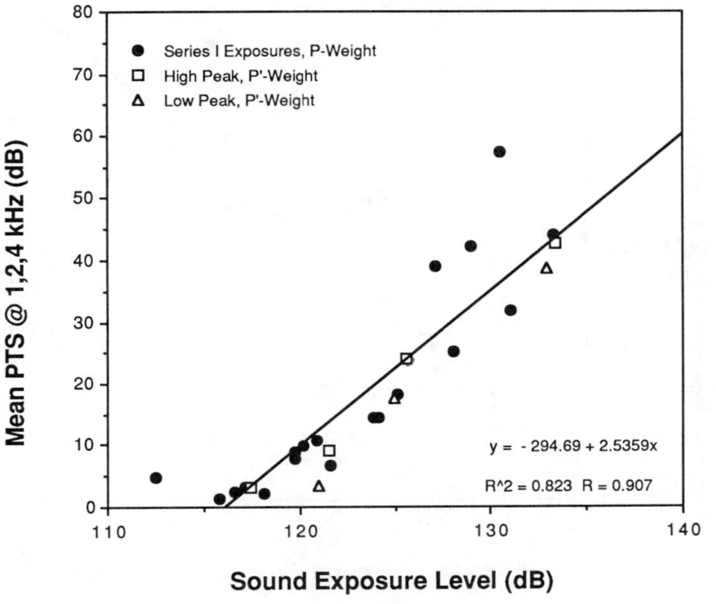

Figure 30-9 Permanent threshold shift at 1, 2, and 4 kHz ($\overline{\text{PTS}}_{1,2,4}$) obtained from the Series I and Series II exposures as a function of P- and P′-weighted sound exposure levels, respectively. The linear regression line was computed using all the points shown plotted in this figure. X-intercept = 116 dB; slope = 2.5.

marginal statistical effects. Thus, a decision was made to evaluate all the PTS data without regard for presentation rate. Also, because relations between PTS and the increasing energy of the stimulus were being sought, presentation rate did not affect the independent variable. This effectively increased the number of animals at each SEL to 15 except for the 1-impulse exposure conditions. Total sound exposure or exposure level is increased by increasing the peak SPL or the number of impulse presentations.

For each audiometric test frequency, the individual animal PTS at that frequency was plotted as a function of the total unweighted SEL in the octave band centered on that test frequency. Two examples of this analysis at 2 kHz and 4 kHz for Source II are shown in Figure 30-10. For impact Sources I, II, and III, 105 individual data points for each source at each audiometric test frequency were plotted over a range of SELs of approximately 30 dB. The actual number of data points in each panel of Figure 30-10 is less than 105, because a number of animals had the same data coordinate. Using data sets such as those shown in Figure 30-10, the 90th percentile hearing loss (PTS_{90}) was computed for each SEL at each octave frequency from 0.5 to 16 kHz. The PTS_{90} at any frequency was computed as follows:

$$PTS_{90} = \overline{x} + st_{.10}$$

where x is the group mean PTS; $t_{.10}$ is the value of t below which 90 percent of the PTS

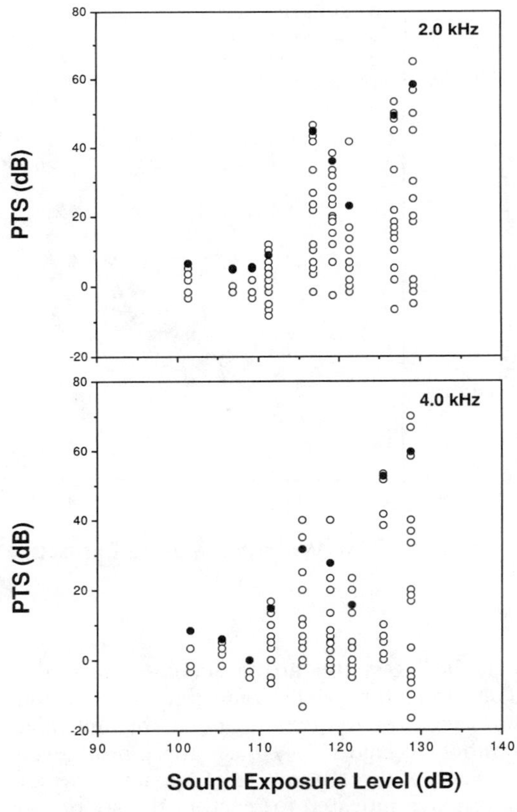

Figure 30-10 Two examples that illustrate the individual animal permanent threshold shift (PTS) values at 2 and 4 kHz following the Series III exposures to Source II. The solid symbols represent the 90th percentile values of the PTS at the various exposure energies.

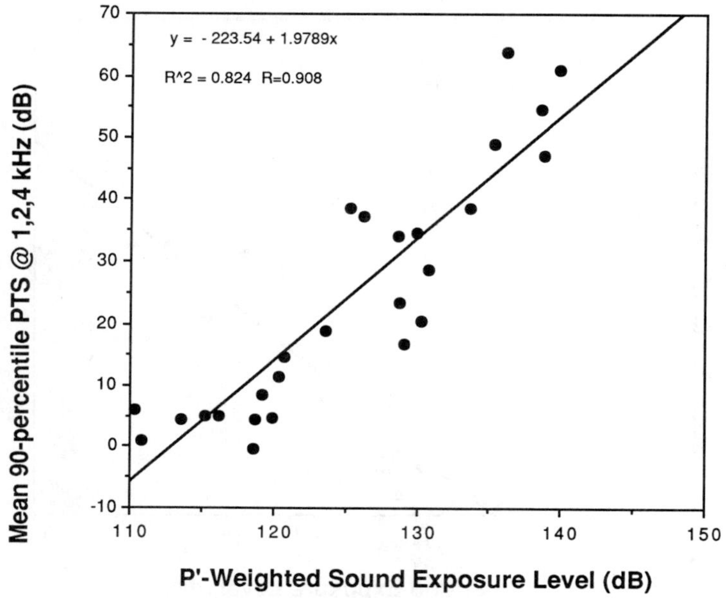

Figure 30-11 The mean of the 90th percentile permanent threshold shift (PTS) measured at 1, 2, and 4 kHz for all of the groups exposed to the Series III impulses as a function of the P′-weighted sound exposure level. A linear regression analysis (solid line) yields a slope of approximately 2.0 and an X-intercept of 113 dB.

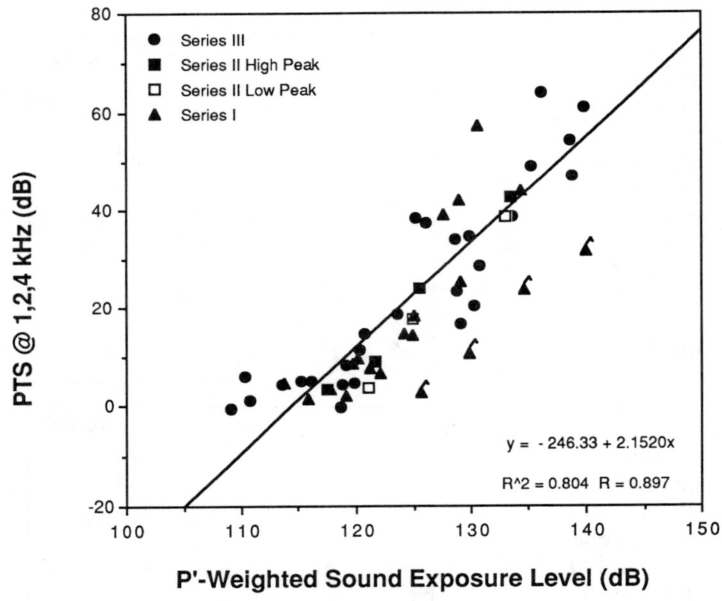

Figure 30-12 The mean permanent threshold shift (PTS) produced by exposures to the Series I, II, and III impulses as a function of the P′-weighted sound exposure level. The equation for the linear regression line (solid line) is also given.

data lies; s is the group standard deviation. This procedure yields nine percentile points for each test frequency, shown by the filled symbols in Figure 30-10, i.e., three peak levels for each of three numbers of impacts. This exercise was repeated for each of the six octave test frequencies and for each of the three sources.

From this set of frequency-specific 90th percentile points, a 90th percentile $\overline{PTS}_{1,2,4}$ was computed for each exposure group and plotted as a function of the P′-weighted SELs (P′-SELs). These results are shown in Figure 30-11. The P′-weighting has the effect of collapsing all the shock tube data into a reasonably cohesive pattern for which a linear regression produces a relation between $\overline{PTS}_{1,2,4}$ and P′-SEL whose correlation coefficient is

0.91. A threshold for the onset of $\overline{\text{PTS}}_{1,2,4}$ of 113 dB SEL and a slope of approximately 2 dB $\overline{\text{PTS}}_{1,2,4}$ for each decibel of P′-SEL describes the equation of this regression line.

Figure 30-12 shows the entire data set from the Series I, II, and III exposures plotted as a function of the P′-SEL. As a first approximation the P′-weighting function has the desired effect of unifying the PTS/SEL relation following a diverse series of impulse noise exposures. The correlation coefficient between the PTS and weighted SEL variables is approximately 0.9.

Conclusion

We have presented a preliminary analysis of a large experimental database obtained from 475 chinchillas that were exposed to a variety of impulse/blast wave noise transients. This analysis, although encouraging in its ability to unify the PTS data, is considered preliminary because only a portion of the data that will eventually be available have been analyzed. In addition to the results presented, the following data sets will ultimately be entered into the database for a final analysis: (1) nonreverberant, high-frequency, Series III–type impulses (N = 105); (2) a more detailed exploration of the 1- to 8-kHz region of the empirical weighting function using the Series I narrow-band impulses (N = 50); (3) highly-reverberant Series III–type impulses (N = 300); and (4) all sensory cell loss data from the above exposures.

The surprising order that is imposed on the PTS data by the P′-weighting function is encouraging and tends to lend some validity to the methods used in the analysis, i.e., the organization of group mean data averaged over several frequencies and, in the Series III exposures, the use of a 90th percentile PTS. The analysis presented would indicate that despite the problems and inconsistencies in some of the data obtained from high-level impulse noise that have been described in the literature, the use of large samples and the systematic variation of exposure conditions can yield a database that reflects some underlying order and can be useful in developing exposure criteria. These data have shown that using electroacoustic methods and narrow-band impulses, a weighting function appropriate for high-level blast waves can be established. This weighting function also may be appropriate for use in the evaluation of industrial impact noise data.

The empirical P′-weighting function presented in Figure 30-7 has a low-frequency segment (i.e., below 1.5 kHz) with a slope of approximately 10 dB per octave, which is greater than the low-frequency slope of either the A-weighting function or the "relative susceptibility" curve presented by Price (1983). This indicates a much smaller hazard from the lower-frequency components of the impulse noise spectrum than previously believed. Above 1.5 kHz the A-weighting function is relatively flat, whereas the Price susceptibility curve rises monotonically at about 18 dB per octave above 3 kHz. The P′-weighting curve provides no evidence relevant to this part of the spectrum. The unusual feature of the empirical P′-weighting function is the 2,450-Hz point. When the weighting indicated by this point is applied to the 2-kHz octave band energy of the impulse of the Series II or Series III data, the effect is to decrease the correlation coefficient between the $\overline{\text{PTS}}_{1,2,4}$ and the P-SEL. (The actual weighting used at the 2-kHz octave band is the value obtained by linear interpolation between the 1,350-Hz and 2,450-Hz data points.) Although the 2,450-Hz point appears to be inconsistent with the rest of the P′-weighting function, it should be noted that this point is the result of a consistent set of data that was obtained from four different exposure groups (N = 24). If, however, the P′-weighting function is used—i.e., an attenuation factor of −5 dB is applied to the 2-kHz octave band energy of the Series II and Series III impulses—the correlation coefficient between $\overline{\text{PTS}}_{1,2,4}$ and the weighted exposure level increases to more than 0.9 (see Figures 30-9 and 30-11). This result seems to indicate that the appropriate weighting function to be applied to an impulse spectrum is not a simple monotonic function, as implied by A-weighting or the Price susceptibility curve, but rather a more complex function (at least in the chinchilla) at frequencies above approximately 1 kHz. The data of von Bismarck (1967) on the external ear transfer function and the multifrequency impedance data of Henderson (personal communication), along with the intracochlear pressure measurements of Patterson et al (1988), would indicate that such nonmonotonic behavior is to be expected.

In conclusion, if a suitable weighting function can be established empirically it could then be applied to the spectrum of an impulse to develop an energy-based approach to the establishment of criteria for exposure to a wide variety of noise transients.

Bases Expérimentales Relatives à l'Estimation des Risques de l'Exposition aux Bruits Impulsionnels

L'analyse des résultats de deux séries expérimentales portant sur l'exposition à deux types de bruits impulsionnels très différents est présentée. Les valeurs sont basées sur des résultats obtenus sur plus de deux cents animaux de laboratoire (chinchillas) chez lesquels les pertes auditives (PTS) et les pertes de cellules sensorielles (SCL) ont été mesurées. Les premières séries d'expositions furent réalisées en utilisant des impulsions réalistes caractéristiques des tirs de trois armes différentes (type Friedlander). Ces impulsions sont produites en utilisant trois sources différentes actionnées à l'air comprimé (tubes à choc). Elles comportent une distribution spectrale d'énergie de large bande avec des pics de bandes d'octave pondérés A situés à 0,25; 1,0; et 2,0 kHz. Les niveaux de crête vont de 150 à 160 dB SPL. Les secondes séries d'impulsions étaient synthétisées par ordinateur à partir de bandes étroites ($\approx$ 250 Hz) reproduites par un haut-parleur de forte puissance. Ces impulsions, dont le niveau crête variait de 124 à 146 dB SPL avaient des fréquences centrales de six valeurs différentes situées entre 0,15 et 3,50 kHz. A partir de chacun des deux groupes de résultats, un niveau lésionnel constant, défini en termes de PTS et de SCL fut mis en relation avec le spectre d'énergie et les niveaux d'exposition globaux de chaque exposition. Les différences et les similitudes trouvées parmi l'ensemble des relations de ce type obtenues avec l'une et l'autre sources d'impulsions ainsi que la valeur prédictive de ces relations sont discutées.

ACKNOWLEDGMENTS

The support of the U.S. Army Medical Research and Development Command through contracts DAMD-17-86-C-6172 and DAMD-17-86-C-6139 is gratefully acknowledged. We would like to thank C.E. Hargett, Jr. and Dr. W.A. Ahroon for their assistance with the audiometric protocol; G. Turrentine for his patience and skill in preparing the figures; and Renee Johnston and Sandy Nease for preparing the manuscript.

References

Coles RRA, Garinther GR, Rice CG, Hodge DC. Hazardous exposure to impulse noise. J Acoust Soc Am 1968; 43:336-343.

Gold B, Rader CM. Digital processing of signals. New York: McGraw-Hill, 1969.

Hamernik RP, Ahroon WA, Hsueh KD. The energy spectrum of an impulse: Its relation to hearing loss. J Acoust Soc Am 1991; 90 (In press).

Hamernik RP, Hsueh KD. Impulse noise: Some definitions, physical acoustics and other considerations. J Acoust Soc Am 1991; 90 (In press).

Henderson D, Hamernik RP. Asymptotic threshold shift from impulse noise. In: Hamernik RP, Henderson D, Salvi RJ, eds. New perspectives on noise-induced hearing loss. New York: Raven Press, 1982:265.

Henderson D, Hamernik RP, Salvi RJ, Ahroon WA. Comparison of auditory-evoked potentials and behavioral thresholds in the normal and noise-exposed chinchilla. Audiology 1983; 22:172-180.

Kryter KD, Garinther GR. Auditory effects of acoustic impulses from firearms. Acta Otolaryngol Suppl 1965; 211.

Kryter KD. The effects of noise on man. New York: Academic Press, 1970.

OSHA, Dept of Labor. Occupational noise exposure. Proposed requirements and procedures. Federal Register 1974; 39(207):155-159.

Patterson JH Jr, Lomba-Gautier IM, Curd DL, Hamernik RP. The effect of impulse intensity and the number of impulses on hearing and cochlear pathology in the chinchilla. USAARL Report No 85-3, 1985.

Patterson JH Jr, Lomba-Gautier IM, Curd DL, Hamernik RP. The role of peak pressure in determining the auditory hazard of impulse noise. USAARL Report No 86-7, 1986.

Patterson JH Jr, Hamernik RP, Hargett CE, et al. The hazard of exposure to impulse noise as a function of frequency. USAARL Report 1991 (In press).

Pfander F, Bongartz H, Brinkmann H, Kietz H. Danger of auditory impairment from impulse noise: A comparative study of the CHABA damage-risk criteria and those of the Federal Republic of Germany. J Acoust Soc Am 1980; 67:628-633.

Price GR. Loss of auditory sensitivity following exposure to spectrally narrow impulses. J Acoust Soc Am 1979; 66:456-465.

Price GR. Relative hazard of weapons impulses. J Acoust Soc Am 1983; 73:556-566.

Price GR. Hazard from intense low-frequency acoustic impulses. J Acoust Soc Am 1986; 80:1076-1086.

Smoorenburg GF. Damage risk criteria for impulse noise. In: Hamernik RP, Henderson D, Salvi RJ, eds. New perspectives on noise-induced hearing loss. New York: Raven Press, 1982:471.

Smoorenburg GF. Effects of Impulse Noise. NATO Document AC/243 (Panel 8/RSG.6) D/9, 1987.

von Bismarck GV. The sound pressure transformation function from free-field to the eardrum of chinchilla. MS thesis, Massachusetts Institute of Technology, Cambridge, MA, 1967.

Young RW. On the energy transported with a sound pulse. J Acoust Soc Am 1970; 47:441-442.

CHAPTER 31

Importance of Spectrum for Rating Hazard: Theoretical Basis

G. RICHARD PRICE

Raising the question of the importance of spectrum in rating auditory hazard may at first glance seem like the resurrection of an issue long since put to rest. More than a century ago, Helmholtz would have been comfortable with the idea that the ear is spectrally tuned; contemporary textbooks introduce students to the familiar U-shape of the audiogram, which clearly demonstrates that the human ear is most sensitive in the mid-frequencies. Furthermore, regulatory bodies in the governments of many countries have accepted the idea of using A-weighting in the assessment of auditory hazard, testimony to the notion that spectrum is a useful concept in rating hazard.

On the other hand, scientific interest in spectrum and hazard continues (see for example Decory and Dancer; Hamernik and Patterson; Hetu et al; Liang; and Smoorenburg). For industrial noises, there is the question of whether a simple A-weighted measure of energy is adequate to rate hazard, given that it "explains" so little of the variance in the data. And for really intense sounds, like gunfire, only France uses a frequency-weighted measure of hazard (Ministry of Defense, 1982a), whereas the rest of the world's impulse noise criteria depend on measures of peak pressure and duration (CHABA, 1968; Cheng et al, 1987; Ministry of Defense, 1982a,b; Pfander, 1975). At the same time, research with intense impulsive sounds seems to indicate that spectrum has a major effect on susceptibility (Dancer et al, 1985; Price, 1986). The issue of the importance and use of spectrum in rating noise hazard is in fact far from settled.

The major proposition of this chapter is that approaching hazard assessment in spectral terms may be useful. Calculation of spectral information can be thought of as a sort of mathematical model of important processes associated with hazard. Insofar as a model matches the behavior of the system being described, the application of the model should be simple. If, on the other hand, the model behaves differently than the system in important ways, then the application of the model should be constrained to allow for such mismatches. Therefore, I examine the relationship between the calculated spectrum of a sound and the prediction of the ear's response to it in order to identify the range of conditions in which spectral information might be useful and to identify those areas in which the spectrum may not be related to the ear's behavior and thus not be a useful predictor of hazard.

This chapter is focused on developing the relationship between spectral measures of sound and the application of those measures to the assessment of noise hazard. I make no pretense of developing the mathematical basis for spectral analysis or of preparing a guide to the practical application of spectral analysis to specific noise measurements. This chapter should promote insight into the problems associated with the application of spectral concepts to the interpretation of the effect of intense sound on the ear and establish some range of conditions over which spectral analysis might be useful.

A Spectral Model

Most of us have an intuitive, albeit imprecise, appreciation of spectrum, perhaps because of the association between the spectrum of a sound and the auditory experience of pitch and timbre. Spectrum can be defined precisely in the mathematical realm by means of the Fourier integral; but as a formula it remains something of an abstraction. As an aid in thinking about spectrum, a mechanical analogy may be useful, at least for those of us who find mechanical analogies intellectually congenial. An image put forward by Trent (1960) and further developed by Kalb (1982) is that of a bar from which are suspended undamped, tuned oscillators, represented in Figure 31-1 as a graded series of weights suspended from springs. If the bar moves so that its velocity is proportional to the instantaneous pressure during an analysis period, then the oscillator amplitudes at the end of the analysis period match the components of the pressure spectral density. At this point we can see the "spectrum" of the noise in the amplitude of each of the oscillators (the size of the envelope drawn at the limit of the balls' travel in Fig. 31-1). But this insight has been gained at a price. Specifically, we have lost track of the instantaneous events that resulted in the final pattern we see when the analysis interval is ended. Patterns of vibration could have built up and canceled; but the spectrum shows only the final result. For some purposes this loss of temporal detail inherent in moving from the time domain into the frequency domain may be of no consequence; but if, for instance, the instantaneous displacements of the oscillators were an issue, the spectrum might not reveal essential information or it could distort important details. Succeeding sections of this chapter identify situations in which these considerations might be relative to predicting hazard from intense sounds.

Utility of Spectrum

The Problem of Linearity and Continuity

In applying spectral analysis to a system, we implicitly assume that the system is linear. With a linear system, a transfer function is a powerful way to describe the behavior of the system as it responds to complex time-varying stimulation. On the other hand, nonlinearities or discontinuities can lead to gross misrepresentations. This is a major problem with the application of spectral analysis to the ear in two areas. Specifically, the conductive path becomes nonlinear for large displacements (Price, 1974; Price and Kalb, 1986) and, perhaps more debatable, the loss mechanisms operating within the cochlea go through a change of mode, also at high levels (Price, 1981). Much might be debated about the specifics of these points, but their general impact will be apparent in appropriate sections of the discussion.

Range of Application

Where might we expect spectrum to be a useful concept, and over what range of conditions might we expect it to provide useful insights?

Conductive Path

The most obvious point is that the mechanisms that conduct sound to the cochlea are spectrally tuned and therefore play a major role in determining cochlear input. A great deal of research and time has been invested over the last 50 years in determining the acoustic properties of mammalian external and middle ears. As a result, it was determined that they function collectively to transmit energy to the cochlea best in the mid-range of frequencies and to be essentially linear with respect to amplitude over essentially the entire normal physiologic range. The middle ear transmits most efficiently at its resonant frequency, near 1.0 kHz for the human. At frequencies below resonance, the efficiency of transmission falls off primarily because structures are not sufficiently compliant; at frequencies above resonance, sensitivity declines primarily because the structures are too massive. The external ear acts as a resonator and extends the region of maximum sensitivity upward about two octaves, so that the ear is an efficient collector of energy for perhaps a 3- or 4-octave range; but it rapidly becomes less sensitive at both higher and lower frequencies. This pattern of sensitivity is reflected in psychoacoustic functions such as the minimum audible pressure and equal loudness contours, from which the A-weighting curve is derived. The theoretical basis for the spectral tuning of the ear (at least from the free field to the stapes) is thus well established, at least for the range of intensities for which the middle ear is linear.

An additional element in the conductive chain, the middle-ear muscle system, also tends to reinforce the same pattern of stimulation. The middle-ear muscles are active during noise exposures, the pattern of action varying over time in a complex fashion; but they have long been known to have their greatest attenuating effect on the low frequencies and to leave the mid-range much less affected (Wiggers, 1937). Therefore, the middle-ear muscle system acts to further sharpen the tuning of

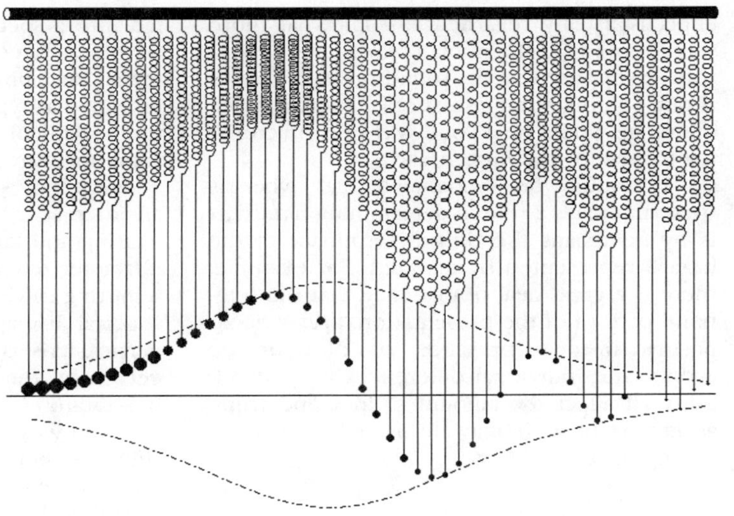

Figure 31-1 Model spectral analyzer at the end of the analysis interval showing the pattern of response in the graded series of oscillators.

the ear by selectively attenuating the sounds below the resonant frequency.

Cochlea

Actual damage to the ear, however, is primarily a function of changes inside the cochlea. How do spectral concepts fit at that level? Given that the intracochlear structures are uniformly graded from base to apex with no apparent discontinuities, it is reasonable to expect that when the auditory system is stimulated with loud sounds, the effect on the inner ear will reflect the spectral shaping of the middle and external ears. And this is essentially the case. Kryter et al (1966) plotted the ear's susceptibility to continuous and intermittent noise, incorporating a great deal of noise research in which ears had been exposed to bands of noises at different frequencies. Their plot of tolerable exposures specifically took spectrum into account by allowing the lowest exposure to bands of noise in the mid-range, where the ear is tuned best, and progressively more exposure at higher and lower frequencies, where the ear is tuned less well. A simpler and more popular approach to the same end has of course been the use of A-weighting in the assessment of auditory hazard.

Another way of looking at the same phenomenon is to consider the pattern of loss when an ear is exposed to intense sounds in the workplace. One of the early audiologic observations was of the "4,096 cycle notch" in the audiogram, now commonly taken as a sign of noise-induced hearing loss. Two circumstances act to produce this effect. In essence, the spectral tuning of the ear is relatively sharp compared to the spectra of the noises commonly found in the workplace. The steepest spectral slopes found in real settings are about ± 6 dB per octave, but the tuning of the ear is very much sharper than that. Therefore, the middle of the cochlea customarily receives the maximum stimulation. This combination of conditions forms the physical basis for explaining the common finding of the greatest damage occurring in the midrange.

Loss Mechanisms Within the Cochlea

The discussion thus far has not specifically addressed the fit of spectral information to specific loss mechanisms within the cochlea. At this point the discussion becomes highly speculative because, despite excellent research on the mechanisms of loss operating within the cochlea, we still know relatively little about the specific effects of intense stimulation on intracochlear structures, the recovery processes, etc. With that caveat, the following speculations are offered.

It is reasonable to suppose that for noises that are commonly present in the workplace, the loss mechanism might be thought of as extreme metabolic demand on the cochlea. In that case, some quantity like energy might do reasonably well in representing the stress. In fact, Ward et al (1983) have shown that, for the chinchilla, the percentage of outer hair cells destroyed by continuous exposure to a 2-octave band of noise (700 to 2,800 Hz) is a linear function of the square root of the energy in the exposure, as long as sound pressures are below 114 dB. Given that the chinchilla is usually regarded as somewhat more susceptible than the human being, it is reasonable to suppose that for sound pressures up to about 115 dB, some measure of energy in the midrange would be a good way of characterizing hazard for the human ear.

It should be recognized that whereas spectrum plays a role in determining hazard, it is by no means the *only* determinant of the hazard represented by a sound. For example, there is a great deal of evidence that the temporal pattern of the presentation, previous exposure history, presence of ototraumatic agents, and individual differences in susceptibility all affect the amount of loss. Spectrum, as important as it may be, is only one issue among many.

Practical Application

Calculating the Spectrum

When we examine the practical details of calculating spectra, then additional questions arise. In theory, the analysis interval is infinitely long, and the displacements of our infinite number of undamped oscillators could grow forever. However, in the modern world of digital frequency analysis, the analysis interval is finite and there are a limited number of oscillators (the analyzer has only so much memory). These practical issues influence the number and spacing of the bumps and dips in the spectral display, which as a result may or may not match the behavior of the ear. Consider our imaginary frequency analyzer. We could suspend 19,981 oscillators tuned at 1-Hz intervals from 20 Hz to 20 kHz along the bar, or we could place 30 of them at ⅓-octave intervals, or we might put 10 of them at 1-octave intervals. All three approaches are commonly used in spectral analysis. However, the critical question is: which of these three "displays" would be expected to match just what structures in the ear? Would other analysis intervals or frequency spacings or both do better? Does this analysis work at all sound pressure levels, or does the behavior of the ear change as a function of level? Unraveling these issues is not a simple matter.

Interpreting the Spectrum

With modern technology, spectral analysis can be performed with deceptive ease. In its most elemental form, a microphone samples pressure in the free field and its output is fed into a spectrum analyzer. Shortly thereafter one is faced with the problem of interpreting an intriguing series of bumps and dips on a display that typically portrays frequency along the horizontal axis (usually a linear scale) and some measure of spectral amplitude, often on a logarithmic scale, on the vertical axis. Given an interest in the effect of intense sound on hearing and knowing that the cochlea can be characterized as a frequency analyzer, it is tempting to visualize the horizontal axis of the spectral display as an unrolled cochlea and the vertical axis as an analog of the stimulation received by the various sections of the basilar membrane.

And why not interpret the spectral plot in such a fashion? Several transformations would make sense if the spectral plot were to be conformal with the cochlea. Given that the waveform analyzed was a free-field sound pressure, it would be necessary to account for the transformations of the external and middle ears to arrive at an estimate of the actual input to the cochlea. In response to sound pressures up to 120 or 130 dB, the middle and external ears are known to be essentially linear and the transfer functions are known; hence, for sound pressures below these levels such a transformation would accurately indicate the spectrum at the stapes.

The second transformation that moves us from input at the stapes to activity on the basilar membrane is more tenuous. What should the horizontal axis show or, in terms of our model, how many oscillators should be on the bar and how should they be spaced? Within the cochlea, frequencies array themselves along the basilar membrane in an essentially logarithmic fashion; but spectra are often calculated for 1-Hz bandwidths or ⅓-octave bandwidths. The problem of finding conformality between the calculated spectrum and the ear is not trivial, and the choice is somewhat arbitrary. The 1-Hz bands provide greater resolution (more bumps and dips), and ⅓-octave bands are reasonably close to critical bands or approximately constant distances along the basilar membrane. The important issue is how our choice relates to the behavior of the ear. If we think in terms of the distribution and absorption of energy in the cochlea, then it is reasonable to argue that something like a ⅓-octave integration is analogous to what actually happens in the ear. Of course, in the ear the ⅓-octave bands are not fixed or even exactly ⅓-octave wide, but the general logarithmic "compression" of energy at higher frequencies is paralleled.

But having made all the right choices, just

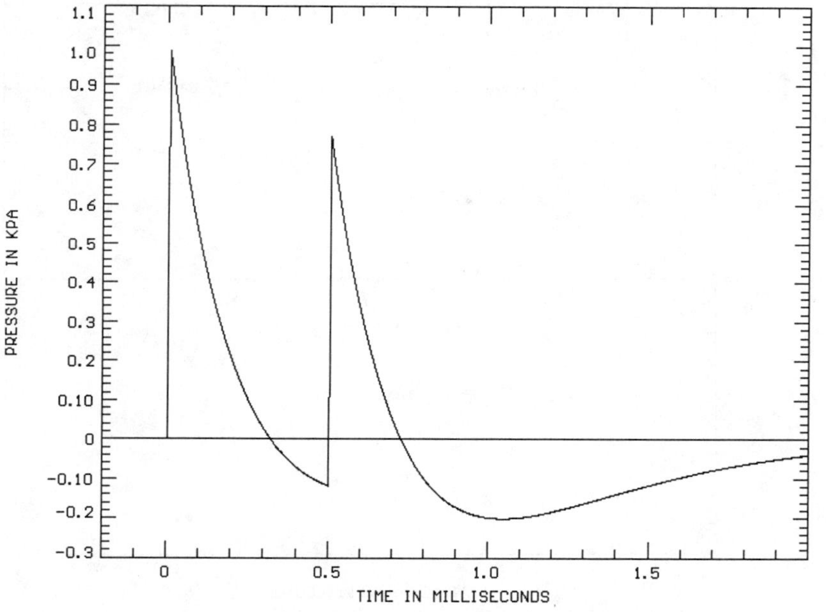

Figure 31-2 Friedlander waveforms simulating a rifle impulse and its ground reflection.

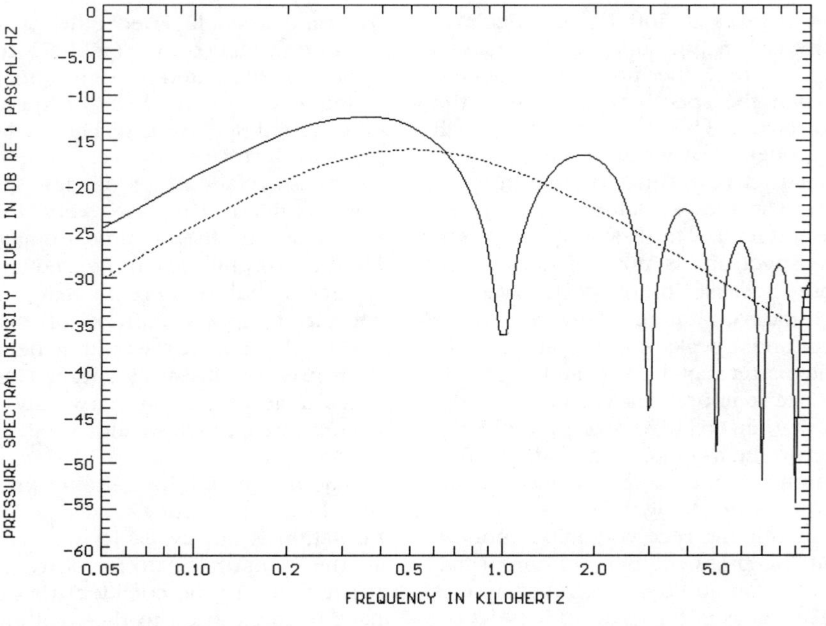

Figure 31-3 Spectra of the Friedlander waveforms in Figure 31-2. The dotted spectrum is for one of the impulses taken alone; the solid spectrum is for the two impulses combined.

how should we view those bumps and dips in the spectrum? The specific form the spectrum takes is a function of many elements that may or may not relate to specific events in the ear. Consider, for instance, the problem in Figure 31-2. A weapon's impulse (simulated by a Friedlander waveform) is almost always accompanied by a reflected impulse from the ground. If the analysis interval includes only the directly transmitted impulse or just the reflection from the ground (here taken to be a relatively good reflector), the two spectra would each be like that shown as the dotted line in Figure 31-3. The spectrum rises

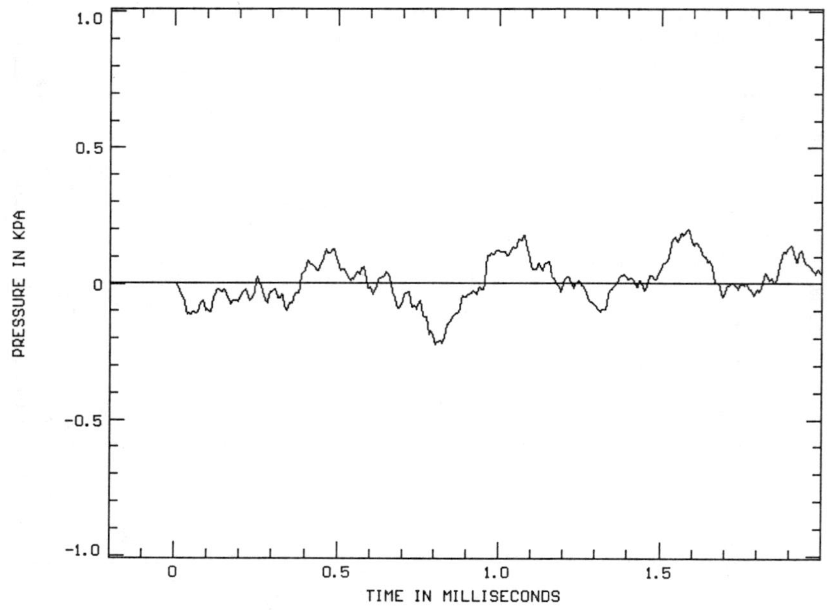

Figure 31-4 Pressure history of an impulse that has the same amplitude spectrum as the Friedlander waveform in Figure 31-3 (dotted line) but with a differing phase spectrum.

smoothly to a peak at 500 Hz and declines smoothly thereafter. But suppose the analysis interval includes *both* the direct and reflected impulses. Then the spectrum appears as the solid line in Figure 31-3. In terms of our ball and spring model, what we are seeing are patterns of constructive and destructive interference that exist in the oscillators at the end of the analysis interval. The low-frequency portion of the spectrum is now higher, which makes sense because there were two impulses, each carrying energy. However, there are now prominent peaks and dips at intervals. The specific pattern of bumps and dips is a function of the temporal spacing between the impulses and their relative sizes. Should the dips be interpreted as indicating relatively quiescent sections of the basilar membrane, or should the peaks be thought of as sections of the basilar membrane receiving maximum excitations? At this point the issue of conformality between the ear and the spectral analysis is apparent. The ear is not a series of lossless oscillators, as is our spectrum analyzer; consequently the analogy between the spectrum and activity within the ear breaks down. Patterns of interference and reinforcement would not be expected to develop within the cochlea for these impulses because in effect they would not be present simultaneously at the oscillator locations.

A variation on this same theme can be seen in Figure 31-4. The waveform in Figure 31-4 and a single Friedlander waveform like the one in Figure 31-3 (without the reflected impulse) are related to each other in an interesting way. Namely, their spectra are identical (the dotted spectrum in Fig. 31-3); but their pressure histories look very different because the phase relationships of their spectral components differ. Thus, two very different pressure histories in the time domain can have identical magnitudes in the frequency domain. If such impulses were to drive the ear, the specific temporal pattern of displacements within the cochlea would generally parallel their pressure histories, the first one having a quick large oscillation or two and the second having many much-smaller oscillations over a longer time.

So in the end, how should the bumps and dips be interpreted? Given that the phase information is not available, we can only guess at the temporal pattern of response. Even though we may be confident that the ear may have been exposed to the total energy represented by the spectrum, we cannot assert, in the case posed in Figure 31-2, that within the cochlea a particular place oscillated appreciably more or less than some other place, matching the bumps and dips in the spectrum. From these illustrations, it is apparent that in the absence of phase information, which would allow examination of the data in the time domain, extreme restraint should be used in interpreting frequency domain data. A final comment on a more positive note: In a general sense, spectrum does indicate energy in different frequency regions, and over the long term in the workplace, the bumps and dips will average out and the spectrum may still retain its utility as a predictor of hazard.

Changes at High Intensities

As the intensity of stimulation rises above 130 dB, as it often does for impulse and impact sounds, additional complexities arise in the calculation, interpretation, and application of the spectrum. Several lines of inquiry are developing a picture of an intricate interplay of loss mechanisms and conductive nonlinearities at high sound pressure levels, which we will attempt to put in a conceptual framework.

To assist in maintaining a frame of reference for relative intensities, it may be worth noting that peak pressures of industrial impulses, cap guns, and even cordless telephones, often rise above 130 dB; small arms (pistols, rifles, shotguns) produce impulses with peak pressures of about 150 to 160 dB, and large-caliber weapons and shoulder-fired rockets can produce levels of nearly 190 dB. Sound pressures well above 130 dB are not at all rare in modern life.

I have argued that at very high sound pressure levels the middle ear becomes nonlinear with respect to amplitude, and the mechanism or mechanisms of loss within the cochlea also undergo a change. In both cases, instantaneous displacement of the structures is hypothesized to be critical; hence there is a fundamental analytical question as to whether a frequency domain analysis (spectrum) is an adequate descriptor of a time domain problem (mechanical stress).

A few calculations will demonstrate the nature of the problem. In the illustrations that follow, the figures are largely the result of calculations done with an integrated mathematical model of the ear that I have been developing with my colleagues at our laboratory (Kalb and Price, 1987; Price and Kalb, 1990). Input to the model is free-field sound pressure, and the model carries energy through the full transmission path to the stapes and ends by calculating hazard within the cochlea. Unfortunately, a full discussion of this model's development is beyond the scope of this chapter. However, the reader may be reassured to know that the model's structure parallels the ear's physiology, and that the external and middle ear sections closely reproduce the transfer functions and impedances that have been measured in real ears. The calculations reported here are made with values appropriate to the cat ear.

Nonlinearities in the Middle Ear

A nonlinearity in the middle ear implies that at some combination of frequency and intensity spectral calculations of energy in the free field will correlate poorly with cochlear input. Therefore it is important to establish the amplitudes and frequencies for which such an error becomes an issue. Various parts of the middle ear could impose a displacement limit; however, some have argued that on anatomic grounds it seems probable that the annular ligament of the stapes would be likely to pose an absolute limit to displacement of about 40 to 50 μm peak to peak (Price, 1974; Price and Kalb, 1986). At any rate, the model embodies this displacement limitation, and it has been used to calculate the level for Friedlander waveforms and tone pips at which the nonlinearity would have affected their amplitudes by 3 dB. The results are shown in Figure 31-5 for both the tone pips and Friedlander waveforms. For the Friedlander waveforms the clipping becomes significant at just over 140 dB for low-frequency impulses, and the clipping occurs at progressively higher levels as the waveforms get shorter (less low-frequency energy). Tone pips, on the other hand, are peak-limited in a pattern that roughly parallels the transfer function for the external and middle ears, which is what one might expect. Clipping becomes significant for them in the upper 140s for low-frequency tones and in the upper 130s where the ear is tuned best. The specific levels would of course be different for different species; but middle-ear nonlinearity is a major influence in high-level stimulation.

A middle-ear clipping nonlinearity would imply that an exposure would have less effect than expected when the middle-ear displacements rose to such amplitude that the nonlinearity was encountered. A pattern consistent with this idea can be seen in data from the chinchilla. When chinchillas were exposed to 100 impulses at 1.4 kHz spectral peak and at peak SPLs between 131 and 139 dB, losses grew rapidly as sound pressure increased, about 7 dB of threshold shift for every decibel of increase in peak pressure (Patterson et al, 1986). This is a spectral region in which the chinchilla is sensitive, and although we have

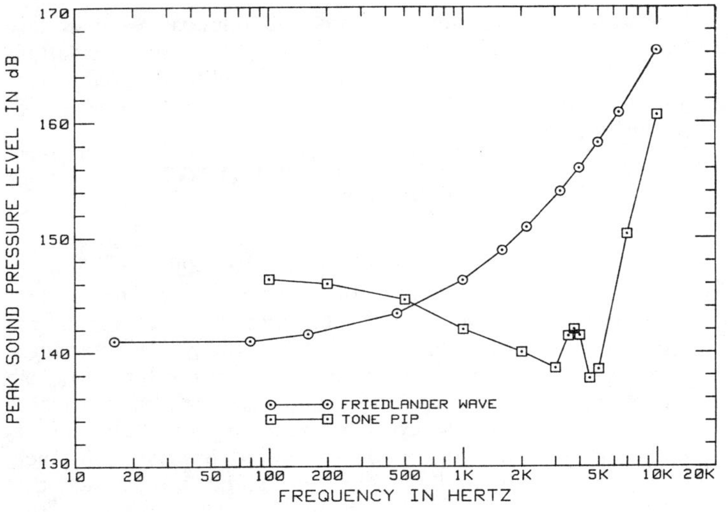

Figure 31-5 Free-field sound pressures at which a mathematical model of the ear (see Kalb and Price, 1987) indicates that Friedlander waveforms and tone pips would experience a 3-dB clipping effect.

no specific data, it seems likely that their middle-ear displacements would not be highly nonlinear at these levels. On the other hand, when chinchillas were exposed to impulses with peak pressures between 150 and 160 dB and spectral peaks below 125 Hz, the growth of threshold shift to 100 impulses had a slope of about 3.0 dB for every decibel of increase in peak pressure (Hamernik et al, 1990). This reduced slope is consistent with the possibility of amplitude limitation at the stapes. Or consider data from an experiment in which cat ears were exposed to one round from a recoilless rifle fired within a room (Price, 1978). The peak pressure was 186 dB, and the energy in the exposure was about 36 kJ per square meter (equivalent to 10 or *more* years of exposure in the workplace), but the average permanent losses were only about 10 dB. These data from the chinchilla and cat are not definitive; but they are consistent with a middle ear that transmits less well at high levels.

Calculations with the mathematical model of the ear have suggested a variation on the same mechanism that could have a major effect on the transmission of energy into the cochlea (Price and Kalb, 1990). At least part of the reason for the smaller-than-expected losses from intense, low-frequency impulses, such as those produced by large-caliber weapons, lies in the modulation of cochlear input by clipping of the stapes. Sommer and Nixon (1973) conducted an experiment that was particularly well suited to demonstrating this effect. They were trying to test auditory hazard from different acoustic components of air bag deployment in an automobile. They simulated air bag deployment by combining a hiss, a 153-dB band of noise at about 1.0 kHz (noise of the bag filling), with a relatively long positive pressure pulse (165 dB peak, simulating the pressure in the car as the bag filled). The low-frequency pulse produced no threshold shift by itself, and the hiss produced a modest threshold shift by itself; but together, they produced *less* threshold shift than the hiss by itself. By means of the mathematical model, the basis for this effect can be discerned. In the lower panel of Figure 31-6 we see the free-field pressure history of a simulated air-bag-deployment pulse consisting of a trapezoidal pedestal (160 dB peak pressure) combined with a tone pip (160 dB peak to peak). In the upper panel we see the calculated stapes response to the combined pulses. The lower-frequency impulse clearly modulates the cochlear input to the tone pip, reducing it by approximately 20 dB. Calculations with the mathematical model and with real weapons impulses suggest that exactly the same thing happens with them as well. In Figure 31-7 note, for example, the calculated stapes displacement in the lower panel in response to the impulse in the upper panel. The clipping is apparent. During the initial 4 or 5 ms the pressure is relatively high, but the stapes is relatively immobile and is held in position by the high pressure. However, stapes displacements are large whenever the waveform passes through ambient pressure. The relatively small pressure oscillations present in the last 10 ms of the period produce surprisingly large stapes displacements.

Upon consideration of the foregoing arguments we can conclude that there is a reasonable physical basis for the ear to be surprisingly resistant to damage at very high levels.

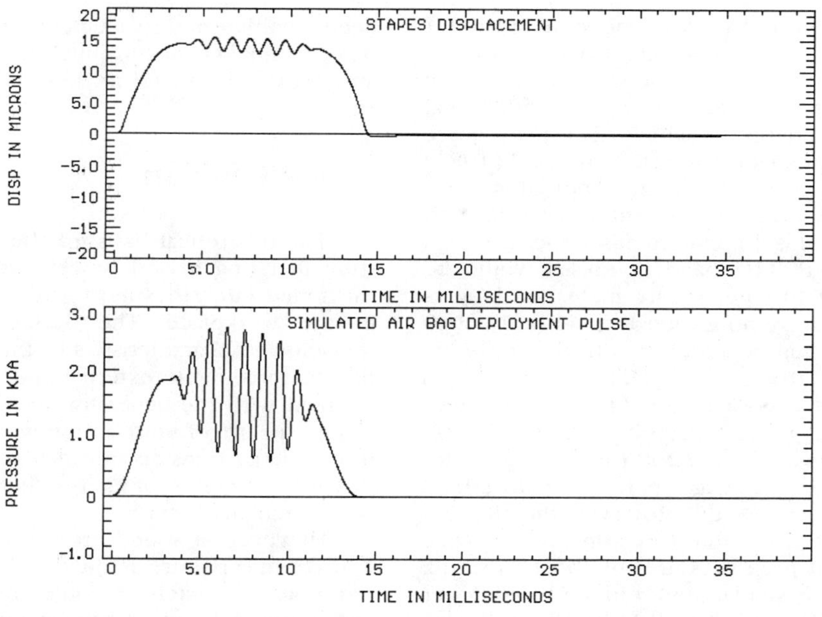

Figure 31-6 Demonstration of co-modulation at the stapes. The lower panel shows the pressure history of a simulated air-bag-deployment pulse. The upper panel shows the mathematical ear model's calculation of stapes displacement response, showing modulation of the tone pip by the lower-frequency pedestal.

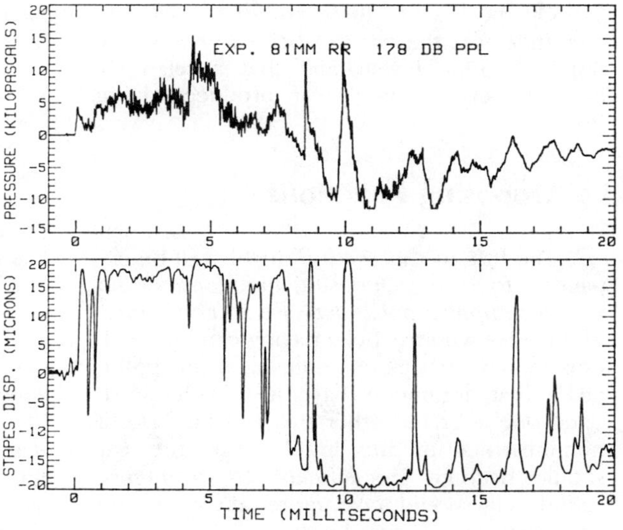

Figure 31-7 Pressure history of an experimental recoilless rifle (upper panel) and the calculated stapes displacement to the impulse (bottom panel).

A Change in the Mechanism of Loss

An additional complexity at high levels is that hazard to the ear rather suddenly becomes very sensitive to level (Patterson et al, 1986; Price, 1981; Ward, 1988). A change of intensity of about 10 dB in level for a given number of impulses could result in an increase ranging from no measurable loss to a total loss of hair cells. Presumably this is a result of the basic loss mechanism becoming some form of mechanical stress within the cochlea. The level at which this change occurs is important because it affects the range over which energy calculations at different spectral locations might be useful as a means of assessing hazard. Perhaps the most complete data pertaining to this issue are now available for the chinchilla ear. Data from Patterson et al (1986) are available for chinchillas exposed to impulses (a damped sinusoid from a speaker) with the spectral peak of the stimulus at 1.4 kHz. Exposure levels ranged from 131 to 147 dB. Such impulses produced an approximate 30 percent loss of outer hair cells, with a total exposure energy of about 2 J per square meter. In dramatic contrast, Ward et al (1983) calculated that the energy required to produce a 30 percent loss of outer hair cells with their stimulus (a continuous exposure to a 700- to 2,800-Hz band of noise) would be about 22,500 J per square meter (as long as the levels were no greater than 114 dB). Similar results can be adduced with data from exposure of the cat ear. Miller et al (1963) found that exposure to a 115-dB continuous broad-band noise (spectral peak at 1.5 kHz) for 2 hours at about 2,200 J per square meter produced an average permanent threshold shift (PTS) of 38 dB. However, the rifle impulse, with a spectral peak in nearly the same region, but peak pressures of 145 to 155 dB, produced a similar loss with only 10 J per square meter (Price, 1986). Clearly, on the basis of data from the cat and chinchilla, there is reason to suspect that there is a significant difference in the response of the ear as a function of level.

On the basis of these arguments, we can conclude that the ear can become extremely fragile at high levels, and that a relatively small amount of energy can produce a large loss.

Opposing Functions

The title to this section might well be expanded to read: *"Opposing functions, or no wonder impulse noise data are so confusing."* The reader who has been paying careful attention should perhaps be confused at this point, given that arguments have just been developed one after the other that (1) because of nonlinearities in the middle ear, the ear should become *less* susceptible to intense sounds (it should take more energy to do damage); and (2) that because of a change in loss mechanism within the cochlea, the ear should become *more* susceptible at high levels, and a relatively small amount of energy could do a great deal of damage. Although the arguments appear to be contradictory, they are not, and in fact go a long way toward explaining both the unusual fragility and robustness of the ear.

The critical question posed in this chapter is whether a frequency domain analytical method is useful for dealing with what are essentially time domain questions, e.g., instantaneous, nonlinear displacements of structures. It seems unlikely at this juncture that spectral analysis will be useful at these very high levels.

Conclusion

The theoretical basis for the use of spectrum in rating hazard is well established for the sound intensities most often encountered in the workplace. The frequency-selective transmission characteristics of the conductive mechanisms of the external and middle ears, coupled with the generally broad and gently sloped spectra of noise in the workplace, promote energy transmission in the midrange so that some measure of energy there should do well at ranking hazard.

However, at sound pressure levels above 130 dB, the picture is much more complex. Important mechanisms come into play that can result in the ear becoming either very resistant or extremely susceptible to particular temporal patterns of stimulation. These mechanisms are not well characterized in the frequency domain; consequently, spectrum is likely to have only marginal utility in rating hazard for really intense sounds.

Importance de la Composition Spectrale des Bruits pour l'Estimation des Risques Lésionnels: Bases Théoriques

L'hypothèse du rôle important joué par le spectre dans l'évaluation du risque lié à l'exposition aux bruits intenses est admise de manière générale. Les bases théoriques des effets du spectre sont à rechercher dans divers aspects de la réponse de l'oreille aux bruits intenses. En premier lieu, la façon dont l'énergie est transmise du champ libre jusqu'à l'étrier conditionne celle qui atteint effectivement la cochlée, où se produisent la plupart des lésions associées aux pertes auditives. Il est maintenant bien établi, empiriquement et théoriquement, que l'oreille externe et moyenne agissent comme un filtre passe-bande, la meilleure transmission de l'énergie ayant lieu dans les fréquences moyennes.

Un facteur additionnel, qui se présente sur une base variable et qui peut jouer un rôle majeur, est constitué par l'atténuation produite par les muscles de l'oreille moyenne. Ces derniers peuvent provoquer une atténuation atteignant 40 dB aux basses fréquences, et un peu moins aux fréquences élevées, mais leur action est complexe. Des facteurs spectraux, temporels et même psychologiques conditionnent leur déclenchement, ainsi que leur importance et leurs effets.

Le risque est non seulement fonction de la susceptibilité du système, mais aussi des caractéristiques de la fonction excitatrice. Comme nous l'avons vu, l'oreille externe et moyenne constituent un filtre passe-bande étroitement accordé. Par ailleurs les bruits en milieu industriel tendent à avoir une distribution spectrale d'énergie large, avec des pentes comprises entre plus et moins 6 dB/oct. Par conséquent le filtrage dû à l'oreille externe et moyenne couplé à l'effet des muscles de l'oreille moyenne agit normalement de manière à produire à l'entrée de la cochlée, un pic spectral situé dans la gamme des fréquences moyennes.

A des niveaux dépassant 120-130 dB, nous pensons que l'oreille moyenne cesse d'être linéaire et qu'elle commence à écrêter, limitant ainsi les déplacements de l'étrier qui dépassent environ 20 microns (cette valeur étant quelque peu fonction de l'espèce). Par la limitation du déplacement, il se produit un décalage additionnel de l'énergie vers les fréquences élevées au niveau de l'entrée de la cochlée.

Finalement il reste la cochlée proprement dite, qui réalise une analyse spectrale du signal d'entrée entre sa base et son apex; ceci nous amène à nous intéresser à la susceptibilité des structures internes à la cochlée. A ce niveau, le raisonnement est beaucoup plus spéculatif. Cependant, on peut noter que les propriétés physiques de la membrane basilaire et de l'organe de Corti varient uniformément en fonction de sa longueur; l'existence de discontinuités dans sa susceptibilité est donc peu probable. Par ailleurs, la susceptibilité dépend du mécanisme spécifique lié aux pertes auditives. Par exemple, un calcul basé sur l'effet provoqué par l'énergie acoustique en un endroit donné, différera de celui basé sur la contrainte mécanique. Et, bien évidemment, les pertes cellulaires peuvent être reliées aux processus mécaniques de manière stochastique. Une analyse définitive du rôle du spectre est tributaire de l'acquisition d'informations nouvelles dans ce domaine.

ACKNOWLEDGMENT

I would like to recognize the considerable assistance of Joel Kalb in the development of these ideas, from his discussions of many technical issues to the preparation of the figures.

References

CHABA. Proposed damage-risk criterion for impulse noise (gunfire). Report of Working Group 57, NAS-NRC Committee on Hearing, Bioacoustics and Biomechanics, Washington, D.C., 1968.

Cheng M, Liang Z, Meng Z, Li X. Investigation of military standard for impulse noise. Proc Inter-Noise 87, 1987; 2:913-916.

Dancer A, Buck K, Vassout P, Lenoir M. Influence du niveau de crete et de la duree d'ondes de choc (bruits d'armes) sur l'audition du cobaye. Acustica 1985; 59:21-29.

Guinan JJ, Peake WT. Middle-ear characteristics of anesthetized cats. J Acoust Soc Am 1967; 41:1237-1261.

Hamernik RP, Ahroon WA, Davis RI, et al. The effects of blast trauma (impulse noise) on hearing: A parametric study. Source II. Report No. ARL 90-2, U.S. Army Medical Research and Development Command, Ft. Detrick, Frederick, MD, 1990.

Kalb JT. Spectral analysis of blast-overpressure pulses. In: Technical proceedings of the blast overpressure workshop. Dover, NJ: USAARADCOM, 1982:163.

Kalb JT, Price GR. Mathematical model of the ear's response to weapons impulses. In: Proceedings of the third conference on weapon launch noise blast overpressure. Special Publication BRL-SP-66. Aberdeen Proving Ground, MD: U.S. Army Ballistics Research Lab, 1987.

Kryter K, Ward WD, Miller JD, Eldredge DH. Hazardous exposure to intermittent and steady-state noise. J Acoust Soc Am 1966; 39:451-464.

Miller JD, Watson CS, Covell WP. Deafening effects of noise on the cat. Acta Otolaryngol Suppl 1963; 176:91.

Ministry of Defense. Recommendation on evaluating the possible harmful effects of noise on hearing. Technical Coordination Group. Human factors and ergonomics. Direction Technique des Armaments Terrestres, 9211 Saint-Cloud Cedex, France, 1982a.

Ministry of Defense. Acceptable limits for exposure to impulse noise from military weapons, explosives and pyrotechnics. Interim Def Stan 00-27/1, Ministry of Defense, Directorate of Standardization, First Avenue House, London, WC1V6HE, England, 1982b.

Patterson JH, Lomba-Gautier I, Curd DL, et al. The role of peak pressure in determining the auditory hazard of impulse noise. USAARL Report No. 86-7, U.S. Army Aeromedical Research Laboratory, Fort Rucker, AL, 1986.

Pfander F. Das Knalltrauma. New York: Springer-Verlag, 1975.

Price GR. Impulse noise hazard as a function of level and spectral distribution. In: Salvi RJ, Henderson D, Hamernik RP, Colletti V, eds. Basic and applied aspects of noise-induced hearing loss. New York: Plenum Press, 1986:379.

Price GR. Implications of a critical level in the ear for assessment of noise hazard at high intensities. J Acoust Soc Am 1981; 69:171-177.

Price GR. Firing from enclosures with 90 mm recoilless rifle: Assessment of acoustic hazard. Technical

Memorandum 11-78, U.S. Army Human Engineering Laboratory, Aberdeen Proving Ground, MD, 1978.

Price GR. Upper limit to stapes displacement: Implications for hearing loss. J Acoust Soc Am 1974; 56:195-197.

Price GR, Kalb JT. Impulse noise model and its implications. J Acoust Soc Am In press.

Price GR, Kalb JT. Mathematical model of the effect of limited stapes displacement on hazard from intense sounds. J Acoust Soc Am 1986; 80:S123.

Price GR, Kim HN, Lim DJ, Dunn D. Hazard from weapons impulses: Histological and electrophysiological evidence. J Acoust Soc Am 1984; 85:1245-1254.

Sommer HC, Nixon CW. Primary components of simulated air bag noise and their relative effects on human hearing. AMRL-TR-73-52, Aerospace Medical Research Laboratory, Wright-Patterson Air Force Base, OH, 1973.

Trent HM. Physical equivalents of spectral notions. J Acoust Soc Am 1960; 32:348-350.

Ward WD. The critical exposure in acoustic trauma. J Acoust Soc Am 1988; 83:S115.

Ward WD, Turner CW, Fabry DA. The total-energy and equal-energy principles in the chinchilla. In: Rossi G, ed. Proceedings of the fourth international congress on noise as a public health problem, Turin: Minerva Medica, 1983:399.

Wiggers HC. The functions of the intra-aural muscles. Am J Physiol 1937; 120:771-780.

CHAPTER 32

The Spectrum of Impulse Noise and Human Ear Response

RAYMOND HÉTU
CHANTAL LAROCHE
HUNG TRAN QUOC
BERNADETTE LEPAGE
JOSÉE ST-VINCENT

A considerable amount of data has been collected on the audiometric and histologic effects of impulse noise. However, there is no agreement among hearing scientists on which descriptors of an exposure best predict these effects on hearing (Henderson and Hamernik, 1986). Among the various physical parameters studied, the frequency spectrum of the impulse noise has only recently been considered. Studies by Price (1983, 1986) have demonstrated the strong contribution of this factor in the prediction of damage to the ear from weapon noises. His results, obtained with small numbers of consecutive nonreverberant impulses presented at high peak levels, can be accounted for by an A-weighted energy measure, when this measure is extrapolated from the cat to the human ear. His results supported the use of this A-weighted energy as a descriptor not only for continuous noise but also for impulse noise, as proposed by ISO-1999 (1990). The inclusion of impulse noise exposure was considered valid for peak levels below 145 dB SPL. This standard was designed for estimating the risk of permanent threshold shift (PTS) from occupational exposures.

In our laboratory, a series of studies was undertaken to characterize the human ear response to spectral variations of impulses at exposure levels and durations compatible with the occupational setting. In particular, the validity of the A-weighting curve for characterizing the effects of impulse noise was examined. However, instrumental problems had to be solved before obtaining systematic variations of the frequency content of impulses while keeping the other characteristics of the noise relatively constant. This led to the design of a digitally controlled impulse-noise generation system (Nicolas et al, 1990). This system operates by means of a computerized digital signal fed into a high-power electroacoustic system operated in a semi-anechoic room. A two-step numeric calculation controls the output signal to obtain the desired time and frequency characteristics. In the first step, the equipment transfer function is computed numerically. In the second step, the input signal is corrected using the previously determined transfer function to obtain the desired output signal. The digitally controlled impulse-noise generation system presently allows control of the spectral input characteristics within a bandpass extending from 100 to 10,000 Hz. The maximum peak pressure level that can be obtained with appropriate nonlinear distortion control varies with the frequency content of the signal from 145 dB SPL at 1 kHz to 125 dB at 8 kHz. To achieve such control over the acoustic signals when conducting psychoacoustic experiments, the subjects are seated facing the loudspeaker at a distance of 25 cm; the height of the chair is adjusted to ensure that the subject's head is always centered on the vertical and horizontal planes of the exponential horn to which the compression driver is coupled. Using this generation system, experiments were conducted to compare the effect of different cutoff and center frequencies of narrow-band impulses on temporary threshold shift (TTS) and on loudness.

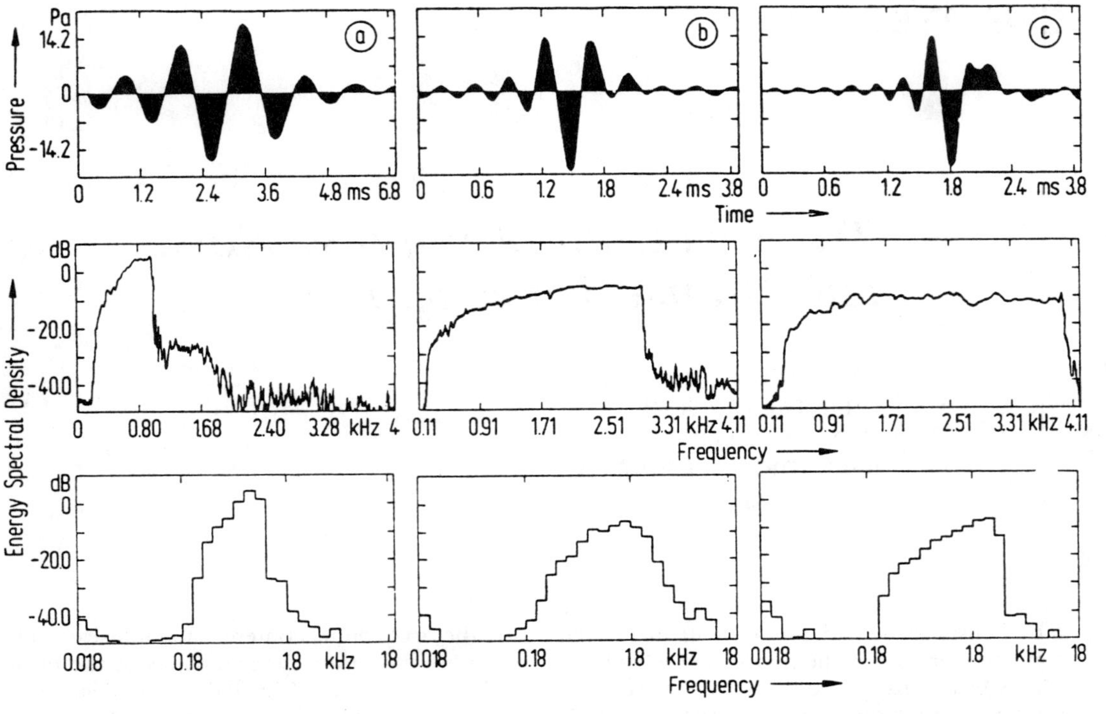

Figure 32-1 Acoustic pressure-time profile, Fourier analysis, and third-octave-band analysis of signals a, b, and c used to induce temporary threshold shift (TTS). (From Nicholas J, Sawan M, Hétu R, Laroche C. A digitally controlled impulse-noise generation system for the study of the ear response to impulses. Acustica 1990; 70:121.)

TTS Studies

Methods

The effect of systematic variations in the spectral content of impulses was quantitatively assessed by finding the corresponding variations in the peak pressure level that induced a predetermined effect on hearing thresholds. Moreover, different exposure durations were tested in order to obtain growth curves of TTS that approached or reached an asymptotic level. This procedure was based on the observation that, with impulses presented at 1 pulse per second (pps), asymptotic threshold shifts (ATS) can be measured within 30 to 60 minutes of exposure (Laroche et al, 1989). Knowing that there is only one possible value of asymptotic threshold shift for a given set of exposure parameters, this approach provides a reliable measure of the effect on human hearing of the noise under study. It provides an anchor point that allows the comparison of results from different studies, including those conducted using animal models (Saunders et al, 1985). Furthermore, it can reasonably be assumed that asymptotic threshold shift predicts the upper bound of PTS for a given noise condition (Mills et al, 1981; Bohne and Clark, 1982).

However, studying ATS in human subjects imposes severe constraints. TTS had to be as low as possible. A maximum amount of TTS measured 2 minutes after exposure (TTS_2) of 15 dB was adopted in these investigations. The minimum amount was determined by the measurement error, which was ± 2.5 dB or less using insert earphones (Etymotic, ER-3A) with subjects well trained to respond to Békésy audiometry (Grason-Stadler 1703B). Within these upper and lower boundaries, the target amount of ATS was set at 10 dB. First of all, this implied identification of the audiometric frequency most affected by the noise under study for each subject tested. Then the target effect was obtained by progressively increasing the exposure level in successive experimental sessions (Laroche et al, 1986). This procedure involved a large number of trials, separated by 24-hour recovery periods. This allowed us to obtain a 10-dB TTS_2 after 45 to 60 minutes of exposure, that is, after a series of 2,700 to 3,600 consecutive impulses presented at a rate of 1 per second.

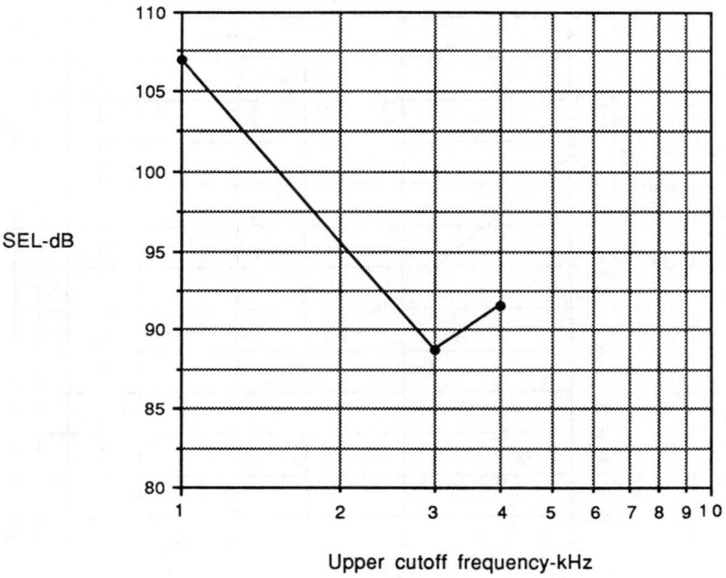

Figure 32-2 Median equal asymptotic threshold shift (ATS) contour as a function of the upper cutoff frequency for signals a, b, and c. SEL-dB, sound exposure level in decibels.

Results

Effect of Increasing the Upper Cutoff Frequency of a Low-Pass Filtered Impulse

In a first investigation, the effect of increasing the upper cutoff frequency of a low-pass filtered impulse was tested using three (sin x)/x digital signals. The lower cutoff frequency was set at 300 Hz and the upper cutoff was set at 1,000, 3,000, and 4,000 Hz for signals a, b, and c, respectively (Fig. 32-1). Three normal listeners participated in the experiment. All had hearing threshold levels better than 15 dB (ANSI S3.6, 1989) between 500 and 6,000 Hz, normal tympanograms, and no history of ear disease.

As we attempted to determine the peak level of signal a (with an upper cutoff of 1,000 Hz) that would induce the target amount of TTS_2, all three subjects reported strong annoyance at levels that induced only 4 to 6 dB of TTS_2 after 24 minutes of exposure (Laroche et al, 1986). Increasing the peak level to induce more TTS would have made the exposure intolerable. Thus, the comparison between the effect of this signal with that of the two others could not be obtained as precisely as expected. For all three subjects, however, after 24 minutes of exposure (1,440 impulses), signal a had to be at least 14 dB SEL higher to induce 4 to 6 dB TTS_2 than signals b and c, which induced TTS_2 of 10 dB or so. Assuming that the asymptotic level was approached in all three conditions and that ATS grows at a rate of 1.7 dB per decibel increase of the sound level (Mills et al, 1979), the median equinoxious levels would be as depicted in Figure 32-2. A difference of 18 dB SEL is obtained between the signal limited at 1,000 Hz and the one limited at 3,000 Hz; this corresponds to a slope of −11 dB per octave. In terms of peak pressure levels, this difference amounts to 12 dB (137 dB versus 125 dB SPL). These results strongly disagree with what would be predicted using the equal A-weighted energy level. Although limited by the number of subjects and the range of signals tested, these results provide a preliminary quantitative estimate of the effect of the frequency content of nonreverberant signals on human subjects.

Effect of Increasing the Center Frequency of a Narrow-Band Impulse

Using the same type of digital signals, four 1-octave-band-wide impulses were designed to test the effect of the following center frequencies: 1,000, 2,000, 3,000, and 4,000 Hz. Four normal-hearing listeners participated in this second investigation. Individual results were fairly comparable, although one subject showed an unexpected sensitivity to the 4,000-Hz signal as compared to the one centered at 3,000 Hz, indicating that a slight variation in the frequency content in this range of frequencies can induce dramatic changes (Laroche and Hétu, 1990a, p. 36). Figure 32-3 de-

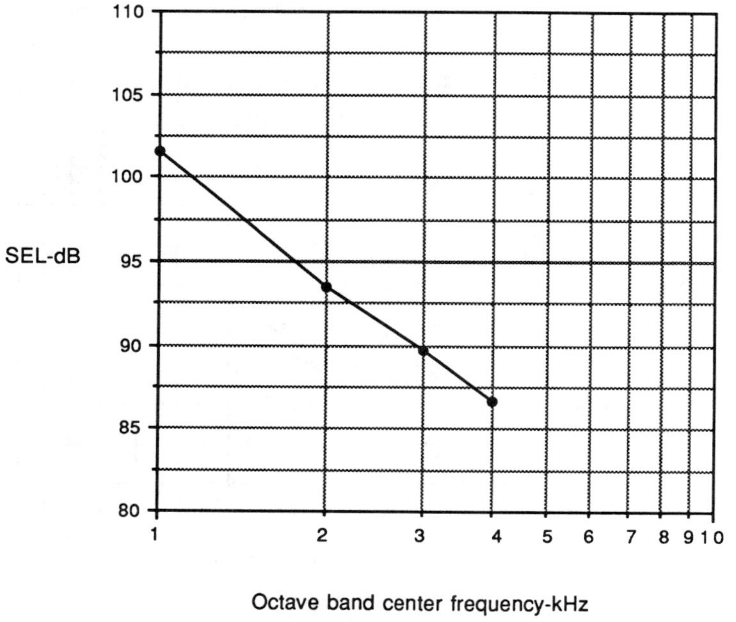

Figure 32-3 Median equal asymptotic threshold shift (ATS) contour as a function of the center frequency of the four-octave-band-wide impulses. SEL-dB, sound exposure level in decibels.

picts the median results in sound exposure level (SEL) associated with an amount of ATS of approximately 10 dB at the frequency most affected. The ATS value was derived using a Gompertz function (Laroche et al, 1989) from measures of TTS_2 made after 15 to 60 minutes of exposure (900 to 3,600 consecutive impulses). It can be seen that to achieve the same effect with the noise centered at 3,000 Hz, the SEL (for one impulse) was 12 dB below that of the impulse centered at 1,000 Hz. Between 1,000 and 4,000 Hz, the slope is −7.5 dB per octave. Again, these results contradict the predictions of the A-weighted energy level, which involves a 1-dB-level difference between 1,000 Hz and the higher three frequencies tested here.

The results presented in Figure 32-3 represent the median values for a small number of individuals. It is only an approximation of the effect of the frequency content of nonreverberant impulses on the human ear. Nevertheless these results are consistent with those obtained with the low-pass filtered impulses (Fig. 32-2). In the latter case, however, the lower-frequency portion of the signal limited to 1,000 Hz appeared to be protective for threshold shifts measured around and above the cutoff frequency of the noise, provided that this effect is not merely a sampling artifact. There is a difference of 5 dB between the median SEL to obtain the same effect, namely 107 dB for the 300- to 1,000-Hz band-pass noise as compared to 102 dB for the 1-octave band noise. The results shown in Figure 32-3 resemble the combined transfer function of the human external and middle ear. Because there was little doubt that the frequency range of maximum sensitivity to impulses, as with any other type of noise, falls near 3,000 Hz, we decided to characterize the distribution of exposure levels that would induce the target effect at this particular frequency for a larger group of subjects. This could serve as an anchor point to define tolerable exposure limits for this type of noise.

A group of 18 normal-hearing subjects participated in an experiment aimed at determining the level of the 1-octave-band-wide impulse centered at 3,000 Hz that induces an ATS of approximately 10 dB. As in the previous experiment, ATS was estimated from growth curves of TTS with exposures lasting 15, 30, 45, and 60 minutes. Figure 32-4 shows the resulting distribution of the SELs associated with the target effect for 18 subjects. Note that the peak level of this particular noise was 37 dB above the SEL. It can be seen from Figure 32-4 that there are very large individual differences in the sensitivity to this narrow-band impulse. At one extreme, there was one subject who had an ATS of 10 dB at an SEL of 78 dB (115 dB peak). At the other extreme, the asymptotic level of 10 dB could not be reached at 97 dB (134 dB peak), although it was reported by that subject to be relatively annoying. Consequently, a range of exposure levels of at least 20 dB is needed in order to

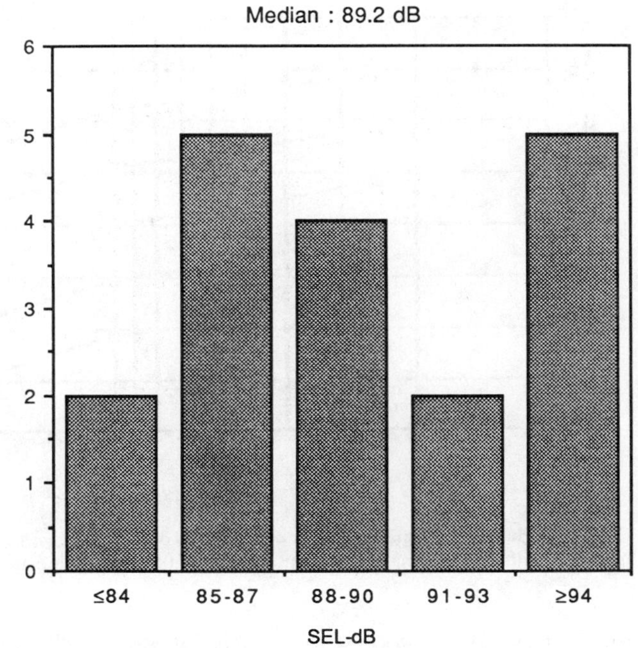

Figure 32-4 Distribution of the sound exposure level needed to induce an asymptotic threshold shift (ATS) of approximately 10 dB with an octave-band-wide impulse centered at 3,000 Hz among 18 normal-hearing subjects. SEL-dB, sound exposure level in decibels.

achieve the same effect with the most- and the least-sensitive subjects. Despite the fairly large number of subjects, the distribution shown in Figure 32-4 bears no resemblance to a gaussian function. It is interesting to note that the median value was 89 dB SEL (126 dB peak) in this group, as was the case for the group of four subjects involved in the previous experiment, indicating that the previous experiment gave an adequate representation of the sensitivity of average normal listeners.

If the hypothesis that ATS is a valid predictor of the upper bound of PTS is correct, exposure limits can be derived from the above results for daily exposure to large numbers (1,800 or more) of nonreverberant impulses centered at 3,000 Hz. Thus, at least 10 percent of the individuals could sustain a measurable PTS even if the SEL is limited to 84 dB or the peak level to 121 dB SPL. If the noise is centered at 1,000 Hz, this limit could be raised to at least 96 dB SEL (127 dB peak). It is worth mentioning that the present limit for the 3,000-Hz signal is close to what would be allowed by a regulation based on $L_{Aeq,8h}$ of 85 dBA that would cover exposure to impulses (Laroche and Hétu, 1990b). Application of the A-weighting curve to such a limit for an impulse centered at 1,000 Hz would result in a conservative estimate of the safe exposure level.

Strictly speaking, the above results apply only to impulses having mid-range frequency spectra. As would be expected from the results obtained with the noise centered at 1,000 Hz, as well as those from the band-pass impulse filtered above 1,000 Hz reported earlier, our procedure precluded any attempt to extend the equinoxious contour presented in Figure 32-3 to frequencies lower than 1,000 Hz. Moreover, because of the rather poor accuracy of audiometric measurements above 6,000 Hz, it is difficult to test the effect of signals centered at frequencies above 4,000 Hz. For these reasons, the above results were complemented by measures of equal-loudness contours for the same type of impulses over a wider range of frequencies. Obviously, loudness is not a direct measure of noxiousness, but it is reasonable to assume that, as for ATS, the effect of the frequency content of nonreverberant impulses is basically governed by the transfer function of the outer and middle ear.

Loudness Studies

Methods

The method of adjustment was used to measure the loudness level of narrow-band impulses. It is easier to compare the loudness of an impulse noise with that of a noise of comparable bandwidth than with a pure tone. For this reason, the loudness level of a narrow-band 500-ms noise (30 ms rise/decay time) centered at 1,000 Hz was first determined us-

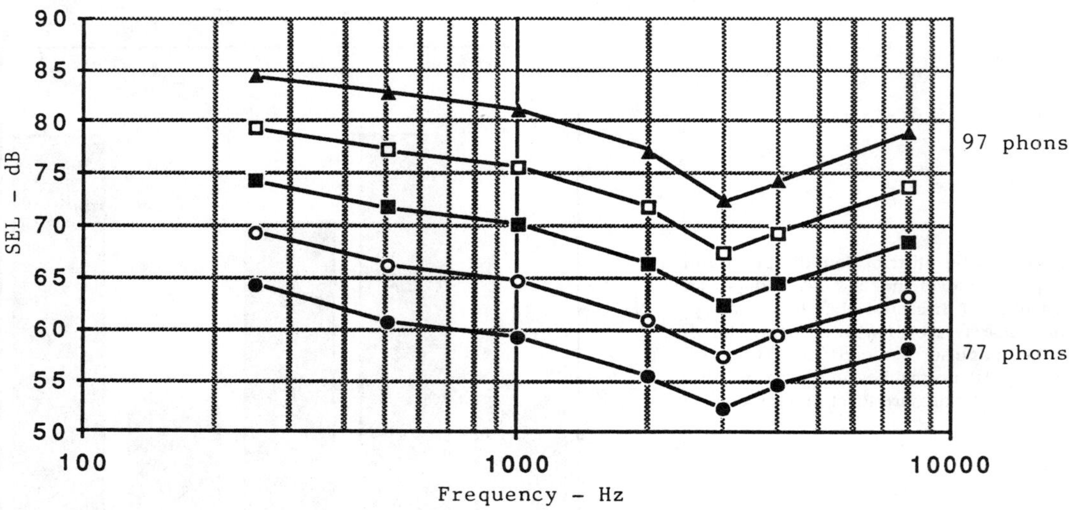

Figure 32-5 Median equal loudness contours of one-octave-band-wide impulses presented at five loudness levels, obtained with nine normal-hearing subjects. SEL-dB, sound exposure level in decibels.

ing a 1,000-Hz reference pure tone of the same temporal characteristics. The reference signal presented at a preset constant level was followed 250 ms later by the test signal. The level of the signal was adjusted by the subject by means of a 30-dB potentiometer. A delay of 500 ms separated two pairs of reference and test signals. The level of the test signal was set randomly at the beginning of each adjustment trial. The subject was asked to adjust the test signal to appear alternatively louder and then softer than the reference until both signals appeared equally loud. A switch was then activated by the subject to indicate that the trial was completed.

Keeping in mind the tendency to judge the second signal louder than the first one of a pair (Stevens, 1956), the procedure described above was reversed; the noise served as the reference and the tone served as the test signal. The same was done with the impulse noises compared to the 500-ms noise centered at 1,000 Hz. Five sound levels were tested, allowing us to obtain an unbiased estimate of the loudness level from the least square solution combining the results of using the 500-ms noise as the reference and as the test signal.

Prior to conducting the experiments on equal loudness contours of narrow-band impulses, a study of the effect of the duration of the impulses on loudness had been conducted (Tran Quoc and Hétu, 1990). It allowed us to verify that the decrease in the duration of narrow-band impulses with the increase of its center frequency is well accounted for by its effect on the total energy of the signal. It also indicated that, with the time sequence of the signal presentation used and at levels between 75 and 95 phons, the measure of the loudness level of impulses was not affected by the sound pressure level. This gave us a good indication that the subjects' responses were not influenced by the acoustic reflex or by auditory fatigue.

Two series of loudness level measurements were conducted, one with 1-octave-band-wide and another with ⅓-octave-band-wide impulses centered at different frequencies.

Results

Equal Loudness Contours of One-Octave-Band-Wide Impulses

One-octave-band-wide impulses were digitally constructed, as in the previous experiments, using the computer-controlled generation system. The loudness level of impulses was measured at seven center frequencies (250, 500, 1,000, 2,000, 3,000, 4,000, and 8,000 Hz) and at five levels of presentation (77, 82, 87, 92, and 97 phons). Nine normal-hearing listeners participated in this experiment, and their hearing threshold levels were better than 15 dB (ANSI S3.6, 1989) between 250 and 8,000 Hz.

The equal loudness contours obtained at the five presentation levels were strictly parallel, as shown in Figure 32-5. Each data point is the median of 27 adjustments made by nine subjects. It can be seen that the sensitivity reaches a maximum at 3,000 Hz, decreasing progressively as the frequency is lowered. The estimated slope is equal to −5 dB per octave between 1,000 and 3,000 Hz, and −4.5 dB per octave between 250 and 1,000 Hz. The slope is approximately +4 dB per octave between 3,000 and 8,000 Hz. Using 1,000 Hz as a reference, one must decrease the SEL by 8 dB to obtain the same loudness level at 3,000 Hz. This difference is similar to, although somewhat smaller than, what was observed with ATS. But, again, these contours clearly depart from the A-weighting curve.

Equal Loudness Contours of One-Third-Octave-Band-Wide Impulses

To assess the individual differences in the response to the frequency content of narrow-band impulses, equal loudness contours were obtained with 20 normal-hearing listeners, 10 men and 10 women. These subjects did not participate in the experiment reported above with the 1-octave-band-wide signals. Impulses were digitally constructed, as explained earlier, for each adjacent normalized ⅓-octave band between 1,000 and 8,000 Hz. The rise and decay time ranged from 3 ms at 1,000 Hz to 0.3 ms at 8,000 Hz; the B-duration (see Coles et al, 1968) ranged from 23 to 3 ms. Figure 32-6 illustrates the type of signal generated: the acoustic pressure time profile and the result of the Fourier analysis of the impulse centered at 1,000 Hz are depicted. The level of this impulse was 90 dB SEL and 116 dB peak. Five presentation levels were tested: 74, 79, 84, 89, and 94 phons.

There were no statistical differences between the results for the women and the men, but the individual configurations varied considerably. These will be analyzed elsewhere. Figure 32-7 presents the five median equal loudness contours that were obtained. As expected, the maximum sensitivity is located at 3,150 Hz. The slope between 1,000 and 3,000 Hz is steeper than with the octave-band impulses, approaching −8 dB per octave. The difference in level to achieve the same loudness at these two frequencies is −11 dB. These results are compared in Figure 32-8 with those from two studies on steady-state signals of comparable bandwidth (Bauer and Torick, 1969; Stevens, 1971). At 3,150 Hz, our results differ slightly from those of the other studies, the relative loudness level being 3 dB lower. There is also a difference of 2 to 3 dB at 6,300 Hz. In view of the differences in the experimental procedures and the type of signal tested, it can be concluded that there is still a close agreement between the present results and the results from studies using continuous noise, especially the results of Stevens. This similarity strongly suggests that the effect of the center frequency for these two types of narrow-band signals is controlled by the same mechanism, namely the transfer function of the external and middle ear. As for continuous noises, the equal loudness contour clearly departs from the A-weighting curve. This is further emphasized by means of direct comparison, as shown in Figure 32-9. The median results from Figure 32-7 are presented in terms of the relative sensitivity of the ear to signals of different frequency content (I). The A-, D-, and E-weighting curves are also reproduced. The D-weighting curve better accounts for the relative response to frequency based on the present results.

Conclusion

Using two lines of evidence, namely TTS and loudness measurements, we have shown that the spectral content of nonreverberant impulses has a major effect on the human ear response at levels below 135 dB peak. The data reported earlier suggest that this influence varies according to the bandwidth of the noise. The general rules for predicting this influence could be derived from the equal loudness contours, which accurately characterize the relative sensitivity of the ear to both transients and steady-state sounds of different frequency content, as proposed two decades ago by Johnson and Robinson (1967, 1969). The shape of such contours appears, in our experiments, to be little influenced by the sound level in the range of 85 dB to at least 120 dB peak. They serve better than the A-weighting curve to account for the effect of the energy spectrum of impulse noises found in the occupational setting.

It is worth recalling that impact noise exposure in industry may very well involve relatively great concentrations of sound energy in narrow frequency bands centered at the resonant frequency of the impacted structure. One typical example is the noise found in bottling plants; the empty bottle shocks generate impulses of very narrow bands whose center frequency generally varies between 2,000 and 4,000 Hz, depending on the size and shape of the bottle (Hétu and Parrot, 1978, Figs. 1 and 2). This phenomenon could explain the increased noxiousness of impact noise, as com-

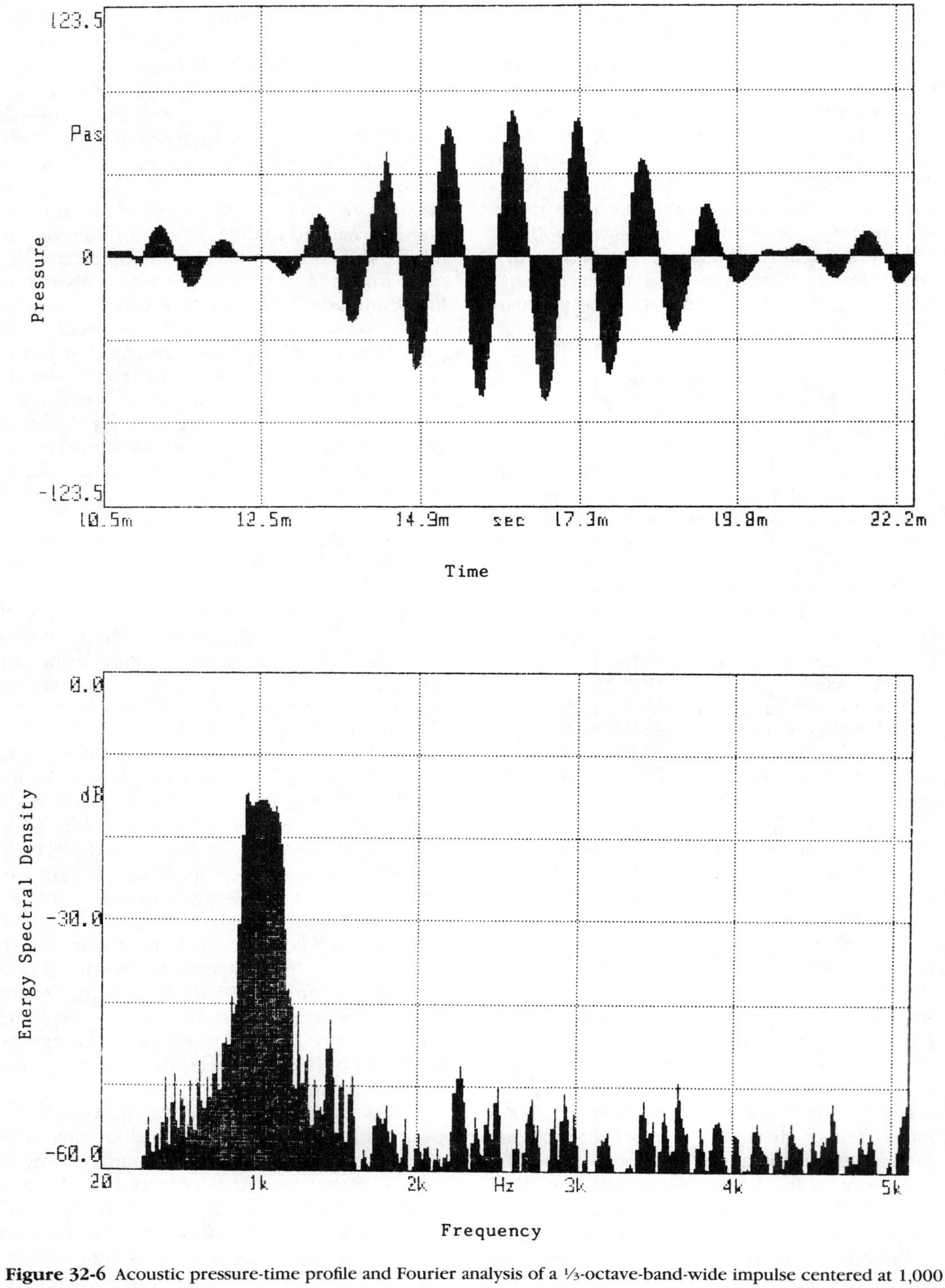

Figure 32-6 Acoustic pressure-time profile and Fourier analysis of a ⅓-octave-band-wide impulse centered at 1,000 Hz.

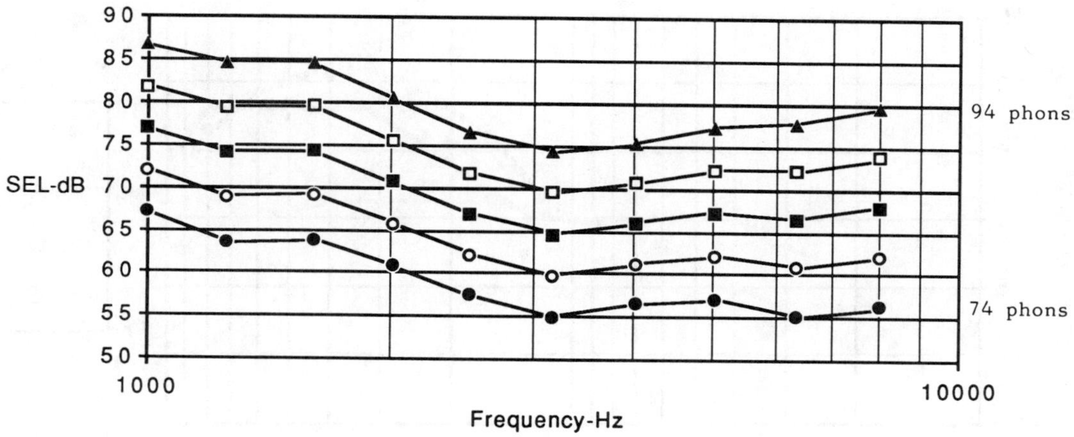

Figure 32-7 Median equal loudness contours of ⅓-octave-band-wide impulses presented at five loudness levels (20 normal-hearing subjects). SEL-dB, sound exposure level in decibels.

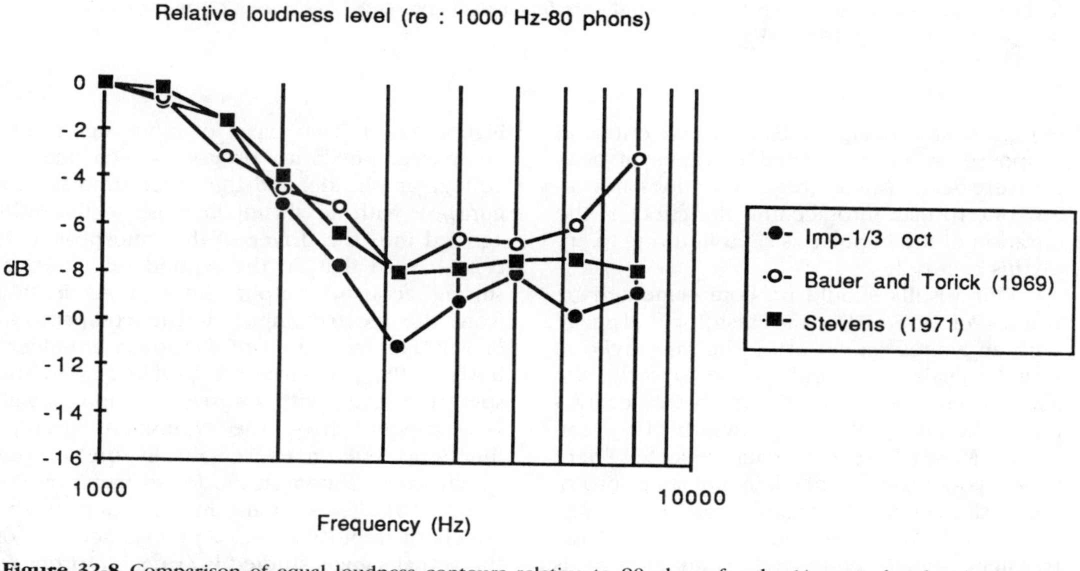

Figure 32-8 Comparison of equal loudness contours relative to 80 phons for the ⅓-octave-band-wide impulses (Imp-⅓ oct) derived from Figure 32-7 and the steady-state noises of the same bandwidth as reported by Bauer and Torick (1969) and Stevens (1971).

pared to steady-state noise of the same amount of A-weighted energy, as reported in several epidemiologic studies of PTS among industrial workers (Sulkowski and Lipowczan, 1982; Taylor et al, 1984; Thiery and Meyer-Bisch, 1988). In other words, the use of the A-weighting could have led to an underestimation of the effect of impact noises with spectral peaks around 3,000 Hz and above, because the energy associated with such peaks is treated as being nearly as noxious as that of noises whose maximum energy is around 1,000 Hz. Such a possibility could be examined in future field studies on the auditory effects of impulse noise.

The present results agree with the general hypothesis put forward by Price (1983) that the spectral content strongly determines the damaging power of impulse noise on the ear. But our results are not directly comparable to those of Price because (1) they do not refer to the same ranges of sound levels and numbers of consecutive impulses and (2) they do not refer to the same type of pressure-time profiles. Differences of the latter parameter imply variations in the duration of the two types of

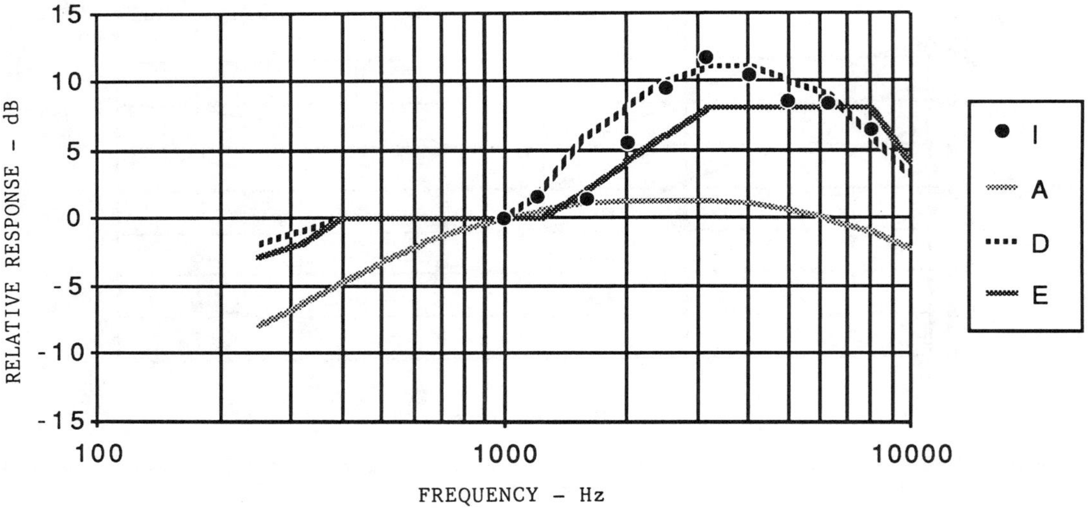

Figure 32-9 Relative response of the ear as a function of the frequency content of sound derived from the equal loudness contours obtained with ⅓-octave-band-wide impulses (I) presented in Figure 32-7 and from the normalized A-, D-, and E-weighting curves.

impulses. Moreover, the damage-risk criterion proposed by Price, defined in terms of peak pressure level versus frequency, does not allow one to take into account the effect of the duration of the impulse as such in trying to apply his criterion.

Our results should be complemented by studies of ATS, PTS, and histologic damage with an animal model using the same type of sound signals. This could serve to verify the above conclusions and also to better characterize the effect of the bandwidth of the impulse. Meanwhile, the data reported here strongly indicate the need, in any study protocol of the effects of impulse noise on hearing, to strictly control the spectral content of the transient signals employed. Such control is particularly crucial for impulses artificially generated in the laboratory using electroacoustic devices. If a study design involves the systematic variation of the peak pressure level, then the effect of nonlinear distortion in the generation system should be assessed. Otherwise, the increased amount of energy in the higher frequencies due to distortion could confound the effect of the peak pressure level (Nicolas et al, 1990, Figs. 10 and 11). Even if the spectrum as such is not investigated, it should be determined from the *acoustic* output of the generation system and should be explicitly reported in any published account of the study. Reporting only the characteristics of the input signals can be misleading. This is illustrated by the examples shown in Figure 32-10. Two types of input signals are compared, one with progressive changes in voltage amplitude, and the other simulating a gunshot, with an abrupt increase in the voltage fed into the driver of the loudspeaker. It can be seen that, in the second case, the resulting acoustic output differs considerably from the electric input to the compression driver (i.e., the output of the power amplifier) both in the pressure-time profile and in the spectrum. Even with a corrected input signal, as computed from the equipment transfer function, differences remain in the output spectrum, as shown in the lower panel of Figure 32-10*C*. Thus, in any investigation on the effects of impulse noise, a precise account of the actual signals studied is crucial in order to properly validate a hypothesis and to compare results with those from other sources.

Le Spectre des Bruits Impulsionnels et la Réponse de l'oreille Humaine

La description des bruits impulsionnels dans le domaine fréquentiel offre vraisemblablement une base de prédiction des effets de ce type de bruit sur l'oreille humaine. Cela est particulièrement le cas des impulsions non-réverbérées pour lesquelles le spectre

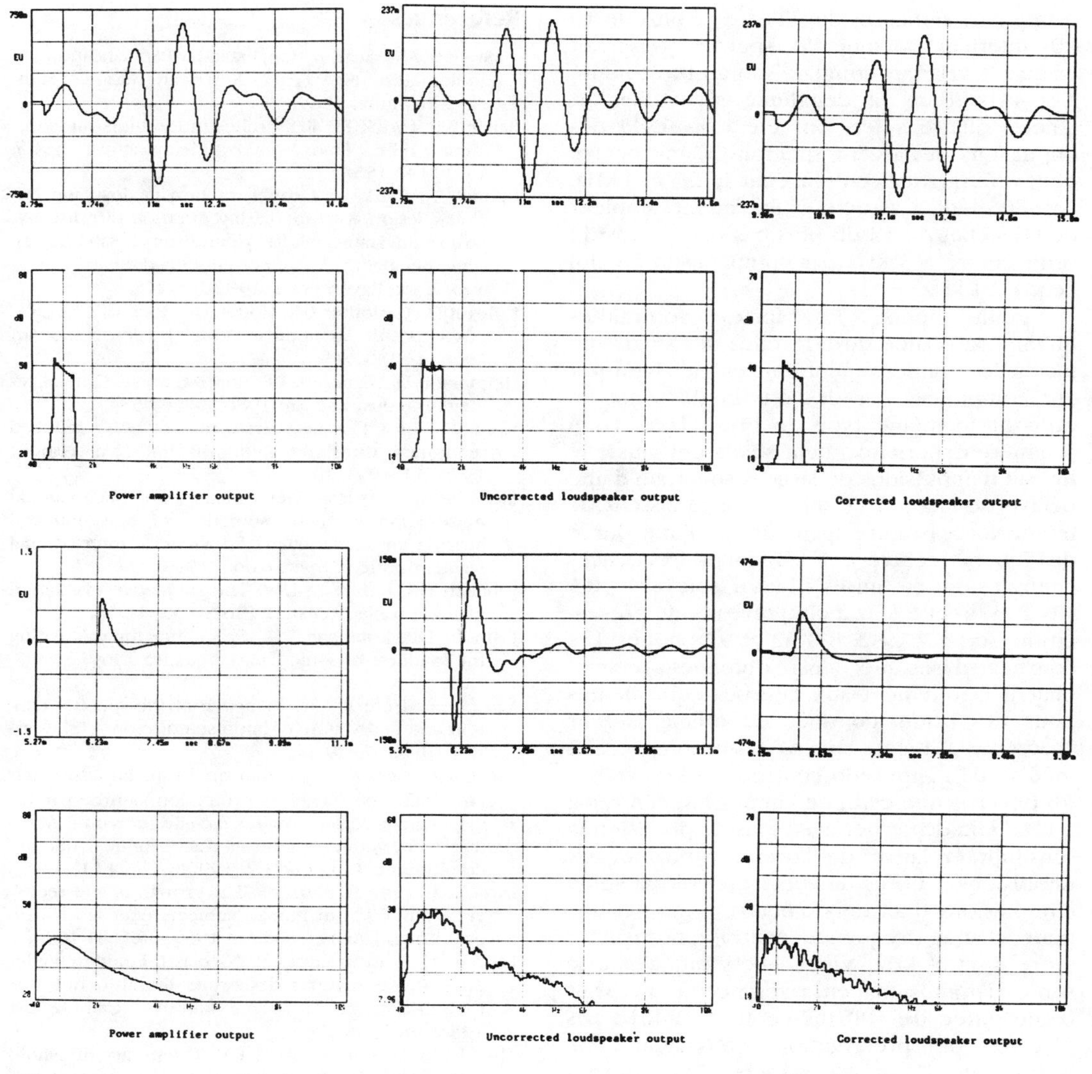

Figure 32-10 Pressure-time profile and Fourier analysis of a (sin x)/x numeric signal (upper panels) and of a simulated gunshot (lower panels) recorded from the impulse-noise generation system used in the experiments reported in the text. *A,* Power amplifier output. *B,* Uncorrected loudspeaker output. *C,* Corrected loudspeaker output.

peut prendre en compte l'influence de paramètres temporels tels que la durée de montée et la durée totale du signal. Toutefois, très peu d'études ont porté sur la contribution du spectre à la prédiction des effets des bruits impulsionnels sur l'oreille humaine, principalement à cause des difficultés associées au contrôle expérimental de ce paramètre. Grâce au développement d'un générateur d'impulsions contrôlé par ordinateur nous avons mené des études ayant pour but d'évaluer l'importance du spectre dans la prédiction (a) du décalage temporaire des seuils d'audition (DTS) provoqué par des impulsions sonores et (b) de la sonie de ce type de bruit.

Deux séries de travaux ont été réalisées sur l'acquisition du DTS consécutif L à l'exposition à des impulsions non-réverbérées présentées à une cadence de 1 par seconde durant des intervalles de 4 à 60 minutes. Dans la première série, on a varié de 1 à 3 et à 4 kHz la fréquence supérieure de coupure d'une impulsion en maintenant constante la fréquence inférieure de coupure à 0,3 kHz. Pour les trois sujets participants à l'expérience, le SEL du bruit permettant d'induire des DTS d'ampleurs similaires devait être de plus de 10 dB inférieur lorsque le spectre s'étendait jusqu'à 3 kHz par comparaison au bruit limité à 1 kHz. Dans la deuxième série d'expériences, quatre sujets ont été exposés à des impulsions de largeur spectrale d'une octave dont la fréquence centrale était 1, 2, 3 et 4 kHz. Le SEL médian associé à une même ampleur de DTS était de 12 dB plus bas dans le cas du bruit centré à 3 kHz par comparaison à celui centré à 1 kHz.

Etant donné les fortes contraintes qu'impose l'étude du DTS chez des sujets humains, les données mentionnées plus haut ont été complétées par des études de sonie en utilisant le même type de bruit. Lors d'une première expérience, neuf sujets ont ajusté le niveau d'impulsions de largeur spectrale d'une octave de façon à ce qu'elles apparaissent de même force sonore qu'un bruit d'une durée de 500 ms centré à 1 kHz. Sept fréquences centrales ont été mises à l'essai, soit 0,25 - 0,5 - 1- 2- 3- 4- et 8 kHz à cinq niveaux de présentation, soit à 77, 82, 87, 92 et 97 phones. Les courbes d'isosonie ainsi obtenues ressemblaient étroitement aux courbes équivalentes pour des bruits continus de même largeur spectrale. A même niveau d'isosonie, le SEL médian de l'impulsion centrée à 3 kHz était 8 dB plus bas que celui de l'impulsion centrée à 1 kHz. Afin de cerner avec plus de précision la sensibilité relative de l'oreille humaine aux impulsions sonores de spectre étroit, la sonie d'impulsions d'un tiers d'octave a été évaluée pour chaque fréquence centrale normalisée entre 1 et 8 kHz. Vingt sujets ont ajusté la sonie d'impulsions en référence à un bruit d'une durée de 500 ms centré à 1 kHz. Les niveaux de présentation couvraient une gamme de 74 à 94 phones. Les courbes d'isosonie variaient considérablement d'un sujet à un autre. Mais encore une fois, les résultats médians montrent une sensibilité maximale à 3 kHz; à même niveau d'isosonie, le SEL à 3,15 kHz était 11 dB plus bas qu'à 1 kHz.

Tous les résultats convergent pour montrer que la fonction de transfert de l'oreille externe et moyenne semble bien gouverner la réponse aux impulsions non-réverbérées de niveaux inférieurs à 140 dB crête. Par conséquent, le contenu spectral peut être considéré comme un prédicteur puissant des effets auditifs des bruits impulsionnels.

ACKNOWLEDGMENT

This research has been financially supported by the Institut de recherche en santé et en sécurité du travail du Québec.

References

ANSI S3.6. American national standard specification for audiometers. New York: American National Standards Institute, 1989.

Bauer BB, Torick EL. Researches in loudness measurement. IEEE Trans Audio Electroacoust 1966; 14(3):141-155.

Bohne BA, Clark W. Growth of hearing loss and cochlear lesion with increasing duration of noise exposure. In: Hamernik RP, Henderson D, Salvi R, eds. New perspectives on noise-induced hearing loss. New York: Raven Press, 1982:265-275.

Coles RRA, Garinther GR, Hodge DC, Rice CG. Hazardous exposure to impulse noise. J Acoust Soc Am 1968; 43:336-343.

Henderson D, Hamernik RP. Impulse noise: Critical review. J Acoust Soc Am 1986; 80:569-584.

Hétu R, Parrot J. A field evaluation of noise induced temporary threshold shift. Am Ind Hyg Assoc J 1978; 39:301-311.

ISO-1999. Acoustics—Determination of occupational noise exposure and estimation of noise-induced hearing impairment. 2nd Ed. Geneva: International Standardization Organization, 1990.

Johnson DR, Robinson DW. The subjective evaluation of sonic bangs. Acustica 1967; 18:241-258.

Johnson DR, Robinson DW. Procedure for calculating the loudness of sonic bangs. Acustica 1969; 21:307-318.

Laroche C, Hétu R. The influence of the spectral content and decay time of impulse noise on ATS. Acustica 1990a; 70:29-44.

Laroche C, Hétu R. Exposition aux bruits impulsionnels en milieux de travail: la protection assurée par les dispositions règlementaires est-elle suffisante? Actes du premier congrès français d'acoustique, Colloque de physique, Colloque C2, 1990b; 51(2):147-150.

Laroche C, Hétu R, Poirier S. The growth of and recovery from T.T.S. in human subjects exposed to impact noise. J Acoust Soc Am 1989; 85:1681-1690.

Laroche C, Hétu R, Sawan M, Nicolas J. Etude de l'effet du contenu spectral des bruits impulsionnels sur l'acquisition de la fatigue auditive. Can Acoust 1986; 14(3):30-47.

Mills JH, Adkins WY, Gilbert RM. Temporary threshold shifts produced by wideband noise. J Acoust Soc Am 1981; 70:390-396.

Mills JH, Gilbert RM, Adkins WY. Temporary threshold shifts in humans exposed to octave bands of noise for 16 to 24 hours. J Acoust Soc Am 1979; 65:1238-1248.

Nicolas J, Hétu R, Sawan M, Laroche C. A digitally controlled impulse-noise generation system for the study of the ear response to impulse noise. Acustica 1990; 70:122-126.

Price GR. Relative hazard of weapons impulses. J Acoust Soc Am 1983; 73:556-566.

Price GR. Impulse noise hazard as a function of level and spectral distribution. In: Salvi R, Henderson D, Hamernik RP, Colletti V, eds. Basic and applied aspects of noise-induced hearing loss. New York: Plenum Press, 1986:372.

Saunders JC, Dear SP, Schneider ME. The anatomical consequences of acoustic injury: A review and tutorial. J Acoust Soc Am 1985; 78:833-860.

Stevens SS. Calculation of loudness of complex noise. J Acoust Soc Am 1956; 28:807-832.

Stevens SS. Perceived level of noise by Mark VII and decibels (E). J Acoust Soc Am 1971; 51:575-601.

Sulkowski WJ, Lipcowczan A. Impulse noise-induced hearing loss in drop forge operators and the energy concept. Noise Contr Eng J 1982; 18(1):24-28.

Taylor W, Lempert B, Pelmear P, Hemstock I, Kershaw J. Noise levels and hearing thresholds in the drop forging industry. J Acoust Soc Am 1984; 76:807-819.

Thiery L, Meyer-Bisch C. Hearing loss due to partly impulsive industrial noise exposure at levels between 87 and 90 dB(A). J Acoust Soc Am 1988; 84:651-659.

Tran Quoc H, Hétu R. L'influence de la durée sur la sonie de bruits impulsifs de spectre étroit présentés à haut niveau de pression acoustique. J Acoust 1990; 3:59-67.

SECTION SIX

Hearing Protection

CHAPTER 33

Current Issues in Hearing Protection

ELLIOTT H. BERGER
FREDRIK LINDGREN

There was an explosion of literature on hearing protection devices (HPDs) and hearing conservation in the 1980s. By one count (Berger, 1990a) the number of English-language articles in the 1980s (approximately 800 citations) was more than twice those appearing in the 1970s, and in the 1970s the published articles exceeded twice the number that had appeared prior to that decade (Berger, 1990a). This chapter neither analyzes nor summarizes that vast body of literature, but rather highlights key areas of current research and discusses the unanswered questions which, when resolved, will hold the greatest promise of benefit to those requiring protection from hazardous noise exposures. Although active and nonlinear hearing protectors are topics that might well be included under the above criteria, they will not be covered in this chapter because they are dealt with by other authors in this book.

HPDs of Better Sound Quality

One of the principal problems faced by hearing conservationists is overcoming employee resistance to the use of hearing protection devices. The causes of such resistance are varied, but a dominant one is the noise reduction of the hearing protector interfering with or distorting the sounds the wearer wishes to hear. Although this problem can be addressed in part by an effective educational and motivational program, a potentially more successful approach is the design of improved HPDs—devices that provide uniform attenuation across frequency, and that provide an optimized rather than a maximized amount of attenuation.

The attenuation of traditional HPDs increases with frequency as a result of the basic physics of sound transmission loss through a sealed orifice or a solid shell (Shaw, 1982). This characteristic is more pronounced for earmuffs than for earplugs. The disadvantage of attenuation increasing with frequency is that sounds become distorted. Workers with noise-induced hearing loss are especially disadvantaged. Speech appears muffled and may be harder to understand. Machine sounds are altered and may be more difficult to evaluate. The world sounds different, strange, or unpleasant. An HPD with uniform attenuation, i.e., possessing a flat frequency response, can overcome or reduce many of these problems (Alberti, 1987; Coleman et al, 1984; Gorman, 1982). As summarized by Lazarus (1983), "To ensure the least possible adverse effect on the recognition of acoustic signals, hearing protectors whose sound attenuation is largely independent of frequency in the frequency range of the masking noise and the acoustic signals should be used."

Likewise, the problem of overprotection has been discussed in the literature (Abel et al, 1982), and at least one national standard (Canadian Standards Association Z94.2) indicates that moderate- or low-attenuation HPDs may be preferable for certain noise exposures (CSA, 1984). Consider too, that equivalent daily exposures in about 90 percent of noisy industries in the United States are less than or equal to 95 dBA (OSHA, 1983), and the required protection under such conditions amounts to only about 10 dB of actual delivered on-the-job noise reduction.

In response to these problems, some manufacturers have introduced HPDs providing moderate, flat attenuation across the important audio frequencies (Allen and Berger, 1990; Killion et al, 1988), and other designs

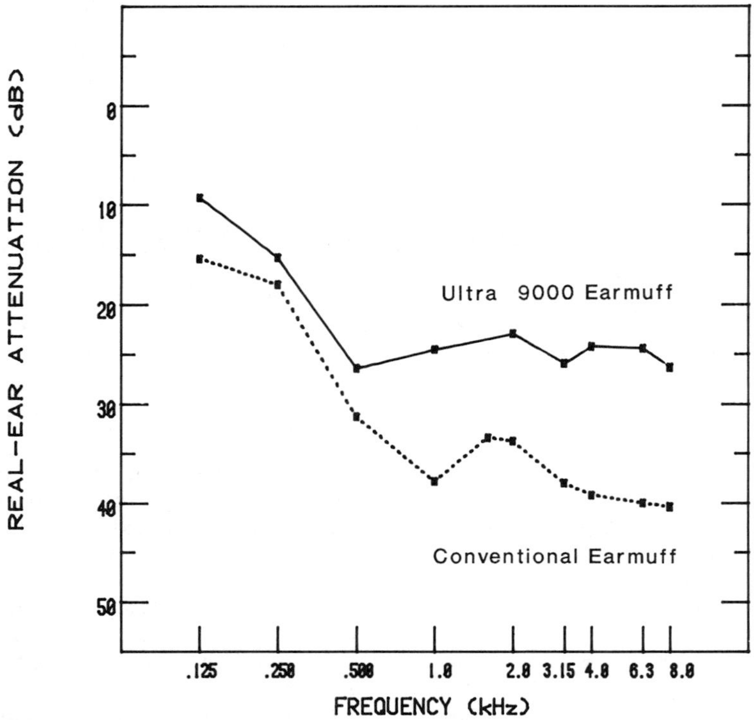

Figure 33-1 Real-ear attenuation of a moderate- and relatively flat-attenuation earmuff (E-A-R Ultra 9,000 muff) compared to a conventional earmuff.

are expected to follow. Examples of the attenuation of a currently available earmuff and earplug are shown in Figures 33-1 and 33-2, respectively, where their performance is compared to conventional products. The desired attenuation in these new designs is achieved by providing a controlled sound path through the hearing protector. In the case of the earmuff the path is through an orifice into a duct-and-earpad assembly, which communicates directly with the canal entrance. In the case of the earplug, the path is through a thin diaphragm, an acoustical network, and into a large-diameter bore through the canal portion of the earplug.

Additional devices like those described above, but with various tailored attenuation characteristics, degrees of complexity, and costs, must be developed and distributed, and research quantifying their performance advantages must be conducted. Of equal importance, users as well as manufacturers of HPDs must be educated regarding the value of products that are matched to particular noise exposures instead of simply purchased for maximum protection.

Strategies for Training and Motivation

Although the literature provides guidance in training and motivation of those required to wear HPDs (Royster and Royster, 1986b) and demonstrates the value (primarily in the short term) of certain educational and motivational approaches (Fleming, 1980; Harvey, 1981; Sadler and Montgomery, 1982; Zohar et al, 1980), ample evidence exists to demonstrate that the majority of industrial and military hearing conservation programs are not effective for the prevention of noise-induced hearing loss (ANSI, 1990; Royster and Royster, 1988).

Reasons for resistance to the use of hearing protectors have been identified. For example, Herberg (1984) interviewed 210 employees in the metal-working, mining, and textile industries, and found that the reasons that the employees resisted the use of hearing protectors included a subjective tolerance for noise, a concern that HPDs would make it harder to hear their machines and to work effectively

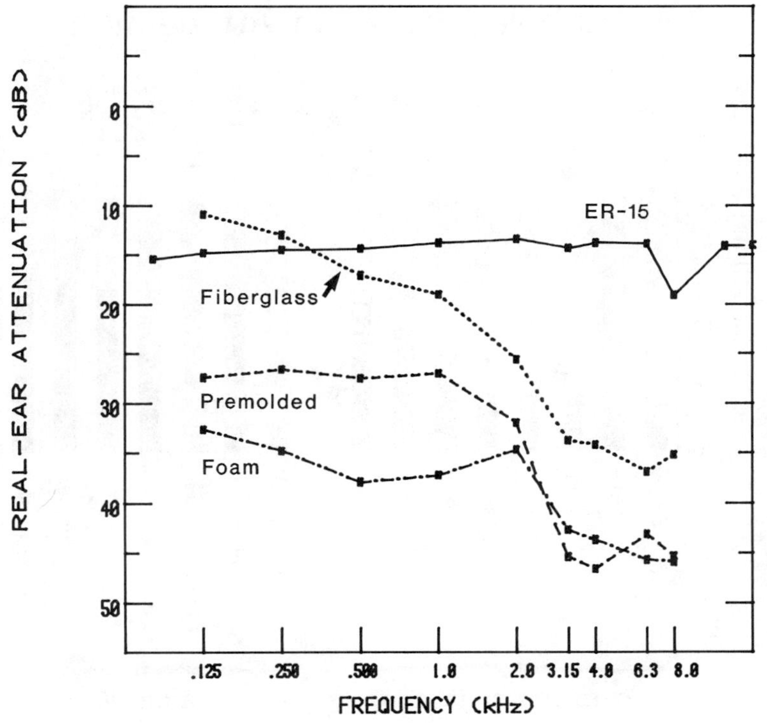

Figure 33-2 Real-ear attenuation of a moderate- and extremely flat-attenuation earplug (Etymotic ER-15 earplug) compared to conventional foam, fiberglass, and premolded earplugs.

and that use of HPDs would interfere with communications, an intolerance for the isolation they felt while wearing hearing protection, an altered body image, a physical intolerance for the subjective tactile and aural sensations they felt while wearing HPDs, a lack of concern for future consequences (i.e., hearing loss), and response to peer pressure.

Not only must existing training and motivational strategies be more widely implemented, but available approaches must be more fully validated (especially with regard to long-term effectiveness), and additional techniques should be developed. Large-scale in-field experiments demonstrating the short-term and long-term effects on both the percentage of exposed individuals wearing HPDs and their achieved protection, would be of particular value. Finally, methods are needed for training those persons within the hearing conservation program (HCP) whose responsibility it is to instruct the actual users in the proper use of, because there is evidence that the trainers' HPD knowledge and fitting skills are sorely lacking (Royster and Royster, 1990).

Real-World Attenuation

Since Regan (1977) published one of the first quantitative studies of real-world attenuation (i.e., attenuation achieved in practice by employees in an HCP), at least 15 additional studies conducted in more than 75 different industries, in 6 different countries, including 2,247 employee/subjects, have been conducted. Portions of those data have been previously summarized by Berger (1983, 1988). The current results on the complete database closely parallel the earlier findings, which demonstrated that current laboratory data reported in the United States provide neither an accurate indicator of the absolute magnitude of field attenuation nor a useful tool to estimate the rank ordering of such results.

The real-world data are summarized in terms of a single number rating, the noise reduction rating (NRR; see EPA, 1979), in Figure 33-3, where they are compared to laboratory data currently reported for products sold in North America. The real-world NRRs are computed with a one–standard deviation correction to represent values obtained by about 84

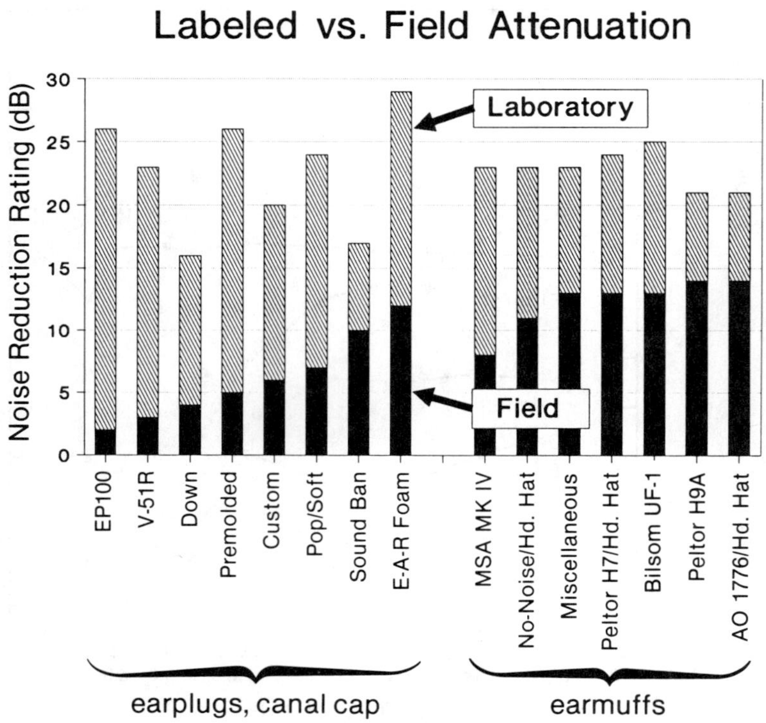

Figure 33-3 Comparison of real-world ("field") noise-reduction ratings (NRRs) to manufacturers' laboratory values published in North America. Field NRRs are computed with a one–standard deviation correction, whereas the laboratory NRRs include a two–standard deviation correction. The minimum sample size for each field data point is 25 subjects.

percent of the wearers. Products are shown individually for all cases with a subject count of greater than 25; otherwise the results were averaged together into generic earplug categories or into one earmuff category labeled "Miscellaneous."

The average real-world NRRs for insert and semi-insert devices range from 2 to 12 dB, averaging 6 dB. As a percentage of laboratory values, the field results vary widely across devices from 8 to 56 percent (averaging 26 percent), and are thus not amenable to a precise derating value that would be appropriate for all products. For earmuffs the real-world NRRs show greater uniformity, ranging from 8 to 14 dB, with an average value of 12 dB. As a percentage of laboratory data the values range from 35 to 67 percent with an average of 50 percent.

Although the sample size is large for certain products shown in Figure 33-3, additional data, especially on semiaural devices, would be of value to provide more accurate product-specific information. Of equal interest are studies to demonstrate achievable attenuation in optimized HCPs as well as the evaluation of the real-world performance of earmuffs and earplugs worn in combination.

More-Representative Laboratory Methods

As discussed above, typical laboratory-derived attenuation values provide poor estimates of real-world attenuation. The problem primarily lies in the subject selection, supervision, training, and fitting procedures used in the laboratory, which are developed with the intention of yielding optimum attenuation results, highly reproducible data, or both rather than values that reflect real-world use and wearing conditions (Berger, 1988). To be able to better match HPDs to their intended applications, laboratory protocols are required that provide data that is more representative of actual field performance.

Currently, an American National Stan-

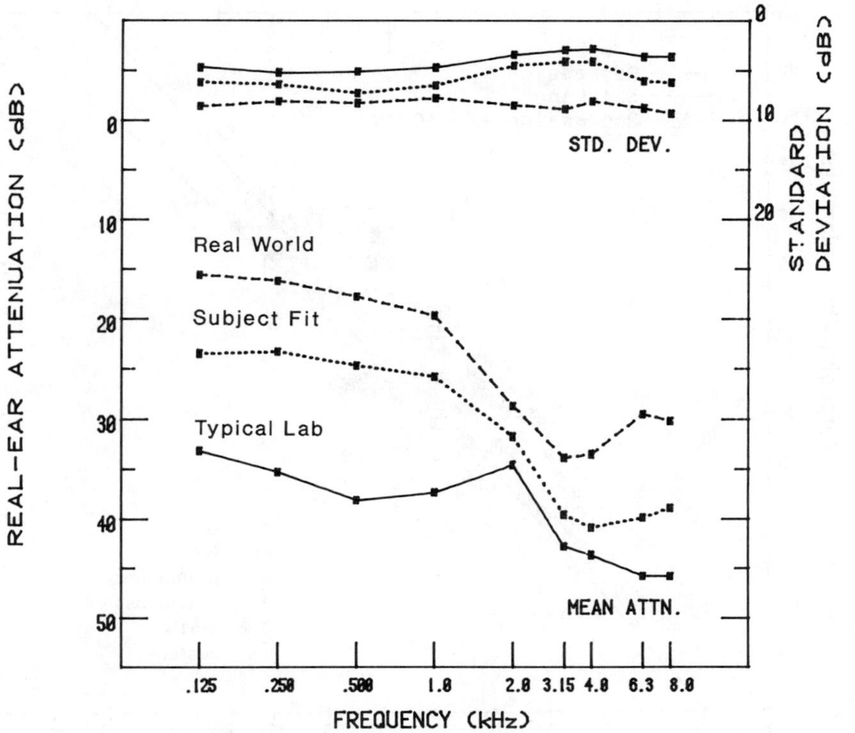

Figure 33-4 Comparison of three procedures for measuring real-ear attenuation of foam earplugs. Typical laboratory data are an average of 18 10-subject tests per ANSI S12.6, as practiced in one laboratory in the United States. Subject fit included 100 subjects tested using procedures like those under development by ANSI S12/WG11; average real-world data included 11 studies with 471 subjects. (Data from Berger EH. Can real-world attenuation be estimated using laboratory data? Sound and Vib 1988; 22(12):26-31.)

dards Institute (ANSI) working group (WG)—ANSI S12/WG11—is addressing this problem and has devised a test protocol that will be evaluated by a number of North American laboratories (Berger, 1990b). The feasibility of using the resultant data to estimate actual field performance will be assessed by comparing the results, averaged across laboratories, to the real-world database cited above. The goal is to estimate the protection that can be, or is being, obtained in the top 10 to 20 percent of today's industrial and military hearing conservation programs. WG11's interlaboratory data will also be compared between laboratories to determine whether the reproducibility is within acceptable limits and how it compares to the results of previous interlaboratory comparisons.

One example of the influence of laboratory procedures on attenuation data is shown in Figure 33-4 (Berger, 1988). The typical laboratory data are indicative of current test practices in the United States as embodied in ANSI S12.6-1984 (ANSI, 1984), whereas the subject-fit data are based on a protocol in which primarily naive subjects were given the HPDs along with written instructions, but with no experimenter assistance whatsoever. Such a protocol is closely modeled after the one under development by WG11. The real-world data are an average of 11 separate field studies. Note how the subject-fit data correspond much more closely with the real-world data than do the values based on the typical laboratory protocol.

The influence of fitting procedure illustrated in the preceding example is considerably greater for earplugs than for earmuffs. This is not only because earplugs are more difficult to fit and more liable to be misused, but because there is also a greater range of options on how to fit them correctly in the laboratory and how they may be misfitted in the field. Also, it should be noted that the "typical laboratory" results pertain to data from the United States, because as Berger (1988) has observed, certain facilities in Australia and Europe already use test protocols that yield results that more nearly approximate real-world data.

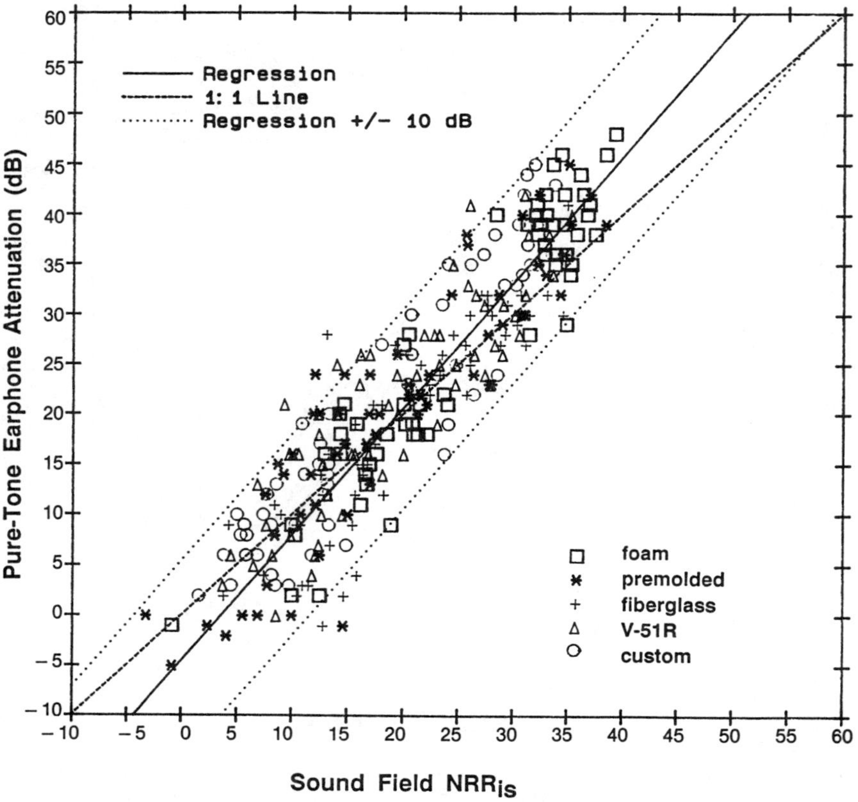

Figure 33-5 Scattergram of pure-tone earphone attenuation at 500 Hz versus the NRR_{is} computed from sound-field attenuation measurements for 300 measurements (15 subjects × 2 types of fit × 5 types of earplugs × 2 replications). The subscript on the NRR indicates a value calculated for each test on each individual subject (is).

Quantitative Fit Tests

Numerous existing methods for developing group attenuation data, either in the field or in the laboratory, have been described and are available (Berger, 1986). However, field methods and statistical techniques applicable to individual users for quantitative fit tests have not been established. Such techniques would aid in developing better procedures for dispensing, fitting, training, and motivating employees in the use of their devices. The methods might include the use of circumaural test devices to test earplugs (Berger, 1989), probe microphones to test earmuffs (Liu et al, 1989), or even evoked-response audiometry to test all types of HPDs (Wilde and Humes, 1987).

The method of using a circumaural test device consists of measuring real-ear attenuation at threshold in a manner directly analogous to the electroacoustic procedures of ANSI S12.6 or International Standards Organization (ISO) 4869-1, except that the incident sound field is created inside circumaural earcups instead of within a room. Berger (1989) has shown that with use of this method, pure tones can be substituted for ⅓-octave-band signals, and a reasonable estimate of overall attenuation can be derived by testing only one or two frequencies such as 500 or 1,000 Hz, or both.

One example of the type of data resulting from the use of circumaural test devices is shown in Figure 33-5, which is a scattergram of the pure-tone attenuation at 500 Hz measured with the circumaural device versus an overall average attenuation rating, the NRR. The NRR was computed from ⅓-octave-band sound-field attenuation measurements (per ANSI S12.6) on the same subjects for the same fitting of the device. Note the excellent correlation between the two types of measurements and the agreement for the averaged results (coefficient of determination, $r^2 = 0.88$). However, in five of the 300 cases the pure-tone headphone-measured attenuation exceeded the sound-field NRR by more than 10 dB and thus, in those cases, predictions of attenuation based on the headphone measures would be substantially in error. Suitable procedures to handle such situations as well as additional data demonstrating the degree and extent of the errors are required before such techniques can be recommended for general application in industry.

Audiometric Database Analysis Techniques

The three preceding sections call for data to better rate HPDs and prescribe them for particular applications, but once they are in use, methods must be devised to determine if in fact the HPDs are working—i.e., protecting the individuals who are wearing them from incurring noise-induced hearing losses (NIHLs). In the United States at least, the data for such determinations are available, because annual audiometric evaluations are required for all employees working in time-weighted average (TWA) exposures equal to or greater than 85 dBA (OSHA, 1983). Although the data have been primarily collected with the intent of monitoring the effects of the noise on individuals, they are a powerful tool for program analysis (Royster and Royster, 1986a) and even for the evaluation of HPD effectiveness (Royster et al, 1984).

ANSI working group S12/WG12 has developed a draft national standard (ANSI S12.13) based on evaluation of numerous industrial and military audiometric databases. It describes procedures by which individual annual audiograms are sequentially compared (i.e., test 2 to test 1, test 3 to test 2, etc.) to determine the number of individuals whose hearing has changed by specified amounts. The values are then compared to proposed reference values, and the HCP is evaluated as acceptable, marginal, or unacceptable.

The draft standard is the culmination of years of data collection and analysis, and yet in some ways it still represents a beginning. What is now required is for industry and the military to apply these procedures to their HCPs, and to evaluate and provide comments on the draft standard. An important goal of the use and comment period is the development of additional reference databases (those which a priori are known to be effective) that can be used to more precisely delimit the boundaries between HCPs that are considered acceptable, marginal, and unacceptable.

Effects of HPDs on Communications

The literature on the effects of HPDs on the ability to communicate and detect warning sounds is extensive. Comprehensive overviews have been published by Lazarus (1983), Wilkins and Martin (1987), and Suter (1989). In general, the results show that those with normal hearing who wear HPDs in noise levels greater than about 85 dBA demonstrate an ability to hear speech, machinery, and warning sounds that is either relatively unaffected or slightly improved. For others, the effects will depend on many factors, including their hearing loss, the noise level, the signal-to-noise ratio, the temporal characteristics of the signal, the HPD attenuation, the visual cues, and the message set. Additional research is called for to better quantify these effects and their interactions.

Of particular interest is the development of predictive techniques to aid in specifying HPDs for particular user groups and applications, and even more importantly for individual wearers, based on their own hearing sensitivity. Various computational schemes incorporating measures of hearing sensitivity, signal levels, and HPD attenuation have been reported (Durkin, 1979; Pfeiffer, 1989), but only two studies include empirical data comparing speech intelligibility measures from human listeners with computational predictions (Coleman et al, 1984; Wilde and Humes, 1990).

Wilde and Humes measured speech intelligibility using the revised speech perception in noise (SPIN) test (sentence materials) on 12 normal and 12 hearing-impaired listeners under 21 different combinations of varying noise level, noise type, and protection or lack of protection. For each condition, the articulation index (AI) values were computed, taking into account the individual's hearing impairment. In Figure 33-6 the measured speech discrimination scores are plotted versus the AI values. Each point represents the average results for either the normal or hearing-impaired subjects. Wilde and Humes found that both sets of mean data points could be described by the same AI transfer function (root-mean-square error of about 10 percent), but predic-

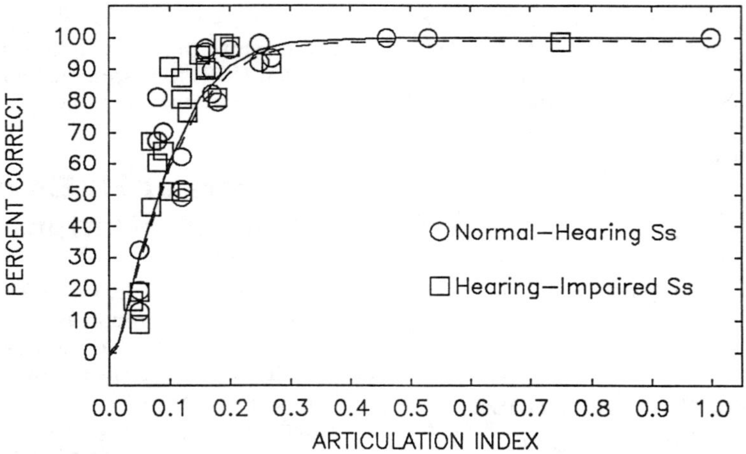

Figure 33-6 Scattergram of mean speech-recognition scores versus computed Articulation Index values. Each point represents the average data for 12 normal or 12 hearing-impaired listeners measured in one of 21 different combinations of varying noise level, noise type, and protection or lack of protection. (From Wilde GL, Humes LE. Application of the articulation index to the speech recognition of normal and impaired listeners wearing hearing protection. J Acoust Soc Am 1990; 87(3):1192-1199.)

tions for individuals varied widely. Obviously, further research is warranted in these areas.

Recreational Earphones and Personal Music Systems

Listening to music while at work, especially when the job is repetitive and otherwise boring, is pleasurable to many employees. However, it may be hazardous as well, and few reports are yet available to properly evaluate the problem. Employees may choose to use recreational earphones, usually of the Walkman variety, or circumaural or supra-aural devices with built-in earphones, or even specially designed noise-attenuating earmuffs with internal earphones. The attenuation of such devices varies from virtually nothing at all with the Walkman-type units to values approaching those of conventional earmuffs (Karlovich, 1988; Skrainar et al, 1985; Waugh and Murray, 1989). Representative data are shown in Figure 33-7.

Regardless of the protection music systems may or may not provide, the more complex issues regarding them include (1) the increased hearing risk that employees may experience from the amplified music superimposed on the partly-attenuated ambient noise, (2) the additional isolation from their auditory environment that employees may experience because of masking caused by the music, and (3) the effects of music on productivity, safety, absenteeism, and the employee willingness to wear hearing protection. Some data are available, as discussed below, but these topics represent an area almost devoid of reported research.

Skrainar et al (1987) evaluated earphone usage in one industrial environment with a TWA of 87 dBA. Use of the earphones increased the employees' TWAs by less than 2 dBA on the average, leading to a predicted increase of NIHL for the most sensitive 5 percent of the population after 20 years of exposure of about 4 dB at 4 kHz. The authors recommended allowance of continued usage with certain restrictions. In a laboratory study, Waugh and Murray (1989) found an increase in listening levels in high ambient noise of about 5 dBA and recommended that such devices should not be worn when exposures equivalent to 8 hours exceeded 80 dBA.

With respect to item (2) above—additional isolation from the auditory environment—only one reported article has directly addressed the problem (Acton and Childs, 1974). The authors recommended playing music in one ear only, which in their study reduced the masking effect from 13 to 3 dB. Although there is much literature on item (3), the effects of music on employee behavior, for noise environments that pose no auditory haz-

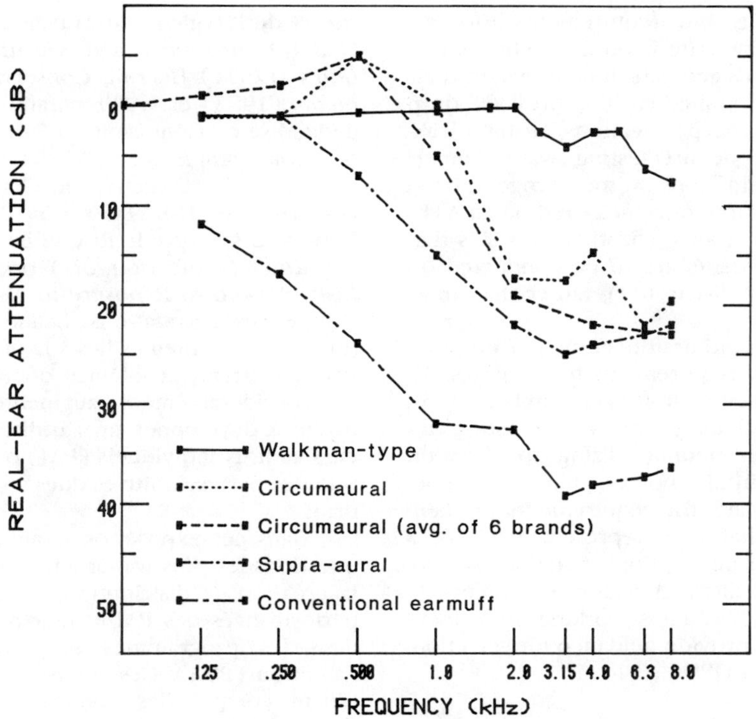

Figure 33-7 Attenuation of various recreational earphones compared to a representative small-volume noise-attenuating earmuff. Walkman-type data from Skrainar et al, 1985; circumaural data from Skrainar et al, and Waugh and Murray, 1989 (average of six brands); supra-aural data from Karlovich, 1988.

ard (Fox, 1983), the literature is sparse for environments with higher-level noise. One Russian study (Derevyanko et al, 1977) examined the issue in a cannery with noise levels above 90 dBA, and employees wearing radio-equipped earmuffs with the music either on or off. Their 165 subjects reported fewer subjective complaints when listening to the music. The results correlated well with objective measures of muscle endurance, strength, and the visual flicker frequency.

International Standards

International standards for hearing protection are the responsibility of the ISO. There are two ISO groups working in this area. The most prolific and the older of the two groups is WG 17, which deals with the measurement of sound attenuation of HPDs. WG 17 is part of Technical Committee (TC) 43, Acoustics. The other group is Subcommittee (SC) 12, which is part of TC 94, Personal Safety—Protective Equipment and Clothing.

WG 17 is responsible for ISO 4869, Acoustics—Hearing Protectors, which is divided into three parts (ISO 1989, 1990a,b). Part 1 describes a real-ear attenuation at threshold (REAT) method of measuring attenuation and is an update and minor revision of the previous version of that standard. Part 2 describes use of the data from Part 1, i.e., how to compute effective exposures when HPDs are worn. It includes an octave-band method as well as two alternative simplified procedures, the HML (high-medium-low) method and the SNR (single number rating). The SNR requires use of only C-weighted noise measurements; the HML requires C- and A-weighted measurements; and the octave-band method obviously requires a full octave-band noise analysis. Part 3 is entitled "Simplified method for the measurement of insertion loss of ear-muff type protectors for quality inspection purposes." It describes the use of a cylindrical steel acoustic test fixture (ATF), which can be placed in a free sound field (established in a room or tunnel) or diffuse field.

As of this writing, SC 12 has no published standards, although it is currently working on three draft documents. The first describes physical testing and requirements for earmuffs. It contains criteria on the ability of earmuffs to fit heads and ears, limitations on their band force and applied cushion pressure, drop tests, flammability specifications, cushion leakage tests, band flexure testing, water immersion testing, limitations on the change in band force and insertion loss (measured on an ATF) after durability testing, and then specifies that REAT measurements are to be conducted on the used (durability-tested), rather than new, samples.

SC 12's second draft document is on physical testing and requirements for earplugs. Although the document lists a number of requirements, including flammability testing and provision for a nominal sizing specification based on 10 circular holes of different diameter in a thin plate, the requirements are general enough that they represent more of a wish list and a description of the status quo, rather than specific technical requirements.

And finally, SC 12 is working on a document that will provide guidance for selection, use, and care of HPDs.

Conclusion

We have come a long way since the development of serious interest in hearing conservation following World War II, and yet there remains much fertile ground for continuing research. Because of the constraints on funding and the abundance of questions, research will be most beneficial if focused on key areas. The nine issues discussed in this chapter are, in our opinion, hearing-protection topics of substantial concern and controversy, and those worthy of this focus. They are not the only issues requiring investigation, but are the areas that we believe will prove the most fruitful for future investigative efforts.

Principaux Problèmes Posés par la Protection Contre le Bruit

Dans le domaine de la protection auditive, la technologie a proliféré depuis le début des années 1970 et l'attention portée à la conservation de l'audition s'est accrue considérablement dans les années 1980. L'intérêt durant ces dix dernières années a été stimulé par l'avènement de nouvelles recommandations comme "l'Amendement pour la Conservation de l'Audition" de "l'Administration de la Sécurité et de l'Hygiène du Travail des Etats-Unis" *(U.S. Occupational and Health Administration's (OSHA) Hearing Conservation Amendment)* (1983) et la "Préparation Européenne de la Mise en Conformité" *(European Préparation for Compliance)* qui débute en janvier 1990 avec la "Directive du Conseil *(Council Directive)* 96/188/EEC sur la Protection des Travailleurs contre le Risque lié à l'Exposition au Bruit" *(Protection of Workers from the Risks Related to Exposure to Noise at Work).* Malgré ces orientations, beaucoup de questions et de problèmes liés à la protection auditive subsistent, problèmes dont la résolution va considérablement augmenter notre capacité à développer et à utiliser les protecteurs auditifs individuels (PAI) pour la prévention des pertes auditives dues à l'exposition au bruit.

Dans cet exposé, on examinera neuf des questions les plus importantes qui intéressent la création, la distribution, l'utilisation et les performances des PAI et leur mise en oeuvre dans les programmes de conservation de l'audition (PCA). Ces sujets seront traités en tenant compte des connaissances actuelles, des problèmes qui subsistent et des questions restant sans réponse.

1) Le développement de PAI de meilleure qualité acoustique, conçus pour procurer une atténuation optimale et pas nécessairement maximale. Ceci pourrait amener les travailleurs à mieux accepter les protecteurs auditifs et à améliorer leur capacité à communiquer et à détecter des signaux critiques dans certaines conditions de bruit, plus spécialement chez ceux qui sont atteints de troubles auditifs préexistants.

2) Le développement de méthodes d'entraînement et de motivation, et la documentation concernant leur efficacité à long terme. Ces méthodes sont nécessaires non seulement pour l'entraînement des utilisateurs proprement dit, mais également pour entraîner les instructeurs eux-mêmes.

3) Des mesures additionnelles de l'atténuation procurée par les PAI à des travailleurs effectivement exposés au bruit, de manière à ce que davantage d'informations deviennent disponibles pour l'évaluation des résultats obtenus grâce à l'utilisation des procédures définies au paragraphe 4 ci-dessous.

4) Des méthodes de mesure en laboratoire de l'atténuation des PAI, méthodes pouvant fournir des résultats qui permettront de prédire avec une meilleure précision la valeur des performances sur le terrain.

5) Le développement de tests objectifs de la mise en place des protecteurs, par exemple

de méthodes de mesure de l'atténuation obtenue chez des utilisateurs individuels, de manière à ce que les techniques de distribution, de pose et d'entraînement deviennent plus précises et plus efficaces.

6) Des méthodes objectives d'évaluation de l'efficacité des PAI pendant le travail, basées sur l'examen des audiogrammes annuels d'une population exposée au bruit.

7) L'acquisition de données complémentaires concernant les nombreux paramètres qui influencent la capacité d'une personne portant un PAI à communiquer et à écouter dans le bruit, en même temps que le développement de procédures permettant de prédire l'intelligibilité de la parole dans des conditions spécifiées.

8) Des études concernant l'utilisation d'écouteurs récréatifs (par exemple du type baladeur), et de serre-tête renfermant un dispositif musical, chez des travailleurs en environnement bruyant. Jusqu'à quel niveau sonore ces dispositifs peuvent-ils être utilisés sans augmentation du risque de pertes auditives induites par le bruit? A quel point les sons ambiants sont-ils masqués et quelle est l'augmentation du risque créée par chaque type de dispositif? Sont-ils utilisables en tant qu'outils motivants?

9) Tendances ressortant des normes internationales liées au développement et à l'utilisation des PAI.

References

Abel SM, Alberti PW, Haythornthwaite C, Riko K. Speech intelligibility in noise: Effects of fluency and hearing protector type. J Acoust Soc Am 1982; 71(3):708-715.

Acton WI, Childs J. Background music as an incentive to wearing ear muffs. Protection 1974; 11(10):16-18.

Alberti PW. Hearing conservation—Past, present and future? Sound Vib 1987; 21(1):46-49.

Allen CH, Berger EH. Development of a unique passive hearing protector with level-dependent and flat attenuation characteristics. Noise Control Eng J 1990; 34(3):97-105.

ANSI. Method for the measurement of the real-ear attenuation of hearing protectors. Am Natl Stds Inst S12.6-1984, New York, 1984.

ANSI. Draft American National Standard, Evaluating the effectiveness of hearing conservation programs. Am Natl Stds Inst S12.13-1991, New York, 1991.

Berger EH. Using the NRR to estimate the real world performance of hearing protectors. Sound Vib 1983; 17(1):12-18.

Berger EH. Review and tutorial—Methods of measuring the attenuation of hearing protection devices. J Acoust Soc Am 1986; 79(6):1655-1687.

Berger EH. Can real-world hearing protector attenuation be estimated using laboratory data? Sound Vib 1988; 22(12):26-31.

Berger EH. Exploring procedures for field testing the fit of earplugs. In: Proceedings, 1989 Industrial Hearing Conservation Conference. Lexington, KY: Office of Engineering Services, University of Kentucky, 1989:7-10.

Berger EH. Bibliography on hearing protection, hearing conservation, and aural care, hygiene and physiology, 1909–1989 (1,337 entries). Indianapolis: E-A-R Report 82-6/HP, 1990a.

Berger EH. Proposed procedures for an interlaboratory comparison: Modified REAT protocols to provide improved estimates of the field attenuation of hearing protectors. Indianapolis: E-A-R Tech. Report 89-14/HP, 1990b.

Coleman GJ, Graves RJ, Collier SG, Golding D, Nicholl AGM, Simpson GC, Sweetland KF, Talbott CF. Communications in noisy environments. Edinburgh, England: Inst. Occup. Med., Rept. TM/84/1, 1984.

CSA. Hearing protectors. Rexdale, Ontario: Canadian Stds. Assoc., Z94.2-M1984, 1984.

Derevyanko EA, Lisichtina ZS, Perrote AA, Khukhlaev VK. The effectiveness of using radio equipped ear protectors for defense against noise [in Russian]. Gig Tr Prof Zabol 1977; 9:44-46.

Durkin J. Effect of electronic hearing protectors on speech intelligibility. Washington, D.C.: U.S. Dept. of the Interior, Bureau of Mines, Report 8358, 1979.

EPA. Noise labeling requirements for hearing protectors. Environmental Protection Agency, 40CFR Part 211, 56120-56147. Fed Reg 1979; 44(190).

Fleming RM. A new procedure for field testing of earplugs for occupational noise reduction. PhD Thesis, Harvard School of Public Health, Boston, MA, 1980.

Fox JG. Industrial music. In: Oborne DJ, Gruneberg MM, eds. The physical environment at work. Chichester, UK: Wiley & Sons, 1983.

Gorman AG. New design concepts in personal hearing protectors. In: Alberti PW, ed. Personal hearing protection in industry. New York: Raven Press, 1982:427-446.

Harvey DG. A method to increase the effectiveness of ear protection. Sound Vib 1981; 15(5):24-27.

Herberg KW. Investigation of the motives for wearing or not wearing hearing protectors [in German]. Die BG 1984; March:174-177.

ISO. Acoustics—hearing protectors—Part 3: Simplified method for the measurement of insertion loss of ear-muff type protectors for quality inspection purposes. Int. Std. Org. ISO/TR 4869-3:1989, Switzerland, 1989.

ISO. Acoustics—hearing protectors—Part 1: Subjective method for the measurement of sound attenuation. Int. Std. Org. 4869-1:1990, Switzerland, 1990.

ISO. Acoustics—hearing protectors—Part 2: Determination of effective A-weighted sound pressure levels when hearing protectors are worn. Int. Std. Org. ISO/DIS 4869-2.2:1990, Switzerland, 1990.

Karlovich R. Hearing damage risk in mail-sorting operations. Sound Vib 1988; 22(12):16-20.

Killion MC, DeVilbiss E, Stewart J. An earplug with uniform 15-dB attenuation. Hear J 1988; 41(5):14-17.

Lazarus H. The effects of hearing protectors on the perception of acoustic signals. Kent, England: Defence Research Information Centre Translation DRIC-T-6786, 1983.

Liu CC, Pekkarinen J, Starck J. Application of the probe microphone method to measure attenuation of

hearing protectors against high impulse sound levels. Appl Acoust 1989; 27(1):13-25.
OSHA. Occupational noise exposure; Hearing conservation amendment. Occupational Safety and Health Administration. Fed Reg 1983; 48(46):9738-9785.
Pfeiffer BH. Hearing protectors for railroad track workers [in German]. Tiefbau BG 1989; 3:148-157.
Regan DE. Real ear attenuation of personal ear protective devices worn in industry. Audiol Hear Educ 1977; 1:16-18.
Royster JD, Royster LH. Audiometric data base analysis. In: Berger EH, Ward WD, Morrill JC, Royster LH, eds. Noise and hearing conservation manual. 4th ed. Akron, OH: Am Ind Hyg Assoc 1986a:293-317.
Royster JD, Royster LH. Data presented to S12/WG12, Evaluation of hearing conservation programs. Report No 6, 1988.
Royster LH, Royster JD. Education and motivation. In: Berger EH, Ward WD, Morrill JC, Royster LH, eds. Noise and hearing conservation manual. 4th ed. Akron, OH: Am Ind Hyg Assoc 1986b:383-416.
Royster LH, Royster JD. Hearing conservation programs: Essential elements. In: Berglund B, Lindvall T, eds. Noise as a public health problem. Vol 4. Stockholm: Swedish Council for Building Research, 1990:59-78.
Royster LH, Royster JD, Cecich TF. An evaluation of the effectiveness of three hearing protection devices at an industrial facility with a TWA of 107 dB. J Acoust Soc Am 1984; 76(2):485-497.
Sadler OW, Montgomery GM. The application of positive practice overcorrection to the use of hearing protection. Am Ind Hyg Assoc J 1982; 43(6):451-454.
Shaw EAG. Hearing protector design concepts and performance limitations. In: Alberti PW, ed. Personal hearing protection in industry. New York: Raven Press, 1982:51-68.
Skrainar SF, Royster LH, Berger EH, Pearson RG. Do personal radio headsets provide hearing protection? Sound Vib 1985; 19(5):16-19.
Skrainar SF, Royster LH, Berger EH, Pearson RG. The contribution of personal radios to the noise exposure of employees at one industrial facility. Am Ind Hyg Assoc J 1987; 48(4):390-395.
Suter AH. The effects of hearing protectors on speech communication and the perception of warning signals. Aberdeen Proving Ground, MD: U.S. Army Human Eng Lab Tech Mem 2-89, 1989.
Waugh R, Murray N. The auditory hazards of using muff-like personal radio headsets in high ambient noise levels. Aust J Audiol 1989; 11(2):107-114.
Wilde GL, Humes LE. Measurement of the attenuation characteristics of nonlinear hearing protective devices using auditory brain stem response. J Acoust Soc Am 1987; 81(3):730-733.
Wilde G, Humes LE. Application of the articulation index to the speech recognition of normal and impaired listeners wearing hearing protection. J Acoust Soc Am 1990; 87(3):1192-1199.
Wilkins PA, Martin AM. Hearing protection and warning sounds in industry—A review. Appl Acoust 1987; 21(4):267-293.
Zohar D, Cohen A, Azar N. Promoting increased use of ear protectors in noise through information feedback. Hum Factors 1980; 22(1):69-79.

CHAPTER 34

Performance of Active Noise Reduction Headsets

CHARLES W. NIXON
RICHARD L. McKINLEY
JOSEPH W. STEUVER

Personal hearing protection devices have been in widespread use for over five decades. The vast majority of these devices are passive units or assemblies that reduce noise by the application of attenuating and absorptive materials. Traditional earmuffs that perform well provide about 20 to 40 dB of sound attenuation at frequencies above about 1,000 Hz, which is adequate high-frequency protection for the majority of acoustic exposures. However, these same earmuffs provide little or no attenuation, 0 dB to about 20 dB, at frequencies from 125 Hz to 1,000 Hz.

Often, the overall A-weighted sound pressure level of a noise at the ear under an earmuff is determined by the amount of acoustic energy in the 125-Hz to 250-Hz frequency region. Hearing damage risk is defined in terms of A-weighted sound level in several noise exposure criteria for hearing. Increasing the sound attenuation in this low-frequency region beyond that which is available with current passive devices would reduce the A-weighted sound levels under the devices as well as the associated risk of noise-induced hearing loss.

The state of the art of passive circumaural hearing protection devices has remained essentially unchanged over the past two decades. Some special devices have been developed that provide nonlinear and "flat" attenuation performance, but the maximum amount of attenuation has not been increased in any frequency region. Additional performance gain in the passive earmuff device is possible, but the increased mass, volume, headband tension, or combinations thereof have rendered such devices impractical. Past efforts to increase attenuation by incorporating these features have resulted in devices that were judged to be uncomfortable and unacceptable to users.

Significant improvements in the attenuation and comfort provided by insert hearing protection devices have been realized with the development of slow-recovery foam materials. These improvements are most evident in the frequency region below 1,000 Hz, where the amount of attenuation is highly associated with the depth of insertion of the device. However, insert devices are not suitable or are not the items of choice for many applications involving voice communications in noise with conventional headset units.

Active noise reduction (ANR) technology (also called active noise cancellation or active attenuation) attempts to reduce the overall level of noises by wave addition or cancellation techniques. The feasibility of this approach has been demonstrated in earmuff and headset devices with good active attenuation of the low-frequency sounds. Integration of active noise reduction with the traditional passive earmuff provides additional attenuation at the low frequencies. This combination passive/active attenuation could have additional benefits of reduced size, reduced headband tension, and increased comfort, particularly for advanced ANR systems.

Background

The original patent on active noise cancellation was awarded to Paul Leug in 1936. The basic technique of reducing noise by the addition of an inverted copy of the noise was described in that patent. The addition of out-of-phase signals resulted in wave cancellation that reduced the amplitude of the resulting noise. Under ideal conditions, this technique would be expected to allow all noise to be completely canceled to produce quiet. However, the reality of physics as currently understood does not allow the earphone, the system microphone, and the eardrum of the listener to be in the same point in space at the same time (propagation with zero time delay). The physical separation of these components in current systems requires a delay for the canceling signal to travel from the earphone to the system microphone to the eardrum of the listener. This delay, which also can be considered a phase delay, limits the maximum frequency at which active attenuation can occur with a given transducer geometry.

The bandwidth of the electronic circuitry in an active attenuation system also limits performance, as reported in 1958 and 1959 by Willard Meeker, who was working under contract to the U.S. Air Force (Meeker, 1958, 1959). Meeker's effort involved a paper design and a working model of active attenuation technology applied to a circumaural earmuff. The active attenuation had a bandwidth of approximately 500 Hz and a maximum attenuation of about 15 dB. The electronics package was "a little larger than a breadbox," required AC voltage for operation, and was nonportable. This hardware was not practical for field use; however, the active cancellation of noise was impressive and it demonstrated the feasibility of the ANR headset concept.

The first practical system used outside the laboratory was developed by P.D. Wheeler (Wheeler and Halliday, 1981) at the University of Southampton, under contract to Graham Rood, Royal Aircraft Establishment, United Kingdom. Numerous flight tests with the helmet were accomplished during this development effort. The ANR system had a cancellation bandwidth of about 800 to 1,000 Hz and a maximum attenuation of approximately 18 dB. This system was the forerunner of the active cancellation systems being produced today in the United Kingdom.

In the early 1980s, the U.S. Air Force, under contract with the Bose Corporation, initiated development of an ANR system for use in headsets and helmets (Carter, 1982). This program produced helmet and headset models that were extensively evaluated in the laboratory and during flight tests in various aircraft. These evaluations demonstrated the effectiveness of the ANR systems in decreasing crew member noise exposure at the ear, in improving speech intelligibility, and in increasing comfort.

This improved sound attenuation and speech intelligibility performance as demonstrated by active attenuation systems over passive systems has resulted in increased interest in, inquiries about, and applications of ANR headset technology. In 1989, at least seven different firms had one or more working models of an ANR headset. Most of these firms provided samples of their devices for evaluation in the effort described in this report.

Objective

The objective of this effort was to examine the state of ANR headset technology in 1989 by acquiring available ANR systems and measuring under laboratory conditions their sound attenuation, speech communications effectiveness, bandwidth, and dynamic range. Attention was directed to attenuation performance, constraints on performance, areas of potential improvement through additional research and development, and the requirement for standard methods and procedures appropriate for evaluating active attenuation headset system technology performance.

Approach

The majority of ANR headset units known to be operational were acquired for use in this study. Almost all were developmental items. Some did not remain functional throughout all the measurements, and these are not included in this report because of incomplete data on their performance.

The total and the passive sound attenuation was measured for each of the headset units. The active attenuation was calculated as the difference between the total and passive attenuation at each of the test signals. The sound attenuation was measured using an acoustic manikin by Knowles Electronics Inc., an artificial ear with a laboratory flat-plate coupler, and a miniature microphone placed under the earcup of the ANR headset while it was worn by a human subject. The subject acted as a test fixture and did not respond during the measurements.

The overall active attenuation was measured for three of the headsets at selected sound pressure levels ranging from 120 to 135 dB. Overall active attenuation is the single-number difference between the overall sound pressure levels under the earcup for the active (total) and the passive modes of operation.

Speech intelligibility was measured on

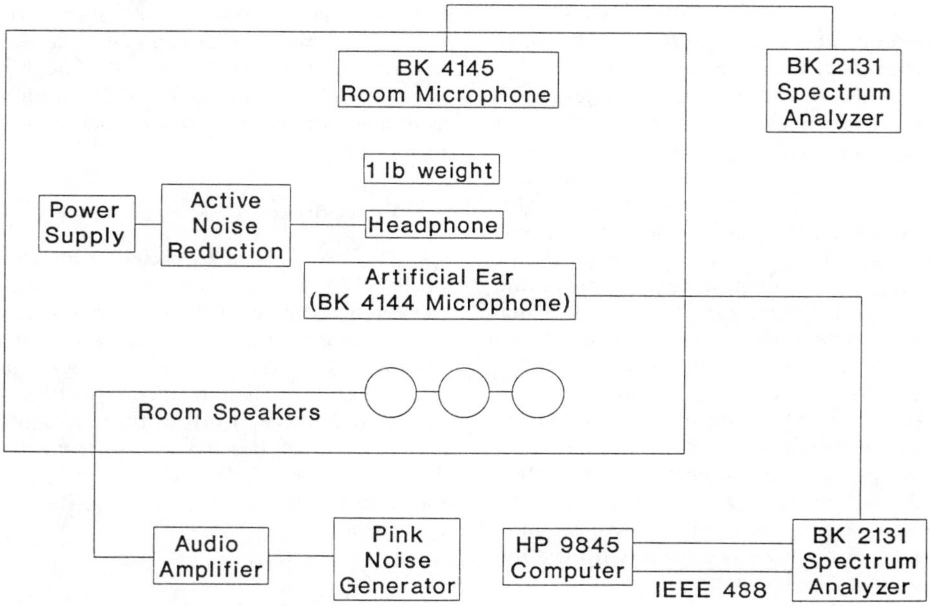

Figure 34-1 Active noise reduction instrumentation arrangement for artificial ear/flat-plate measurements.

three of the active attenuation headset units in four different levels of a broad-band noise inside a reverberation chamber. Intelligibility was measured with the units in the passive mode and again in the active mode.

Method

Sound Attenuation

Acoustic Measurement Systems

The attenuation provided by the ANR headsets was determined from measurements made in a large 8,000 ft^3 acoustic reverberation chamber equipped with a programmable sound system capable of generating levels as high as 135 dB SPL. A pink noise spectrum was generated at the appropriate sound pressure levels for all attenuation measurements. The noise spectra and levels at the locations of the subjects or test fixtures in the chamber were monitored at all times by a B&K 4144 1-inch pressure microphone and a B&K 2131 spectrum analyzer.

Three different measurement procedures and systems were used to obtain the attenuation performance data. (1) A B&K 4152 artificial ear and a flat-plate coupler with a B&K 4144 1-inch pressure microphone made up one measurement system. The configuration of instrumentation as arranged for the artificial ear/flat-plate measurements is displayed in Figure 34-1. (2) The KEMAR acoustic manikin was equipped with a B&K 4134 ½-inch pressure microphone in a Zwislocki coupler. The coupler unit was imbedded in the manikin so that the microphone was positioned at the approximate location of the eardrum. (3) Human subjects were used as test fixtures in that the headset devices were worn by them but only physical measurements were taken with a miniature microphone under the headset; the subjects made no responses at any time. A Knowles 1834 miniature microphone and preamplifier provided signal input to the spectrum analyzer. The measurement systems for all procedures were controlled by a Hewlett-Packard 9845 computer. All measured data were analyzed with a B&K 2131 ⅓-octave band spectrum analyzer.

Procedures

A set of three noise-level measurements was taken with each of the systems described above for each ANR headset device. These measurements were made in a pink noise field of the test fixture system without a headset in place, of the system with the headset in place and in the passive mode, and of the system with the headset in place and in the active, noise-canceling mode. The same test-room noise spectrum and level were maintained for each set of these three measurements for an individual device. The sound pressure level of each ⅓-octave band from 100 to 10,000 Hz was recorded, stored, and plotted by the computer for each measurement condition.

The artificial ear/flat-plate coupler measurements were made with a 1-lb weight on the earcup to provide a constant pressure and "good" acoustic seal. The KEMAR and real-head (human) measurements were made with the headbands of the various headsets at normal tension. The real-head measurements were taken with the miniature microphone positioned at the entrance to the ear canal with the canal occluded. An EAR foam earplug served as the microphone mounting platform. After insertion of the EAR earplug, a small plastic rod attached to the back of the microphone was inserted into a tube imbedded in the foam earplug. The microphone was then oriented to be on the axis with the ear canal. The three noise measurements with an individual headset device were made with the microphone in this same position.

The various attenuation values were then calculated from each set of measurements. The passive attenuation was calculated by spectrally subtracting the measured passive headset noise levels from the open test-fixture noise levels. The total attenuation was calculated by spectrally subtracting the measured active headset noise levels from the open test-fixture noise levels. The active attenuation was calculated by spectrally subtracting the passive attenuation from the total attenuation.

The artificial ear/flat-plate system was also used to measure the overall active attenuation of headset devices at selected sound pressure levels ranging from 120 to 135 dB. The overall active attenuation was calculated by subtracting the overall sound pressure level of the passive condition from the overall sound pressure level of the total condition.

Speech Intelligibility

Measurement System

A computer-controlled voice communications research facility housed in a reverberation chamber was used for these measurements. The facility contained all of the operator, system, and environmental variables important for voice communications except whole-body motion, as might be experienced in a noisy aircraft or in a highway vehicle. Ten individual listening stations housed trained communicators who responded to the Modified Rhyme Test instrument in four different levels of a pink noise spectrum (about 75 dB, 95 dB, 105 dB, and 115 dB) (House et al, 1965). These measurements were taken in compliance with American National Standards Institute (ANSI), S3.2-1989, Method for Measuring the Intelligibility Over Communication Systems (American National Standards Institute, 1989).

Procedure

The subjects were fitted with the ANR headsets. A round-robin procedure was used in which the role of talker was passed to the next subject for each 50-word Modified Rhyme list so that all subjects performed as both talker and listener. This procedure was repeated until each of the three headsets was measured with the active electronics in the "off" (passive) mode and in the "on" (active) mode in the presence of each of the four levels of the noise.

Results

Attenuation

The active noise reduction of the headset devices is summarized for each of the three measurement systems and procedures in Figure 34-2. All were circumaural headsets except for one supra-aural device. In general, the circumaural device response patterns exhibited various amounts of active attenuation at frequencies below about 900 Hz with essentially no attenuation at 1,000 Hz and above. Almost all of the active circumaural devices displayed some negative attenuation of the noise under the headset in the frequency region between 500 to 600 Hz and about 1,500 Hz. The exception to these patterns is the supra-aural device, which shows no attenuation around 100 Hz, about 5 dB attenuation at 1,000 Hz, zero attenuation at about 2,000 Hz, and no amplification of the signal at the ear.

Although performance of the devices varies among the three measurement systems, similarities can be observed in the response patterns. The real-ear/miniature microphone and artificial-ear/flat-plate data show this similarity among the devices as a group. All of the real-ear data below 1,000 Hz fall within a range of only about 5 to 10 dB with one or two exceptions. The flat-plate data show the same general profile, but the range of the data almost doubles to 10 to 20 dB.

The KEMAR data are variable and range from about 20 dB attenuation to amplification of the sound under the earcup. The effects of poor acoustic seals and corresponding losses

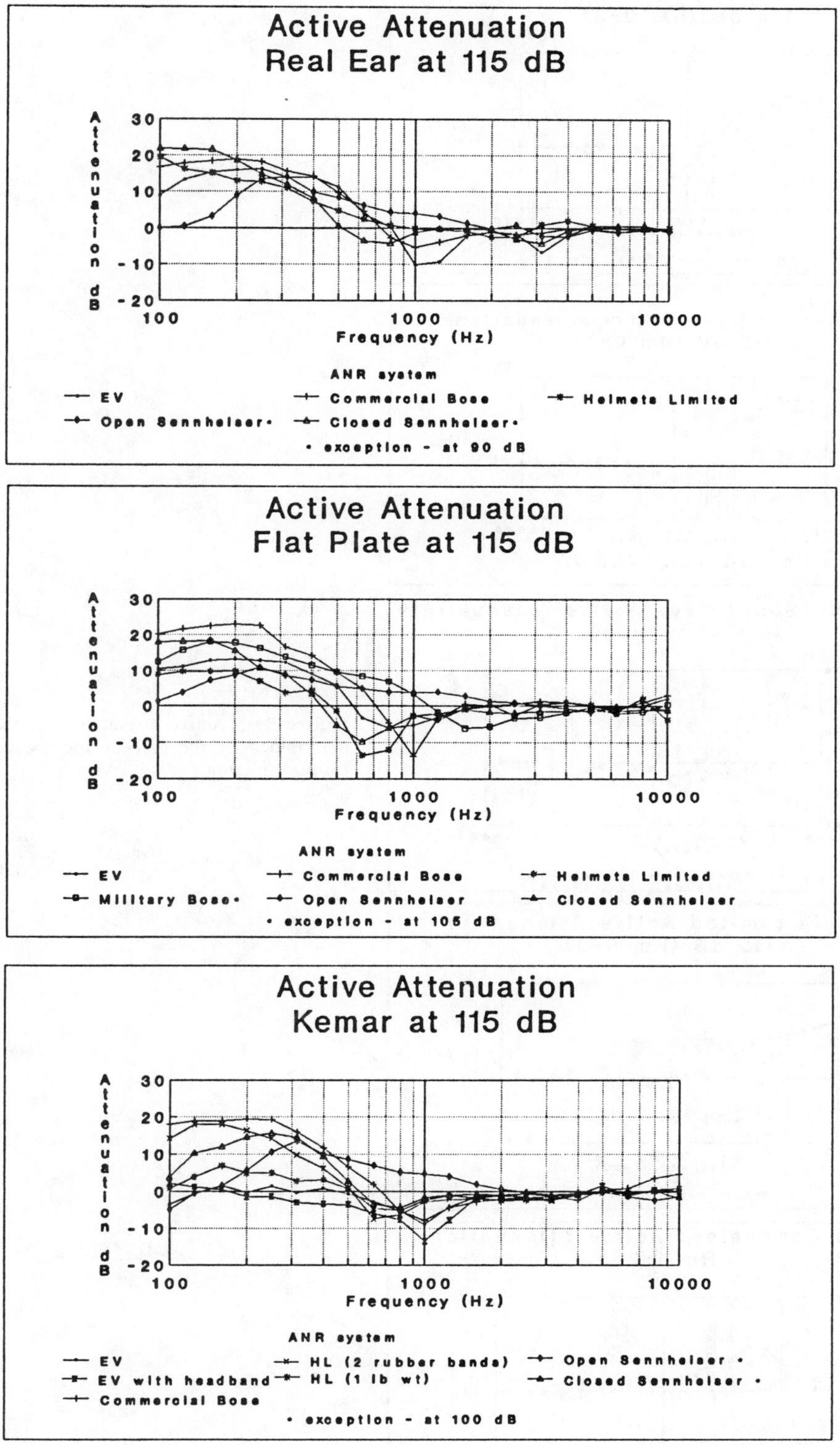

Figure 34-2 Active attenuation of the headsets determined by three different instrumentation procedures.

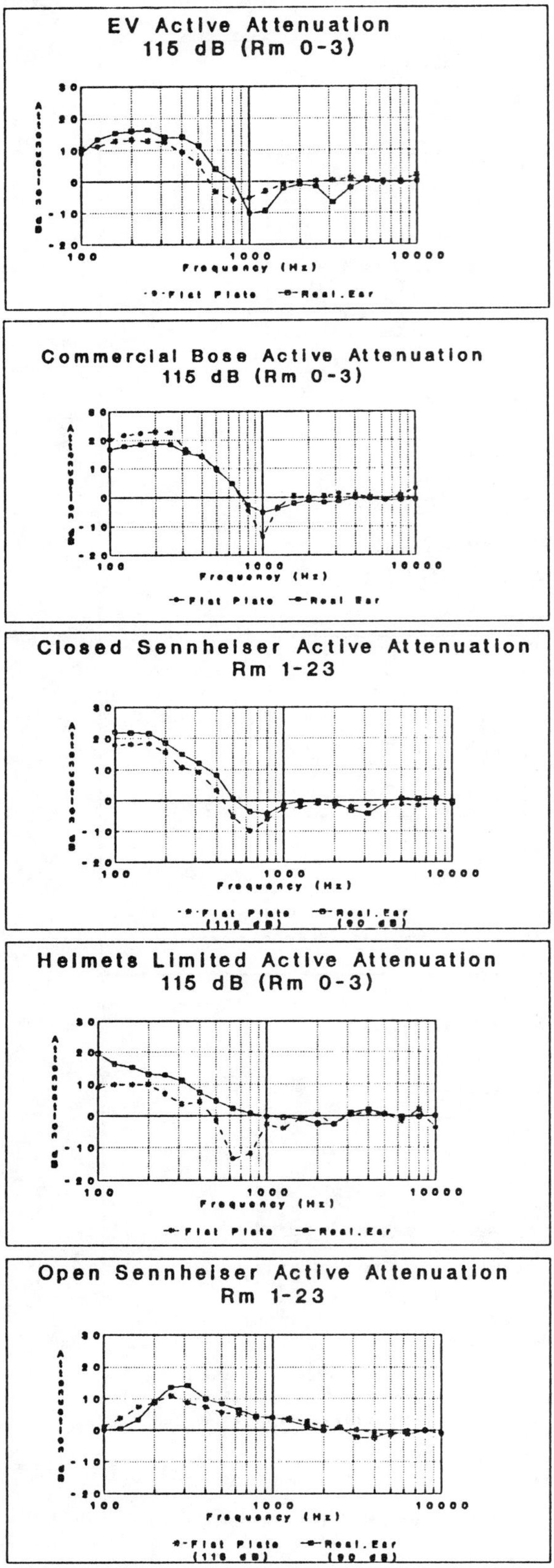

Figure 34-3 Active attenuation of the headsets determined by the real-ear and the artificial-ear/flat-plate methods.

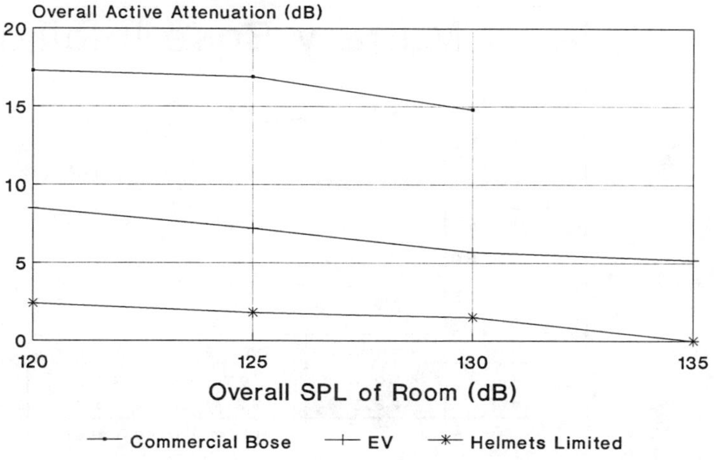

Figure 34-4 Active attenuation in overall sound pressure levels (SPLs) ranging from 120 to 135 dB.

of attenuation with these current-technology ANR systems are evident in these data. An acoustic seal could not be obtained on the manikin with some of the headset devices. The fitting problem was attributed to both the manikin and the headset devices. Some of the headset devices were properly fit on the manikin without acoustic leaks, whereas those that did not fit the manikin were satisfactorily fit to the flat-plate system and the human subjects.

The relative performances of the flat-plate and real-ear methods for each headset are summarized in Figure 34-3 and show differences in attenuation of only about 5 dB or less, with few exceptions. Information derived from these measurements shows that the maximum attenuation across devices occurs at 250 Hz and below, with the maximum at 100 Hz for two of them. The maximum amount of attenuation is about 17 to 22 dB and differs among devices. The flat-plate system showed less attenuation than the real-ear system for most of the devices. Zero crossover occurs between 500 and 1,000 Hz, with no useful attenuation above 1,000 Hz, with the exception of the supra-aural device. The total bandwidth cannot be determined for the circumaural devices because of the 100-Hz cutoff of the measurement system, although minimum bandwidths of 500 to 1,000 Hz are evident. The bandwidth of the supra-aural device is estimated to be about 1,800 to 1,900 Hz.

Performance of the supra-aural headset was essentially independent of the measurement method. The response curves are similar except that the maximum attenuation at about 250 Hz is a couple of decibels less with the flat-plate system. These data clearly demonstrate that supra-aural configurations of ANR do not require an acoustic seal or a circumaural earcup.

The performance of three of the ANR headsets was examined in very high sound pressure levels. Measurements were taken using the artificial-ear/flat-plate coupler system in a pink noise at overall sound pressure levels of 120 dB, 125 dB, 130 dB, and 135 dB (Fig. 34-4). Two of the three headsets continued to operate at the 135 dB level, however, the amount of noise reduction was zero to 5 dB. The third headset provided larger amounts of noise reduction at the lower sound pressure levels but ceased to function above 130 dB.

Speech Intelligibility

The percentages of correct speech intelligibility of three of the circumaural headsets are summarized in Figure 34-5. Intelligibility was measured in the voice communications research facility with trained subjects in the presence of pink noise at sound pressure levels of about 75 dB (ambient), 95 dB, 105 dB, and 115 dB. Although all three headsets in the active mode showed improvements in intelligibility at the higher noise levels, considerable variation is apparent from the data. One of the systems showed improvements of about 5 to 9 percent in the three high-level noises. Another showed only a negligible amount of change at two frequencies, and the third showed a 10 percent increase but only in the highest-level noise. All three devices showed an increase or a trend toward an increase in intelligibility in the 115-dB noise. All three systems should provide satisfactory voice communications in broad-band noises at the levels examined.

The articulation index (AI) is a computational procedure based on physical measures for estimating speech intelligibility and is highly correlated with group intelligibility of

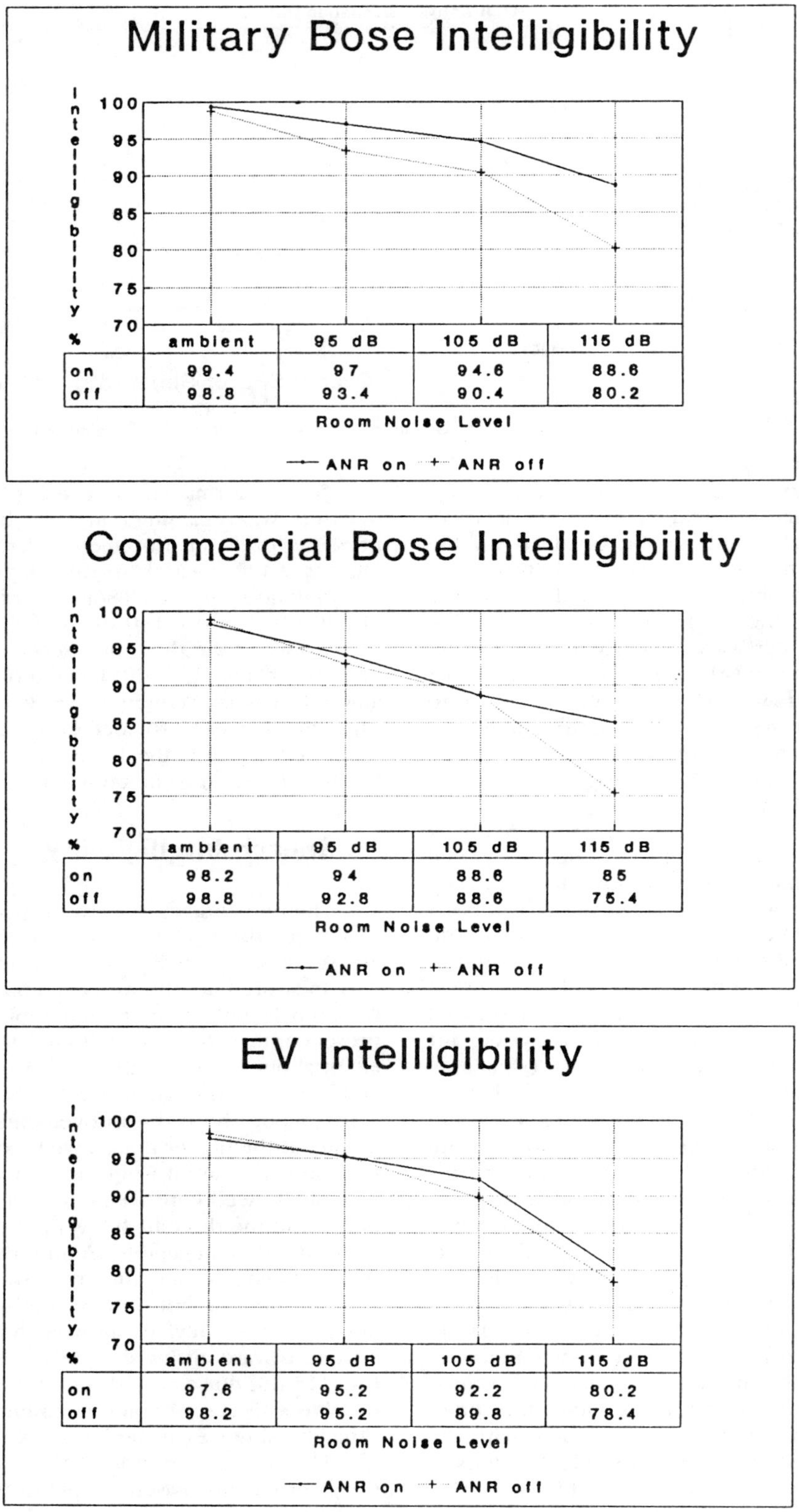

Figure 34-5 Speech intelligibility of active noise reduction (ANR) headsets in the passive and active modes.

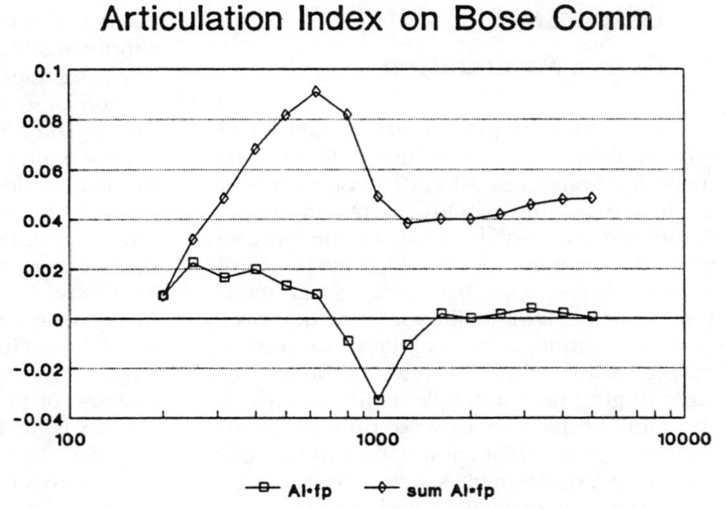

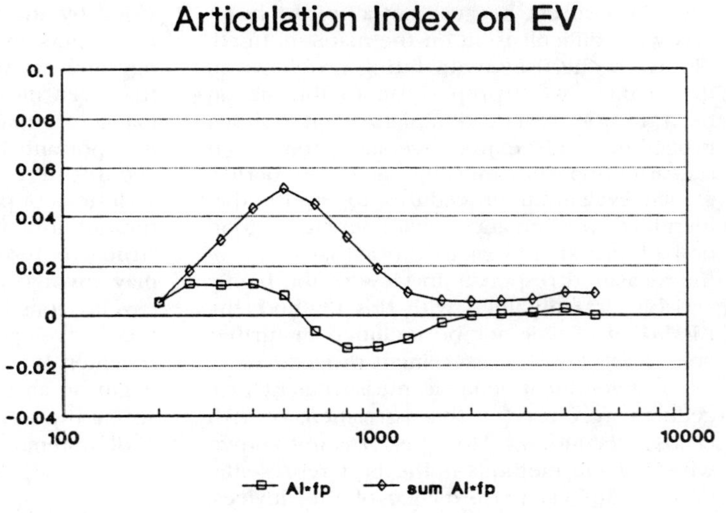

Figure 34-6 Calculations of the articulation index for two active noise reduction systems; Bose Commercial and Electrovoice.

speech as evaluated by standardized speech tests. The AI procedure as described in ANSI S3.5-1969 (R 1986) returns a value between 0 and 1, which is a weighted sum of the signal-to-noise ratios in individual bands of speech that correlate highly with measured intelligibility scores in linear systems (American National Standards Institute, 1986). The ⅓-octave band method of calculating AI was used to evaluate two of the active attenuation headsets. The products of the AI ⅓-octave band weighting values and the signal-to-noise ratio increases (or decreases, represented by the negative numbers) due to the active cancellation are shown in Figure 34-6. These products are labeled "AI · fp" (fp = flat plate). The cumulative sum of the products is shown as "sum AI · fp."

The negative portion of the active cancellation significantly impacts the predicted overall intelligibility gain around 1,000 Hz. If the zero crossover point in these active headset systems could be moved one or two octaves higher in frequency, or if the negative cancellation could be substantially reduced, outstanding gains in intelligibility could be realized. The AI calculation for one of the headsets in Figure 34-6 displays an increase of 0.049, whereas the other displays an increase of 0.009, both of which correspond within experimental error to the intelligibility gains seen in Figure 34-5.

Discussion

Active Attenuation

The ANR performance data varied widely with the different test fixtures and measurement methods. The KEMAR data were contaminated by the inability to obtain an adequate acoustic seal of some of the headsets with the manikin head. The effects of the acoustic leaks range from very small reductions in active attenuation for some devices to zero attenuation; some amplification even occurred with other devices. Although the KEMAR head has limited flexibility and plasticity, some of the devices were properly fit and provided good attenuation. Other items could not be fit even though special effort was put forth to obtain an acoustic seal. This fitting difficulty is related to both the manikin and the affected headsets, because not all of the headsets were difficult to fit on the manikin. In addition, the headsets with fitting problems on the manikin were properly fit to the human head in the real-head/miniature-microphone procedure. This experience also points out the attention that must be given to performance evaluation procedures to ensure that identified performance characteristics, good or bad, are attributed to the actual cause of the measured response. In view of the highly variable data obtained with this method, the KEMAR data will not be included in further considerations of measurement procedures.

Conventional acoustic measurement procedures were used in this assessment of ANR headset technology. However, it is not known which of the methods is the best representation of the real performance of the devices. The objective of a measurement system/method of this type is to obtain a "true" representation of the performance that allows valid extrapolations of the performance to nonlaboratory situations. The ranges of responses obtained in this study show large differences in data obtained on the same devices by different but widely accepted and commonly used acoustic measurement schemes. It is obvious that the potential for inaccuracies is increased when it is necessary to draw conclusions and make decisions based on such data. This is particularly true when it is obtained with only one of these measurement schemes known to provide data that differ from that of other schemes. At this time, we prefer the real-ear/miniature-microphone method of those used in this study.

The scientific community is similarly concerned with the question of a predictive measurement scheme that will allow accurate and "true" extrapolations of passive hearing protection performance to real-world situations. The current national and international standard schemes for measuring personal hearing protection device performance are appropriate only for linear, passive devices; ANR systems do not fall within the scopes of the standards. The ANSI Real Ear Attenuation at Threshold Method, S12.6, was considered for inclusion as a method in this study, but will instead be included in a future study that will examine procedures for assessing the effectiveness of personal ANR (American National Standards Institute, 1984).

The data collected and reported in this study leaves many questions unanswered. One of the questions concerns the accurate and valid measurement of the attenuation provided by these devices. The interest of both developers and potential users of this technology appears to continue to grow, indicating that even more studies of attenuation performance are being and will be accomplished. It is important that a standard procedure or procedures be established to ensure uniform descriptions of performance, to minimize opportunities for confusion, and to determine the "true" representation of performance. These may involve conventional physical methods, psychoacoustic methods, or both, or require the development of new measurement schemes. It is expected that work should soon begin on an investigation of methods of measuring the sound attenuation characteristics of ANR systems.

Speech Intelligibility

Early evaluations with a military ANR headset were accomplished under various laboratory conditions and during in-flight use (headset was mounted in a military flight helmet) in a variety of different aircraft. Laboratory measurements demonstrated consistent 10% increases in active mode speech intelligibility over that measured in the passive mode. Subjective reports from the numerous air crews who flew with the device were surprising in their experiences of dramatic improvements in voice communications effectiveness over that obtained with the standard flight helmet. In some situations the speech communications were changed from unintelligible to intelligible. Although some improvement in voice communications in the active mode was suggested by the early measurements, the magnitude of the reported real-world improvements was not expected.

The speech intelligibility data collected on the three ANR headsets in both the passive and active modes in this study were not generally impressive. Some gain in speech intelligibility was measured for each of the headsets in the active over the passive mode. The type of headset used in the in-flight assessments provided the most improvement (about 5 to 9 percent) and best communications. Although some intelligibility gains attributed to ANR were observed, the amount of the intelligibility gains was less than we were led to believe they would be from the earlier laboratory and flight test experiences. However, the intelligibility of all three of the active attenuation headsets would be expected to provide satisfactory voice communications in operational noise environments.

An evaluation of the comfort or wearability of the active attenuation headsets was not within the scope of this study. However, some wearers voluntarily reported that most of the ANR headsets, with some exceptions, worn in high levels of noise in both laboratory and flight situations provided increased comfort in the active over the inactive mode. This aspect of comfort is attributed primarily to the attenuation of low-frequency noise under the earcup and the perception of a dramatic reduction of the noise at the ear, and is not due to the wearability or mechanical properties of the headset or ear cushion. It is estimated that this lowered acoustic energy at the ear will reduce noise-induced fatigue over long exposures. The magnitude of this low-frequency attenuation is also expected, over time, to reduce noise-induced hearing loss.

Some attention has been given to the comfort of the headset systems in terms of specific mechanical properties. Efforts are ongoing to minimize factors such as weight and headband pressure on both passive and active systems. One of the active attenuation systems evaluated in the study was equipped with a new earcup cushion that was judged to be more comfortable than those on existing headset systems. These cushions are fabricated with "new" materials that provide a good acoustic seal in addition to comfort. The headset fitted with these cushions obtained the best fit among all the headsets on the KEMAR manikin, whereas poor acoustic seals caused measurement problems with some other headset systems.

Conclusion

Numerous personal ANR systems are and will be under development for several years. The capabilities and performance of these systems will continue to expand as knowledge and experience with their development and operation are gained. The objectives of this study have been met by assessing the state of the technology of these ANR headsets through measures and analyses of available systems. Performance was evaluated in terms of active attenuation, dynamic range, and speech communications effectiveness. Consideration was given to constraints on performance, areas of potential growth, and the requirement for standard methods and procedures for evaluation of ANR headset systems.

ANR technology is moving rapidly towards production, with one system in the United States and others in the United Kingdom currently available to the commercial market. ANR development and application projects are now under way in several nations. The potential applications of these systems are extremely wide, covering the full spectrum of activities from military applications to entertainment.

Suggestions for Future Activities

The number of different methods to measure the attenuation of ANR headsets equals or may exceed the number of headsets available at this time. A standard method for measuring and reporting the attenuation of these devices would greatly benefit research, development, and use. The method could include both a physical measurement procedure using real and dummy heads and a psychoacoustic measurement procedure for determining total and active attenuation. This method could become the basis for a national or international standard.

The utility of ANR headsets would be improved if performance was increased in two areas. First, the bandwidth should be extended to include higher frequencies, initially to about 2,500 Hz and increasing later to 4,000 Hz. The 4,000-Hz bandwidth would cover the majority of the speech band and should significantly reduce the passive attenuation requirements at 1,000 Hz, making the design of a comfortable, high-performance hearing protector possible. Second, research should focus on realizing more of the intelligibility that should be available from the reduced noise levels. Possible areas for investigation are speech spectrum shaping, reduction of distortion of the speech signal by the active circuitry, treatment of nonlinear acoustics in the earcup, and other presently unknown causes.

The issue of comfort is important because users will not wear uncomfortable hearing protection devices. Active noise cancellation allows hearing protectors to be designed and produced that have significantly increased comfort while providing excellent hearing protection. There is no standard method for quantifying the comfort feature of earmuff hearing protection devices and headsets. A uniform method to quantify and compare the absolute and relative comfort of devices would be a welcome tool.

Although not a consideration of this study, it is noted that the power consumption of some of the devices is an issue that could limit their applications. Power consumption requirements should enable battery operations for 8 to 16 hours before recharging or replacement. This type of battery-powered system provides applications for mobile users who are not in a stationary location or attached to a vehicle.

Performances des Casques à Atténuation Active du Bruit

Des évaluations portant sur 6 casques à atténuation active du bruit ont été réalisées dans les laboratoires de Biocommunication de l'US Air Force à Dayton, Ohio. Quatre de ces dispositifs étaient des serre-tête étanches et les deux autres semi-ouverts. Certains étaient analogiques d'autres étaient des systèmes hybrides analogique-digital.

Dans le mode actif ou dans le mode passif, sur une tête artificielle ou sur un sujet humain, on prenait comme atténuation du son, la différence de niveau de pression, avec ou sans casque, en un point de référence de l'oreille. L'intelligibilité de la parole avec des serre-tête portés par des auditeurs expérimentés, ayant une audition normale, a été évaluée en utilisant les systèmes MRT (Modified Rhyme Test) pour 4 niveaux de bruits de bande qui simulaient le bruit existant dans le cockpit d'un avion de combat.

L'intelligibilité du langage analogique et de 3 types différents de language digital, entendus chacun avec des serre-tête a été mesurée pour 4 niveaux de bruit. Quoique les performances dans le bruit diffèrent quelque peu selon les matériels, les résultats indiquent que ceux-ci peuvent procurer un meilleur confort, une meilleure communication de la parole et une meilleure réduction du bruit (moins de pertes auditives) que ceux procurés par les systèmes les plus couramment utilisés actuellement.

References

American National Standards Institute. S3.2-1989, Method for measuring the intelligibility of speech over communication systems. New York: ANSI, 1989.

American National Standards Institute. S3.5-1969 (R-89), Methods for the calculation of the articulation index. New York: ANSI, 1986.

American National Standards Institute. S12.6-1984, Method for the measurement of real-ear attenuation of hearing protectors. New York: ANSI, 1984.

Carter J. Active noise reduction. Framingham, MA: Bose Corp., 1982.

House AS, et al. Articulation testing methods; Consonantal differentiation with a closed-response set. J Acoust Soc Am 1965; 37(1):158-166.

Leug P. Process of silencing sound oscillations. U.S. Patent No. 2,043,416. 1936.

Meeker WF. Active ear defender systems component considerations and theory, Part I, WADC TR Wright-Patterson AFB, Dayton, OH, 1957; 57-368.

Meeker WF. Active ear defender systems development of a laboratory model, Part II, WADC TR Wright-Patterson AFB, Dayton, OH, 1957; 57-368.

Wheeler PD, Halliday SD. An active noise reduction system for aircraft helmets. Southampton, U.K.: University of Southampton, 1981.

CHAPTER 35

Objective Methods for Evaluating Conventional, Nonlinear, and Active Hearing Protector Attenuation

PER-ANDERS HELLSTRÖM

Different methods for measuring hearing protector (HP) attenuation have been used during the last decade—for example, the standardized "real ear attenuation at threshold" (REAT) method (ISO 4869, 1981; ANSI S12.6, 1984). These methods use the differences in subjects' hearing thresholds with or without the HP being tested. The test signal is white noise filtered through ⅓-octave bands with center frequencies in accordance with International Electrotechnical Commission (IEC) publication No. 225. The acoustic test signal is presented in a diffuse sound field in accordance with standards. The two methods most frequently used to achieve a diffuse field are the multiple speaker and signal system, installed in an anechoic test chamber (with the sound direction pointed to the test site), or a speaker system consisting of one or more speakers in a reverberation chamber provided with diffusers.

To measure the insertion loss of HPs, the acoustic test fixtures (ATF) method is frequently used. This technique is often used for quality control of earmuffs in HP factories (Pfretzschner and Moreno, 1986).

The use of artificial heads with and without a torso has also been described. A great deal of effort has been expended to construct artificial heads acoustically similar to the average human head (Schroeter, 1982, 1986; Giguère and Kunov, 1989; Kunov and Giguère, 1989; Ivey et al, 1987; Pösselt and Schroeter, 1985).

All these methods have advantages and disadvantages, depending on the aims of the measurements. The REAT method is accepted to be the one that gives "true" data on the measured attenuation from both earmuffs and earplugs. However, this method has been criticized for producing some minor errors in attenuation at low frequencies, depending on the masking effects from physiologic noise. Another disadvantage is the variability of the measured attenuation. This is due to the well-known variability of hearing threshold measurements, the problem of proper fitting of the HP, the selection of trained subjects, and the difference in the dimensions between subjects' heads and ear canals. Further, it is time-consuming, and the measured attenuation is limited to low-exposure sound levels.

The use of metal ATFs (ISO DP 6290, 1983) is only applicable for quality control of earmuffs; the measured insertion loss is not comparable to the measured attenuation using the REAT method. The HP attenuation measured on artificial heads with artificial ears (Maxwell et al, 1987) is more comparable to the results from human subjects, but there are still some disadvantages. One is the lack of human soft tissue on the artificial head; another is the normal variability of head dimensions between subjects, which also influences attenuation. Still another is the lack of any sound transfer by bone conduction, which limits the HP attenuation. This limit is accounted for when measuring with the REAT method (Berger, 1983).

During the past 10 years, the use of microphones in real ears for measurement of HP attenuation has become increasingly common (Baines, 1982; Liu et al, 1989; Gerling et al, 1989; Hellström and Axelsson, 1990; Humes and Ahlstrom, 1983; Preves and Pehringer, 1983; Rood, 1982; Shenoda et al, 1987; Traynor et al, 1989). Some of these authors have used probe microphones outside the earmuff with the probe opening inside the muff;

muff; others have used ¼-inch microphones mounted through a hole in the earmuff. Further, some studies describe the use of a two-microphone technique, one on the inside and one on the outside of the muff, and still others have used a mini-microphone inside the muff. Although all these methods have advantages compared to the methods described above, they also have some disadvantages that may cause errors.

The use of a probe-microphone outside the earmuff, with the probe inserted between the muff-seal and the skin, may cause sound leakage to the inside. Further, the sound reduction of the microphone housing, placed outside the muff, has to be greater than the HP attenuation in order to achieve an accurate measurement. The use of a two-microphone system, one outside and one inside the muff, will give data on the insertion loss but not the attenuation and must be recalculated for the sound transfer function between the two microphone positions without the HP.

We have tried the following different kinds of microphone measuring techniques in order to gain the advantages and to eliminate the disadvantages mentioned above.

1. In the first experiment we determined the optimal microphone position in the external ear. By optimal we mean a position in which the measurement results are least sensitive to small movements.
2. In the second experiment we compared the results from the mini-microphone (MMP) measuring technique of HP attenuation with the results from the subjective REAT method.
3. In the third experiment we studied the attenuation from five nonlinear HPs with the MMP technique for different sound exposure levels.
4. In the fourth experiment we studied the attenuation produced by an active noise reduction (ANR) system mounted in pilot helmets.

Method

Subjects

Experiment I: 10 subjects (25 to 50 years old) participated

Experiment II: 10 subjects (16 years old) were tested two times

Experiment III: 10 subjects (16 to 45 years old) participated

Experiment IV: 4 subjects (25- to 40-year-old helicopter pilots) participated

All subjects' external auditory canals and tympanic membranes (TMs) were normal and free from wax before the start of each experiment. All subjects had normal acoustic reflexes, middle-ear pressure, and compliance. The subjects participating in the second experiment also had a hearing threshold better than 10 dB HL at the tested ear (right), and were all trained in Békésy audiometry.

Equipment

All experiments, except for the fourth one, were performed in a semianechoic chamber provided with a movable speaker system covering 360 degrees in the horizontal plane and 0, +45, and −45 degrees in the vertical plane (Fig. 35-1). The MMPs (Knowles EA1842) used in these experiments were provided with silicon probes with a length of 26 mm (outer diameter 1.5 mm, inner diameter 0.8 mm). The MMP cable was elastic and soft (outer diameter less than 1 mm). The signal, white noise, was produced by a noise generator (Bruel & Kjaer 1405) and filtered through a ⅓-octave band equalizer (Technics SH-8065). The electric signal was amplified (Adyton XP3) and converted into an acoustic signal by broadband loudspeakers (Tannoy T165). The microphone signal was analyzed in a real-time analyzer (Norwegian Electronic 830). The audiometer was a computerized Békésy type (Entomed SA-260) and was set for Fix Békésy with pulsed tones in the second experiment. The subjects and the measurement setup in the test chamber were visually observed during the experiments via television camera and screen.

Hearing Protectors

In the second experiment the hearing protector used was an earmuff type (Bilsom Comfort), and the earplug was a foam type (EAR). The nonlinear hearing protectors tested in the third experiment were Bilsom Impact stereo, Ceotronic stereo, EAR-Ultra 9000, Hellberg Active stereo, Peltor Tactical mono, and Peltor Tactical 7 stereo.

Experiment I

To find the optimal microphone position in the external auditory canal, the sound transfer function was measured from free field to the TM at 12 different positions, 2 mm apart. The subject was seated in a chair in the middle of the test chamber, facing the speaker,

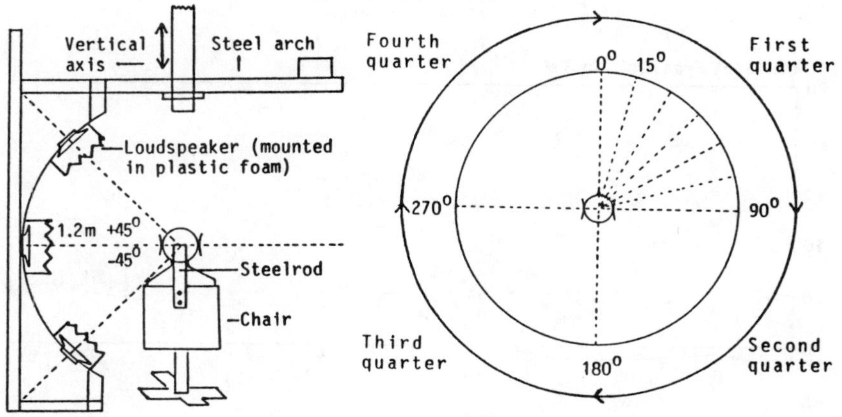

Figure 35-1 *A,* The movable loudspeaker arrangement in the experimental chamber. *B,* Top view of the sound incidence angles in the horizontal plane.

with the neck against a headrest. The probe provided with the MMP was held in position by a fixture arrangement (Fig. 35-2). The probe was inserted into the external auditory canal until the opening was 1 mm from the TM. In this position the sound pressure level was recorded in ⅓-octave bands from 200 to 20,000 Hz. The probe was then moved 2 mm outwards and the measurement was repeated. These measurements were recorded at 12 positions (24 mm from the first position) in 10 subjects. Further, the SPL was measured in a position corresponding to the center of the subject's head.

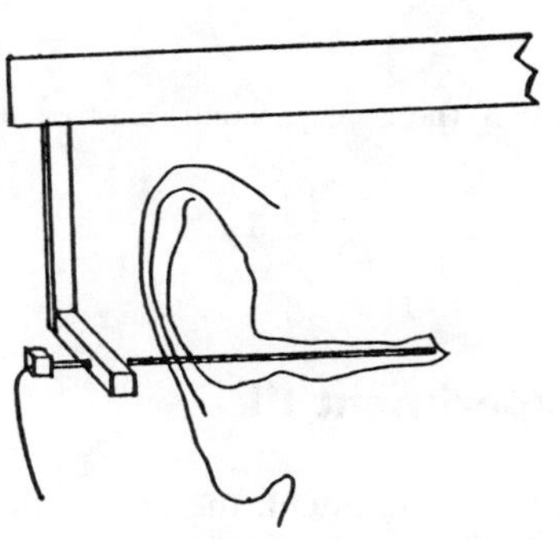

Figure 35-2 The fixture arrangement of the minimicrophone (MMP) probe.

Experiment II

To compare measurements of HP attenuation using the MMP method and the subjective method, the two methods were used simultaneously with two different directions of sound incidence. The directions were selected from the averaged data of sound transfer functions (STF) showing greatest differences (Hellström and Axelsson, 1990). The first position was 60 degrees and the second was 240 degrees in the horizontal plane, and both positions were at −45 degrees in the vertical plane. The difference in STFs at these two positions was up to 17 dB (Fig. 35-3).

The subject was seated in a chair as in Experiment I. The MMP probe was inserted into the right ear canal with its opening 1 mm from the TM and fixed in this position by taping the MMP cable above and in front of the tragus. To ensure that the hearing threshold measurement was limited to the right ear, the left ear canal was plugged with a well-inserted foam plug. The hearing thresholds were then recorded without HP using fixed Békésy audiometry for both directions of sound incidence. The HP was then carefully placed on the subject's head and new hearing threshold measurements were recorded in both positions. Without moving the HP, SPL measurements were taken at the same speaker positions used for the hearing threshold measurements but using white noise. The HP was then removed from the subject and the SPL measurements were repeated. Each subject participated four different times. The attenuation from both methods was then calculated for each of the 10 subjects. Further, the mean attenuation as well as the intersubject and intrasubject variability was calculated from the four measurements and from all subjects for the two methods and for the two directions of sound incidence.

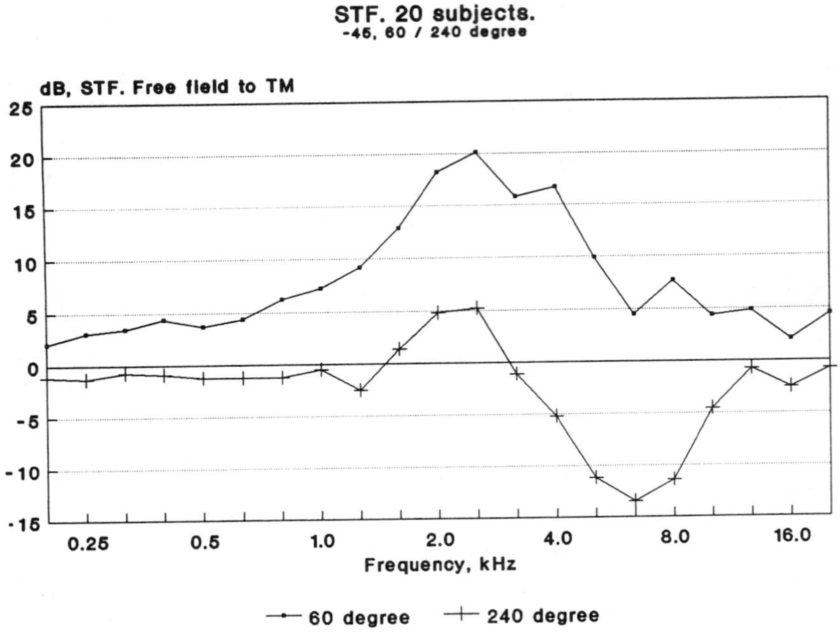

Figure 35-3 The average sound transfer functions from free field to the TM for two incidence angles, 60° and 240°.

Experiment III

In this experiment, the attenuation/amplification from five electronic nonlinear HPs and one passive nonlinear HP was studied. The noise exposure (white noise) was calibrated to give 60 dBA in the free field at a position corresponding to the center of the subject's head when seated. The preamplifier-attenuator was calibrated in six steps to give a difference of 10 dBA between each step at the center position (60 to 110 dBA).

The subject was seated in a chair facing the speaker; the MMP probe was inserted into the ear canal as described under Experiment II. The HP was placed on the subject's head, and the sound level adjustment of the electrically equipped HPs was set to maximum. The noise stimulus was turned on at the first level (60 dBA) and the first SPL measurement was recorded. The measurement was repeated and stored at each of the other five levels. The HP was removed, the next HP was put on, and the measurement was repeated for each exposure level. When the six HPs had been tested, the measurements were repeated without HP at each level. The exposure time was decreased from 10 seconds to 5 seconds in the situation without HP at the highest sound level. The six SPL measurements without HPs were compared for each subject in order to control for any level dependence that might have occurred in the unprotected situation as a result of changes in impedance due to the acoustic reflex. The attenuation/amplification was calculated for each HP, exposure level, and subject. The mean attenuation was then calculated for each HP and exposure level.

Experiment IV

This was a field experiment with MMP measurements in real HP user situations. The users were helicopter pilots. The helicopters were twin rotary-wing vehicles (Vertol). Four different helmets with HPs (earmuffs) and communication systems were tested in different flying situations. Two situations were of primary interest: normal transport speed with and without the communication system turned on. One of the helmets was provided with an ANR system. This rather simple system was phase-locked to the fundamental frequency.

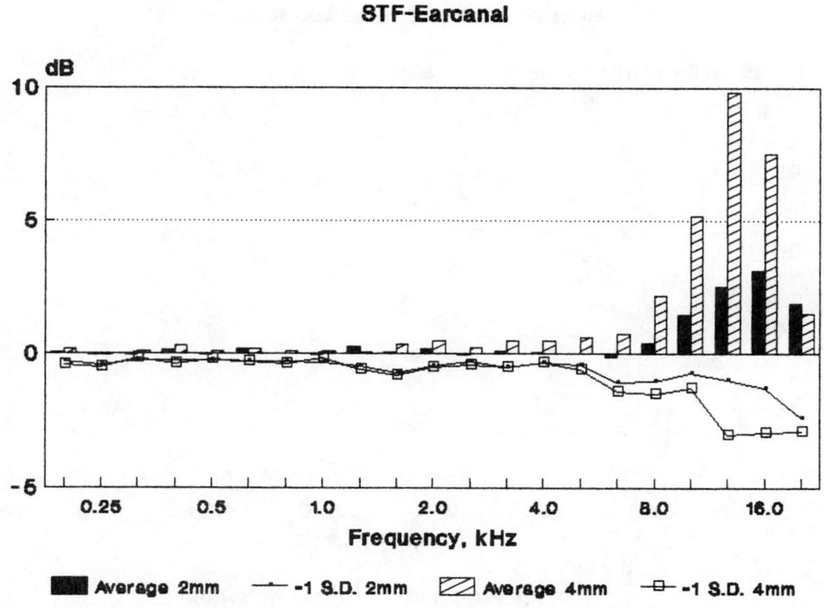

Figure 35-4 The average sound transfer functions (STFs) of 10 subjects between the tympanic membrane (TM) position and two other positions, 2 mm and 4 mm, in the external auditory canal as well as the variability expressed by 1 standard deviation (S.D.).

Results

Experiment I

Figure 35-4 illustrates the difference in the average ⅓-octave band STFs between the MMP probe position 1 mm from the TM (x) and two other positions, 2 and 4 mm from x. The difference in STF between the positions x and 2 mm is not significant for frequencies up to 10 kHz. The maximum shift occurs in the 16 kHz band where the 95 percent confidence interval is less than 4 dB. At the next position, 2 mm further outwards in the canal (4 mm from x), the maximum shift is located in the 12.5 kHz band (less than 10 dB). For frequencies up to 10 kHz, the 95 percent confidence interval is less than 3.5 dB.

Experiment II

Figure 35-5 shows attenuation measured using the MMP and HT methods with the speaker position at 60 degrees. Figure 35-6 illustrates the differences and standard deviations of results from data in Figure 35-4. The MMP method results in higher attenuation in the frequency area from 0.25 to 2 kHz and at 4 kHz. The most pronounced difference appears at 8 kHz. The variability in the results is greater with the HT method at all frequencies except for 8 kHz and reaches its maximum at 6 kHz. The differences are significant at all frequencies except for 6 kHz. Figure 35-7 shows the resulting attenuation using both methods with the speaker position at 240 degrees. The differences are less than 2.5 dB at frequencies up to 6 kHz. The MMP method results in higher attenuation at all frequencies except for 3, 6, and 8 kHz. The differences are significantly separated at 0.25, 0.5, 6, and 8 kHz. The difference is 10.4 dB at 8 kHz.

Experiment III

Figure 35-8 shows the average HP (Bilsom Impact Stereo) attenuation/amplification for six different exposure levels from 60 dBA to 110 dBA. At the two lowest exposure levels there is amplification at frequencies between 1 and 3 kHz. The other frequencies are attenuated with a maximum (25 dB) in the 12.5-kHz ⅓-octave band. The attenuation increases with increasing exposure level and is 35 dB at 6 kHz when the exposure level is 110 dBA.

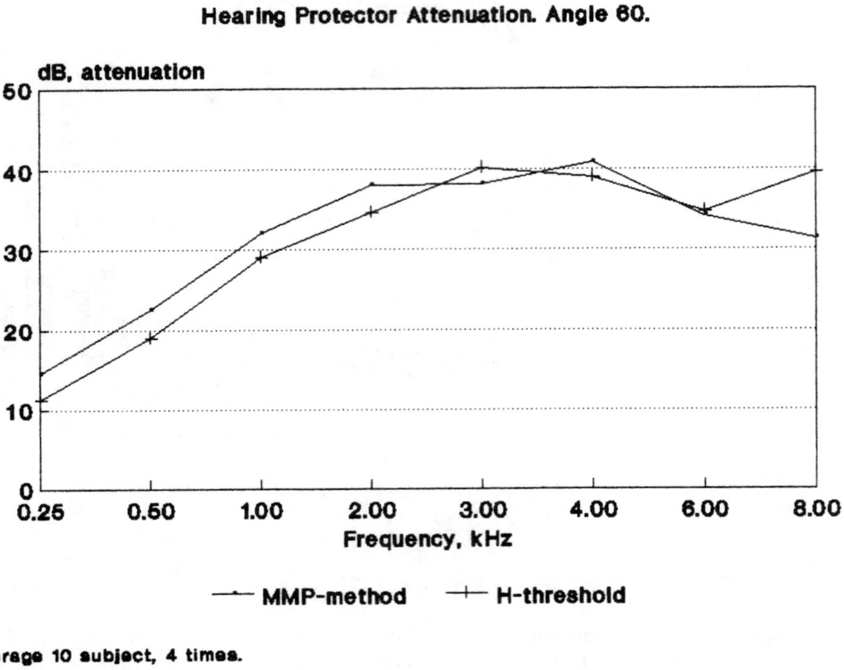

Figure 35-5 The average hearing protector (HP) attenuation measured with the mini-microphone (MMP) and hearing threshold (HT) methods at 60 degrees.

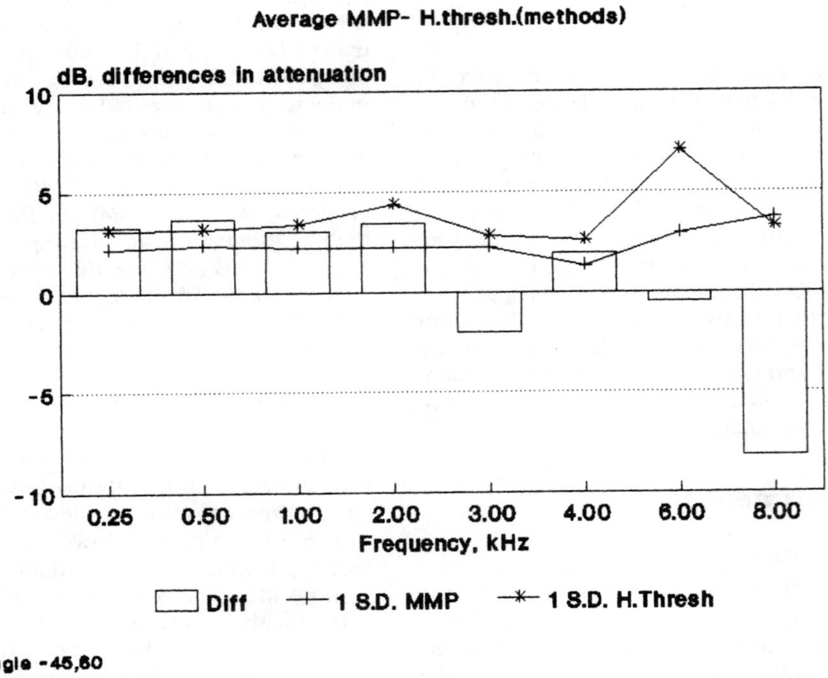

Figure 35-6 The difference in hearing protector (HP) attenuation between the mini-microphone (MMP) and hearing threshold (HT) methods, based on the data in Figure 35.4. The lines display the variability in both methods.

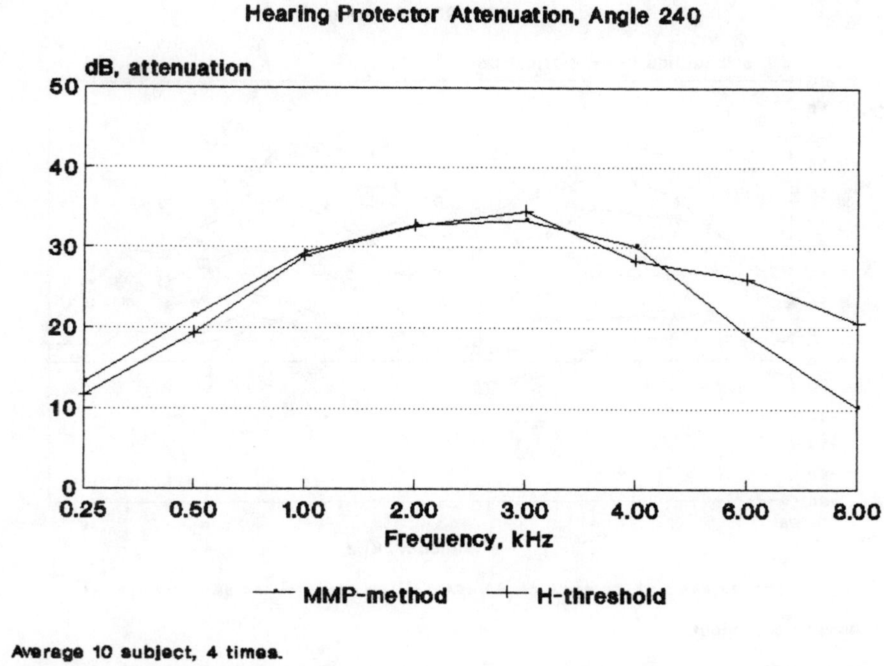

Figure 3-7 The average hearing protector (HP) attenuation measured with the mini-microphone (MMP) and hearing threshold (HT) methods at 240 degrees.

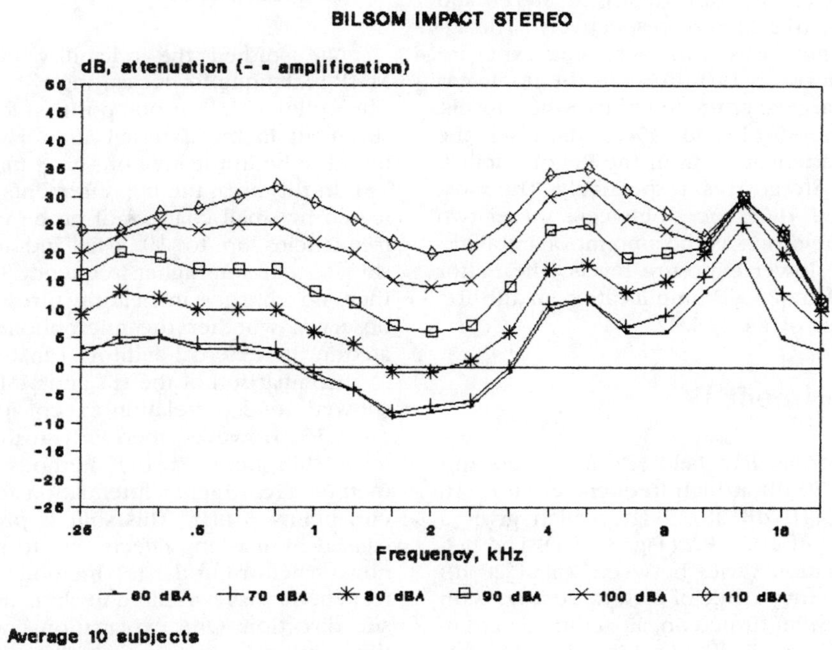

Figure 35-8 The nonlinear effect for the Bilsom Impact Stereo hearing protector. Each line indicates the attenuation/amplification at different exposure levels from 60 to 110 dBA.

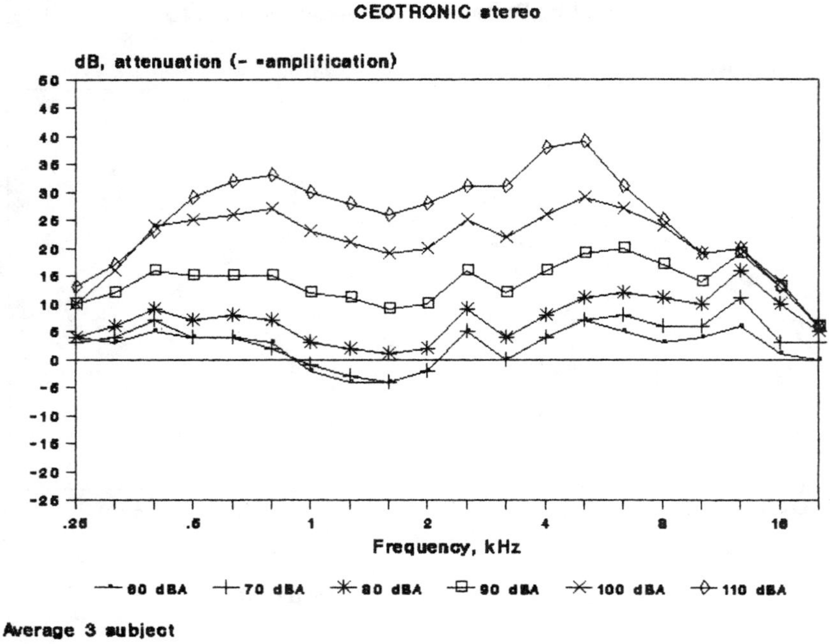

Figure 3-9 The nonlinear effect for the Ceotronic Stereo hearing protector. Each line indicates the attenuation/amplification at different exposure levels from 60 to 110 dBA.

Figures 35-9 and 35-10 illustrate the corresponding results from Ceotronic Stereo and Hellberg Active Stereo, respectively. The attenuation increases with increasing exposure levels from 60 to 110 dBA, but the nonlinear effect is marginal at the lower exposure levels.

Figures 35-11 and 35-12 illustrate the nonlinear attenuation from the Peltor Tactical Mono and Stereo HPs, respectively. The most pronounced difference between these two HPs and the others is the amount of amplification at the lower exposure levels. The Peltor HP has 20 to 25 dB amplification in the frequency area of 1 to 2 kHz.

Experiment IV

The normal free field SPL in the cockpit was about 70 dB at high frequencies (6 to 10 kHz) and 110 dB at 25 Hz, which gives a sound level of 100 dBA (Fig. 35-13). The helmet attenuation varies between 7 and 28 dB in the frequency range of 0.16 to 10 kHz. With the ANR system turned on, an additional attenuation of 7 to 17 dB is achieved in the frequency range of 40 to 400 Hz.

Conclusion

We studied the reliability of using an MMP technique for measuring HP attenuation. The optimal MMP probe position for SPL measurement in the external auditory canal was found to be in the area of 1 to 3 mm from the TM. In this area, the measurements are not affected by small changes of probe position for frequencies up to 10 kHz, and only minor shifts occur for higher-frequency bands. Further, no changes in hearing thresholds were observed whether the microphone was situated in the external auditory canal or not.

Comparison of the HT and MMP methods showed good correlation except for high frequencies. However, there is a small but significant shift between the methods; the MMP method gives higher attenuation for frequencies below 3 kHz. This shift is probably not caused by masking effects due to physiologic noise when using the HT method. Such an effect should have resulted in shifts in the opposite direction. One explanation could be the different exposure signals being used. The HT measurement signals were pulsed pure tones,

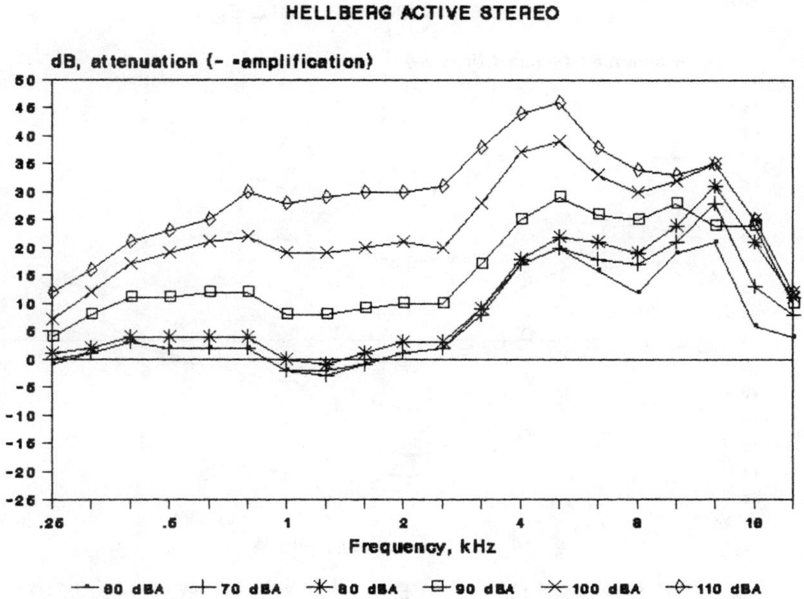

Average 10 subjects

Figure 35-10 The nonlinear effect from the Hellberg Active Stereo hearing protector. Each line indicates the attenuation/amplification at different exposure levels from 60 to 110 dBA.

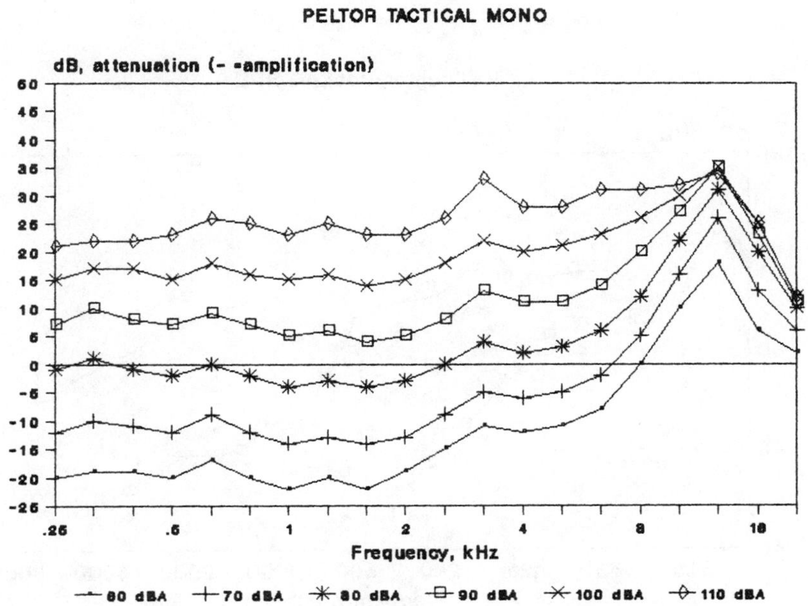

Average 10 subject

Figure 35-11 The nonlinear effect for the Peltor Tactical Mono hearing protector. Each line indicates the attenuation/amplification at different exposure levels from 60 to 110 dBA.

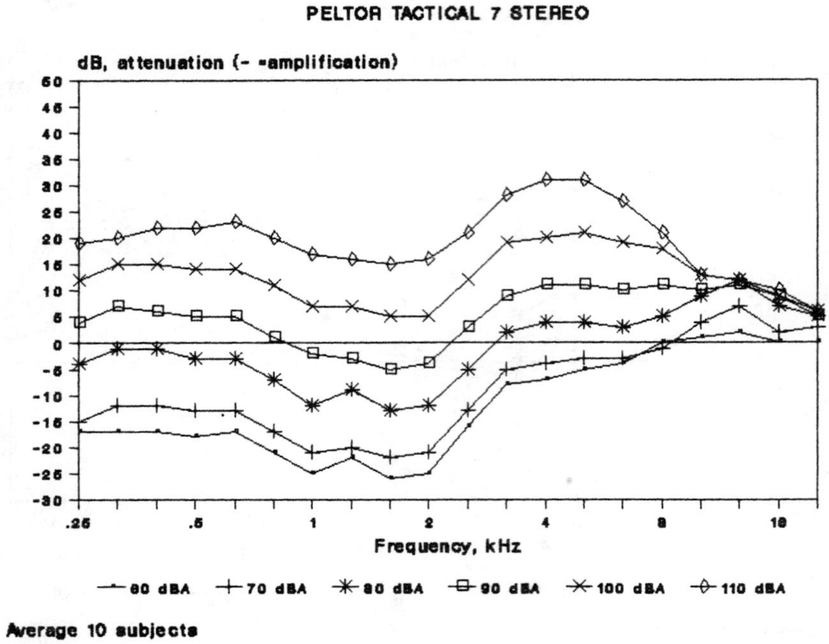

Figure 35-12 The nonlinear effect for the Peltor Tactical Stereo hearing protector. Each line indicates the attenuation/amplification at different exposure levels from 60 to 110 dBA.

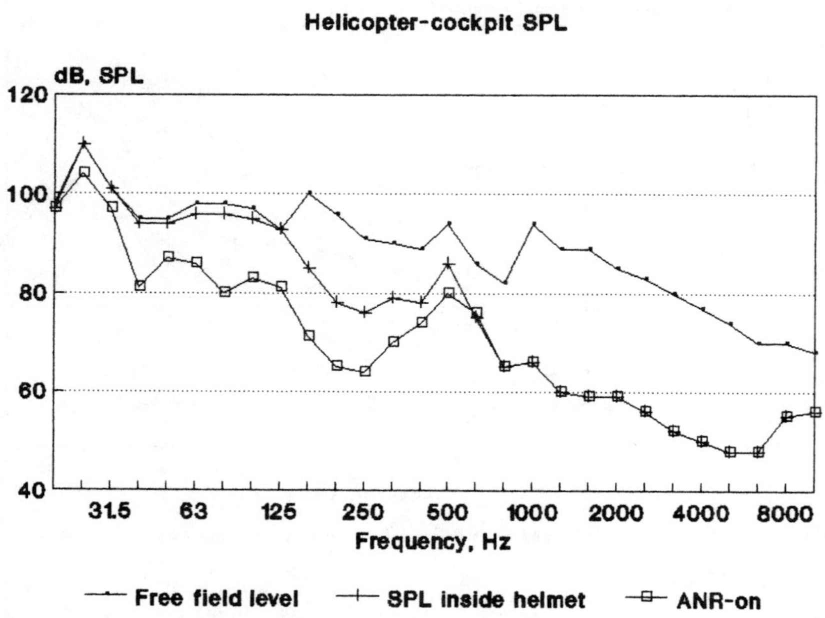

Figure 35-13 The average sound pressure level (SPL) in the helicopter cockpit measured inside pilot helmets with the active noise reduction (ANR) turned on and off, and in free field.

and the signal used for the MMP measurement was white noise. Another explanation is the monaural listening situation at the HT measurement. The contralateral ear was plugged with a well-inserted foam plug that should produce enough attenuation to eliminate binaural listening. If the plug did not attenuate enough, the measured attenuation with the HT method should have been less. The difference in results using the two methods was larger at 8 kHz. This difference could be explained by the two different exposure signals.

The nonlinear attenuation effect from the electrically equipped HPs worked well for the exposure level range used. The passive nonlinear HP did not show any nonlinear effect for these exposure levels. In an earlier study this effect started at an SPL of 118 dB. The ANR system we tested caused an attenuation of at most 17 dB. The attenuation covered frequencies from 25 to 630 Hz. These systems can be functional in HPs of the future. With lower pressure of the earmuffs and thus better comfort, the low-frequency attenuation will decrease. This can be compensated by the effect of the ANR system.

The MMP method was found to be an alternative to the HT method for measuring HP attenuation, especially the attenuation from nonlinear HPs and in real user situations.

Méthodes d'Évaluation Objectives des Protecteurs Auditifs Conventionnels, Non-Linéaires et Actifs

La méthode conventionnelle pour la mesure de l'atténuation de protecteurs auditifs (ISO-4869) n'est pas utilisable dans tous les cas. L'un des problèmes réside dans l'évaluation de l'atténuation de protecteurs non linéaires. Ces protecteurs sont supposés avoir une faible atténuation aux niveaux de bruit faibles et une atténuation plus importante aux niveaux élevés.

Au cours de l'année passée, le nombre de protecteurs auditifs non linéaires commercialisés s'est accru mais les caractéristiques chiffrées de l'effet non linéaire ne sont pas disponibles. Il est cependant possible de mesurer l'atténuation de ces protecteurs à l'aide de la méthode subjective, l'amplification étant soit coupée soit réglée à sa valeur maximale. Mais ces valeurs ne nous apprendront rien sur l'effet non linéaire ou sur la valeur de l'atténuation aux niveaux sonores élevés. Nous avons étudié la possibilité d'utiliser des microphones miniatures pour mesurer les niveaux de pression acoustique dans le conduit auditif externe avec et sans protecteurs auditifs.

Différents types de microphones miniatures ont été comparés en ce qui concerne leur gamme dynamique, la fréquence et la linéarité du niveau sonore. Les microphones retenus furent ensuite placés dans des conduits auditifs humains de manière à contrôler toute influence éventuelle sur l'impédance acoustique. Nous avons décidé d'utiliser le microphone miniature Knowles (EA-1842) équipé d'une sonde en silicone.

Pour trouver la meilleure position pour le microphone, la fonction de transfert de l'entrée du conduit auditif à la membrane tympanique fut mesurée par pas de 2 mm. Par meilleure position on entend une zone à l'intérieur de laquelle les résultats sont affectés le moins possible par de faibles déplacements du microphone.

La fonction de transfert du champ libre à la membrane tympanique fut mesurée chez 20 sujets pour 24 angles d'incidence sonore dans le plan horizontal et pour chacun de ceux-ci, pour 3 angles dans le plan vertical, soit au total pour 72 incidences.

Les résultats moyens constituent un outil pour le calcul des niveaux de pression acoustique en champ libre à partir de ceux mesurés dans le conduit auditif.

Pour deux angles d'incidence sonore, l'un avec une forte amplification l'autre avec une faible amplification dues à la forme du corps et à la résonance du conduit auditif, les différences de seuils subjectifs furent comparées avec les valeurs obtenues à partir de mesures effectuées avec les microphones miniatures.

L'étude fut réalisée et répétée quatre fois sur 10 sujets avec et sans protecteurs auditifs.

L'atténuation des protecteurs auditifs mesurée à l'aide de la technique des microphones miniatures s'avéra être en bon accord avec les résultats obtenus à partir de la méthode subjective et l'on constata que la technique de mesure était valable avec néanmoins quelques limitations.

L'atténuation de cinq protecteurs auditifs non linéaires (serre-tête) fut étudiée pour 6 niveaux d'exposition différents (entre 60 et 110 dBA) chez 10 sujets.

L'effet non linéaire de protecteurs équipés de systèmes électroniques a fonctionné conformément aux prévisions.

L'atténuation de trois protecteurs non linéaires (serre-tête) fut évaluée dans des situations d'utilisation réalistes en régime de bruits impulsionnels et en régime de bruit continu.

Dans le cas de bruits impulsionnels, l'effet non-linéaire fonctionnait aussi bien que dans le cas de bruits continus.

L'atténuation de casques équipés de dispositifs à atténuation acoustique active du bruit et destinés au personnel navigant fut étudiée en situation réelle à bord d'hélicoptères. On a observé une atténuation active dans le domaine des fréquences comprises entre 40 et 600 Hz.

ACKNOWLEDGMENTS

This work was supported by grant 86-0241 from The Swedish Work Environment Fund.

References

ANSI S12.6. Method for the measurement of the real-ear attenuation of hearing protectors. New York: Acoustical Society of America, 1984.

Baines DC. Developments in the use of Knowles miniature microphones to measure conditions inside the ear muffs. Appl Acoust 1982; 15:117-131.

Berger EH. Laboratory attenuation of earmuffs and earplugs both singly and in combination. Am Ind Hyg Assoc J 1983; 44(5):321-329.

Gerling IJ, Metz DA, Roemer-Bonko J, Rowsey LM. Real ear attenuation with a probe tube system. Hear Instr 1989; 40(2):34-55.

Giguère C, Kunov H. An acoustic head simulator for hearing protector evaluation. II: Measurements in steady-state and impulse noise environments. J Acoust Soc Am 1989; 85(3):1197-1205.

Hellström PA, Axelsson A. Sound transfer function characteristics from free field to tympanic membrane. Submitted for publication.

Humes LE, Ahlstrom JB. New procedures for the evaluation of hearing protectors. Noise as a public health problem. Proc of the 4th Int Congr 1983; (1):257-260.

ISO 4869. Acoustics—Measurement of sound attenuation of hearing protectors—Subjective method. Genève, Switzerland: International Organization for Standardization, 1981.

ISO DP 6290. Acoustics—Simplified method for measurement of insertion loss of hearing protectors of ear-muff type for quality-control purposes. Genève, Switzerland: International Organization for Standardization, 1983.

Ivey ES, Nerbonne GP, Tolhurst GC. Measuring helmet sound attenuation characteristics using an acoustic manikin. J Acoust Soc Am 1987; 81(2):370-375.

Kunov H, Giguère C. An acoustic head simulator for hearing protector evaluation. I: Design and construction. J Acoust Soc Am 1989; 85(3):1191-1196.

Liu C-C, Pekkarinen J, Starck J. Application of the probe microphone method to measure attenuation of hearing protectors against high impulse sound levels. Appl Acoust 1989; 27:13-25.

Maxwell DW, Williams CE, Robertson RM, Thomas GB. Performance characteristics of active hearing protection devices. Sound and Vibration, May 1987, pp. 14-18.

Pfretzschner J, Moreno A. Anamorphical measurements on ear-muffs. Proc ICA 12. B Toronto, 10-8, July 24-31, 1986.

Preves DA, Pehringer JL. Calculating individual NRR's in situ using subminiature probe microphones. Hear Instr 1983; 34(3):10-14.

Pösselt C, Schroeter J. Objective measuring technique for hearing-protective devices including bone-conduction effects. Proc Inter-Noise 85, Munich, 1985; 1255-1258.

Rood GM. The in-situ measurement of the attenuation of hearing protectors by the use of miniature microphones. In: Alberti PW, ed. Personal hearing protection in industry. New York: Raven Press, 1982:175.

Schroeter J. Improvements in measuring the attenuation of personal earprotectors with artificial heads. J Acoust Soc Am 1982; 71(suppl 1):552.

Schroeter J. The use of acoustical test fixtures for measurement of hearing protector attenuation. Part I: Review of previous work and the design of an improved test fixture. J Acoust Soc Am 1986; 79(4):1065-1080.

Shenoda FB, Ising H, Fischer R. Sound attenuation of earmuffs under conditions of impulsive noise—laboratory measurements. Appl Acoust 1987; 21:295-307.

Traynor RM, Ackley RS, Wiersbowsky L. Probe tube microphone measurement of hearing protection devices. Hear Instr 1989; 40(2):32-60.

SECTION SEVEN

Role of the Acoustic Environment

CHAPTER 36

Medial Efferents and Acoustic Trauma

JEAN-LUC PUEL
PATRICK VASSOUT

It is well documented that hearing deficits may result from exposures to relatively intense acoustic stimulation. When threshold shift is produced by tonal stimuli, the maximum hearing loss is measured at half an octave above the exposure frequency, and the loss recovers if the threshold depression is no greater than 40 dB (McFadden, 1986). In addition, it has been shown that exposure to high-intensity sound results in various structural changes (Saunders et al, 1985). Recent studies have focused on two major structural changes in the cochlea to explain the hearing losses: (1) stereocilia lesions (Tilney et al, 1982; Robertson, 1982; Slepecky et al, 1982; Engstrom et al, 1983; Liberman and Dodds, 1984; Nielsen and Slepecky, 1986; Canlon et al, 1987), and (2) swelling of afferent dendrites at the level of inner hair cells (IHCs) (Beagley, 1965; Spoendlin, 1971; Robertson, 1983). In a previous study (Puel et al, 1988), we investigated the possibility that an intense sound produces damage at the level of IHC afferent synapses by an excessive release of neurotransmitter. Because intracochlear perfusion of kynurenate, which is known to block the action of the afferent neurotransmitter postsynaptically (Bobbin and Ceasar, 1987), did not reduce the traumatic effect of the intense sound, we concluded that the active processes were affected first.

One current hypothesis is that the fast motility of the isolated outer hair cells (OHCs) is related to these active processes (Brownell et al, 1985; Ashmore, 1987), whereas the chemically-induced slow motility of the OHCs is related to the modulation of the active processes, modulation that is probably driven in vivo by the efferent fibers. The only efferents connected to the outer hair cells are the medial olivocochlear (MOC) efferents coming from the medial nuclei of the superior olivary complex (Warr et al, 1986). Because electrical stimulation of the crossed olivocochlear bundle (COCB), which essentially activated the MOC efferents, has been demonstrated to reduce the effect of intense sound on the cochlear potentials (Rajan, 1988a,b), one suggestion is that the MOC efferents might protect the cochlea against the damaging effects of intense sound exposure.

Because strychnine has been shown to block the effects of an electrical stimulation of the COCB (Wiederhold, 1986), we decided to test the protective role of MOC efferents by comparing the effect of intense sound exposure during intracochlear perfusion of artificial perilymph with or without strychnine. In addition, Buck et al (1984) observed in anesthetized and curarized animals that for isoenergetic exposure to burst noise, the greatest threshold shift occurred at a repetition rate of one per second, whereas almost no threshold shift was observed when the repetition was set at 17 per second. At this time, they proposed that there might be a protective mechanism, different from a middle-ear reflex, which minimizes the effect of stimulation on the organ of Corti. Therefore, we designed a second series of experiments to test the hypothesis that the absence of threshold shift observed at a rate of 17 per second might result from a protective mechanism driven by the MOC efferents, by testing strychnine applied intraperitoneally and by sectioning the crossed MOC efferents at the floor of the fourth ventricle.

Methods

First Series of Experiments

The method used was the same as previously described (Puel et al, 1988). Briefly, 15 pigmented guinea pigs of both sexes were anesthetized with pentobarbital and chlorprothixene, and the middle-ear muscles were sectioned. In five animals, contralateral ear destruction was carried out after the animal was anesthetized by physically destroying the cochlea with a blunt probe about 2 hours before the exposure to the intense sound. Three groups of animals were studied. Group 1 underwent intense sound exposure during perfusion with artificial perilymph. Group 2 underwent contralateral ear destruction before intense sound exposure during perfusion with artificial perilymph. Group 3 underwent intense sound exposure during perfusion with artificial perilymph containing strychnine.

The potentials were average responses (20 samples) to 6,000-, 8,484-, and 10,000-Hz tone bursts of 0.25 ms exponential rise/fall time, 10 ms duration, and 200 ms interstimulus interval, presented in a closed acoustic delivery system. Intensity functions were obtained by varying tone burst intensities (14 to 110 dB SPL, in 6-dB steps).

Artificial perilymph was infused into the basal turn of scala tympani and allowed to flow out of the basal turn of scala vestibuli at 2.5 μl per minute through holes made in the cochlea. The artificial perilymph solution had the following composition: 137 mm NaCl; 5 mm KCl; 2 mm $CaCl_2$; 1 mm $MgCl_2$; 10 mm Hepes; 10 mm glucose, pH 7.4. Three consecutive intracochlear perfusions of different durations were carried out in all animals, the first lasting 10 minutes, a second lasting 35 minutes, and a third lasting 10 minutes. In all 15 animals artificial perilymph was perfused for 10 minutes. This was then followed by the second perfusion of 35 minutes, which in 10 animals (five normal animals and five with contralateral ear destroyed) consisted of artificial perilymph alone and in five other animals consisted of artificial perilymph containing 10 μm strychnine sulfate. Starting 10 minutes after the beginning of the second perfusion period, a 6-kHz, 95-dB SPL, 15-minute continuous tone was presented to the ipsilateral ear. In all animals after the second perfusion period, the third perfusion was finally carried out with artificial perilymph. Intensity functions to the tone bursts were recorded before any perfusion and immediately after each perfusion (within 2 minutes).

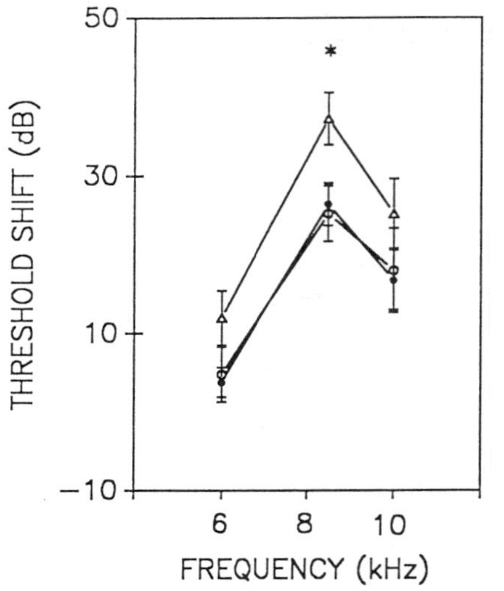

Figure 36-1 Compound action potential (CAP) threshold shift in decibels (mean ± SEM) as a function of tone frequency after acoustic trauma (6 kHz, 95 dB SPL, 15 minutes) recorded after the end of the third perfusion in the first series of experiments. The threshold shift was recorded as the difference from the recording after the first perfusion with artificial perilymph and the recording after all perfusions. Shown are data obtained after intense sound exposure during perfusion with artificial perilymph alone (n = 5, open circle), after contralateral ear destruction before intense sound exposure during perfusion with artificial perilymph (n = 5, filled circle), and after intense sound exposure during perfusion with artificial perilymph containing 10 μm strychnine (n = 5, open triangle). Analysis of variance and the Newmann-Keuls multiple range test were used to determine significance (asterisk, *p* less than 0.001).

Treatment effects were defined by comparing potentials recorded after the various treatments to those recorded after the first perfusion. Analysis of variance and Newmann-Keuls multiple range test were used to determine significance (*p* less than 0.05). The data are expressed as means ± SEM.

Second Series of Experiments

Thirty-four pigmented guinea pigs were anesthetized with ketamine. Tone bursts of 8 kHz (10 ms duration) were presented in a closed acoustic delivery system with a repetition rate of either 1 per second for 17 minutes (n = 8) or 17 per second for 1 minute (n = 14). This paradigm represents isoenergetic exposures of 10 seconds in total effective duration. The duration of the tone burst (10 ms) was chosen to be shorter than the latency of the efferent fiber's response as recorded by

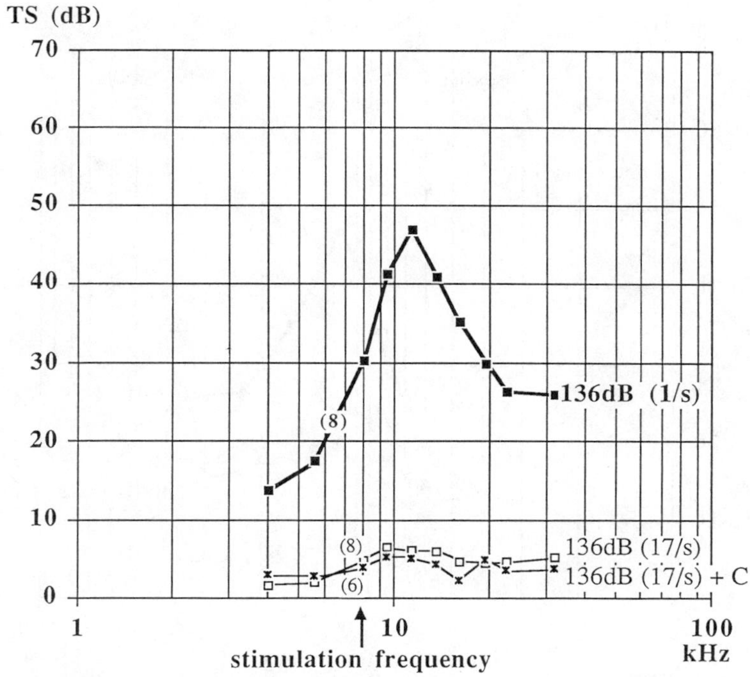

Figure 36-2 Compound action potential (CAP) threshold shift in decibels (mean ± SEM), as a function of tone frequency, induced by a 136-dB SPL stimulus for isoenergetic tone burst exposure at a repetition rate of 1 per second for 17 minutes (heavy lines) and at a repetition rate of 17 per second for 1 minute (light lines). C, The group of animals that were curarized. The number of animals in each group is indicated in parentheses.

Robertson and Gummer (1985) and Liberman and Brown (1986).

The threshold shifts were measured ipsilaterally by electrocochleography at the level of the round window, 20 minutes after the end of the exposure for frequencies ranging from 4 to 32 kHz.

Two different drugs were used to try to block the normal function of the MOC efferents: strychnine (n = 5) and scopolamine (n = 4). The drugs were injected intraperitoneally (2 mg per kilogram) 10 to 30 minutes before the exposure to tone bursts presented at a repetition rate of 17 per second. In addition, in three animals a section of the brain stem at the floor of the fourth ventricle was also performed in order to eliminate the crossed part of the MOC efferents.

Results

First Series of Experiments

The greatest effect of the intense sound on compound action potential (CAP) threshold during perfusion with artificial perilymph alone was observed at 8,484 Hz, with less of an effect occurring at 10,000 Hz, and the least effect occurring at 6,000 Hz (Fig. 36-1). The results in the group of animals with contralateral ear destruction did not differ from the above group (Fig. 36-1). However, in the group of animals exposed to an intense sound during perfusion with artificial perilymph containing 10 μm strychnine, the shift in CAP threshold at 8,484 Hz exposure was significantly greater (about 12 dB) than that observed in animals exposed to intense sound during perfusion with artificial perilymph alone.

Second Series of Experiments

For the same stimulation level (136 dB SPL), exposure to a tone burst presented at a repetition rate of 17 per second for 1 minute induced a slight threshold shift, whereas with a repetition rate of 1 per second for 17 minutes a threshold shift of about 50 dB was observed at a frequency half an octave above the exposure frequency (Fig. 36-2). No modification of the responses could be observed when anesthetized animals exposed to the repetition rate of 17 per second were injected with

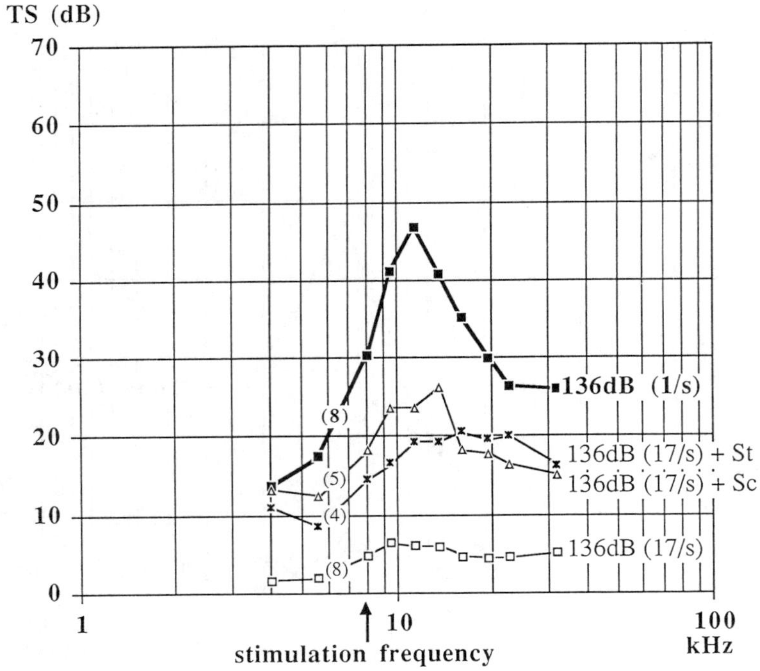

Figure 36-3 Compound action potential (CAP) threshold shift in decibels (mean ± SEM), as a function of tone frequency, induced by a 136-dB SPL stimulus for isoenergetic tone burst exposure at a repetition rate of 1 per second for 17 minutes (heavy lines) and at a repetition rate of 17 per second for 1 minute (light lines). St and Sc, Animals that respectively received intraperitoneal injections of strychnine and scopolamine (2 mg per kilogram) 10 to 30 minutes before the exposure to tone bursts presented at a repetition rate of 17 per second for 1 minute. The number of animals in each group is indicated in parentheses.

curare (Fig. 36-2). In contrast, administration of strychnine or scopolamine induced an increase in the threshold shift in animals exposed to the repetition rate of 17 per second (about 12 dB), but still far less than the value measured with a repetition rate of 1 per second (Fig. 36-3). The same result was obtained after the section of the brain stem at the floor of the fourth ventricle (Fig. 36-4).

Conclusion

The main result of both series of experiments is that the effects of an intense sound were about 12 dB greater in the presence of strychnine applied either directly to the cochlea or intraperitoneally. In addition, the largest threshold shift was always observed at a frequency half an octave above the exposure frequency, which is consistent with results obtained in different species of mammals (Mitchell et al, 1977; Lonsbury-Martin and Meikle, 1978; Cody and Johnstone, 1981; McFadden and Plattsmier, 1982)

The function of the efferents on the cochlea has been generally studied by electrical stimulation of the COCB (Wiederhold and Kiang, 1970; Desmedt and Robertson, 1975). The major effect of such stimulation was to reduce the amplitude of the CAP; this effect could be blocked by strychnine (Desmedt, 1975). In both series of experiments, the effect of an intense sound was greater in the presence of strychnine. This suggests that one effect of the efferents may be to act as protectors against an intense sound.

Consistent with this interpretation, electrical stimulations of the COCB attenuate the effect of an intense sound on the cochlear potentials (Rajan, 1988a,b). In addition, sound stimulation of the contralateral ear attenuates the effect of intense sound on the ipsilateral ear (Cody and Johnstone, 1982). Because this effect was blocked by an intramuscular injection of strychnine, Cody and Johnstone proposed that this desensitization could be the result of acoustically-evoked contralateral efferent activity. The same reduction of the effect of intense sound was also shown after destruc-

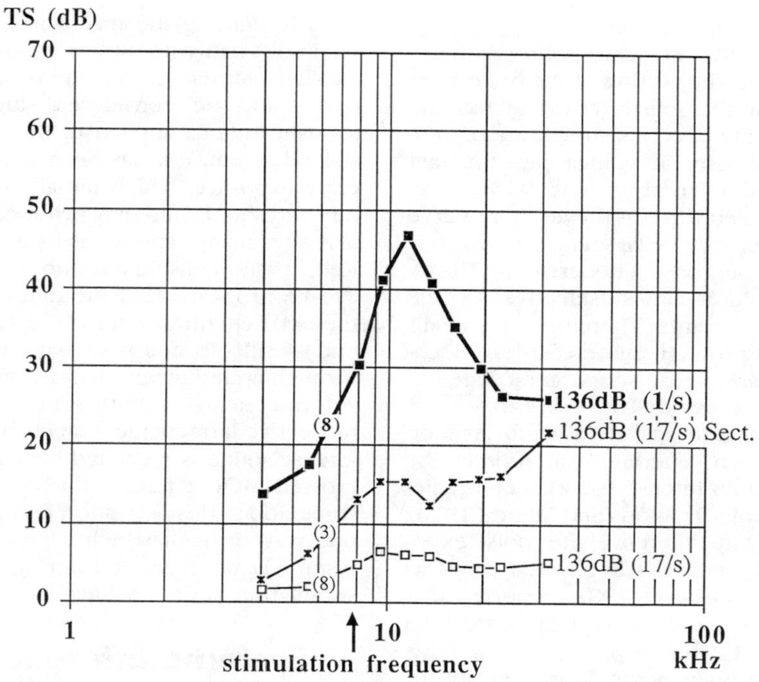

Figure 36-4 Compound action potential (CAP) threshold shift in decibels (mean ± SEM), as a function of tone frequency, induced by a 136-dB SPL stimulus for isoenergetic tone burst exposure at a repetition rate of 1 per second for 17 minutes (heavy lines) and at a repetition rate of 17 per second for 1 minute (light lines). Sect, Animals in which a section of the brain stem at the floor of the fourth ventricle was performed before the exposure to tone bursts presented at a repetition rate of 17 per second for 1 minute. The number of animals in each group is indicated in parentheses.

tion of the contralateral cochlea (Rajan and Johnstone, 1983). However, in our first series of experiments, no difference was found between the animals with and without contralateral destruction. This apparent contradiction may be explained by (1) the effect of the contralateral destruction possibly dissipating over a 2-hour period before the noise exposure, or (2) the different duration and intensity of sound exposure, or (3) both. In any case, our results suggest that no contralateral components are involved in the present study. Therefore, the potentiation of the ipsilateral intense sound by strychnine observed in the first series of experiment in which the middle-ear muscles were severed suggests that (1) an ipsilateral cochlear efferent loop is activated by the ipsilateral intense sound, and (2) these fibers suppressed the damaging effects of the intense sound in the animals not treated with strychnine.

The second series of experiments shows that for an isoenergetic exposure level, the greatest effect of intense sound upon CAP threshold was obtained at a repetition rate of 1 per second, whereas almost no threshold shift was observed when the repetition rate was set at 17 per second. Because the results remained unchanged when the exposed animals were curarized, it is unlikely that an acoustic reflex of the middle-ear muscles is involved in this phenomenon. One interpretation is that the repetition rate of 1 per second might give time to the cochlea to return to its original condition before the occurrence of the following tone burst. In this way, tone bursts presented at a repetition rate of 1 per second could be considered isolated stimuli in which no significant efferent-induced phenomenon exists. On the contrary, the repetition rate of 17 per second could correspond to a condition in which the protective mechanism driven by the efferents is fully efficient. Indeed, an intraperitoneal injection of strychnine or scopolamine 10 minutes before an exposure of 17 tone bursts per second induced a larger threshold shift; this potentiation was about the same as that observed in the first series of experiments (about 12 dB). Here again, these results suggest that an ipsilateral cochlear efferent loop is involved in a protective mechanism of the cochlea against intense sound. Moreover the section of the brain stem at the floor of the fourth ventricle has the same potentiating effect as strychnine or scopolamine. Especially in guinea pig, the fact that the lateral efferent system, which synapses with the dendrites of the auditory nerve below the inner hair cells, seems to have few contralateral neurons (Robertson, 1985), makes this section almost selective for the crossed MOC efferents. Therefore, this result suggests that a protective intracochlear mechanism against an intense sound is mediated at least in part by crossed MOC efferents.

Evidence that an ipsilateral cochlear loop mediated by MOC efferents can protect the cochlea against an intense sound is contradictory. For example, Trahiotis and Elliott (1970) failed to show any difference after noise exposure in animals with COCB severed, whereas Handrock and Zeisberg (1982) reported that both temporary and permanent threshold shifts increased after severing all efferents within the vestibular nerve. Moreover, in our second series of experiments, pharmacologic or surgical efferent manipulations failed to completely cancel the protective effect (see Figs. 36-3 and 36-4). The intraperitoneal administration of strychnine or scopolamine, or the section of the brain stem at the floor of the fourth ventricle, induced an increase of threshold shift in animals exposed at the repetition rate of 17 per second, but this threshold shift was far less than the shift that occurred with a repetition rate of 1 per second. Of course, one can speculate that the mode of administration, the doses, the drugs, the type of section we used, or a combination thereof, were not adequate to completely cancel the protective mechanism. Nevertheless, other alternative explanations can be proposed. For example, in addition to MOC efferent activation, the OHCs themselves might also exhibit a protective mechanism against intense sound that cannot be expressed when using a repetition rate of 1 per second. Brundin et al (1990) reported that mechanical responses of isolated OHCs in vitro can be induced by acoustic stimulation of the lateral wall of the cells, but not of the stereocilia. Ding et al (1990) proposed that these mechanical (acoustic) responses may result from the opening of stretch-activated channels. This could allow calcium to enter the cell, leading to a shortening of the OHCs through the interaction of actin and myosin. Therefore, it might be possible that, at such intensities of stimulation, the OHCs respond by contracting and consequently limiting the mechanical input to the organ of Corti without any action of the MOC efferents. Moreover, the rate of 1 tone per second could be considered single moderate acoustic trauma applied to the cochlea every second. Because it has been shown that moderate exposure, which initially causes temporary threshold shift, may produce a permanent loss after many repetitions (Taylor et al, 1965; Kell, 1975; Lonsbury-Martin et al, 1987), it can be proposed that the difference between the two repetition rates (1 versus 17 per second) results from a potentiation phenomenon through an unknown mechanism.

In conclusion, both studies suggest that a protective intracochlear mechanism against an intense sound is mediated by activation of the crossed MOC efferents during intense sound stimulation. This activation constitutes at least one way through which a protective mechanism may be expressed during intense sound stimulation of the cochlea.

Système Efférent Médian et Traumatisme Sonore: Pharmacologie et Electrophysiologie

Dans une étude précédente (Puel et coll., 1989), nous avons testé la possibilité selon laquelle une libération excessive de neurotransmetteur induite par une sur-stimulation sonore pouvait provoquer des dégâts au niveau des fibres afférentes des cellules ciliées internes. Etant donné qu'une perfusion intracochléaire de kynurénate ne réduisait pas l'effet du traumatisme acoustique utilisé dans cette étude, nous en avons conclu que seules les structures impliquées dans la transduction avant la synapse afférente étaient affectées. Ces structures sont: (1) les cellules ciliées internes (CCI), véritables cellules sensorielles et (2) les cellules ciliées externes (CCE) qui modulent de manière mécanique l'activité des CCI (mécanismes actifs). Les seules efférences des CCE sont celles du système efférent médian. La stimulation électrique de ces fibres pendant une exposition sonore réduit l'effet du traumatisme acoustique (Rajan and Johnstone, 1988). Aussi, nous avons étudié l'effet d'un traumatisme acoustique en présence ou en absence de strychnine, drogue connue pour bloquer l'activité des fibres efférentes.

Dans une première série d'expériences, nous avons pu montrer qu'une sur-stimulation sonore provoquait une réduction du potentiel d'action composite (PAC) et du potentiel de sommation plus importante une demie octave au-dessus de la fréquence du son traumatique, et peu de changement du potentiel microphonique. Une perfusion intracochléaire de strychnine potentialisait les dégâts occasionnés par une même sur-stimulation sonore. Ce résultat montre qu'une boucle de rétroaction cochléaire est activée pendant une sur-stimulation sonore et qu'elle est bloquée par une perfusion intracochléaire de strychnine.

Dans une seconde série d'expériences, le traumatisme sonore était induit par des bouffées tonales (8 kHz, 0.4 ms de front de montée/descente, 10 ms de durée), à une cadence de 17 coups par seconde durant une minute ou de 1 coup par seconde durant 17 minutes. Les dégâts les plus importants étaient obtenus pour une cadence de stimulation 1 coup par seconde. Le même résultat était obtenu chez des animaux curarisés, excluant donc la mise en jeu du réflexe stapédien. Par contre, une injection intrapéritonéale de strychnine (2 mg/kg) administrée 10 mn avant l'expérience entraînait une potentialisation de l'effet traumatique de l'exposition à une cadence de 17 coups par seconde durant une minute. Ces résultats sont en accord avec la première série d'expériences suggérant que les fibres du système efférent médian pourraient jouer un rôle protecteur contre les sur-stimulations sonores.

ACKNOWLEDGMENTS

We wish to thank Prof. R.P. Bobbin and Dr. A. Dancer, who initiated this work, and Drs. G. Rebillard and M. Lenoir for helpful discussions concerning the manuscript. We also thank P. Sibleyras for photographic work, and Dr W.R. Lippe, E. Mayat, and A. Bara for editorial assistance.

References

Ashmore JF. A fast motile response in guinea-pig outer hair cells: The cellular basis of the cochlear amplifier. J Physiol 1987; 388:323-347.

Beagley HA. Acoustic trauma in the guinea pig. Acta Otolaryngol 1965; 60:479-495.

Bobbin RP, Ceasar G. Kynurenic acid and gamma-D-glutamyl-aminoethylsulfonic acid suppress the compound action potential of the auditory nerve. Hear Res 1987; 25:77-81.

Brownell WE, Bader CR, Bertrand D, de Ribeaupierre Y. Evoked mechanical responses of isolated cochlear outer hair cells. Science 1985; 227:194-196.

Brundin L, Flock Å, Canlon B. Sound induced motility of cochlear outer hair cells shows tuning. Abstract 260 of the 13th A.R.O. Midwinter Research Meeting, St. Petersburg, FL, 1990:227.

Buck K, Dancer A, Franke R. Effect of the temporal pattern of a given noise dose on TTS in guinea pigs. J Acoust Soc Am 1984; 76:1090-1097.

Canlon B, Miller J, Flock Å, Borg E. Pure tone overstimulation changes the micromechanical properties of the inner hair cell stereocilia. Hear Res 1987; 30:65-72.

Cody AR, Johnstone BM. Acoustic trauma: Single neuron basis for the "half-octave shift." J Acoust Soc Am 1981; 70:707-719.

Cody AR, Johnstone BM. Temporary threshold shift modified by binaural acoustic stimulation. Hear Res 1982; 6:199-205.

Desmedt JE. Physiological studies of the efferent auditory system. In: Keidel WD, Neff WD, eds. Handbook of sensory physiology. Berlin: Springer Verlag, 1975:219.

Desmedt JE, Robertson D. Ionic mechanisms of the efferent olivo-cochlear inhibition studied by cochlear perfusion in the cat. J Physiol (Lond) 1975; 247:407-428.

Ding JP, Salvi RJ, Sachs F. Stretch activated ion channels in outer hair cells from guinea pig cochlea. Abstract 258 of the 13th A.R.O. Midwinter Research Meeting, St. Petersburg, FL, 1990:226.

Engstrom B, Flock Å, Borg E. Ultrastructural studies of stereocilia in noise-exposed rabbits. Hear Res 1983; 12:251-264.

Handrock M, Zeisberg J. The influence of the efferent system on adaptation, temporary and permanent threshold shift. Arch Otol Rhinol Laryngol 1982; 234:191-195.

Kell RL. Hearing loss in female jute weavers. Ann Occup Hyg 1975; 18:97-109.

Liberman MC, Dodds LW. Single-neuron labeling and chronic cochlear pathology. III. Stereocilia damage and laterations of threshold tuning curves. Hear Res 1984; 16:55-74.

Liberman MC, Brown MC. Physiology and anatomy of single olivocochlear neurons in the cat. Hear Res 1986; 24:17-36.

Lonsbury-Martin BL, Meikle MB. Neural correlates of auditory fatigue: Frequency-dependent changes in activity of single nerve fibers. J Neurophysiol 1978; 41:987-1006.

Lonsbury-Martin BL, Martin GK, Bohne BA. Repeated TTs exposures in monkeys: Alterations in hearing, cochlear structure, and single-unit thresholds. J Acoust Soc Am 1987; 81:1507-1518.

McFadden D. The curious half-octave shift: Evidence for a basalward migration of the traveling-wave envelope with increasing intensity. In: Salvi RJ, Henderson D, Hamernik RP, Colletti V, eds. Basic and applied aspects of noise-induced hearing loss. New York: Plenum Publishing, 1986:295.

McFadden D, Plattsmier HS. Exposure-induced loudness shifts and threshold shifts. In: Hamernik RP, Henderson D, Salvi R, eds. New perspectives on noise-induced hearing loss. New York: Raven Press, 1982:363.

Mitchell C, Brummett RE, Vernon JA. Frequency effects of temporary N1 depression following acoustic overload. Arch Otolaryngol 1977; 103:117-123.

Nielsen DW, Slepecky N. Stereocilia. In: Altschuler RA, Bobbin RP, Hoffman DW, eds. Neurobiology of hearing: The cochlea. New York: Raven Press, 1986:23.

Puel J-L, Bobbin RP, Fallon M. The active process is affected first by intense sound exposure. Hear Res 1988; 37:53-64.

Rajan R. Effect of electrical stimulation of the crossed olivocochlear bundle on temporary threshold shifts in auditory sensitivity. I. Dependence on electrical stimulation parameters. J Neurophysiol 1988a; 60:549-568.

Rajan R. Effect of electrical stimulation of the crossed olivocochlear bundle on temporary threshold shifts in auditory sensitivity. II. Dependence on the level of temporary threshold shifts. J Neurophysiol 1988b; 60:569-579.

Rajan R, Johnstone BM. Crossed cochlear influences on monaural temporary threshold shifts. Hear Res 1983; 9:279-294.

Robertson D. Effects of acoustic trauma on stereocilia structure and spiral ganglion cell tuning properties in the guinea pig cochlea. Hear Res 1982; 7:55-74.

Robertson D. Functional significance of dendrite swelling after loud sounds in the guinea pig cochlea. Hear Res 1983; 9:263-278.

Robertson D. Brainstem location of efferent neurons projecting to the guinea pig cochlea. Hear Res 1985; 20:79-84.

Robertson D, Gummer M. Physiological and morphological characterization of efferent neurones in the guinea pig cochlea. Hear Res 1985; 20:63-77.

Saunders JC, Dear SP, Schneider ME. The anatomical consequences of acoustic injury: A review and tutorial. J Acoust Soc Am 1985; 78:833-860.

Slepecky N, Hamernik R, Henderson D, Coling D. Correlation of audiometric data with changes in cochlear hair cell stereocilia resulting from impulse noise trauma. Acta Otolaryngol 1982; 93:329-340.

Spoendlin H. Primary structural changes in the organ of Corti after acoustic overstimulation. Acta Otolaryngol 1971; 71:166-176.

Taylor W, Pearson J, Mair A, Burns W. Study of noise and hearing in jute weaving. J Acoust Soc Am 1965; 38:113-120.

Tilney LG, Saunders JC, Egelman E, DeRosier DJ. Changes in the organization of actin filaments in the stereocilia of noise-damaged cochleae. Hear Res 1982; 7:181-197.

Trahiotis C, Elliott DN. Behavioral investigation of some possible effects of sectioning the crossed olivocochlear bundle. J Acoust Soc Am 1970; 47:592-596.

Warr WB, Guinan JJ, White JS. Organization of the efferent fibers: The lateral medial olivocochlear system. In: Altschuler RA, Bobbin RP, Hoffman DW, eds. Neurobiology of hearing: The cochlea. New York: Raven Press, 1986:333.

Wiederhold ML. Physiology of the olivocochlear system. In: Altschuler RA, Bobbin RP, Hoffman DW, eds. Neurobiology of hearing: The cochlea. New York: Raven Press, 1986:349.

Wiederhold ML, Kiang NY-S. Effects of electrical stimulation of the crossed olivocochlear bundle on single auditory-nerve fibres in the cat. J Acoust Soc Am 1970; 48:950-965.

CHAPTER 37

Does Olivocochlear Feedback Protect the Cat's Inner Ear from Acoustic Injury?

M. CHARLES LIBERMAN

In recent years, a number of published studies from one laboratory have suggested a protective role for the olivocochlear efferent system (Rajan, 1988a,b; Rajan and Johnstone, 1988a, b; see Chapter 38). In these experiments, the effects of acoustic overstimulation in guinea pigs are compared with and without activation of the olivocochlear bundle (OCB). It is reported that, when groups of animals are exposed to a 10-kHz tone for 1 minute at intensities of roughly 100 dB SPL, animals in which the OCB is electrically stimulated during the exposure show significantly less threshold shift than animals exposed without electric stimulation. The protective effects of this electric stimulation disappear when animals are treated with systemic strychnine, a known blocker of efferent function (Desmedt and Monaco, 1961). It has been suggested that this protective effect is mediated via the so-called medial olivocochlear (MOC) system, i.e., the OC projection to the outer hair cells (Cody and Johnstone, 1982; Rajan, 1988a; Rajan and Johnstone, 1988a).

Although a protective effect is unequivocally demonstrated in the guinea pig studies, ambiguities remain as to the mechanisms underlying the effect. The electric stimulation applied in these studies, either at the floor of the fourth ventricle or at the round window, could be activating other feedback pathways to the inner ear, such as the middle-ear muscle reflex or autonomic fiber systems, or, alternatively, could be changing systemic variables such as blood pressure or temperature, which might, in turn, affect the vulnerability of the ear to acoustic overstimulation. The widespread central and peripheral effects of strychnine (Franz, 1985) make the systemic injection of this drug a nonspecific test for olivocochlear involvement.

The present series of experiments was designed to probe the underlying basis for the protective effects reported. The major differences in experimental design were that (1) cats were used rather than guinea pigs; (2) the middle-ear muscles were cut bilaterally; (3) the olivocochlear bundle was sectioned surgically to one ear only; and (4) both ears of each animal were simultaneously exposed to high-intensity tones. The resultant database includes measurements of threshold shifts from a control (efferents intact) and an experimental (efferents cut) ear from each animal. The simultaneity of the binaural exposures ensures that all systemic variables are matched, and that, to the maximum extent possible, the *only* difference between the two ears is the status of the OCB.

Methods

Young adult cats weighing between 1.5 and 2.5 kg were anesthetized with diallyl barbiturate in urethane. Both ear canals were severed close to the tympanic rings to allow for insertion of closed, calibrated acoustic systems (Kiang et al, 1965). The bulla cavities were opened bilaterally and bony septa removed. Once a clear view of the middle ear was achieved, the tendon of the stapedius muscle was cut with electrocautery, and the attachment of the tensor tympani muscle was cut with iris scissors. The skin, muscles, and bone overlying the cerebellum were removed, and the cerebellum over the fourth ventricle was removed by aspiration. The OCB was

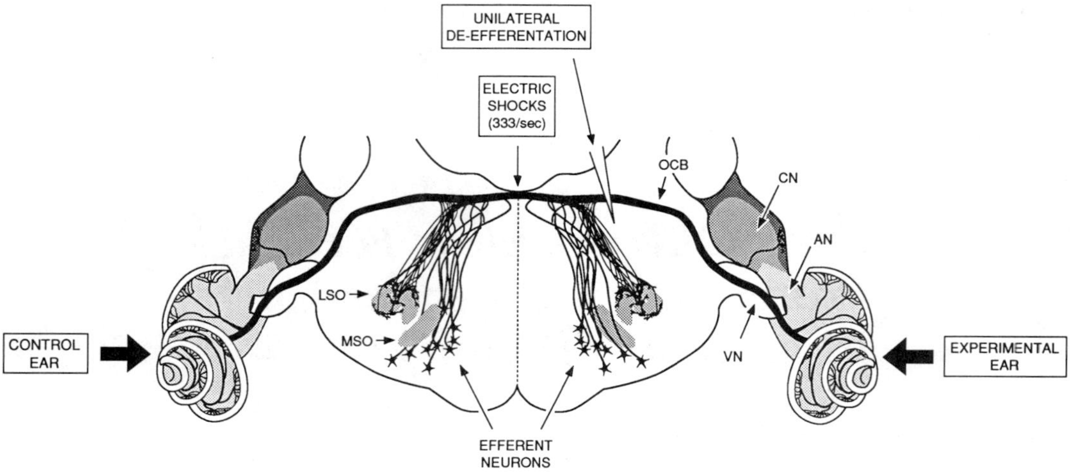

Figure 37-1 Schematic of a transverse section through the cat's brain stem illustrating the cells of origin of the olivocochlear bundle (OCB) and the brain-stem course of their cochlear projections. Efferent cell bodies are found near the medial superior olive (MSO) and the lateral superior olive (LSO). Their axons coalesce near the floor of the fourth ventricle and exit the brain stem with the vestibular nerve (VN), finally crossing to the auditory nerve (AN) within the internal auditory meatus. The OCB also sends projections to the cochlear nucleus (CN). The position of the knife cut used to unilaterally de-efferent each animal is illustrated, as is the midline position at which the OCB was electrically stimulated in certain experiments.

transected with a small knife cut positioned at the lateral margin of the brain-stem surface (Fig. 37-1).

The auditory-function test used in these studies was the "threshold" for compound action potentials (CAPs) recorded at the round window to 4-ms tone pips at a number of test frequencies. A computerized procedure automatically determined the sound pressure required, at each test tone frequency, to produce a peak-to-peak CAP of 10 microvolts (minimum step size of 1 dB). Testing proceeded from high to low frequencies, alternating between the two ears at each frequency.

The completeness of the knife cuts in transecting the entire OCB was assessed by one of two functional tests. In some animals, a "contrasound suppression" test was used. In the cat, it has been shown that the addition of moderate-level noise to the contralateral ear raises the thresholds for test tones presented ipsilaterally, as measured either in the responses of single auditory-nerve fibers or in the CAP (Liberman, 1989; Warren and Liberman, 1989). This contrasound suppression of the CAP disappears completely after sectioning the OCB. Thus, after placing the knife cut, it could be shown that the control ear (opposite the lesion) could still be suppressed by contralateral sound, whereas the experimental ear (same side as the lesion) could not. In other animals, the OCB was electrically stimulated at the floor of the fourth ventricle. After a successful unilateral de-efferentation, OCB shocks delivered at the brain-stem midline (Fig. 37-1) elevated CAP thresholds to the control ear by as much as 20 dB, while having no measurable effect on CAP thresholds to the lesioned side.

After the functional tests demonstrated that unilateral de-efferentation had been achieved, the baseline CAP thresholds were measured at least three times at each test frequency, and the average pre-exposure thresholds were determined. The two ears were then exposed simultaneously to the same tone at the same intensity for the same duration. During the exposure, the sound pressure at each ear was monitored and adjusted, if necessary (in 0.25-dB steps), to maintain the desired value. In some experiments, the OCB was shocked (at 333 per second) during the acoustic overexposure. Immediately after the exposure, CAP threshold testing was resumed and continued without interruption for the next 1 to 2 hours.

Results

Sound-Evoked Efferent Activity

It is well known that single fibers of the OCB respond to sound, even in anesthetized animals (Liberman, 1988). If shock-evoked

OCB activity can protect the ear, sound-evoked activity should have an effect as well. In the first series of experiments, this hypothesis was tested by comparing the threshold shift caused by simultaneous binaural overexposure when one ear is de-efferented, without electric stimulation of the OCB to either ear.

The choice of exposure frequency was dictated by the desire to stimulate the cochlear region most richly endowed with efferent innervation. Recent anatomic studies in the cat have shown that those regions of the basal turn tuned to frequencies between 6 and 10 kHz have significantly more efferent terminals on the OHCs than other regions (Liberman et al, 1990). Given the half-octave shift between exposure frequency and the frequency of maximum damage commonly seen in such experiments, an exposure frequency of 6 kHz was chosen (rather than the 10 kHz used in the guinea pig experiments). The choice of exposure intensity and duration was dictated by the desire to match the amount of threshold shift to that seen in the guinea pig studies, because it has been reported that the size of the protective effect is proportional to the size of the threshold shift in control animals (Rajan, 1988b). Because the cat is, in general, less vulnerable to acoustic injury than the guinea pig (see Chapter 7), either the intensity or the duration had to be increased. We chose to increase the latter (to 10 minutes) so as to minimize the stimulus distortions that occur at higher intensities.

As illustrated in Figure 37-2*A*, the lack of efferent feedback in nine unilaterally de-efferented animals had no significant effect on the average threshold shift from a 6-kHz tone at 100 dB for 10 minutes. Although the mean threshold shift for the de-efferented ears was slightly higher at several test frequencies, the standard errors are very large, and the differences are not statistically significant. Identical results were obtained in another series of animals in which the OCB was cut unilaterally by sectioning the inferior vestibular nerve in the internal auditory meatus (Liberman, 1990).

Shock-Evoked Efferent Activity

Based on existing physiologic studies of OC neurons, it is likely that the ensemble discharge rate in the OCB during these binaural acoustic exposures is not as great as could be achieved with electric stimulation of the OCB (Liberman and Brown, 1986). Thus, in the next series of experiments the sound-evoked activity was supplemented by a shock train (333 per second) delivered to the OCB at the floor of the fourth ventricle. The shocks were delivered simultaneously with the binaural exposure, after each animal had been unilaterally de-efferented. As illustrated in Figure 37-2*B*, even with this maximal activation of the OCB to the control ear, there was no difference in the mean threshold shift between control and de-efferented ears. Identical results were obtained for this experimental paradigm in another group of animals when the exposure frequency was moved to 1.5 kHz (Fig. 37-2*C*): once again, there is no significant difference in average threshold shift in control versus de-efferented ears.

Note that in all the threshold shift data (Fig. 37-2*A–C*) the standard errors of the mean are large, significantly larger than in Rajan's studies (e.g., Rajan, 1988a; Rajan and Johnstone, 1988a). These errors reflect the great interanimal variability in the response to these exposures. In contrast to the large *inter*-animal variability, the *intra*-animal variability was low, i.e., the threshold shifts in the two ears were always similar, even though the OCB was cut to one side (Liberman, 1990).

Conclusion

The results of the present study suggest that, in the cat, for the types of acute exposures and temporary threshold shifts studied, feedback activity in the OCB does not play a role in protecting the ear from acoustic injury. Thus, at the least, these results limit the generality of the conclusions reached by others concerning the protective actions of the OCB (see Chapter 36).

The obvious discrepancies between the present results and those of Rajan and coworkers could arise in many ways. It might be, for example, that 10-kHz exposures (as studied by Rajan) are different from 6.0- or 1.5-kHz exposures used in the present study; or that 10-minute exposures (as used here) involve different processes than those impaired by 1-minute exposures (as used by Rajan) and that only the latter are OCB-sensitive. If we have learned anything about acoustic injury in the last decades, it is that the reaction of the inner ear to acoustic overexposures involves a host of different degenerative processes and that, depending on the exposure conditions, different subsets of these processes may be involved.

Another obvious hypothesis to explain the discrepancies is that cats are different

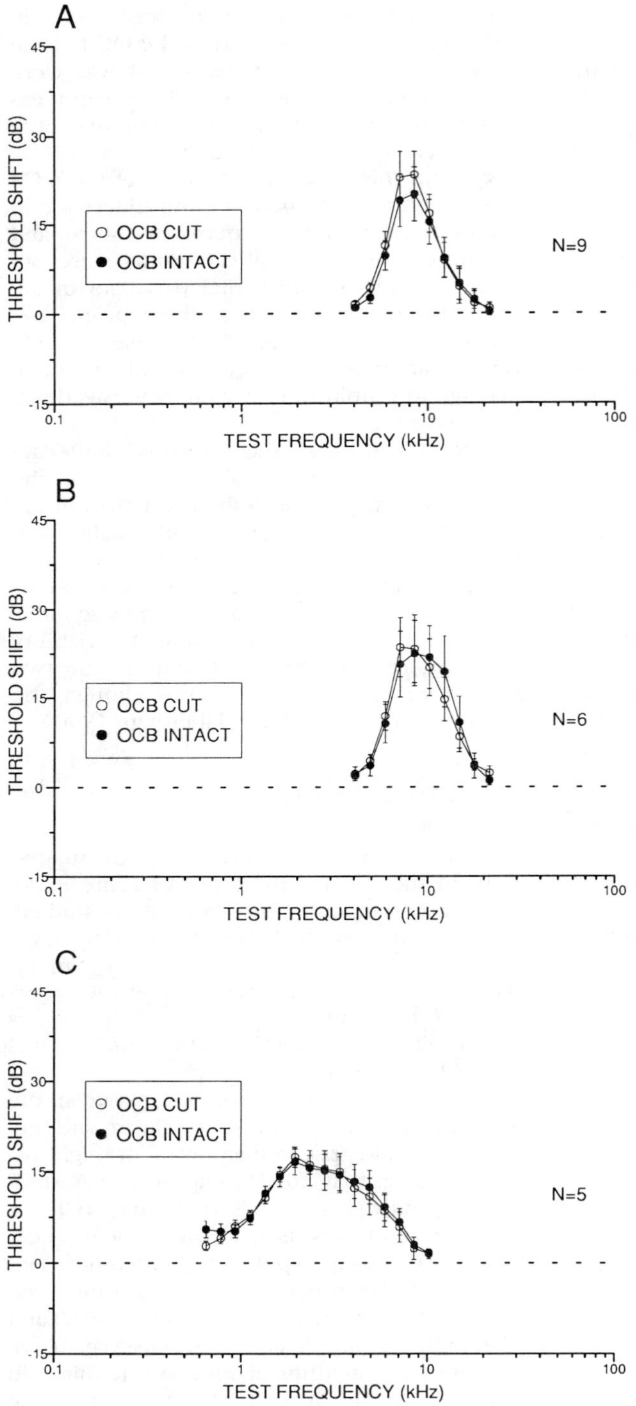

Figure 37-2 *A,* Comparison of average threshold shift seen in experimental versus control ears of nine animals unilaterally de-efferented and then binaurally exposed to a 6-kHz tone at 100 dB for 10 minutes. There was no electric stimulation of the olivocochlear bundle (OCB) in this series of experiments. Error bars denote standard error of the mean. *B,* Comparison of average threshold shift seen in six animals unilaterally de-efferented and then binaurally exposed to the same stimulus as in *A,* except that during the acoustic overexposure the OCB was shocked at 333 per second. *C,* Comparison of average threshold shift seen in five animals unilaterally de-efferented and exposed binaurally to a 1.5-kHz tone at 95 dB for 10 minutes with simultaneous electric stimulation of the OCB.

from guinea pigs. Arguing against this suggestion is the wealth of anatomic and physiologic data on the OC system in these two species demonstrating extensive similarities in projection patterns and response patterns (Brown, 1987, 1989; Liberman, 1988; Liberman and Brown, 1986; Robertson, 1984; Robertson and Gummer, 1985, 1988). Indeed, based on existing information, the effects in the cat should be greater than in the guinea pig, because (1) sound-evoked discharge rates are greater in the cat and (2) in the present study, the contrast in OCB activity levels was maximized by de-efferenting one ear, whereas the control ears in Rajan's experiments always had an intact efferent system and thus a moderate level of sound-evoked activity during the exposures. Thus, to attribute the discrepant results to interspecies differences, at present, one can only speculate about undiscovered qualitative differences, for example, in the OCB transmitters released in the periphery or in their postsynaptic effects.

A third way to view the differences in the two sets of results is to suggest that the protective effects seen in the guinea pig studies were due to mechanisms other than the OCB. In the guinea pig studies, the middle-ear muscles were not cut. These muscles can easily be stimulated with electrodes in the brain stem or round-window area, and if stimulated electrically can attenuate even at frequencies near 10 kHz by as much as 10 dB (Pang and Peake, 1986). According to Rajan's control data (Rajan, 1988b), a stimulus attenuation of only 3 dB is required to explain all of the protective effects of the electric shocks. Although the guinea pigs were paralyzed during the exposures, it is hard to rule out residual activation of the muscles by the high-level electric stimulation.

It is also possible that the effects seen in guinea pigs were due to activation of the autonomic nervous system or some as yet undiscovered feedback pathway to the inner ear. At present, it is impossible to decide which of the multitude of possible explanations is correct. However, the issue is an important one, and well worth future study. If nature has designed a way to protect the inner ear from acoustic overstimulation, understanding how that protection comes about should teach us a great deal about the basic mechanisms underlying acoustic injury.

Rôle du Faisceau Efférent dans la Protection de l'Oreille Interne contre les Bruits

Il a été démontré, chez le cobaye, que l'activation du faisceau olivocochléaire (FOC) par une stimulation électrique ou sonore réduit les pertes auditives temporaires induites par une surstimulation (Cody et Johnstone, 1982). Le but de la présente série d'expériences est d'étudier l'éventuel effet protecteur du FOC chez le chat.

Dans chaque expérience, les fibres efférentes étaient sectionnées d'un seul côté et les deux oreilles étaient ensuite exposées simultanément à un même stimulus traumatique (6 kHz, 100 dB, 10 minutes). Ce stimulus traumatique est connu pour provoquer un maximum de déficit auditif dans la région du 10 kHz, et c'est précisément cette région qui possède la plus grande densité d'efférences (Liberman, résultats non publiés). Dans la première série d'expériences, le FOC était activé par une stimulation sonore (stimulation traumatique binaurale), dans la seconde série d'expériences, le FOC était activé par une stimulation électrique délivrée durant le son traumatisant. Les déficits auditifs étaient évalués grâce à l'enregistrement sur la fenêtre ronde du potentiel d'action global en réponse à une bouffée tonale. Un algorithme permettait de faire varier l'intensité du stimulus jusqu'à ce que l'amplitude de l'onde N1 atteigne 10 μV. Les animaux étaient anesthésiés à l'uréthane et les tendons des muscles de l'oreille moyenne étaient sectionnés bilatéralement.

L'état fonctionnel du FOC était estimé par deux méthodes: (1) L'activation du FOC induite par une stimulation sonore controlatérale était estimée par la mesure des seuils auditifs dans l'oreille ipsilatérale. Une stimulation controlatérale d'environ 80 dB SPL entraînait une élévation des seuils auditifs d'environ 4 ou 8 dB. Cet effet, induit par une stimulation controlatérale, disparaissait complètement après section du FOC (Liberman, 1989); (2) l'efficacité des chocs électriques induisant l'activation du FOC était estimée en comparant les seuils auditifs avec et sans stimulation électrique. Cette stimulation était opérée grâce à l'implantation de deux électrodes dans la ligne médiane du plancher du 4ème ventricule. Une cadence de 333 chocs électriques par seconde augmentait les seuils auditifs de 20 dB dans la gamme des fréquences moyennes.

La section des fibres efférentes était opérée au scalpel au niveau du bord latéral du plancher du 4ème ventricule. Cette section est connue pour éliminer la majeure partie des terminaisons efférentes cochléaires. Les tests fonctionnels du FOC étaient répétés afin de démontrer l'absence d'effet du côté opéré. La section du FOC n'entraînait jamais d'altération des seuils auditifs.

Les 26 animaux ayant subi une section latérale furent exposés bilatéralement à un son traumatique de 6 kHz: chez 16 d'entre eux l'activation du FOC était évoquée par un son controlatéral; chez 10 animaux, une stimulation électrique du FOC était effectuée en plus de l'activation sonore. Les déficits auditifs temporaires étaient enregistrés durant les 120 minutes consécutives à cette exposition sonore. Trente minutes après l'exposition les déficits auditifs temporaires se situaient entre 10 et 50 dB. Il n'y avait aucune différence statistiquement significative entre les animaux ayant subi une section et les animaux contrôles que le FOC soit activé acoustiquement ou électriquement. L'apparente contradiction de nos résultats avec les précédentes études sera discutée.

ACKNOWLEDGMENTS

This research was supported by NIH grant DC0188. The surgical skill of L.W. Dodds, who prepared the animals and cut the middle-ear muscles, is gratefully acknowledged.

References

Brown MC. Morphology of labeled efferent fibers in the guinea pig cochlea. J Comp Neurol 1987; 260:605-618.

Brown MC. Morphology and response properties of single olivocochlear fibers in the guinea pig. Hear Res 1989; 40:93-110.

Cody AR, Johnstone BM. Temporary threshold shift modified by binaural acoustic stimulation. Hear Res 1982; 6:199-206.

Desmedt JE, Monaco P. Mode of action of the efferent olivocochlear bundle on the inner ear. Nature 1961; 192:1263-1265.

Franz DN. Central nervous system stimulants. In: Gilman AG, Goodman LS, Rall TW, Murad F, eds. The pharmacological basis of therapeutics. New York: Macmillan, 1985.

Kiang NYS, Watanabe T, Thomas EC, Clark LF. Discharge patterns of single auditory nerve fibers in the cat's auditory nerve. Cambridge, MA: MIT Press, 1965.

Liberman MC. Response properties of cochlear efferent neurons: Monaural vs. binaural stimulation and the effects of noise. J Neurophysiol 1988; 60:1779-1798.

Liberman MC. Rapid assessment of sound-evoked olivocochlear feedback: Suppression of compound action potentials by contralateral sound. Hear Res 1989; 38:47-56.

Liberman MC. The olivocochlear bundle and susceptibility of the inner ear to acoustic injury. J Neurophysiol 1991; 65:123-132.

Liberman MC, Dodds LW, Pierce S. Afferent and efferent innervation of the cat cochlea: Quantitative analysis using light and electron microscopy. J Comp Neurol 1990; 301:443-460.

Liberman MC, Brown MC. Physiology and anatomy of single olivocochlear neurons in the cat. Hear Res 1986; 24:17-36.

Pang XD, Peake WT. How do stapedius contractions alter the acoustic properties of the ear? In: Allen JB, Hall JL, Hubbard A, Neely ST, Tubis A, eds. Peripheral auditory mechanisms. Berlin: Springer-Verlag, 1986:36.

Rajan R. Effect of electrical stimulation of the crossed olivocochlear bundle on temporary threshold shifts in auditory sensitivity. I. Dependence on electrical stimulation parameters. J Neurophysiol 1988a; 60:549-568.

Rajan R. Effect of electrical stimulation of the crossed olivocochlear bundle on temporary threshold shifts in auditory sensitivity. II. Dependence on the level of temporary threshold shifts. J Neurophysiol 1988b; 60:569-579.

Rajan R, Johnstone BM. Electrical stimulation of cochlear efferents at the round window reduces auditory desensitization in guinea pigs. I. Dependence on electrical stimulation parameters. Hear Res 1988a; 36:53-74.

Rajan R, Johnstone BM. Electrical stimulation of cochlear efferents at the round window reduces auditory desensitization in guinea pigs. II. Dependence on level of temporary threshold shifts. Hear Res 1988b; 36:75-88.

Robertson D. Horseradish peroxidase injections of physiologically characterized afferent and efferent neurons in the guinea pig spiral ganglion. Hear Res 1984; 15:113-121.

Robertson R, Gummer M. Physiological and morphological characterization of efferent neurons in the guinea pig cochlea. Hear Res 1985; 20:63-77.

Robertson R, Gummer M. Physiology of cochlear efferents in the mammal. In: Syka J, Masterton RB, eds. Auditory pathway. New York: Plenum Press, 1988:269.

Warren EH, Liberman MC. Effects of contralateral sound on auditory-nerve responses. I. Contributions of cochlear efferents. Hear Res 1989; 37:89-104.

CHAPTER 38

Protective Functions of the Efferent Pathways to the Mammalian Cochlea: A Review

RAMESH RAJAN

Recent studies have provided strong evidence that the efferent pathways to the mammalian cochlea can protect the cochlea from damage caused by loud sounds. Previous studies had mooted a protective role for these olivocochlear pathways (Filogamo et al, 1967); these studies observed that human susceptibilities to losses in threshold sensitivities caused by loud sounds in one ear could be modified by sounds in the other ear. The effects in these studies were attributed to the crossed olivocochlear bundle (COCB) (Rasmussen, 1960), originating in the brain stem contralateral to the test ear that was presented the loud sound. However, as noted by Ward (1965), these effects could have been more reliably attributed to the middle-ear reflex, especially as most of the crossed effects were seen when using low-frequency sounds that can elicit the middle-ear reflex (Møller, 1972), either ipsilaterally or contralaterally. In contrast to the human studies, the more recent studies used anesthetized animals, allowing confirmation that the observed protective effects were attributable solely to the olivocochlear pathways. This chapter reviews the significant features of some of my own studies of the protective functions of the olivocochlear pathways.

The basic experimental preparation and procedures in these studies in barbiturate-anesthetized guinea pigs have been detailed elsewhere (Rajan, 1988a; Rajan and Johnstone, 1983a,b). Cochlear damage was produced by loud pure-tone exposures presented at a specified intensity for a fixed duration. The exposure frequency was always 10 kHz, within the area of greatest neural sensitivity for the guinea pig and producing significant damage at the frequencies of greatest sensitivity. Damage to cochlear neural sensitivities was monitored in the compound action potential (CAP) audiogram (Dallos et al, 1978), constructed from visual detection thresholds for the N1 component of the CAP (Johnstone et al, 1979) and was measured as temporary threshold shifts (TTSs) in N1 thresholds. Results presented here are almost always the N1 losses from 10 to 24 kHz measured 5 minutes after exposure. Statistical significances are based on Student's t-tests.

Involvement of the Crossed Olivocochlear Bundle in the Protective Effects of Brain-stem Electric Stimulation

Basic Features of the Protective Effects

Electric stimulation at the floor of the fourth ventricle in the brain stem exerts a variety of effects at the cochlea through the olivocochlear pathways (Desmedt, 1975; Fex, 1962; Galambos, 1956; Klinke and Galley, 1974; Weiderhold, 1986). To determine if these pathways were protective, bipolar electric stimulation at this site was tested on the TTS caused by loud sound exposures (Rajan, 1988a,b). The effect of brain-stem electric stimulus (BES) on the TTS caused by a standard monaural exposure (at 10 kHz, 103 dB SPL for 1 minute) is illustrated in Figure 38-1*A*. In the control group only the standard

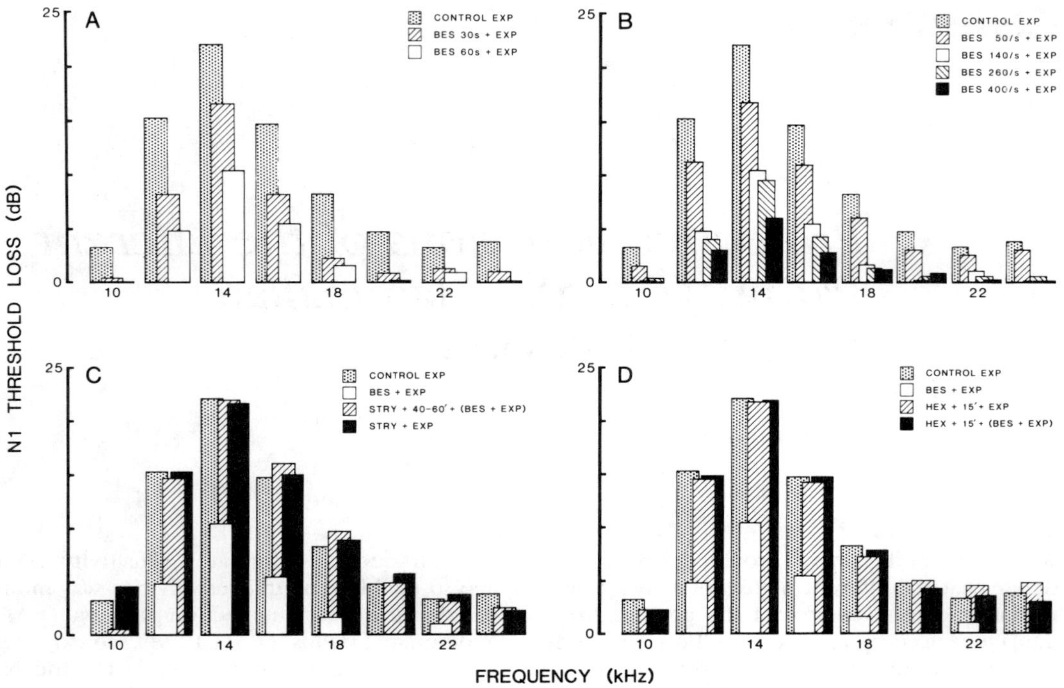

Figure 38-1 Protective effect of an electric stimulus delivered at the floor of the fourth ventricle in the brain stem (BES). In this figure, as in all figures in this chapter except 38.4 and 38.6, the results are mean threshold losses from 10 to 24 kHz, in 2-kHz steps, measured 5 minutes after the standard ipsilateral exposure (see text). In the control group only this exposure was presented. *A,* Basic protective effects of the BES. In the test groups, the standard exposure (EXP) was combined with a BES at 400 μA, with 150-μs pulses delivered at 140 pulses per second as a continuous burst (the "standard" BES), simultaneous with and lasting either the full 60-second duration of the exposure (BES 60s + EXP) or only the first 30 seconds of the standard exposure (BES 30s + EXP). *B,* Effect of varying the rate of pulses in the standard BES on protection from the standard exposure. Rates of 50 per second, 140 per second, 260 per second, and 400 per second were tested in different groups. The BES was always simultaneous with the exposure and presented for the duration of the exposure. *C,* Effect of strychnine. In the "BES + EXP" test group, the standard BES was applied simultaneously with and for the duration of the exposure with no other treatment. In the "STRY + 40-60 + (BES + EXP)" group, 4 mg per kilogram of strychnine was injected intraperitoneally 40 to 60 minutes before the standard BES was tested on the standard exposure. In the "STRY + EXP" group, 10 mg per kilogram of strychnine was injected intraperitoneally 15 minutes before the exposure alone. *D,* Effect of hexamethonium perfused into scala tympani. In the "HEX + 15′ + (BES + EXP)" group, 1 μl of 3.44 mM hexamethonium was perfused 15 minutes before testing the effect of the standard BES simultaneous with the standard exposure. In the "HEX + 15′ + EXP" group, the same hexamethonium dose was perfused 15 minutes before the exposure alone.

monaural exposure was presented. In the test group, the same exposure was combined with the BES (bipolar 150-μs pulses at 400 μA, presented at a rate of 140 pulses per second as a continuous burst) presented simultaneously with and for the 1-minute duration of the exposure. Threshold losses from 10 to 24 kHz in the test group were significantly lower (p less than 0.05) than control group losses at the corresponding frequencies. In a second test group, the same BES was presented for only the first 30 seconds of the 1-minute exposure. The TTS in this group was reduced (Fig. 38-1*A*), but only by about half the reduction in the previous test group. Threshold losses in the second test group were significantly higher (p less than 0.05) than losses in the first test group, but significantly lower (p less than 0.05) than control group losses.

The dependence of the protective effects on the rate of stimulation was investigated in groups in which rates of 50, 260, or 400 pulses per second were used. All other electric parameters were kept constant, and the continuous BES burst was presented simultaneously with and for the duration of the standard monaural exposure. In general, increasing stimulus rates resulted in greater reductions in the maximum TTS (Fig. 38-1*B*). With a rate of 50 pulses per second, some TTS reductions were obtained, but only from 12 to 18 kHz, and they were not as large as with stimulation at 140 pulses per second. With a rate of 260 pulses per second, TTS reductions from 10 to 24 kHz were slightly greater than with 140 pulses per second, but not significantly so (*p* greater than 0.10). Finally, the highest rate of 400 pulses per second enhanced the reductions at 14 kHz, the frequency of greatest loss, but did not produce more widespread TTS reductions compared to stimulation at 260 pulses per second.

In later experiments, the standard continuous BES was one with bipolar 150-μs pulses at 400 μA applied at 140 pulses per second as a continuous burst for 1 minute.

The BES could activate three auditory efferent pathways—the facial nerve motor units to the stapedius muscle, the uncrossed OCB (UOCB), and the COCB. Activating the facial nerve produces contractions of the stapedius that could reduce the efficiency of ossicular transmission (Irvine and Wester, 1974; Møller, 1972) and reduce the (damaging) input. Three factors exclude the stapedius muscle: (1) effective curarization to block the middle-ear muscles (Desmedt et al, 1971; Fex, 1962; Galambos, 1956; Klinke and Galley, 1974) was obtained before testing the BES on TTS (Rajan, 1988a); (2) the exposure frequency was outside the range affected by contractions of the muscles in the guinea pig (Møller, 1972; Nuttal, 1974); and (3) drugs that blocked the classic effects of the olivocochlear pathways also blocked the temporary threshold shift reductions, as detailed below.

Effect of Intraperitoneal Administration of Strychnine

Strychnine, the classic olivocochlear antagonist (Desmedt and Monaco, 1962), was injected intraperitoneally in three test groups. The drug's action was always monitored with regard to the classic efferent effects on the amplitude of the N1 to tone bursts, clicks, or both. The efferents were stimulated from the fourth ventricle by pulsed, gated, short electric trains (Rajan, 1988a).

In the first test group, injection of strychnine (4 mg per kilogram) totally blocked, within 40 to 60 minutes, the olivocochlear pathway–mediated reductions in tone burst/click N1 amplitudes caused by the pulsed electric trains, without affecting N1 thresholds from 6 to 24 kHz or N1 intensity functions to tone bursts or clicks. Then, when the standard loud sound exposure (10 kHz, 103 dB SPL for 1 minute) was presented simultaneously with the standard continuous BES burst, no TTS reductions occurred. Except at 10 kHz, threshold losses in this group (Fig. 38-1*C*) were not significantly different from control group losses (*p* greater than 0.10), but were significantly higher (*p* less than 0.05) than the TTS in the original test group with the same standard BES, but without strychnine pretreatment.

The specificity of the strychnine block on the efferent pathways involved in the TTS protection was confirmed by testing the drug on monaural TTS alone. Strychnine, injected at a much higher dose (10 mg per kilogram) 15 minutes prior to the standard exposure alone, did not affect heart rates, N1 thresholds, intensity functions, or—just as significantly—monaural TTS (Fig. 38-1*C*). Threshold losses from 10 to 24 kHz in this strychnine-treated control group were not significantly different (*p* greater than 0.10) from losses in the standard control group presented the same exposure without any strychnine pretreatment (Fig. 38-1*C*).

In two other test groups, the strychnine block of the protective effects of the BES was more closely allied to the drug's blocking action on the N1 amplitude reductions produced by pulsed, gated, short electric trains at the floor of the fourth ventricle. The results are briefly described here, but are not illustrated (see Rajan, 1988a for details).

In the first group, only 15 minutes elapsed between intraperitoneal injection of strychnine (4 mg per kilogram) and testing of the effects of the standard BES on the standard monaural exposure. In this interval strychnine had no significant effects on the N1 amplitude reductions produced by pulsed trains at the floor of the fourth ventricle. Now, presenting the standard continuous BES simultaneously with and for the duration of the exposure resulted in TTS reductions. Threshold losses in this group were significantly lower (*p* less than 0.05) than those in the control group (monaural exposure alone), but were comparable to the reduced TTS in the original test group with the same conditions of exposure and electric stimulation but no strychnine.

In the second group, strychnine at 2 mg per kilogram blocked, over about an hour, the N1 amplitude reductions caused by pulsed trains in the brain stem, again without affecting N1 thresholds or intensity functions. This block reversed over the course of another hour, and pulsed trains once again reduced N1 amplitudes. Then the standard continuous BES was presented simultaneously with the standard exposure. TTS reductions were again obtained and threshold losses were significantly lower (*p* less than 0.05) than those in the control group or in the first strychnine-treated test group in which the continuous BES was tested on TTS when strychnine had blocked the cochlear effects of the pulsed trains.

Effect of Intracochlear Perfusion of Hexamethonium

Testing was also done with intracochlear perfusion of hexamethonium, because this effectively blocks the classic efferent effects on N1 amplitudes elicited by pulsed electric trains at the fourth ventricle (Galley et al, 1973; Bobbin and Konishi, 1974). The action of hexamethonium was always monitored with regard to the classic effects.

Perfusion of 1 μL of 3.44 mM hexamethonium into scala tympani blocked, within about 15 minutes, the N1 amplitude reductions elicited by pulsed trains at the floor of the fourth ventricle, without affecting N1 thresholds and amplitudes (Rajan, 1990a). Then the standard monaural sound was presented simultaneously with the standard continuous BES. The results for this group are illustrated in Figure 38-1*D* with the results for the control group and for the test group with the same exposure and BES conditions but without hexamethonium pretreatment. Threshold losses from 10 to 24 kHz in the hexamethonium-treated test group were similar (*p* greater than 0.10) to losses in the control group, but were significantly higher than losses in the untreated test group (*p* less than 0.05).

As a control, hexamethonium was tested on TTS alone. As before, intracochlear perfusion of 1 μl of 3.44 mM hexamethonium had no deleterious effects on the N1 audiogram or intensity functions (Rajan, 1990a). As importantly, 15 minutes later, the drug had not altered the normal susceptibilities of the cochlea to the standard monaural loud sound exposure (Fig. 38-1*D*): threshold losses from 10 to 24 kHz 5 minutes after exposure were similar (*p* greater than 0.10) to those in the standard control group presented only during the exposure.

Thus, the protective effects are mediated by pathways terminating within the cochlea. The blocking action of both drugs on the protective effects of the continuous BES paralleled their blocking action on olivocochlear-mediated N1 effects of pulsed, gated, short electric trains at the floor of the fourth ventricle. With strychnine, for which more complete testing was done, it was found that if the drug's block of the classic olivocochlear effects had not yet occurred, then the protective effects of the standard continuous BES were also not blocked. When the drug's blocking action on the classic effects was allowed to reverse, protection was again obtained with the continuous BES.

These results do not differentiate between the COCB and the UOCB pathways. However, there are many reasons for attributing the reductions to the COCB (see Rajan, 1988a), principally related to electrode location in the midline of the brain stem and the extent of current spread. It is unlikely that, at the level used here, there was any significant current spread to the UOCB fibers. Concordant with this is the fact that strychnine acted in parallel on the TTS reductions and the large N1 amplitude reductions associated with COCB, not UOCB, stimulation with pulsed trains (Desmedt, 1975; Fex, 1967; Klinke and Galley, 1974; Sohmer, 1966). Finally, a lesion placed at the floor of the fourth ventricle to disrupt the COCB (see below), with possibly only marginal effects on the UOCB, prevented the BES from reducing TTS.

Memory Component of the Protective Effects of the BES

Time Course of the Protective Effects

To study the time course of the protective effects, the standard BES was presented by itself for 1 minute; presentation of the standard exposure alone was delayed either 5 or 10 minutes. The results from these groups are compared in Figure 38-2*A* with the results from the earlier test group in which the same standard BES was presented simultaneously with the standard exposure. The BES was most effective in reducing TTS when it was simultaneous with the exposure, and was less effective with increasing delay. When the BES preceded the exposure by 5 minutes, the TTS reductions were not as large as when the BES was simultaneous with the exposure. Losses from 12 to 24 kHz in the group delayed 5 minutes were still significantly lower (*p* less than 0.05) than control group losses; however, losses from 12 to 16 kHz were significantly higher than those in the no-delay test group. When the BES preceded the exposure by 10 minutes, no TTS reductions were obtained and, except for 20 kHz, losses from 10 to 24 kHz were not different (*p* greater than 0.10) from control group losses. Compared to the intermediate-delay group, the long-delay group had significantly higher losses (*p* less

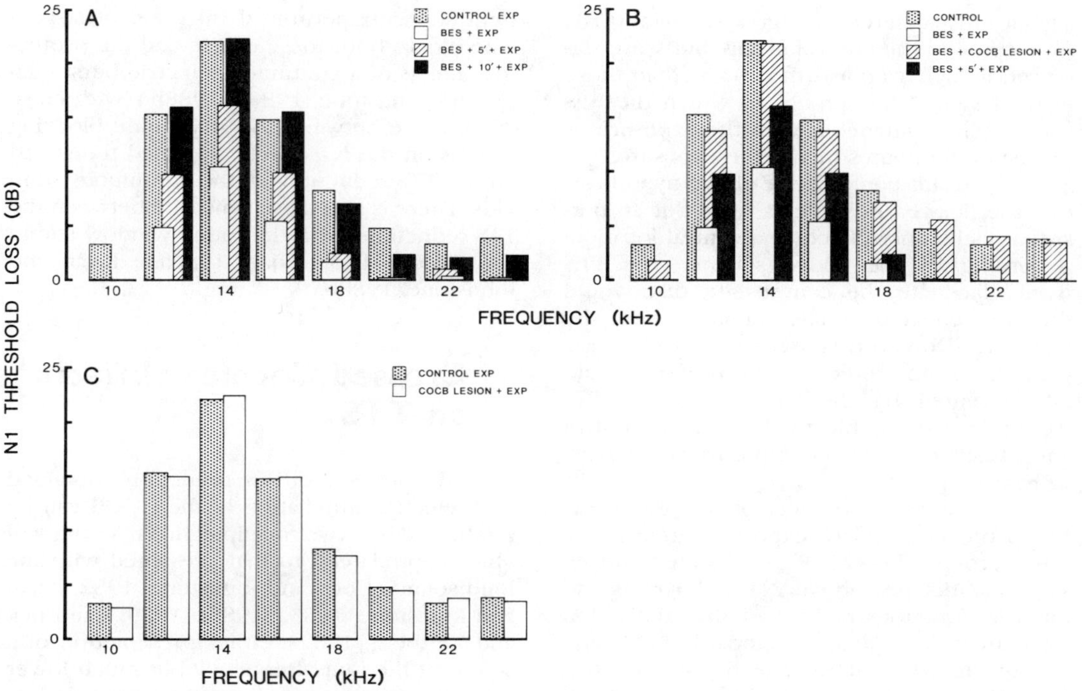

Figure 38-2 Time course of the brain-stem electric stimulus (BES) protective effects. *A,* In the control group (the same as in Fig. 38.1), only the standard exposure (EXP) was presented. In the test groups the standard BES was presented either simultaneously with the exposure or by itself 5 or 10 minutes before the standard exposure alone. *B,* Test of the hypothesis of persistent central effects of the BES in the delay experiments. In the new test group (BES + COCB LESION + EXP), the standard BES was presented by itself. Then the crossed olivocochlear bundle (COCB) fibers were lesioned with the stimulating electrodes. Finally, the exposure was presented by itself 2 minutes after the BES. The results are compared to the results from the control group, from the test group in which the same BES and exposure were simultaneous (BES + EXP), and from the test group in which the BES preceded the exposure by 5 minutes (BES + 5′ + EXP). *C,* Effect of COCB lesions on temporary threshold shift (TTS). In the "COCB LESION + EXP" group, the COCB fibers were lesioned at the floor of the fourth ventricle before the standard exposure.

than 0.05) at all frequencies from 12 to 24 kHz, except 22 kHz.

Central and Peripheral Sites of Action of the BES in the Delay Experiments

In the two test groups with delays between the BES and the exposure, a number of cochlear responses were remeasured within the first 2 to 3 minutes following the BES, commencing 10 to 15 seconds after the end of the BES (Rajan, 1988a). None of these responses were altered from initial values. Thus, the BES had no apparent persistent cochlear effects; yet, with a 5-minute delay between the BES and the exposure, TTS reductions still occurred. A working hypothesis for this result was that, in the delay experiments, the long-lasting BES effects occurred not at the cochlea, but centrally. Because the BES was applied to the COCB fibers along their length, it could stimulate the fibers both orthodromically and antidromically. The antidromic stimulus may have had a persistent effect at some central location, facilitating its activation by the subsequent exposure and producing reductions in TTS through COCB action at the cochlea.

This hypothesis was tested in a new test group in which the standard continuous BES alone was presented for 1 minute. The COCB fibers were then lesioned by moving the electrodes a number of times only in the dorsoventral plane. After removing the electrodes, N1 thresholds from 10 to 20 kHz were quickly rechecked, but were never altered from initial values. Two minutes after the end of the BES, the standard loud sound exposure was presented. No TTS reductions occurred in this lesion group (Fig. 38-2*B*), and losses were not significantly different (p greater than 0.10) from those in the control group, but were significantly higher (p less than 0.05) than those in nonlesioned test groups in which the BES was either simultaneous with the exposure or presented 5 minutes before the exposure.

This result confirms the above hypothesis that the delayed BES effects were due to persistent facilitatory effects at a central location. According to the above scheme, the BES would facilitate the central site that would then be activated by afferent input from the exposure. However, subsequent cochlear expression of the protective COCB effect would be prevented by the lesion, and the TTS would be comparable to the TTS in control animals subjected to the exposure alone—exactly as seen here.

As a control, the effect of the lesion was tested on the standard exposure alone in another group. The COCB was located and lesioned as detailed above. N1 audiograms and intensity functions rechecked after the lesion were unaltered. Then the standard loud sound was presented by itself. The threshold losses from 10 to 24 kHz (Fig. 38-2*C*) were not significantly different (p greater than 0.10) from losses at the corresponding frequencies in the original control group, which were presented only with the standard exposure with no brain-stem lesions.

Postmortem histology confirmed that the lesions were always placed between the facial genua, the area of decussation of the COCB, and extended rostrally at least to the lateral lemnisci and caudally to the nucleus of cranial nerve VII. The efferent cell bodies in the guinea pig are located well within this area (Aschoff and Ostwald, 1988; Robertson et al, 1987; Strutz and Bielenberg, 1984), and similar lesions in guinea pigs are known to interrupt most if not all of the COCB and perhaps even some of the UOCB (Kimura and Wersäll, 1962; Terayama and Yamamoto, 1971; Wright and Preston, 1973). Some of our restricted lesions would have interrupted only the COCB; in fact, depending on the exact coursing of the fibers, a few COCB fibers may even have been spared.

Almost all the features of COCB-mediated protection obtained by the brain-stem stimulus have been duplicated by similar electric stimuli applied at the round window (Rajan and Johnstone, 1988b,c). Pulsed, gated, short electric trains at the latter site also activate the efferent pathways (Rajan and Johnstone, 1983c) and can produce N1 amplitude reductions similar to those produced by pulsed trains in the brain stem. As with the brain stem site, intraperitoneal injection of strychnine blocks both these effects and the protective effects of a continuous electric burst (Rajan and Johnstone, 1983c, 1988b), with close congruence between the strychnine blocking actions on the N1 effects of pulsed trains and on the TTS reductions of the continuous stimulus. There is also close similarity between the TTS reductions with the round window stimulus and the BES (Rajan, 1988a,b; Rajan and Johnstone, 1988b,c).

Crossed Cochlear Effects on TTS

The protective TTS reductions obtained with electric stimulation of the COCB can be duplicated by two manipulations at the cochlea contralateral to that presented with the loud sound (Cody and Johnstone, 1982; Rajan and Johnstone, 1983a, 1988a, 1989; Handrock and Zeisberg, 1982): either presentation of a sound of the same frequency but much lower intensity (contralateral acoustic stimulation, or CAS) or destruction of the cochlea (contralateral cochlear destruction, or CCD). The protective effects of these manipulations on the ipsilateral TTS produced by the standard monaural exposure (10 kHz, 103 dB SPL for 1 minute) are illustrated in Figure 38-3*A* (CAS) and 38-3*C* (CCD). In the CAS test group, the CAS was at 10 kHz, 80 dB SPL, and was presented for 1 minute simultaneously with the ipsilateral exposure. In the CCD test case, the contralateral cochlea was destroyed 2 minutes prior to the ipsilateral exposure. Threshold losses from 12 to 24 kHz (CAS) and from 10 to 24 kHz (CCD) were significantly lower in the test groups (p less than 0.05) than in the control group.

Two tests confirmed that the protective effects of CAS and CCD were due to the COCB: (1) intraperitoneal injection of strychnine prior to testing the effects of the contralateral manipulations on TTS, and (2) lesioning at the floor of the fourth ventricle. In all groups, the ipsilateral exposure was always the standard one.

Intraperitoneal Administration of Strychnine

Strychnine was injected intraperitoneally at 2 mg per kilogram in two groups. In the next 15 minutes, ipsilateral N1 thresholds from 8 to 24 kHz and N1 intensity functions to 10-kHz or 14-kHz tone bursts (or both), or

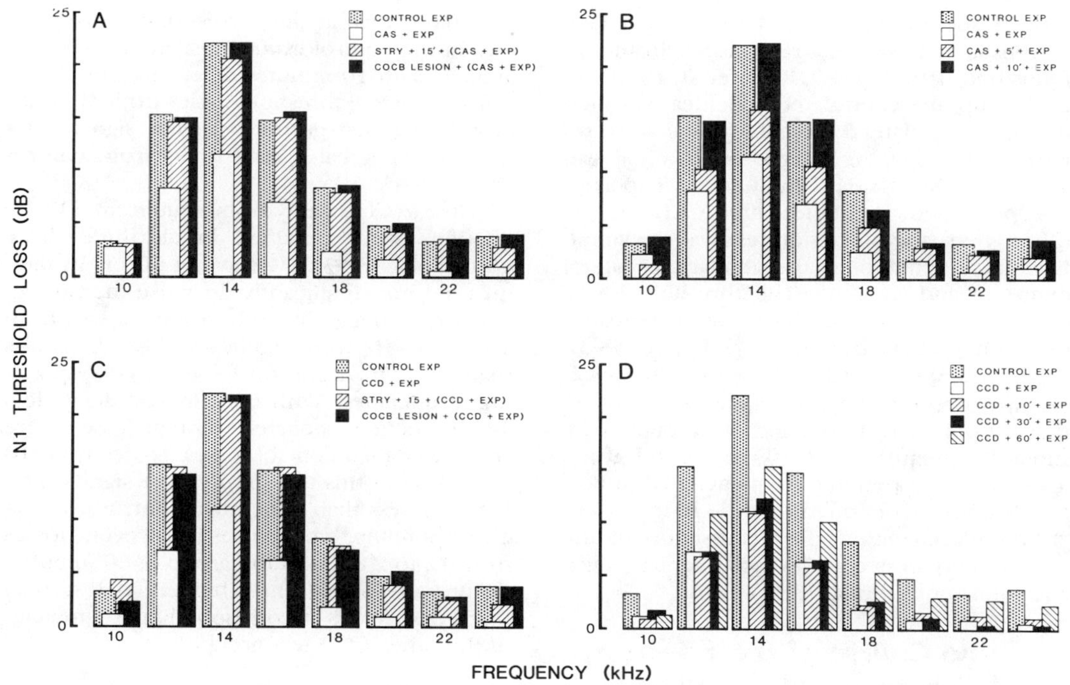

Figure 38-3 Protective effect of contralateral cochlear manipulations on temporary threshold shift (TTS) to the standard ipsilateral exposure. The contralateral manipulations were either a contralateral acoustic stimulus (CAS) at 10 kHz, 80 dB SPL, for 1 minute, or destruction of the contralateral cochlea (CCD) prior to the ipsilateral exposure. *A,* Effect of CAS. In the control group (the same as in Fig. 38.1), only the standard ipsilateral exposure (EXP) was presented. In the test groups, this exposure was simultaneous with the CAS. In the "CAS + EXP" group, there was no other treatment. In the "STRY + 15′ + (CAS + EXP)" group, strychnine (2 mg per kilogram) was injected intraperitoneally 15 minutes before the test. In the "COCB LESION + (CAS + EXP)" group, the crossed olivocochlear bundle (COCB) was lesioned at the floor of the fourth ventricle before the test. *B,* Time course of the protection by CAS. The CAS was presented either simultaneously with the exposure (the same group as in *A*), or by itself 5 minutes or 10 minutes before the ipsilateral exposure alone. *C,* Effect of CCD. The control group was the same as before. The test condition was destruction of the contralateral cochlea 2 minutes before the ipsilateral exposure. In the "CCD + EXP" group, this was the only test condition. In the "STRY + 15′ + (CCD + EXP)" group, strychnine (2 mg per kilogram) was injected 15 minutes before the test. In the "COCB LESION + (CCD + EXP)" group, the COCB was lesioned at the floor of the fourth ventricle before the test. *D,* Time course of protection by CCD. In the test groups, the CCD was destroyed 2 minutes (the same group as in *C*), 10 minutes, 30 minutes, or 60 minutes before the exposure.

to a click, or to both the bursts and a click were monitored and were always unaltered from initial values (Rajan and Johnstone, 1983a, 1989; unpublished observations). Heart rates, monitored continuously, were also unaltered. In one group the contralateral cochlea was then destroyed. In the next 2 minutes, ipsilateral N1 thresholds were rechecked and found to be unaltered. Then the standard ipsilateral exposure was presented. In the other group, 15 minutes after the strychnine injection, the standard ipsilateral exposure was presented simultaneously with the CAS (10 kHz, 80 dB SPL for 1 minute). The results for these groups are presented in Figure 38-3*A* (CAS) and 38-3*C* (CCD). Strychnine pretreatment prevented CAS and CCD from having any protective effects. Threshold losses from 10 to 24 kHz in both strychnine-treated test groups were not significantly different (p greater than 0.10) from losses at corresponding frequencies in the control group.

As discussed earlier, intraperitoneal injection of a much-higher dose of strychnine did not alter the TTS to the standard monaural exposure alone. Thus, the blocking action of strychnine was not due to any nonspecific effect of the drug.

Lesioning at the Floor of the Fourth Ventricle

In two test groups, bipolar electrodes located at the floor of the fourth ventricle were used to lesion the COCB in the manner described above. The lesion did not affect normal ipsilateral cochlear responses (Rajan and Johnstone, 1988c, 1989; Rajan et al, 1990). In one group, the contralateral cochlea was then destroyed. Ipsilateral N1 audiograms were remeasured and never altered from initial values. Then the standard loud sound exposure was presented 5 minutes after CCD. In the other group, the postlesion test was the simultaneous presentation of the standard ipsilateral exposure and the CAS. The threshold losses from 10 to 24 kHz 5 minutes after exposure for both groups, presented in Figure 38-3*A* (CAS) and 38-3*C* (CCD), show that the COCB lesion prevented the protective effects of either CAS or CCD. Losses in both groups were similar (*p* greater than 0.10) to control group losses at corresponding frequencies. Postmortem histology confirmed that the lesions were always placed about the decussation of the COCB fibers between the facial genua (Rajan and Johnstone, 1988a, 1989).

Time Course of the Effects of Contralateral Cochlear Manipulations

The time course of the protective effects of CAS or CCD was examined in groups in which either manipulation alone was carried out some time before the standard ipsilateral exposure alone. In CAS test groups, 5- or 10-minute delays were interposed between CAS and ipsilateral exposure, whereas in CCD test groups, the delays were 10, 30, and 60 minutes.

Even with a delay of 5 minutes after CAS, smaller but significant TTS reductions were obtained (Fig. 38-3*B*). Threshold losses from 12 to 18 kHz (where losses were greater than 5 dB in the control group) were significantly lower in the group of 5 minutes' delay (*p* less than 0.05) than at the corresponding frequencies in the control group (ipsilateral exposure alone). With 10 minutes delay, no TTS reductions occurred: threshold losses from 10 to 24 kHz in this test group were not significantly different (*p* greater than 0.10) from control group losses.

In the CCD delay tests, significant TTS reductions were obtained in all three delay groups (Fig. 38-3*D*). Delays of 10 or 30 minutes did not significantly decrease the protective CCD effects. In both groups, losses from 10 to 24 kHz were significantly lower (*p* less than 0.05) than control losses at corresponding frequencies. With 60 minutes' delay, less TTS reduction occurred, though losses were still lower than control losses. Losses from 10 to 24 kHz in this test group were significantly lower (*p* less than 0.05) than control losses at corresponding frequencies; however, losses from 12 to 24 kHz in the group of 60 minutes' delay were significantly higher (*p* less than 0.05) than losses at corresponding frequencies in the other CCD test groups.

Mode of Activation of the COCB in Crossed Cochlear Protection

In many animals with delays between the contralateral manipulation and the ipsilateral exposure, a number of ipsilateral responses were measured before the contralateral manipulation and again in the delay period. In the CAS-test animals, ipsilateral N1 audiograms and intensity functions to tone bursts and clicks were measured. Remeasures commenced 10 to 15 seconds after the CAS and were completed in 2 to 3 minutes. A wider variety of ipsilateral responses was measured in the CCD test groups. Some of these responses are illustrated in Figure 38-4. Measurements

Figure 38-4 Effect of contralateral cochlear destruction (CCD) on other responses from the ipsilateral cochlea. *A,* N1 audiograms and tuning curves. For the N1 audiogram the open symbols are initial values, and the half-filled circles are repeat measures made 15 seconds to 2 minutes after CCD. For N1 tuning curves the test 10-ms, 10-kHz tone was set 10 dB higher than threshold. The criterion was always a 25 percent reduction in the N1 amplitude. For simultaneous masking curves (crosses), the test tone was presented 80 ms after the onset of the 100-ms masker. Full lines show the initial tuning curve; dotted lines show the tuning curve determined after CCD. For forward masking (squares), the test tone was presented 3 to 5 ms after the 100-ms masker. Open squares show the initial tuning curve; filled squares show values recorded within 5 minutes of CCD. *B,* The upper panel presents input-output functions for the onset N1 to a click. The lower panel presents input-output functions for onset (left side) and termination responses (right side) to 300-ms tone bursts at 10 kHz. Crosses show initial values, and circles show values recorded within 5 minutes of CCD. *C,* Modulation of N1 sensitivity by a 40-Hz tone. 10-kHz N1 thresholds were determined while cycling a 30-ms tone burst at 10 kHz through a continuous 40-Hz tone set at levels below that needed to elicit an N1 itself. The 40-Hz tone level is expressed as attenuation regarding input voltage to

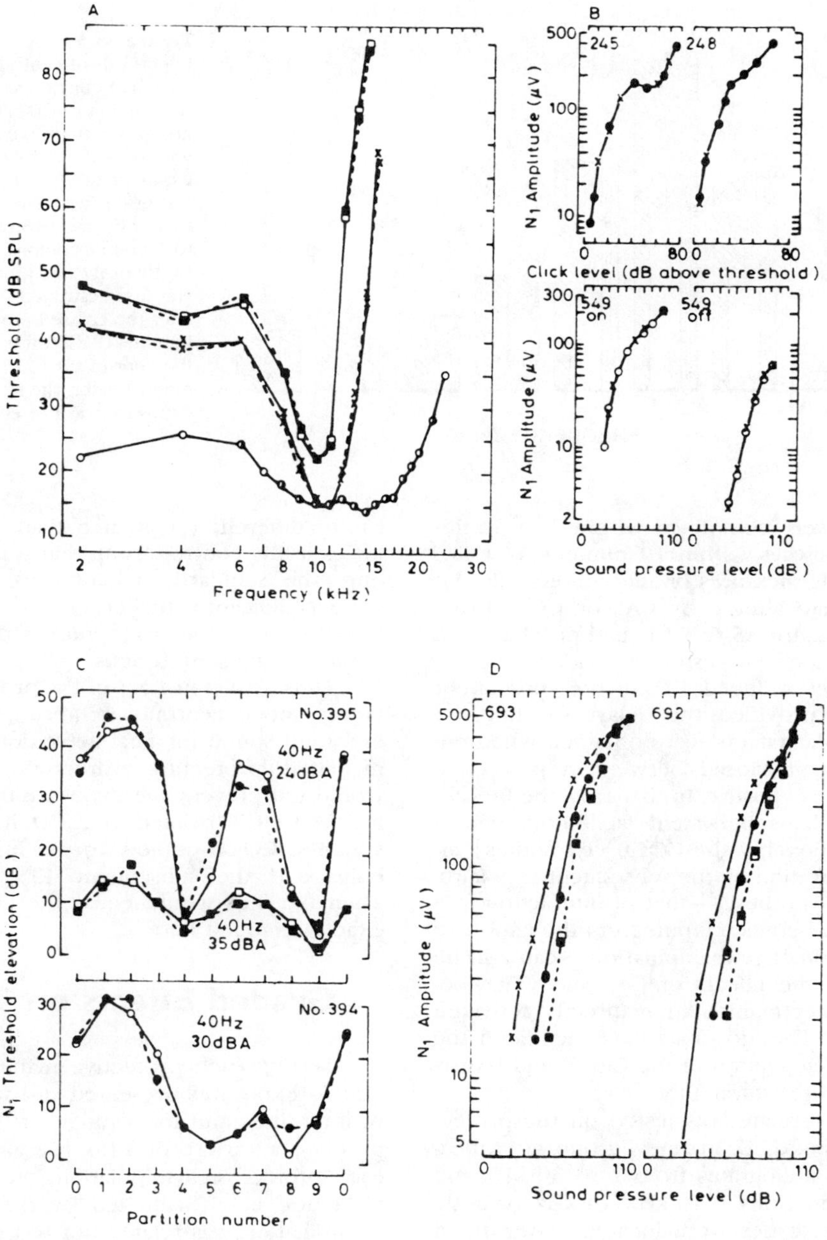

the speakers. Each partition number represents 36 degrees of 40-Hz phase. Open symbols show initial recordings; closed symbols show measures made between 15 seconds and 5 minutes after CCD. *D,* Crossed olivocochlear bundle (COCB) effects on the N1 amplitude. Crosses are input-output functions for the N1 to 50-ms tone bursts at 10 kHz. Open symbols show functions recorded, prior to CCD, when a COCB stimulus (one per second, 300-ms train of bipolar 150-µs pulses, delivered at a set rate at 400 µA) preceded the 10-kHz tone burst by 10 ms. Closed symbols show repeat measures made between 15 seconds and 5 minutes after CCD. Circles show values recorded when the rate of COCB pulses was 140 per second; squares show values when the rate was 260 per second. The N1 amplitude was always determined by averaging 32 responses; corrections for this procedure have been made. For clarity, the input-output function without COCB stimulation redetermined after CCD is not presented, because no changes were ever found in these functions. From Rajan R, Johnstone BM. Contralateral cochlear destruction mediates protection from monaural loud sound exposures through the crossed olivocochlear bundle. Hear Res 1989; 39:263-278.

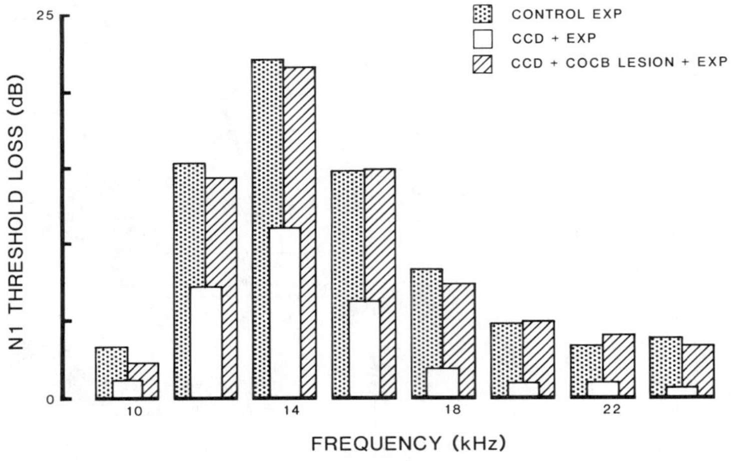

Figure 38-5 Test of the hypothesis of central facilitatory effects of controlled cochlear destruction (CCD). The control group was the same as before, with only the standard ipsilateral exposure (EXP). The first CCD test group was also the same as that in Figure 38.3, with CCD 2 to 5 minutes before the exposure. In the other test group, the CCD was first destroyed. Five minutes later the crossed olivocochlear bundle (COCB) was lesioned at the floor of the fourth ventricle; 2 minutes later, the standard exposure was presented.

generally were completed within 2 to 3 minutes, and always within 10 minutes, of CCD. None of the measures of afferent and efferent activity were altered by CAS or CCD. However, although CAS or CCD had no effects on ipsilateral cochlear responses prior to the exposure, they reduced TTS to the subsequent exposure (provided the delay was not too long). Similar effects were obtained when delays were interposed between a protective BES and the exposure. In that case, the BES appeared to have persistent facilitatory effects centrally (possibly the COCB cell bodies), allowing activation by the subsequent exposure. A similar hypothesis—that of interaction at a central site between inputs from the exposure and the protective manipulation—can also be applied to the effects of CAS and CCD, because neither manipulation directly activated the COCB. They too may have facilitated the exposure's activation of the COCB and reduction of the ipsilateral TTS.

This postulate was tested on the protective effects of CCD. In a new group, after measuring N1 audiograms from 2 to 30 kHz and intensity functions at 10 kHz, 14 kHz, or both, bipolar electrodes were located in the brain stem such that pulsed, gated electric trains produced N1 amplitude reductions equal to those in previously tested animals. The contralateral cochlea was destroyed, and N1 audiograms from 8 to 24 kHz and intensity functions were remeasured, and always found unaltered. The electrodes were used to lesion the COCB, as discussed previously. N1 audiograms were remeasured, and were again unaltered. Then the standard ipsilateral exposure was presented (7 minutes after CCD). The TTS in this group (Fig. 38-5) was not reduced, and losses from 10 to 24 kHz were not significantly different (p greater than 0.10) from losses in the control group that was presented only the standard monaural exposure, but were significantly higher (p less than 0.05) than losses in the test group with CCD but without brain-stem lesions.

Thus, CCD must act in the proposed facilitatory mode centrally, requiring the ipsilateral loud sound for final activation of COCB-mediated protection. Although the lesion would not prevent the exposure from activating the COCB "primed" by CCD, it would prevent the COCB outflow to the ipsilateral cochlea and the subsequent TTS reductions. Then the TTS would equal the control TTS, exactly as found here.

Graded Effects on TTS

Testing each protective manipulation on 10-kHz exposures presented at a wide variety of intensities and for a range of durations to produce a variety of TTSs revealed that, for each protective manipulation, the amount of reduction in TTS elicited by the protective manipulation was related not to the exposure intensity or duration per se, but rather to the amount of TTS. The results are summarized in Figure 38-6, which was constructed using the threshold losses caused by the exposure, allowing all exposures to be represented regardless of intensity or duration of exposure.

When low levels of maximum TTS, of about 25 dB or less, occurred immediately after the exposure, neither CAS nor CCD had any significant effect on TTS. With increasing TTS, increasing protection resulted. A plateau in protection was reached with maximum losses of about 40 dB or more.

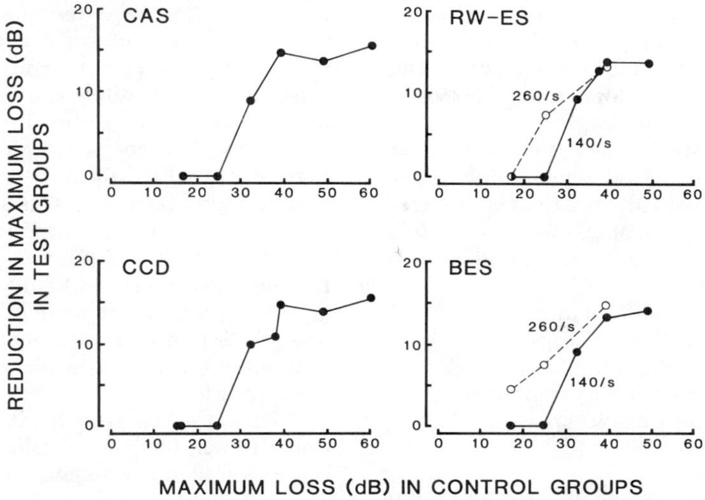

Figure 38-6 Dependence of the temporary threshold shift (TTS) reductions obtained with application of protective manipulations in test groups on the amount of TTS occurring in the corresponding control groups. The amount of TTS in the control groups is represented by the maximum TTS recorded in each group (the 14-kHz loss 10 seconds after exposure). The TTS reductions were calculated as the difference between maximum TTS in the control group and maximum TTS in the test group (both maxima occurred at 14 kHz 10 seconds after exposure). Left panels, Tests with contralateral acoustic stimulation (CAS) and contralateral cochlear destruction (CCD). The CAS was always at the same frequency as the ipsilateral exposure, and at 80 dB SPL simultaneous with and for the same duration as the exposure. In CCD tests, the contralateral cochlea was destroyed 2 to 10 minutes prior to the ipsilateral exposure. Right panels, Test with electric stimulation either at the round window (RW-ES) or at the floor of the fourth ventricle (BES). The exposures were identical to those tested with CAS or CCD except that an exposure at 110 dB SPL for 1 minute was not tested with electric stimulation. The test bipolar stimulus was always at 400 μA, with continuous 150-μs pulses presented at a rate of 140 or 260 per second, simultaneous with and for the duration of the exposure.

Similar effects were obtained with electric stimulation of the COCB either in the brain stem or at the round window. The results for two stimulation rates (140 and 260 pulses per second) are summarized in Figure 38-6 as they were for the contralateral manipulations. The effects of the contralateral manipulations are similar to the effects of COCB stimulation at 140 pulses per second at either stimulation site. No significant differences (p greater than 0.10) were found between the test groups with either contralateral manipulation or electric stimulation at that rate. With stimulation at the higher rate, slightly greater TTS reductions were obtained; with the brain-stem site, exposures that had not been protected before were now protected. It is possible that the effects of a higher stimulation rate may have been duplicated by using a higher CAS intensity, although Cody (1982) has indicated that above 80 dB SPL the CAS does not exert any greater protective effect on a fixed monaural high-intensity exposure.

In summary, the protective effects of the COCB pathway to the test cochlea appeared to depend on the TTS, the integrated effect of intensity and duration of exposure, rather than either one of the two variables of the exposures.

Comparison Between the Protective Manipulations

As shown above, CAS and CCD reduced TTS as much as electric stimulation of the COCB did at a moderate rate. Over a wide range of exposures, there were no significant differences in the TTS reductions over most of the affected frequency range. There was a graded relationship between the TTS reductions obtained with each protective manipulation and the TTS that would otherwise have occurred.

Further, all modes offered tonic protection, always without any persisting effects at the cochlea. The duration of persistence of protection depended on the nature of the manipulation. Manipulations (CAS, BES, and round-window stimulation) presented for the same period showed the same persistence of protection with 5 minutes' delay, but not with 10 minutes' delay. In contrast, a manipulation

(CCD) with no finite period of application had protective effects that persisted considerably longer. Perhaps if the CAS or the electric stimuli had been presented for a longer period or at a higher level, their protective effects would have persisted longer. It must be noted that the 5-minute period over which reductions could be obtained after the CAS or electric stimuli still represents a long-term facilitation of the central locus for stimuli of relatively short duration.

Finally, the crossed cochlear effects were also blocked by the same drugs that blocked the effects of electric stimulation, and were prevented if the COCB was transected at the floor of the fourth ventricle.

Pathways and Interactions Involved in the Protective Effects

Lower Brain-Stem "Reflex" Mechanisms

As shown earlier, CAS and CCD appeared to provide a facilitation at the COCB cell bodies to allow the loud sound to activate the COCB where the exposure alone did not do so. The inferior colliculus (IC) can also act through the COCB to reduce the cochlear TTS caused by a monaural exposure (Rajan, 1990a). IC stimulation does not appear to directly activate the COCB, but may facilitate the exposure's activation of the COCB (Rajan, 1990a). Thus, the two peripheral manipulations may exercise their effect through the IC, allowing the IC to act through the COCB to reduce TTS.

To examine this possibility, the effect of isolating the COCB cell bodies in the lower brain stem from more central structures, with an upper pontine lesion, was tested on the protective effects of a CAS (Rajan, 1990b). The lesion did not affect N1 audiograms and intensity functions (Rajan, 1990b) or the cochlear susceptibilities to the standard monaural exposure (Fig. 38-7). Threshold losses in the decerebrated control group, presented only by the standard monaural exposure, were similar (*p* greater than 0.10) to losses in the former control group with the same monaural exposure but without decerebration. Just as significantly, decerebration did not prevent the protective CAS effects (Fig. 38-7). Threshold losses from 10 to 24 kHz in the decerebrated test group, in which the standard ipsilateral exposure and the standard CAS were presented together after decereberation, were significantly lower (*p* less than 0.05) than losses at corresponding frequencies in the decerebrated control group. There were also no significant differences (*p* greater than 0.10) between the TTSs from 10 to 24 kHz in the two test groups with the same binaural test conditions, with or without decerebration. Threshold losses in both test groups were significantly lower (*p* less than 0.05) than TTS at all corresponding frequencies from 12 to 24 kHz in the two control groups presented with only the monaural exposure with and without decerebration).

Thus, CAS exercised its protective effects only through the lower brain stem without intercession from any higher centers. As shown above, lesioning the COCB blocked the protective effects of CAS. Therefore, the protective action of the CAS appears to be exerted through a lower brain-stem "reflex" arc involving input from both ears being integrated by the COCB neurons to the traumatized cochlea. It is parsimonious to assume that CCD also acts through the same pathways. The action of these protective manipulations through such a pathway does not preclude any descending influence on this COCB action. Low-rate electric stimulation of the IC also protects the cochlea by providing a facilitatory influence at the olivocochlear cell bodies that allows activation by a loud sound (Rajan, 1990a). The descending pathways from the midbrain could exert significant modulatory effects on the protective actions of the contralateral cochlear manipulations.

Involvement of Two Strychnine-Sensitive Sites in Protection

The time courses of the blocking actions of strychnine on the protective effects reveal an interesting result. Strychnine, injected intraperitoneally at 2 or 4 mg per kilogram, blocked both the protective effects of the continuous electric burst and the N1 amplitude reductions of pulsed gated trains, either at the brain stem or at the round window, only within about 40 to 60 minutes. In contrast, intraperitoneal injection of strychnine at 2 mg per kilogram blocked the protective effects of the two contralateral manipulations within 15 minutes. Because, across a wide range of exposures, both contralateral manipulations protected as much as did electric stimulation at

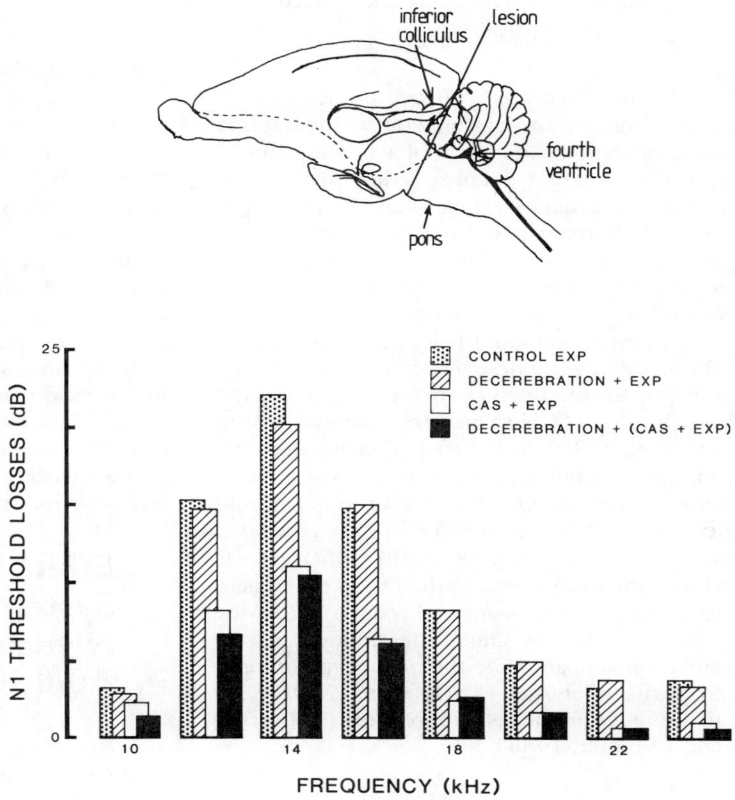

Figure 38-7 Lower brain-stem "reflex" actions of the protective effects of controlled acoustic stimulation (CAS). The upper drawing shows the location of the lesion made in two new groups to remove all descending influences to the crossed olivocochlear bundle (COCB). In the control groups only the standard ipsilateral exposure (EXP) was presented either after decerebration (DECEREBRATION + EXP) or without any decerebration (CONTROL + EXP—the same control group as in all the other figures). In the test groups, the test conditions were the simultaneous presentation of the CAS and the exposure, either after decerebration—DECEREBRATION + (CAS + EXP)—or without any decerebration (CAS + EXP; the same group as in Fig. 38-3*A*).

140 pulses per second, the difference cannot be due to any differences in the efficacy of reducing TTS. Rather, it suggests that the strychnine block was exercised at different sites in the case of the electric stimuli as compared to the contralateral manipulations.

This result is explained when it is noted that, in the case of COCB electric stimulation simultaneous with the exposure, the protective effects must be exercised through the stimulus' directly producing COCB action at the cochlea. Thus, these protective effects can only be blocked if the COCB terminals in the cochlea are blocked. In contrast, CAS and CCD do not directly activate the COCB, but may provide a facilitatory influence at the COCB cell bodies to allow the exposure to then activate the COCB. Then the protective effects of the contralateral manipulations can be blocked by blocking either the COCB terminals in the exposed cochlea or the input (or inputs) to the central site at which the proposed interaction occurs. The differences in time courses of the strychnine blocks therefore suggest that, in the case of CAS and CCD, it must be the inputs that were blocked within 15 minutes, because the results with COCB stimulation show that strychnine injected intraperitoneally blocks the COCB terminals only after about 40 to 60 minutes.

Thus, at least two sets of strychnine-sensitive sites are involved in the protective effects of the contralateral manipulations. One set consists of the COCB terminals in the ipsilateral cochlea at which COCB action reduces TTS. The other set, located centrally, is involved in providing input to the locus (suggested to be the COCB cell bodies) at which interaction occurs between the facilitatory input from the contralateral manipulation and the input from the ipsilateral exposure. This interaction finally leads to activation of the COCB to the cochlea that is presented the exposure. Because the protective CAS effects are exercised only through the lower brain stem, the second site must be located in this part of the brain. It is not known if the second site synapses directly on to the central locus at which the proposed interaction occurs or is a site from which originates input to the integrating locus. It is also unknown whether it is the facilitatory contralateral input or the input from the exposure that is blocked by strychnine.

Binaural Interactions Leading to Protection

Efferent neurons with cell bodies located in the brain stem contralateral to their target cochlea respond to monaural acoustic stimulation of the target cochlea rather than of the nontarget cochlea (Liberman and Brown, 1986; Robertson and Gummer, 1988). Thus, the COCB neurons to the cochlea exposed to loud sound must respond to monaural input from the traumatized target cochlea rather than to monaural input from the nontarget cochlea. However, these neurons appear to be subject to modulatory influences from the nontarget ear (Liberman, 1988; Robertson and Gummer, 1988). In the case of protection, the nontarget cochlea appears to provide a facilitatory influence to the COCB (Rajan and Johnstone, 1983a, 1988a, 1989). Low-level sound in, or destruction of, the nontarget ear allows the loud sound in the target ear to activate the COCB neurons and reduce TTS in the target cochlea. In single efferent neurons, facilitation appears to be the major type of input from the nontarget ear (Liberman, 1988), or to be as common as suppression (Robertson and Gummer, 1988).

Site of the Protective Action at the Ipsilateral Cochlea

Other than TTS, the (protective) continuous CAS was also tested on ipsilateral N1 audiograms from 6 to 30 kHz and on intensity functions at 10 and 14 kHz, recorded from the round window, or on DC potentials (the endocochlear potential, or EP, and the summating potential, or SP) recorded from scala media of the basal turn. The SP was recorded with a variety of tones, including 10-kHz tones as used for the exposures and 20-kHz tones more appropriate to the basal turn recording site, at intensities from about 90 to 110 dB SPL. None of these responses was ever altered by the CAS (Rajan and Johnstone, 1988a). Similarly, CCD had no effect on a wider variety of ipsilateral responses (see Fig. 38-4). (The latter results can be applied here because CCD provided equal protection over a long duration.) The (protective) continuous BES was also tested on the DC potentials (Rajan, 1988a). The SP was again evoked by 10-kHz and 20-kHz tones. Although the BES always decreased the EP and increased the SP, the effects decayed rapidly over about 10 to 20 seconds (Rajan, 1988a), especially at the higher stimulus rates most effective in reducing TTS. Konishi and Slepian (1971) also found that the effects of continuous COCB stimulation on DC potentials (paralleling N1 and CM effects) decayed totally within a few seconds of the start of the stimulus.

Thus, these results do not reveal the ipsilateral site of protection. However, recent work of Robert Patuzzi and his colleagues has shown that TTS appears to occur because of a reduction in the probability of opening of transduction channels on outer hair cell stereocilia (Patuzzi et al, 1989). CAS appears to negate this effect, at least partially (Patuzzi, personal communication). This raises the intriguing question of how efferent terminals along the sides and the base of the outer hair cells can affect events at the apex of the hair cells. Further work by these investigators should answer this question.

Effets Protecteurs du Système Efférent au Niveau de la Fatigue Auditive chez le cobaye

Des études récentes chez le cobaye ont montré que les efférences cochléaires pouvaient agir en réduisant les dommages occasionnés par une exposition de la cochlée à des sons intenses. Nous présenterons ici des informations plus précises concernant cet effet protecteur.

La stimulation électrique des efférences cochléaires, au niveau du tronc cérébral ou de la fenêtre ronde, réduit les déficits auditifs transitoires occasionnés par une exposition à un son intense. Cet effet protecteur a un effet maximum quand les chocs électriques ont une cadence élevée et lorsqu'ils sont présentés durant toute la durée de l'exposition sonore. Toutefois, le même effet peut être obtenu lorsque cette stimulation électrique est effectuée 5 minutes avant l'exposition traumatique. Cet effet protecteur est bloqué par l'administration intrapéritonéale ou intracochléaire de drogues connues pour inhiber l'action des efférences cochléaires et avec une cinétique comparable aux autres études. Cet effet peut être aussi bloqué par une section du faisceau olivocochléaire croisé (FOC).

Cet effet protecteur a été aussi obtenu par des manipulations au niveau de l'oreille controlatérale. Ces effets cochléaires croisés peuvent être aussi supprimés en utilisant les mêmes drogues que précédemment ou par des sections du FOC. L'effet protecteur de ces manipulations controlatérales persiste pendant la durée de la manipulation. Ces manipulations controlatérales n'activeraient pas directement le FOC, mais pourraient avoir des influences facilitatrices.

Quelles que soient la durée et l'intensité de l'exposition sonore, les manipulations effectuées réduisent les pertes auditives transitoires. Cet effet protecteur est maximum pour des déficits auditifs d'environ 15 à 17 dB enregistrés à la fréquence la plus affectée par l'exposition traumatique.

Les stimulations acoustiques controlatérales semblent agir uniquement au niveau des voies "réflexes" du tronc cérébral. En effet une décorticalisation ne supprime pas l'effet protecteur. Toutefois des influences modulatrices plus centrales pourraient s'exercer, étant donné que la stimulation électrique du colliculus inférieur (CI) a aussi un effet protecteur contre les effets d'un traumatisme acoustique. Cet effet est aussi bloqué par les mêmes perfusions intracochléaires de drogues, et persiste de la même manière que la stimulation électrique du FOC ou celle de la stimulation acoustique controlatérale. Toutefois, un même niveau de protection peut être obtenu pour des cadences de stimulation électrique plus faibles que celles du FOC.

La stimulation électrique du colliculus inférieur ipsilatéral réduit aussi les déficits auditifs transitoires, dans des proportions moindres et pour des cadences de stimulations électriques plus élevées. Ces différences pourraient être attribuées au nombre de fibres croisées et non croisées du système efférent médian innervant les régions cochléaires affectées par le son intense. Le colliculus inférieur pourrait aussi avoir des influences à la fois sur les voies croisées et non croisées du système efférent olivocochléaire.

ACKNOWLEDGMENTS

I thank Professor B.M. Johnstone for his guidance during the course of this work. The study was supported by grants from the National Health and Medical Research Council of Australia and the Australian Research Grants Scheme.

References

Aschoff A, Ostwald J. Distribution of cochlear efferents and olivo-collicular neurons in the brainstem of rat and guinea pig. Exp Brain Res 1988; 71:241-251.

Bobbin RP, Konishi T. Action of cholinergic and anticholinergic drugs at the crossed olivocochlear bundle–hair cell junction. Acta Otolaryngol 1974; 77:56-65.

Cody AR. Temporary and permanent threshold shifts: An electrophysiological and histological study of the effects of acoustic overstimulation on the guinea pig cochlea. Ph.D. thesis, University of Western Australia, 1982.

Cody AR, Johnstone BM. Temporary threshold shift modified by binaural acoustic stimulation. Hear Res 1982; 6:199-206.

Dallos P, Ozdamar O, Ryan A. Behavioral, compound action potential, and single unit thresholds: Relationship in normal and abnormal ears. J Acoust Soc Am 1978; 64:151-157.

Desmedt JE. Physiological studies of the efferent recurrent system. In: Keidel WD, Neff WD, eds. Handbook of sensory physiology. Berlin: Springer-Verlag, 1975:219.

Desmedt JE, Monaco P. The pharmacology of a centrifugal inhibitory pathway in the cat's acoustic system. Proc 1st Int Pharm Meeting, Stockholm, 1962; 1:183-188.

Desmedt JE, LaGrutta V, LaGrutta G. Contrasting effects of centrifugal olivocochlear inhibition and of middle ear muscle contraction on the response characteristics of the cat's auditory nerve. Brain Res 1971; 30:375-384.

Fex J. Auditory activity in centrifugal and centripetal cochlear fibres in cat. A study of a feedback system. Acta Physiol Scand 1962; 55(Suppl 189):1-68.

Fex J. Efferent inhibition in the cochlea related to hair-cell dc activity: Study of post-synaptic activity of the crossed olivocochlear fibres in the cat. J Acoust Soc Am 1967; 41:666-675.

Filogamo G, Candiollo L, Rossi G. The morphology and function of auditory input control. In: Tonndorf J, ed. Translations of the Beltone Institute for Hearing Research, No. 20. Chicago: The Beltone Institute for Hearing Research, 1967:1.

Galambos R. Suppression of auditory nerve activity by stimulation of efferent fibres to cochlea. J Neurophysiol 1056; 19:424-437.

Galley N, Klinke R, Oertel W, Pause M, Storch WH. The effect of intracochlearly administered acetylcholine-blocking agents on the efferent synapses of the cochlea. Brain Res 1973; 64:55-63.

Handrock M, Zeisberg J. The influence of the efferent system on adaptation, temporary and permanent threshold shift. Arch Otorhinolaryngol 1982; 234:191-195.

Irvine DRF, Wester KG. Middle ear muscle effects on cochlear responses to bone-conducted sound. Acta Physiol Scand 1974; 91:482-496.

Johnstone JR, Alder VA, Johnstone BM, Robertson D, Yates GK. Cochlear action potential and single unit thresholds. J Acoust Soc Am 1979; 65:254-257.

Kimura R, Wersall J. Termination of the olivocochlear bundle in relation to the outer hair cells of the organ of Corti in guinea pig. Acta Otolaryngol 1962; 55:11-32.

Klinke R, Galley N. Efferent innervation of the vestibular and auditory receptors. Physiol Rev 1974; 54:316-357.

Konishi T, Slepian JZ. Effects of electrical stimulation of the crossed olivocochlear bundle on cochlear potentials recorded with intracochlear electrodes in guinea pigs. J Acoust Soc Am 1971; 49:1762-1769.

Liberman MC. Response properties of cochlear efferent neurons: Monaural vs. binaural stimulation and the effects of noise. J Neurophysiol 1988; 60:1779-1798.

Liberman MC, Brown MC. Physiology and anatomy of single olivocochlear neurons in the cat. Hear Res 1986; 24:17-36.

Møller AR. The middle ear. In: Tobias JV, ed. Foundations of modern auditory theory. New York: Academic Press, 1972:133.

Nuttal AL. Tympanic muscle effects on middle-ear transfer characteristics. J Acoust Soc Am 1974; 56:1239-1247.

Patuzzi RB, Yates GK, Johnstone BM. Changes in cochlear microphonic and neural sensitivity produced by acoustic trauma. Hear Res 1989; 39:189-202.

Rajan R. Effect of electrical stimulation of the crossed olivocochlear bundle on temporary threshold shifts in auditory sensitivity. I. Dependence on electrical stimulation parameters. J Neurophysiol 1988a; 60:549-568.

Rajan R. Effect of electrical stimulation of the crossed olivocochlear bundle on temporary threshold shifts in auditory sensitivity. II. Dependence on the level of temporary threshold shifts. J. Neurophysiol 1988b; 60:569-579.

Rajan R. Electrical stimulation of the inferior colliculus at low rates protects the cochlea from auditory desensitization. Brain Res 1990a; 506:192-204.

Rajan R. The effects of upper pontine transection upon normal cochlear responses and on the protective effects of contralateral acoustic stimulation in barbiturate-anaesthetised normal-hearing guinea pigs. Hear Res 1990b; 45:137-144.

Rajan R, Johnstone BM. Crossed cochlear influences on monaural temporary threshold shifts. Hear Res 1983a; 9:279-294.

Rajan R, Johnstone BM. Residual effects in monaural temporary threshold shifts to pure tones. Hear Res 1983b; 12:185-197.

Rajan R, Johnstone BM. Efferent effects elicited by electrical stimulation at the round window of the guinea pig. Hear Res 1983c; 12:405-417.

Rajan R, Johnstone BM. Binaural acoustic stimulation exercises protective effects at the cochlea that mimic the effects of electrical stimulation of an auditory efferent pathway. Brain Res 1988a; 459:241-255.

Rajan R, Johnstone BM. Electrical stimulation of cochlear efferents at the round window decreases auditory desensitization in guinea pigs. I. Dependence on electrical stimulation parameters. Hear Res 1988b; 36:53-73.

Rajan R, Johnstone BM. Electrical stimulation of cochlear efferents at the round window decreases auditory desensitization in guinea pigs. II. Dependence on level of temporary threshold shifts. Hear Res 1988c; 36:75-88.

Rajan R, Johnstone BM. Contralateral cochlear destruction mediates protection from monaural loud sound exposures through the crossed olivocochlear bundle. Hear Res 1989; 39:263-278.

Rajan R, Robertson D, Johnstone BM. Absence of tonic activity of the crossed olivocochlear bundle in determining compound action potential thresholds, amplitudes and masking phenomena in anaesthetised guinea pigs with normal hearing sensitivities. Hear Res 1990; 44:195-208.

Rasmussen GL. Efferent fibers of the cochlear nerve and cochlear nucleus. In: Rasmussen GL, Windle WF, eds. Neural mechanisms of the auditory and vestibular systems. Springfield: Charles C Thomas, 1960:105.

Robertson D, Gummer M. Physiology of cochlear efferents in the mammal. In: Syka J, Masterton RB, eds. Auditory pathway. New York: Plenum, 1988:269.

Robertson D, Cole KS, Harvey AR. Brainstem organization of efferent projections to the guinea pig cochlea studied using the fluorescent tracers fast blue and diamidino yellow. Exp Brain Res 1987; 66:449-457.

Sohmer H. A comparison of the efferent effects of the homolateral and contralateral olivo-cochlear bundles. Acta Otolaryngol 1966; 60:59-70.

Strutz J, Bielenberg K. Efferent acoustic neurons within the lateral superior olivary nucleus of the guinea pig. Brain Res 1984; 299:174-177.

Terayama Y, Yamamoto K. Olivo-cochlear bundle in the guinea pig after central transection of the crossed bundle. Acta Otolaryngol 1971;72:385-396.

Ward WD. Temporary threshold shifts following monaural and binaural exposure. J Acoust Soc Am 1965; 38:121-125.

Weiderhold ML. Physiology of the olivocochlear system. In: Altschuler RA, Hoffman DW, Bobbin RP, eds. Neurobiology of hearing: The cochlea. New York: Raven Press, 1986:349.

Wright CG, Preston RE. Degeneration and distribution of efferent nerve fibres in the guinea pig organ of Corti. A light and scanning electron microscopic study. Brain Res 1973; 58:37-59.

CHAPTER 39

Effects of Periodic Rest on Cochlear Damage and Hearing Loss

WILLIAM W. CLARK
BARBARA A. BOHNE

One of the major unresolved issues concerning the effects of noise exposure on the auditory system is how intermittence affects hearing loss and cochlear damage produced by the exposure. Although several studies have addressed intermittence in both laboratory (Eldredge et al, 1959; Ward, 1970) and industrial environments (Sataloff et al, 1983), few have addressed the issue of threshold shifts observed after repeated exposures for more than a few days (Johnson et al, 1976). Saunders et al (1977) evaluated threshold shifts produced by exposure to an octave band of noise (OBN) centered at 4.0 kHz, 57 to 92 dB SPL, 6 hours per day for 9 days in groups of trained chinchillas. They interpreted their findings as supporting the idea that threshold shifts reached an asymptote (asymptotic threshold shift, or ATS) after 2 to 3 days of exposure on this schedule, and suggested the "equivalent power hypothesis," which predicts that ATS will be reduced from that produced by continuous exposure by the reduction of power (with a period of integration of 24 hours) times 1.7 dB (1.7-dB decrease in ATS for every 1-dB decrease in equivalent power of noise). For the 25 percent duty cycle utilized by Saunders et al, ATS values were close to those predicted.

However, Clark et al (1987), using behaviorally-trained chinchillas, measured threshold shifts produced by an exposure to an OBN centered at 0.5 kHz, 95 dB SPL, 6 hours per day for 36 days or 15 minutes per hour for 144 days. They found that both exposures initially produced threshold shifts of 35 to 45 dB, but as the exposure continued, thresholds began to decline and eventually recovered to within 10 to 15 dB of baseline values even though the exposure continued. The behavioral and anatomic data indicated that these intermittent exposures produced less temporary and permanent hearing loss and less cochlear damage than continuous exposures of equal energy. In a follow-up physiologic experiment, Sinex et al (1987) demonstrated similar recovery phenomena in whole nerve action potentials and single auditory nerve fiber recordings from groups of chinchillas exposed to the 500 Hz OBN at 95 dB SPL, 15 minutes per hour, for 4 or 40 days. Taken together, these studies showed that auditory thresholds could recover by as much as 30 dB during exposure, and that the locus of the recovery phenomenon is peripheral, probably at the level of the hair cell. This finding has recently been confirmed and extended by another laboratory (Henderson et al, 1990). It also supports findings originally reported by Miller et al for interrupted exposures in the cat (Miller et al, 1963).

Bohne and her colleagues (e.g., Bohne et al, 1985, 1987) have shown that the apical and basal turns of the chinchilla cochlea are damaged differently by noise exposure. Damage in the apical turn is usually restricted to scattered losses of outer hair cells (OHCs) that can reach 30 to 50 percent without elevating thresholds for low-frequency tones. In contrast, damage in the basal turn of the cochlea from exposure to low- or high-frequency noise usually begins as a discrete lesion in which there is a severe loss of inner hair cells (IHCs), OHCs, or both. Similar findings from human ears have been reported by Bredberg (1968).

It is possible that the different types of damage or different mechanisms of damage produced by low- or high-frequency exposure to noise determine whether recovery occurs during exposure on an interrupted schedule. The objective of the study reported here was to determine if the recovery seen in repeated exposure to low-frequency noise also occurs after exposure to a high-frequency band of noise on similar schedules.

Methods

Subjects

Subjects for these studies were chinchillas born and reared in a low-noise animal colony; they were 1 to 2 years old at the start of the experiments. All subjects were made monaural by removing the ossicles on the left side; this technique provides approximately 60 dB of attenuation for signals reaching the left ear, but preserves the cochlea for histologic analysis (Clark and Bohne, 1987). Ossicular removal was completed prior to behavioral training in group 1; after 36 days of noise exposure for group 2; and after 72 days of exposure in group 3.

Behavioral Technique

Audiometric data were obtained from the chinchillas using a food-reward, operant-conditioning technique (Clark et al, 1974, 1987; Clark and Bohne, 1978; Bohne and Clark, 1982). Briefly, the animal initiated a trial sequence by depressing and holding a response key/feeder chute (an observing response). After a variable period (1 to 9 seconds) a 2-second trial was presented; 67 percent of the trials contained tones, whereas the rest were silent. The chinchillas were trained to report the presence of a tone by releasing the response key. Absence of a tone was correctly reported when the animal continued to hold the response key throughout the 2-second trial. These correct responses ("hits" or "correct rejections") were rewarded by delivery of a food pellet. Incorrect responses ("misses" or "false alarms") were not punished; however, they delayed the opportunity for the next pellet.

An adaptive tracking procedure was used to measure pure-tone thresholds for as many as 23 frequencies daily. Threshold tests were begun with stimuli presented at 60 to 80 dB SPL. Each correct response to the tone (hit) reduced the stimulus by 10 dB until the first failure to respond to the tone (miss) occurred. The attenuation step size was reduced to 5 dB, and the stimulus was increased in 5-dB steps until the next hit occurred. Subsequent hits and misses adjusted the stimulus intensity in 2.5-dB steps until six alternations had occurred at the 2.5-dB step size. Threshold was defined as the mean of these intensities. Each threshold test required 2 to 3 minutes, during which time about 15 45-mg food pellets were obtained by the chinchilla. Well-trained animals generated a full audiogram (23 frequencies tested) and consumed about 350 pellets during each daily, 1-hour session.

Thresholds were determined at quarter-octave frequency intervals from 0.125 to 16.0 kHz. At least five threshold determinations at each frequency (typically 25 to 30) were used to establish the animal's pre-exposure baseline. Behavior during silent trials was used to determine the existence of any conditions that could interfere with the threshold determinations; pellets delivered for correct rejections also served to maintain the key holding behavior of the animal. Changes in the animal's criteria for reporting tones near threshold were reflected in its false alarm (FA) rate (No. FAs/No. silent trials). By monitoring false alarm behavior, one can determine if thresholds have been altered by any nonauditory effects of the experimental treatment. Although training time varied among individual animals, approximately 1 month was required to train a young animal to report tones near threshold, and at least two additional months of training were required before the animal became a reliable observer (i.e., the false alarm rate was 5 to 20%; standard deviation of threshold measures <3 dB).

Noise Exposure

After training was completed, subjects were exposed to an OBN centered at 4.0 kHz. The octave band level (OBL) of the noise was 86 dB re 20 μPa. Animals in group 1 were exposed 6 hours per day for 36 days; the exposure for group 2 was 6 hours per day for 72 days. Group 3 was exposed for 15 minutes per hour for 144 days. The schedule of ossicular removal in groups 2 and 3 resulted in exposures of 36 and 72 days for the left and right cochleas, respectively, of animals in group 2, and 72 and 144 days for the left and right cochleas, respectively, of animals in group 3. Measures of hearing sensitivity were obtained twice daily for all groups. Animals exposed 6 hours per day were tested immediately before and again after each day's exposure (i.e., threshold shift [TS] 1 hour and TS 18 hours after the previous day's exposure). Those exposed on the 15 minute per hour schedule were also tested twice daily, in the morning and afternoon, and data were plotted by day of exposure.

Anatomic Technique

The cochleas of the experimental animals were prepared for examination after a recovery period of at least 90 days. Briefly, under deep pentobarbital anesthesia, the cochleas were preserved by gently perfusing the fixative (1% OsO4 in Dalton's buffer) through the perilymphatic spaces. After perfusion of both cochleas, the animals were sacrificed, the temporal bones were removed, and fixation was continued for 2 hours. Leaving most of the bone intact, the cochleas were washed, dehydrated, and passively infiltrated with araldite. After polymerization of the plastic, the cochleas were dissected and trimmed in order to obtain whole mount preparations of the entire cochlear duct. The length of the organ of Corti was measured and the number of missing cells was counted in each control and experimental cochlea; these data were plotted as cytocochleograms. The position and extent of damage to the stria vascularis and the location and amount of degeneration of the dendritic processes of the spiral ganglion cells were also reported on each cytocochleogram.

Results

Group I (6 hours per day, 36 days)

Average TS functions for these animals are shown in Figure 39-1. Filled symbols represent the TS functions measured just after each daily exposure (TS 1 hour); open symbols are the TSs measured just before each daily exposure (TS 18 hours from previous day's exposure). Because the exposure band was restricted to the basal half of the cochlea, little TS was noted for the low-frequency tones, as expected (Fig. 39-1*A*). However, the TS 1-hour functions for the frequencies encompassed by the noise exposure, 3.35 to 5.7 kHz, all showed initial shifts of 40 to 55 dB over the first 5 to 10 days of exposure. Comparison with the last 10 days of exposure indicated recovery of 10 to 17 dB at all test frequencies (Fig. 39-1*B* through *E*).

The TS 18-hour measures for the frequencies 3.35 to 5.7 kHz indicated a growth of shift with exposure duration; that is, less recovery was observed as the exposure period lengthened. For example, at 5.7 kHz (Fig. 39-1*E*), TSs recovered by 26 dB on the average during the first 10 days of exposure; the last 10 days of exposure TSs recovered less than 0.5 dB during 18-hour quiet periods between noise exposures.

After 36 days, the noise was terminated and the animals were allowed to recover. Permanent threshold shifts (PTSs) were observed in all animals; they averaged 15 to 20 dB for the high frequencies (3.35 to 5.7 kHz; data not shown). Cytocochleograms for these animals indicated small basal-turn lesions; cochlear damage was less than that observed with equal-energy continuous exposures (cytocochleograms not shown).

Group 2 (6 hours per day, 72 days)

Average TS functions for these animals are shown in Figure 39-2. The malleus/incus complex was removed from the left ears after the thirty-sixth exposure, and is denoted by the arrows on the figure. Otherwise, the format of the figure is the same as that of Figure 39-1. Threshold-shift functions for 0.715 kHz are shown in Figure 39-2*A*. Although there was no shift of thresholds during the first 36 days of exposure, thresholds increased by 10 to 15 d*B* in the days immediately after ossicular removal, and the average TS over the last 10 days of exposure was 5 dB.

Threshold shifts for the test frequencies within the exposure band are shown in Figure 39-2*B* through *E*. The TS 1-hour functions are characterized by an initial shift of 40 to 50 dB and a sloping recovery function that displayed recovery of 10 to 20 dB after the first 5 to 10 days of exposure. For test frequencies of 3.35, 4.0, and 4.8 kHz, no changes were noted after ossicular removal. However, at 5.7 kHz the TS 1-hour function became elevated by 10 dB between days 37 and 41 of exposure and stabilized for the duration of the 72-day exposure.

Like the data shown in Figure 39-1, the TS 18-hour measures for the frequencies 3.35 to 5.7 kHz indicated a growth of shift with exposure duration; that is, less recovery was observed as the exposure period lengthened. For all frequencies, the TS 18-hour thresholds converged toward the TS 1-hour measures; after 25 to 30 days of exposure, little recovery occurred during the 18-hour quiet period between noise exposures. An elevation of TS 18-hour measures was observed for the 5.7-kHz test frequency after ossicular removal.

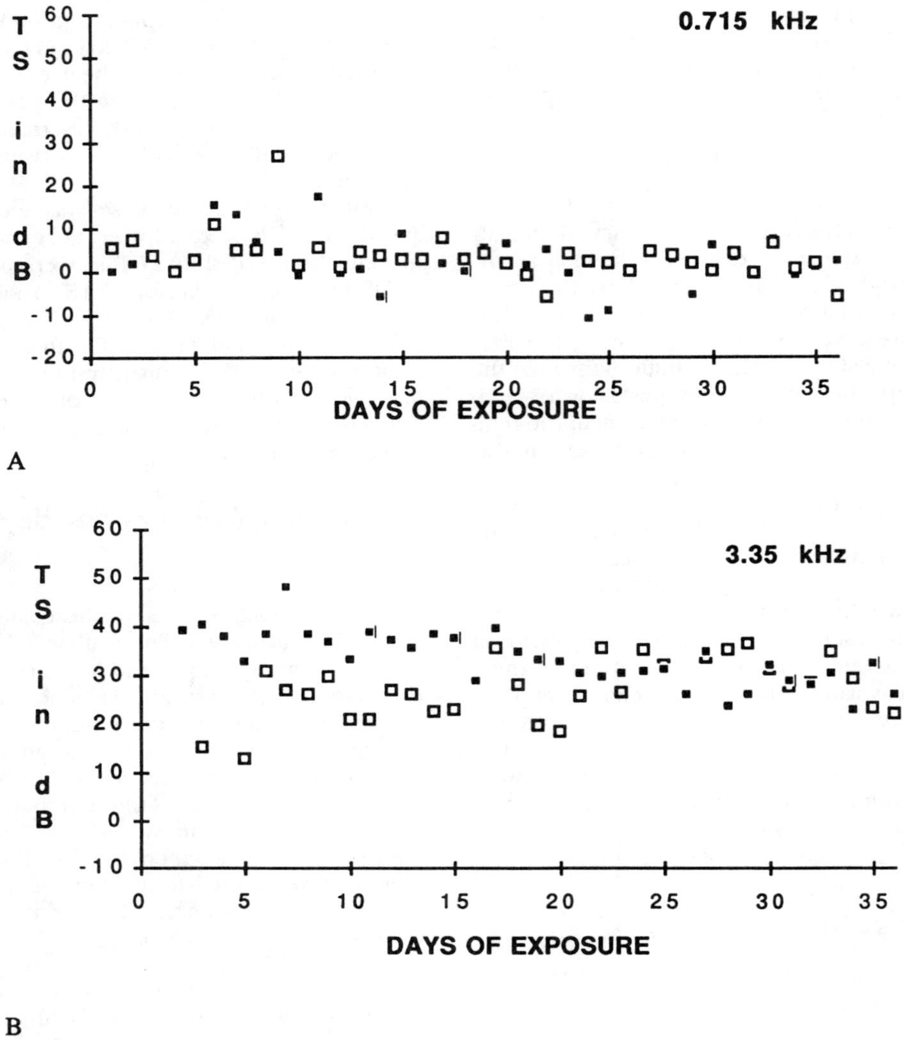

Figure 39-1 Threshold shift (TS) as a function of days of exposure for animals exposed to an OBN centered at 4.0 kHz, 86 dB SPL, 6 hours per day for 36 days (group 1). Filled symbols denote thresholds obtained immediately after each daily exposure (TS 1 hour); Closed symbols denote thresholds obtained 18 hours after each exposure (TS 18 hours). Panels *A* through *E* represent thresholds at 0.715, 3.35, 4.0, 4.8, and 5.7 kHz, respectively.

Group 3 (15 minutes per hour, 144 days)

Average TS functions for these animals are shown in Figure 39-3. Because approximately 1 hour of testing was needed to complete the audiogram, the animals were tested twice daily during 45-minute quiet periods between exposures. Therefore, all data shown in Figure 39-3 are TSs measured within 45 minutes of noise exposure.

Two characteristics of these data are noteworthy. The post–ossicular removal elevations in thresholds observed in group 2 were not confirmed in these animals. Average TSs from days 20 to 50 (before ossicular removal) and 80 to 110 (after ossicular removal) of exposure were compared and are displayed in Figure 39-4. For the frequencies 3.35 to 5.7 kHz, generally there were no significant differences in TS before and after ossicular removal. Only the 4.0-kHz comparison reached signifi-

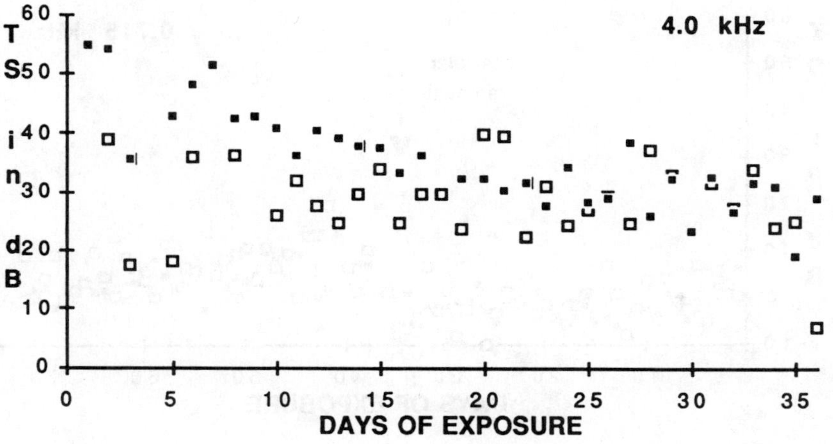

C

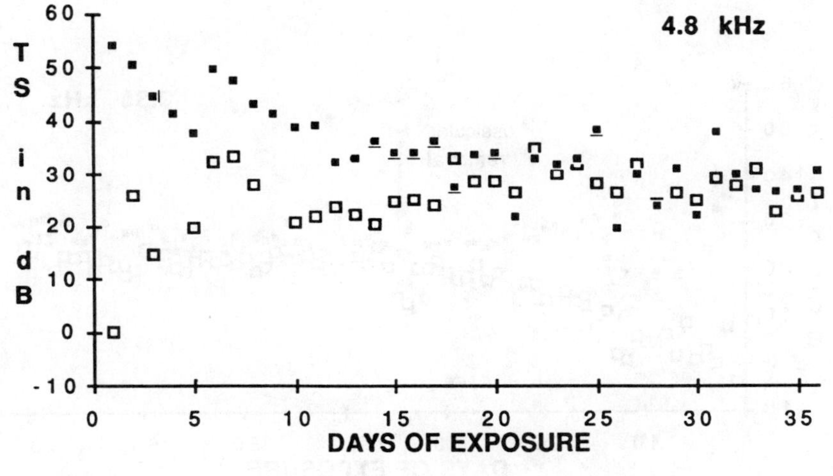

D

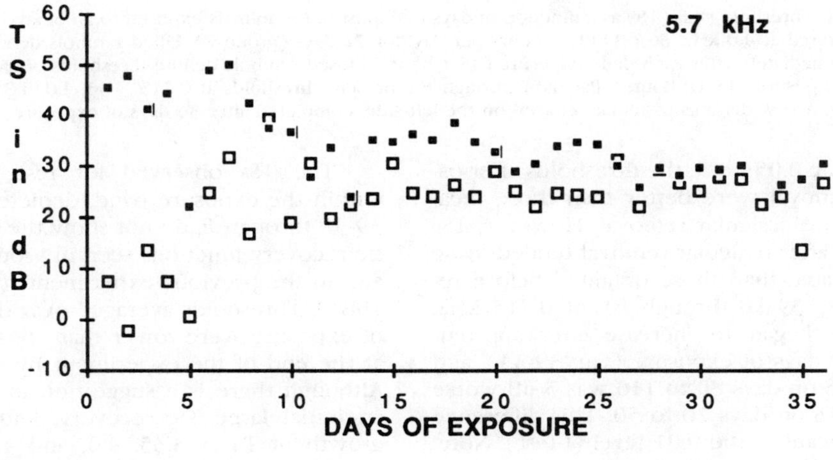

E

Figure 39-1 *Continued*

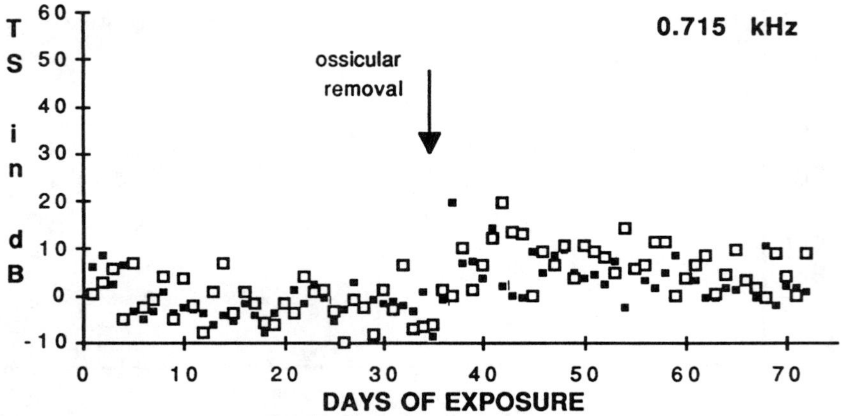

A

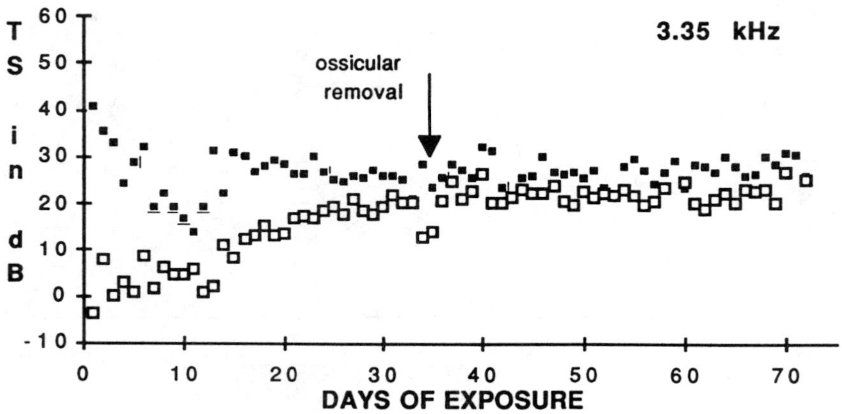

B

Figure 39-2 Threshold shift (TS) as a function of days of exposure for animals exposed to an octave band of noise (OBN) centered at 4.0 kHz, 86 dB SPL, 6 hours per day, for 72 days (group 2). Filled symbols denote thresholds obtained immediately after each daily exposure (TS 1 hour); Closed symbols denote thresholds obtained 18 hours after each exposure (TS 18 hours). Panels *A* through *E* represent thresholds at 0.715, 3.35, 4.0, 4.8, and 5.7 kHz, respectively. Arrow denotes ossicular removal on the left side, completed after 36 days of exposure.

cance at the 0.05 level; the thresholds after ossicular removal were better than those measured before ossicular removal. However, TSs measured after ossicular removal tended to be more variable than those obtained before removal (Fig. 39-3*B* through *E*). At 0.715 kHz, thresholds began to increase after approximately 40 days of exposure (Fig. 39-3*A*), and average TS on days 80 to 110 was 5 dB worse than the TS on days 20 to 50. This difference was significant at the 0.01 level (t-test). Note, however, that the time course of threshold elevation was unrelated to ossicular removal.

The TSs observed for test frequencies within the exposure band, depicted in Figure 39-3*B* through *E*, do not show the characteristic recovery functions seen in groups 1 and 2, and in the previous experiments (Clark et al, 1987). Thresholds averaged over days 1 to 10 of exposure were *lower* than those observed at the end of the experiment by 4 to 13 dB. Although there is a suggestion in the data of an initial large TS, recovery, and secondary growth of TS at 3.35, 4.0, and 4.8 kHz, the time course of the effect is much shorter than for the other exposures reported, and the general trend is qualitatively different.

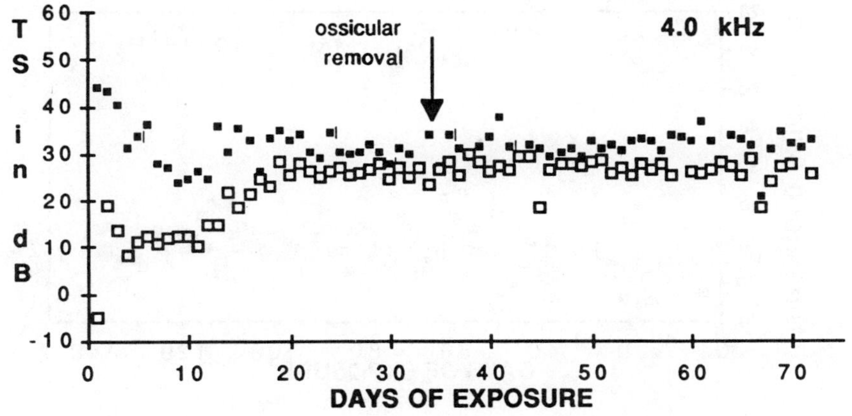

C

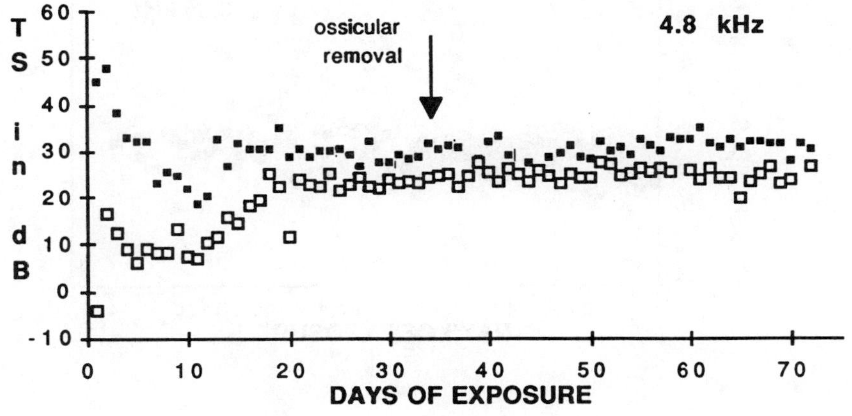

D

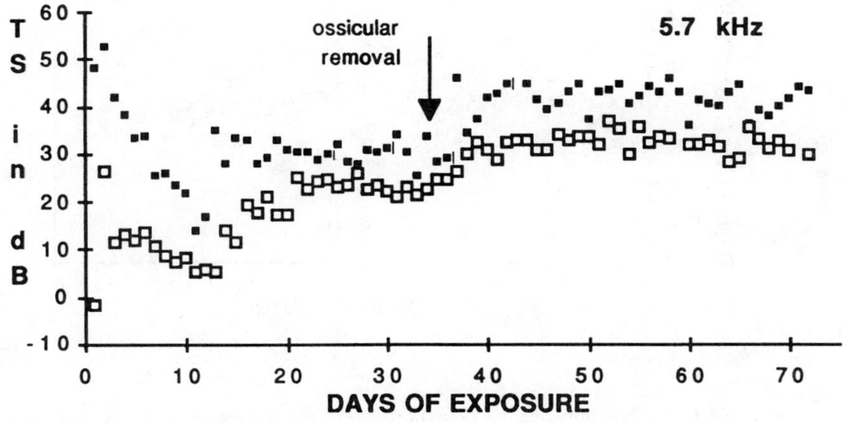

E

Figure 39-2 *Continued*

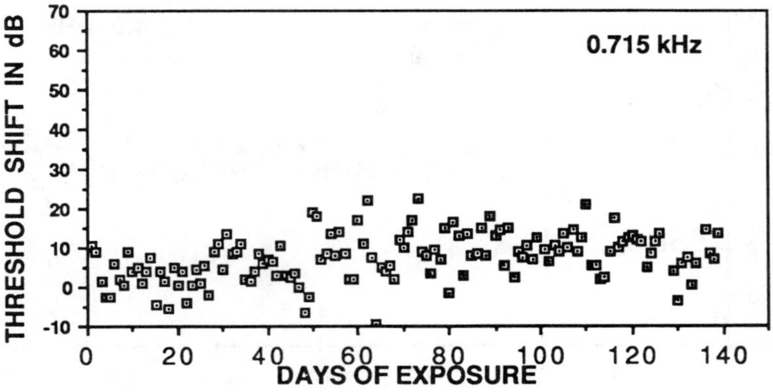

A

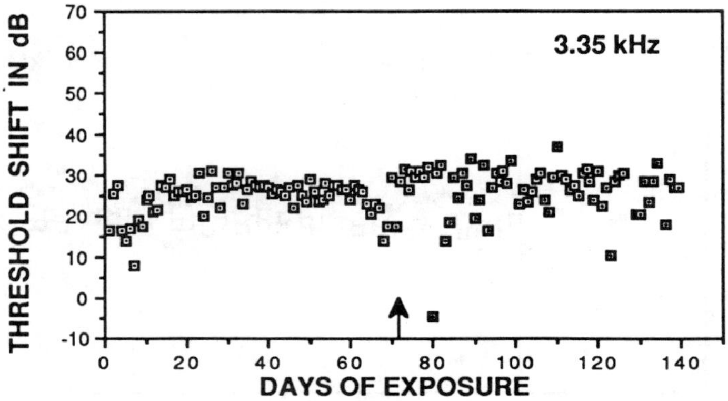

B

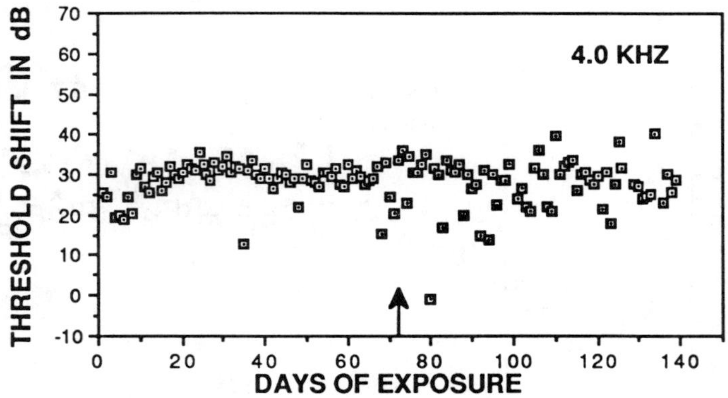

C

Figure 39-3 Threshold shift as a function of days of exposure for animals exposed to an octave band of noise (OBN) centered at 4.0 kHz, 86 dB SPL, 15 minutes per hour for 144 days (group 3). Panels *A* through *E* represent thresholds at 0.715, 3.35, 4.0, 4.8, and 5.7 kHz, respectively. Arrow denotes ossicular removal on the left side, completed after 72 days of exposure.

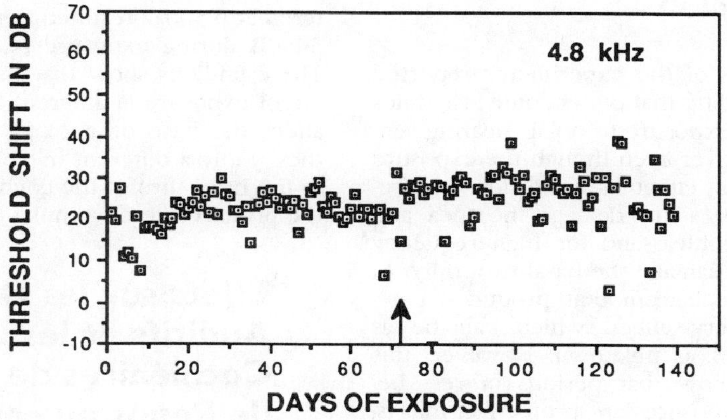

D

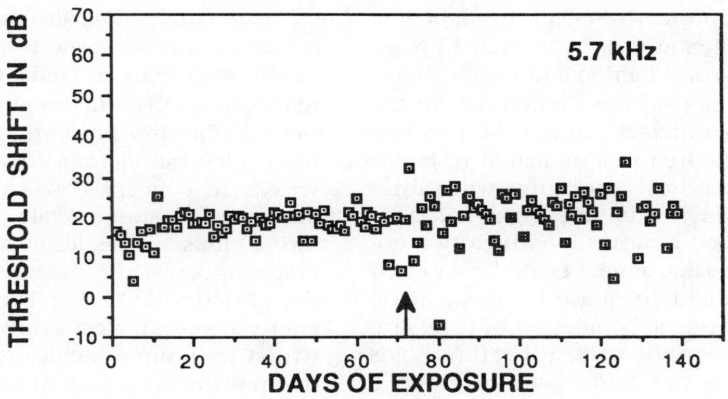

E

Figure 39-3 *Continued*

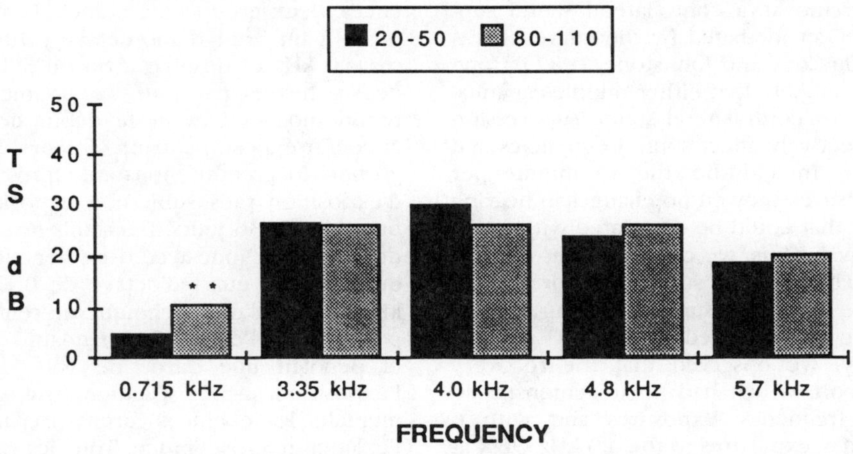

Figure 39-4 Comparison of threshold shifts (TSs) averaged over days 20 to 50 (before ossicular removal) and 80 to 110 (after ossicular removal) for animals in group 3. Significant differences, identified by single or double asterisks, represent the 0.05 and 0.01 levels, respectively.

Conclusion

The results of the experiments reported confirm the finding that under some schedules of interrupted exposure to noise, hearing sensitivity can recover even though the exposure continues. This effect is seen for low-frequency exposures that damage the apex and base of the cochlea, and for high-frequency exposures that damage the basal turn only. At present the mechanism that produces a peripheral recovery effect, which can be as much as 30 dB, is unknown. However, this finding does show that periods of rest between noise exposures are protective; that is, they produce less hearing loss and cochlear damage than equal-energy continuous exposures. This finding is also consistent with recent findings of protective effects produced by the "training phenomenon" reported by Canlon et al (1988) and Canlon and Borg (1990).

Ossicular removal was carried out on the left ears of experimental subjects for two reasons. First, it resulted in a monaural response from the subjects for correlation with histopathologic findings from the right ear. Secondly, it provided a means by which two cochleas from the same animal could be exposed to different amounts of noise for comparison of cochlear damage as a function of exposure duration. However, the finding that thresholds were elevated at two frequencies in group 2 after ossicular removal was troubling. There are several potential explanations for this finding. In addition to the obvious possibility of artifact, ossicular removal may have altered the middle-ear muscle reflex for the contralateral ear. Another possibility is that by eliminating the binaural nature of the stimulus after ossicular removal, a contralateral sound suppression effect mediated by the efferents was eliminated (Cody and Johnstone, 1982). However, it is unlikely that either middle-ear muscle effects or contralateral sound suppression would selectively affect some frequencies and not others. In addition, the 15 minute per hour exposures showed no changes in hearing sensitivity that could be correlated with ossicular removal. Thus, we conclude that there is no contralateral sound suppression or middle-ear muscle effects produced by binaural exposure in the data reported here.

Finally, we observed that the recovery phenomenon, which had been demonstrated with low-frequency exposures and with 6 hour per day exposures to the 4.0 kHz OBN at 86 dB SPL, did not occur when the period of exposure was 15 minutes (group 3). However, 15-minute exposures to an OBN centered at 0.5 kHz resulted in recovery of nearly 30 dB during exposure (Clark et al, 1987). These findings show that the effect of schedule of exposure is different for exposures that affect the base or apex of the cochlea, and they imply a different mechanism of recovery in the basal turn of the cochlea, depending on the primary site of stimulation.

Effets sur les Déficits Auditifs et les Lésions Cochléaires de Périodes de Repos au cours d'une Stimulation Acoustique

L'une des principales questions non résolues en ce qui concerne les effets du bruit sur l'audition a trait à l'influence de l'intermittence sur les éventuelles pertes auditives et lésions cochléaires produites par l'exposition au bruit. Bien que certains résultats semblent favoriser le concept d'iso-énergie, dans lequel l'énergie acoustique totale permettrait de prédire à elle seule les lésions, il est évident que l'interruption d'une dose donnée de bruit par des périodes de "calme effectif" constitue un effet protecteur, c'est-à-dire que la perte auditive et les lésions cochléaires sont plus faibles que pour une exposition iso-énergétique continue.

Les effets de différentes séquences comportant une succession de périodes de bruit et de repos sur l'atteinte cochléaire et la perte auditive ont été étudiés dans nos laboratoires chez des chinchillas ayant subi un entraînement comportemental. Dans l'une des expériences, deux groupes de chinchillas furent exposés à un bruit d'une octave (OBN) centré sur 4,0 kHz et de niveau 86 dB SPL, à raison de six heures par jour. Le premier groupe, rendu monaural avant le début de l'expérience, fut exposé pendant 36 jours. Le second groupe fut rendu monaural après 36 jours d'exposition puis subit une exposition additionnelle de 36 jours. Les seuils furent relevés deux fois par jour avec des intervalles de fréquence d'un quart d'octave de 0,125 à 16,0 kHz à l'aide d'une technique de renforcement positif, avant l'exposition, pendant l'exposition et pendant une durée de 100 jours après l'exposition. Après l'audiométrie comportementale, les cochlées furent préparées pour l'examen microscopique. Tous les sujets montraient une élévation de seuil initiale de 45-55 dB à des fréquences de test comprises dans le domaine des fréquences de stimulation (3,35 -

8,0 kHz); après 5 à 10 jours, les élévations de seuils commencèrent à décliner et l'on observa une récupération d'environ 20 dB au cours des 10 jours d'exposition suivants (25-35 dB d'élévation de seuil). Les seuils se stabilisèrent après environ 20 jours d'exposition aussi bien pour le groupe "36 jours" que pour le groupe "72 jours". De faibles déficits permanents furent observés, dans le domaine des fréquences de stimulation, pour les deux groupes d'animaux: 15 -20 dB pour l'exposition la plus courte et 20-25 dB pour la plus longue. Les cochlées exposées pendant 36 jours avaient des lésions faibles mais significatives dans le tour basal; celles exposées pendant 72 jours montraient des atteintes légèrement plus importantes.

Un groupe additionnel de chinchillas fut exposé à un OBN de 86 dB SPL centré sur 4,0 kHz pendant 144 jours. Le plan d'exposition était de 15 minutes par heure. Ces animaux furent rendus monauraux après les 72 premiers jours d'exposition. Les seuils d'audition étaient mesurés quotidiennement pendant la période d'exposition et jusqu'à stabilisation après la fin de cette période.

Les résultats de ces deux séries d'exposition à des bruits de fréquences élevées confirment le fait que l'oreille peut récupérer au cours d'une exposition intermittente au bruit et que des mesures de la fatigue auditive ne sont pas toujours de bons indicateurs des pertes auditives ou des lésions cochléaires ultérieures.

ACKNOWLEDGMENT

This work was supported by grants OH 02128 from the National Institutes for Occupational Safety and Health, and DC 00071 from the National Institute for Deafness and other Communication Disorders.

References

Bohne BA, Clark WW. Growth of hearing loss and cochlear lesion with increasing duration of noise exposure. In: Hamernik RP, Henderson D, Salvi R, eds. New perspectives on noise-induced hearing loss. New York: Raven Press, 1982:283.

Bohne BA, Zahn S, Bozzay D. Damage to the cochlea following interrupted exposure to low frequency noise. Ann Otol Rhinol Laryngol 1985; 94:122-130.

Bohne BA, Yohman L, Gruner MM. Cochlear damage following interrupted exposure to high-frequency noise. Hear Res 1987; 29:251-264.

Bredberg G. Cellular pattern and nerve supply of the human organ of Corti. Acta Otolaryngol Suppl 1968; 236:1-135.

Canlon B, Borg E, Flock Å. Protection against noise trauma by pre-exposure to a low level acoustic stimulus. Hear Res 1988; 34:197-200.

Canlon B, Borg E. Current findings on the functional and morphological aspects of the training phenomenon. Proceedings of the 4th International Conference on the Effects of Noise on the Auditory System, A. Dancer, ed., May 31-June 4, 1990, Beaune, France.

Clark WW, Bohne BA. Animal model for the 4 kHz tonal dip. Ann Otol Rhinol Laryngol 1978; 88(Suppl 51):pp. 1-16.

Clark WW, Bohne BA. Attenuation and protection provided by ossicular removal. J Acoust Soc Am 1987; 81:1093-1099.

Clark WW, Bohne BA, Boettcher FA. Effect of periodic rest on hearing loss and cochlear damage following exposure to noise. J Acoust Soc Am 1987; 82:1253-1264.

Clark WW, Clark CS, Moody DB, Stebbins WC. Noise-induced hearing loss in the chinchilla as determined by a positive reinforcement technique. J Acoust Soc Am 1974; 56:1202-1209.

Cody AR, Johnstone BM. Temporary threshold shift modified by binaural acoustic stimulation. Hear Res 1982; 6:199-206.

Eldredge DH, Covell WP, Gannon RP. Acoustic trauma following intermittent exposure to tones. Ann Otol Rhinol Laryngol 1959; 68:723-733.

Henderson D, Campo P, Subramanian M, Fiorino F. Development of resistance to noise. Proceedings of the 4th International Conference on the Effects of Noise on the Auditory System, A. Dancer, ed., May 31-June 4, 1990, Beaune, France.

Johnson DL, Nixon CW, Stephenson MR. Long-duration exposure to intermittent noises. Aviat Space Environ Med 1976; 47:987-990.

Miller JD, Watson CS, Covell WP. Deafening effects of noise on the cat. Acta Otolaryngol 1963; Suppl; 176:pp. 1-91.

Sataloff J, Sataloff RT, Menduke H, et al. Intermittent exposure to noise: Effects on hearing. Ann Otol Rhinol Laryngol 1983; 92:623-628.

Saunders JC, Mills JH, Miller JD. Threshold shift in the chinchilla from daily exposure to noise for six hours. J Acoust Soc Am 1977; 61:558-570.

Sinex DG, Clark WW, Bohne BA. Effect of periodic rest on physiological measures of auditory sensitivity following exposure to noise. J Acoust Soc Am 1987; 82:1265-1273.

Ward WD. Temporary threshold shift and damage-risk criteria for intermittent noise exposures. J Acoust Soc Am 1970; 48:561-574.

CHAPTER 40

Intermittent Noise and Equal Energy Hypothesis

PIERRE CAMPO
ROBERT R. LATAYE

In recent decades, exposure to intense noise has become an important occupational problem. Consequently, in most industrial settings, the need for prevention of noise-induced hearing loss is receiving ever increasing attention. One of the most important problems is to develop a practical indicator to estimate the auditory hazards encountered by noise-exposed employees. The Equal Energy Principle (EEP) has been proposed as a comprehensive strategy to rate the hazard of noise exposures over a wide range of exposure conditions. The EEP was initially proposed by Eldred et al (1955) and assumes that hearing damage is function of the total acoustic energy received. The EEP assumes a reciprocal trading relationship between the intensity of the noise and the duration of the exposure, the product of time and intensity being a measure of the total acoustic energy received. Hence, for the total energy to remain constant, the exposure intensity must decrease by 3 dB SPL for each doubling of the exposure duration. Thus, any interrupted noise exposure can be equated to the level of a continuous noise of equal energy, i.e., the equivalent continuous level (Leq).

The Leq is an attractive concept that can be incorporated with ease into instrumentation and into normalization rules, but there are some questions as to whether the Leq is a good indicator of the auditory hazard associated with fluctuating noise exposures. Indeed, most of the industrial exposures are not continuous, but rather intermittent or fluctuating. So it is important to determine if the Leq takes into account the effects of rest periods on auditory threshold shifts.

One approach to evaluating the EEP is to determine the amount of hearing loss or hair cell loss that occurs in an animal model after different noise exposures. The permanent threshold shift (PTS) is probably the most important single metric for evaluating the EEP. Although many noise-exposure studies have been carried out with animals, only a few of the studies have attempted to simulate acoustic conditions similar to those encountered in industry, i.e., interrupted noise exposures of moderate intensity emitted daily during at least 2 weeks (Sinex et al, 1987; Clark et al, 1987). By contrast, most studies of acoustic trauma have dealt with short exposure (a few minutes or a few hours) using high noise intensities, typically 110 dB and over (Buck and Franke, 1986; Cody and Johnstone, 1982; Sataloff et al., 1983; Goulios and Robertson, 1983). In such conditions, the cochlear injuries observed and the underlying mechanisms of hearing loss due to noise exposure could be different than those generated by a moderate-intensity exposure emitted over a long period of time. Moreover, the effect of intensity in the studies of Ward et al (1981) and Roberto et al (1985) showed that Leq, especially as it applies to impulse noises, is not a good indicator of the hazard of the noises (Henderson and Hamernik, 1978; Hamernik et al, 1980). Given the paucity of data, we felt that it was important to determine if 8-hour noise exposures at levels similar to those encountered in the work place (moderate intensity) would produce the same amount of hearing loss as shorter exposures of higher intensity. Hence, the primary goal of the present study was to find the sound pressure level of an 8-hour continuous noise that would generate a similar magnitude of PTS as that generated by a short continuous or intermittent noise with the same spectrum. If the EEP is an appropriate measure of hearing hazard, then the degree of hearing loss should be the same in groups of animals exposed to continuous and intermittent exposures with the same Leq. A second objective was to compare the amount of hearing loss with the levels of cochlear damage from two exposure schedules that had the same total acoustic energy, but a different temporal distribution, specifically short continuous noises versus intermittent noises.

Materials and Methods

Subjects

Subjects for these experiments were young, female, pigmented guinea pigs with melanotic eyes. All animals were at least 2 months old (400 to 500 g) at the start of the experiment and between 4 and 5 months old at the end of the experiment. The animals were selected on the basis of a preliminary audiologic test: Preyer reflex and direct observation of the outer ear.

Electrocochleography

Auditory thresholds were estimated using electrocochleography. The electrodes were implanted under anesthesia. A levomepromazine premedication (Nozinan, 2 mg per 100 g body weight) was administered a half an hour before the anesthesia. The ketamine anesthesia (Clorketam 1000, 15 mg per 100 g body weight) was administered by intraperitoneal injection. The core temperature of the animal was maintained at 38°C using a heating pad control system regulated with a rectal probe sensor.

A retroauricular incision of about 1.5 cm in length was made under sterile surgical conditions. The otic capsule was exposed by cutting through the connective tissue and the neck musculature. The recording electrode (insulated platinum wire) was inserted through a guide hole under visual control by way of an operating microscope. When the electrode tip was on the edge of the round window membrane, the electrode was anchored onto the otic capsule with dental cement (Taab 2000). The reference and ground electrodes were inserted onto the vertex of the animal's skull. The electrodes were connected to an electrical connector anchored to the skull by means of dental cement. With this technique, the compound action potential (CAP) can be recorded over a period of a least 3 months (Aran and Erre, 1979; Walger et al, 1985).

The audiometry was performed in an audiometric room (Amplisilence, G11). Awake animals were restrained in holders so that the audiometric tests were repeated under constant acoustic conditions. The sound stimuli were produced by a speaker (JBL 2405) positioned 15 cm from the pinna of the outer ear.

The stimulus used to elicit the CAP was trapezoidally gated (9 ms duration, linear rising and falling ramps of 1 ms). Each tone burst was repeated at a rate of 20 per second. To cancel the microphonic potential, a tone burst was emitted with a positive phase, the following one with a negative phase. The audiometry test was always performed in the following order: 2, 3, 4, 5, 6, 8, 10, 12, 16 kHz.

The CAP threshold was averaged (N = 256) to enhance the signal-to-noise ratio. CAP magnitude was measured from baseline to the bottom of the first negative deflection (N_1). The CAP N_1 was measured by decreasing the intensity of the tone bursts to obtain a wave magnitude of 8 μV.

Noise Exposure

The awake animals were exposed in an open field acoustic chamber (340 × 340 × 250 cm). Four loudspeakers were placed in the corners of the acoustic chamber, 120 cm in front of the wire mesh cages (individual cage: 35 × 25 × 21 cm). The cages were positioned at the center of the acoustic chamber. Each subject was housed in a separate cage during the entire exposure period. During the noise exposure, the animals were not restricted and they had free access to food and water. No feeding problems were observed.

The noise was a ⅓-octave band centered at 8 kHz (8 kHz, ⅓ OBN). The center frequency of the noise was chosen to generate noise-induced hearing loss in the cochlear partition area where auditory sensitivity is the best. The spectrum of the noise is shown in Figure 40-1. The sound pressure level of the noise was checked inside the individual cages and was found to vary by 1 dB or less within the cages. Moreover, the exposure cages were rotated to ensure equivalent exposure to all animals. The exposure period lasted 14 days for all noise exposure conditions.

Experimental Paradigm

Two weeks after the electrode implantation, the CAP N_1 thresholds (T_1) were mea-

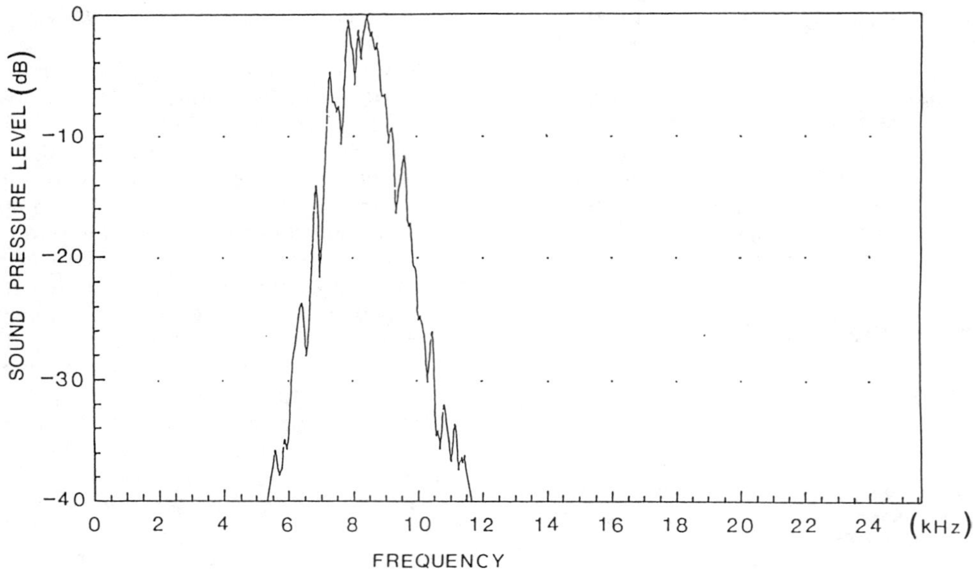

Figure 40-1 Relative amplitude of the spectrum acoustic of the exposure. Analysis bandwidth of 32 Hz.

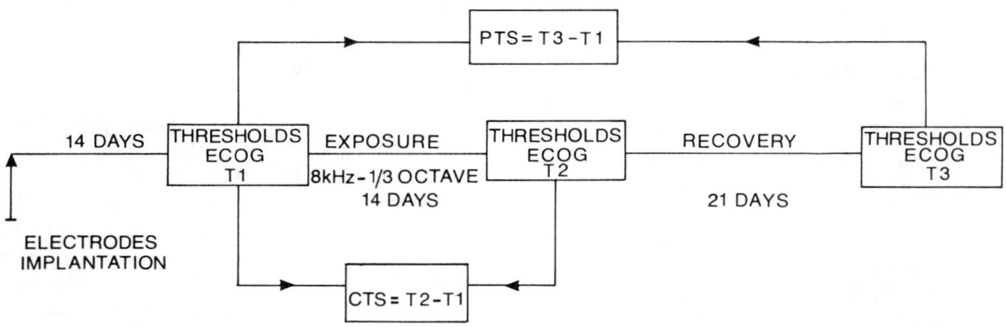

Figure 40-2 Experimental paradigm to measure the permanent threshold shift (PTS). T1, T2 correspond to the audiograms. T1, Pre-exposure threshold; T2, Threshold measured after the exposure period; T3, Threshold measured 21 days following exposure; ECoG, Electrocochleography; CTS, Compound threshold shift.

sured. The animals were exposed to 8-kHz, ⅓ OBN for 14 days, 8 hours per day. After the exposure, CAP N_1 thresholds were remeasured (T_2). The difference ($T_2 - T_1$) corresponds to the CTS (compound threshold shift). Electrocochleographic measures were performed every day during the recovery period in order to determine the daily threshold shifts and to determine the PTS value in our experimental paradigm. A recovery period of 21 days was considered more than sufficient to measure the PTS (Buck and Franke, 1986; Cody and Johnstone, 1982; Cody and Robertson, 1983; Mills, 1973; Syka and Popelar, 1980). The last audiogram (T_3) was carried out 21 days after the exposure. The difference $T_3 - T_1$ corresponds to the PTS.

A representation of the experimental paradigm is shown in Figure 40-2. Groups of guinea pigs (n_x = number of animals) were sound exposed (8 kHz, ⅓ OBN) for 8 hours at sound pressure levels of 85 dB ($n_1 = 18$), 87.5 dB ($n_2 = 13$), 90 dB ($n_3 = 14$), or 95 dB ($n_4 = 17$). The magnitude of PTS measured 21 days after exposure was related to the sound pressure level of the continuous 8-hour exposure period.

Four other groups of animals were exposed daily for 14 days to four different noises (8 kHz, ⅓ OBN) with the same Leq value of 92 dB. We chose a 92-dB Leq to use the linear part, and only the linear part, of the function relating PTS to Leq obtained with the 8-hour noise exposures. One group ($n_5 = 15$) was

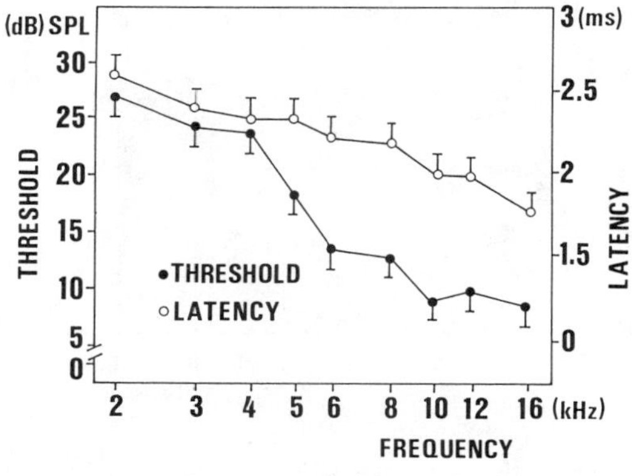

Figure 40-3 Pre-exposure mean thresholds (n = 29, filled circles) and latencies (open circles) of N_1 CAP as a function of frequency. The N_1 threshold was a visual detection level of 8 μV magnitude from N_1 to the baseline potential. The bars represent half of the 95 percent confidence intervals.

exposed continuously for 4 hours at 95 dB. A second group (n_6 = 12) was exposed to an intermittent noise for 8 hours with the following noise/rest schedule: a 2-minute noise at 95 dB followed by a 2-minute rest period. A third group (n_7 = 23) was exposed to a 48-minute noise at 102 dB. The fourth group (n_8 = 12) was exposed for 8 hours to an intermittent noise in which a 2-minute noise at 102 dB was followed by an 18-minute rest period.

Results

Electrocochleography

The mean thresholds and the 95 percent confidence interval for normal N_1 thresholds calculated with 29 guinea pigs are shown in Figure 40-3. There was little interanimal variation in threshold over the range 2 to 16 kHz. The most sensitive region in the pigmented guinea pig audiogram was from 8 to 16 kHz, with decreasing sensitivity for the frequencies below this range.

Recovery After the Exposures of 85, 87.5, 90, and 95 dB SPL

Figure 40-4 shows the recovery of CTS after the continuous noise exposures. In general, the maximum recovery was observed at the most damaged frequencies, ½ octave above the center frequency of the noise exposure. The data from the 85-dB group showed the greatest recovery. By contrast, the data from the highest level (95 dB) showed the least recovery. Following the exposure at 85 dB, the guinea pig's ear recovered 15 dB at 10 to 12 kHz by the fifth day. After the fifth day, the threshold shift showed little recovery. The lack of recovery suggests that the thresholds measured at 21 days after exposure can be used to estimate the PTS without making a large error.

PTS After the Exposures of 85, 87.5, 90, and 95 dB SPL

The mean PTS values are shown in Figure 40-5. The greatest variation in the threshold between the four different exposures occurred above 8 kHz. The peak losses occurred in the 10 to 12 kHz frequency range, or approximately half an octave above the exposure frequency. For instance, with the 95-dB exposure, the maximum magnitude of the PTS (PTS max) was 40.5 dB around 10 to 12 kHz. At the 90-dB exposure, the PTS max was 33 dB around 10 to 12 kHz. At the 87.5 dB exposure, the PTS max was 27 dB at 10 kHz. At the 85-dB exposure, the PTS max was 9.5 dB at 10 kHz. Note that the PTS measured at the 8-kHz frequency was relatively low: 0 dB at 85 dB, 9 dB at 87.5 dB, 18 dB at 90 dB, and 26 dB at 95 dB exposure level. Data for the test frequencies below 8 kHz show no evidence of threshold shift.

Figure 40-6 shows the mean PTS at 8, 10, 12, and 16 kHz as a function of exposure level (85, 87.5, 90, 95 dB SPL) for the 8-hour continuous noise (8 kHz, ⅓ OBN). With the aid of the four curves in Figure 40-5 we are able to find the sound pressure level of an 8-hour continuous noise that generates the same amount of PTS as a short-duration continuous or intermittent noise.

Nocivity of the Four Noises with the Same Leq Value: 92 dB

Short, Continuous Noises

Figure 40-7 shows the PTS as a function of frequency for a 4-hour exposure of 95 dB SPL (n_5 = 15) and a 48-minute exposure of 102 dB SPL (n_6 = 12). The PTS magnitudes generated by the 4-hour continuous noise at 95 dB were consistent with the EEP because the values 18.2, 32.1, 33.9, and 29.4 dB at 8, 10, 12, and 16 kHz, respectively, correspond to the PTS generated by an 8-hour continuous expo-

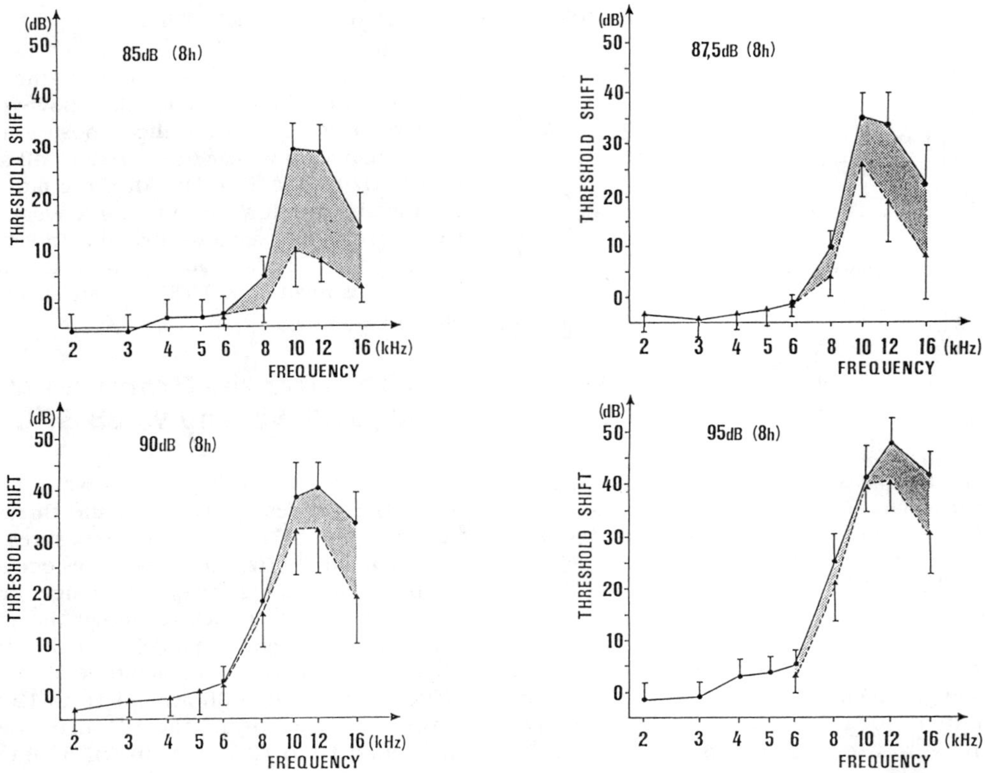

Figure 40-4 Mean threshold shifts (TSs) as a function of test frequency. Permanent threshold shift (PTS) was measured 21 days after a 14-day exposure to a ⅓ OBN centered at 8 kHz. Bars represents half of the 95 percent confidence interval. The triangles represent the PTS values; the circles represent the compound threshold shift (CTS) values. The exposure levels were 85 (n_1 = 18), 87.5 (n_2 = 13), 90 (n_3 = 14) or 95 dB SPL (n_4 = 17).

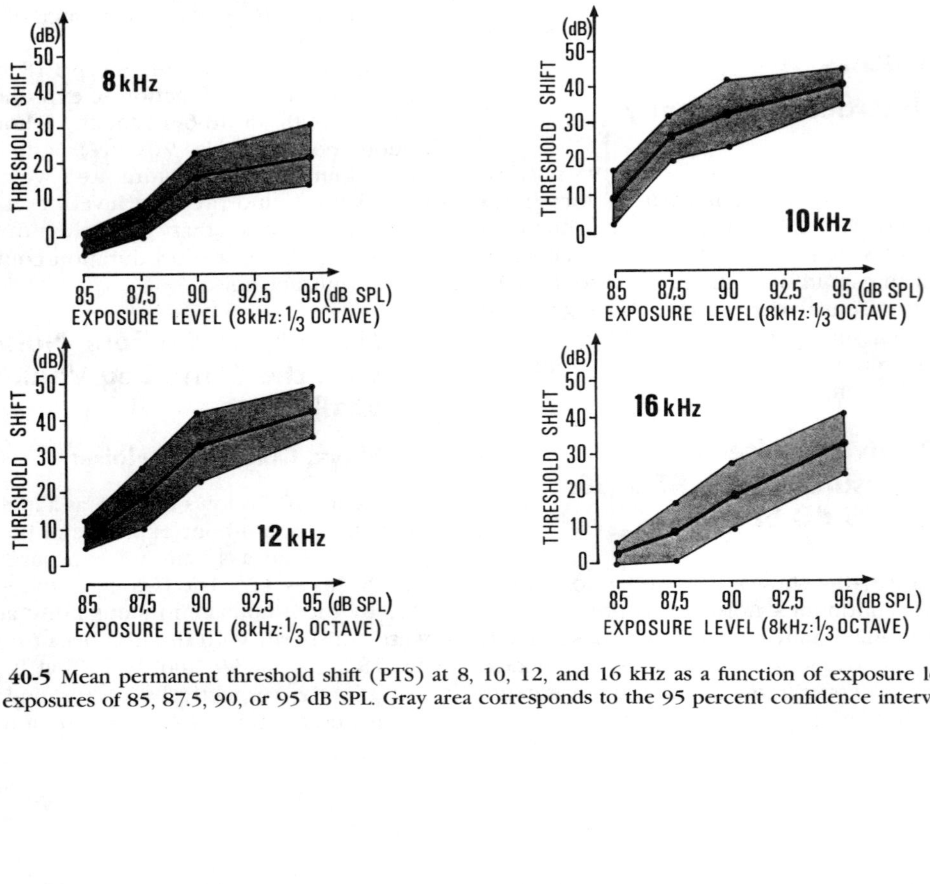

Figure 40-5 Mean permanent threshold shift (PTS) at 8, 10, 12, and 16 kHz as a function of exposure level for 8-hour exposures of 85, 87.5, 90, or 95 dB SPL. Gray area corresponds to the 95 percent confidence interval.

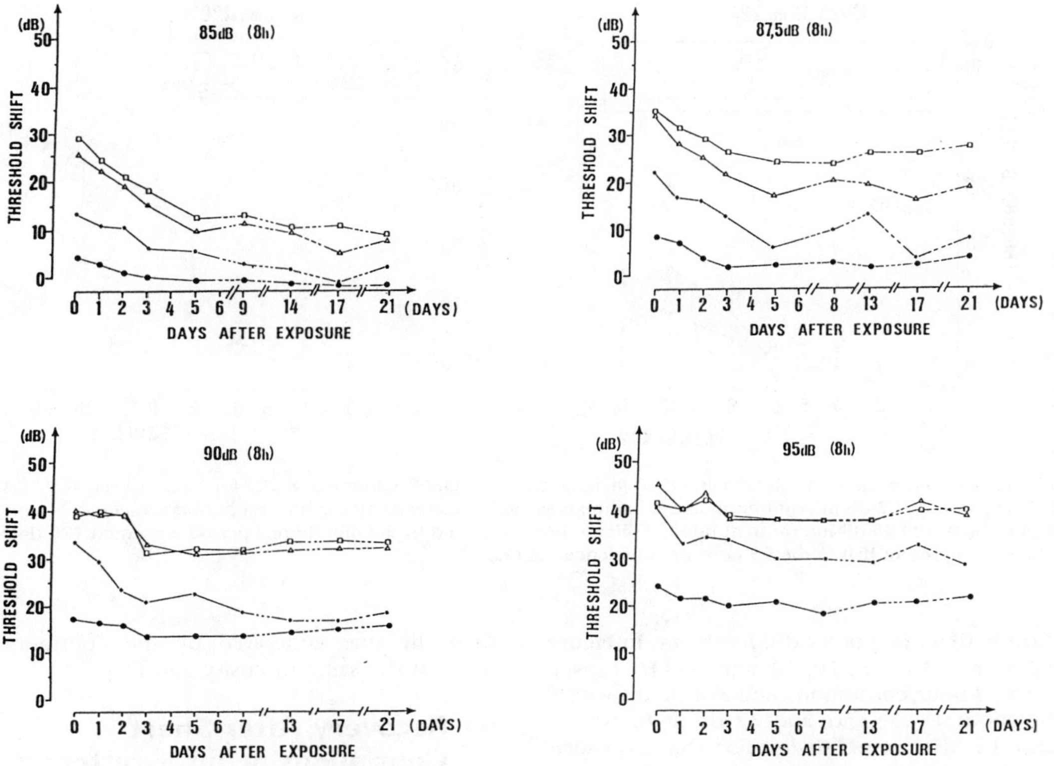

Figure 40-6 Recovery of threshold after a 14-day exposure to a ⅓ OBN centered at 8 kHz. Each noise lasts 8 hours daily. Circles, 8 kHz; squares, 10 kHz; triangles, 12 kHz; stars, 16 kHz.

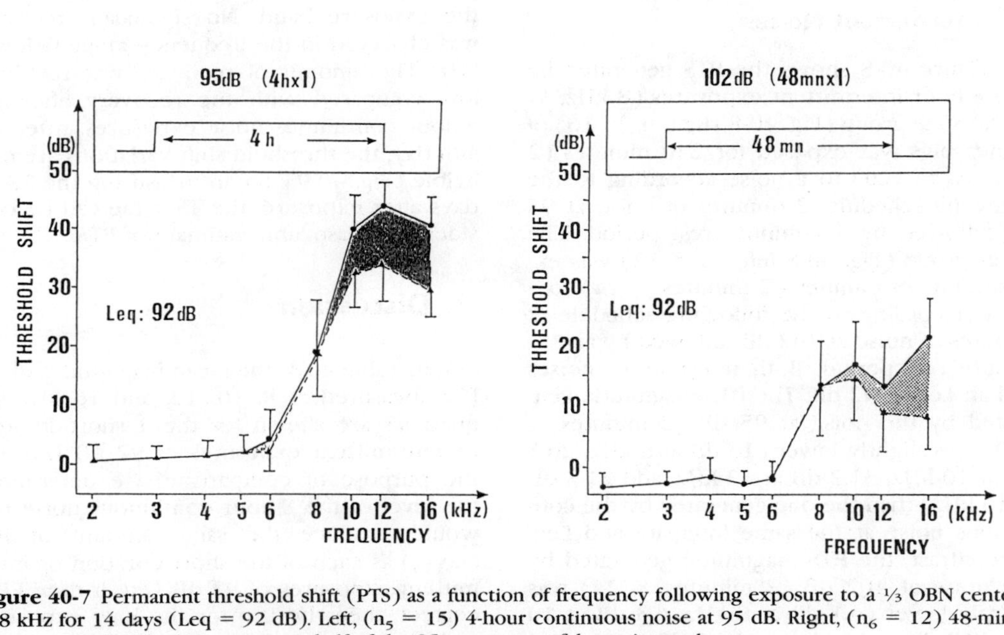

Figure 40-7 Permanent threshold shift (PTS) as a function of frequency following exposure to a ⅓ OBN centered at 8 kHz for 14 days (Leq = 92 dB). Left, (n_5 = 15) 4-hour continuous noise at 95 dB. Right, (n_6 = 12) 48-minute noise at 102 dB. The bars represent half of the 95 percent confidence interval.

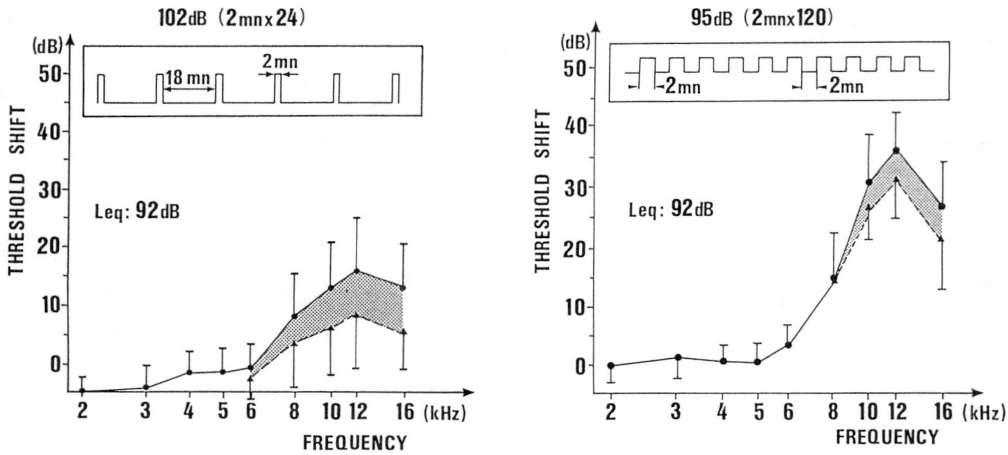

Figure 40-8 Permanent threshold shift (PTS) generated by a ⅓ OBN centered at 8 kHz for 14 days (Leq = 92 dB). Left, (n_6 = 16) 102-dB intermittent noise: 2-minute noise followed by an 18-minute rest period presented 24 times. Right, (n_8 = 12) 95 dB intermittent noise: 2-minute noise followed by a 2-minute rest period presented 120 times. The bars represent half of the 95 percent confidence intervals.

sure with an Leq of 92 dB. As shown in Figure 40-6, the PTS at 8, 10, 12, and 16 kHz caused by an 8-hour continuous noise of 92 dB would be about 18, 35, 36, and 22 dB at 8, 10, 12, and 16 kHz, respectively. For this exposure, the Leq is a reasonable predictor of acoustic trauma. The PTS generated by the 48-minute continuous noise at 102 dB was relatively low. The PTS max was about 13 to 15 dB at 8 to 10 kHz. In this case, the Leq overestimates the hazards for a 48-minute exposure of 102 dB.

Intermittent Noises

Figure 40-8 shows the PTS generated by two 8-hour intermittent exposures (8 kHz, ⅓ OBN). One group (Fig. 40-8 right, n_6 = 16) of guinea pigs was exposed for 240 minutes (2 minutes × 120) to a noise according to the following schedule: 2 minutes of noise at 95 dB followed by a 2-minute rest period. The other group (Fig. 40-8 left, n_8 = 12) was exposed for 48 minutes (2 minutes × 24) to a noise according to the following schedule: 2 minutes of noise at 102 dB followed by an 18-minute rest period. Both intermittent noises had an Leq of 92 dB. The PTS magnitude generated by the noise at 95 dB (2 minutes × 120) was slightly lower (16 dB at 8 kHz, 26.5 dB at 10 kHz, 31.2 dB at 12 kHz, and 21.3 dB at 16 kHz) than the one generated by the continuous noise at the same intensity and Leq. By contrast, the PTS magnitude generated by the noise at 102 dB (2 minutes × 24) was sharply lower (4.1 dB at 8 kHz, 6.3 dB at 10 kHz, 8.2 dB at 12 kHz, and 6.7 dB at 16 kHz) than the one generated by the continuous noise at the same intensity and Leq.

Recovery After Short Continuous or Intermittent Exposures

Figure 40-9 shows CTS as a function of recovery time. The maximum amount of recovery occurred at the most damaged frequencies, ½ octave above the center frequency of the exposure band. No significant recovery was observed in the frequency range below 8 kHz. The amount of recovery was relatively low compared with the recovery after the 8-hour continuous noise exposures. After the fifth day, the threshold shift variations are negligible (Fig. 40-9). So, in measuring the TS 21 days after exposure, the TS value can be considered a reasonable estimate of PTS.

Discussion

In Table 40-1, the mean magnitudes of the PTS measured at 8, 10, 12, and 16 kHz frequencies are shown for the 4 short-duration or intermittent exposures of 92 dB Leq. For the purpose of comparison, we determined the level of the 8-hour continuous noise that would produce the same amount of PTS (Le_{PTS}) as each of the short duration or intermittent exposures of 92 dB Leq. If the EEP is correct, then the Leq for the long exposures and the Le_{PTS} for the short and fluctuating

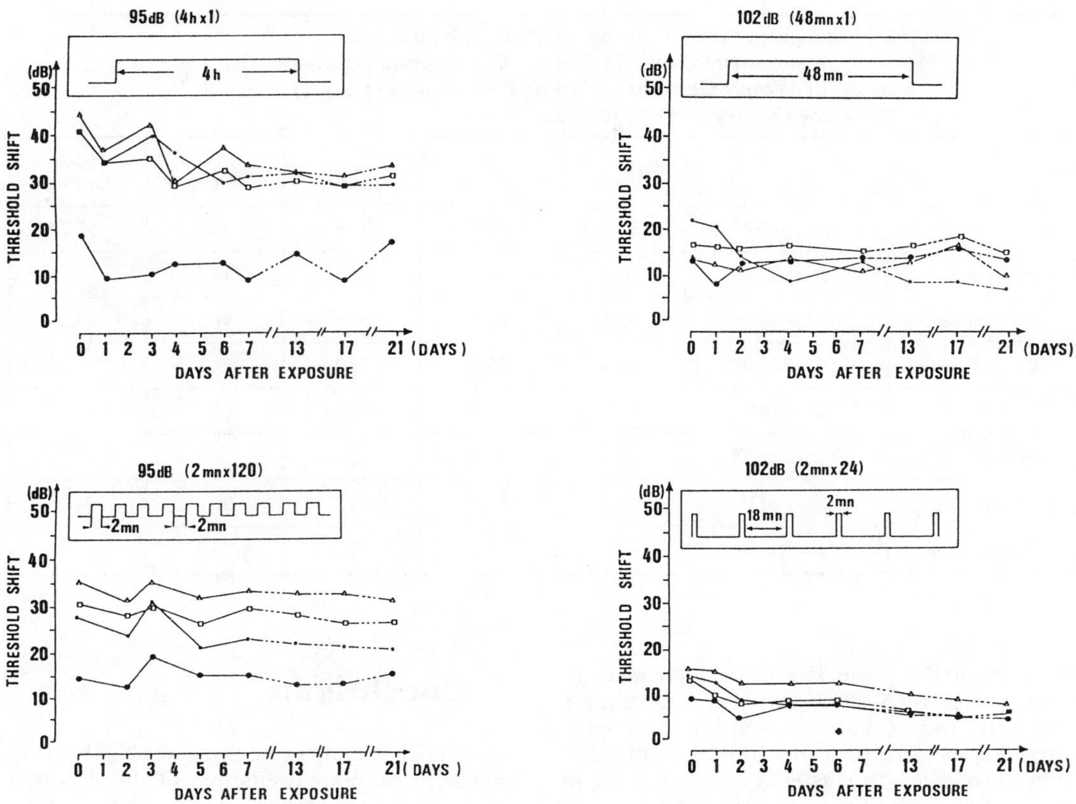

Figure 40-9 Recovery of threshold following exposure to a ⅓ OBN centered at 8 kHz. Upper left, 240 minutes × 1 at 95 dB; upper right, 48 minutes × 1 at 102 dB; lower left, 2 minutes × 120 at 95 dB; lower right, 2 minutes × 24 at 102 dB; Circles, 8 kHz; squares, 10 kHz; triangles, 12 kHz; stars, 16 kHz.

noise exposures should all be the same. Futhermore, the Le_{PTS} for such exposures should also be the same.

Table 40-1 shows that the Le_{PTS} values for short and fluctuating noise exposures differed by as much as 6 dB (2 minutes × 24) of the Leq value of 92 dB, except for the 240-minute exposure of 95 dB, in which the value of the Le_{PTS} is 92.2 dB, very close to the theoretical value of Leq—92 dB.

In light of the present study, the Leq_{8h} appears to overestimate the PTS from short-duration continuous (48 minutes at 102 dB) and intermittent noise exposures (2 minutes × 24 at 102 dB; 2 minutes × 120 at 95 dB). According to the EEP, the mean magnitudes of the PTS presented in Table 40-1 would be produced by 8-hour exposure levels lower than those actually used for the present exposures. In spite of the generally negative findings related to the EEP, the concept does appear to have some predictive value for moderate-intensity noises emitted during a relatively long period (4-hour exposure at 95 dB). This point is in agreement with the findings of Martin et al (1970) and Atherley and Martin (1971) who, however, worked on the effects of impulse noises. Whatever the nature of moderate-intensity noises tested in this present study, the Leq has the advantage of assuming overprotection for employees' ears. From a practical standpoint, the Leq affords a safe means of estimating the hazard of short-duration, moderate-intensity noise exposures that are continuous or intermittent. According to the literature (Henderson and Hamernik, 1986; Roberto et al, 1985; Ward et al, 1981), the EEP might be also appropriate for impact noises at lower intensities; however, above a "critical intensity" of 115 to 119 dB, the amount of damage increases significantly enough that the EEP would be inappropriate for high-level exposures.

Concerning the effect of the distribution of the temporal noise or the rests on hearing, our data indicate that the 95-dB intermittent exposures (2 minutes × 120) produce slightly less PTS than the 95-dB short, continuous ex-

TABLE 40-1 **PTS Magnitudes Generated by the Intermittent and Short Continuous Noises and 8-Hour Continuous Noise Levels that Would Generate Similar PTS Values (Le $_{PTS}$) at the Most Damaged Frequencies**

		8 kHz	10 kHz	12 kHz	16 kHz	Means Le PTS
Leq 92 dB 95 dB 240 min × 1	Le_{PTS} (dB)	93.0	90.7	91.5	93.4	92.2
	PTS value (dB)	18.2	32.1	33.9	29.4	
Leq 92 dB 95 dB 2 min × 120	Le_{PTS} (dB)	89.7	87.8	89.6	91.0	89.5
	PTS value (dB)	16.0	26.5	31.2	21.3	
Leq 92 dB 102 dB 48 min × 1	Le_{PTS} (dB)	89.3	85.8	85.2	87.7	87
	PTS value (dB)	13.4	14.7	8.5	7.9	
Leq 92 dB 102 dB 2 min × 24	Le_{PTS} (dB)	87.3	84.7	85.2	86.6	86
	PTS value (dB)	4.1	6.3	8.2	6.7	

posures of the same intensity and equal energy (Le_{PTS} 89.5 dB versus Le_{PTS} 92.2 dB). Similarly, the 102-dB intermittent exposures produce less PTS than the 102-dB continuous noise (Le_{PTS} 86 dB versus Le_{PTS} 87 dB). So, in agreement with the results of Sataloff et al (1983) and Clark et al (1987), the intermittent noise exposures cause less damage to hearing than continuous noise exposures of the same intensity and equal energy. The slight reduction in PTS could be partly explained by the fact that the auditory system has time to recover between the noise phases. Thus, the cochlea does not seem to react to noise as a passive receptor, but instead may profit from a rest period to recover from hearing fatigue and to improve its resistance. Basically, the interstimulus interval is an important variable that, by definition, the EEP fails to take into consideration.

Moreover, recent findings allow us to think that an intracochlear mechanism would be able to protect the cochlea against intermittent or short continuous noises at high intensities. Such a phenomenon could be controlled by the crossed olivocochlear bundle (COCB) (Bonfils et al, 1986; Brown, 1988; Brown et al, 1983; Puel et al, 1988a,b; Siegel and Kim, 1982). These particular studies show a decrease of the inner hair cell potentials (Brown et al, 1983) and a punctual modification of cochlear mechanics (Guinan, 1986; Siegel and Kim, 1982). It is not yet clear whether the protection afforded by the COCB could be effective for long-lasting exposures.

Conclusions

The EEP and, more specifically, the Leq, appear to be poor predictors of the PTS that results from moderate-intensity, short-duration continuous and intermittent noise exposures. However, the error in the prediction of acoustic hazards is consistent with the protection of employees. Indeed, for the intermittent or short-duration continuous exposures, the Leq overestimates the encountered hearing hazards. At the same acoustic energy, the effects of rest periods seem to allow for exposures with higher levels of noise. If the duration of the recovery period partly could explain the better cochlear resistance to these particular noises, the role of the efferent system could give us new insights into the phenomenon of cochlear resistance.

Exposition Intermittente et Principe d'Isoénergie

Dans le milieu industriel, la prévention des pertes auditives engendrées par le bruit reçoit une attention toujours croissante. Un des problèmes importants est de disposer d'un indicateur pratique pour estimer le risque de lésion cochléaire encouru par le personnel exposé au bruit.

Le Leq_{8h}, basé sur le principe d'égale énergie, est utilisé comme critère d'exposition

	Nombre d'animaux	Niveau (dB SPL)	Durée/8 h		Cycles/jour	Leq_{8h} (dB)	Nocivité équivalente (dB)
			Bruit	silence			
G_1	15	95	4 h	4 h	1	92	92,2
G_2	12	95	2 mn	2 mn	120	92	89,5
G_3	23	102	48 mn	442 mn	1	92	87,0
G_4	12	102	2 mn	18 mn	24	92	86,0

pour prédire le traumatisme acoustique. En utilisant ce principe, Clark et al. (1987) et Sinex et al. (1987) ont montré que la nocivité des bruits continus est supérieure à celle des bruits intermittents. La surestimation de la nocivité des bruits intermittents par le Leq n'est cependant pas bien connue et le but de la présente étude est de la quantifier.

Des cobayes tricolores ont été exposés dans un champ acoustique homogène, à un bruit de bande d'un tiers d'octave centrée sur 8 kHz. La durée d'exposition était de 14 jours. Les amplitudes des déplacements permanents des seuils ont été mesurées à l'aide d'une technique électrophysiologique chronique, 21 jours après l'exposition.

Quatre groupes d'animaux (G_1 à G_4) ont été exposés selon le plan expérimental présenté dans le tableau.

Par ailleurs, quatre autres groupes d'animaux ont été exposés à des bruits de 85 - 87,5 - 90 et 95dB pendant 8 heures par jour. Les courbes des PTS en fonction du niveau d'exposition ont été utilisées pour déterminer le niveau du bruit continu de "Nocivité équivalente" (tableau I). La comparaison des amplitudes des PTS engendrés par les expositions, aux bruits de 8 heures, aux bruits continus de courte durée (4 h et 48 mn) et aux bruits intermittents, montre que, excepté pour le bruit de 4h, le Leq_{8h} surestime la nocivité des bruits continus de courte durée et intermittents. En effet, pour les bruits intermittents (G_2 et G_4), les "nocivités équivalentes" respectives sont 89,5 et 86 dB alors qu'elles sont de 87 et 92,2 dB pour les bruits continus de courte durée émis avec la même énergie acoustique (tableau I).

Pour l'exposition continue de 4 h à 95 dB SPL, le Leq_{8h} (92 dB) semble un bon indicateur puisque le niveau de bruit continu de nocivité équivalente est d'environ 92 dB. La meilleure résistance de la cochlée aux bruits intermittents ou continus de faible durée peut s'expliquer en partie par la durée de la période de récupération mais le rôle du système efférent pourrait apporter un nouvel éclairage sur les phénomènes de résistance cochléaire.

ACKNOWLEDGMENTS

We wish to thank Dr. Richard J. Salvi and Dr. Donald Henderson for their ideas, criticisms and supporting discussions, and for their help in writing this paper.

References

Aran JM, Erre JP. Long-term recording of cochlea-neural potentials in the guinea pig. In: Beagley HA, ed. Auditory investigation: The scientific and technological basis. Oxford: Oxford University Press, 1979:233.

Atherley GRC, Martin AM. Equivalent continuous noise level as a measure of injury from impact and impulse noise. Ann Occup Hyg 1971; 14:11-19.

Bonfils P, Remond MC, Pujol R. Efferent tracts and cochlear frequency selectivity. Hear Res 1986; 24:277-283.

Brown AM. Continuous low level sound alters cochlear mechanics: An efferent effect? Hear Res 1988; 34:27-38.

Brown MC, Nuttall AL, Masta RI. Intracellular recordings from cochlear inner hair cells: Effects of stimulation of the crossed olivocochlear efferents. Science 1983; 222:69-72.

Buck K, Franke R. Can TTS be an indicator for individual susceptibility to PTS? In: Salvi R, Henderson D, Hamernik RP, Colletti V, eds. Basic and applied aspects of noise-induced hearing loss. New York: Plenum Press. 1986; 441-456. Published in cooperation with NATO Scientific Affairs Division.

Clark WW, Bohne B, Boettcher FA. Effect of periodic rest on hearing loss and cochlear damage following exposure to noise. J Acoust Soc Am 1987; 82:1253-1264.

Cody AR, Johnstone BM. Reduced temporary and permanent hearing losses with multiple tone exposures. Hear Res 1982; 6:291-301.

Cody AR, Robertson D. Variability of noise induced damage in the guinea pig cochlea: Electrophysiological and morphological correlates after strictly controlled exposures. Hear Res 1983; 9:71-78.

Eldred KM, Gannon W, von Gierke HE. Criteria for short time exposure of personnel to high intensity jet aircraft noise. W.A.D.C. TN, Aero Space Medical Lab A.F.B., 1955:55-355.

Goulios H, Robertson D. Noise-induced cochlear damage assessed using electrophysiological criteria: An examination of the equal energy principle. Hear Res 1983; 11:327-341.

Guinan JJ. Effect of efferent neural activity on cochlear mechanics. Scand Audiol Suppl 1986; 25:53-62.

Hamernik RP, Henderson D, Salvi RJ. Contribution of animal studies to our understanding of impulse noise. Scand Audiol Suppl 1980; 12:128-146.

Henderson D, Hamernik RP. Impulse noise-induced hearing loss. In: Lipscomb DM, ed. Noise and audiology. Baltimore: University Park Press, 1978:143.

Henderson D, Hamernik RP. Impulse noise: Critical review. J Acoust Soc Am 1986; 80:569-584.

Martin AM, Atherley GRC, Hempstock TI. Recurrent impact noise from pneumatic hammers. Ann Occup Hyg 1970; 13:59-67.

Mills JH. Temporary and permanent threshold shifts produced by nine-day exposures to noise. J Speech Hear Res 1973; 16:426-438.

Puel JL, Bobbin RP, Fallon M. The active process is affected first by intense sound exposure. Hear Res 1988a; 37:65-71.

Puel JL, Bobbin RP, Fallon M. An ipsi-lateral cochlear efferent loop protects the cochlea during intense sound exposure. Hear Res 1988b; 37:65-71.

Roberto M, Hamernik RP, Salvi RJ, et al. Impact noise and the equal energy hypothesis. J Acoust Soc Am 1985; 77:1514-1520.

Sataloff J, Sataloff RT, Menduke H, et al. Intermittent exposure to noise: Effects on hearing. Ann Otol Rhinol Laryngol 1983; 92:623-628.

Siegel JH, Kim DO. Efferent neural control of cochlear mechanics? Olivocochlear bundle stimulation affects cochlear biomechanical nonlinearity. Hear Res 1982; 6:171-182.

Sika J, Popelar J. Hearing threshold shifts from prolonged exposure to noise in guinea pigs. Hear Res 1980; 3:205-213.

Sinex DG, Clark WW, Bohne B. Effect of periodic rest on physiological measures of auditory sensitivity following exposure to noise. J Acoust Soc Am 1987; 82:1265-1273.

Walger M, Schmiedt U, von Wedel H. The influence of moderate-intensity noise on the compound action potential evoked by tone bursts in the guinea pig, Cavia porcellus. Hear Res 1985; 19:143-149.

Ward WD, Duvall AJ, Santi PA, Turner C. Total energy and critical intensity concepts in noise damage. Ann Otolaryngol 1981; 90:584-590.

CHAPTER 41

Individual Variability of Noise-Induced Hearing Loss

ERIK BORG
BARBARA CANLON
BERIT ENGSTRÖM

Individual variability in noise-induced permanent threshold shift (NIPTS) has been a puzzle and a nuisance for the researcher as well as those responsible for occupational noise environments and individual risk evaluation. There are numerous possible sources for the observed variability; some of these sources are listed in Table 41-1.

To address the problem of variability, a series of experiments were performed in the same animal species (the small chinchilla rabbit), with a specified set of exposure and recording conditions. The aim of the present study was to describe and analyze the individual variability of NIPTS in rabbits, specifically:

1. To determine the dependence of hearing loss on the level of a standardized exposure noise
2. To determine individual variability under different exposure conditions
3. To assess the relative contribution of measurement error with respect to threshold determination
4. To determine whether individual variability was stable or varied with time
5. To study the nature of possible fluctuations in susceptibility over time

Material and Methods

Animals

Adult rabbits of the small chinchilla strain of both sexes were used. The animals were in the age range 3 to 10 months at the time of exposure. Between tests they were kept in a quiet animal room with free access to food and water.

Hearing Threshold Determination

Frequency-specific electrophysiologic auditory thresholds were obtained using the auditory brain-stem response (ABR). The technique has been described in detail earlier (Borg and Engström, 1983, 1989). Thresholds were obtained at 0.5, 1.0, 2.0, 3.15, 4.0, 6.3, 8.0, 12.5, 16.0, and 20.0 kHz with narrow-band-filtered single, full-cycle sine waves. The average of 2,000 epochs with a time window of 10 or 15 ms was evaluated for threshold determination.

Noise Exposure

Four different exposure conditions were used:

A. Long-term, binaural sound-field exposure
B. Short-term and high-level, unilateral sound-field exposure
C. Short-term, monaural exposure with a closed delivery system
D. Short-term, monaural exposure with a closed delivery system fitted with an ear canal microphone

The sound-field exposures (A and B) have been described earlier (Engström and Borg, 1981; Borg and Engström, 1989). The animals

TABLE 41-1 **Sources of Individual Variability of Noise-Induced Permanent Threshold Shift**

1. Inaccurate or inappropriate description of the exposure noise
2. Individual variation of performance at the work place leading to individually different exposures in individual ears—variation in quantity and quality of ear protector use
3. The sound transmission system of the ear canal, middle ear, and stapedius muscle function, including pathologic middle-ear conditions
4. Specific susceptibility of the critical structures and processes in the inner-ear (e.g., hair cell sensory hairs, supporting cells, blood vessels, membranes)
5. Physiologic factors influencing the function of the inner ear, e.g., blood flow, sympathetic innervation, efferent innervation, hormones, and endolymphatic and perilymphatic physiology
6. Other causes of hearing loss, e.g., infections, toxic substances, drugs, and spontaneous inner-ear degeneration due to heredity or aging
7. Interaction with other ergonomic factors such as work load, vibration, temperature, toxic substances, and radiation
8. Errors in determination of hearing threshold; hearing threshold is an inadequate and incomplete measure of the physiologic and morphologic damage actually present

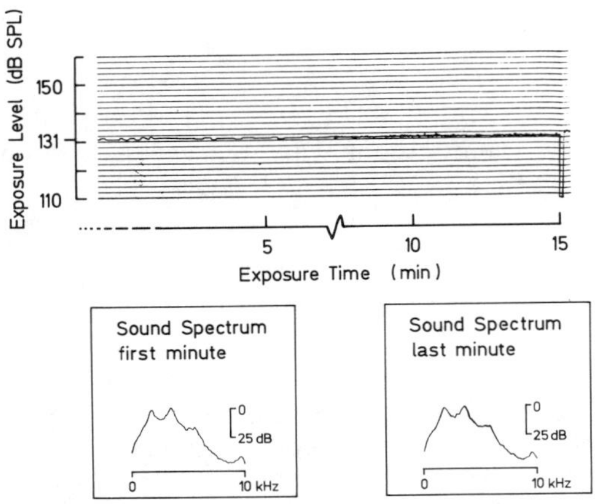

Figure 41-1 Closed exposure system with electret microphone control. Continuous recording of exposure-noise level (top) and spectrum in the ear canal of an awake animal exposed at 131 dB SPL.

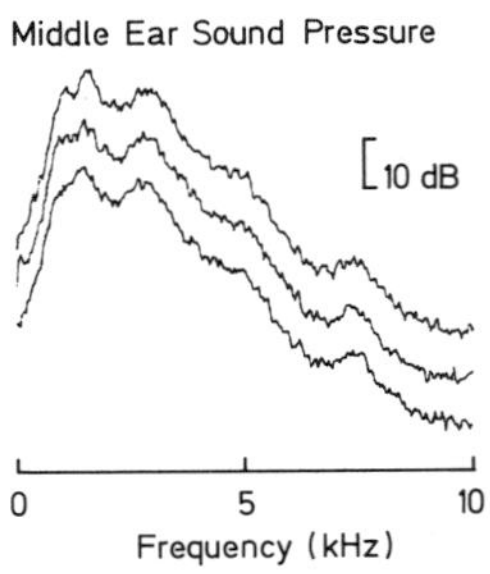

Figure 41-2 Spectrum of the exposure noise obtained with a probe microphone sealed to the middle ear of a freshly-killed animal. The different curves are obtained at repeated replacements of the exposure ear phone. They are displayed with a 10-dB vertical shift.

were exposed in a large box for 512 hours at 85 dB SPL (condition A) or in a small box for 30 minutes at 115 dB SPL (condition B). Both ears were exposed in condition A, whereas one ear was plugged in condition B. Maximum noise energy was between 2 and 7 kHz in both cases. In both conditions, sound level varied within a maximal range of 3 to 4 dB.

The closed acoustic system (conditions C and D) consisted of an Oticon Power body-worn hearing-aid telephone connected to a 4-cm tube. The tube was anchored to the ear canal and sealed with Xantoprene. In condition D, a Knowles electret microphone was embedded in the proximal end of the tube, near the eardrum. The exposure noise was generated by a General Radio 1385 noise generator and a Fonema attenuator-amplifier. The level and spectrum of the noise are illustrated in Figure 41-1, which shows a continuous level recording during the exposure and the spectrum obtained with the electret microphone at the beginning and at the end of the exposure. Figure 41-2 shows the spectrum obtained with a probe microphone introduced into the ear canal of a freshly killed animal. The stability, as well as the frequency of maximum energy, is illustrated.

Results

Dependence on Sound Level

The growth of loss of ABR threshold as a function of increasing exposure noise level is shown in Figure 41-3. Figure 41-3A shows the average audiograms of groups of 10 to 20 ears exposed with the closed system for 15 minutes between 122 and 137 dB SPL. With exposures of 122 and 125 dB the threshold loss exceeds 10 dB at only one frequency. At levels of 128 dB and higher, the threshold loss is significant and increases in proportion to the exposure level. The frequency for maximum loss

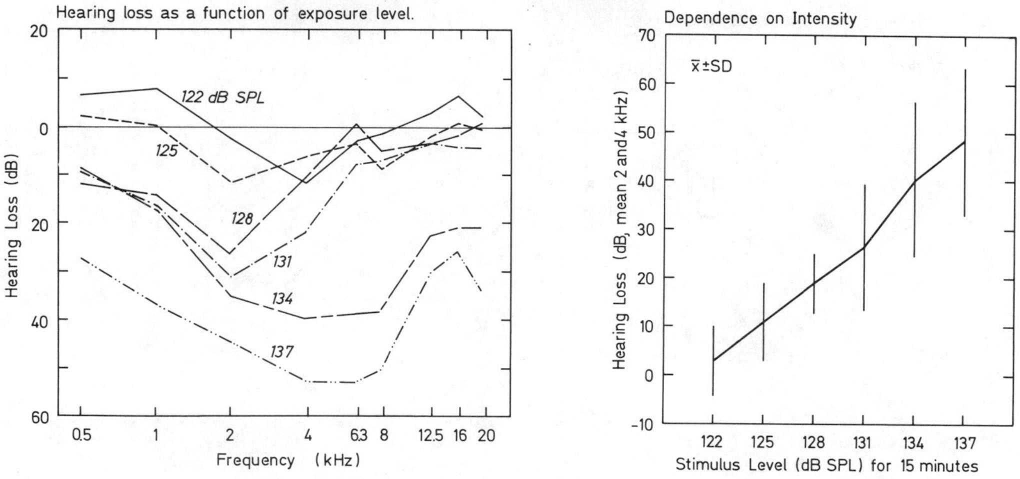

Figure 41-3 *Left,* Average auditory brain-stem response (ABR) threshold loss (re normal controls) for groups of animals exposed with a closed system at different levels for 15 minutes. *Right,* Growth of threshold loss (average of 2 and 4 kHz) as a function of exposure-noise level.

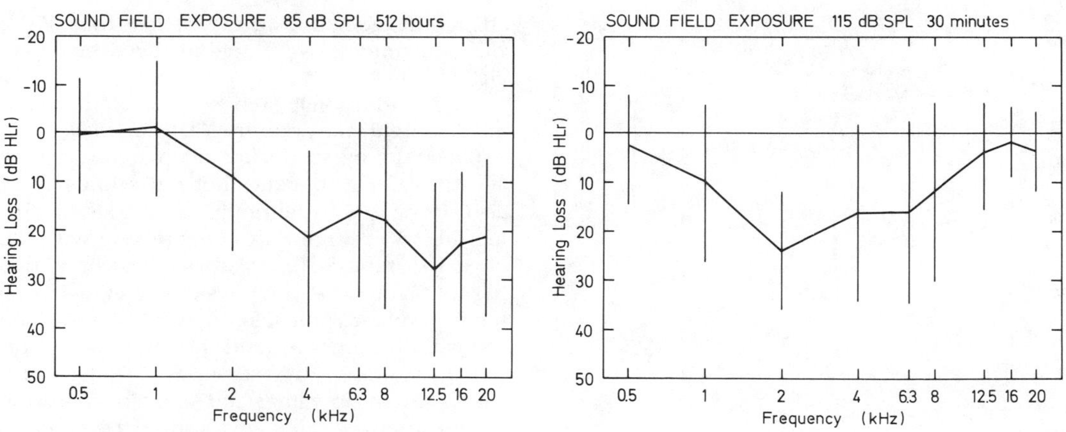

Figure 41-4 *Left,* Average (±SD) auditory brain-stem response (ABR) threshold loss for rabbits exposed to low-level (85 dB SPL) long-term noise. *Right,* Average (±SD) ABR threshold loss for rabbits exposed to high-level (115 dB SPL) short-term noise with the same frequency composition and total energy.

is shifted from 2 kHz at the lower exposure levels to 4 and 6.3 kHz at the highest exposure levels. Figure 41-3*B* shows the mean value of the hearing loss at 2 and 4 kHz as a function of exposure sound level between 122 and 137 dB SPL. The increase in threshold with noise level is roughly linear, with about a 45-dB increase in hearing loss for the 15-dB increase in exposure sound level. Furthermore, the variance is larger the higher the exposure level ($p < 0.01$). It can be seen from Figure 41-3*A* that it is important which frequencies are used for quantification of the hearing loss. If, for instance, 6.3 kHz was chosen, there would be a threshold for damage at 134 dB SPL and a rapid rise above that level. The quantification at 2 and 4 kHz, on the other hand, indicates a threshold at 122 dB SPL for 15 minutes of exposure.

Individual Variability Under Different Exposure Conditions

The average and standard deviation of loss of ABR threshold for four different exposure conditions are shown in Figures 41-4 and 41-5. Figure 41-4*A* shows the group exposed in a sound field at 85 dB SPL for 512 hours,

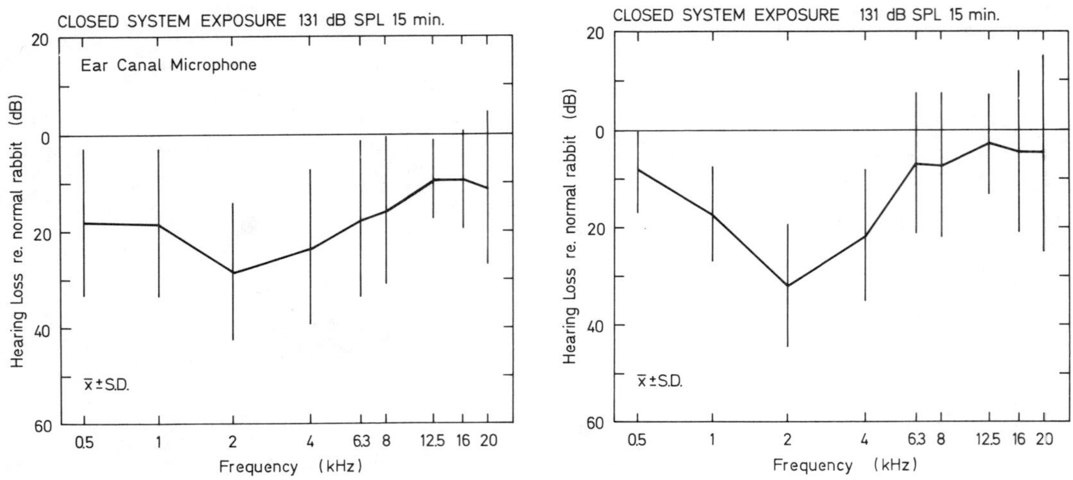

Figure 41-5 *Left,* Average threshold loss for rabbits exposed with a hearing-aid telephone connected to the ear with a 4-cm tube. Level and spectrum control was via an electret microphone in proximal end of tube. *Right,* Average threshold loss using the same exposure system without electret microphone control.

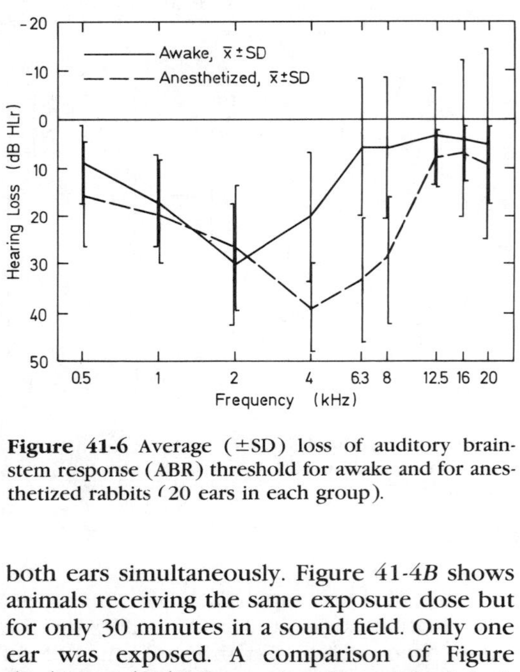

Figure 41-6 Average (±SD) loss of auditory brainstem response (ABR) threshold for awake and for anesthetized rabbits (20 ears in each group).

both ears simultaneously. Figure 41-4*B* shows animals receiving the same exposure dose but for only 30 minutes in a sound field. Only one ear was exposed. A comparison of Figure 41-4*A* and 41-4*B* shows that the standard deviation is slightly larger for the data shown in Figure 41-4*A*.

Figure 41-5 shows the threshold loss after exposure in a closed sound system to 131 dB SPL for 15 minutes. This better-controlled exposure was tested in two conditions, with (A) and without (B) electret microphone control over the sound level and spectrum. Although the sound level could be adjusted only in case A, there was no difference in the standard deviation between the two groups. In fact, the change in the sound level was less than 1 dB, and adjustments were seldom necessary (see Fig. 41-1).

One additional step was taken to minimize individual variability. The animals were exposed to noise during deep pentobarbital anesthesia. The nonanesthetized rabbits were also sitting quietly, although unrestrained, during the 15 or 30 minutes of exposure with the closed system. With anesthesia, however, one has to assume that the physiologic control systems, middle-ear muscle reflexes, efferents and sympathetic nerves, and possibly also hormonal systems, are stabilized. Figure 41-6 shows the mean values and standard deviation of anesthetized and unanesthetized animals exposed to the same noise. It can be seen that the region of maximum damage is shifted one octave and increased in the anesthetized animals (significant at 4, 6.3, and 8 kHz; $p < 0.01$).

The variance within the different groups was analyzed statistically (ANOVA), and all exposure groups showed a larger standard deviation than the anesthetized animals exposed under closed conditions; the nonanesthetized rabbits exposed with the y system closed ($p < 0.05$, $F = 5.1$), short-term sound-field exposed animals ($p < 0.01$, $F = 7.9$), and long-term sound-field-exposed animals ($p < 0.01$, $F = 10.5$). The gradual increase of the F-values shows that the variability in the exposure increases the more "natural" the exposure conditions are, i.e., the more naturally active and less controlled the exposure conditions are. Even though the animals were anesthetized, there was substantial individual variability.

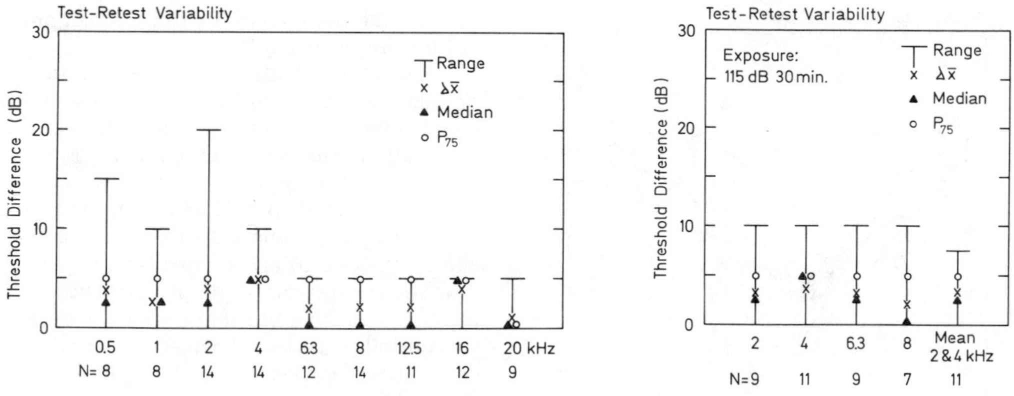

Figure 41-7 Test-retest variability in normal-hearing rabbits *(left)* and noise-exposed rabbits *(right)*. Two measurements were taken for each animal.

Sources of Variability

Hearing Threshold Assessment. The ABR thresholds were determined on two occasions, each for one group of normal-hearing animals and one group of noise-damaged animals. The thresholds were assessed without knowledge of the previous results, only whether the animal was exposed or not. The results are shown in Figure 41-7. The range, median, mean, and semi-interquantile range (P75) are illustrated. At no frequency did P75 exceed 5 dB; the median was 2.5 dB or less for all but two test frequencies. The range of threshold shift was 5 or 10 dB for most frequencies and did not exceed 10 dB for any frequency in the exposed animals. The range of the test-retest difference was less than 7.5 dB for the mean value of the two usually affected frequencies, 2 and 4 kHz.

We also investigated whether the variability was smaller when individually determining pre-exposure and postexposure thresholds than when relating the postexposure threshold to the mean of a normal population of nonexposed animals. The standard deviations for the two procedures were practically identical, which means that we could use the simpler and safer procedure of relating thresholds to a normal population. The normal threshold for rabbits was assessed earlier in a separate group of 30 rabbits (Engström & Borg, 1983). Therefore, in our standard procedure, only assessment of pre-exposure thresholds at 2, 4, and 12 kHz were included in order to identify animals presenting with ear problems (a very unusual condition in our rabbits). Statistical analysis showed that less than 20 percent of the standard deviation of the hearing loss (3 percent of variance) between animals could be explained by uncertainty in threshold determination. Other factors must play a considerably greater role in individual variability after noise exposure.

Method for Quantification of the Noise-Induced Lesion. The threshold loss can be quantified as the value at one particular frequency, mean value in a certain frequency range, or across the whole audiogram. Ten groups of rabbits exposed at high level (115 to 137 dB SPL) for short duration (15 to 334 minutes) were used for an analysis of the value of the coefficient of variance (SD divided by mean) for different combinations of evaluated audiometric frequencies. A total of 164 animals were evaluated. In the different groups, the maximum loss was seen at 2 or 4 kHz. The coefficient of variance was largest when the whole frequency range of the audiogram was evaluated. The next largest value was seen at 4 kHz. The coefficient of variance was nearly the same for 2 kHz and for the mean value 2 and 4 kHz. In order to get the best stability, a small coefficient of variance, and independence from shift of the peak of hearing loss, the mean value of 2 and 4 kHz was selected for standard evaluation of the audiograms in the present series of studies.

Postexposure Time. Obviously, if the threshold determination is made too close to the end of the exposure, there will be a component of TTS. In this study, TTS was avoided by making measurements approximately 3 weeks after the end of the exposure.

Exposure Level and Frequency. The most obvious source of variability is the exposure stimulus and the measurement thereof. In an occupational situation, the exposure is usually measured at a standardized position in relation to the noise sources, or with a dosime-

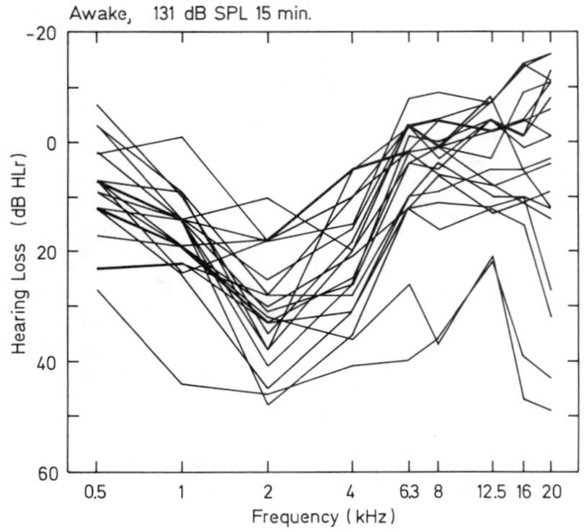

Figure 41-8 ABR threshold loss relative to normal controls from 20 different ears exposed to 131 dB SPL for 15 minutes.

ter placed on the subject. In animal experiments, better control of the exposure is usually possible. As shown in the previous section, there is a significant decrease in the standard deviation in closed exposure conditions, implying somewhat better control of the exposure. However, even in the closed system with sound calibration in the ear canal, there is very large individual variability. The individual values can be recalculated to equivalent exposure levels assuming a one-to-one relation between exposure level and hearing loss. For the animals exposed to 131 dB for 15 minutes with the closed system, the individual threshold curves are shown in Figure 41-8. The animals with the least hearing loss have a threshold curve corresponding to the mean threshold for the group exposed to 122 dB, and the animals with the largest hearing loss have a threshold curve corresponding to the mean value for the group exposed to 134 dB. There is thus a 12-dB range. It is highly unlikely that such a large variability could be caused by variations in the exposure sound itself. Only very small adjustments of the attenuator were needed to obtain 131 dB SPL in the ear canal of each animal. Furthermore, we measured sound-pressure level in the middle ear with an acoustic probe. The exposure system was replaced several times and manipulated. We found variations in the total sound pressure in the middle ear of less than 1.5 dB and minor deviations of the spectrum (Fig. 41-2). The relatively low exposure frequency chosen, with maximum energy between 2 and 4 kHz, also makes the ear-canal resonances and directional effects for these small animals of little importance.

Specific Individual Susceptibility. The animals participating in the present study were obtained from the same breeder and were all of the small chinchilla strain. This means that the range of inherent susceptibility can be expected to be lower than in an unselected animal population or in a human population exposed to an occupational noise.

The main issue of the present analysis was to identify a possible stable individual-specific susceptibility factor. Because we used unilateral noise exposure and a nontraumatic method for evaluation of hearing, it was possible to expose and test the two ears independently and repeatedly. The stable individual susceptibility factor would appear as a larger or a smaller amount of damage to both ears of each animal, even if the two ears were exposed at a time interval of several days. In two series of experiments in the closed system with and without the ear-canal microphone, the variances within and between animals were compared for ears exposed on different days. In none of the two series was there a significant difference in variance between the ears of the same or between different individuals.

In the long-term, sound-field exposed animals (condition A), the variance between animals was 197; the variance between ears was 117, substantially (but not significantly) lower. This smaller difference between the ears than between the individuals in the long-term exposed animals might indicate that there is also an individual-specific susceptibility factor that is stable over time, but not evident in the short-term exposures. These findings can be explained by individual susceptibility to noise damage that varies with time.

The results can also be explained by a stable *ear* factor that differs between the two ears of the same individual as much as between different individuals in this homogeneous group of animals. One obvious ear-specific factor is the individual auditory threshold of the ear before the exposure. Good hearing (e.g., a low threshold) may mean that the effective sound pressure in the inner ear will be large upon exposure, and thereby cause a greater loss. However, the threshold of ABR before exposure showed only a slight (insignificant) negative correlation with the final size of the loss. Furthermore, there was no difference in the hearing loss between the right and the left ear, no difference between males and females, and no difference as a function of age (which ranged from 3 to 10 months).

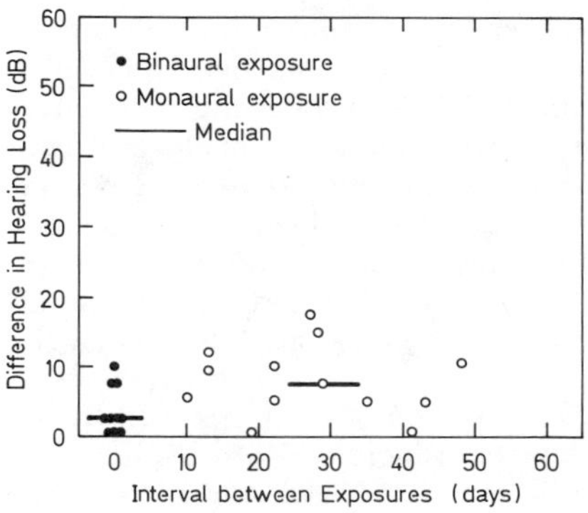

Figure 41-9 Difference in auditory brain-stem response (ABR) threshold loss between the two ears as a function of interval between exposures (131 dB SPL for 15 min).

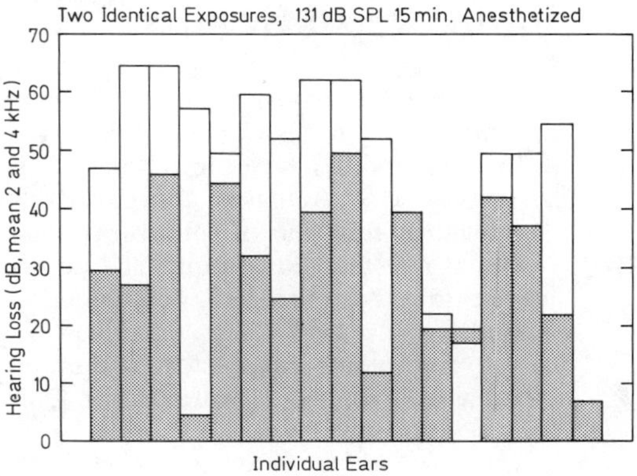

Figure 41-10 Threshold loss for individual ears exposed to identical noise on two different occasions at least 3 weeks apart. Shaded areas show loss after first exposure; light areas show loss after the second exposure. For two animals no additional loss was seen, and for one animal the loss after the second exposure was smaller than the loss after the first exposure.

Time-Varying Susceptibility

The time between exposure and measurement of threshold was 7 to 50 days, with most animals measured approximately 3 weeks after exposure. There was no difference in the mean values for those measured between 7 and 10, 10 and 20, and >20 days after exposure. To avoid temporary threshold shift, most of the animals were measured between 2 and 3 weeks after the exposure.

The degree of the hearing loss might be related to time of year during exposure. The hormonal cycles of rabbits have a time variation, which, however, has not been assessed for our animals. We have, however, not been able to identify any seasonal variation in the size of the hearing loss. The variance was not larger for females than for males, indicating a minimal influence of female hormonal cycles.

A temporal variation in the susceptibility might be studied more closely in animals, the ears of which were separately exposed with different time intervals. One would expect the difference between the ears to be smallest if the ears were exposed simultaneously and gradually increasing with increasing time interval. Figure 41-9 shows the absolute value of the difference in hearing loss between the two ears. Animals exposed at an interval of 10 to 50 days show a larger variation and a significantly larger mean difference than the animals exposed simultaneously. It is, however, not clear in this material if there is any cyclic variation or a random variation in noise susceptibility as a function of time.

Repeated Exposures of the Same Ear

Because the NIPTS after the 131-dB 15-minute exposure was rather small, the exposure could be repeated without the risk of reaching a ceiling. Figure 41-10 shows the NIPTS (mean value of 2 and 4 kHz) after two exposures of the same ear with an interval of more than 3 weeks between exposures. The shaded bars show the NIPTS after the first exposure, and the light bars show the loss after the second exposure. The general impression is of a large difference between first and second exposure for most animals—thus, no stable susceptibility factor. Four animals showed no increase of threshold loss after the second exposure. If they were excluded as "dropouts," the variance after one exposure was 190, and after two exposures, 39. The additional exposure alone had a variance of 192. There was a strong negative correlation between the sizes of the losses from the first and the second exposures ($r = -0.9$). There was an insignificant (negative) correlation between the size of the threshold loss produced by the first and the second (additional) exposures, if all animals were included. This experiment failed to show a stable individual susceptibility factor, but the observations could be explained by a time-varying susceptibility. These results differ from the results obtained from the training experiments (Canlon et al, 1988), because the present animals had a substantial permanent threshold shift after the first exposure. In the training experiments, Canlon et al selected parameters which would produce neither a temporary nor a permanent shift of the threshold after the training exposure.

Summary of Results

1. Intense noise exposure yields a permanent hearing loss, which becomes stable after about 1 week in rabbits.
2. Hearing loss increases approximately as a linear function of sound level and shows a distinct knee-point at low energy for the parameter combination used.
3. The frequency range for maximum damage is shifted upwards for higher noise-exposure level.
4. It is not appropriate to evaluate the threshold shift at any single frequency.
5. Variance increases as a function of exposure dose, compatible with the effect of an individual susceptibility factor (stable or varying over time).
6. The standard deviation of the auditory threshold determination explains only 3 percent of the variance between animals.
7. Improved control over exposure conditions decreases the variability to some extent, but leaves considerable variability despite continuous control of sound pressure and spectrum in the ear canal.
8. There is only a small *stable* individual-specific susceptibility factor. The pre-exposure hearing threshold does not correlate with the size of the hearing loss.
9. There is evidence that susceptibility to NIPTS varies over time.

Conclusion

The main finding is the lack of a dominating *stable* individual-specific susceptibility factor, but there is evidence that noise susceptibility varies over time.

The minimal role of a stable individual-susceptibility factor is interesting. It might be caused by the use of a homogeneous animal strain from the same breeder. However, despite the genetic homogeneity, the individual variability was substantial. The hypothesis presented on the basis of our findings is that susceptibility is time-varying. A temporal variation in a critical noise intensity has earlier been suggested by Rüedi, 1954. More recently, Saunders et al (1985) came to a similar conclusion on the basis of a literature survey and suggested the possible existence of a probabilistic damaging process. Davis et al (1950) reported results compatible with fluctuations in susceptibility over time in studies on repeated TTS in the same individuals. In a series of experiments with binaural exposure to impact or continuous noise, Grenner et al (1990) found a high left-right correlation, but a large interindividual variability. These findings are in accordance with our finding of a small intraindividual variability when the two ears were exposed simultaneously. Conversely, Lindgren and Axelsson (1983) found a highly reproducible TTS in humans. The details of the temporal variations in susceptibility have not been possible to identify, e.g., whether the susceptibility varies randomly or with a regular cyclic pattern. A much larger sample is needed to settle this question.

Although the underlying mechanisms behind the temporal variability of susceptibility are not known, the steadily growing body of information about the active nature and biologic properties of hair cells and neural control of the inner ear is relevant. Such mechanisms are likely to be capable of temporal variations in function and resistance to damage like other complex somatic and mental functions. We know that mental and physical fitness varies in a way that is only partly predictable and that is influenced by numerous external and internal processes. The recent findings of changes of susceptibility after earlier "training" support the view that NIPTS is a dynamic process (Canlon et al, 1988).

Variabilité dé la Susceptibilité Inter et Intra-Individuelle des Déficits Auditifs: Étude chez l'Animal

La variabilité de l'importance des pertes auditives dues au bruit est un problème pour l'application de critères de risques de dommages, aussi bien que pour les recherches expérimentales sur le bruit. D'autre part, la variabilité peut indiquer la présence de processus biologiques inconnus, dont la connaissance peut avoir son importance à la fois pour ce problème, pour les pertes auditives induites par le bruit, et pour la biologie de l'oreille interne. Dans des séries d'expériences sur des lapins, nous avons analysé plusieurs aspects de la variabilité et de la perte de seuils, ainsi que les dommages aux cellules ciliées. Les animaux ont été exposés de façon unilatérale ou bilatérale dans un système acoustique fermé ou dans un "champ de bruit," avec ou sans anesthésie. 2 variétés de lapins ont été utilisées, de petits chinchillas et des lapins albinos. De plus un groupe de cobayes tricolores et de rats albinos ont été inclus dans l'expérience à des fins de comparaison. L'exposition standard était un bruit de bande de 2 kHz et délivré par un système "Oticon Power Hearing Aid" directement dans le conduit auditif pendant 15 minutes à 131 dB SPL. Une grande variabilité individuelle a été observée. La variabilité entre les deux oreilles d'un même animal exposé à différentes occasions était la même que la variabilité entre différents animaux. L'influence d'une variation contrôlée dans le "champ de bruit" et dans l'exposition au son a été étudiée en comparant les expositions dans le "champ de bruit" et celles en circuit fermé. La variance était légèrement mais significativement plus petite dans l'exposition en circuit fermé. L'influence des facteurs sensibles à l'anesthésie a été analysée en comparant la variabilité après exposition, avec ou sans anesthésie. L'exposition avec anesthésie donnait une petite mais significative diminution de la variance.

L'écart de variabilité correspondait à une variation équivalente du niveau d'exposition de 12 dB, plus élevée que la variation mesurée dans le niveau d'exposition. La contribution de la variabilité d'évaluation du seuil était seulement de 3% de la variance totale. La variance pour les expositions binaurales simultanées était plus petite que la variance entre les oreilles exposées avec un décalage de temps. On n'a pas remarqué d'influence ni du sexe ni de l'âge (pour les animaux adultes). Les lapins albinos montraient des pertes auditives significativement plus grandes que les chinchillas. Les animaux avec les muscles de l'oreille moyenne coupés ou les animaux sous anesthésie montraient des pertes auditives exagérées. Ces résultats montrent que la variabilité de la susceptibilité au bruit est un phénomène variant avec le temps, avec des contributions de mécanismes actifs de contrôle physiologiques, et des composantes génétiques et métaboliques.

ACKNOWLEDGMENTS

This study was supported by grants from the Swedish Work Environmental Fund and Swedish Medical Research Council, the Knut and Alice Wallenberg Foundation, and the Tysta Skolan Foundation.

References

Borg E, Engström B. Hearing threshold in the rabbit. A behavioral and electrophysiological study. Acta Otolaryngol (Stockh) 1983; 95:19-26.

Borg E, Engström B. Noise level, inner hair cell damage, audiometric features, and equal-energy hypothesis. J Acoust Soc Am 1989; 86:1776-1782.

Canlon B, Borg E, Flock Å. Protection against noise trauma by preexposure to a low level acoustic stimulus. Hear Res 1988; 34:197-200.

Davis H, Morgan CT, Hawkins JE, et al. Temporary deafness following exposure to loud tones and noise. Acta Otolaryngol Suppl 1950; 88:1-57.

Engström B, Borg E. Lesions to cochlear inner hair cells induced by noise. Arch Otorhinolaryngol 1981; 230:279-284.

Engström B, Borg E. Cochlear morphology in relation to loss of behavioural, electrophysiological, and middle ear reflex thresholds after noise exposure. Acta Otolaryngol (Stockh) 1983; Suppl 402:1-23.

Grenner J, Nilsson P, Katbamna B. Right-left correlation in guinea pig ears after noise exposure. Acta Otolaryngol (Stockh) 1990; 109:41-48.

Lindgren F, Axelsson A. Temporary threshold shift after exposure to noise and music of equal energy. Ear Hear 1983; 4:197-201.

Rüedi L. Different types and degrees of acoustic trauma by experimental exposure of the human and animal ear to pure tones and noise. Ann Otol Rhinol Laryngol 1954; 63:702-726.

Saunders JC, Deer SP, Schneider ME. The anatomical consequences of acoustic injury: Review and tutorial. J Acoust Soc Am 1985; 78:833-860.

CHAPTER 42

Development of Resistance to Noise

DONALD HENDERSON
PIERRE CAMPO
MALINI SUBRAMANIAM
FRANCESCO FIORINO

The wide range of individual susceptibility to noise-induced hearing loss (NIHL) has been a puzzle to scientists for at least 40 years. Reviews by Ward (1965) and later by Chung et al (1982) discuss a number of potential factors contributing to an individual's susceptibility to noise, e.g., gender, eye color, age, smoking, and life style. Although some of these factors undoubtedly play a role in the acquisition of NIHL, none can account for the extreme intersubject variability in populations exposed to noise.

In the last few years it has become apparent that history of exposures to noise may be a factor in determining a subject's susceptibility to NIHL. Although this is a relatively recent hypothesis, data supporting this idea can be traced through a number of experiments leading back to the classic paper of Miller et al (1963). In one of their experiments, monaural cats were exposed to broad band noise of 115 dB for 7.5 minutes per day for 17 days. As can be seen in Figure 42-1, the first day's exposure produced 35 dB of temporary threshold shift (TTS) at 4 kHz, but by the end of the tenth day, the same exposure produced only 15 dB of TTS. Miller et al discussed a number of possibilities for these unexpected results, including the idea that the system's response to noise could be moderated by prior exposure, but unfortunately this interpretation was neglected for the next 25 years. Recently, several investigators—Clark et al (1987), Sinex et al (1987), and our laboratory—have all reported similar trends.

Figure 42-2 shows the results from Byrne et al (in press), for monaural chinchillas exposed to octave band noise (OBN) centered at 500 Hz at 100 dB SPL for 6 hours a day for 20 days. Again there is a systematic decrease in threshold shift (TS) across the days of exposure. What is interesting is that all the test frequencies showed this trend, thereby raising some puzzling questions about the biologic changes responsible for the reduced TS.

Although reduced TS with repeated exposures is an interesting observation, it would be even more important if prior exposure also reduced the susceptibility to permanent threshold shift (PTS). Canlon et al (1988) exposed guinea pigs to a 1,000-Hz tone at 81 dB for 21 days and then exposed the subjects to 105 dB for 48 hours (Fig. 42-3). Subjects that received the "conditioning" exposure developed substantially less PTS (approximately 20 to 25 dB) and hair cell losses than the control group exposed only at 105 dB for 48 hours. These are intriguing results that require clarification, particularly about the changes in auditory functioning during the 21 days of exposure. In the Canlon et al experiment the "conditioning" exposure was at a single frequency for 21 days continuously. This exposure is unlikely to be found in nature or in the work place. Also, the use of the whole nerve action potential to assess auditory sensitivity yields thresholds substantially above the guinea pig's behavioral threshold, and the action potential (AP) measures might have precluded observation of any residual hearing loss prior to the traumatic exposure.

Thus, the purpose of this research is to begin to understand the relationship between the conditioning exposure and the resultant changes in vulnerability to NIHL, when the conditioning exposure approximates more typical industrial exposures. Two sets of experiments are reported. The first is a system-

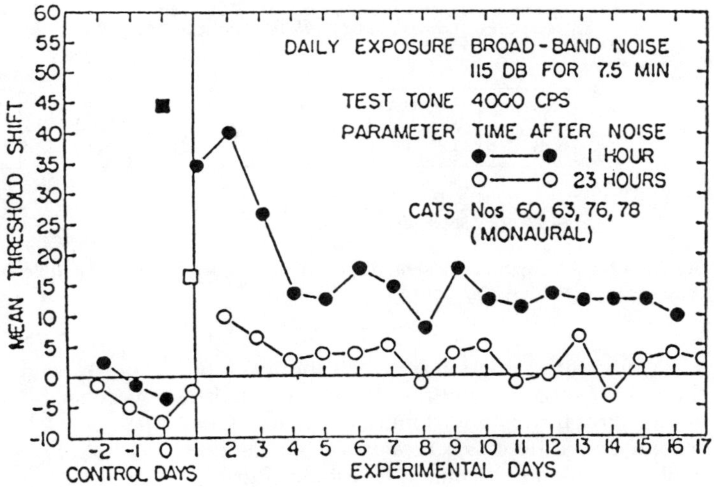

Figure 42-1 Threshold shift before and after exposure to a broad-band noise at 115 dB SPL. Modified from Miller JD, Watson CS, Covell WP. Deafening effects of noise on the cat. Acta Otolaryngol Suppl 1963; 176:1-91.

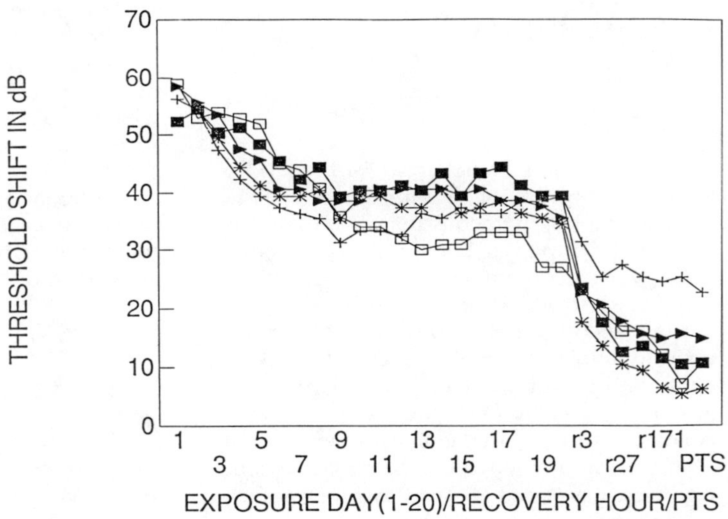

Figure 42-2 Postexposure threshold shift and recovery following exposure to an octave band of noise (OBN) at 500 Hz at 100 dB SPL for 6 hours per day for 10 days. From Byrne C, Henderson D, Saunders S, et al. Interaction of noise and whole body vibration. J Acoust Soc Am (submitted).

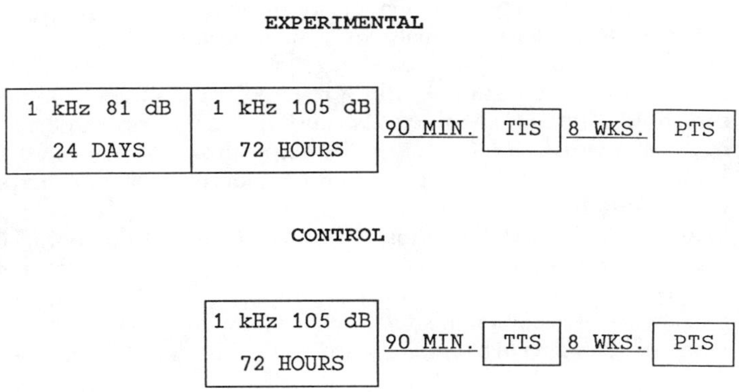

Figure 42-3 Schematic representation of the exposure conditions in Canlon et al's (1988) experiment. TTS, temporary threshold shift; PTS, permanent threshold shift.

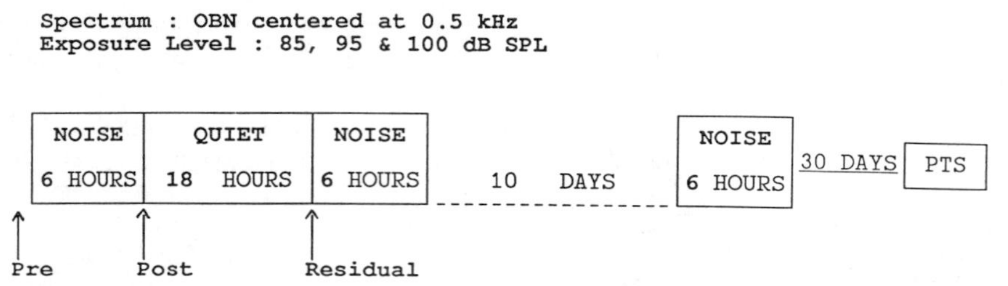

Figure 42-4 Schematic representation of the exposure and test schedule employed in experiment I. OBN, octave band of noise; PTS, permanent threshold shift.

atic study of the relation between the level of the noise exposures and the degree of "toughening" during the conditioning exposure. The second experiment is a replication of Canlon et al's, in which the shifts in thresholds during the conditioning exposure are documented and the traumatic exposure is given when there is no residual hearing loss.

Experiment I

Methods

Subjects

Twenty adult chinchillas (500 to 700 g) served as subjects. Each animal was anesthetized with a subcutaneous injection of acepromazine (0.56 mg per kilogram) and ketamine (36 mg per kilogram) and made monaural by surgical destruction of the left cochlea. A chronic recording electrode was then stereotaxically implanted in to the left inferior colliculus, and a ground electrode was implanted just below the dura (Henderson et al, 1973). Following surgery, the animals were given antibiotics (chloramphenicol palmitate twice a day for 4 days) and allowed to recover for at least 2 weeks prior to testing.

Evoked Response Testing

After the 2-week recovery period hearing thresholds of all the animals were measured on 5 consecutive days. The average of these five measures constitutes the pre-exposure threshold. The animals were also tested each day just before and just after the exposure. Each animal was tested separately in a sound-treated booth. A yoke-like harness kept the animal's head in a fixed position within the calibrated sound field.

Test stimuli consisted of tone pips (5 ms Blackman rise/fall ramp) in the frequency range of 0.5 to 16 kHz at octave intervals. The signals were generated and the responses were analyzed using a personal computer.

Noise Exposure

All the animals were exposed to the same spectrum of noise (OBN centered at 0.5 kHz) for 6 hours a day for 10 days. Three levels of exposures were used: 85, 95, and 100 dB SPL. The exposure schedule and the test schedule are shown schematically in Figure 42-4.

The animals were exposed in groups of two or three. Each animal was housed in a separate cage (8″ × 8½″ × 8″) and given free access to food and water. The cages were placed just below the loudspeaker such that the difference, if any, in the sound pressure across the cages was within 1 dB. Further, the animals were rotated to different cages during the course of the exposure.

Results

Pre-Exposure Thresholds

The mean pre-exposure thresholds for the three groups of animals are presented in Figure 42-5. The mean thresholds of all the three groups were consistent with both the laboratory reference standards and the thresholds reported by Miller (1970).

Postexposure Threshold Shift

The difference between the threshold obtained at the end of each exposure and the pre-exposure threshold at a given frequency constituted the postexposure threshold shift. The postexposure threshold shifts recorded in the three groups at the six test frequencies are depicted in Figure 42-6.

Certain trends are clear from Figure 42-6. The largest hearing loss occurred within the first 2 days for the 100-dB group, and then the hearing loss was progressively smaller on en-

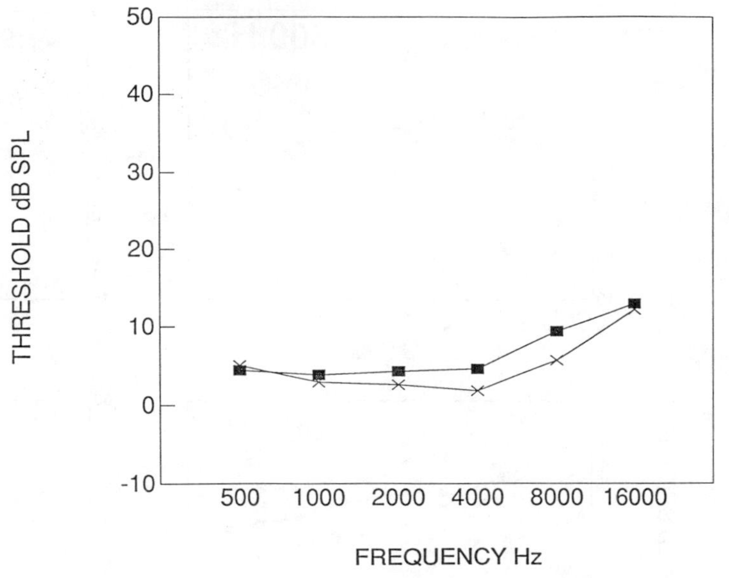

Figure 42-5 Pre-exposure thresholds (filled squares) of animals in experiment I. Results from Miller (1970) are presented for comparison (crossed lines).

suing days. For some frequencies, particularly in the 85-dB group and also in the 95-dB group, the maximum hearing loss did not occur until after 2 to 4 days of the exposure. At high frequencies, i.e., above 4 kHz, the 85-dB exposure did not cause a significant threshold shift.

The toughening effect varied with frequency and level. There was a significant reduction in the postexposure threshold shift at 0.5 and 1 kHz at all the three exposure levels, with the maximum reduction in TS occurring in the 100-dB SPL group. The threshold shifts of the 85- and 95-dB groups showed considerable overlap at 500 and 1,000 Hz. At 2 kHz there is a reversal in the threshold curves. The 95-dB group showed the greater shift on day 1, but as the exposure continued the threshold shift in the 95-dB group decreased with repeated exposures, and the threshold shift actually dropped below the threshold for the 85-dB group by day 4.

The progressive reduction in the threshold shift or toughening appeared to depend on the level of exposure. Although at the lowest level the toughening was restricted to frequencies between 0.5 and 2 kHz, significant reduction in threshold shift was observed even at the higher frequencies for the higher exposure levels. The toughening effect seen with exposure to 100 dB was greater than such effects with 95-dB exposures at 4 and 8 kHz.

In general, for any combination of level and audiometric test frequency, if there was a significant threshold shift (TS greater than 20 dB), then there was a trend for decreased threshold shift with repeated exposures. The actual size of the toughening effect is not clear because at some frequencies and levels the amount of TS was still decreasing after 10 days of exposure. Thus the magnitude of the toughening effect is probably underestimated from Figure 42-6.

Recovery from Daily Exposures

The threshold prior to each exposure was subtracted from the postexposure threshold at the end of the previous exposure, to obtain a measure of how much recovery occurred over the 16 hours of quiet. These differences are plotted in Figure 42-7 to monitor how the process of recovery changed over the course of the 10 days of exposure.

In contrast to the decreasing threshold shifts as seen in Figure 42-6 the amount of recovery in Figure 42-7 appears to be less than 10 dB across the 10 days of exposure. The amount of residual hearing loss in the 100-dB group on the tenth day of exposure was about 25 to 30 dB across all frequencies, suggesting the possibility that the animals in the 100-dB group might develop some permanent threshold shift. When animals were exposed at 100 dB to the same noise and exposure schedule for 20 days, they developed 15 to 20 dB of permanent threshold shift at the high frequencies (Byrne et al, to be published). The 95-dB exposures did not produce any permanent

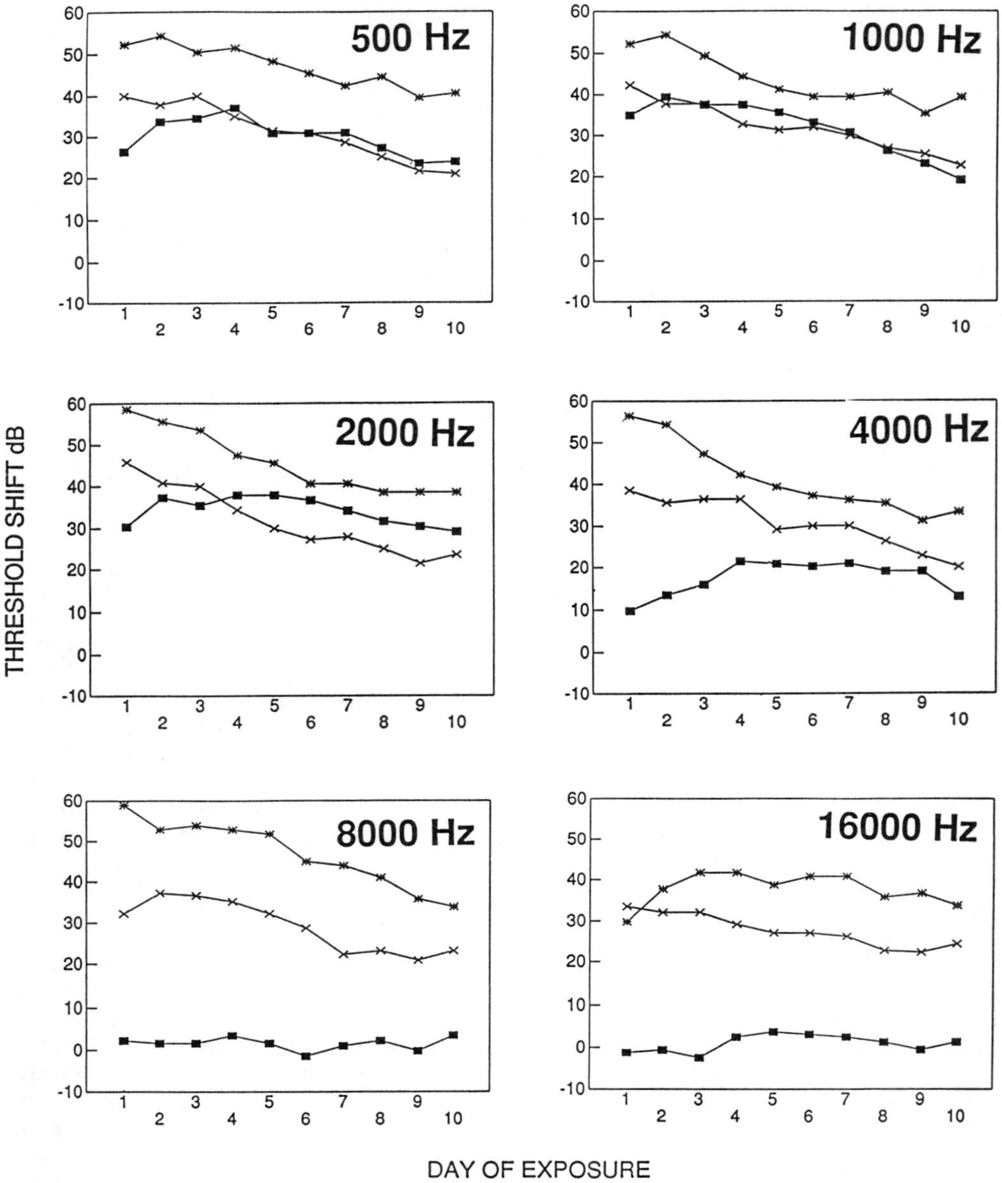

Figure 42-6 Postexposure threshold shifts at the six test frequencies for each of the exposure levels: 85 dB (filled squares), 95 dB (crossed lines), and 100 dB (asterisks).

threshold shifts, and sensitivity recovered to pre-exposure values within 4 to 5 days after the cessation of exposure (see Fig. 42-9).

Experiment II

Methods

Two groups of adult chinchillas served as subjects. The experimental group consisted of six chinchillas, and the control group consisted of seven chinchillas. The surgical procedure and the evoked response audiometry were carried out as described under experiment I. The noise exposure schedule is schematically represented in Figure 42-8.

Hearing thresholds were determined five times for each animal before the exposures were begun. The average of these five measures constituted the pre-exposure threshold for a given animal and served as the baseline with which the results of postexposure tests

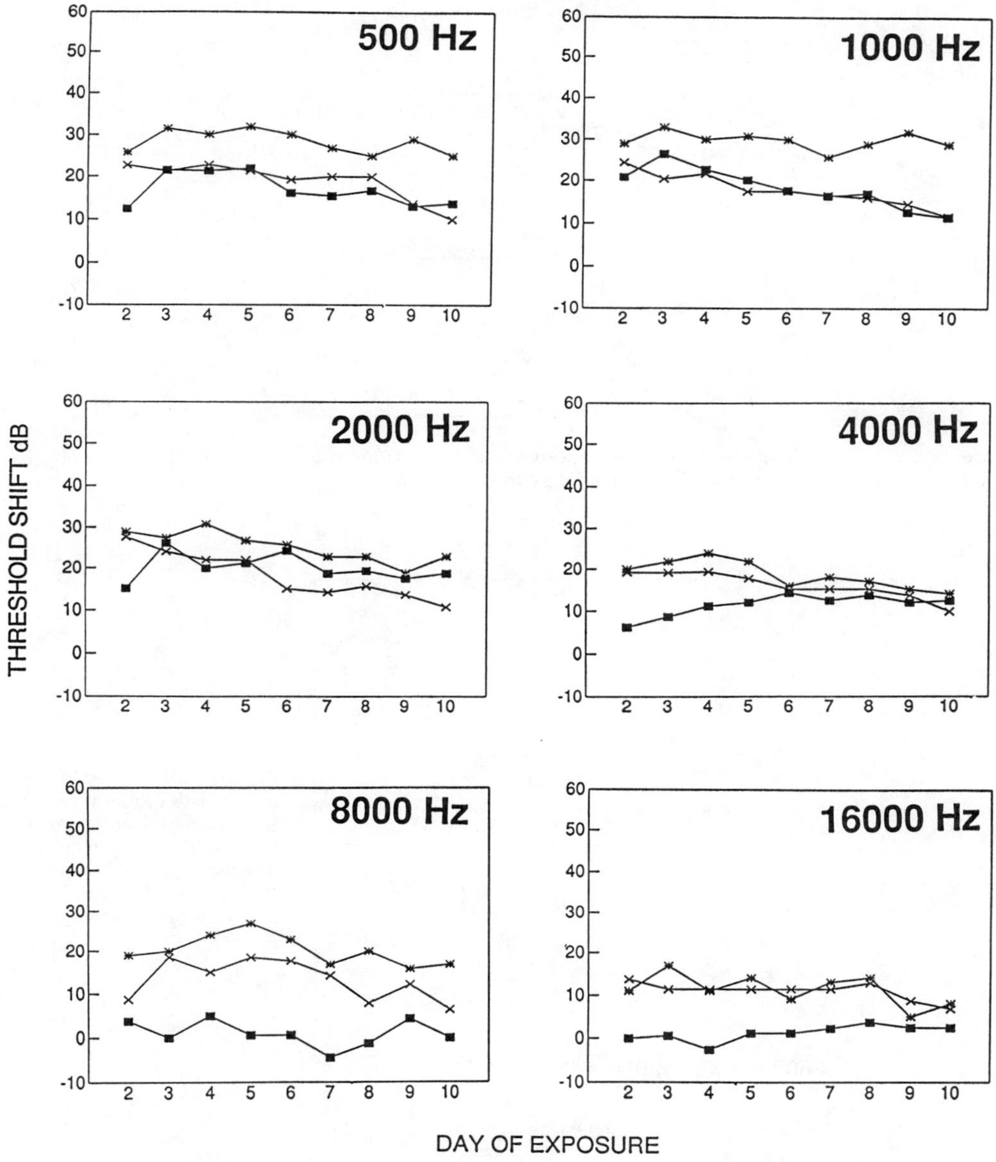

Figure 42-7 Recovery from hearing loss measured at the end of the 18 hours of recovery. 85 dB, filled squares; 95 dB, crossed lines; 100 dB, asterisks.

were compared. Animals in the experimental group were tested on each day before and after the 95-dB exposure, and tested at the end of the 5-day recovery period, just before the 106-dB exposure began. Animals in both groups were tested immediately after the 106-dB exposure and periodically thereafter. At 4 weeks after the last exposure, threshold measurements were repeated for 5 days. The difference between the average of these five measures and the pre-exposure thresholds constituted the permanent threshold shift.

Results

Pre-Exposure Thresholds

As reported for experiment I, the mean pre-exposure thresholds of the two groups were normal and in good agreement with the laboratory norms and with previously published norms (Miller, 1970).

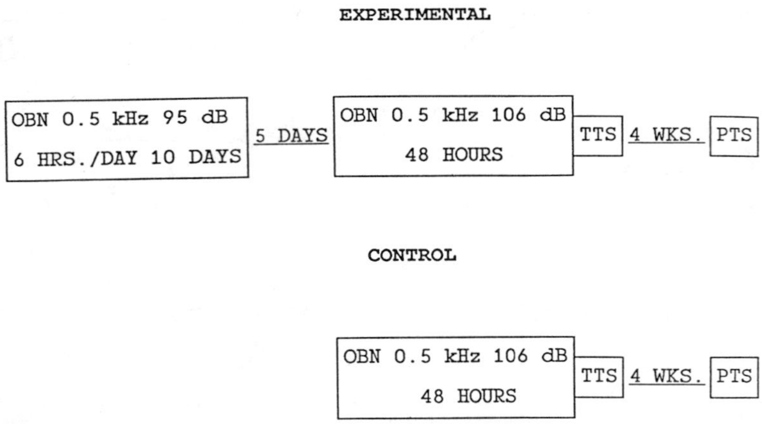

Figure 42-8 Schematic representation of the exposure schedule employed in experiment II. OBN, octave band of noise; PTS, permanent threshold shift; TTS, temporary threshold shift.

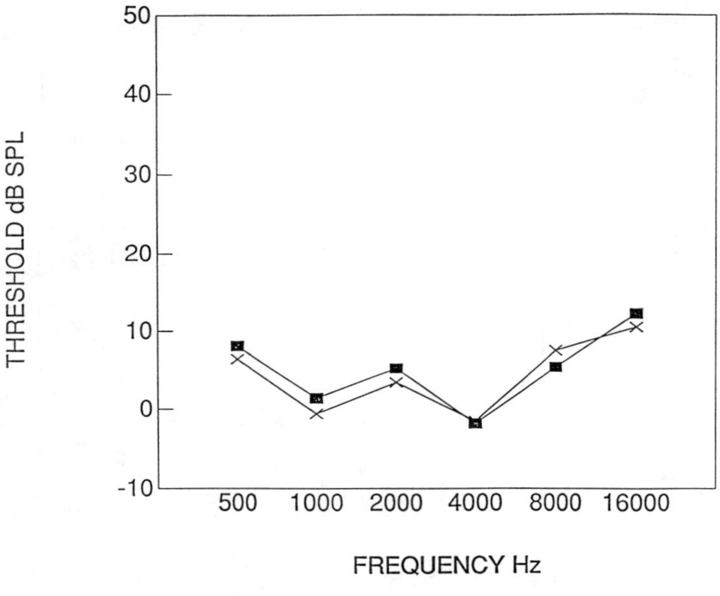

Figure 42-9 Thresholds recorded after 5 days of recovery following the 95-dB exposure (crossed lines) in the experimental group. The mean pre-exposure thresholds (filled squares) are plotted for comparison.

Threshold Shift from "Conditioning" Exposure

The results of the conditioning experiment have been discussed in-depth under experiment I. In general, the animals showed decrease in the threshold shift with repeated exposures. They also showed greater recovery with increase in the number of days of exposure. Further, the thresholds recorded at the end of the 5-day recovery period, just before the onset of the 106-dB 48-hour exposure, were close to the pre-exposure thresholds, indicating complete recovery at all the frequencies (Fig. 42-9).

Threshold Shift from Traumatic Exposure

The threshold shifts recorded at various recovery times following exposure to the noise at 106 dB are depicted in Figure 42-10.

The figures indicate that the animals in the experimental group incurred less threshold shift (about 20 to 30 dB between 500 and 4,000 Hz) initially when compared to the control group. The recovery functions run almost parallel up to 5 days, and most of the recovery was completed within 5 days after the exposure, so that the thresholds were within 5 dB of the PTS at most of the test frequencies. This

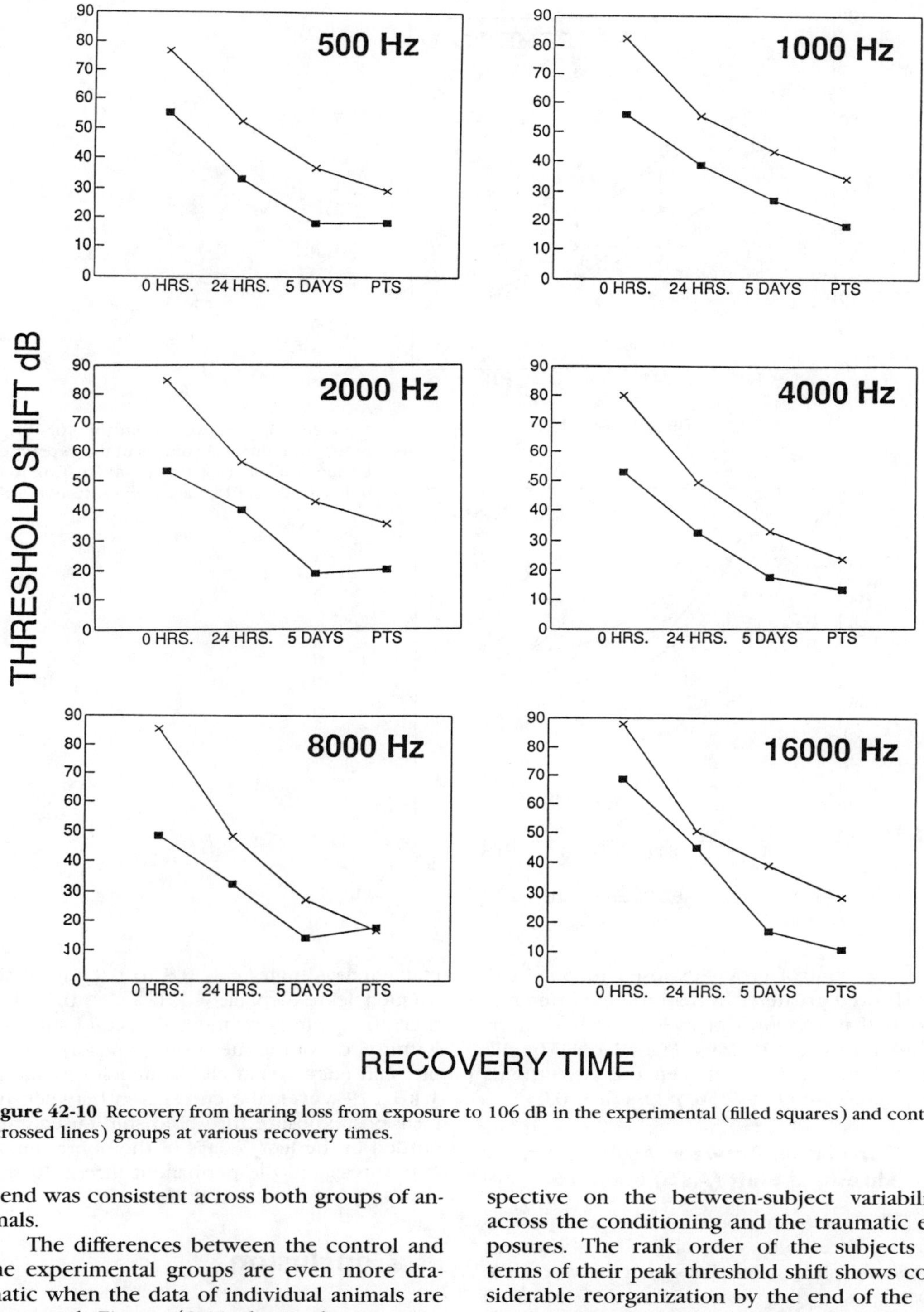

Figure 42-10 Recovery from hearing loss from exposure to 106 dB in the experimental (filled squares) and control (crossed lines) groups at various recovery times.

trend was consistent across both groups of animals.

The differences between the control and the experimental groups are even more dramatic when the data of individual animals are compared. Figure 42-11 shows the recovery curves at 1 kHz. The individual animals show a monotonic recovery process, and they maintain their rank order within their respective groups.

Figure 42-12 provides an interesting perspective on the between-subject variability across the conditioning and the traumatic exposures. The rank order of the subjects in terms of their peak threshold shift shows considerable reorganization by the end of the 10 days' conditioning exposure, but the rank ordering then is held reasonably closely through the following phases of the experiment, including the measurement of PTS. This is an interesting observation that deserves future study.

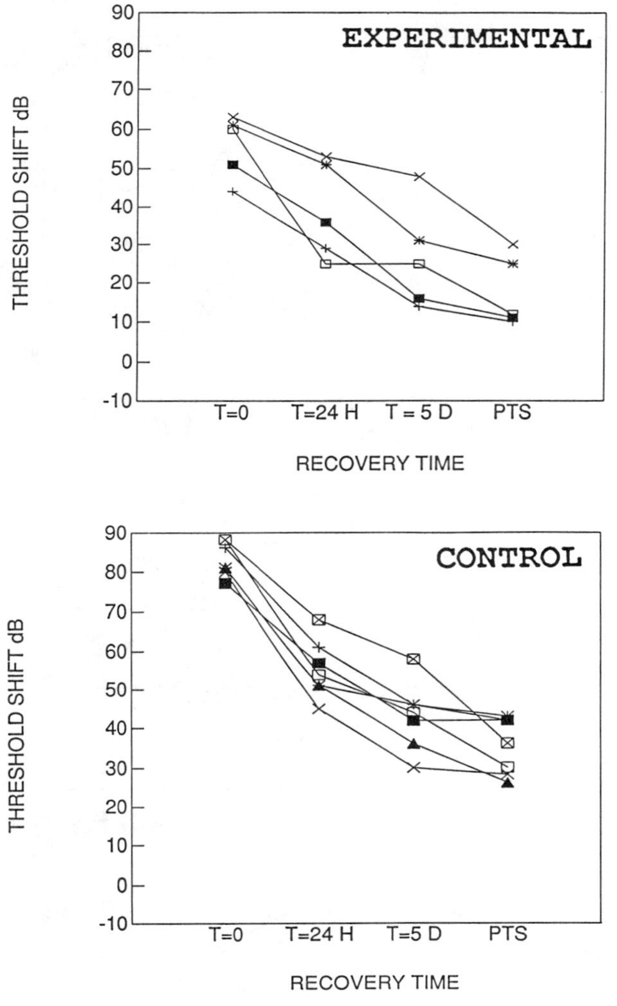

Figure 42-11 Recovery from the 106-dB exposure in individual animals in the experimental and control groups, at 1,000 Hz. T, time; H, hours; D, days; PTS, permanent threshold shift.

The control group exposed to only 106 dB showed greater PTS than the experimental group that was previously exposed to intermittent noise for 10 days (Fig. 42-13). The difference in the PTS between the two groups was significant ($F = 7.56$, p less than 0.05).

Correlation Between Asymptotic Threshold Shift (ATS) and PTS

The correlation between the peak postexposure threshold shift and the permanent threshold shift, as well as that between the postexposure threshold shift at the end of 10 days of the nontraumatic exposure and the permanent threshold shift, were computed in the case of the experimental group. The results indicated a high correlation between the postexposure threshold shift (day 10) and the permanent threshold shift. The correlation coefficient was high ($r = 0.8$ to 0.9) at all the frequencies except at 1 kHz ($r = 0.5$). Further, the mean permanent threshold shift was within 5 dB of the mean postexposure threshold shift (day 10) at all frequencies including 1 kHz. However, the correlation between the peak postexposure threshold shift (usually recorded in the first 3 days of the nontraumatic exposures) and the permanent threshold shift was high only at 4 and 8 kHz.

Conclusion

The results of experiment 1 showed a systematic decrease in TS with repeated exposure. The clearest exception to the current results comes from an experiment by Saunders et al (1977), who reported stable threshold shifts over 9 days of exposure to an octave

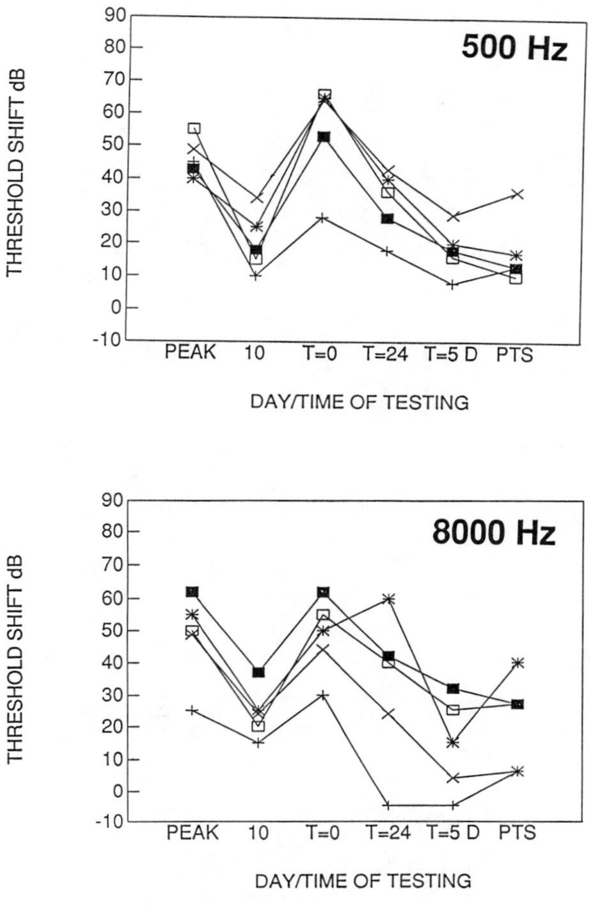

Figure 42-12 Recovery from the 95-dB and the 106-dB exposures in five of the experimental animals at two test frequencies. Symbols represent individual animals. T, time (time is in hours unless otherwise specified); D, days; PTS, permanent threshold shift.

band noise centered at 4,000 Hz for 6 hours per day. The results are, however, completely consistent with previous results reported by Miller et al (1963), Clark et al (1987), and Byrne et al (in press). Each of these experiments clearly showed that the auditory system can become resistant to repeated daily exposures to noise. By contrast, exposure to a continuous noise for periods of 2 days to 1 year often produces the maximum threshold shift in 1 or 2 days, after which the TS is reduced by 5 to 10 dB and remains relatively stable over the course of the exposure. An interesting question to pursue is the relation between the amount of toughening and the percentage of off-time during the intermittent exposure.

The size of the toughening phenomenon (decrease in TS of 30 dB or more) and the fact that a low-frequency exposure can produce the toughening effect across the entire audiometric range raise interesting questions about the biologic basis of the phenomenon. In a pilot study, Fiorino et al (1989) severed the COCB at the floor of the fourth ventricle and repeated the 500-Hz (OBN), 100-dB exposure outlined in experiment I. Figure 42-14 shows that the low-frequency region of the audiogram (500 to 2,000 Hz) show the "toughening process," but there is no evidence of reduced threshold shift at 4 and 8 kHz. Although there are data only for two animals, in the previous experiment (Byrne et al, in press) 23 subjects showed toughening at all frequencies tested except at 16,000 Hz.

The fact that the conditioning exposures can render the subject less susceptible to PTS raises a number of practical and theoretical questions: (1) Over what intensity range is the "conditioning" exposure effective? (2) What is the time course of the conditioning effect, i.e., is the system more resistant after a short exposure or does it require the 10 or 20 days as reported here and by Canlon et al? (3) How persistent is the change? (4) What is the bandwidth of the effect, i.e., is the conditioning effect specific to the spectrum of the conditioning sound or is it a more generalized response to stimulation? (5) Does the condi-

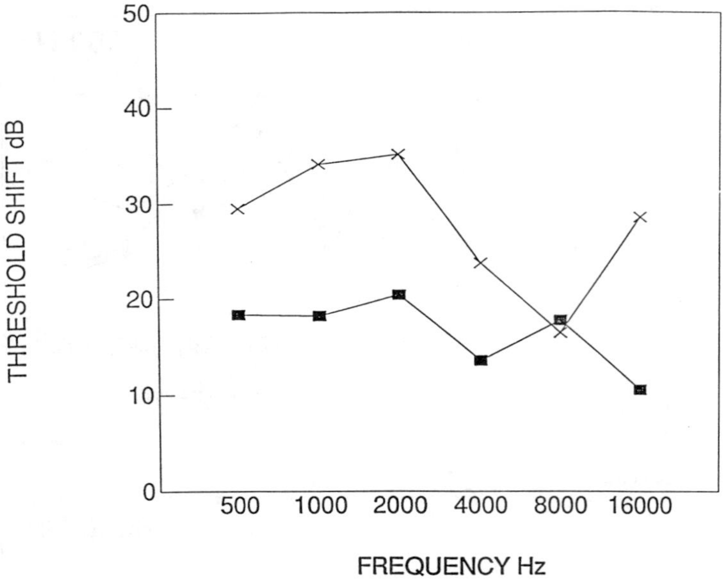

Figure 42-13 Permanent threshold shifts recorded in the experimental (filled squares) and control (crossed lines) groups following the 106-dB exposure.

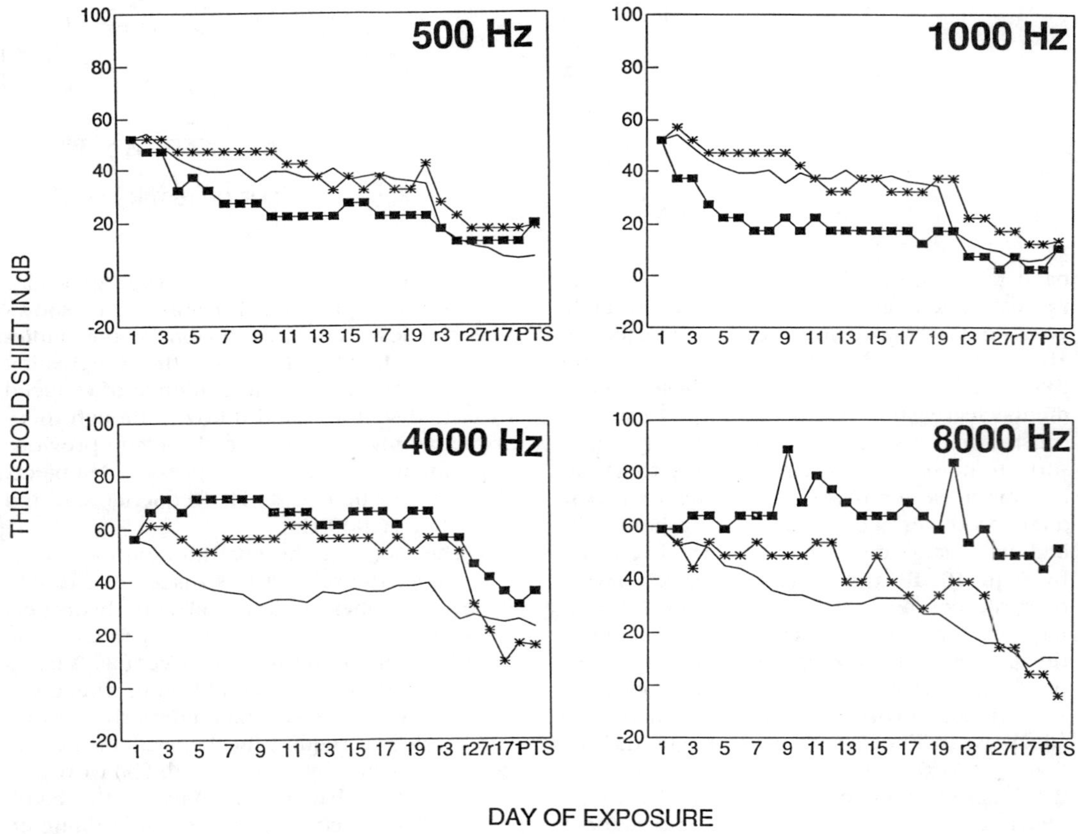

Figure 42-14 Postexposure threshold shifts in two animals following section of the crossed olivocochlear bundle (COCB). The data are normalized with reference to Byrne et al's (in press) data. Symbols represent the data from the two individual animals, and the line shows the results from Byrne et al's experiment.

tioning effect protect the system from the mechanical trauma associated with impulse or impact noise? and (6) What is the biologic basis of the conditioning effect, i.e., does the acoustic reflex become more effective or is there a fundamental change in the cochlea, perhaps mediated by the efferent system?

Développement de la Résistance au Bruit

Dans l'étude des traumatismes auditifs engendrés par le bruit, l'un des aspects les plus étonnants demeure la grande variabilité des résultats. Certaines données récentes suggèrent que les déficits auditifs engendrés par le bruit dépendent, en partie, des expositions sonores préalablement subies par les sujets. Des études mettant en oeuvre des expositions répétées, ont montré que les déficits auditifs pouvaient être réduits, jusqu'à 30 dB, par des expositions quotidiennes pendant 10 à 20 jours. D'autres études ont montré que des expositions préalables à de faibles niveaux de bruit pouvaient réduire les déplacements de seuils permanents. Cet article apporte des données complémentaires, obtenues à l'aide d'une technique de potentiels évoqués, quant à l'importance des expositions sonores préalables subies par des sujets pour déterminer leur susceptibilité au bruit.

La première exposition s'attache au niveau sonore dans le développement de la résistance au bruit. Deux groupes de chinchillas ont été exposés quotidiennement à un bruit de bande centré à 500 Hz (0,5 dB OBN) à des intensités sonores de 85, 95 et 100 dB SPL pendant 10 jours. Les déplacements de seuils ont été mesurés pour une gamme de fréquence allant de 500 Hz à 16 kHz, au début et à la fin de chaque jour d'exposition. Les résultats montrent pour chaque groupe d'animaux la tendance à la diminution des déplacements de seuils pendant les 10 jours d'exposition. Cependant, le groupe d'animaux exposés à 100 dB montre une résistance à toutes les fréquences tandis que pour les plus faibles niveaux, la résistance est moins prononcée aux fréquences élevées.

La seconde exposition a été réalisée dans le but de vérifier si l'augmentation de la résistance aux TTS observée dans la première expérience, pouvait apporter une protection contre le PTS engendré par une exposition traumatique. Dans cette expérience, deux groupes d'animaux ont été utilisés. Le premier groupe a été exposé quotidiennement, pendant 10 jours, à raison de 6 heures par jour à un bruit d'une bande d'octave de 0,5 kHz et de niveau sonore de 95 dB. Une période de récupération de 5 jours leur était accordée. Au terme des 5 jours, tous les animaux avaient quasiment retrouvé leurs seuils auditifs initiaux (+5 dB). Au sixième jour, les animaux ont été exposés au même bruit à un niveau de 106 dB pendant 48 heures. Un groupe témoin constitué d'animaux n'ayant pas subi d'exposition préalable, a été exposé au même bruit à un niveau de 106 dB pendant 48 heures. A ce jour, les résultats semblent indiquer qu'une exposition sonore préalable-non traumatique protége les animaux d'une exposition traumatique.

La troisième expérience avait pour but de déterminer si l'existence préalable d'un PTS peut protéger lors d'une exposition ultérieure au bruit. Deux groupes d'animaux, l'un ayant un PTS de 27 à 40 dB engendré par une exposition préalable au bruit, l'autre, groupe témoin, sans PTS préalable, sont exposés à un bruit de 106 dB pendant 48 heures. Les seuils étaient enregistrés pour une gamme de fréquence allant de 0,5 à 16 kHz avant et après l'exposition.

Les résultats indiquent que les animaux ayant un déficit auditif pré-existant, présentent une amplitude de PTS plus faible que celle des animaux témoins. Cela suggère qu'un déficit pré-existant pourrait offrir une protection contre des expositions sonores ultérieures

ACKNOWLEDGMENTS

We thank Mr. Samuel S. Saunders for his technical assistance and Mrs. Jingui Wu for her assistance in data collection. This research was supported by a grant from NIOSH (5R010H0115209).

References

Byrne C, Henderson D, Saunders S, Powers N, Farzi F. Interaction of noise and whole body vibration. J Acoust Soc Am (Submitted).

Canlon B, Borg E, Flock Å. Protection against noise trauma by pre-exposure to a low level acoustic stimulus. Hear Res 1988; 34:197-200.

Chung D, Wilson GN, Gannon RP, Mason K. Individual susceptibility to noise. In: Hammernik RP, Henderson D, Salvi RJ, eds. New perspectives on noise induced hearing loss. New York: Raven Press, 1982.

Clark WW, Bohne BA, Boettcher FA. Effect of periodic rest on hearing loss and cochlear damage following exposure to noise. J Acoust Soc Am 1987; 82:1253-1264.

Fiorino F, Gratton M, Subbanna M, Bianchi L, Henderson H. Physiological mechanism underlying the progressive resistance to noise induced hearing loss. VALSALVA LXV, Supplement to 1, 1989; 36-41.

Henderson D, Hamernik RP, Woodford C, Sitler RW, Salvi R. Evoked-response audibility of the chinchilla. J Acoust Soc Am 1973; 54:1099-1101.

Miller JD. Audibility curve of the chinchilla. J Acoust Soc Am 1970; 54:1099-1101.

Miller JD, Watson CS, Covell WP. Deafening effects of noise on the cat. Acta Otolaryngol Suppl 1963; 176:1-91.

Saunders JC, Mills JH, Miller JD Threshold shift in the chinchilla from daily exposure to noise for six hours. J Acoust Soc Am 1977; 61:558-570.

Sinex DG, Clark WW, Bohne BA. Effects of periodic rest on physiological measures of auditory sensitivity following exposure to noise. J Acoust Soc Am 1987; 82:1265-1273.

Ward WD. The concept of susceptibility to hearing loss. J Occup Med 1965; 7:595.

CHAPTER 43

Physiologic and Morphologic Aspects to Low-Level Acoustic Stimulation

BARBARA CANLON
ERIK BORG
PAULA LÖFSTRAND

One of the most intriguing problems in noise research concerns the auditory system's capacity to modulate the adverse effects of acoustic stimulation. An understanding of the auditory system's means of modulating these effects would help to elucidate the relationship between permanent and temporary hearing losses. At present, the underlying physiologic, morphologic, and biochemical mechanisms that distinguish a temporary hearing loss from a permanent hearing loss are not known.

Since the pioneering, and to say the very least, courageous experiments of Hallowell Davis and co-investigators (1943), the concept of a temporary threshold shift was introduced. These investigators exposed themselves to a rather intense noise generated by a bull horn and then determined the degree of hearing loss with the recently developed pure-tone audiometer. Thresholds were generally reported to return to pre-exposure levels. The principal finding from this study was that the degree of hearing loss depended on the frequency, the intensity, and the duration of the exposure. In addition, the phenomenon of the half-octave shift was first noted. The greatest threshold shift occurred at frequencies one-half octave above the stimulating frequency, whereas thresholds for frequencies below were generally not affected. Extensions of this first report on the half-octave shift have shown that exposures of moderate intensity yield thresholds in the same region as the exposure, yet when the intensity is systematically increased the half-octave shift becomes apparent (Ward et al, 1973; Mitchell et al, 1977; Lonsbury-Martin and Meikle, 1978; Salvi et al, 1982). Unfortunately, there are no physiologic or morphologic features to indicate when a temporary threshold shift might develop into a permanent lesion. Threshold shifts as large as 80 dB can be completely revesible, whereas in other cases a shift of 60 dB can result in as much as a 30-dB permanent loss (Robertson et al, 1980; Cody and Robertson, 1983).

Morphologic changes induced from a temporary hearing loss have been primarily associated with the stereocilia (Hunter-Duvar, 1977; Tilney et al, 1982; Liberman et al, 1986). The pathology includes floppy stereocilia, depolymerization of the actin filaments at the base of the stereocilium, a loss in the crossbridges between adjacent actin filaments in the stereocilium, and reductions in the length of the supracuticular portion of the rootlets. Moreover, experiments with the isolated guinea pig cochlea coil have shown micromechanical changes in stereocilia following overstimulation. These changes were reversible and metabolically dependent (Saunders et al, 1986). The functional consequences of these temporary alterations in morphology are suggested to decrease the stiffness of the stereocilia and thus change the sensitivity and tuning properties of the auditory system.

Modulation of Auditory Sensitivity

One means of better understanding the relationship between a temporary and a permanent noise-induced threshold shift is to experimentally manipulate the sensitivity of the auditory system in such a way as to increase or decrease the effects of noise. Interesting results have been obtained with respect to experimentally induced manipulations of cochlear metabolism. Noise-induced hearing loss can be either increased or decreased by altering the body temperature (Drescher, 1976; Henry and Chole, 1984). These changes are reversible, do not affect the pre-exposure thresholds, and are believed to be of cochlear origin.

Protection from noise trauma can also occur through the activation of either the middle-ear muscles or the olivocochlear bundle. The middle-ear muscles control the amount of sound energy entering the cochlea by increasing the stiffness of the ossicular chain as they contract. The stapedius reflex, a bilateral reflex, is activated at a sound level of approximately 85 dB hearing level in humans and slightly lower in animals. The middle-ear muscles are known to adapt rapidly during exposure to high-frequency tones, yet are more stable at frequencies lower than 2 kHz and in time-varying noise (Borg and Nilsson, 1984). The stapedius muscle has been shown to influence the susceptibility of the ear to permanently-induced threshold shifts in experimental animals (Borg and Nilsson, 1984). Furthermore, in patients suffering from Bell's palsy with total unilateral paralysis of the stapedius muscle, there is a greater threshold shift in the affected ear compared to the normal ear after a temporary threshold shift is induced (Zakrisson and Borg, 1974).

The efferent innervation to the cochlea is supplied by the olivocochlear bundle. The olivocochlear bundle originates in the superior olivary complex in the brain stem and terminates on the outer hair cells or the afferent dendrites under the inner hair cells. Although many efforts have been made to delineate the functional role of the efferent system, no functional role has yet been determined. One of the various roles proposed for the efferent system has been to diminish the deleterious effects of noise trauma. Indeed, Cody and Johnstone (1982) showed that protection of the ipsilateral ear occurred when the contralateral ear was simultaneously stimulated at the same frequency but at a lower intensity. This effect was blocked by strychnine, a known blocker of the olivocochlear bundle. Furthermore, high rates of electrical stimulation of the crossed olivocochlear bundle presented simultaneously with acoustic overstimulation reduced the magnitude of a temporary threshold shift (Rajan, 1988).

Another means of reducing the susceptibility to noise trauma is by exposing experimental animals to interrupted noise. Miller et al (1963) demonstrated that when cats were exposed to interrupted noise for 16 days, threshold shifts declined during the latter part of the exposure compared to thresholds obtained after the first day. Another interesting study has shown that intermittent exposures result in a reduced threshold shift as well as less cochlear damage compared to chinchillas exposed to continuous exposures of equal energy (Clark et al, 1987).

Given these observations, it is apparent that the degree of hearing loss induced by noise can be modulated by a variety of means. The anatomic site responsible for these changes in sensitivity of the auditory system to noise is not known and can lie either in the periphery or in the central nervous system. These findings provide a foundation on which to further assess and experimentally test the differences between temporary and permanent noise-induced hearing loss.

Outer Hair Cells

Current concepts of auditory physiology include an active mechanism in order to counteract the high degree of viscous damping caused by the cochlear fluids (Neely and Kim, 1983). The demonstration that the outer hair cells contain contractile proteins (Zenner, 1986) and that they exhibit motile behavior in response to electrical stimulation (Brownell et al, 1985; Ashmore, 1987), chemical manipulations (Zenner et al, 1985; Flock et al, 1986), or mechanical stimulation (Canlon et al, 1988b) suggest that the outer hair cells are the active elements.

In light of these recent developments, it is interesting to point out that it is the outer hair cells that are most susceptible to acoustic trauma. Morphologic studies have repeatedly illustrated that the outer hair cells are more susceptible to noise trauma than the inner hair cells. Because the postulated function of the outer hair cells is to modify cochlear sensitivity and frequency selectivity, it is essential to have a basic understanding as to why the outer hair cell is the underdog of noise trauma. By applying the analogy that the outer hair cells have a "muscle-like" role, we attempted to exercise or "train" the guinea pig cochlea to tolerate higher levels of acoustic stimulation.

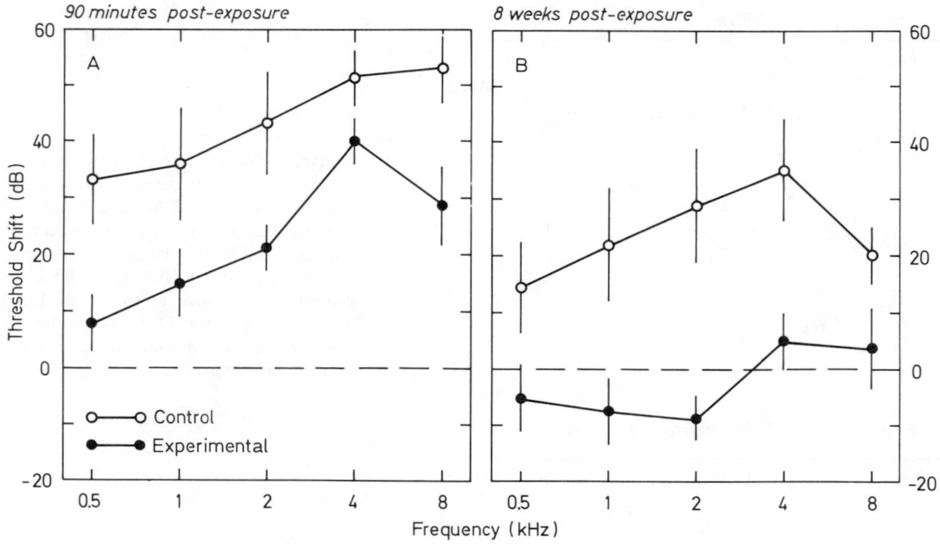

Figure 43-1 Protection from noise trauma in the guinea pig. The control group (open circles) was exposed to 1 kHz, 105 dB SPL for 72 hours; the experimental group (closed circles) was pre-exposed to 1 kHz, 81 dB SPL for 24 days followed by the 1 kHz, 105 dB SPL for 72 hours. *Left,* Auditory brain-stem response thresholds measured 90 minutes after exposure to 1 kHz, 105 dB SPL, 72 hours. *Right,* Auditory thresholds measured after an 8-week recovery period.

Training Paradigm

In an attempt to reduce the damaging effects of noise, guinea pigs (200 to 350 g body weight) were exposed continuously to a 1-kHz tone at 81 dB SPL for 21 days in free field. This level was chosen in the following fashion: It was determined that a continuous exposure to a 1-kHz tone at 105 dB SPL for 72 hours creates a permanent hearing loss between 30 and 50 dB (Canlon et al, 1987). By reducing the intensity and time of exposure systematically and experimentally testing the consequent brain-stem audiometry response, an exposure of 90 dB SPL at 1 kHz for 72 hours was found to be a "safe" level in that no threshold shift could be detected. By maintaining equal energy, the intensity of the exposure was decreased to 81 dB SPL and the duration increased to 576 hours, or 24 days. The duration and intensity of this exposure were considered sufficient to stimulate the auditory system without damaging cochlear structures.

The auditory brain-stem response (ABR) threshold was determined prior to and immediately after exposure (n = 10). A threshold shift could not be detected. It remains possible that a temporary threshold shift may have been induced by the low-level exposure, but it either recovered rapidly before the threshold measures could be made, or it was too small to be detected with this measuring technique. Under the test conditions, there was a 5- to 10-dB standard deviation of the threshold values, indicating that a threshold shift of less than 10 dB would not have been detected. The test-retest reliability of the procedure for both the experimental group (trained) and the control group (not trained) neither differed significantly between the two measurements within each group nor differed between the groups.

After recovery from the anesthesia, animals were exposed to the traumatizing tone (1 kHz, 105 dB SPL, 72 hours). At the end of this exposure, auditory thresholds were determined. Animals were then maintained in ambient noise for either 3 days, 1 month, or 2 months for yet another threshold determination.

Protection from Noise Trauma by Pre-Exposure to Low-Level Acoustic Stimulation

One hour after acoustic overstimulation to the 1-kHz tone at 105 dB SPL for 72 hours, the ABR thresholds for the control group (n = 10) and the experimental group (n = 10) were elevated at all frequencies (Fig. 43-1). The control group showed a 30- to 50-dB

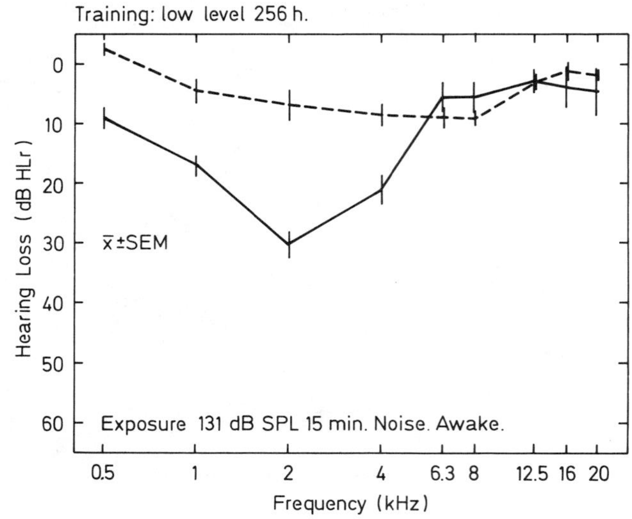

Figure 43-2 Protection from noise trauma in the rabbit. The control group (solid line) was exposed to a 2- to 4-kHz noise, 131 dB SPL for 15 minutes; the experimental group (dashed line) was pre-exposed to a 2- to 7-kHz noise at 79 dB SPL for 256 hours followed by exposure to the 2- to 4-kHz noise at 131 dB SPL for 15 minutes. Hearing loss was measured 3 weeks after exposure to the 131-dB SPL exposure.

threshold shift, whereas the experimental group showed a 10- to 40-dB shift across frequency. The difference in threshold shift between the two groups was statistically significant at the 5 percent level for all frequencies (Students' t-test). When both groups were allowed an 8-week recovery period, the auditory thresholds improved at all frequencies. Although the experimental group showed complete recovery, the control group continued to show a 20- to 30-dB threshold shift. In fact, already by 3 days after exposure, the experimental group showed complete recovery, whereas the control group exhibited a slightly higher threshold shift than that found after 8 weeks.

Comparative Studies in the Rabbit

To determine if protection against noise trauma by pre-exposure to a low-level acoustic stimulus was a unique feature to the guinea pig auditory system, a study was designed to test the rabbit. One group of rabbits (n = 4) was pre-exposed to a 2- to 7-kHz noise at 79 dB SPL for 256 hours prior to a high-intensity noise exposure (2 to 4 kHz, 131 dB SPL, 15 minutes). This second exposure is known to cause a permanent hearing loss. The second group of rabbits (n = 12) were exposed only to the damaging noise. The auditory thresholds for all rabbits were tested prior to exposure and 3 weeks after the damaging exposure. Both groups were exposed in the awake state. Figure 43-2 illustrates the brain-stem response threshold shifts obtained 3 weeks after exposure to the damaging noise (131 dB SPL, 15 minutes). Threshold shifts differ for the two groups by 10 to 25 dB between 0.5 and 4 kHz. Thresholds did not differ in the region of 6.3 to 20 kHz. The group of rabbits exposed to the low-level stimulus prior to the damaging tone showed a threshold shift that was under 10 dB for the frequencies between 0.5 and 4 kHz. Furthermore, it was found that the training effect is relatively long-lasting. When rabbits are maintained in ambient noise for either 2 weeks or 1 month after being trained, and then exposed to the high-intensity stimulation, protection against noise trauma is still evident. Under these conditions, the threshold shifts are similar to when the rabbits were exposed to the damaging noise immediately after the training exposure.

Morphologic Analysis

Neither the mechanisms nor the sites responsible for these changes are known. Several different mechanisms located throughout the auditory pathway could account for the protection against noise trauma. Participation of the middle-ear muscles, inner or outer hair cells, afferent or efferent nerve endings, sympathetic influences, and modulation by the central nervous system are all likely candidates.

To begin to address these questions, an electron microscopic study was undertaken to determine if morphologic differences could be detected between the control animals and the two groups of noise-exposed guinea pigs. The first group was only exposed to the 1-kHz tone at 81 dB SPL for 21 days, and the second group was exposed to the 81-dB SPL tone for 21 days followed by the 105-dB SPL tone for 72 hours. After each exposure, auditory thresholds were determined with the auditory brain-stem response. Cochleas were then fixed in either 1.0 percent or 6.0 percent glutaraldehyde and 0.2 percent tannic acid in 0.1 M phosphate buffer. After dehydration and embedding in Agar 100 epoxy resin (Agar Scientific, Ltd.), the cochleas were then cleaved axially, and the areas around 14, 16, 17, and 18 mm from the round window were cut out and remounted on blocks that were sectioned and finally examined in a Zeiss EM 109 electron microscope. Analysis of the electron micrographs was performed at a final magnification of 27,600 ×.

Outer Hair Cell Afferent Synapse

The two morphologically distinct spiral ganglion cells, type I and type II, innervate the inner and outer hair cells, respectively, in all mammalian species studied. The typical outer hair cell afferent synapse is a small bouton-type ending arising from the outer spiral fiber. The representation of outer spiral fibers on the outer hair cell is graded in such a fashion that the third-row outer hair cell shows a greater number of boutons than the first- or second-row outer hair cells (Brown, 1987). These small afferent nerve endings contain microtubules, mitochondria, and a few vesicles relative to the efferent synapse, in a filamentous matrix. In the presynaptic region, in the infranuclear region of the outer hair cell, there are mitochondria, vesicles, coated vesicles, and tubulovesicular cisternae (Fig. 43-3*A*). Of the control cells studied (n = 9), the total membrane content at the base of the cell (vesicles + coated vesicles + tubulovesicular cisternae) per afferent synapse has a range of 15 to 26 and a mean value of 19.2 ± 3.5 S.D. (Fig. 43-4).

Two animals were exposed to the 1-kHz tone at 81 dB SPL for 21 days. Auditory thresholds were measured prior to the exposure and at the end of the exposure, and a threshold shift could not be detected. When the total membrane content per afferent synapse at the base of the cell was counted, there was nearly a two-fold increase over the control cells. An overall increase in all the membrane components, vesicles, coated vesicles, and tubulovesicular cisternae was found (Fig. 43-3*B*). Of the two animals studied, animal number 196 had a range of 20 to 47 vesicles per afferent synapse with a mean value of 34.0 ± 7.0 S.D. (n = 14 outer hair cells), and animal number 204 had a range of 32 to 48 with a mean value of 39.0 ± 4.5 S.D. (n = 6 outer hair cells). These values are illustrated in Figure 43-4.

After the combined exposure to 81 dB SPL for 21 days and to 105 dB SPL for 3 days, auditory thresholds were measured, and the protective effect against the high-intensity exposure was apparent. The pretreatment resulted in approximately a 20-dB reduction in the threshold shift relative to animals not preexposed. The cochlea of this animal was studied at the electron microscopic level, and the total membrane content in the infranuclear region of the outer hair cells was determined to be almost two-fold that of the control outer hair cell (Fig. 43-3*C*). This animal had a range of vesicles per afferent synapse of 25 to 49 and a mean value of 36.6 ± 7.8 S.D. (n = 9 outer hair cells) (Fig. 43-4). Although the total number of vesicles per afferent synapse did not differ from the animals exposed only to the 81-dB tone, the number of tubulovesicular cisternae had increased. The 1.5-fold increase is marginal, but because the diameter of these cisternae had increased, these changes are more apparent.

According to the widely accepted hypothesis of Heuser and Reese (1973), after fusion of the synaptic vesicle with the presynaptic membrane and release of the transmitter into the synaptic cleft, the vesicular membrane is incorporated into the plasmalemma. The vesicular membrane then diffuses laterally within the plasma membrane and is eventually retrieved at the periphery of the active zone through coated vesicles. The coated vesicles lose their coats and coalesce to form smooth cisternae. The coated vesicles and smooth cisternae are endocytic organelles able to generate and refill new vesicles with transmitter. An analogous scheme is apparent for the outer hair cell afferent synapse and has either directly or indirectly been suggested by various investigators (Saito, 1983; Nadol, 1983; Ekström von Lubitz, 1981). Figure 43-5*A* illustrates the scheme for the unstimulated outer hair cell. Vesicles, coated vesicles, and tubulovesicular cisternae are shown undergoing membrane recycling in a manner similar to that described for the neuromuscular junction (Heuser and Reese, 1973). Figure 43-5*B* illustrates an outer hair cell after acoustic stimulation. An increased turnover of the membrane components at the base of the outer hair cell in the presynaptic region is depicted. The

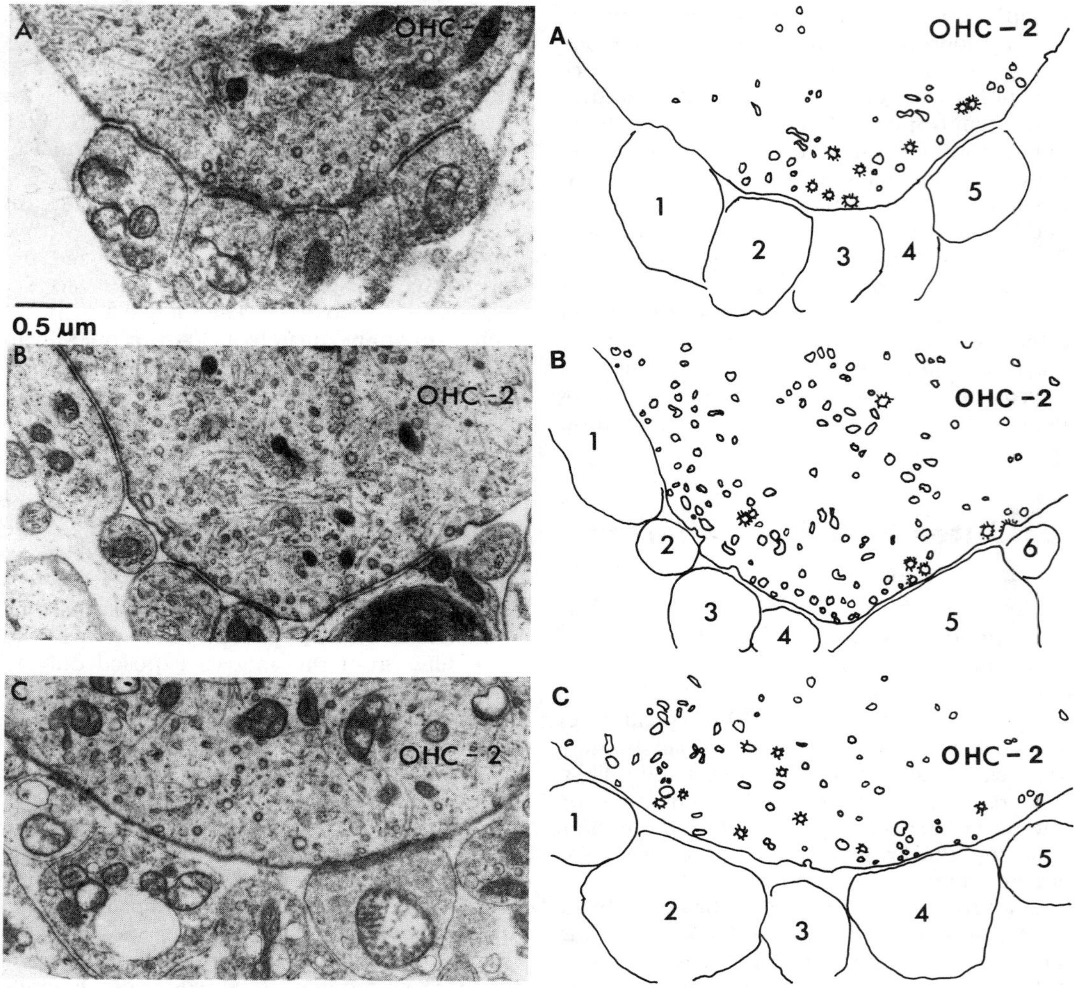

Figure 43-3 *Left,* Electron micrographs of the infranuclear region of outer hair cells with nerve endings from the outer spiral fibers. *A,* Control outer hair cell. *B,* After exposure to 81 dB SPL for 24 days. *C,* After exposure to 81 dB SPL for 24 days followed by exposure to 105 dB SPL for 72 hours. An increase in the total membrane content (vesicles, coated vesicles, and tubulovesicular cisternae) is noted in *B* and *C. Right,* Tracings from the electron micrographs shown on the left to illustrate more clearly the increase in membrane components in *B* and *C* compared to *A.*

finding that all the membrane components at the base of the outer hair cell are increased after stimulation is in contrast to the effect of stimulation at the neuromuscular junction (Heuser and Reese, 1973). After either 1 minute or 15 minutes of stimulation of the motor nerve terminal, the total amount of membrane components remained constant. Even though the total membrane remained constant, there was a depletion of vesicles and an increased number of cisternal membranes and coated vesicles. The depletion of vesicles is believed to be a reflection of the decrease in the postsynaptic potential that was monitored during stimulation of the muscle. In contrast, when the auditory system was stimulated with a low-level tone (81 dB SPL, 21 days), the membrane components in the infranuclear region, the area opposing the afferent synapse of outer hair cells, increased, yet changes in auditory sensitivity could not be detected. There was an overall increase in all membrane components—i.e., vesicles, coated vesicles, and tubulovesicular cisternae. However, when the auditory system was stimulated with the low-level tone followed by the high-intensity tone of 105 dB SPL for 72 hours, the increase in membrane components was not uniformly distributed amongst all of the membrane components. That is, the tubulocisternae showed an

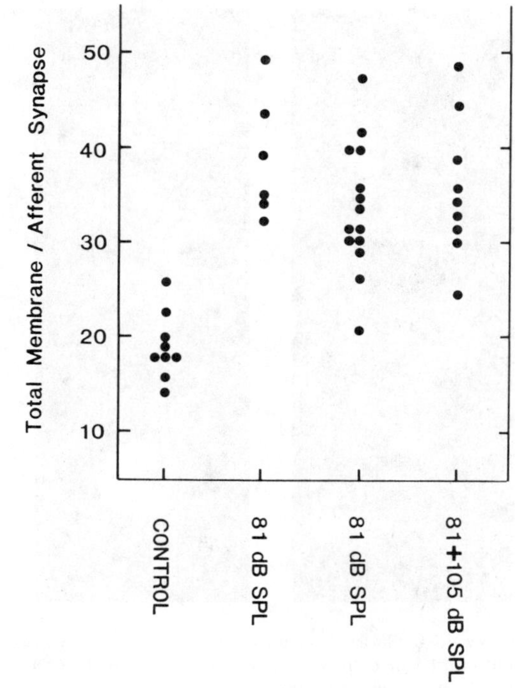

Figure 43-4 Total membrane content per afferent synapse for individual outer hair cells after different noise conditions. Total membrane content is the sum of all vesicles, coated vesicles, and tubulovesicular cisternae at the base of the outer hair cell. The total membrane content is normalized to the number of afferent synapses in contact with the outer hair cell. Each point is obtained from a single outer hair cell from a control animal, two animals exposed to 81 dB SPL for 24 days, and one animal exposed to 81 dB SPL for 24 days followed by 105 dB SPL for 72 hours.

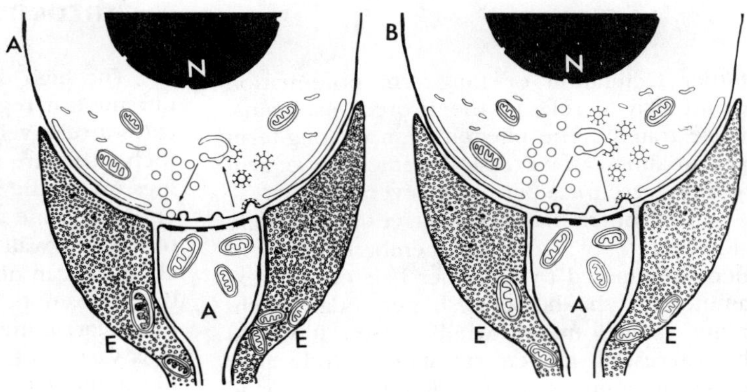

Figure 43-5 Schematic illustration showing the recycling of the membrane components at the base of an outer hair cell in an unstimulated outer hair cell *(A)* and after exposure to a low-level, long-term, nondamaging acoustic stimulus *(B)*. A two-fold increase in the turnover of the membrane components is apparent in *B*. Afferent nerve endings *(A)*, Efferent nerve endings *(E)*.

increase in number and a decrease in the number of vesicles, whereas the number of coated vesicles remained the same.

These findings indicate that the presynaptic region of the outer hair cell has the capacity to undergo increased membrane recycling during long-term, low-level acoustic stimulation. This includes recycling of vesicles as well as the resynthesis of the transmitter substance. Short-term acoustic stimulation apparently does not cause similar changes in the region of the afferent synapse in the outer hair cell, at least in the cat (Liberman and Dodds, 1987). It has been previously reported that the total membrane components at the base of the outer hair cell vary in an inconsistent fashion. It is therefore important to emphasize that it is essential to normalize the total membrane components to the total number of afferent synapses in contact with the cell. When the total membrane components are normalized, it is found that the membrane values are fairly constant for each outer hair cell.

The increase in membrane recycling after exposure to low-level stimulation could be one underlying mechanism for the protection against noise trauma. Activity-dependent improvement of synaptic efficiency, as suggested from the present study, would perhaps enhance the response to a second stimulation.

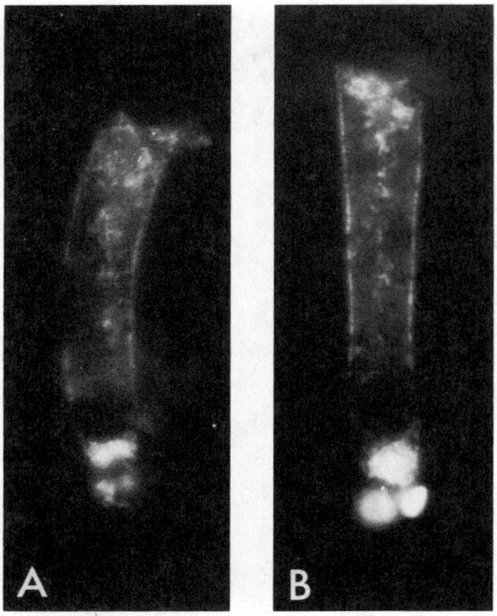

Figure 43-6 Fluorescent mitochondrial activity in isolated outer hair cells from a control outer hair cell *(A)* and an outer hair cell after exposure to 81 dB SPL for 24 days *(B)*. There is no qualitative difference in the staining pattern.

Either facilitation or long-term potentiation could play a role in the protection against noise trauma. The phenomenon of long-term potentiation can increase the efficiency of synaptic release for a period of several weeks.

The outer hair cells have a relatively slower rate of recycling membrane components compared to the inner hair cells as examined by the horseradish peroxidase technique (Siegel and Brownell, 1986). It would be interesting to perform such a study after exposing animals to the low-level acoustic stimulation.

Outer Hair Cell Efferent Synapse

The large efferent nerve endings at the base of the outer hair cell of the control group and the two groups of noise-exposed animals showed no consistent difference in the density of vesicles. It has been suggested that an increase in the density of vesicles in the efferent nerve ending increased following noise exposure (Spoendlin, 1971). In the present study, however, a reduction in the density of the vesicles as well as an increase in the diameter of the vesicles occasionally was found after noise exposure. This finding was sporadic and it is difficult to know if it was a normal variation in the efferent synapse or if it was the result of the noise exposure.

Other morphologic changes that were studied include the character of the subsynaptic cisternae and its distance to the synaptic cleft. No obvious alterations were noted. It may be possible that short-term stimulation influences primarily the efferent system (Cody and Johnstone, 1982; Rajan, 1988). Protection against noise trauma was found by stimulating the efferents for a short duration, either acoustically or by electrically stimulating the crossed olivocochlear bundle prior to noise exposure. The effects could be blocked by applying known inhibitors of the efferent system. To find a morphologic correlate to these findings may be difficult because the protective effect after these short durations of stimulation could occur at the level of the ion channel. It seems unlikely that these changes could also be related to an increase in membrane recycling because the synthesis of new protein and transmitter is not a rapid process.

Mitochondria

The high density of mitochondria in the infranuclear region of the outer hair cell indicates a relatively high-energy metabolism. Mitochondria are also present in the nerve endings under the hair cells as well as under the cuticular plate and along the longitudinal axis of the cell wall. It has been shown that mitochondria can undergo configurational changes due to osmotic shock or to an altered metabolic state either through increased activity or by a variety of chemical agents such as 2,4-dinitrophenol (Rydzynski and Cieciura, 1980). Swollen mitochondria have also been shown to be a common feature after acoustic overstimulation (Omata and Schätzle, 1984). Some of these mitochondrial configurational changes are reversible, but if the insult is severe enough they can undergo necrosis.

Qualitative Measures of Mitochondrial Activity

The cationic fluorescent probe, $DiOC_2[3]$, a dicarbocyanine dye, has been shown to stain the mitochondria of living cells (Johnson et al, 1981). The specific interaction of the dye with mitochondria is related to the high transmembrane potential of mitochondria. This fluorescently labeled dye was used to determine if the long-term, low-level acoustic stimulation had altered the metabolic capacity of the mitochondria of outer hair cells. The activity of the mitochondria in isolated outer hair cells of the control group (no noise) (n = 24 cells) and the experimental group (81 dB, 21 days) (n = 28 cells) was studied. Outer hair cells from the 15-, 16-, and 17-mm distance from the round window were isolated and incubated for 10 minutes in 5 μM 3,3′diethyloxacarbocyanine [$DiOC_2(3)$], rinsed, and examined by epifluorescence microscopy. No qualitative difference could be discerned between the staining pattern of the outer hair cells from the two groups. Figure 43-6 shows a control outer hair cell and an outer hair cell from the experimental group. Fluorescence is noted under the cuticular plate, along the longitudinal axis of the plasma membrane, beneath the nucleus, and within the synapses contacting the outer hair cell. To test the sensitivity of the dye to detect changes in mitochondrial activity, control cells were preincubated in 4 mM sodium cyanide for 30 minutes prior to the incubation with the fluorescent dye, $DiOC_2(3)$. Under this condition, there was neglible staining of the mitochondria of the outer hair cells. Thus, if major metabolic differences exist between the two conditions, it is most probable that the technique is sensitive to detect such changes.

Conclusion

The results from the present study show that guinea pigs and rabbits can be protected against noise trauma by pre-exposure to a low-level, long-term acoustic stimulus. The low-level acoustic stimulus affords long-lasting protection for up to several weeks. Electron micrographs suggest that after the long-term acoustic stimulation, the outer hair cells undergo increased membrane recycling in the presynaptic region opposing the nerve endings of the outer spiral fibers. Although the mechanism for the protective effect against a second, damaging acoustic stimulus is not known, one possibility is an increased neurotransmitter pool allowing the system to tolerate longer durations of stimulation. Other possibilities for the protective effect include modulation of ion channels, rearrangements of the synaptic complex, changes in the cytoskeletal framework of the cell, and the involvement of second messengers.

Aspects Fonctionnels et Morphologiques du Phénomène d'Entraînement à L'Exposition au Bruit

Le montant des pertes auditives induites par le bruit peut être modifié par différentes manipulations expérimentales. Dans cette étude nous avons essayé de réduire les effets lésionnels du bruit en pré-exposant des cobayes à un stimulus acoustique de bas niveau avant une exposition à un bruit traumatisant. Cette idée a été développée à partir des concepts habituels de la physiologie cochléaire, et entre autres, celui selon lequel les cellules ciliées externes auraient le même rôle qu'un muscle. En appliquant cette analogie nous comptions exercer ou "entraîner" la cochlée à être capable de tolérer des expositions sonores de plus haut niveau. Un groupe de cobayes a été exposé, pendant une longue durée, de façon continue, à un bruit non traumatisant (1 kHz, 81 dB SPL, 24 jours), préalablement à une exposition connue pour provoquer un déplacement permanent de seuil auditif (PTS) (1 kHz, 103 dB, 3 jours). Le second groupe de cobayes n'a pas été pré-exposé à la stimulation de bas niveau, mais seulement au bruit traumatisant. La réponse à chaque exposition était évaluée en déterminant le seuil de sensibilité auditive par audiométrie au niveau du tronc cérébral. Après exposition au son de 1 kHz à 105 dB SPL pendant 3 jours, le groupe qui avait été pré-exposé (entraîné) montrait approximativement une réduction du niveau de seuil de 20 dB par rapport aux animaux non pré-exposés. Deuxièmement, le groupe pré-exposé récupérait totalement ses fonctions auditives après un repos de 2 mois. Le groupe qui n'avait pas été pré-exposé au stimulus préalable continuait de montrer un déplacement de seuil de 20 à 30 dB.

Suite à ces résultats nous avons étendu nos recherches en manipulant: (1) les paramètres de la pré-exposition (2) l'intervalle de temps entre la pré-exposition et l'exposition traumatisante. Nous avons également élargi la gamme de tests électrophysiologiques pour déterminer la sensibilité auditive, et également étudié la nature du phénomène d'entraînement chez le lapin. De plus, les résultats préliminaires obtenus au microscope électronique indiquent que des changements morphologiques non traumatiques apparaissent dans la région post-synaptique à la base des cellules ciliées externes, suggérant que "l'entraînement" peut influencer leurs capacités métaboliques. Les résultats mettent en évidence qu'après "l'entraînement" la sensibilité de la cochlée au trauma acoustique peut être modifiée par les cellules ciliées externes. Il faut cependant souligner que le mécanisme sous-jacent de l'effet "d'entraînement" est inconnu. Il reste encore à déterminer le rôle que jouent, les muscles de l'oreille moyenne, la circulation sanguine cochléaire, la mécanique de la membrane basiliaire, dans l'effet "d'entraînement."

References

Ashmore JF. A fast motile response in guinea pig outer hair cells: The cellular basis of the cochlear amplifier. J Physiol 1987; 388:323-347.

Borg E, Nilsson R. Acoustic reflex in industrial noise. In: Silman S, ed. The acoustic reflex: Scientific aspects and clinical application. New York: Academic Press, 1984:413.

Brown MC. Morphology of labeled afferent fibers in the guinea pig cochlea. J Comp Neurol 1987; 260:591-604.

Brownell WE, Bader CR, Bertrand D, Ribaupierre Y. Evoked mechanical responses of isolated cochlear hair cells. Science 1985; 227:194-196.

Canlon B, Miller J, Flock Å, Borg E. Pure tone overstimulation changes the micromechanical properties of the inner hair cell stereocilia. Hear Res 1987; 30:65-72.

Canlon B, Borg E, Flock Å. Protection against noise trauma by preexposure to a low level acoustic stimulus. Hear Res 1988a; 34:197-200.

Canlon B, Brundin L, Flock Å. Acoustic stimulation causes tonotopic alterations in the length of isolated outer hair cells from the guinea pig hearing organ. Proc Natl Acad Sci 1988b; 85:7033-7035.

Clark WW, Bohne BA, Boettcher FA. Effects of periodic rest on hearing loss and cochlear damage following exposure to noise. J Acoust Soc Am 1987; 82:1253-1264.

Cody AR, Johnstone BM. Temporary threshold shift modified by binaural acoustic stimulation. Hear Res 1982; 6:199-205.

Cody AR, Robertson D. Variability of noise-induced damage in the guinea pig cochlea: Electro-physiological and morphological correlates after strictly controlled exposures. Hear Res 1983; 9:55-70.

Davis H, Morgan CT, Hawkins JE Jr et al. Temporary deafness following exposure to loud tones and noise. Acta Otolaryngol Suppl 1943; 88.

Drescher DG. Effect of temperature on cochlear responses during and after exposure to noise. J Acoust Soc Am 1976; 59:401-407.

Ekström von Lubitz DKJ. Subsurface tubular system in the outer sensory cells of the rat cochlea. Cell Tissue Res 1981; 220:787-795.

Flock Å, Flock B, Ulfendahl M. Mechanisms of movement of outer hair cells and a possible structural basis. Arch Otorhinolaryngol 1986; 243:83-90.

Henry KR, Chole RA. Hypothermia protects the cochlea from noise damage. Hear Res 1984; 16:225-230.

Heuser JE, Reese TS. Evidence for recycling of synaptic vesicle membrane during transmitter release at the frog neuromuscular junction. J Cell Biol 1973; 57:315-344.

Hunter-Duvar IM. Morphology of the normal and the acoustically damaged cochlea. SEM 1977; 2:421-428.

Johnson LV, Walsh ML, Bockus BJ, Chen LB. Monitoring of relative mitochondrial membrane potential in living cells by fluorescence microscopy. J Cell Biol 1981; 88:526-535.

Liberman MC, Dodds LW, Learson DA. Structure-function correlation in noise-damaged ears. In: Salvi RJ, Henderson D, Hamernik RP, Colletti V, eds. Basic and applied aspects of noise-induced hearing loss. New York: Plenum Press, 1986:163.

Liberman MC, Dodds LW. Acute ultrastructural changes in acoustic trauma: Serial-section reconstruction of stereocilia and cuticular plates. Hear Res 1987; 26:45-64.

Lonsbury-Martin BL, Meikle MB. Neural correlates of auditory fatigue: Frequency-dependent changes in activity of single cochlear nerve fibers. J Neurophysiol 1978; 41:987-1006.

Miller JD, Watson CS, Covell WP. Deafening effects of noise on the cat. Acta Otolaryngol Suppl 1963; 176.

Mitchell C, Brummett RE, Vernon JA. Frequency effects of temporary N_1 depression following acoustic overload. Arch Otolaryngol 1977; 103:117-123.

Nadol JB. Serial section reconstruction of the neural poles of hair cells in the human organ of Corti. II. Outer hair cells. Laryngoscope 1983; 93:780-791.

Neely ST, Kim DO. An active cochlear model showing sharp tuning and high sensitivity. Hear Res 1983; 9:123-130.

Omata T, Schätzle W. Electron microscopical studies on the effect of lapsed time on the nerve endings of the outer hair cells in acoustically exposed rabbits. Arch Oto-Rhino-Laryngol 1984; 240:175-183.

Rajan R. Effect of electrical stimulation of the crossed olivocochlear bundle on temporary threshold shifts in auditory sensitivity. I. Dependence on electrical stimulation parameters. J Neurophysiol 1988; 60:549-568.

Robertson D, Johnstone BM, McGill TJ. Effects of loud tone on the inner ear: A combined electrophysiological and ultrastructural study. Hear Res 1980; 2:39-53.

Rydzynski K, Cieciura L. Modification of the configuration states of mitochondria of the choroid plexus ependyma in vivo. J Ultrastruct Res 1980; 70:118-127.

Saito K. Fine structure of the sensory epithelium of guinea-pig organ of Corti: Subsurface cisternae and lamellar bodies in the oute hair cells. Cell Tissue Res 1983; 229:467-481.

Salvi R, Perry J, Hamernik RP, Henderson D. Relationship between cochlear pathologies and auditory nerve and behavioral responses following acoustic trauma. In: Hamernik RP, Henderson D, Salvi R, eds. New perspectives on noise-induced hearing loss. New York: Raven Press, 1982.

Saunders JC, Canlon B, Flock Å. Changes in stereocilia micromechanics following overstimulation in metabolically blocked hair cells. Hear Res 1986; 24:217-225.

Siegel JH, Brownell WE. Synaptic and Golgi membrane

recycling in cochlear hair cells. J Neurocytol 1986; 15:311-328.

Spoendlin H. Primary structural changes in the organ of Corti after acoustic overstimulation. Acta Otolaryngol 1971; 71:166-176.

Tilney LG, Saunders JC, Egelman E, DeRosier DJ. Changes in the organization of actin filaments in the stereocilia of noise-damaged lizard cochleae. Hear Res 1982; 7:181-197.

Ward WD, Glorig A, Sklar DL. Dependence of temporary threshold shift at four kc on intensity and time. J Acoust Soc Am 1973; 30:944-954.

Zakrisson JE, Borg E. Stapedius reflex and auditory fatigue. Audiology 1974; 13:231-235.

Zenner HP. Motile responses in outer hair cells. Hear Res 1985; 22:83-90.

Zenner HP. Molecular structure of hair cells. In: Hoffmann DW, Altschuler RA, Bobbin RP, eds. Neurobiology of hearing—The cochlea. New York: Raven Press, 1986.

CHAPTER 44

Physical Exercise and Active Protection from Temporary Threshold Shift

VITTORIO COLLETTI
FRANCESCO G. FIORINO
GIUSEPPE VERLATO
GIANCARLO Z. MONTRESOR

A common finding in all studies of noise-induced hearing loss (NIHL) is significant individual variability in susceptibility (Burns, 1973; Ward, 1973; Robinson, 1976; Melnick, 1978). The reasons for this variability are still unknown, although several endogenous and exogenous factors have been proposed. Endogenous factors reported to contribute to variability include age, sex, resonance of the external ear, middle-ear impedance, acoustic reflex properties, body temperature, physical effort, stress sensitivity, cochlear blood supply, cochlear pigmentation, and ovarian cycle (Borg, 1968; Sanden and Axelsson, 1981; Dengerink et al, 1984; Humes, 1984). Exogenous factors, such as ambient temperature, vibrations, drug intake, smoking, and physical activity, can also influence susceptibility to processes that damage hearing (Hamernik et al, 1981; Humes, 1984; Manninen and Ekblom, 1984; Dengerink et al, 1984; Drettner et al, 1985; Byrne et al, 1989).

A recent study stressed the importance of the interaction between noise and physical activity on the amount of temporary threshold shift (TTS) (Lindgren and Axelsson, 1988). Normal-hearing youngsters were exposed to a narrow-band noise at 105 dB SPL for 10 minutes. The results indicated that the combination of noise and simultaneous physical exercise (40 percent of the maximum work load capacity) elicited a larger amount of TTS when compared with test conditions of noise alone, noise before exercise, and noise during recovery. The investigators attributed the greater TTS to increases in whole-body metabolic demand and in blood temperature, which depleted cochlear reserve capacity.

One of the most important endogenous variables in susceptibility to NIHL is the middle-ear transfer function. Small differences in the resonant frequency or in sound transformation across individuals may have a significant influence on the spectrum of noise intensity reaching the inner ear. In this context, differences in the amount of attenuation provided by the acoustic reflex (AR) over time may play an important role in individual susceptibility (Colletti and Sittoni, 1986; Borg, 1968).

The effectiveness of AR in acoustic trauma protection has been debated for several years. Certain features of the reflex, mainly its rapid decay, suggest that the sound attenuation provided by stapedius contraction is of minor importance. However, studies performed in real or simulated industrial conditions show that the AR decay can be prevented by changing the spectral or temporal characteristics (or both) of the eliciting stimuli (Zakrisson and Borg, 1974; Kaplan et al, 1977; Lutman and Martin, 1978; Borg et al, 1979; Nilsson et al, 1980). In addition, it has been demonstrated that when the AR is not operating, the amount of TTS is not only greater in the 4-kHz region but also extends to the speech frequencies (Zakrisson et al, 1980; Nilsson et al, 1980). In fact, the observations that a low-frequency

(0.5 kHz) exposure can yield injuries several octaves above the exposure frequency (Fried et al, 1976), and that a conductive loss in the low-frequency range decreases the amount of the permanent threshold shift (PTS) at 4 kHz (Nilsson et al, 1980), suggest that even though the attenuation provided by the AR is primarily in the low frequencies, the AR can also decrease the risk of damage at high frequencies.

On the basis of these considerations, it has been suggested that the measurement of an individual's reflex characteristics may be useful to predict susceptibility to NIHL (Johansson et al, 1967; Colletti and Sittoni, 1986). However, this simple approach does not take into account simultaneous factors that can interact with AR efficiency, such as drug intake, physical effort, inner ear disorders, and toxic substances.

In addition, other studies suggest that AR response is affected by mental tasks requiring attention, such as selecting words in a passage of writing (Corcoran et al, 1980), solving a visual maze, or mathematical problems (Robinette and Snyder, 1982). Interestingly, when attention is concentrated on auditory stimuli, AR depression is nearly absent. Corcoran et al (1980) also observed that simple eye closure increased the amplitude of the AR response, possibly as a consequence of a general enhancement in muscle tone.

If such simple tasks are able to modify the AR activity, it can be argued that physical activity is a major factor of AR response modification. To investigate this hypothesis, we conducted two experiments with the following aims: (1) to clarify whether dynamic physical exercise is able to modify AR activity and (2) to evaluate whether the modification of the AR by physical exercise influences the amount of TTS.

Materials and Methods

Subjects

The experimental subjects were 10 male volunteers, aged 27 to 34 years (mean 30.8). They were staff or students of the University of Verona. Each subject showed normal hearing sensitivity (less than 20 dB HL) at all test frequencies (250 to 8000 Hz) with pure-tone audiometry (Amplaid A 455 with TDH-39 headphones in MX-41/AR) and normal middle-ear pressure (± 25 daPa). Threshold of the contralateral or ipsilateral AR for tonal or noise stimuli was less than 90 dB SPL. Subjects had no history of ear disease or exposure to hazardous noise and presented normal tympanic membrane on otoscopic examination.

Work Capacity Determination

Prior to beginning the experiment, each subject's maximum work capacity was established on an ergometer cycle (Monark, Stockholm, Sweden). After a rest period of at least 30 minutes the subjects performed a maximal incremental test to exhaustion. The work load was increased every 2 minutes in 25-watt steps, and the wattage value of the last completed step was considered the maximum work capacity. The amount of physical exercise performed by each subject during the 10-minute experimental session was then fixed at 50 percent of the individual maximum work capacity.

Test Conditions

Subjects were randomly submitted to the following five test conditions on different days for a total test period of 5 days. (1) During the exercise, the AR morphology in the right ear was recorded following white noise (WN) stimuli to the contralateral ear at 15 dB SL (re AR threshold). Measurements were taken immediately before exercise (time 0), at 1, 2, 4, 6, 8, and 10 minutes of exercise, as well as at 2, 5, and 10 minutes of recovery. (2) As a control, AR morphology was also assessed during a 20-minute period of rest. The test procedure was identical to test 1, the only difference being the absence of physical activity. (3) The third condition was the evaluation of the amplitude/intensity function of AR at the same time intervals as tests 1 and 2; WN stimuli were used, with an intensity increasing from 60 to 115 dB in 5-dB steps. Only five subjects were submitted to this test. (4) In the fourth condition, the AR decay was measured during noise exposure to the left ear, and the amount of TTS following exposure was studied. During a 10-minute period of exercise, a 105-dB SPL white noise was continuously presented to the left ear. Reflex amplitude was monitored in the right ear at the onset of noise and at 1, 2, 4, 6, 8, and 10 minutes of exposure. Pure-tone audiometry in the left ear (3, 4, 6, and 8 kHz) was performed immediately before and after (2, 5, 10, and 20 minutes) noise exposure. (5) For the final condition, the same protocol as test 4 was repeated in the absence of exercise, so that each subject served again as his own control.

Impedance and Audiometric Testing

Acoustic impedance measurements were carried out with a commercial instrument (Amplaid 720 clinical admittance meter) equipped with an X-Y recorder. The contralateral stapedius reflex was elicited by acoustic stimuli of 1 second duration and 30 seconds rise-fall time, administered to the left ear through TDH-39 earphones. To evaluate AR morphology, four time-domain parameters of the AR were examined according to Colletti (1974) and Borg (1976). *(A) Onset latency:* Time interval between stimulus onset and 10 percent of the maximum amplitude of the response. *(B) Delay time:* Time required for the response to reach 50 percent of maximum amplitude. *(C) Rise-time:* Time required for the response to rise from 10 to 90 percent of its final value. *(D) Amplitude:* Height of the response at steady state expressed as relative admittance changes.

To study the amplitude/intensity function of AR, the reflex amplitude was recorded at different stimulus intensities as the absolute change of admittance in cubic centimeters (cc). Experimental data were fitted with the following sigmoidal logistic function (Mendelowitz and Scher, 1980):

$$Y = \frac{Y\ max}{1 + A \cdot e^{-x/k}}$$

To evaluate the fit, we calculated correlation coefficients and standard error of estimates (Spiegel, 1961).

Subsequent analysis was centered on the following parameters: threshold, defined as stimulus intensity at which the increase in slope, i.e., the second derivative of curve, is maximum; maximal slope; and Y max, defined as the range of AR amplitude (Mendelowitz and Scher, 1980).

During noise exposure to the left ear performed in tests 4 and 5, the contralateral AR response was continuously monitored and changes in compliance with respect to the baseline values were recorded. Percentage modifications with respect to onset amplitude were reported at 1, 2, 4, 6, 8, and 10 minutes.

The static pressure in the external ear was continuously monitored and maintained at the point of maximum compliance. The subject's hearing thresholds before and after noise exposure were established for the left ear with a manual audiometer (Amplaid A 155 with TDH-39 earphones in MX-41/AR) at the frequencies of 3, 4, 6, and 8 kHz. TTS was defined as the difference in decibels between post- and pre-exposure hearing thresholds at the frequencies given above.

Statistical Analysis

Two-way analysis of variance (ANOVA) for repeated measurements was performed for statistical comparison. Sources of variability were represented by time, presence or absence of exercise, and interaction between time and exercise. Simple contrasts were also performed at corresponding intervals between exercise and no exercise conditions. Regression analysis was used to evaluate the relationship between TTS and AR amplitude during tests 4 and 5. A significance level of 0.05 was chosen.

Results

Work Capacity

The subjects' maximum work capacity ranged from 125 to 225 W, with a mean of 185 W. Therefore, the actual work load performed during the experimental sessions at 50 percent of the maximum work capacity ranged from 62.5 to 112.5 W (mean: 92.5).

Effect of Exercise on AR Parameters

Table 44-1 displays the means and the standard errors of time-domain AR parameters recorded before, during, and after exercise (test 1). Figures 44-1 and 44-2 compare the outcome obtained for each time-domain parameter, expressed respectively as absolute changes and percent changes, for the conditions of "noise with exercise" and "noise only." These parameters remained fairly constant during time control experiments, but changed markedly during exercise.

The onset latency was 111.2 ± 10.2 ms (mean ±SEM) at rest, rapidly increased at the onset of exercise (reaching 131 ±7.5 ms at 4 minutes), and slowly decreased thereafter. However, the difference between experimental and control conditions was not significant for either percentage or absolute values.

The time course of delay time was approximately parallel to that of the onset latency just described. Delay time was 179 ±15.3 ms before the onset of the "exercise" and reached peak values of about 205 ms 1 to 4 minutes after the onset of exercise. The dif-

TABLE 44-1 **Modification of AR Parameters During the Exercise and Recovery (Absolute Values)**

TIME (MIN)	LATENCY-TIME (MS)	DELAY-TIME (MS)	RISE-TIME (MS)	AMPLITUDE (CC)
0	111.2 (±10.2)	179 (±15.3)	183.5 (±13.9)	0.075 (±0.008)
1	127 (±9.1)	203 (±15.2)	242.5 (±21.2)	0.067 (±0.008)
2	124 (±12.2)	208 (±18.9)	245 (±22.4)	0.055 (±0.006)
4	131 (±7.5)	205.5 (±12.6)	236.5 (±20.4)	0.056 (±0.007)
6	118 (±9.1)	186.7 (±13.7)	242.5 (±22.7)	0.065 (±0.008)
8	120 (±8.8)	187.5 (±11.3)	222 (±14.8)	0.064 (±0.007)
10	121.5 (±7.1)	189 (±11.5)	235.5 (±14.6)	0.065 (±0.006)
12	126 (±9.6)	196.5 (±11.5)	248.5 (±16.4)	0.069 (±0.008)
15	121.5 (±9.2)	196.5 (±14.6)	231 (±10)	0.070 (±0.009)
20	117 (±10.1)	190.5 (±14.1)	189.5 (±19.6)	0.070 (±0.009)

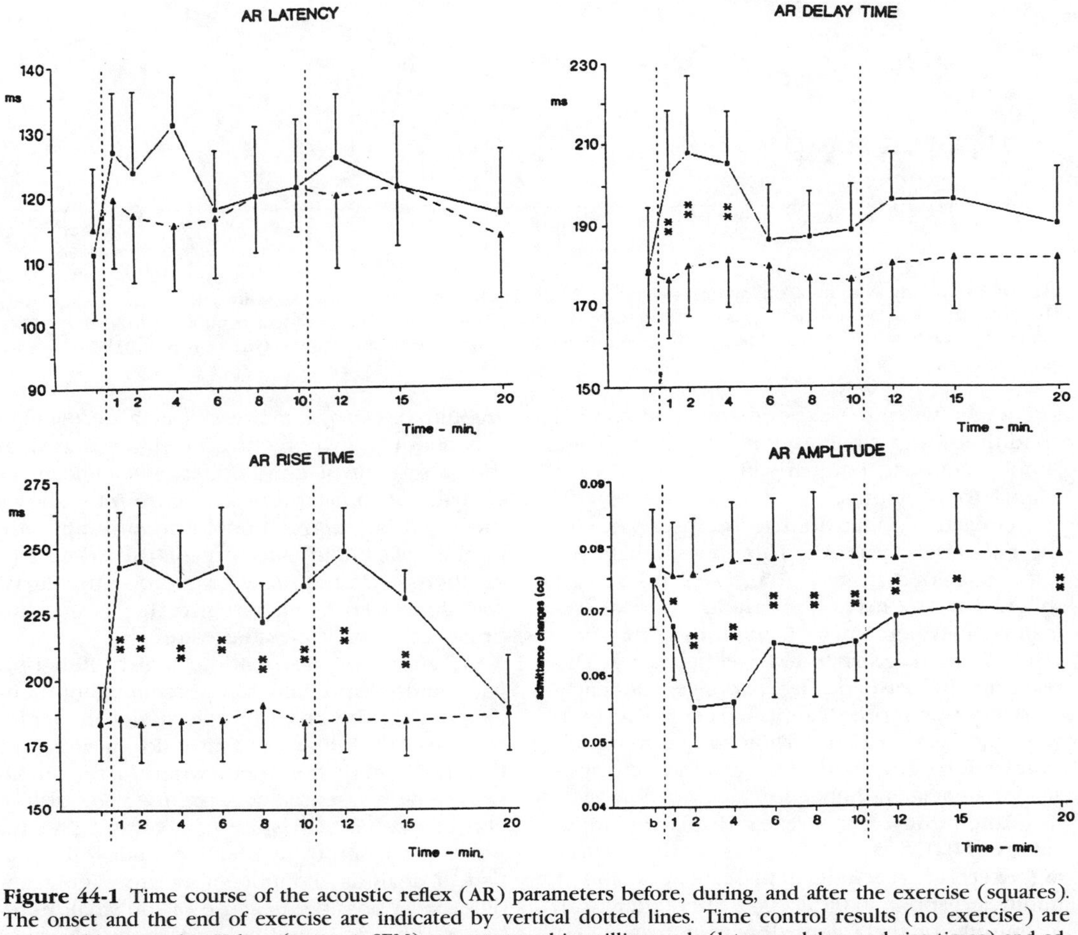

Figure 44-1 Time course of the acoustic reflex (AR) parameters before, during, and after the exercise (squares). The onset and the end of exercise are indicated by vertical dotted lines. Time control results (no exercise) are indicated by triangles. Values (mean ± SEM) are expressed in milliseconds (latency, delay, and rise times) and admittance changes in cubic centimeters (amplitude). One star: $p < 0.05$; two stars: $p < 0.01$.

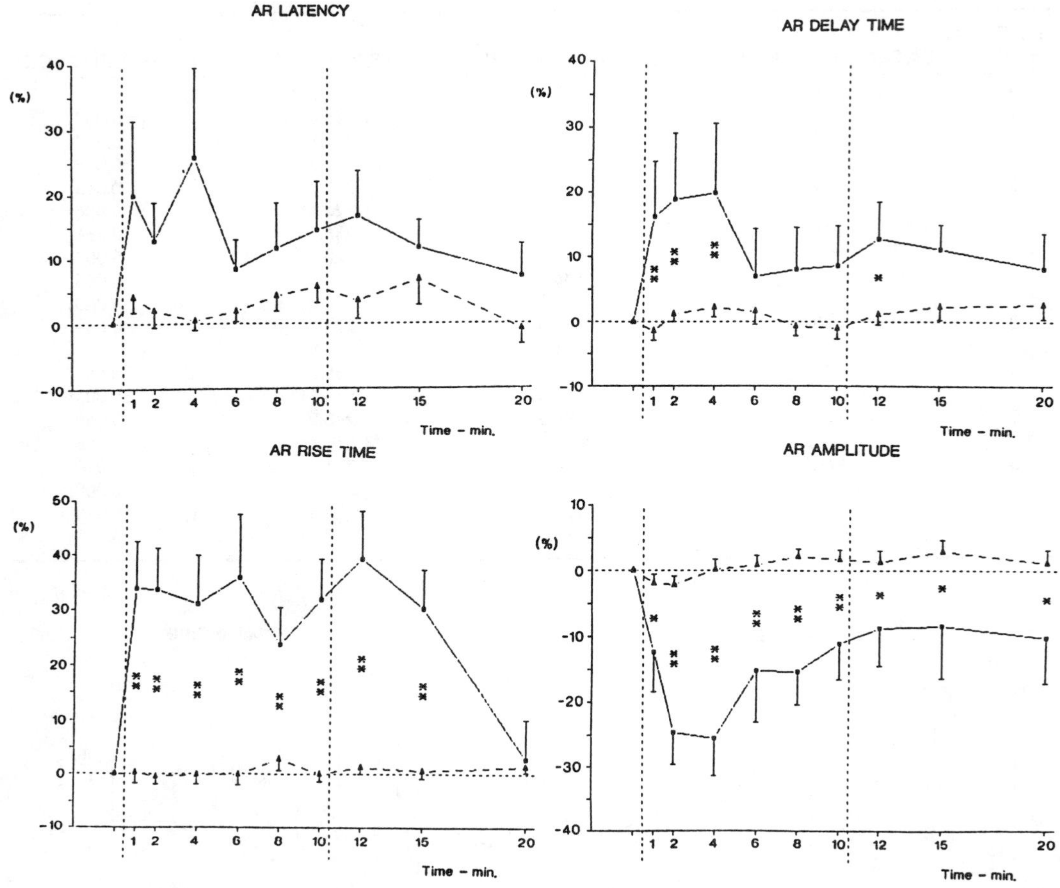

Figure 44-2 Time course of the acoustic reflex (AR) parameters before, during, and after the exercise (squares). The onset and the end of exercise are indicated by vertical dotted lines. Time control results are indicated by triangles. The vertical axis corresponds to the percentage of change of the basal values. One star: $p < 0.05$; two stars: $p < 0.01$.

ference between the experimental and control conditions was significant at the 0.05 level. Simple contrast comparison was significant from 1 to 4 minutes.

Greater modifications were observed with the rise-time of the AR. This time-domain parameter shifted from 183.5 ±13.9 ms at rest to 242.5 ±21.2 ms at 1 minute of exercise, remained elevated up to 5 minutes after exercise, and then returned to baseline values. The rise-time increase during exercise and early recovery was more than 30 percent. The two-way analysis of variance showed highly significant differences, both for absolute changes and percentages of change.

Amplitude of the reflex displayed initial values of 0.075 ±0.008 cc and decreased during exercise, reaching a plateau at 2 and 4 minutes (about 0.055 cc). Thereafter, the magnitude of the reflex slowly increased but did not reach the initial value. The maximal amount of change expressed as a percentage was about −25 percent. The difference with the time control condition was significant at virtually all time intervals. Figure 44-3 shows the input-output relation between amplitude of the reflex and intensity of the stimuli in decibels SL. At the onset of exercise the curve was depressed at all intensity levels and approached basal values thereafter.

Figure 44-4 displays the logistic function parameters expressed as a percentage of modification. At the onset of exercise, a moderate decrease in Y-max and a mild increase in threshold were observed, whereas the maximal slope presented a large increase at the end of exercise. In spite of a clear trend towards a change from baseline values, the statistical analysis did not show any significant difference, possibly because of the small number of subjects submitted to this test (N = 5) or because of the lack of temporal controls.

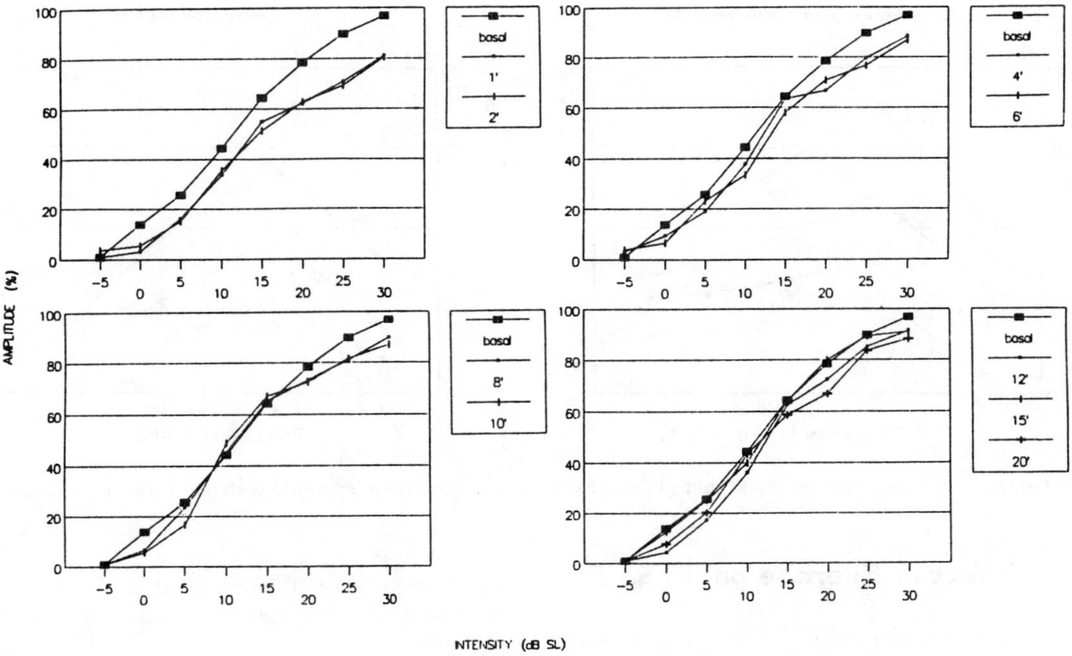

Figure 44-3 Input-output function of the acoustic reflex (AR) before, during, and after the exercise. The curve obtained at rest is reported for comparison in each figure. Values are expressed in decibels SL (re AR threshold) and as a percent of the maximal amplitude obtained at rest.

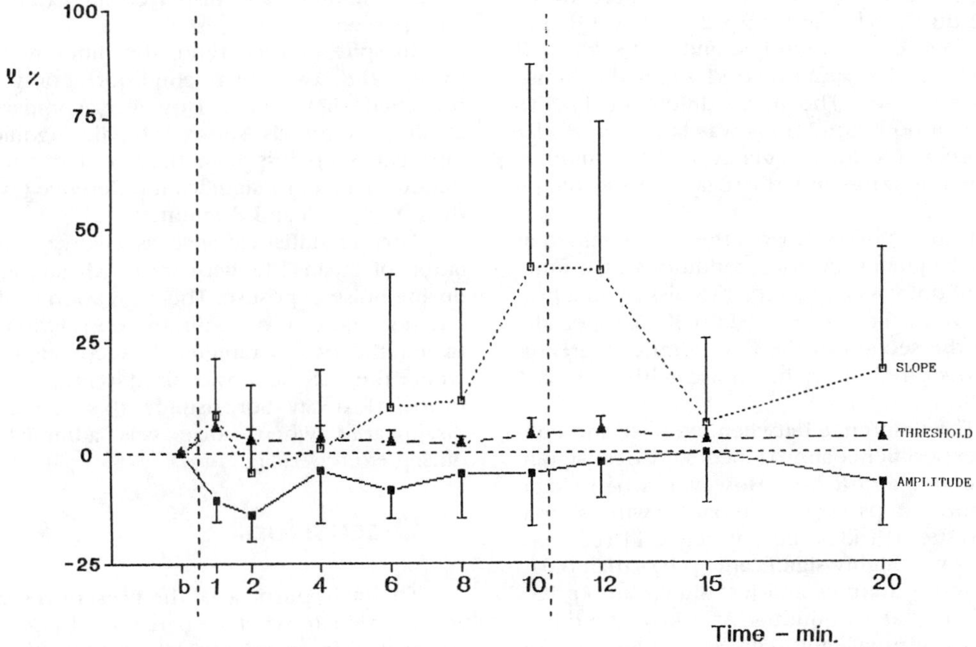

Figure 44-4 Logistic function parameters of the acoustic reflex (AR) input-output curves, expressed as a percentage of modification of the basal values. Vertical bars correspond to 1 S.D.

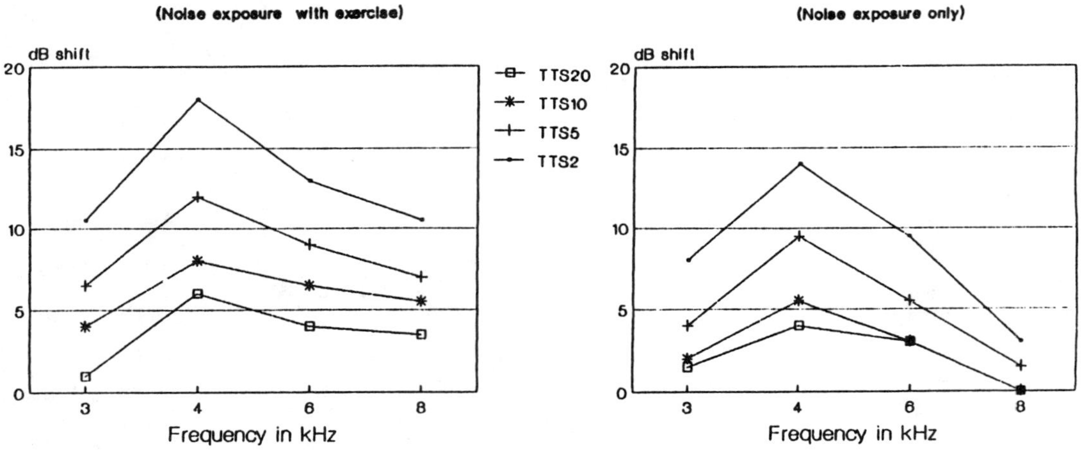

Figure 44-5 Temporary threshold shift (TTS) 2 to 20 minutes after noise exposure with and without exercise.

Effect of Exercise on TTS

The second purpose of the present study was to investigate the effect of physical exercise on the amount of TTS and the role of AR depression in the interaction between noise and exercise. Figure 44-3 shows the temporary threshold shifts from 2 to 20 minutes after the exposure as a function of frequency. The frequencies of 4 and 6 kHz displayed the greatest TTS in both conditions. Two minutes after the exposure, the TTS amounted to 14 ±1.8 dB (4 kHz) and 9.5 ±2.6 dB (6 kHz) in the "noise only" condition, and to 18 ±1.7 dB (4 kHz) and 13 ±2 dB (6 kHz) for the "noise with exercise." The mean difference in TTS between both conditions was largest at 8 kHz with regard to the frequency, and at 2 minutes following exposure with regard to the recovery time.

Figure 44-6 compares the TTS obtained at each frequency in both conditions as a function of time. As expected, TTS displayed a progressive decline (*p* less than 0.001), especially from the second to the fifth minute. A greater TTS occurred after the "noise with exercise" condition.

The difference between exercise and control experiments approached statistical significance at 4 and 8 kHz. However, when single temporal steps were compared with simple contrasts, at 3 kHz the difference in recovery curves was highly significant (*p* less than 0.01) at 2 and 5 minutes and just significant (*p* less than 0.05) at 10 minutes. At 4 kHz, the difference was significant only at 2 minutes. The recovery curves at 6 and 8 kHz displayed highly significant differences at 2, 5, and 10 minutes and a just-significant difference at 20 minutes.

AR amplitude was continuously monitored during noise exposure. As may be seen from Figure 44-7, AR decayed faster when subjects were exercising. The mean half-life time of the AR recorded at rest occurred at about 6 minutes, and the final mean amplitude was 34.2 percent of the initial value. AR recorded during exercise reached the half-life time at about 4 minutes and displayed final values of 24.7 percent.

In spite of this trend, the difference between the two test conditions only approached significance. However, comparison at single intervals showed highly significant differences (*p* less than 0.001) at 4 and 10 minutes and a just-significant difference (*p* less than 0.05) at 6 and 8 minutes.

Further statistical analysis involved correlation of mean TTS with mean AR amplitude during noise exposure. The regression analysis did not show any significant correlation between the two parameters, except at 4 kHz where the TTS value was directly proportional to the AR decay. Surprisingly, this correlation disappeared when noise was administered during exercise (Fig. 44-8).

Discussion

The main purpose of the present research was to evaluate whether dynamic physical exercise is able to modify AR activity. In addition, the possibility that physical activity could

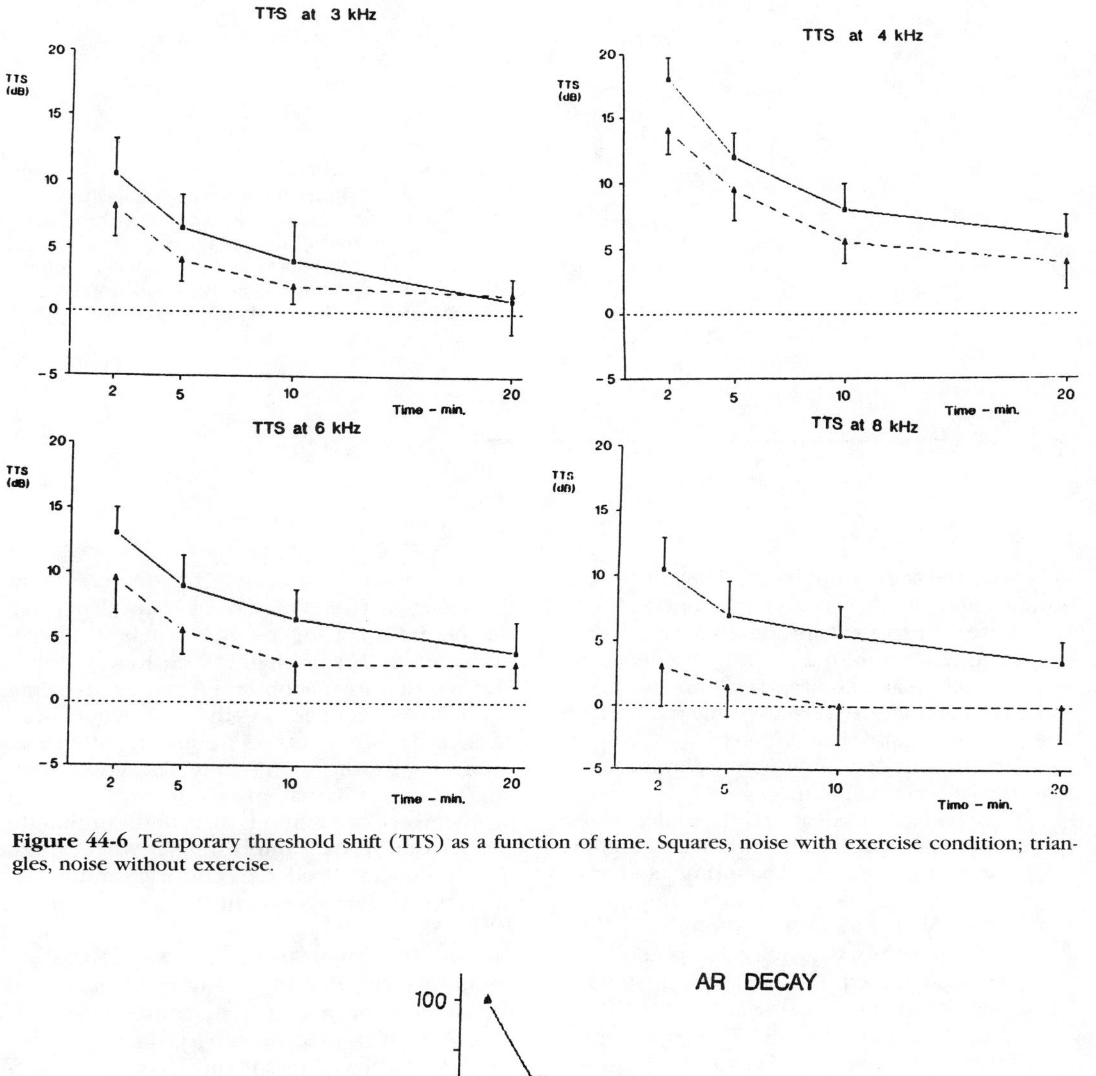

Figure 44-6 Temporary threshold shift (TTS) as a function of time. Squares, noise with exercise condition; triangles, noise without exercise.

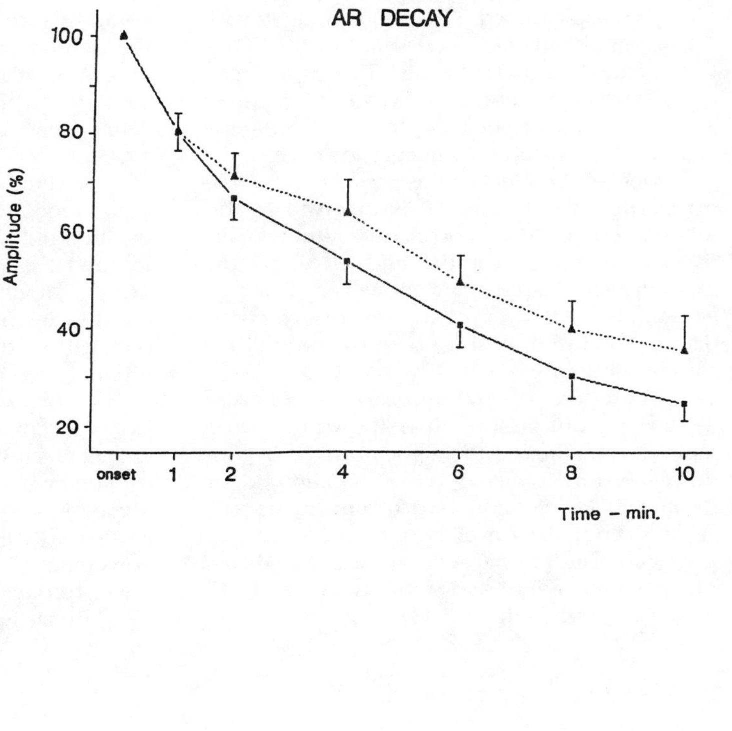

Figure 44-7 Acoustic reflex (AR) decay during noise exposure. Squares, noise with exercise condition; triangles, noise without exercise.

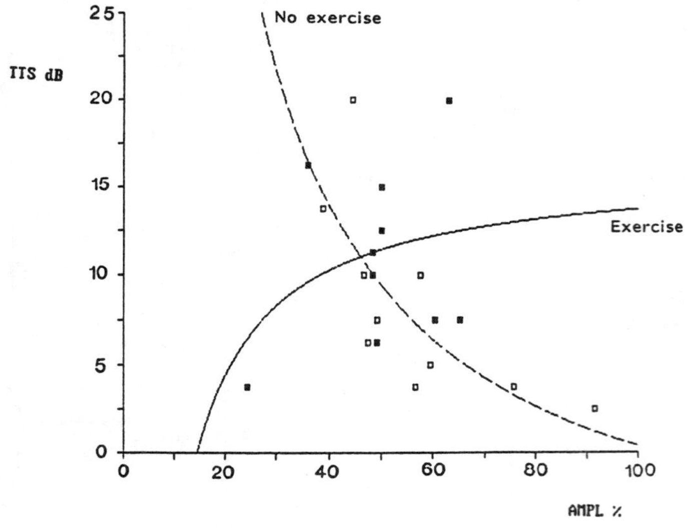

Figure 44-8 Regression analysis between mean temporary threshold shift (TTS) and mean acoustic reflex (AR) decay at 4 kHz, obtained during both test conditions (noise exposure with and without exercise).

influence the susceptibility to TTS through a modification of AR was also examined. These issues are of practical interest because workers are often submitted to noise when performing physical activity. For this purpose, some AR parameters were investigated both at rest and during physical exercise.

The present data, although preliminary, allow the following conclusions:

1. Dynamic physical exercise depresses the AR. Specifically, there is a significant increase in delay time and rise time as well as a decrease in amplitude, mainly at the onset of exercise.
2. Dynamic physical exercise potentiates noise-induced TTS, in agreement with Lindgren and Axelsson (1988). They attributed the "extra" TTS to a depletion in cochlear reserve, possibly caused by increase in blood temperature, metabolic changes, or both.

One of the aims of the present study was to clarify whether the AR is involved in this phenomenon. The correlation studies between the amount of TTS and AR decay did not furnish clearcut data, however. The perstimulatory AR decay was statistically correlated with TTS only at 4 kHz for the condition "noise without exercise."

There are several possible mechanisms underlying our findings. It is known that exercise can modulate other types of reflexes; for instance, the soleus H reflex is inhibited by isometric leg flection (Gritti and Schieppati, 1989). Arterial baroreflexes and reflexes arising from cardiac baroceptors are attenuated by dynamic exercise (Staessen et al, 1987; Ludbrock and Graham, 1985).

The exercise-induced AR depression at the onset of exercise may be caused by central neural mechanisms, reflex neural mechanisms, or both (Mitchell, 1985; Kjaer, 1989). The AR depression observed during dynamic exercise is similar to the AR depression caused by mental tasks requiring attention, such as selecting words in a passage of writing, solving a visual maze, or mathematical problems (Corcoran et al, 1980; Robinette and Snyder, 1982). Interestingly, when attention is concentrated on auditory stimuli, depression is nearly absent (Corcoran et al, 1980).

On the other hand, the AR depression could be attributed to inhibitory influences in the brain stem arising from contracting muscles. A similar mechanism has been demonstrated for the arterial and cardiac baroreflexes depression during exercise (Mitchell, 1985).

Dynamic exercise causes biochemical blood modifications, such as an increase in potassium and lactate, a decrease in free fat acids, and changes in pH (Wahren et al, 1971). These modifications could underlie the changes in AR response observed in the second half of the exercise and following exercise.

The reason for TTS potentiation during dynamic physical effort remains unexplained. Our data showed the largest effect at 8 kHz, a frequency not thought to be attenuated by AR. Metabolic factors, as advocated by Lingren and Axelsson (1988), could be the cause, but involvement of the AR cannot be ruled out for lower frequencies.

To clarify some unresolved questions, we

plan to study the AR and TTS values under static exercise, such as the Jendrassix hand-clenching maneuver and handgrip. This future research will probably allow a better interpretation of the present findings and of their practical implications.

Influence de l'Activité Physique sur la Protection contre la Fatigue Auditive

Les déficits auditifs temporaires (TTS) après une exposition au bruit sont potentialisés, chez l'homme, par un exercice physique (Lindgren et Axelsson, 1988). Puisque le réflexe stapédien exerce un rôle protecteur vis-à-vis des traumatismes acoustiques, il est possible qu'une baisse de son efficacité soit responsable de TTS plus élevés. Cinq volontaires, entendant correctement, âgés de 29 à 34 ans ont été testés pour vérifier cette hypothèse.

Avant chaque expérience, chaque sujet était testé avec un maximum d'exercices, par ordre croissant d'un cycle ergométrique. Dans le jour qui suivait, les paramètres du réflexe stapédien étaient évalués (latence et amplitude) avant, pendant et après un exercice test réalisé à 50% de la capacité de travail maximale pendant 10 minutes.

Le réflexe stapédien était passagèrement diminué au début de l'exercice. La latence était augmentée de 11,1 + 7,4 % après 1 minute et l'amplitude diminuée de 18,7 + 9,3 % après 4 minutes. Ces variations, cependant, n'étaient pas statistiquement significatives et disparaissaient par la suite.

Ces résultats préliminaires indiquent qu'une interaction entre une activité physique et l'efficacité du reflexe stapédien peut exister mais demande des investigations supplémentaires.

References

Borg E. A quantitative study of the effect of the acoustic stapedius reflex on sound transmission through the middle ear of man. Acta Otolaryngol 1968; 66:461-472.

Borg E. Dynamic characteristics of the intra-aural muscle reflex. In: Feldman AS, Wilber LA, eds. Acoustic impedance and admittance: The measurement of middle ear function. Baltimore: Williams & Wilkins, 1976:236-299.

Borg E, Nilsson R, Liden G. Fatigue and recovery of the human acoustic stapedius reflex in industrial noise. J Acoust Soc Am 1979; 65:846-848.

Burns W. Temporary effects of noise on hearing. In: Murray J, ed. Noise and man. London: W. Cloews & Son, 1973.

Byrne C, Henderson D, Saunders S, et al. Interaction of noise and whole body vibration. Paper presented at the Twelfth Midwinter Research Meeting of the Association for Research in Otolaryngology, St. Petersburg Beach, Florida, Feb. 5–9, 1989.

Colletti V. Biometric aspects of the stapedius reflex. Acta Otorhinolaryngol Belg 1974; 28:545-552.

Colletti V, Sittoni V. Noise history, audiometric profile and acoustic reflex responsivity. In: Salvi RJ, et al, eds. Basic and applied aspects of noise induced hearing loss. New York: Plenum Press, 1986; 247.

Corcoran AL, Cleaver VCG, Stephens SDG. Attention, eye closure and the acoustic reflex. Audiology 1980; 19:233-244.

Dengerink JE, Dengerink HA, Swanson S, et al. Gender and oral contraceptive effects on temporary auditory effects of noise. Audiology 1984; 23:411-425.

Drettner B, Hedstrand H, Klockhoff I, Svedberg A. Cardiovascular risk factors and hearing loss. A study of 1000 fifty-year old men. Acta Otolaryngol 1975; 79:366-371.

Fried MP, Dudek SE, Bohne B. Basal turn cochlear lesions following exposure to low-frequency noise. Trans Am Acad Ophthalmol Otolaryngol 1976; 82:285-298.

Gritti I, Schieppati M. Short-latency inhibition of soleus motoneurones by impulses in Ia afferents from the gastrocnemius muscle in humans. J Physiol 1989; 416:469-484.

Hamernik RP, Henderson D, Coling D, Salvi R. Influences of vibration on asymptotic threshold shift produced by impulse noise. Audiology 1981; 20:259-269.

Humes LE. Noise induced hearing loss as influenced by other agents and by some physical characteristics of the individual. J Acoust Soc Am 1984; 76:1318-1329.

Johansson B, Kylin B, Langfy M. Acoustic reflex as a test of individual susceptibility to noise. Acta Otolaryngol 1967; 64:256-262.

Kaplan H, Gilman S, Dirks DD. Properties of acoustic reflex adaptation. Ann Otol Rhinol Laryngol 1977; 86:348-354.

Kjaer M. Ephinephrine and some other hormonal responses to exercise in man, with special reference to physical training. Int J Sports Med 1989; 10:2-15.

Lindgren F, Axelsson A. The influence of physical exercise on susceptibility to noise-induced temporary threshold shift. Scand Audiol 1988; 17:11-17.

Ludbrook J, Graham WF. Circulatory responses to onset of exercise: Role of arterial and cardiac baroreflexes. Am J Physiol 1985; 248:H457-H467.

Lutman ME, Martin AM. Adaptation of the acoustic reflex to combination of sustained steady state and repeated pulse stimuli. J Sound Vibrat 1978; 56:137-150.

Manninen O, Ekblom A. Single and joint actions of noise and sinusoidal whole body vibration on TTS2 values and low frequency upright posture sway in men. Int Arch Occup Environ Health 1984; 54:1-17.

Melnick W. Temporary and permanent threshold shifts. In: Lipscomb DM, ed. Noise and audiology. Baltimore: University Park Press, 1978.

Mendelowitz D, Scher AM. Pulsatile pressure can prevent rapid baroreflex resetting. Am J Physiol 1980; 258:H92-H100.

Mitchell J. Cardiovascular control during exercise: Central and reflex neural mechanisms. Am J Cardiol 1985; 55:340D-410D.

Nilsson R, Borg E, Liden G. Fatigability of the stapedius reflex in industrial noise. Acta Otolaryngol 1980; 89:433-439.

Robinette MS, Snyder KS. Effect of eye closure, mental concentration, and nonauditory sensory stimulation on the threshold and magnitude of the acoustic reflex. Ear Hear 1982; 3:220-226.

Robinson DW. Characteristics of occupational noise induced hearing loss. In: Henderson D, et al, eds. Effects of noise on hearing. New York: Raven Press, 1976.

Sanden A, Axelsson A. Comparison of cardiovascular responses in noise resistant and noise sensitive workers. Acta Otolaryngol Suppl 1981; 337:75-83.

Spiegel MR. Theory and problems of statistics. New York: McGraw-Hill, 1961:343.

Staessen J, Fiocchi R, Fagard R, et al. Progressive attenuation of the carotid baroreflex control of blood pressure and heart rate during exercise. Am Heart J 1987; 114:765-772.

Wahren J, Felig P, Ahlborg G, Lennart J. Glucose metabolism during leg exercise in man. J Clin Invest 1971; 50:2715-2725.

Ward WD. Adaptation and fatigue. In: Jerger J, ed. Modern developments in audiology. New York: Academic Press, 1973:301.

Zakrisson JE, Borg E. Stapedius reflex and auditory fatigue. Audiology 1974; 13:231-235.

Zakrisson JE, Borg E, Liden G, Nilsson R. Stapedius reflex in industrial impact noise: Fatigability and role for the temporary threshold shift (TTS). Scand Audiol Suppl 1980; 12:326-334.

SECTION EIGHT

Conclusions

CHAPTER 45

Status and Shortcomings of Military Noise Standards

ARMAND L. DANCER

In the military environment, noise is a severe hazard to hearing and can be a limiting factor in the use of some weapons. Two different types of noise can be found in these environments:

Continuous or intermittent noises. Inside vehicles (e.g., tank, army personnel carrier, helicopter) the acoustic level can exceed 120 dB SPL. The hazard resulting from exposure to these noises can be evaluated by using the same procedures that are used in the case of exposure to industrial noise (e.g., measurement of the A-weighted energy, measurement of the equivalent level, use of earmuffs or earplugs with or without active noise reduction systems).

Impulse noises. Impulse noises are produced by the weapons themselves and consist generally of an advancing shock wave. The pressure-time history can be simple in the free field or complex in a reverberant field (Fig. 45-1).

To evaluate the hazard of exposure to impulse noises a number of criteria have been proposed (Coles et al, 1968; CHABA, 1968; Pfander et al, 1980; Smoorenburg, 1982; for reviews see Dancer and Franke, 1986; NATO, 1987). Most of these criteria are derived from temporary threshold shift (TTS) measurements performed after exposure to the noise produced by small weapons (rifle noises). The criteria for the evaluation of hazard are based on the measurement of some of the physical parameters of the impulse—i.e., "duration" of the impulse, number of impulses, and peak pressure. Figure 45-2 presents a comparison of these various criteria, taking into account the different definitions of the "duration" of the impulse (Smoorenburg, 1982; NATO, 1987). The fact that these criteria are very close to each other does not imply that they are comprehensive or reliable.

On behalf of the French Military, the French Committee for Weapon Noises (FCWN) and the "Direction des Armements Terrestres" (DAT) established another criterion that was derived from the criterion used for industrial noises. This new criterion corresponds to an A-weighted equivalent level of 90 dB over 8 hours (DTAT, 1983). It allows us to evaluate in a simpler way the hazard of combined exposures of continuous and impulse noises as well as the efficiency (which is frequency-dependent) of hearing protectors (Dancer, 1982).

Shortcomings of the Criteria

All of these criteria can be considered at least partially obsolete and not applicable to the impulses produced by present-day weapons. The following section elaborates on this statement.

Large-Caliber Versus Small-Caliber Weapons

Let us consider two Friedlander waves of the same peak pressure but of different durations. The longer one (large-caliber weapon) contains as much acoustic energy as the shorter one (small-caliber weapon) at the medium and high frequencies, but more at low frequencies (Kryter, 1970a). If any of the current weighting functions are applied to the two impulses, the measured acoustic energy

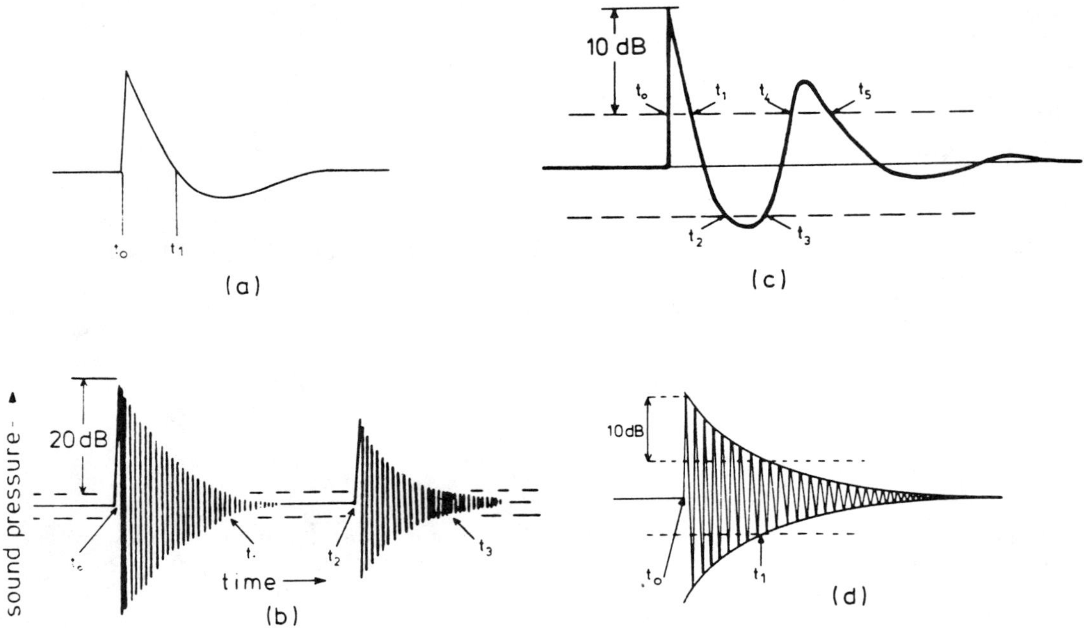

Figure 45-1 Some definitions of impulse duration. *a,* A-duration $(t_1 - t_0)$. *b,* B-duration $(t_1 - t_0) + (t_3 - t_2)$ (from Coles et al, 1968). *c,* C-duration $(t_1 - t_0) + (t_3 - t_2) + (t_5 - t_4)$ (from Pfander et al, 1980). *d,* D-duration, τ_{-10} $(t_1 - t_0)$ (from Smoorenburg, 1982). From NATO. Effects of impulse noise. Research Study Group on the Effects of Impulse Noise, AC/243 (Panel 8/RSG.6) D/9, 1987.

will always be greater for the longer shock wave, and all existing criteria will predict a greater hazard for exposure to the long-duration shock wave and hence the larger weapon. However, experiments conducted on two different animal species, the cat (Price, 1982) and the guinea pig (Dancer et al, 1985), showed that this was not the case. When all other parameters are kept the same, the longer the duration of the impulse, the smaller the threshold shift (TS).

To study this problem in man, the FCWN compared the TTS induced in soldiers following exposure to 20 noise impulses of the same peak pressure (about 160 dB SPL)* presented at the same interval (30 seconds) but having either an A-duration of 0.3 ms (D-duration: 1.4 ms) or 8 ms (rifle and howitzer). Two groups of 12 soldiers (selected as having hearing thresholds not larger than 25 dB at any frequency from 0.25 to 8 kHz) were exposed in the free field/grazing incidence) without any hearing protection to each of the two classes of impulsive noise. In all cases, recovery of TS was complete by at most 24 hours after the end of the exposure. Table 45-1 shows that TTS occurred more frequently and was larger following the exposures to the short duration impulses. This result contradicts the predictions of all the usual criteria (Fig. 45-2). The exposure to the longer-duration impulses exceeds more the limits of the criteria than does the exposure to the short-duration impulses but produces less TTS. Nonlinear transmission mechanisms at the level of the middle ear and especially of the annular ligament, as proposed by Price (1990), could explain this phenomenon.

If we consider now the French criterion (DTAT, 1983), the exposure to the short impulses corresponds to an L_{Aeq8} of 92 dB (level of a continuous A-weighted signal applied during 8 hours and containing the same total acoustic energy), whereas the exposure to the long impulses is equivalent to an L_{Aeq8} of 88 dB. In these experimental conditions, this criterion exhibits a better predictive efficiency than the others.

Two additional observations were also made during this study: (1) In some subjects the maximum TTS did not occur immediately after the end of the exposure but rather 1 or 2 hours later. This phenomenon was described by Luz and Hodge (1971) and Hamernik et al (1988) and seems to be specific to impulse

*According to the French criterion (DTAT, 1983), this peak pressure corresponds to the limit (critical level) for the exposure of unprotected ears in the free field (even for a single round).

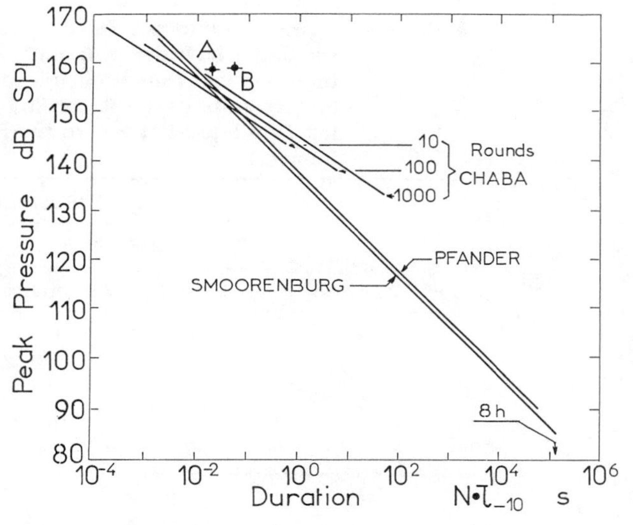

Figure 45-2 Comparison of damage risk criteria taking into account the different definitions of impulse duration. The abscissa gives the total duration of all impulses, given by the number, N, of impulses multiplied by the D-duration of each impulse. *A* corresponds to the exposure to 20 rifle rounds; *B* corresponds to the exposure to 20 howitzer rounds (at 70 meters from the muzzle). Pfander: Damage risk criterion of Pfander et al, 1980; Smoorenburg: Damage risk criterion of Smoorenburg, 1982; CHABA: Damage risk criterion of CHABA, 1968. Adapted from NATO. Effects of impulse noise. Research Study Group on the Effects of Impulse Noise, AC/243 (Panel 8/RSG.6) D/9, 1987.

TABLE 45-1 **Number of Subjects (of 24 Total) Presenting a Maximum TTS Greater than 10 dB and 20 dB in at Least One Ear at Any Audiometric Frequency (in Practice, Between 3 and 8 kHz)**

TTS	SHORT-DURATION IMPULSE (RIFLE)	LONG-DURATION IMPULSE (HOWITZER)
> 10 dB	10	4
> 20 dB	7	2

From Comité "Bruits d'Armes." Effets des bruits d'armes sur l'audition: Campagne audiométrique de Bourges (18–22 Septembre 1989). ISL Report SR-905/90, 1990.

noise exposures. This growth of TS represents a real problem for criteria that are based on the measurement of TTS immediately after the end of an impulse noise (typically TTS_{2min}); and (2) A significant improvement in the auditory threshold is observed in some cases at the same time that the first smallest TTS appear.

Daily Exposures

The criteria previously described were established for daily exposures. There is some evidence (Comité "Bruits d'Armes," 1990) that daily exposure could induce larger TS than anticipated.

Spacing Between the Impulses

The criteria previously described do not take into account the spacing between the impulses; i.e., the inter-impulse interval. There is no special evaluation procedure for distinguishing between single-shot exposures and multiple rounds.

Table 45-2 summarizes the results of a study conducted by Reid (1946) on subjects exposed to machine gun noises (28 rounds). In some instances (two subjects out of four) the differences in TS are very large between rounds fired at intervals of from 10 to 20 seconds and rounds fired rapidly (500 per minute). We found similar results in a subject who was exposed first to 25 rifle impulses at intervals of 5 seconds and 3 days later (after complete TS recovery) to the same 25 impulses presented in 1.7 second (see also Kryter, 1970b). These differences in TS resulting from different impulse presentation rates are probably due to the protective effect of the acoustic reflex of the middle ear or to some "intracochlear acoustic reflex" partially mediated by the efferent innervation of the cochlea (Brundlin et al, 1989; Vassout et al, 1990).

In fact all these criteria (established for unprotected ears) are not very useful in practice. Even the noises produced by the small-

TABLE 45-2 **Comparison of the TS (dB) Measured After Exposure to the Same Number of Rounds Either with a Spacing of 10 to 30 seconds (Single) or Fired Rapidly (500 to 900 per Minute Automatic) According to Reid (1946) (Average TS for Two Subjects) and to the FCWN (1988) (TS for One Subject)**

	THRESHOLD SHIFT (DB)			
	Reid (1946)		FCWN (1988)	
AUDIOMETRIC FREQUENCY	Single	Automatic	Single	Automatic
0.5 kHz	5	0	0	0
1	10	0	5	0
2	40	0	15	0
4	64	5	40	0
6	57	10	35	0
8	50	0	30	0

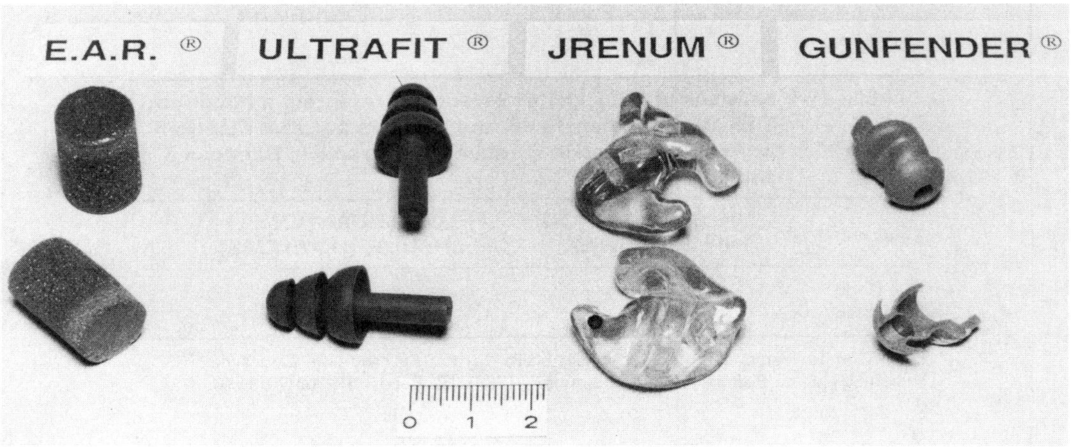

Figure 45-3 Earplugs used in this study.

caliber weapons (rifle) are too hazardous (especially in reverberant areas) for the soldiers who are using them and can induce permanent threshold shift (PTS) in the case of repeated exposures on unprotected ears. Therefore it is imperative to establish criteria that take into account the use and the actual efficiency of hearing protection devices.

Hearing Protection Devices

In the present criteria there are no provisions for evaluating the risk of hearing loss from impulse noise exposure when hearing protection devices are being employed. Nonlinear conductive phenomena, which occur at very high stimulation levels and affect the properties of hearing protectors themselves as well as influence the transmission of the acoustic energy by the middle ear and its dissipation inside the inner ear, complicate this area.

Generally speaking the protective effect of earplugs and earmuffs, when correctly used and well fitted, is underestimated (NATO, 1987), and soldiers are very often obliged to wear cumbersome and uncomfortable hearing protectors that isolate them from their comrades and from the acoustic environment, with potentially dangerous consequences.

The FCWN decided to test the efficiency of minimal and simple hearing protectors that are able to protect the ear against PTS while allowing good speech intelligibilty and good sound localization (Fig. 45-3). The following protective devices were used: EAR foam earplug; an EAR earplug prototype (similar to the Ultrafit); JRENUM (filter LD03) molded earplugs; and the GUNFENDER earplug.

Groups of 10 to 12 soldiers were exposed, in the crew position, to the impulses produced by a 155-mm howitzer. All the exposure conditions were tested by the members of the FCWN equipped with the same hearing protection devices prior to the exposure of the different groups of soldiers.

The peak pressure of the impulses was about 175 dB SPL, and the A-duration was equal to 7 ms. For a single exposure, the A-weighted acoustic energy corresponded to an equivalent 8-hour level of 95 dB. The number of rounds was either 10 or 20, fired at 30-second intervals. All soldiers were equipped for each exposure with the different earplugs mentioned above. These earplugs were deeply inserted and fitted by an experienced individual.

The attenuation afforded by the various hearing protection devices (measured by classic methods using threshold measurements) differs considerably (Fig. 45-4). The best attenuation is provided by the EAR foam earplug, and the worst by the GUNFENDER.

For these earplugs the Speech Transmission Index was roughly evaluated using the RApid Speech Transmission Index method (RASTI) (Bruël & Kjaer 4225 and 4419) by the "Groupement Ergonomie" of the "Section Technique de l'Armée de Terre" (STAT). The results of this evaluation are shown in Table 45-3.

TABLE 45-3 **Speech Transmission Index (STI) Evaluated Using the RASTI Method for the Unprotected Ear and for Different Earplugs (1985)**

EAR PROTECTION	GLOBAL STI
Unprotected	0.78
EAR foam earplug	0.28
EAR prototype	0.7 (approximate)
Molded earplug JRENUM (LD03)	0.69
GUNFENDER	0.76

From Comité "Bruits d'Armes." Effets des bruits d'armes sur l'audition: Campagne audiométrique de Bourges (18–22 Septembre 1989). ISL Report SR-905/90, 1990.

These results show that the STI of the GUNFENDER is equivalent to that of an unprotected ear. The EAR prototype with an STI of approximately 0.7 and the molded earplug JRENUM (LD03) with an STI of 0.69 are satisfactory. The EAR foam earplug has a relatively poor STI.

Audiometric thresholds were measured as described earlier, with the help of a Békésy audiometer (continuous frequency sweep from 0.125 to 8 kHz) before and after (either 10, 20, or 40 minutes) the impulse noise exposures. The TTS measured with the EAR foam earplugs correspond to the results obtained from 24 soldiers exposed to 20 rounds; those measured with the EAR prototypes correspond to the results obtained from four soldiers exposed to 20 rounds and from 2 soldiers exposed to 10 rounds; those measured with the molded earplugs (JRENUM LD03) correspond to the results obtained from eight soldiers exposed to 10 rounds; and those measured with the GUNFENDER earplugs correspond to the results obtained from 11 soldiers exposed to 10 rounds (Comité "Bruits d'Armes," 1990).

In all cases the earplugs were efficient and no significant TTS (greater than 10 dB) was found at any frequency in any subject. This was a surprising result, especially considering the poor attenuation of some of the earplugs when measured by using real ear at threshold (REAT) test data (Fig. 45-4). Nonlinear phenomena such as the transition from laminar to turbulent flow through the small openings of the EAR prototype, molded earplug JRENUM LD03, and GUNFENDER are probably partially responsible for these results. The actual attenuation properties for a Friedlander wave of 175 dB peak pressure are probably greater than those presented in Figure 45-4 (Forrest and Coles, 1970; Forrest, 1971; Parmentier, 1988). Nevertheless the attenuation achieved at very high peak pressure levels is probably not large enough to explain the hearing protective efficiency of the earplugs that were measured in our study. This is especially true if we take only into account, according to the classic criteria, the peak pressure attenuation measured under a hearing protector (Ylikoski et al, 1987; Price et al, 1990). Other nonlinear mechanisms occurring at the level of the middle or the inner ear could also play an important role (Price, 1990).

Based on these results, it is difficult to assess the efficiency of hearing protectors (earplugs, earmuffs, or both) for actual weapon noises by only measuring their attenuation as a function of frequency with the help of REAT methods. Measurements performed on head and ear simulators at very high levels could provide useful information about nonlinear attenuation phenomena and provide a better understanding of the actual performance characteristics of earplugs and earmuffs. Moreover, carefully conducted studies on human subjects, such as those performed in our experiments, are necessary to determine the most

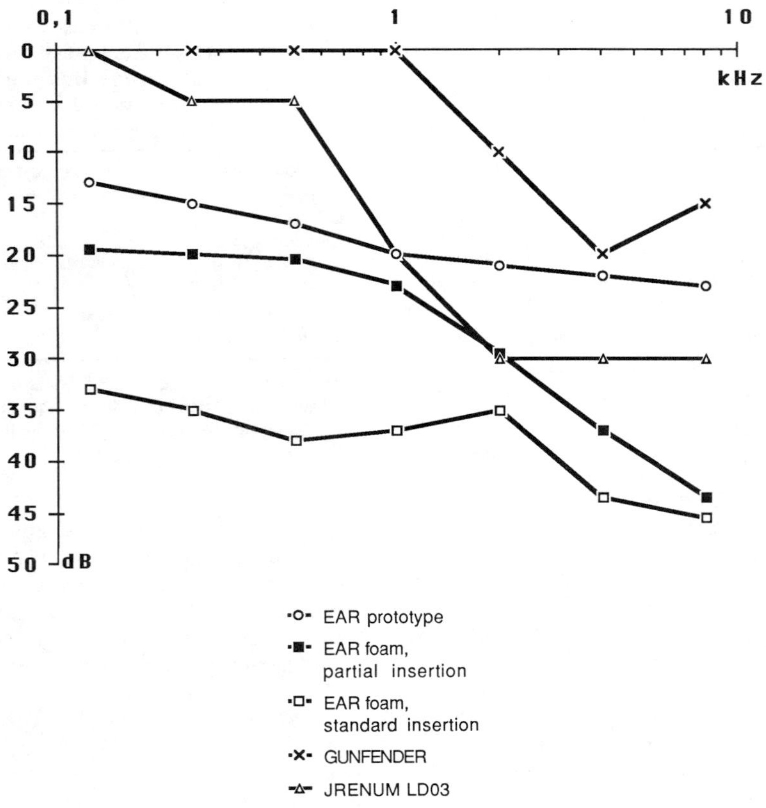

Figure 45-4 Attenuation provided by different earplugs. The results corresponding to the EAR earplugs are from Berger, 1989, and those of the GUNFENDER and the JRENUM LD03 are from the Comité "Bruits d'Armes," 1990.

convenient hearing protection devices, to avoid overprotection when unnecessary, and to preserve speech communication and sound localization (Mosko and Fletcher, 1971).

We have shown here that it is possible to protect the ear from high-level impulses produced by large weapons, through the use of simple devices that still allow good communication between individuals wearing hearing protectors.

Conclusion

We would like to stress that as a result of studies performed in several countries, it is possible to protect the ear from the noise of various weapons (up to the threshold of the nonauditory injuries) by using well-fitted single or double hearing protection but at the cost of isolating the subject from his acoustic environment.

The challenge for the future, in the case of exposure to impulse (weapon) noise, is to develop a light, simple, nonexpensive and comfortable device (earplugs for example) that will protect the ear against TS even in the case of severe impulse noise exposures and that will also allow the soldier to communicate and be aware of his acoustic environment.

Practical solutions to this problem seem to be within reach with the use of nonlinear devices derived from some molded earplugs or from the GUNFENDER or the EAR prototype earplugs, provided that these devices are well fitted and correctly worn.

The French Committee on Weapon Noises in cooperation with other research teams in Europe and in the United States will continue to work toward the development of an earplug that can be used in all impulse noise exposure conditions and will preserve the ability to communicate and to localize acoustic sources in an operational environment.

Etat Actuel et Insuffisances des Critères d'Exposition aux Bruits d'Armes

"La question de savoir quels sont les bruits d'armes dangereux pour l'audition est l'objet de recherches dans un grand nombre de pays. Les études visent tout d'abord à déterminer une méthode de mesure satisfaisante des caractéristiques physiques des bruits et évaluer les risques représentés par ces bruits." Cette constatation faite par des scientifiques Anglais et Américains (Coles et al., 1968) est toujours d'actualité.

La plupart des critères d'exposition aux bruits d'armes en service dans les différentes armées de l'OTAN sont basés sur la mesure de la pression crête, de la durée et du nombre des bruits. Dans l'armée Française, un critère basé sur la mesure de l'énergie acoustique pondérée A et le principe d'isoénergie a été mis en place (DTAT 1983). Ce critère permet d'évaluer les effets lésionnels relatifs des armes lourdes et des armes légères aussi bien que ceux des expositions combinées (bruits continus et bruits impulsionnels). Il permet également de mieux estimer la protection acoustique apportée par les serre-tête et les bouchons d'oreilles en prenant en compte leurs caractéristiques d'atténuation en fonction de la fréquence.

Néanmoins **tous** les critères existants présentent de nombreuses imperfections. Les problèmes liés au rythme de répétition des bruits, aux expositions quotidiennes, aux effets des ondes de longue durée, au niveau critique, à la protection effective apportée par les serre-tête ou les bouchons d'oreilles aux niveaux correspondant à ceux des bruits d'armes . . . ne sont pas résolus.

Des observations réalisées en France sur des soldats effectuant des tirs d'entraînement montrent que les critères classiques surestiment l'effet lésionnel des armes lourdes. Ces observations ont également permis de mesurer la protection apportée par divers bouchons d'oreilles au cours de l'exposition à des bruits d'armes lourdes et laissent espérer la mise au point d'un bouchon d'oreille capable de protéger l'audition tout en préservant la communication parlée et la localisation des sources sonores.

ACKNOWLEDGMENTS

This study was performed on the authority of the presidents of the French Committee on Weapon Noises, Professors Borredon and Grateau, and with the participation of all the members of this committee, especially Cdt Cabanis and M. Vaillant.

I would like to thank Dr. E.H. Berger and M. Forrest for their scientific and technical support, and Professor R.P. Hamernik for his valuable advice on the writing of this manuscript.

References

Berger EH. Personal communication, 1989.

Brundlin L, Flock Å, Canlon B. Sound-induced motility of isolated cochlear outer hair cells is frequency-specific. Nature 1989; 342:814-816.

CHABA. Proposed damage-risk criterion for impulse noise (gunfire). National Academy of Sciences, National Research Council, Committee on Hearing, Bioacoustics and Biomechanics. Ward WD, ed. Report of Working Group 57, 1968.

Coles RR, Garinther GR, Hodge DC, Rice CG. Hazardous exposure to impulse noise. J Acoust Soc Am 1968; 43:336-346.

Comité "Bruits d'Armes." Effets des bruits d'armes sur l'audition: Campagne audiométrique de Bourges (18–22 Septembre 1989). ISL Report SR–905/90, 1990.

Dancer A. Isoenergy principle and A-weighting in the rating of the hazard of noise exposure in the military environment. In: Borchgrevink HM, ed. Hearing and hearing prophylaxis. Scand Audiol Suppl 1982; 16:49-52.

Dancer A, Buck K, Vassout P, Lenoir M. Influence du niveau de crête et de la durée d'ondes de choc (bruits d'armes) sur l'audition du cobaye. Acustica 1985; 59:21-29.

Dancer A, Franke R. Effects of weapon noise on hearing. In: Salvi RJ, Henderson D, Hamernik RP, Colletti V, eds. Basic and applied aspects of noise-induced hearing loss. NATO ASI Series, Series A: Life Sciences, Vol. 111. New York and London: Plenum Press, 1986:425.

DTAT. Recommendation on evaluating the possible harmful effect of noise on hearing. Direction Technique des Armements Terrestres, GCT "Facteurs Humains—Ergonomie," Comité "Bruits d'Armes," AT–83/27/28, 1983.

Forrest MR, Coles RRA. Problems of communication and ear protection in the royal marines. J R Nav Med Serv 1970; 56:162-169.

Forrest MR. Occupational hearing loss. In: Robinson DW, ed. British Acoustical Society Special Vol. 1. London: Academic Press, 1971:151.

FWCN. Personal communication, 1988.

Hamernik RP, Ahroon WA, Patterson JA. Threshold recovery functions following impulse noise trauma. J Acoust Soc Am 1988; 84:941-950.

Kryter KD. The effects of noise on man. New York and London: Academic Press, 1970a:20.

Kryter KD. The effects of noise on man. New York and London: Academic Press, 1970b:188.

Luz GA, Hodge DC. Recovery from impulse noise induced TTS in monkeys and men: A descriptive model. J Acoust Soc Am 1971; 49:1770-1777.

Mosko JD, Fletcher JL. Evaluation of the Gunfender earplug: Temporary threshold shift and speech intelligibility. J Acoust Soc Am 1971; 49:1732-1733.

NATO. Effects of impulse noise. Research Study Group on the Effects of Impulse Noise, AC/243 (Panel 8/RSG.6) D/9, 1987.

Parmentier G. Etude du protecteur auditif EAR Ultra 9000 à atténuation non linéaire en régime de bruits continus et impulsionnels. ISL Report RT–514/88, 1988.

Pfander F, Bongartz H, Brinkmann H, Kietz H. Danger of auditory impairment from impulse noise: A comparative study of the CHABA damage-risk criteria and those of the Federal Republic of Germany. J Acoust Soc Am 1980; 67:628-633.

Price GR. Relative hazard of weapons impulses as a function of spectrum. J Acoust Soc Am Suppl 1982; 1:579.

Price GR. Importance of spectrum for rating hazard: Theoretical basis; to be published in the same book.

Price IR, Walles EJ, Ward T. Noise levels at the ears of marksmen wearing conventional and non-linear ear muffs. Proceedings Inter Noise, August, Gothenburg, Sweden, 1990.

RASTI. Technical Review, Bruël & Kjaer, No. 3, 1985.

Reid G. Further observations on temporary deafness following exposure to gunfire. J Laryngol Otol 1946; 61:609-633.

Smoorenburg GF. Damage risk criteria for impulse noise. In: Hamernik RP, Henderson D, Salvi RJ, eds. New perspectives on noise-induced hearing loss. New York: Raven Press, 1982:471.

Vassout P, Dancer A, Rebillard G. Study of the ipsilateral intracochlear acoustic reflex. In: Abstracts of the 13th Midwinter Meeting of the Association for Research in Otolaryngology, St Petersburg, FL, February 4–8, 1990:324.

Ylikoski J, Pekkarinen J, Starck J. The efficiency of earmuffs against impulse noise from firearms. Scand Audiol 1987; 16:85-88.

CHAPTER 46

Occupational Noise Standards: Status and Critical Issues

WILLIAM MELNICK

Only the status of the occupational noise standards and hearing conservation programs of the United States are considered here. There is not an attempt to exhaustively cover the subject of noise standards. It would be presumptuous to be critical of the standards and practices of other nations. However, it is likely that some of the conditions applicable to the occupational noise programs in the United States will be found in other industrial countries of the world and subject to the same concerns.

In the United States, Congress enacts the laws of the country. The Executive Branch of the government administers these laws. This administration frequently requires the issuing of regulations. Agencies of the Federal Administration, such as the Occupational Safety and Health Administration (OSHA) of the Department of Labor (DoL), promulgate and enforce regulations. Although government agencies may originate standards for regulations implementation, they often make use of consensus (voluntary) standards in this formulation. In this context, a standard is a codified set of rules or a set of procedural guidelines. The term "standard" is frequently used synonymously with the term "regulation" (Suter, 1988).

Because the effects of noise are such a pervasive problem, there are noise-related programs in many federal agencies of the United States. Some agencies such as the National Institute of Occupational Safety and Health (NIOSH) are mainly concerned with research. Agencies such as the Environmental Protection Agency (EPA) are involved in both research and regulation. Other agencies such as OSHA are mainly regulatory.

The OSHA estimates that slightly more than 1 million Americans have a "material hearing impairment" resulting from exposure to noise in manufacturing industries. More than 9 million employees are exposed to hazardous levels of noise in their occupational environments. Approximately 5 million manufacturing workers are exposed to daily average noise levels of 85 dBA; more than 2 million experience exposures between 85 and 90 dBA; about 1.5 million are exposed to levels between 90 and 95 dBA; over 800,000 endure levels from 95 to 100 dBA; and about 425,000 are exposed to occupational noise levels exceeding 100 dB (Suter, 1989). Table 46-1 provides a perspective on the magnitude of the problem of noise exposure for specific occupational categories as estimated by the EPA in 1981.

During the decade of the 1970s, the EPA and OSHA made progress in reducing or limiting noise exposure in the workplace as well as in the general environment. In 1969, the DoL began to regulate occupational noise exposure for employers who held federal contracts. In 1971, the regulatory standard was expanded to cover practically all employers in the United States. Enforcement of these noise standards was hesitant at first but was conducted with increasing rigor with changes in presidential administrations. As part of this regulatory fervor, Congress passed the Noise Control Act of 1972, which gave the EPA powers to regulate major sources of environmental noise with a strict schedule for accomplishing its assigned task (Noise Control Act, 1972). The act instructed other federal agencies to minimize the harmful effects of noise and gave the EPA the responsibility for coordinating all federal noise activities (Suter, 1989).

This is the background of conditions that existed when the current occupational noise standards in the United States were initiated.

TABLE 46-1 **Summary of U.S. Population Exposed to Daily Average Noise Levels of 85 dBA and Above**

EMPLOYMENT AREA	TOTAL EMPLOYED	NUMBER EXPOSED TO 85 dBA AND ABOVE
Agriculture	3,600,000	323,000
Mining	957,000	400,000
Construction	4,644,000	513,000
Manufacturing and Utilities	21,781,000	5,124,000
Transportation	4,345,000	1,934,000
Military	3,019,000	976,000
Totals	38,346,000	9,270,000

From Environmental Protection Agency, Office of Noise Abatement and Control. Noise in America: The extent of the noise problem. (EPA Report No. 550/9-81-191). Washington, D.C.: EPA, 1981.

The details of these regulations, the extent of their coverage, and their current status are considered in the following section.

U.S. Occupational Noise Standards

The fundamental responsibility of the United States Department of Labor (DoL) is to promote the welfare of working people. One of the major objectives of DoL regulations is to protect people at work. Prior to 1936, there were no occupational safety and health regulations enforceable by the federal government. In that year, Congress passed the Walsh-Healey Public Contracts Act. Under this act, the Secretary of Labor was given the ability to set safety and health standards enforceable on employers who contracted with the United States government in excess of $10,000 per year. Failure to comply with these standards could lead to termination of the contract.

The DoL first attempted to regulate workplace noise in 1960 when the Secretary of Labor decided to set minimum levels of noise exposure that could serve as criteria for compliance with the Walsh-Healey Public Contracts Act (Barry, 1989). The noise provisions were added to the Walsh-Healey Act in 1969 (U.S. DoL, 1969).

Shortly after the Walsh-Healey Noise Standard took effect, Congress passed Public Law 91-596, the Occupational Safety and Health Act of 1970 (OSH Act). The Secretary of Labor was directed to adopt as occupational safety and health standards any existing national consensus standards or established federal standards as OSHA standards. As a consequence, the Walsh-Healey Noise Standard was adopted as the OSHA General Industry Noise Standard (29 CFR 1910.95), together with the Construction Noise Standard (29 CFR 1926.52). With passage of the OSH Act, the only change in the noise standard was its coverage. This standard now covers all general industry, construction, and maritime employees in the United States. Another DoL agency, the Mine Safety and Health Administration (MSHA), also applied the former Walsh-Healey Noise Standard to mining operations. Only agricultural workers were left exempt from the occupational noise standards (29 CFR 1928.21).

All the noise limits found in current occupational noise standards derive from those proposed by the American Conference of Industrial Hygienists (ACIH) in 1968, which were adopted under the Walsh-Healey Act in 1969. The standard requires employers to limit workers' exposures to daily average noise levels of 90 dBA for 8-hour exposures. For durations shorter than 8 hours, the noise level can be increased by 5 dB for every halving of the exposure duration as shown in the (familiar) Table 46-2. The relationship between allowable level and duration is known as the exchange rate. Other exchange rates have been and are being used (3 dB, 4 dB, variable rates). The simplicity of the constant exchange rate was appealing to the ACIH. Ostensibly the 5-dB rate was selected over 3 dB to allow for the effect of intermittency during a typical work day on hearing.

The time-intensity exchange relationship had an upper limit of 115 dBA for 15 minutes. Levels exceeding 115 dB required conservation practices regardless of duration. Impulsive noises were considered only generally. Impulsive noises were not to exceed 140 dB peak sound pressure level. If the specified time-weighted average (TWA) of 90 dB for 8 hours or the 115 dB ceiling value were exceeded, or if impulses of greater than 140 dB peak were experienced, then the computed noise dose would exceed unity.

Two other provisions in the OSHA standard adopted from the earlier Walsh-Healey Standard should be mentioned (Suter, 1988).

TABLE 46-2 **Permissible Noise Exposures**

DURATION PER DAY (HOURS)	SOUND LEVEL (dBA SLOW RESPONSE)
8	90
6	92
4	95
3	97
2	100
1½	102
1	105
½	110
¼ or less	115

That standard, when considering impulse noise, stated that impulse noise *should* not exceed a peak sound pressure level of 140 dB. Because the standard used the word "should" instead of "shall," the provision regarding impulsive noise has been considered advisory, and has not been enforceable.

The other provision of interest is the section that called for "a continuing, effective hearing conservation program" whenever the noise limits were exceeded. Enforcement of this provision was difficult because of the lack of specifications for what constituted such a program. Even though the DoL issued guidelines for this purpose, this guidance did not have the official (enforceable) status of a regulation.

OSHA Hearing Conservation Amendment

The lack of specifications for an effective hearing conservation program motivated an amendment process that culminated in the Hearing Conservation Amendment (DOL, 1983). This amendment requires that hearing conservation programs be available to all employees whose 8-hour TWAs were 85 dBA or greater. Employers must monitor noise environments suspected of exceeding these levels at least once and remonitor the environment with changes of equipment or work processes that might cause a significant increase in exposure level. All continuous, intermittent, and impulsive noises between 80 and 130 dBA must be included in the exposure assessment. Area monitoring is permitted but employers must use personal exposure monitoring (dosimeters) whenever there is considerable variation of noise level over time.

The amendment requires employers to provide baseline audiograms within the first year of an employee's exposure to noise environments of 85 dBA and above and annual audiograms thereafter. The tests must be conducted by trained and competent personnel, and the testing program must be supervised by a physician or an audiologist. Tests must be conducted in environments that meet or exceed specifications for ambient background noise. Audiometers must meet appropriate American National Standards Institute (ANSI) standard specifications and be calibrated according to prescribed schedules.

TABLE 46-3 **Occupational Noise: Regulatory Agencies**

OCCUPATIONAL AREA	AGENCY
Manufacturing	OSHA
Utilities	OSHA
Construction	OSHA
Mining	MSHA
Transportation	DoT
Petroleum	OSHA
Military	DoD

OSHA, Occupational Safety and Health Administration; MSHA, Mine Safety and Health Administration; DoT, Department of Transportation; DoD, Department of Defense.

Workers identified as showing significant (standard) shifts in threshold hearing levels must be notified in writing and counseled regarding fitting and use of hearing protection and referred to a specialist if necessary. A significant threshold shift is defined as a shift from baseline of 10 dB or more for the average of the threshold levels measured at 2,000, 3,000, and 4,000 Hz.

Hearing protection must be worn by all workers exposed to a TWA of 90 dBA and above. Employers must offer hearing protection to workers exposed to levels above 85 dBA. The amendment recommends using the noise reduction rating (NRR) as an indication of expected performance of hearing protectors.

Training and education sessions must be given annually to workers exposed to 85 dBA or more. Employers are required to keep records of noise measurements, audiograms, audiometer calibration, and background noise level measures for the audiometric test rooms.

Other Noise Standards

Although the noise standards covering occupations in the United States are modeled after those of OSHA, not all aspects of the noise standard have been adopted. Table 46-3 gives an indication of the regulatory agency responsible for the noise standards applicable to particular occupational categories. The regulations covering these occupations are not the same. The manufacturing and utility industries are covered by both the permissible noise section and the hearing conservation amendment of the DoL noise standard (29 CFR 1910.95). The construction industry adopted the noise limits of the OSHA noise standard (29 CFR 1926.52) but not the hearing conservation amendment. Construction adheres to the general statement about continuing effective hearing conservation programs that appeared in the Walsh-Healey standard. In addition, the construction regulation specifies that ear protective devices shall be provided and used, and further that these devices be fitted by competent persons.

The petroleum industry is covered by the provisions of the OSHA standard relating to permissible noise levels. This industry applied for and was granted, by the federal administration, exemption from the provisions of the hearing conservation amendment.

The mining industry is regulated by the Mine Safety and Health Administration (MSHA). Noise standards covering the mining industry are promulgated by the MSHA. The regulations differ depending on whether the mining activity is surface or underground and whether the material mined is coal or another material. Each mining operation has adopted the permissible noise level provisions of Walsh-Healey, but none have embraced the Hearing Conservation Amendment. Underground metal and nonmetal mines (30 CFR 57), as well as surface operations in these types of mines (30 CFR 56), specify use of feasible administrative controls, engineering controls, or both to meet the noise limits. When these methods fail to reduce the noise to permissible limits, personal protection is to be used.

The coal mining industry, both surface (30 CFR 71) and underground mining operations (30 CFR 70), have similar regulations. The noise limits are those of Walsh-Healey. In addition, relatively detailed provisions cover measures of the noise environment including equipment, procedures, and personnel. When noise limits are exceeded, the mine operator is required to institute administrative and engineering controls. Such controls may include hearing protection devices. When a notice of violation has been issued, a plan for effective hearing conservation is to be submitted to the MSHA. These plans should include methods for reducing noise levels, personal ear protection devices, and audiometry, with provisions for pre-employment as well as periodic monitoring.

The Department of Defense (DoD) issued an instruction regarding hearing conservation programs that encompasses all DoD military and civilian personnel (DoD, 1987). Only personnel considered deaf are excluded. The DoD instruction incorporates the OSHA noise limits with a major difference. The time-intensity exchange is specified as 4 dB per doubling rather than 5 dB. Hearing conservation programs are to be implemented when the TWA for 8 hours is 85 dB. The instruction includes guidance in noise measurement and permits both area assessment and evaluation by dosimetry. The limit for impulsive noise is the same as that for the OSHA, 140 dB peak level.

The focus for the DoD noise standard is on engineering controls. Hearing protection is considered an interim strategy while engineering controls are being explored. When noise sources are operating, personnel are required to wear hearing protection. This includes personnel exposed to gun and artillery fire under test or training conditions.

The instructions include programs of audiometric testing that involve pre-placement, annual, and termination hearing tests. Standard specifications for audiometric test equipment are those specified in S3.6-1969 (ANSI, 1969). The background noise levels are more stringent than those in the OSHA standard, requiring limits specified in S3.1-1977 (ANSI, 1977).

The DoD permits development of minimum preselection hearing level criteria for particular occupational specialties. The criteria are permitted to permanently exclude personnel with substantial hearing loss from working in hazardous noise environments provided they are used judiciously to ensure that qualified, trained personnel are not indiscriminately excluded from their careers.

Records for personnel are required to be kept for the period of employment plus 30 years. The DoD further requires the maintenance of a hearing conservation data base for assessing the effectiveness of the hearing conservation program.

The DoD instructions are minimal and permit variation in implementation of the hearing conservation program. Each of the branches of military service has developed its own specific programs which, although generally similar, vary in detail.

The Department of Transportation (DoT) is also involved with occupational noise standards. The United States Coast Guard is responsible for the noise program in the maritime industry. The Navigation and Vessel Inspection Circular No. 12-82 contains recommendations for control of excessive noise. The uniqueness of the occupational environment and the inability, in many instances, to escape noise exposure aboard ship led the Coast Guard to adopt the index of 24-hour effective exposure level. The permissible noise limit is designated as a 24-hour effective level of 82 dBA. The circular further recommends that new ships (1,600 gross tons or more) be designed to achieve levels of 77 dBA. These design specifications would be difficult to achieve in smaller vessels, so other conservation methods may be applied.

The Coast Guard standard considers different permissible levels for living spaces such as crew sleeping and eating areas. For these locations levels should be no more than 75 dBA. Again, these requirements depend on ship size (500 gross tons or more). Sound levels from a vessel's fog horn are not to exceed 110 dBA at listening posts.

Crew members are required to wear hearing protection when entering noise levels of 85 dBA or more. OSHA's limit of 140 dB peak impulsive levels and 115 dB ceiling for continuous noise are part of the maritime standard. Those personnel with 24-hour effective levels exceeding 77 dBA or those who are routinely exposed to noise levels of 85 dBA or more are to be involved in hearing conservation programs including hearing testing and noise education. The owner/operator of the ship is responsible for the conservation program and noise control. Crew members are responsible for complying with the program, particularly with the requirements for wearing hearing protection.

The Federal Aviation Administration (FAA) is authorized to establish and enforce rules and regulations for safety including noise and exhaust emissions from aircraft in cooperation with the EPA. The Noise Control Act of 1972 gave the EPA authority to set national noise standards for commercial products and required the EPA to assist the FAA in developing regulations for airport and aircraft. The focus of this effort is less on the employee and more on the effect of noise on the general public.

The only major occupational category not covered by a noise standard is agriculture. The Agricultural Workers Regulation 1928.21 exempts agricultural workers from the noise standard.

Individual states are authorized under federal regulations to operate their own plan for occupational safety and health providing their plans are judged to be at least as stringent and protective as those required by federal regulations. Twenty-three states have accepted these conditions and have their own program approved by the DoL.

Critical Issues

Fragmentation

The situation in the United States regarding the application of noise standards and the populations covered by the standards is confused and fragmented. The amended noise standard of OSHA, which at present is the most comprehensive, applies only to those involved in manufacturing, utilities, and maritime occupations. Construction workers are handled differently by the administration. Those working in the construction industry are covered by a narrower, less stringent rule that existed prior to the implementation of the hearing conservation amendment and that is rarely enforced. Transportation workers are the responsibility of various bureaus within the U.S. Department of Transportation. Their coverage from the hazards of noise is variable, and the enforcement is spotty. The Mine Safety and Health Administration has standards that differ depending on the type of mining involved. The MSHA applies a standard that is less stringent than that of the OSHA to its constituents. Agricultural workers who are supposed to be covered by the OSHA regulations are in reality not covered at all from the noise hazards of the machinery and equipment they use in farm operations.

The NIOSH and the Association of Schools of Public Health, in their consideration of the national strategies for the prevention of leading work-related diseases and injuries (ASPH/NIOSH, 1988), proposed, as a long-term objective, that the provisions of the OSHA's 1971 noise standard together with the 1983 hearing conservation amendment be extended to cover all industries in which potentially hazardous noise exists. This coverage would include not only the manufacturing and utilities industries but also agriculture, mining, forestry, transportation, oil and gas well drilling, construction, and the service industries. Such an extension would provide protection to an estimated 3 million additional workers.

Prevalence and Compliance

Assessment of the importance of the problem of industrial noise exposure dictates that a realistic estimate of the number of workers who are exposed to hazardous workplace noise be available. Prevalence of noise exposure in industry and the availability of hearing conservation programs were among the items of interest to the National Occupational Hazard Survey (NOHS) conducted in the period from 1974 to 1978. Results from this survey were used by OSHA as an indication of the number of people working in various manufacturing industries and the number of workers exposed to noise in these industries (Franks, 1988).

Although these estimates of the prevalence of workers exposed to hazard may have had some validity in the late 1970s, the appropriateness of extrapolating from these data to arrive at estimates for the 1990s is questionable. Many industries that have been very noisy have become quieter as a consequence of equipment replacement and retooling. In the United States, noisy manufacturing industries, such as primary metals, have had significant reductions in production workers. Other areas such as printing and publishing have had major increases in workers. The initial NOHS indicated that less than 5 percent of those working in the service group were exposed to potentially hazardous noise. Employment in the United States has shifted from the noisy environments of heavy industry to quieter activities in the service sector. There is a distinct possibility that the number of exposed people is not as great as the earlier estimates indicated. The relationship of employment and noise exposure is dynamic and requires continual monitoring to maintain desirable levels of accuracy (Franks, 1988).

The NOHS provided estimates of the number of workers exposed to continuous noise who were involved in some type of audiometric testing. Although hearing testing only represents one element of an effective hearing conservation program, indirectly these data provided estimates of compliance with the requirement for hearing conservation. The NOHS estimated that 37 percent of all workers exposed to continuous noise have their hearing tested. Although these estimates do provide some information regarding hearing conservation, there is no indication of the quality of the program or, for that matter, the quality of the audiometry. Further, how well these data represent the situation as it exists today is subject to the same concerns expressed for the estimates of prevalence of employee noise exposure. Unfortunately, however, these estimates still remain the best available.

There is a need for systemic data collection from occupational hearing conservation programs. These data could provide current estimates of the magnitude of the occupational noise problem as well as provide information regarding the effectiveness of attempts to protect hearing from this noise. Designation of a specific agency to serve as a repository for data gathered by industry would be a definite asset in the assessment of the value and efficacy of occupational noise standards.

Enforcement

In the 1970s the hazardous and undesirable effects of noise received considerable attention in the United States. Regulations were developed and promulgated by OSHA and by the EPA. A number of conferences and seminars were occupied with the subject. Research projects dealing with various aspects of noise were proposed and funded. Professionals with expertise in noise effects and noise control were in demand. A change in the presidency brought with it a change in the policy of the administration with a de-emphasis on regulatory activity of the federal government (Suter, 1989).

OSHA's enforcement of its standards has weakened. The citations issued by OSHA for violations of the provisions of its hearing conservation regulation decreased from 3,572 in 1984 to 2,368 in 1987. A better index of enforcement is the amount of the penalties resulting from these citations. In 1980, prior to the implementation of the hearing conservation amendment, industry in the United States was fined $633,485 for 2,292 violations of the noise standard. In 1987, the fines decreased to $200,880 for 2,259 violations. OSHA frequently adjusts the amount of the penalty following negotiations with the companies involved; consequently the cited firms actually paid only $279,962 in 1980 and $46,236 in 1987 for noise violations. In the year 1987, then, the average cost per citation was $18 and, in reality, could not be considered an economic incentive for complying with OSHA's noise standard (Suter, 1989).

Undoubtedly, the reticence to issue citations and to prosecute violations is due, in part, to the fact that employers are more likely to contest these actions. In 1987, companies contested a quarter of all noise-related citations. The requirement of "feasible engineering controls" of noise has been interpreted as technically feasible. Now the courts are requiring that the procedures be economically feasible as well. Despite the fact that the courts have not defined economic feasibility, the opinion that OSHA must consider the cost of engineering controls legally has been upheld. Lawyers representing the DoL avoid litigating cases involving the stipulation of feasible engineering controls because of the difficulty in proving the test of economic feasibility.

The noise programs of the EPA and OSHA are either weak or have disappeared. Governmental de-emphasis of the problem of noise in the industrial environment and the living environment, in general, needs to be reversed if the hearing of its citizens is to be protected and preserved. There are hopeful signs that this reversal may be under way, because the interest in problems of the environment seems to be returning and pressure again is being exerted on governmental agencies for their solution.

Procedural Focus

The hearing conservation amendment to OSHA's noise regulation served to strengthen these regulations. By requiring initiation of hearing conservation practices for employees exposed to the equivalent of 8 hours at 85 dBA, the amendment provides protection for those who would not be considered under the limits of 90 dBA specified as permissible in the standard.

The administration under President Reagan viewed the amendment as an opportunity to shift OSHA's enforcement from engineering controls to reliance on hearing protection. In 1982, OSHA instructed its field offices to stop issuing citations to companies whose employees were exposed to daily average noise levels of less than 100 dB as long as companies had effective hearing conservation programs. As a consequence of these instructions, OSHA has raised the permissible exposure limit from 90 to 100 dBA without going through the formal rule-making procedure. This policy change has not been tested in the courts despite its questionable legality (Suter, 1989).

The most desirable method for noise control is for reduction of noise from the source. This would require design of equipment and procedures by the manufacturers to operate more quietly at the outset. An expert panel from industrial, academic, and professional consulting firms at a symposium on machinery and construction noise sponsored by the EPA in 1979 was confident that quieter products could be designed provided there was economic incentive. The symposium participants indicated that without incentives, both positive and negative, there would be no technologic development; they further expressed the opinion that the incentives for noise control were weak, uncertain, or absent (Suter, 1989). Focus on hearing protection as the method for reduction of noise exposure serves to subvert efforts and incentives for developing and using engineering procedures for noise reduction. In practice, people generally dislike wearing hearing protectors and are reticent to use them. Even when the protectors are used failure to fit the devices properly limits their effectiveness. Employees may not receive the benefit intended or specified by the manufacturers of this protection and thereby diminish the value of the conservation program.

As one of the short-term objectives, the NIOSH and the Association of School of Public Health (ASPH/NIOSH, 1988) recommended the rescinding of OSHA's instructions that do not require engineering control below 100 dBA and that permit the use of hearing protectors. Further, it was recommended that regulations should require noise specifications in the procurement of new equipment on federally funded projects.

Evaluating Hearing Conservation Programs

The OSHA Hearing Conservation Amendment describes those elements required for an effective hearing conservation program. The amendment does not specify how to implement this program or how to judge whether the program is effectively meeting its objectives. If hearing conservation programs are to succeed in preventing noise-induced hearing loss, those people responsible for the programs must understand how they should be organized and operated. A program cannot be considered effective simply because it contains, in some fashion, the five elements prescribed by the amendment, i.e., sound surveys, engineering/administrative controls, education, audiometric evaluations, and hearing protection.

Efforts are under way to develop procedures for evaluating the effectiveness of hearing conservation programs using techniques of audiometric data base analysis (Royster and Royster, 1988). The Standards Committee,

S12, Noise, accredited by the ANSI through its Working Group 12, has proposed several procedures for using audiometric data base information for the purpose of evaluating program effectiveness. These procedures are being considered for publication as a document for the purposes of trial and comment. The ultimate objective is for one or more of these methods to serve as a consensus standard procedure for program evaluation.

Impulse and Impact Noise

An important issue not adequately addressed in the occupational noise standards of the United States is the criteria for exposure to short, usually intense noises described as impulse and impact noise. None of the current standards contains explicit requirements for these exposures. There are a number of unresolved questions regarding the relations of the acoustic properties of these types of noises to hearing loss. These questions include effect of rise and decay times, the spectrum, and the effect of background level between pulses. Are impulse and impact noises sufficiently different that they should be considered separately? Are there critical levels at which the underlying mechanisms change from those involved in noise-induced hearing loss to those of noise trauma? These questions are being addressed by NIOSH (ASPH/NIOSH, 1988) as well as by a working group of the Committee on Hearing and Bioacoustics/Biomechanics (CHABA) of the National Research Council.

Risk

OSHA has not specified the level of risk for noise-induced hearing loss that would be considered acceptable. Using data compiled by the EPA (EPA, 1974), OSHA chose a level of 90 dBA as the maximum permissible exposure level (PEL), which implies that a risk of from 20 to 29 percent is tolerable. Implementation of the hearing conservation at a level of 85 dBA suggests that a risk of material impairment in 10 to 15 percent of the exposed population is more acceptable to OSHA. There are those who feel that the risk should be reduced still further by moving the PEL to 85 dBA (Suter, 1989).

The debate continues regarding the appropriate exchange rate for time and intensity. OSHA has adopted the 5-dB rule, the DoD a 4-dB rule, and many of the other industrial nations, particularly in Europe, a 3-dB rule. Unquestionably, the 3-dB exchange rate would offer more protection to those exposed to occupational noise.

The present noise standards could be made more protective. However, there can be no doubt that the OSHA noise standard, as it now stands, would offer protection to a significant segment of the population now at risk for incurring occupational noise-induced hearing loss if the requirements are effectively implemented and enforced. Continued debate on whether the standard should be more or less stringent has no value if the standard, whatever its requirements, is given no support by government agencies responsible for its enforcement.

Conclusion

With the exception of the agricultural industry, there are noise standards, federal or state, that apply to all major occupational categories in the United States. All of the existing noise standards have adopted the permissible noise limits that first appeared as part of the Walsh-Healey Act in 1969. The various standards differ in definition and description of effective hearing conservation programs. Authority for implementing and monitoring the noise standard provisions varies depending on the particular industry. Compliance with and enforcement of the standards are less than might be desired. Uniform adoption of the DoL Hearing Conservation Amendment and more vigorous enforcement of existing noise regulations would go a long way toward preserving the hearing of workers from the noxious effects of occupational noise exposure.

Les Normes d'Exposition au Bruit: Etat Actuel et Problèmes en Suspens

Certaines des dispositions de base des textes normatifs sur l'exposition professionnelle au bruit du Ministère du Travail des Etats-Unis *(U.S. Department of Labor)* sont restées inchangées depuis plus de 20 ans. Ces normes concernent environ 5 millions de travailleurs dans les industries de transformation dans plus de 300.000 lieux de travail. La limite d'exposition autorisée est un niveau sonore pondéré A de 90 dB, avec un "taux de doublement" de 5 dB qui constitue la relation entre durée et niveau. La norme appelle à une réduction de l'exposition au bruit des travailleurs surexposés en instituant des mesures applicables ou des contrôles administratifs, techniques ou d'organisation du travail, lorsque c'est faisable.

En 1972, l'Institut National pour la Sécurité et l'Hygiène du travail *(National Institute for Occupational Safety and Health: NIOSH)* a recommandé de réduire la dose d'exposition permise à 85 dB (A) et suggéré une série de mesures pour la sauvegarde de l'audition des travailleurs surexposés qui inclue un contrôle du bruit, des tests audiométriques, le choix de protections auditives et la tenue de fichiers. Le Service de la Sécurité et du l'Hygiène du Travail *(Occupational Safety and Health Administration: OSHA)* du Ministère du Travail a utilisé les recommandations du NIOSH comme ossature de base pour une modification de son ancienne norme sur le bruit. La norme sur le bruit de l'OSHA comporte maintenant des spécifications détaillées pour des programmes de sauvegarde de l'audition, qui furent promulguées en 1981 et révisées en 1983.

D'autres organismes des Etats-Unis qui ont promulgué des normes de bruit en milieu de travail sont le Bureau de Sécurité du Transport Motorisé *(Bureau of Motor Carrier Safety)* du Ministère des Transports *(Department of Transportation)*, la Sécurité Minière *(Mine Safety)* du Ministère du Travail et le Ministère de la Défense *(Department of Defense)*. Certaines questions critiques liées au développement et à l'application des normes sur le bruit sont devenues évidentes durant ces dernières années. L'une des plus importantes et des plus difficiles d'entre elles est constituée par le critère d'exposition aux bruits impulsionnels et d'impacts. Aucune des normes américaines sur le bruit en milieu de travail ne comporte d'exigences explicites en ce qui concerne ce type d'expositions. Parmi les questions non résolues [se trouvent] le rôle des temps de montée et d'extinction, le spectre de fréquence et le niveau de bruit de fond entre les impulsions; la question se pose également de savoir s'il existe un niveau critique au-dessus duquel les lésions auditives augmentent plus rapidement et si, effectivement, les bruits impulsionnels et les bruits d'impact doivent être traités séparément.

D'autres questions importantes concernent le "taux de doublement," la relation entre durée et niveau de bruit (est-il de 3, 4, ou 5 dB, etc.), l'extension des normes de bruit aux populations actuellement non soumises à la réglementation, les méthodes d'évaluation du succès des programmes de sauvegarde de l'audition fondées sur l'analyse de bases de données audiométriques et le degrée de réduction des pertes auditives dues au bruit que l'on peut effectivement attribuer aux normes U.S. sur le bruit.

References

American Conference of Governmental Industrial Hygienists. Physical Agents Threshold Committee. Threshold limit values for physical agents. Cincinnati, OH: 1968.

American National Standards Institute (ANSI). American Standard Specifications for Audiometers, S3.6-1969. New York, ANSI, 1969.

American National Standards Institute (ANSI). Standard Criteria for Permissible Ambient Noise During Audiometric Testing. S3.1-1977. New York: ANSI, 1977.

ASPH/NIOSH. Proposed national strategies for prevention of leading work-related diseases and injuries, part 2. Washington, D.C.: The Association of Schools of Public Health, 1988:51.

Barry JP. Developmental and enforcement history of the occupational noise standards in the USA. Presented to the American Industrial Hygiene Conference.

Environmental Protection Agency. Occupational noise exposure regulation: Request for review and report. Fed Reg 1974; 39:43802-43809.

Environmental Protection Agency, Office of Noise Abatement and Control. Noise in America: The extent of the problem. Washington, D.C.: EPA Report No. 550/9-81-101, 1981.

Franks JR. Number of workers exposed to occupational noise. Semin Hear 1988; 9:287-297.

National Occupational Health Survey. Vol III, National Institute of Occupational Safety and Health. Washington, D.C.: NIOSH Pub. 78-114, 1978.

Noise Control Act. PL92-574. Washington, D.C., 1972.

Occupational Safety and Health Act. PL 91-596. Washington, D.C., 1970.

Royster LH, Royster JD. Getting started in audiometric data base analysis. Semin Hear 1988; 9:325-337.

Safety and Health Standards—Surface Metal and Nonmetal Mines. Part 56.5050. Exposure limits for noise. 30 CFR 56 (7-1-88 edition). p 315.

Suter AH. The development of federal noise standards. In: Lipscomb DM, ed. Hearing Conservation in Industry, Schools and the Military. Boston: College-Hill Press, 1988:45.

Suter AH. Noise wars. Technol Rev 1989; Nov/Dec: 42-49.

U.S. Department of Agriculture. 1928.21. Applicable standards in 29 CFR part 1910. Federal Register 38569. Washington, D.C., 1977.

U.S. Department of Defense. Hearing Conservation Program. Instruction No. 6055.12. Washington, D.C.: DoD, 1987.

U.S. Department of Labor, Bureau of Labor Standards. Occupation noise exposure. Fed. Reg. 34, 7946-7949. Washington, D.C.: DoL, 1969.

U.S. Department of Labor, Mine Safety and Health Administration. Mandatory Health Standards—Surface coal mines and surface work areas of underground mines. Part 71.800-805. Noise Standard. 30 CFR 71

Washington, D.C.: DoL, 1988.

U.S. Department of Labor, Mine Safety and Health Administration. Mandatory Health Standards—Underground coal mines. Parts 70.500-511. Noise Standard. 30 CFR 70. Washington, D.C.: DoL, 1988.

U.S. Department of Labor, Mine Safety and Health Administration. Safety and Health Standards—Underground metal and nonmetal mines. Part 57.5050. Exposure limits for noise. 30 CFR 57. Washington, D.C.: DoL, 1988.

U.S. Department of Labor, Occupational Safety and Health Administration. Construction Noise Standard, Federal Register Parts 1926.52 and 1926.101. Washington, D.C.: DoL, 1971.

U.S. Department of Labor, Occupational Safety and Health Administration. Occupational noise exposure: Hearing conservation amendment; Final rule. Fed Reg 1983; 48:9738-9785.

U.S. Department of Labor, Occupational Safety and Health Administration. Part 1910.95. Occupational noise exposure. 29 CFR 1910. Washington, D.C.: DoL, 1988.

U.S. Department of Labor, Occupational Safety and Health Administration. Office of State Programs. States with approved plans. Washington, D.C.: DoL, 1990.

U.S. Department of Transportation, Coast Guard. Recommendations on control of excessive noise. Navigation and Vessel Inspection Circular No. 19-82. Washington, D.C.: DoT, 1982.

CHAPTER 47

Control of Occupational Noise in the European Economic Community

MARCEL J. VAN DER VENNE

Occupational hearing loss is a major subject of concern to all interested parties (management, labor, and relevant national authorities) within the European Communities. The exact number of workers exposed to various noise levels is not known; however, according to estimates, a total of 25 to 35 million workers are exposed during work hours to continuous noise levels equal to or higher than 80 dBA; for half the cases the average ambient noise exceeds 85 dBA, and for 7 to 9 million of the workers the average noise exceeds 90 dBA.

The number of workers exposed to excessive noise is obviously high, and loss of hearing is a leading occupational disease in industrialized countries. The rising costs of the corresponding compensation have also contributed to a heightened perception of the problem, and it was decided that a minimum level of worker protection had to be achieved in all the Member States, through legislative provisions. A mandatory legal hearing protection instrument was selected, because neither a consensus on objective data (the International Standards Organization, or ISO, recommendation dates back to 1971) nor voluntary agreements (ILO, 1977) succeeded in tackling the problem.

Procedure

To reach common objectives while providing the required flexibility and acknowledging different structures and approaches of our Member States, Council Directives appear as the most appropriate instruments. Council Directives are binding on the Member States as to the result to be achieved, but leave to the national authorities the choice of forms and methods (EEC, 1957).

A Council Directive is a mandatory legal instrument that satisfies the following conditions:

—Proposed by the Commission, which collects the information and associates the interested parties during the preparation

—Discussed by the European Parliament and by the Economic and Social Committee

—Decided on by the Council of Ministers

—Implemented nationally by the Governments

The Commission assures that all the requirements are integrated into each state's legal system; the resulting statutes are then enforced by the national authorities.

The requirements mandated in a directive usually call for technical specifications and supporting documents to assist the final users (designers, manufacturers, employers, controlling authorities) in meeting their duties. According to the "New Approach" (EEC, 1985) this can be done by European standards harmonized that show in operational terms how the objectives fixed by a directive can be achieved. They are developed by the European Committee for Standardization (CEN) and the European Committee for Electrotechnical Standardization (CENELEC). When its reference is published by the Commission, such a harmonized standard enjoys a privileged legal status. Equipment complying with a European harmonized standard is deemed to comply with the corresponding directive's safety requirements; manufacturers thus have a clear incentive to use such a standard, although this is not mandatory.

Controlling Risk Due to Noise

Community action has primarily addressed the risk to hearing caused by occupational noise. A considerable amount of scientific work has resulted in a reasonable understanding of the exposure-effect relationship (ISO, 1990). However, the available data do not permit a similar evaluation of the nonauditory effects and risks. An analysis of international scientific reviews (WHO, 1980; ISO, 1990) led to selection of two parameters used to express the risk: (1) the maximum value of the acoustic pressure likely to result in almost immediate damage; and (2) the amount of A-weighted sound energy reaching the ear that leads to long-term hearing impairment.

Exposure to noise can be limited in a number of ways. Reducing the emission at its source or fixing the maximum allowed values of ambient noise conflicts with technologic and economic factors and often is neither realistic nor reasonable. Objective observations and practical reasons led to the decision that ambient noise levels should be reduced (primarily at the source) whenever it is reasonable, but that mandatory limits will apply only on the noise reaching the ear. Thus, if noisy equipment cannot be avoided, the conditions of the equipment's use are regulated. Hearing protectors certainly can be useful in controlling the risk, but they remain a last resort considering the disadvantages and uncertainties attached to their use. Workers and employers have held strong and differing views on the level to which occupational noise should be limited.

One may argue that a noise-induced permanent threshold shift can be detected at the most sensitive audiometric frequency as soon as the daily noise exposure exceeds 75 dBA; this figure represents a "zero-risk to hearing" (although not socially significant). Any higher value implies a judgment on the amount of hearing impairment that is considered acceptable, and this is not a technical but a political process.

Two specific problems also had to be solved: (1) how to treat short bursts of very intensive noise (impulse-impact), and (2) to what extent acoustic rest should be accounted for (intermittent exposure). Practical considerations played an important role here in addition to available evidence, the aim being an applicable and enforceable regulation that, if errant, errs modestly and on the safe side. It was thus decided that when the ear is exposed to noise bursts, the peak pressure must be limited and the acoustic energy must be included in the allowable daily exposure; this of course requires the use of measuring equipment capable of integrating the rapidly varying sound pressure. We feel that an instrument with an onset time of 100 μs covers at least 99 percent of the noise bursts experienced in industrial situations.

A 3-dB exchange rate was chosen for trading intensity against duration. This is consistent with international standardization and avoids any necessity of controlling level and is simple to apply in industrial practice when a given level of protection must be guaranteed. Larger exchange rates (eg, 5 dB) rely on some hearing recovery during acoustic rest, and selecting such a value assumes that a given pattern of noisy-quiet periods is respected; otherwise the corresponding people will not be granted the assumed protection and, sadly, their underprotection increases with the magnitude of their overexposure. Checking the afforded protection requires monitoring the noise levels and durations of intermittent exposure—complex to implement and hardly enforceable!

The size of the population concerned, the resulting human and social costs, and the economic and technical constraints have led to a two-pronged approach combining safety requirements for equipment with safe working conditions for persons.

Directives on Equipment

Part of the program aimed at protecting the environment and at ensuring the free circulation of goods involves regulation of the noise produced by some types of machinery (e.g., tractors, earth-moving equipment, compressors). Noise emissions must be indicated and maximum accepted figures are specified; this certainly contributes to reducing the noise exposure at work, although it applies only to new equipment and specific uses (e.g., civil engineering and building sites).

A more comprehensive treatment is found in the Council Directive 89/392 EEC (EEC, 1989), which lists emitted noise as one of the risks caused by a machine. Directive 89/392 requires that each machine be designed and constructed so as to limit noise risk to the lowest possible level. Furthermore, each machine must be "labeled" with the peak pressure when it exceeds 63 Pa (130 dB) and with the sound pressure level at the work station when it exceeds 70 dBA. When the latter exceeds 85 dBA, the sound power level must also be indicated. The directive refers to technical standards for the conditions in which the measurements are to be made, and CEN is actively proceeding with the development of European standards covering both the method of noise measurements and machine-specific test codes.

The Noise at Work Directive 86/188

While acknowledging the contribution of quieter equipment to a reduction of the exposure, a specific directive was aimed at protection from the risks related to exposure to noise at work, and was adopted by the Council in 1986 (EEC, 1986). The provisions of the directive had to be implemented by national legislation by 1 January 1990 at the latest (one year later for Greece and Portugal). The directive is concerned essentially with protecting workers against risks to their hearing and lays down the general principle that such risks must be reduced to the lowest level compatible with technical possibilities and economic constraints.

The responsibility of containing the risk belongs primarily to the employer. To assist the employer in containing risks, the directive uses "action levels"—values that, when exceeded, trigger specific actions. The action levels apply to two parameters mentioned earlier: the peak sound pressure (expressed in pascals to avoid confusion with continuous noise levels) and the sound energy received during the actual working day. The latter is expressed as the "daily personal exposure (LEP,d)" and is the same as the noise exposure level normalized to a nominal 8-hour working day (LEX,8 h) used by the recently published ISO 1999 standard. The LEP uses a 3-dB exchange rate and differs from the equivalent continuous A-weighted sound pressure level (LAeq,T) by the fact that the sound pressure is averaged over a fixed duration (8 hours) instead of over the measurement period (T).

Action levels have been specified as 200 Pa peak, 85 and 90 dBA LEP,d. The following actions are taken when noise measurements show that action levels have been exceeded: (1) Above an LEP,d of 85 dBA, workers must be informed of the risk that they can incur and also of the specific locations of risk. Hearing protectors are to be made available, and workers are entitled to hearing examinations in order to diagnose any reduction in hearing due to noise; and (2) If the LEP,d exceeds 90 dBA or if the peak acoustic pressure exceeds 200 pascals, the employer has to draw up and implement a program of technical measures (engineering control) or changes in the work organization (administrative control) with a view to improving the situation. If these means do not make it reasonably possible to reduce the exposure below the action levels, hearing protectors must be worn. The protectors must not, however, increase the risk of accident due, for example, to the nonperception of sounds or to noises signalling a danger.

Installations and equipment, having an essential role to play in the long-term improvement of the working environment, and the need to reduce the risks applies also to the design, construction and putting into service of new installations. Finally, whenever equipment is used that emits a noise that is likely to exceed the action levels, the employer must be informed of that risk so that he can take the necessary measures to meet his duties; the requirement to provide such information will also make manufacturers and users aware of the advantages of quieter devices, and will help to improve the situation through market forces. The directive also deals with the involvement of the work force (as well as their representatives) in protection from noise.

The directive specifies no procedures regarding the measuring of noise and the monitoring of hearing; advisory annexes give indications on how they can be performed.

A considerable amount of leeway is left to national practices for the implementation of the directive, thereby reconciling respect of the aims of the directive—which guarantees protection—with the flexibility and the economy of means made necessary by the diversity of structures and industrial practice. The provisions of the directive will be re-examined on 1 January 1994. The provisions do not apply, however, to sea and air transport personnel on board a ship or aircraft; the possibility of extending the directive to those areas had to be examined before 1 January 1990, and the Commission is currently looking at the problem.

Conclusion

Protection against noise at work, the backbone of which is the Council Directive

86/188EEC, was the subject of hard and long discussions. The directive's provisions inevitably represent a compromise between divergent positions resulting from contradictory requirements. We are convinced that they can be practically applied and will provide an acceptable minimum level of risk control throughout the Community; they also provide a good basis for future improvements whenever these are possible, thus contributing to the social dimension of the single market. However, any text's worth is judged by its implementation, and the Commission has explicitly stated its determination to see all the Community legislation accurately implemented and, when necessary, vigorously enforced in the workplace.

Le Contrôle du Bruit Pendant le Travail dans la CEE

Comme de nombreux pays industrialisés, les Etats membres de la CEE se sont préoccupés des effets nocifs de l'exposition professionnelle au bruit.

Considérant les coûts humains, sociaux et économiques mis en jeu, un accord s'est fait pour assurer à tous les travailleurs dans la Communauté un degré minimum harmonisé de protection contre les risques affectant leur ouïe.

Les Directives du Conseil (qui sont des instruments juridiques contraignants applicables à toute la Communauté) ont donc abordé le problème suivant deux axes.

Les équipements doivent être conçus et construits de façon à réduire le bruit qu'ils produisent; de plus l'exposition des personnes doit être contenue: la limite correspond à 90 dB(A) pendant 8 heures (avec un "taux de doublement" de 3 dB), tandis que la pression crête doit rester au-dessous de 200 Pa (140 dB).

Les travailleurs exposés au-dessus de "niveaux d'action" fixés doivent être informés et formés, et les employeurs ont l'obligation de contenir l'exposition, en agissant prioritairement à la source de bruit, les protecteurs d'ouïe étant un dernier recours.

Les réglementations s'appliquent à tous les secteurs d'activité, à l'exception des travailleurs des transports maritimes et aériens lorsqu'ils sont à bord.

Des normes techniques peuvent être utilisées afin de savoir comment les objectifs fixés dans les Directives peuvent être atteints, et les organisations européennes de normalisation (CEN et CENELEC) préparent activement des normes harmonisées.

On estime que cette réglementation contrôlera les risques principaux et les autorités ont exprimé leur détermination de les voir mises en oeuvre de façon effective.

References

European Economic Community (EEC). Treaty Establishing the European Community, Article 189—Office for Official Publications of the European Communities. Luxembourg: EEC, 1957.

European Economic Community (EEC). Council Resolution of 7 May 1985 regarding a new approach to technical harmonization and standards. Official Journal of the European Communities N° C13, 4 June 1985, p. 1. Office for Official Publications of the European Communities, Luxembourg.

European Economic Community (EEC). Council Directive of 12 May 1986 on the protection of workers from the risks related to exposure to noise at work (86/188 EEC). Official Journal of the European Communities N° L137, 24 May 1986, pp. 28-34. Office for Official Publications of the European Communities, Luxembourg.

European Economic Community (EEC). Council Directive of 14 June 1989 on the approximation of the laws of the Member States relating to machinery (89/392 EEC). Official Journal of the European Communities N° L183, 29 June 1989, pp 9-32. Office for Official Publications of the European Communities, Luxembourg.

International Labour Organization (ILO). Convention No. 148, Working Environment (air pollution, noise and vibration). Geneva, 1977.

International Organization for Standardization (ISO). Recommendation ISO/R 1999. Acoustics—Estimation of Occupational Noise Exposure in View of Hearing Protection. Geneva: ISO, 1971.

International Organization for Standardization (ISO). International Standard ISO 1999:1990. Acoustics—Determination of occupational noise exposure and estimation of noise-induced hearing impairment. Geneva: ISO, 1990.

World Health Organization (WHO). Environmental Health Criteria 12, Noise. Geneva: WHO, 1980.

Index

A *"t"* following a page number indicates a table.
An *"f"* following a page number indicates an illustration.